Student Resource CD-ROM

for

A Massage Therapist's Guide to PATHOLOGY

THIRD EDITION

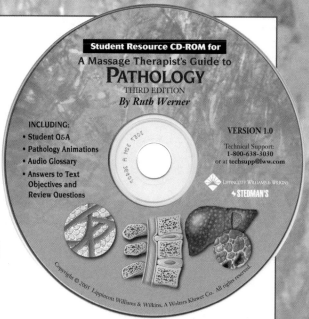

Student Resource CD-ROM for
A Massage Therapist's Guide to
PATHOLOGY
THIRD EDITION
By Ruth Werner

INCLUDING:
• Student Q&A
• Pathology Animations
• Audio Glossary
• Answers to Text Objectives and Review Questions

VERSION 1.0

Technical Support:
1-800-638-3030
or at techsupp@lww.com

LIPPINCOTT WILLIAMS & WILKINS
STEDMAN'S

Copyright © 2005 Lippincott Williams & Wilkins, A Wolters Kluwer Co. All rights reserved.

As a bonus for you, Lippincott Williams & Wilkins has included an interactive CD-ROM with tools to enhance your learning!

This resource is the perfect tool to help you prepare for exams, reinforce what you have learned, and illustrate important concepts.

The CD-ROM includes:

• A quiz tool with approximately 300 multiple-choice questions so you can test your knowledge and study for tests Choose study mode or test mode, and even e-mail your results to your instructor. A comprehensive exam is offered and rationales are given so you can understand the reasoning behind the correct answer.

• The answers to the textbook Chapter Objectives and Chapter Review Questions.

• Animations that demonstrate several disease processes including Cell Cycle, Congestive Heart Failure, Hypertension, Immune System, Nerve Synapse, and Stroke.

• An auditory pronunciation guide of glossary terms from the textbook, as found in *Stedman's Medical Dictionary, 27th edition.*

For technical support, contact 1-800-638-3030 or techsupp@lww.com.

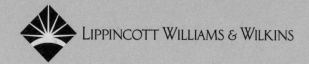

LIPPINCOTT WILLIAMS & WILKINS

A MASSAGE THERAPIST'S GUIDE TO PATHOLOGY
THIRD EDITION

A MASSAGE THERAPIST'S GUIDE TO PATHOLOGY

THIRD EDITION

Ruth Werner, LMP, NCTMB

LIPPINCOTT WILLIAMS & WILKINS
A **Wolters Kluwer** Company

Philadelphia • Baltimore • New York • London
Buenos Aires • Hong Kong • Sydney • Tokyo

Aquisition Editor: Peter J. Darcy
Managing Editor: Karen Gulliver
Development Editor: Nancy Peterson
Project Editor: Jennifer D. Glazer
Marketing Manager: Christen Murphy
Designer: Doug Smock
Compositor: Maryland Composition
Printer: RR Donnelley—Willard

The publisher is not responsible (as a matter of product liability, negligence, or otherwise) for any injury resulting from any material contained herein. This publication contains information relating to general principles of medical care that should not be construed as specific instructions for individual patients. Manufacturers' product information and package inserts should be reviewed for current information, including contraindications, dosages, and precautions.

Printed in the United States of America

Library of Congress Cataloging-in-Publication Data

Werner, Ruth (Ruth A.)
  A massage therapist's guide to pathology / Ruth Werner.—3rd ed.
      p. ; cm.—(LWW massage therapy & bodywork educational series)
  Includes bibliographical references and index.
  ISBN 0-7817-5489-5
  1. Massage therapy. 2. Physiology, Pathological. 3. Diseases. I. Title. II. Series.
  [DNLM: 1. Massage. 2. Diagnosis, Differential. WB 537 W494m 2006]
RM721.M366 2006
615.8'22—dc22

2004016947

The publishers have made every effort to trace the copyright holders for borrowed material. If they have inadvertently overlooked any, they will be pleased to make the necessary arrangements at the first opportunity.

To purchase additional copies of this book, call our customer service department at **(800) 638-3030** or fax orders to **(301) 824-7390**. International customers should call **(301) 714-2324**.

Visit Lippincott Williams & Wilkins on the Internet: http://www.LWW.com. Lippincott Williams & Wilkins customer service representatives are available from 8:30 am to 6:00 pm, EST.

05 06 07 08 09
1 2 3 4 5 6 7 8 9 10

*This book is dedicated to
the memory of my grandmother,
Dora C. Beckhard,
who probably never got
a massage in her life—but she
sure could have used one.*

PREFACE TO THE THIRD EDITION

DEAR STUDENTS AND PRACTITIONERS,

This book is a compilation of years of teaching and doing massage, collaboration with dozens of professionals in the field, a variety of printed resources, hundreds of articles about ongoing research, and *lots* of feedback on the strengths and weaknesses of the first and second editions. I have done my best to make it a useful, accurate source of information, so that bodyworkers can make informed choices when selecting modalities for clients who may not be perfectly healthy.

WHY DO MASSAGE THERAPISTS NEED TO KNOW ABOUT PATHOLOGY?

We all know that the demographics of the average massage client are changing. Every year the percentage of the population that receives massage goes up; every year more people perceive massage as a health care modality rather than (or in addition to) as an occasional indulgence.

The result is that today massage therapists can expect to see clients who struggle with various simple and complex health issues. These clients may seek massage as a special treat, but they are just as likely to be using massage as part of an integrated, proactive, carefully constructed health care plan. This puts a burden on the shoulders of massage therapists that we have never had before. When we work with clients whose bodies may not have the capacity to keep up with the kinds of changes some types of bodywork bring about, we run the risk of doing more harm than good.

Carefully, knowledgeably applied massage has found an important place in hotels, spas, and salons—but also in cancer wards, hospice centers, senior citizen homes, drug rehabilitation clinics, and other settings where the health of the clientele is far from perfect. The only way to work safely in these environments is to engage in a thorough education about the physiology of a healthy human body and the consequences of diseases and disorders that interrupt normal processes. This background is absolutely fundamental to the training of any bodywork professional and is critical for the maintenance of public safety.

The positive power of informed touch is irrefutable. When massage therapists and other bodyworkers have the tools to make educated decisions about how to structure their sessions for maximum benefit with minimum risk, they can help not only themselves, but whole communities of clients who otherwise would be out of their reach.

WHAT IS MASSAGE, AND HOW DO WE MAKE DECISIONS ABOUT IT?

Massage is a notoriously difficult term to define and is open to wide interpretation. I have used the terms "massage" and "bodywork" to mean *the application of informed, educated touch with the consent and participation of the receiver, for the purpose of allowing or promoting positive changes to occur in the receiver's physical and/or energetic state.* For the purposes of this text I have loosely classified bodywork into two different but complementary camps. One involves mechanical types of massage that work through the physical manipulation of skin, fascia, muscles, tendons, ligaments, and fluid flow. The other includes reflexive and energetic types of bodywork that address the flow of energy and/or the parasympathetic nervous system response to create an environment conducive to positive change. In simplified terms, the mechanical approach to bodywork *enacts* change; the reflexive/energetic approach *invites* change. Some modalities defy categorization, of course; manual lymph drainage and other lymph drainage techniques, for instance, work to mechanically influence the direction of lymph flow, but they also enlist the parasympathetic response to encourage the lymphatic capillaries to open fully. Craniosacral therapy influences the flow of cerebrospinal fluid (a mechanical goal), but does so through feather-light touch and reflexive parasympathetic affect. Ultimately, most therapists use both mechanical and reflexive/energetic intention; one could hardly touch another body without doing so!

For massage therapists or bodyworkers to evaluate whether their skills are applicable to the needs of a particular client, they must have a thorough knowledge of three things:

- how the human body works when it is healthy;
- how the body works in the context of disease or dysfunction;
- how a particular bodywork modality may influence those processes, either for good or for ill.

When these questions can be answered clearly, the therapist is in a position to turn positive intention into positive action, evaluating how to minimize any possible risks, and how to derive the best possible benefits from his or her skills.

HOW IS THE BOOK ORGANIZED?

This book has been written for two audiences: massage students who are learning about the body in health and disease for the first time, and practicing therapists working with a wide variety of people who may present a broad spectrum of disorders. It is written to present a wealth of complicated, interrelated, and convoluted material in an orderly fashion, but it can also provide an accurate reference and quick answers to the practitioner who needs to make a fast, well-informed decision.

The conditions that have been chosen to appear in this book are here for one of two reasons: either they occur frequently enough that practicing massage therapists will probably encounter them at some point or because massage may have such a profound effect on certain conditions that practitioners are obligated to be well-informed about them.

The material is presented by body system, following the order most anatomy and physiology texts use. Each chapter begins with a brief overview of how the system works to provide the context for a discussion of what happens when things break down. Then the disorders are arranged by category, so that related conditions will appear together in the text. Each section contains information about the condition, including, where applicable, the demographics of the disorder, the etiology and progression of the disease, signs and symptoms, the standard medical approach to diagnosis and treatment, and the applicability of massage.

Each condition is said to "indicate" or "contraindicate" massage. Where bodywork is contraindicated, guidelines are provided to explain whether this is a local caution, in other words, only the affected area must be avoided, or whether this is a systemic situation, in which case the client needs to be referred to a primary care physician or needs to reschedule his or her appointment. Further qualifications list whether some bodywork modalities are more appropriate than others, or they describe specific phases or stages of healing when massage can be most helpful.

Many of the conditions are said to indicate massage, at least at some stage of the healing process. I want to make very clear that to call massage "indicated" does *not* imply that massage will *fix* something that is wrong. We all know that at times massage can certainly influence the healing process for the better: the subacute stage of a sprained ankle, for instance. In other circumstances massage may have no effect on the severity of a condition whatsoever, for instance, with fibroid tumors. Massage is called "indicated" for both of these situations, which in this case, simply means that massage will not make the situation any worse.

Finally, the appendices provide important peripheral information, including a guide for taking a client history; an overview of Standard Precautions and hygienic methods; illustrations of client endangerment sites; a Quick Reference Guide, and a new piece: a brief discussion of massage in the context of several common classes of medications.

LEARNING RESOURCES

Features in *A Massage Therapist's Guide to Pathology* were designed to organize information in a way to facilitate learning (also see the User's Guide).

- *New full-color design and artwork* to help organize information and clearly illustrate conditions. Cross-references to other conditions that are related in important ways are in bold. Terms that have a pronunciation guide in the glossary appear in color. Beautiful new 4-color drawings were included in this edition.

- *In Brief Boxes* that give a synopsis of the definition, signs and symptoms, and guidelines for bodywork for each condition. All the In Brief Boxes also appear alphabetically in Appendix 4 to provide a valuable Quick Reference Guide.

- *Compare and Contrast Boxes* offer a chance to put key features of closely related disorders side-by-side for a point-by-point comparison.

- *Sidebars* present information that is important, but peripheral to the core discussion. Disease histories, some statistics, and specific cancer staging protocols are provided in the sidebars.

- *Case Histories* provide an inside look at the people who live with a variety of diseases and conditions. They offer a chance to see how some disorders powerfully influence people's lives.

- *Chapter Review Questions* require critical thinking skills and the ability to use information to draw conclusions about the safe practice of bodywork in complicated situations. (Answers to the Chapter Review Questions appear in the Student Resource CD-ROM)

- *Student Resource CD-ROM* includes 6 animations to demonstrate disease processes cross-referenced in the text. It includes all the answers to the Chapter Objective and Chapter Review Questions, Supplementary Questions, and an auditory pronunciation guide of glossary terms found in Stedman's Medical Dictionary.

TEACHING RESOURCES

A useful selection of materials is available to instructors with this edition, including:

- *Instructor Resource CD-ROM* includes an image collection of 162 figures that appear in the text; Power Point slides, Lecture Notes that can be printed; a 60-hour syllabus; a 40-hour syllabus; and the Brownstone Test Generator.

- The *Connection Web Site*, http://connection.LWW.com/go/werner3e, offers the Instructor Resource materials from the CD-ROM.

A NOD TO POLITICAL CORRECTNESS

In this book the terms "therapist" and "practitioner" are synonymous and refer to the person performing bodywork. The people who have conditions are called "patients" in the context of medical care and "clients" in the context of receiving massage. Patients or clients are referred to as "he" or "she" depending on what statistics indicate is the more likely gender to experience the condition. Thus, although it is possible for a woman to have hemophilia, for instance, the large majority of hemophiliacs are male and patients are therefore referred to as males. When there is no particular gender-related risk factor, patients or clients have been referred to as males or females more or less randomly.

IS THIS THE DEFINITIVE TEXT?

This text is more complete and more up-to-date than the first and second editions of *A Massage Therapist's Guide to Pathology*, but it still cannot be a permanent, definitive massage pathophysiology text. Readers of earlier editions will see how our understanding of some conditions has remained static over the past several years, but some others have substantially changed; it will always be so. We all anticipate that future research will reveal much more about massage and disease, perhaps even research that some of you will conduct.

A FINAL NOTE

Every possible effort has been made to make this material as accurate as possible. However, it needs to be said that *nothing* in this book is meant to act as a substitute for a doctor's advice. Massage therapists and bodyworkers with questions about the applicability of their work should consult with their clients' health care team for the best possible results. This consultation cannot occur without the consent of the client. Therefore, the most fruitful relationships happen when a client, the massage therapist, and the other members of the health care team are all informed of each others' activities and all work together toward the same goals.

One of the items on my personal agenda in writing this book is to share with you the wonder of the human body. It is amazing that we work as well as we do. It is even more miraculous that we can recover from injury and disease. As massage practitioners we work to create an internal environment in our clients that fosters healing and recovery. Having conscious intention in our work makes us even better at achieving this goal. My purpose in writing this book is to help each practitioner develop that specific sense of intention: we should know why we are doing what we are doing every minute that we are working with a client.

So, happy reading. Do more research if it interests you, and remember that some of the questions dealt with here will probably never be completely answered. What we think we know now may someday be revised or proved wrong. Isn't that terrific?!

Ruth Werner
Summer 2004

How to Use This Book

USER'S GUIDE

A Massage Therapist's Guide to Pathology gives you the tools to make informed decisions about bodywork for clients who live with a wide variety of diseases and conditions. This User's Guide shows you how to put the book's features to work for you.

CHAPTER OBJECTIVES

These begin every chapter, alerting the reader to important pieces of information that follow, and providing a framework for independent study. Answers to the Chapter Objective Questions are provided on the Student Resource CD-ROM.

CHAPTER INTRODUCTIONS

Each chapter opens with a brief review of the body system under discussion, with special emphasis on factors that may be interrupted by the disease process.

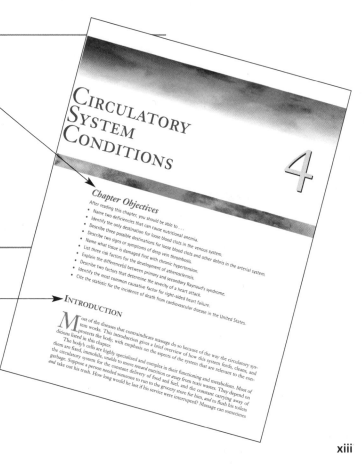

CIRCULATORY SYSTEM CONDITIONS

4

Chapter Objectives

After reading this chapter, you should be able to . . .
- Name two deficiencies that can cause nutritional anemia.
- Identify the only destination for loose blood clots in the venous system.
- Describe three possible destinations for loose blood clots and other debris in the arterial system.
- Describe two signs or symptoms of deep vein thrombosis.
- Name what tissue is damaged first with chronic hypertension.
- List three risk factors for the development of atherosclerosis.
- Explain the difference(s) between primary and secondary Raynaud's syndrome.
- Describe two factors that determine the severity of a heart attack.
- Identify the most common causative factor for right-sided heart failure.
- Cite the statistic for the incidence of death from cardiovascular disease in the United States.

INTRODUCTION

Most of the diseases that contraindicate massage do so because of the way the circulatory system works. This introduction gives a brief overview of how this system feeds, cleans, and protects the body, with emphasis on the aspects of the system that are relevant to the conditions listed in this chapter.

The body's cells are highly specialized and complex in their functioning and metabolism. Most of them are fixed, immobile, unable to move *toward* nutrition or *away* from toxic wastes. They depend on the circulatory system for the constant delivery of food and fuel, and the constant carrying away of garbage. Suppose a person needed someone to run to the grocery store for him, *and* to flush his toilets and take out his trash. How long would he last if his service were interrupted? Massage can sometimes

In Brief Boxes

These give a synopsis of the definition, signs and symptoms, and guidelines for bodywork for each condition discussed. All the In Brief Boxes are then repeated alphabetically in Appendix IV to provide a valuable Quick Reference Chart.

Sidebars

These present information that is important, but peripheral to the core discussion. Disease histories, some statistics, and specific cancer staging protocols are provided in the sidebars.

SNIGLETS

These give extra tidbits of information about word derivations, the people who first named or documented various diseases, and other fascinating details.

CASE HISTORIES

These provide an important voice to the people who live with a variety of diseases and conditions. They offer a chance to see how some disorders powerfully influence people's lives.

4

A Massage Therapist's Guide to Pathology

Boils:

Boils are also called furuncles, from the Latin *furunculus*, which means "petty thief." The association between petty thievery and boils is obscure, unless one refers to the extreme irritation caused by both.

CONTAGIOUS SKIN DISORDERS

Boils

Definition: What Are They?

Boils, also called *furuncles*, are localized staphylococcus infections of the skin.

Boils in Brief

What are they?
Boils are localized bacterial infections of the skin. The causative agent is usually *Staphylococcus aureus*.

How are they recognized?
Boils involve painful, red, hot pustules on the skin. They may occur singly or in interconnected clusters called carbuncles.

Is massage indicated or contraindicated?
Boils contraindicate massage at least locally, and care should be taken to make sure the infection is not systemic (screen the client for other symptoms such as swelling, fever, or discomfort other than at the site of the lesion). The bacteria that cause boils are extremely virulent and communicable. The sheets of a client with boils should be isolated and treated with bleach.

Etiology: What Happens?

Boils are staphylococcus infections of sebaceous glands or hair shafts that are clogged by dirt, dead skin cells, or other debris. They have much in common with acne, but the type of bacterium that usually causes boils, *S. aureus*, is a particularly virulent aggressive variety. It is resistant to temperatures up to 50°C (122°F), salt, and drying.

Boils usually occur in areas where a lot of friction, in combination with sweat, can irritate or injure skin. They are most common in the axilla or groin, where if they are recurrent they may be referred to as *hidradenitis suppurativa*. A specific type of boil, *pilonidal cysts*, occurs around the buttocks.

Signs and Symptoms

Boils are large and painful infections. They usually occur one at a time, or in small groups (Figure 1.2). A cluster of boils connected by channels under the skin is called a *carbuncle* (Figure 1.3).

In the early stages, boils are hard, small, and red. As they mature, they may grow to the size of a golf ball. They soften in the middle, and accumulate pus; this is the site where drainage usually takes place.

Treatment

As long as the infection stays localized, boils are not dangerous, although they are extremely painful. Conservative treatment begins with hot compresses, relieving the pressure and therefore the pain. If compresses are not sufficient, doctors may lance the boil. Antibiotics are sometimes prescribed, but they tend to be slow acting, and have the best effect for people who have a recurring problem.

It is important never to try to squeeze or pop a boil. It could force the infection deeper into tissues, or spread the bacteria over the surface of the skin. This raises the risk of complications brought about by the possibility of the bacteria invading other parts of the body, or even other bodies altogether.

Chronically repeating boils may indicate a compromised immune system. They may also be a warning sign for *diabetes* (Chapter 8) or kidney problems.

235

Massage?

... is a local infection with extremely virulent, hardy bacteria. A client who has a boil ... no signs of systemic infection may receive massage, but not on or near the lesion.

Chapter 3 / Nervous System Conditions

Case History

Eating Disorders

Jessica, Age 19: "Food was the one thing I thought I could control completely."

I think my eating problems began when I was around 12 years old. I was an only child and a gymnast, and working hard in my program. All my coaches wanted muscle, muscle, muscle—no flab. At that time I got in the mindset that the more I worked out, the more muscle I'd have, so I started skipping meals to have more body-building time.

Having muscles and doing my routines perfectly were the only things on my mind. I went on a pretty much just-rice diet. Rice doesn't have any fat, but lots of carbs to burn for energy. I'd have a bowl of rice and some water, which would make me feel really full. I think due to that my stomach shrank; just eating regular foods became really hard. Since I was always by myself, my parents didn't realize my problem. I always wore baggy clothes because I was constantly cold, and if I wore something tighter, my mother would say I looked fat; but in truth I was barely 5 feet tall and about 70 to 75 pounds. When I was in 7th grade I also got food poisoning from a school lunch. I ended up in the hospital. After that I couldn't eat lunch anymore until I was 18.

When I was 15, my grandfather, who had been the center of my life, died. I went into a deep depression. I had already lost gymnastics because of an injury. So I'd just go to school, home, go to sleep, get up for a little bit to eat, and go back to sleep to do it all over again. When I slept I had terrible dreams, and I heard voices when I was awake. I started to lose a lot of hair and have irregular menstrual cycles.

At this time, and up until I turned 18, I felt like my parents controlled everything; what I wore, who I spent time with, where I was, every minute of the day. Food was the one thing I thought I could control completely. Sometimes I'd get up in the middle of the night and eat and eat like I was about to die. I would feel awful later, but I would never make myself throw up. I saw a movie on bulimia once, and saw how much damage it caused, so instead, I would not eat for a day or two after I binged. I still do that sometimes, but not as severely as I used to.

I had always been a straight-A student in school until my senior year in high school. That is when I learned of my eating problem. Several of my friends noticed how I never seemed to eat and started to help me break out of my cycle. The best thing I did was to go to Europe by myself. That gave me a chance to "break out of my box," which opened a whole new world of options to me. I'd say that was when I began to heal from both my depression and my eating problems.

Now I'm in massage school. I eat about 2 1/2 meals every day. I was kind of surprised that getting massage was so easy for me. I did have some fears about laying supine on the table, but I'm over it. I have chronic back pain, and I enjoy deep massage. I did have some fears about long-term problems from anorexia. My periods were irregular then, and they're painful now. I still have some fears about long-term problems from anorexia. My periods were irregular then, and they're painful now. I lose a lot of blood every month; I'm definitely anemic.

Still, I know I was lucky. I was able to control my eating before it got so bad that I needed to be admitted to the hospital. My whole sense of who I am and what makes me feel good is different now. I still really like getting compliments. If I hear, "You look great," or "That shirt looks good on you," then I feel like I can eat a chicken sandwich or a bowl of ice cream without feeling guilty later. But for the most part, for stuff like the grades I get in school, or what courses I take, no one decides what I need now. I am my own person, and I am in control of my life once again. It feels really good.

Treatment

A Massage Therapist's Guide to Pathology

Working with diet and other life habits to cleanse the liver and make its filtering job easier often results in clearer skin, as well as a host of other benefits. Massage of the abdomen and liver may support this process, but it is erroneous to claim that massage will reliably clear up acne; there are too many other factors to consider.

For teenagers with acne, the best advice is the most difficult to follow: *do not touch the face*. Touching, scratching, and popping acne lesions does little except to spread the bacteria and open the possibility of permanent scarring.

Over-the-counter preparations usually use benzoyl peroxide or other similar substances to limit the activity of *P. acnes*.

When medical help is requested for acne, interventions usually take a two-pronged attack: topical steroids are applied for their anti-inflammatory properties, and antibiotics are administered internally to go after the bacteria. The disadvantage is that being on a long-term course of antibiotics can play havoc with intestinal flora and the immune system. One alternative is a line of drugs called *retinoins*, which are effective for acne, but have a list of troubling side effects including joint pain and hair loss. Retinoins are also contraindicated if the patient may be pregnant during treatment, because they are highly implicated in birth defects.

Massage?

Massage of the abdomen and liver can sometimes yield good results. But massage on the lesions themselves is out of the question. Pimples are infections, and they involve a com-

---

Compare and Contrast
ACNE AND BOILS

Boils and acne have a lot in common: they are both localized infections of sebaceous glands in hair follicles; they are both caused by *Staphylococcus* infections; they both have a red base with a pustule. But boils are far more serious than acne and require different precautions from massage therapists. Here are some differentiating features:

BOILS

Pattern of Appearance
One lesion at a time, or a small inter-connected group of pustules

Virulence
Aggressive bacteria that attack living tissue

Symptoms
Extremely painful

Communicability
Highly communicable

Special Precautions
At least a local contraindication, but may be systemic if signs of general infection are present. Isolate and bleach sheets

ACNE

Pattern of Appearance
Spread over large areas (the face, back, or neck)

Virulence
Less aggressive bacteria that simply take advantage of a hospitable growth medium

Symptoms
Mildly painful

Communicability
Not communicable without prolonged contact

Special Precautions
Local contraindication; no other precautions necessary

COMPARE AND CONTRAST BOXES

These offer a chance to put key features of closely connected disorders side-by-side for a point-by-point comparison.

ARTWORK AND PHOTOS

These are rendered in full color throughout the book help to illustrate key points, and provide a valuable resource to help recognize a wide range of skin conditions in various stages of severity.

xvi

CHAPTER REVIEW QUESTIONS

These questions require critical thinking skills and the ability to use information to draw conclusions about the safe practice of bodywork in complicated situations. Answers to the Chapter Review Questions appear on the Student Resource CD-ROM.

- *Peritoneal dialysis* is a method of kidney dialysis for people with advanced kidney failure. It uses the peritoneal membrane as a filter to clean the blood. One of the risks of peritoneal dialysis is the contamination of the tubing that connects to the peritoneum: this can cause peritonitis.

Signs and Symptoms

The symptoms of peritonitis vary, depending on the original cause. Abdominal pain is usually part of the picture. It tends to begin as diffuse pain, but it localizes at the original site of infection. Nausea and vomiting are usually present, and if the infection is untreated, severe dehydration may result. Many patients experience reduced urine output, and difficulty passing gas or bowel movements. After 2 or 3 hours, the abdomen will swell and pain may subside, but this is not a sign of improvement; rather, it is an indication that the intestines have gone into paralysis. At this point, death is not far away unless the patient gets immediate hospital care.

Treatment

Treatment for peritonitis varies according to cause and severity. At the very least, antibiotics are needed. Emergency situations will require abdominal surgery to remove or repair the ruptured organ, and to wash out the peritoneal cavity as fully as possible. When peritonitis is caught early, it usually responds well to treatment, but if it is left too long it can be deadly.

Massage?

Any form of acute peritonitis systemically contraindicates massage until all signs of infection have passed.

CHAPTER REVIEW QUESTIONS

1. Describe how ongoing stress can contribute to digestive system problems.
2. Why is the appendix no longer routinely removed in the course of other abdominal surgery?
3. What is ascites? How can liver dysfunction cause it?
4. Why might someone with ulcerative colitis be at a higher risk of developing colon cancer than the general population?
5. Describe the leading theory behind the development of colon cancer.
6. What is the difference between diverticula and colon polyps?
7. Most people with gallstones never have symptoms. What finally causes symptoms to occur?
8. Why are oral antibiotics often ineffective for dealing with a bacterial infection of the gastrointestinal tract?
9. What is a possible cause of ulcers that does not involve the *Helicobacter pylori* bacterium?
10. A client is recovering from a bout with hepatitis A. His skin has a yellowish tone and the sclera of his eyes is yellow too. What condition is probably present? Is this client a good candidate for circulatory massage? Why?

Answers to these questions can be found on the Student Resource CD-ROM that accompanies this book.

STUDENT RESOURCE CD-ROM

This resource has all the answers to the Chapter Objective Questions and Chapter Review Questions, a student question and answer section, animations to demonstrate several disease processes, and an auditory pronunciation guide of glossary terms found in Stedman's Medical Dictionary.

Items in text that refer the reader to the Student Resource CD-ROM have this icon.

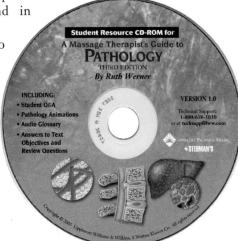

REVIEWERS

The publisher and author gratefully acknowledge the many professionals who shared their expertise and assisted in developing this textbook, appropriately targeting our marketing efforts, creating useful ancillary products, and setting the stage for subsequent editions. These individuals include:

Sameh Abdelaal
Academy of Massage
    Therapy
Englewood, New Jersey

Robert Adams
New Hampshire
    Community Technical
    College
Nashua, New Hampshire

Adedayo Adeeko
Sir Sandford Fleming
    College
Peterborough, Ontario

Elizabeth Aerts
The School of Integrative
    Therapies
Holmdel, New Jersey

Marc Ague
Virginia College of
    Huntsville
Huntsville, Alabama

Chantel Anstine
Education/Coordinator
Rasmussen College
Roseville, Minnesota

Pat Archer
Brenneke School of
    Massage
Seattle, Washington

Robin Archey
Director of Education
Healing Hands Institute
    for Massage Therapy
Montvale, New Jersey

Margaret Avery Moon
Desert Institute of the
    Healing Arts
Tucson, Arizona

Wayne Baiton
Western College of
    Remedial Massage
    Therapies Inc.
Regina, Saskatchewan

Dr. Viktor Benedek
Victoria, British
    Colombia

Patricia Berak
Baker College of Clinton
    Township
Clinton Township,
    Michigan

Susan Bova
Penn Commercial
Washington,
    Pennsylvania

Gary Bruce, NCTMB,
    LMT
Executive Director
Project Special Care
St. Augustine, Florida

Mary Capozzi, MS, RN,
    LMT, NCTMB
Finger Lakes Community
    College
Canandaigua, New York

Paul Chambers
Salter School
Tewksbury,
    Massachusetts

Beverly Chumbley
Massage Institute of
    Memphis
Memphis, Tennessee

Anthony Clapp
Center Point
Minneapolis, Minnesota

Patricia Coe
National University of
    Health Sciences
Lombard, Illinois

Steve Colarusso
Charles of Italy School of
    Massage Therapy
Lake Havasu City,
    Arizona

Laurie Craig, MS
Executive Director;
    Chair, Human Sciences
    Department
Atlanta School of
    Massage
Atlanta, Georgia

David Crozier
Body Wisdom Massage
    Therapy School
Des Moines, Iowa

Vicki Cunningham, DC
Soma Institute of
    Massage Therapy, Inc.
Shawnee, Oklahoma

Nancy Dail
Director
Downeast School of
    Massage
Waldoboro, Maine

Judy Deken
International Professional
    School of Bodywork
Pacific Beach, California

Rod Diehm
Ashmead College
Tigard, Oregon

Marc Ellsworth
Baker College of Jackson
Jackson, Michigan

Darnell Erickson
DoveStar
Orleans, Massachusetts

David Esteppe
Education Chair of
    Massage Therapy
    Department
Kee Business College
Virginia Beach, Virginia

Stan Ewald
West Los Angeles,
    California

Mary Allice Farina
Sandhills Community
    College
Pinehurst, North
    Carolina

Leora Fellus
Western Institute of
    Neuromuscular
    Therapy
Laguna Hills, California

Nadine Forbes, MS
National Director of
    Education
Steiner Education Group
(Florida College of
    Natural Health,
    Baltimore School of
    Massage, Virginia
    School of Massage)
Baltimore, Maryland

Karen Harrison
D.G. Erwin Technical
    Center
Tampa, Florida

Lisa Holk
Pacific College of
    Oriental Medicine
Chicago, Illinois

Amanda Hooten
Cumberland Institute for
    Wellness Education
Brentwood, Tennessee

Connie Jakubcin
Southeastern Career
    College
Nashville, Tennessee

Judith Jamieson
Green Mt Institute for
    Integrative Therapy
North Bennington,
    Vermont

Cora Janzen
Professional Institute of
    Massage Therapy
Saskatoon, Saskatchewan

Kate Jordan
Director
Kate Jordan Seminars
La Jolla, California

Sarita Kalu
Sanford Brown College
St. Louis, Missouri

Rich Kamasinski Sol
The New School for
    Massage
Chicago, Illinois

Carrie Kaye
The Salter School
Tewksbury,
    Massachusetts

Judie Klein
Sarasota School of
    Massage Therapy
Sarasota, Florida

Leslie Knee
TESST College of
    Technology
Beltsville, Maryland

Laura Kwitek
Martin's College of
    Cosmetology
Green Bay, Wisconsin

Vito LaFerrera
Academy of Massage
    Therapy
Englewood, New Jersey

Terry Lancaster
National Institute of
    Massotherapy
Akron, Ohio

Nancy Lankston
Overland Park, Kansas

Jerry Levin
Mercy College of NW
    Ohio
Toledo, Ohio

Stacey Long
Miami Jacobs Career
    College
Dayton, Ohio

Jean Loose
Southwest Academy of
    Natural Therapies
Grand Junction,
    Colorado

Wendy Loren
Lane Community
    College
Eugene, Oregon

Maryagnes Luczak
Career Training Academy
New Kensington,
    Pennsylvania

James MacIntyre
Foothills College of
    Massage Therapy
Calgary, Alberta, Canada

Harlin Magee
New Creation Massage
    Institute
Austin, Texas

Mark Manton
Program Director
Massage Therapy
    Institute of Colorado
Denver, Colorado

Andrea Mariani
Union County College
Plainfield, New Jersey

Terri Martens
Fox Institute of Business
West Hartford,
    Connecticut

Cecile Martin
Bodyworks School of
    Massage
Evansville, Indiana

Jonathan Martine
Faculty Chair
Rolf Institute
Boulder, Colorado

Teresa Matheson
Utah Career College
West Jordan, Utah

Michael Matthews
Miller-Motte Technical
    College
Chattanooga, Tennessee

Mary McCluskey
Director
Wisconsin School of
    Massage Therapy
Germantown, Wisconsin

Leo McElroy
International School of
    Shiatsu
Doylestown,
    Pennsylvania

Cheryn McGillicuddy
Director of Education
Central Florida School of
    Massage Therapy, Inc.
Winter Park, Florida

Maria Mendola
Providence Institute
Tucson, Arizona

Karen Mitchell
St Louis College of
    Health Careers
St Louis, Missouri

Roger Olbrot
Myotherapy College of
    Utah
Salt Lake City, Utah

Joni Olehausen
Director of Schools and
    Clinic; Science
    Instructor
Sister Rosalind Gefre
    School of Massage
Sauk Rapids, Minnesota

Robert Oliver
Curriculum Director
Ralston School of
    Massage
Reno, Nevada

Angela Palmier
Education Director;
    Co-owner
Midwest Institute of
    Massage Therapy
Belleville, Illinois

Aaron Pavlechko
Central Pennsylvania
    School of Massage
State College,
    Pennsylvania

Michael Polon
The Rolf Institute
Boulder, Colorado

Susan Powers
Morrisville State College
Morrisville, New York

Kalyani Premkumar
Mount Royal College
Calgary, Alberta

Graham Rae
Manatee Technical
    Institute
Bradenton, Florida

Holly Rasmusson
Total Look
Cresco, Iowa

Sallye Raymond
Delgado Community
    College
New Orleans, Louisiana

Melissa Reedy
Great Lakes Institute of
    Technology
Erie, Pennsylvania

Laura Reilly
American Institute of
    Massage
Richmond, Virginia

Monica Reno, LMT
Director of Education
Central Florida School of
    Massage Therapy
Winter Park, Florida

Andrea Robins
Daytona Beach
    Community College
New Smyrna Beach,
    Florida

Sharon Round
Kee Business College
Newport News, Virginia

John Schewe
The Rolf Institute
Boulder, Colorado

Dawn Schmidt
Brenneke School of
    Massage
Seattle, Washington

Matthew Schrier
Chair of Health Sciences
Connecticut Center for
    Massage Therapy
Newington, Connecticut

Lorissa Sickmiller
Institute of Therapeutic
    Massage
Ottawa, Ohio

Teressa Sloan, PhD, DD,
    LMT, NCBTMB
Bluegrass Professional
    School of Massage
    Therapy
Lexington, Kentucky

Francesca Stark
Ashmead College School
    of Massage
Everett, Washington

Timothy Starkey
Spa Tech Institute
Westboro, Massachusetts

Sandra Stone
Broward Community
    College
Coconut Creek, Florida

Victoria Stone
Academic Director
Blue Ridge School of
    Massage & Yoga
Blacksburg, Virginia

M. Sullivan
Anne Arundel
    Community College
Arnold, Maryland

Heather Thom, DC
Duluth Business
    University
Duluth, Minnesota

Dale Thomas
Director
Desert Springs Therapy
Desert Hot Springs,
    California

Jeff Thompson
NM Academy of Healing
    Arts
Santa Fe, New Mexico

Elizabeth Upton
Allentown Business
    School
Center Valley,
    Pennsylvania

Marcia Vahila
Chair
National Institute of
    Massotherapy
Akron, Ohio

Charlotte Versagi
Carnegie Institute
Troy, Michigan

Dr. Cheryl M. Ward
Louisville School of
    Massage
Louisville, Kentucky

Wanona Wellspring
Director of Programs
Wellspring Centre of
    Natural Healing Art
Naperville, Illinois

Jean M. Wible, RN,
    BSN, NCTMB,
    CHTP
Adjunct Faculty,
    Community College of
    Baltimore County
Continuing Education
    Faculty, for
    Community College of
    Baltimore County
Community College of
    Allegany County
AMTA Maryland
    Chapter
The Baltimore School of
    Massage
Massage Therapist and
    Healing Touch
    Practitioner at
    Baltimore Centre for
    Wellness
Baltimore, Maryland

Ronda Wimmer
Anaheim, California

Melissa Wollin
Bryman College
San Bernardino,
    California

Brad Yates
Lakeside School of
    Massage Therapy
Madison, Wisconsin

ACKNOWLEDGMENTS

No book is written in a vacuum, although it may sometimes seem that way. Many people contributed to the development of this work, and it is important to recognize them publicly and with gratitude.

To Brian Utting, LMP, teacher, boss, Big Kahuna, commissioner of the original work, and source of inspiration to constantly strive to do something that might be too hard (and to this day one of the most influential people in my life), and to Suzanne Carlson, RN, LMP, who first made it clear to all of us how important it was to know this material—years before we were required to:
The two of you formed the germinal material from which this work grew. My thanks and admiration will always be with you.

To the students of the Brian Utting School of Massage, the Myotherapy College of Utah, the Ogden Institute of Massage Therapy, and those I have encountered in my travels with this material:
I am so grateful to you all. You continue to teach me far more than I could ever hope to teach you, and I dearly hope that it never, ever stops.

To all the people who I pestered and bugged and cornered and button-holed to look at this, or comment on that, or talk to me about the other; and to the very special people who allowed themselves to be interviewed for case histories:
Your generosity will provide a service to many people for many years. Thank you with all my heart.

To Candy Lavicky, my research assistant and never-failing booster, and to the wonderful people at LWW who have unfailingly supported this project:
Thank you, thank you, thank you, thank you. Your shared commitment to excellence has made working on this project a deeply satisfying and fulfilling experience.

Finally, to my wonderful family—Curtis, Nathan, and Lily Anne Rose:
We did it again, and it wouldn't have happened without you. Remember that I love you, all the time, every minute, no matter what.

R. Werner
Summer 2004

I want to express my heartfelt gratitude to Ruth Werner. First my instructor, then my mentor, now my friend. She provided yet another "learning opportunity" for me. This book is invaluable to massage therapists in their professions.

I also want to extend a hug to my husband, Tim Seminoff. Thanks for the many times you rescued me and helped me navigate my way around the computer with your technical knowledge and support.

Candy Lavicky
Summer 2004

The author and publisher wish to acknowledge special gratitude to Jean Wible, whose text, *Pharmacology for Massage Therapy*, served as an important resource, and whose generous input was central to the creation of Appendix V: Medications.

Contents

DETAILED CONTENTS

INTEGUMENTARY SYSTEM CONDITIONS

1

Chapter Objectives

After reading this chapter, you should be able to . . .

- Explain why broken skin contraindicates massage.
- Name three differences between acne and boils.
- Identify three types of fungal infections of the skin.
- Identify the type of bacteria associated with boils.
- Identify the type of bacteria associated with cellulitis.
- State two dangers associated with widespread burns.
- State three dangers associated with the long-term use of corticosteroid creams.
- Recite the ABCDEs of malignant melanoma.
- Describe the cardinal sign of non-melanoma skin cancer.
- Describe a feature that distinguishes plantar warts from callus.

INTRODUCTION: FUNCTION AND CONSTRUCTION OF THE SKIN

Massage practitioners speak in a language of touch. The messages practitioners give are invitations to a number of different possibilities: to enjoy a state of well-being, to heal and repair what is broken, and to reacquaint a client with his or her own body. All of this happens through the skin: a medium that is equipped like no other tissue in the body to take in information and respond to it, mostly on a subconscious level. The goal of massage practitioners is to anticipate these reactions and to set the stage for them in a way that is most beneficial for their clients.

Functions of the Skin

A student once said that the purpose of skin is to keep our insides from falling out. That is true, but it is not all skin does; its functions are manifold. Among them are several devices to keep the body healthy and safe, all wrapped up in one tidy 18- to 30-pound package.

Protection

The skin keeps pathogens *out* of the body, just by being intact, and it discourages their growth on its surface by secreting the acidic lubricants otherwise needed for keeping hair shafts oiled. Furthermore, by constantly sloughing off dead cells, it sloughs off potential invaders too.

The skin is the first line of defense against invasion, and the superficial fascia is especially well supplied with immune system cells that are constantly on the lookout for potential sources of infection. These mast cells and other nonspecific white blood cells can create an extreme inflammatory response very quickly. When these defense mechanisms become hyperactive, they can cause certain types of rashes and other skin problems. For more details on hypersensitivity reactions, see the Introduction to Lymph and Immune Conditions (Chapter 5).

Homeostasis

The skin protects us from fluid loss, a top homeostatic priority, and one of the most dangerous functions to lose when the skin is damaged. The skin is the membrane that connects inner bodies to the outside world. It helps to maintain a constant internal temperature in spite of what is happening outside because blood supply to the skin far exceeds the need for local nutrition: capillaries will dilate or constrict according to what is needed at the time. The fat in the subcutaneous layer also acts as insulation.

Sensory Envelope

With as many as 19,000 sensory receptors in every square inch of skin, obviously this is the organ (or tissue, or membrane, or system—depending on the source of information) that tells us the most about our environment. Eyes and ears appear to be indispensable, but look how far Helen Keller got with just her skin to take in information. Massage therapists must develop the skill of becoming *conscious* of the subtle information their hands pick up when they touch their clients and must understand that every sensation created on a client's skin is also causing ripples of reactions all through the client's body.

Absorption, Excretion

To a small extent, the skin *does* absorb and excrete. Fat-soluble materials can be absorbed through the capillaries in hair shafts. Some massage oil is also absorbed in this way. Compounds such as *DMSO* are completely absorbed, a phenomenon called *transcutaneous absorption*.

The skin can help to excrete metabolic wastes, but it does so only as a last ditch option. When the liver, colon, or especially kidneys are so congested that they cannot handle any more waste products, sweat can carry noxious chemicals out of the body.

Construction of the Skin

Skin varies from being very thin (on the lips) to remarkably thick (on the heels). It remodels according to stresses put upon it. *Callus* is an example of this phenomenon: extra thick, extra hard epidermis on places that take a beating.

The construction of the skin is important to understand because it has relevance for how disease occurs and how easily it might spread. Three basic layers of tissue define the skin, and within those layers are more layers (Figure 1.1). The subcutaneous tissue is probably familiar: it is also called superficial fascia. The dermis, or "true skin," is the location of hair shafts, oil and sweat glands, and some nerve endings. The outermost layer of dermis, the basal layer, lies just below the epidermis and has the best capillary supply. This is where new skin cells are born. Pigment cells (called melanocytes) are here, protecting people from harmful ultraviolet (UV) rays. Some of the worst diseases are born here too, for reasons described later in this chapter. New cells are cloned near the base of the epidermis, and migrate toward the top, dying of starvation and becoming keratinized, or scaly, in the process, which takes approximately 1 month. By the time they reach the surface, they are long dead and will soon be sloughed off to become the major ingredient of household dust.

● *The animation "Cell Cycle" can be found on the Student Resource CD that accompanies this book.* The epidermis is made of epithelium. Epithelium heals faster than any other type of tissue, which is good because no other tissue type is as vulnerable to damage as skin. It would be nice if the central nervous system healed as readily as the skin does, but consider the priorities: compare the number of neurologic traumas a person is likely to experience with the number of cuts, scrapes, scratches, tears, and punctures he will endure. Nevertheless, healing quickly has its disadvantages. Cells that have instructions to replicate at the drop of a hat sometimes replicate *without* the hat dropping, and that causes trouble.

Rules for Massage

Skin conditions have a special relevance for massage therapists because they are in a position to notice lesions and blemishes that clients often do not know are there. Thus, being able to recognize most common skin conditions, at least as far as being able to recommend that clients investigate further with their own doctors, is important. Many skin conditions contraindicate massage because they might be contagious. Beyond that danger, however, the one cardinal rule for skin conditions and massage is: *if the intactness of the skin has been compromised in any way, the client is a*

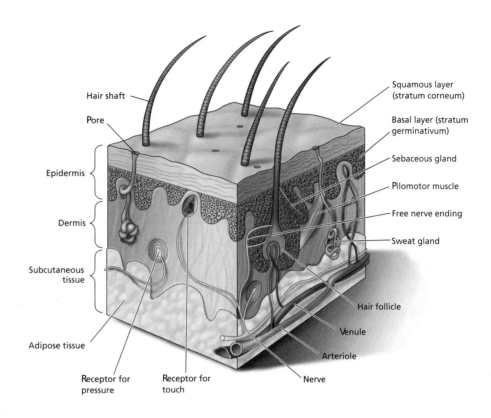

Figure 1.1. Cross-section of the skin.

walking invitation for infection. Open skin, broken skin, scabbed skin, any skin that allows access to the blood vessels inside is a red flag for massage practitioners. No matter how much a person scrubs, pathogens will always be present on the skin. By considering any compromised area of skin at least a local contraindication, practitioners take the responsibility to ensure that their microorganisms do not jump into their clients' vulnerable spots. At the same time, practitioners can prevent *clients'* pathogens jumping into the tiny cracks in the practitioner's skin.

INTEGUMENTARY SYSTEM CONDITIONS

Contagious Skin Disorders

Boils
Cellulitis
Fungal Infections
Herpes Simplex
Impetigo
Lice and Mites
Warts

Noncontagious Inflammatory Skin Disorders

Acne Vulgaris
Acne Rosacea
Dermatitis/Eczema
Hives

Neoplastic Skin Disorders

Moles
Psoriasis
Skin Cancer

Skin Injuries

Burns
Decubitus Ulcers
Open Wounds and Sores
Scar Tissue

Other

Ichthyosis

Boils:

Boils are also called furuncles, from the Latin *furunculus*, which means "petty thief." The association between petty thievery and boils is obscure, unless one refers to the extreme irritation caused by both.

CONTAGIOUS SKIN DISORDERS

Boils

Definition: What Are They?

Boils, also called *furuncles*, are localized staphylococcus infections of the skin.

Etiology: What Happens?

Boils are staphylococcus infections of sebaceous glands or hair shafts that are clogged by dirt, dead skin cells, or other debris. They have much in common with acne, but the type of bacterium that usually causes boils, *S. aureus*, is a particularly virulent, aggressive variety. It is resistant to temperatures up to 50°C (122°F), salt, and drying.

Boils usually occur in areas where a lot of friction, in combination with sweat, can irritate or injure skin. They are most common in the axilla or groin, where if they are recurrent they may be referred to as *hidradenitis suppurativa*. A specific type of boil, *pilonidal cysts*, occurs around the buttocks.

Signs and Symptoms

Boils are large and painful infections. They usually occur one at a time, or in small groups (Figure 1.2). A cluster of boils connected by channels under the skin is called a *carbuncle* (Figure 1.3).

In the early stages, boils are hard, small, and red. As they mature, they may grow to the size of a golf ball. They soften in the middle, and accumulate pus; this is the site where drainage usually takes place.

Boils in Brief

What are they?
Boils are localized bacterial infections of the skin. The causative agent is usually *Staphylococcus aureus*.

How are they recognized?
Boils involve painful, red, hot pustules on the skin. They may occur singly or in interconnected clusters called carbuncles.

Is massage indicated or contraindicated?
Boils contraindicate massage at least locally, and care should be taken to make sure the infection is not systemic. Screen the client for other symptoms such as swelling, fever, or discomfort other than at the site of the lesion. The bacteria that cause boils are extremely virulent and communicable. The sheets of a client with boils should be isolated and treated with bleach.

Treatment

As long as the infection stays localized, boils are not dangerous, although they are extremely painful. Conservative treatment begins with hot compresses, which helps them to burst and then drain, relieving the pressure and therefore the pain. If compresses are not sufficient, doctors may lance the boil. Antibiotics are sometimes prescribed, but they tend to be slow acting and have the best effect for people who have a recurring problem.

It is important never to try to squeeze or pop a boil. It could force the infection deeper into tissues or spread the bacteria over the surface of the skin. Boils also carry a risk of complications brought about by the possibility of the bacteria invading other parts of the body, or even other bodies altogether.

Chronically repeating boils may indicate a compromised immune system. They may also be a warning sign for *diabetes* (Chapter 8) or kidney problems.

Massage?

This is a local infection with extremely virulent, hardy bacteria. A client who has a boil with no signs of systemic infection may receive massage, but not on or near the lesion.

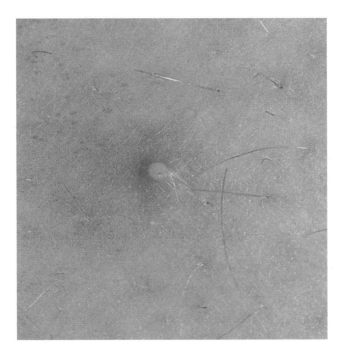

Figure 1.2. Single boil.

If signs of systemic infection are present (fever, swelling at nearby lymph nodes, discomfort anywhere other than the site of the boil), it will be necessary to reschedule the massage.

The sheets of a client with a boil require special treatment: isolate them and wash them at high temperature with extra bleach to ensure that any bacteria are eradicated.

Figure 1.3. A group of interconnected boils is called a carbuncle.

Cellulitis

Definition: What Is It?

Cellulitis is a streptococcal infection of the cells in the skin, usually involving one of the group A class of bacteria, which are also causative factors for strep throat, impetigo, toxic shock syndrome, and necrotizing fasciitis ("flesh-eating bacteria"). One variety of cellulitis, *erysipelas*, is also known as St. Anthony's Fire.

Etiology: What Happens?

It is virtually impossible to remove all the bacteria from a living person's skin; colonies of organisms are always growing on the skin: under the fingernails, between the toes, everywhere. When these organisms get inside the skin, an infection may develop. Staphylococcus is usually responsible for small, localized infections such as boils; it seems to have an affinity for sebum. But once streptococcus gets under the skin, the local infection may become systemic, involving first the lymphatic, then the circulatory systems.

Streptococci must gain access to the body through some portal of entry. In many cases it can be difficult to identify exactly where the bacteria got in, but sometimes the infection can be traced to a specific cut or scratch, athlete's foot (see *ringworm* this chapter), an insect bite, surgery to remove a section of saphenous vein, or some other skin injury. Once the bacteria gain entry, they produce enzymes that destroy cell membranes and inhibit processes that would otherwise limit and localize infection.

Signs and Symptoms

Sometimes signs of systemic infection precede an obvious skin infection with cellulitis, but it usually begins with a tender, red, swollen area (Figure 1.4). The wound soon shows signs of infection, which may include red streaks running toward the nearest set of lymph nodes. If the infection starts on the face, a raised red, hot tender area may develop that spreads laterally across the bridge of the nose. One hallmark of erysipelas is a sharp margin between involved and uninvolved skin; the red edges are usually very clear (Figure 1.5). Other forms of cellulitis have less distinct borders.

Figure 1.4. Cellulitis: a staphylococcus infection of the skin.

Figure 1.5. Erysipelas: note the clear delineation
between involved and uninvolved skin.

When the infection has thoroughly engaged the lymph system, symptoms include fever, chills, and systemic discomfort. Facial infections are particularly dangerous because of the risk of intracranial spreading through lymphatics. If cellulitis is left untreated, the bacteria may get past the lymph system and enter the circulatory system, leading quickly, and perhaps fatally, to septicemia, or blood poisoning.

Treatment

Many varieties of streptococcus have become resistant to antibiotics, so a simple prescription of penicillin is no longer adequate for most cases of cellulitis. Furthermore, the risk of having this infection develop serious complications is high enough that aggressive courses of oral or intravenous antibiotics are usually prescribed.

Massage?

This is a condition involving skin damage, a highly contagious bacterial infection, and the risk of blood poisoning if the infection should spread into the circulatory system. It systemically contraindicates massage until all signs of infection have passed.

Fungal Infections

Definition: What Is It?

The nomenclature for the range of fungal infections people can get is dizzying. Fungal infections of human skin, also called *mycoses*, can involve several different types of fungi (*dermatophytes*). *Dermatophytosis*, then, is another term for mycosis. The lesions the infections create are called *tinea*. And to top it all off, the generic term *ringworm*, although it is misleading because there are no worms involved at all, is frequently used to refer to several types of tinea.

Fungal Infections in Brief

What are they?
Fungal infections of human skin, also called *mycoses*, are caused by fungi called *dermatophytes*. The characteristic lesions caused by dermatophytes are called *tinea*. Several types of dermatophytes cause tinea in different areas; they are typically named by location.

How is it recognized?
Most tinea lesions begin as one reddened circular itchy patch. Scratching the lesions spreads them to other parts of the body. As they get larger, they tend to clear in the middle and keep a red ring around the edges. Athlete's foot, another type of mycosis, involves moist blisters and cracking between the toes. Fungal infections of toenails or fingernails involve thickened, pitted, discolored nails that may detach.

Is massage indicated or contraindicated?
Fungal infections locally contraindicate massage in all stages. If the affected areas are very limited—for instance, only the feet are involved or only one or two small, covered lesions on the body are present—massage may be administered elsewhere. If a large area is involved, and especially if the infection is acute (i.e., not yet responding to treatment), then it systemically contraindicates massage.

Etiology: What Happens?

Dermatophytes live on dead skin cells. They thrive in warm, moist places such as skin folds between toes or around the groin. They tend to infect people with depressed or sluggish immune systems. Fungal infections are transmitted by touch: either skin-to-skin or skin-to-anything that has some fungus on it, such as massage sheets, locker room benches, or the family hairbrush. Dogs and cats can also transmit fungal infections to humans. It takes anywhere from 4 to 14 days for lesions to appear; during that time the carrier is infectious, which makes this condition very hard to control.

Several different types of dermatophytes may create tinea lesions. Most cases of ringworm are related to colonies of *trichophyton*, *epidermophytin*, or *microsporum* varieties of fungi.

Signs and Symptoms

Tinea infections vary considerably depending on the causative agent and where they appear. Several varieties of tinea affect humans; here are descriptions of the most common ones.

- *Tinea corporis*, or *body ringworm*, is relatively common and very contagious, so it deserves special attention. It generally begins as one small round, red, scaly, itchy patch of skin on the trunk. Scratching spreads the fungus to other parts of the body, and so other lesions appear. They heal from the center first, and they soon take on the appearance of red circles, or rings with a scaly edge that may gradually increase in size, as the fungus spreads out for new food sources (Figure 1.6).

- *Tinea capitis*, or *head ringworm*, inhabits the scalp (Figure 1.7). Lesions here result in itchiness and flaking (like bad dandruff), and if scratching and secondary infection result in scar tissue, there may be temporary or permanent hair loss. This variety is as contagious as body ringworm. Some of the dermatophytes that cause tinea capitis fluoresce under black light, so this is sometimes used as a diagnostic tool.

- *Tinea pedis*, or *athlete's foot*, usually grow on the skin between the toes, especially between the 3rd and 4th digits (Figure 1.8). Athlete's foot affects approximately 20% of the population to some degree. It burns and itches and carries the additional complication of weeping blisters, cracking, peeling skin, and the possibility of infection; athlete's foot can even lead to *lymphangitis* (Chapter 5) or *cellulitis* (this chapter). One va-

Figure 1.6. Tinea corporis: body ringworm.

Figure 1.7. Tinea capitis: permanent baldness.

riety of athlete's foot fungus presents as dry, scaly, itchy lesions on the heel and sole of the foot. This is called a "moccasin distribution." Athlete's foot thrives in the growth medium provided by closed shoes. If a person has athlete's foot, it is especially important to make sure his feet and shoes are always as dry as possible because these fungi, like most others, love warm, dark, moist places.

• *Tinea cruris*, or *jock itch*, is probably the least contagious of the group, but it does not stay exclusively in the groin. It can be found also on the upper thigh and buttocks, and lesions may be present that a client is not aware of, but which massage therapists must avoid carefully (Figure 1.9).

• *Other varieties of tinea.* These include ***tinea manus***, ***tinea barbae***, ***tinea versicolor***, and ***tinea unguium***. Tinea manus, or hand ringworm, usually appears on the palm or between the fingers. It often occurs when a person also has athlete's foot. Tinea barbae affects the bearded area of the face; it is often misdiagnosed as bacterial folliculitis (a variety of *boils*, this chapter). Tinea versicolor is a fungal infection frequently picked up from the sand on Caribbean beaches. It creates variegated pigmentation on the skin. Tinea unguium is a fungal infection that invades the skin under finger and toenails. It is also called ***onychomycosis***.

Figure 1.8. Tinea pedis: athlete's foot.

Figure 1.9. Tinea cruris: jock itch.

Treatment

Treatment for fungal infections can be frustrating. Dermatophytes can be resistant to standard fungicides, and when they grow under toenails or fingernails they can be difficult to reach. Furthermore, they can resemble the body's own proteins, which makes it difficult for the immune system to tag them, and it will therefore be slow to fight them off. External applications of fungicide are the normal treatment, but oral medications are recommended for stubborn or hard-to-reach infections.

Prevention

Where any kind of dermatophytosis is concerned, an ounce of prevention is worth a pound of cure. The best way for a massage therapist to avoid getting ringworm is to know what it looks like and to stay away from it. It is also particularly important to maintain one's own health. This gives the body every chance of fighting off any fungal attack.

Massage?

Fungal infections contraindicate massage in every phase (including the invisible gestation period, which can make it difficult). But a small infestation (just one or two lesions) can be considered a *local* caution as long as the lesions are covered and the therapist does a 10% bleach rinse afterwards. For clients with athlete's foot that shows blistering, weepy skin, the feet are a local contraindication. The decision also might depend on the therapist's own state of health; if the therapist is feeling run down and vulnerable, this may not be the week to work with someone with ringworm.

Case History 1.1

Ringworm

Delores G.: "It Wasn't Until I Remembered Petting the Kittens That I Realized Where They Came From."

In June 1994, I was working hard in massage school. I was living in a house where some stray kittens were close by. I wanted to pet them, so I bought them some food. They came out, and I got to pet them while they were eating.

I was sitting down next to them with my knees up. I had shorts on. I was petting them with my left hand, and then I held my legs with the same hand when I was done. I also folded my arms, so my left hand touched my right bicep.

Approximately 9 days later, there were specific round red spots, the size of a half-dollar, on my left calf, and then on my right arm. It was not until I remembered petting the kittens that I realized where they came from. Approximately a week after the spots appeared, they started really burning and keeping me awake.

Having ringworm was awful. It turns out that I had massaged only two people between being exposed and being diagnosed, so it did not spread through the class, but I had to wait until I was cleared up before I could work again. I sat out of practices, which was really depressing, *plus* it was spreading all over me, from my right arm to my right breast, and on my other calf.

I treated it by showering and then putting tea tree oil and antifungal vaginal cream all over me. I did that for 2 or 3 weeks before it started clearing up. I was all cleared up in about 4 weeks. I waited an extra week just to be sure, so I missed a total of 3 weeks of massage school.

When I got ringworm, I was extremely run down from school, which probably made me susceptible. My teacher said it was interesting that my body chose ringworm as the thing that would slow me down, but it worked!

Herpes Simplex

Definition: What Is It?

Among the several different viruses in the herpes family that affect humans, two closely related herpes simplex viruses are especially common. These viruses cause painful blisters around the outside of the mouth and lips (oral herpes) or around the genitals, thighs, and buttocks (genital herpes).

When the herpes simplex viruses were first being documented, it was found that the virus that caused oral herpes (type I) was different from the one associated with genital herpes (type II). Since then, a large amount of crossover has been noted, and so the delineation between a type I and a type II herpes infection has lost much of its significance.

Demographics: Who Gets It?

Estimates of the incidence of herpes simplex vary. Up to 60% of all sexually active adults may carry genital herpes; the number is probably around 80% for oral herpes. Approximately 30 million people in the United States experience at least one outbreak of some variety of herpes every year. Men and women are affected equally.

Herpes:

The name for this collection of viruses, some of which spread on the skin, comes from the Greek word *herpo*, which means "to creep." This is also the root word of *herpetology*: the study of snakes.

Herpes Simplex in Brief

What is it?
Herpes simplex is a viral infection resulting in cold sores or fever blisters on the face or around the mouth, or blisters around the genitals, thighs, or buttocks.

How is it recognized?
Herpes outbreaks are often preceded by 2 to 3 days of tingling, itching, or pain. Then blisters appear gathered around a red base. The blisters gradually crust and disappear, usually within 2 weeks.

Is massage indicated or contraindicated?
Any kind of herpes in the acute stage locally contraindicates massage. Massage is systemically contraindicated if the client is showing any signs of systemic infection. The sheets of clients with herpes must be isolated and bleached. Massage for clients with a history of herpes but no active symptoms is indicated.

When Is a Mouth Sore *Not* Herpes?

Oral herpes causes the familiar lesions we call "fever blisters" or "cold sores," but not all sores around the mouth are caused by the herpes virus.

- *Angular stomatitis* is a condition involving painful, irritated cracks around the corners of the mouth. This is often associated with denture-wearers who may drool while they sleep. The accumulation of saliva around the corners of their mouths provides a rich growth medium for the yeast that causes these lesions.

- *Aphthae, or* "canker sores," are lesions that occur *inside* the mouth, often on the gums and cheeks. These are small, painful ulcers whose cause is unknown. Aphthae may be virally related, but they are not contagious.

Etiology: What Happens?

Oral herpes is transmitted through oral or respiratory secretions. Genital herpes is transmitted through mucous secretions during sexual contact. In either case, a person's first outbreak, which usually occurs 2 to 20 days after exposure, is called *primary* herpes. All subsequent outbreaks are called *recurrent* herpes.

A primary herpes outbreak may be almost unnoticeable. Most cases of oral herpes are picked up during childhood, and the new carrier may never be aware of his or her infection. In some cases, however, the primary infection may be very extreme. It may be accompanied by fever, swollen glands, and painful sores that may last from 2 to 6 weeks.

One of the distinguishing features of the herpes virus is that it is never fully vanquished from the body. After the primary outbreak, the virus goes into hiding in the dorsal root ganglia of the spine. There it will wait for an appropriate trigger, which could be a fever, a systemic infection, a sunburn, stress, a menstrual period, or something that is never completely understood. When the virus reactivates, a recurrent outbreak will occur, usually at or near the site of the original infection.

Communicability

The herpes virus is famous for its communicability. Unlike many pathogens, the herpes virus can remain dormant and healthy outside of a host body for hours at a time; exactly how long is a matter of some debate. This means that the face pad that an infected client used may now pass the virus to another client. Face cloths and towels are also potentially dangerous. Even leaving aside the strong possibility of infecting other people, herpes is notorious for spreading to other parts of the body. Touching a cold sore and then touching the eye can result in a painful and dangerous herpetic infection of the cornea (herpes keratitis).

One of the most dangerous aspects of a herpes infection is that a patient could be shedding the virus even from skin that has no visible lesion. This means that all it takes to catch herpes from another person is skin-to-skin contact with live virus. *No sore or break in the skin is necessary.*

Signs and Symptoms

Whether oral or genital, herpes simplex usually presents in the same way: the affected area may experience some pain or tingling a few days before an outbreak (the *"prodromic"* stage), then a blister or cluster of blisters appears on a red base. The blisters erupt and ooze virus-rich liquid all around the area (Figure 1.10). The blisters scab over after a week to 10 days, ending the most contagious phase of the disease. Altogether the outbreak lasts approximately 2 to 3 weeks.

Oral herpes and genital herpes have different patterns in their presentations:

- *Oral herpes* tends to erupt when immunity is otherwise depressed (they are called "cold sores" or "fever blisters" because they often occur when a person is fighting off some other infection), during hormonal changes as in pregnancy

Figure 1.10. Oral herpes.

or menstruation, after prolonged exposure to sunlight, or after any emotional stress. They appear most often on the lips, and on the skin around the mouth. They may be a lifelong problem.

Herpes simplex type I lesions usually appear on or around the mouth, but it is possible for them to appear elsewhere on the body as well. Of special concern to massage therapists is a variety called *herpes Whitlow* (Figure 1.11), which is an outbreak of

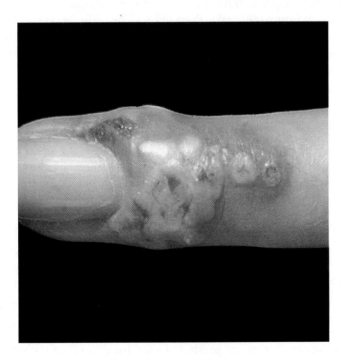

Figure 1.11. Herpes Whitlow.

lesions around the nail beds of the hands. *Herpes gladiatorum* is a variety of herpes simplex that occurs among wrestlers and other athletes who share skin-to-skin contact.

- *Genital herpes* outbreaks also correspond to depressed immunity and general stress levels, but they do seem to run a course of appearing with less and less frequency until finally they simply never come back. These blisters appear on the genitals, but they can also be found on the thighs, buttocks, and on the skin over the sacrum. People who have herpes and are immune-suppressed tend to experience outbreaks over larger areas of the body than others. The lesions are usually quite painful, but if they are inside the vaginal canal, then a woman may be unaware of them, which has important implications for communicability. Genital herpes outbreaks are sometimes accompanied by systemic symptoms: fever, muscular achiness, swelling in the inguinal lymph nodes, and difficult or painful urination.

Complications

Secondary bacterial infection is a common complication of herpes lesions. Immune-suppressed people (especially acquired immune deficiency syndrome [AIDS] and organ transplant patients) are especially susceptible to infections. People who are human immunodeficiency virus (HIV) positive and who have active herpes have a greater risk of communicating HIV to sexual partners as well. Vaginally delivered newborns of mothers with active genital herpes may suffer blindness or brain damage. Genital herpes has also been statistically connected with higher rates of *cervical cancer* (Chapter 10), so infected women are wise to have frequent Pap smears performed. The herpes simplex virus has also been linked to *encephalitis* and *meningitis* (Chapter 3).

Treatment

Herpes is a viral infection, which means there is little to do for it but wait for it to be over. Antiviral drugs may suppress viral activity and shorten the duration of an infection, but they do not prevent future outbreaks. Prevention is the main thrust for treatment of this condition; this means isolating towels, bedding, and clothing, and avoiding sexual contact while lesions are present. Keeping as healthy as possible between outbreaks is an important way to reduce the frequency and severity of herpes episodes.

Massage?

Obviously, acute herpes outbreaks contraindicate massage. If a client has a history of herpes, it is important to explain why it is a bad idea to receive a massage during an outbreak and request that she reschedule if she has prodromic symptoms or blisters on her appointment day. Even after a lesion has scabbed over, herpes is at the very least a local contraindication. Because this virus can survive outside of a host for hours at a time, consider the bed sheets of any client with herpes as "hot": isolate them in a closed container and either have them professionally sterilized or add extra bleach to their wash cycle.

Clients who have active herpes outbreaks are not good candidates to receive massage. Likewise, massage therapists who have active herpes outbreaks need to respect their clients' health by not exposing them to the virus. Scabbed-over cold sores may be very itchy. Massage therapists need to take special care not to inadvertently brush their face with their sleeves, wrists, or hands and then touch a client with a contaminated surface.

Impetigo

Definition: What Is It?

Impetigo is a bacterial infection that is especially prevalent in children. Lesions usually occur around the nose and mouth, sometimes appearing inside the nostrils or ear canals. Although it usually begins somewhere on the head, impetigo can infect the skin anywhere on the body.

This infection is caused by both staphylococcus and streptococcus bacteria.

Signs and Symptoms

Streptococcal impetigo begins as a rash with small blisters or pustules filled with clear or murky fluid. These often occur where the skin has been damaged by some other injury. When the blisters pop, a characteristic honey-colored crust forms (Figure 1.12). Staphylococcal impetigo forms large, delicate blisters that rupture and seep fluid. Impetigo is itchy and is most common in hot, humid climates or in dry, cold areas in the winter when lips and noses become chapped and vulnerable to infection.

Treatment

Mild impetigo can be treated with topical antibiotic cream. However, if the blisters have spread over much of the body, and especially if there are other signs of systemic infection (i.e., fever and chills), then oral antibiotics are prescribed.

Prevention

Impetigo often appears where the skin has already been damaged: scabbed-over mosquito bites, chapped lips or noses, cuts and sores. The first step in prevention is to stop any kind of infection from

Impetigo:

This comes from the Latin words *im* and *peto*, which mean "to rush up, attack." This may refer to the invasive and extremely infectious nature of this type of infection.

Impetigo in Brief

Pronunciation
im-pe-tī′gö

What is it?
Impetigo is a bacterial (staphylococcus or streptococcus) infection of the skin.

How is it recognized?
Streptococcal impetigo is marked by a rash with fluid-filled blisters and honey-colored crusts. It usually begins somewhere on the face, but it can appear anywhere on the body. Staphylococcal impetigo involves large, delicate blisters that may appear anywhere on the body.

Is massage indicated or contraindicated?
Until the lesions have completely healed, this highly contagious condition strictly contraindicates massage.

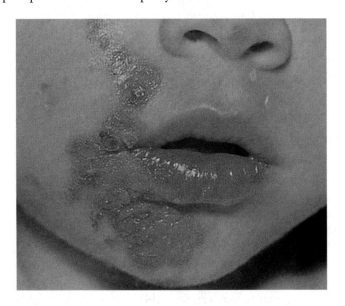

Figure 1.12. Impetigo.

developing at these sites. Chapped skin should be treated with lubricant to prevent damage. All other wounds should be cleaned thoroughly and treated with antibacterial ointment.

This is an extremely contagious condition, and because it is both very itchy and most common in children, special precautions are recommended to prevent its spread. The patient first must be discouraged from touching or scratching his lesions; impetigo can easily be spread to other parts of the body this way. The lesions must be kept clean and dry, and crusts removed as soon as possible because they harbor bacteria in the moistness underneath. The patient's bedding and towels must be strictly isolated while he is infected. Children with impetigo are encouraged to stay home from school and to avoid contact with other children for 1 to 3 days after they begin treatment.

Massage?

This is a contagious bacterial infection of the skin involving very virulent pathogens that can be drug resistant. It systemically contraindicates massage until the lesions have completely healed.

Mites and Lice

Mites and Lice in Brief

What are they?
Lice and mites are tiny animals that drink blood. They are highly contagious and spread through close contact with skin, infested sheets, or clothing.

How are they recognized?
- The mites that cause scabies are too small to see, but they leave itchy trails where they burrow under the skin. They prefer warm, moist places such as the axillae or between fingers.
- Head lice are easy to see, but they can hide. A more dependable sign is their eggs: nits are small white rice-shaped flecks that cling strongly to hair shafts.
- Body lice look very similar to head lice, but they live primarily in clothing and only visit the host for blood meals.
- Pubic lice look like tiny white crabs in pubic and coarse body hair.

All of these parasites create a lot of itching through allergic reactions to the toxins they produce.

Is massage indicated or contraindicated?
Massage is contraindicated for all three infestations until the infestation has been completely eradicated. If a massage therapist is exposed to any of these parasites, every client who he or she works on subsequently will also be exposed even before the therapist shows any symptoms.

Parasitic infestations are something every massage therapist fears; body workers are so very vulnerable to whatever is crawling around on clients' skin. But here, as in all things fearful, the best defense is information.

Mites

Definition: What Are They?

Tiny mites called *Sarcoptes scabiei* are the cause of skin lesions called scabies (Figure 1.13). The female mites burrow under the skin in warm, moist spots, where they drink blood, defecate and urinate, and lay eggs so the next generation can carry on. The mites' waste is highly irritating, which causes an itchy allergic reaction in most hosts. If scratching damages the skin, the risk of secondary infection is high.

How Do They Spread?

Mites spread readily through close personal contact, or through contact with something someone else has worn or lain on—such as massage sheets. Depending on the local conditions, scabies mites can live for several hours or several days when removed from a host.

One type of scabies, called Norwegian scabies, is caused by a different parasite. These lesions tend to be larger and develop crusts, but they tend to itch less. Norwegian scabies tend to be more communicable than the more common *Sarcoptes* species.

Signs and Symptoms

Scabies-causing mites are too small to see with the naked eye, so a visual diagnosis is based on the trails they leave behind. Sometimes their burrows are visible. They look like reddish or grayish lines around the areas scabies favor: the groin, the axilla, elbows, between fingers (Figure 1.14). Mites like skin folds, although they also colonize the skin around the belt line. Other signs of mite

Figure 1.13. Scabies mite.

Figure 1.14. Scabies lesions.

infestation are the irritated blisters and pustules that arise from allergic reactions to their waste and secondary bacterial infection.

This condition is itchiest at night, when the mites are most active, but many skin irritations seem to itch more at night, simply because when a person is trying to sleep he has fewer distractions. The itching caused by mites, however, has a distinctive unrelenting quality. Where eczema or mosquito bites might itch intermittently and then subside, scabies itching gets continually worse and worse.

Diagnosis

Scabies lesions can sometimes be hard to diagnose. Just a few mites can cause a lot of irritation. People can be so miserable with their infestation that they cannot eat or sleep, but the skin tests sometimes do not catch an actual bug, so a definitive diagnosis is difficult to make. It is typically based on the nature of the rash, the person's history, and the possibility that he might have been exposed.

Treatment

Mites, like other parasitic infestations, are treated by bathing with a pesticidal soap. This treatment can be highly toxic and so must be used carefully. Washing and then isolating bedding and towels is important to prevent further outbreaks. It is not usually necessary to fumigate the home, because scabies mites do not stray far from their hosts.

Massage?

Massage is out of the question. If a massage therapist thinks she might have been exposed to mites by accident, she should consider those sheets "hot" (isolate them from other sheets and wash them with extra bleach) and see a doctor about treating herself, right away. The symptoms of scabies sometimes do not show up for 4 weeks or more; it takes that long to build up enough toxins to be irritating. The therapist is certainly contagious the whole time; anyone she works on could become infested too.

Case History 1.2

Scabies

Valerie: "Mystery Rash"

Valerie was a massage student. She worked with a variety of people, including fellow students, friends, and her student internship group, people with AIDS.

One day Valerie noted that she had some areas on the outsides of her elbows that were slightly but persistently itchy during the day. They gradually developed red bumps. Ironically, this occurred while Valerie was studying skin conditions in her massage course. "It's natural to convince yourself that you have symptoms for a lot of things. I knew something was going on, and it seemed like it *could* be scabies, but my symptoms were different from anything I'd seen described," she said. The itching was not particularly worse at night, and there were no tracks or typical signs of infestation. Even the site of the infestation was unusual: scabies mites usually go for warm, moist, protected areas such as skin folds on the *insides* of elbows, but not the outsides.

Eventually Valerie went to her general practitioner, who pronounced her condition a "mystery rash" and suggested a corticosteroid cream to limit the itchiness. In a way, Valerie was relieved by this diagnosis. "You never want to think you have scabies," she said. When her husband also developed symptoms, however, he went straight to a dermatologist, who immediately diagnosed scabies and prescribed enough pesticidal soap for both of them.

The cream was applied all over the body up to the chin; evidently scabies do not infest the head or face. "That night after I washed off the cream, I was really, really, *really* itchy, and then for 4 or 5 weeks my skin was raw and uncomfortable." The cream itself can create symptoms that mimic a scabies infestation for weeks at a time. This can lead to a condition called "scabiosis," in which a person is convinced that he or she needs to medicate for scabies again and again, although he or she is not really infested. Scabiosis can become a life-threatening condition if the person repeatedly self-medicates.

Six to eight weeks passed between the onset of Valerie's symptoms and a final diagnosis. During this time, Valerie had continued to work on friends and clients, as well as to receive massage from other students. Two other classmates were finally infested and diagnosed. "The first few days (after we knew it was scabies) were full of panic and fear. Within a couple of days, people were getting over their fear and paranoia, and there was a lot of support. People had the attitude that this is just one of the things that can happen when you're a bodyworker."

Head Lice

Definition: What Are They?

Head lice are insects (*pediculus humanus capitis*) that live in head hair and suck blood from the scalp. Lice are quite a bit larger than mites and can easily be seen without a microscope (Figure 1.15). Their saliva is very irritating, which causes itching and the accompanying complication of possible infection.

How Do They Spread?

Lice like hats and other soft surfaces. They thrive in batters' helmets that are shared by little league teams and in hairbrushes that are shared by best friends. A person does not

Figure 1.15. Head louse.   **Figure 1.16.** Nits attached to a hair shaft.

need close contact to an infected person to catch lice; *no* contact is needed. All he needs to do is try on a hat at the local hat store, hang his coat on the same hook that an infested person used, or take a ride in a car with an infested headrest.

Signs and Symptoms

If a client has lice, the actual parasites may or may not be obvious; they are quite mobile and can hide. But they lay eggs called *nits*. (This is the source of the term "nitpicky.") Nits cling to hair shafts and look like tiny grains of rice (Figure 1.16). They hatch after about a week. If nits are dark, they may not yet have hatched. White nits are usually the empty eggshells that are still sticking to the hair. Nits are a prime diagnostic feature for pediculosis; anything else of that size and color (like dandruff) would brush out easily.

Lice lay their eggs right at the base of the hair shaft, mostly behind the ears and along the base of the neckline. One way to determine how long an infestation has been present is to observe how far the nits have grown away from the scalp.

A person with an active infestation of lice experiences itchiness and the sensation of movement on the scalp. Rigorous scratching can damage the skin and open the door to secondary infection or *dermatitis* (this chapter).

Treatment

Repeated applications of pesticidal shampoo to kill adults and eggs is the first step in treating lice. Some types of lice are becoming resistant to the standard pesticides, so it is now recommended that applications of the medicine be followed by systematically combing every section of hair with a very fine-toothed comb.

Persons averse to bathing in the toxic pesticides that are prescribed for lice infestations may choose to "smother" the lice with petroleum jelly or mayonnaise. These treatment options are slightly less effective than medicated shampoos, and so it is especially important to combine them with the systematic removal of nits with a nit comb.

Washing bedding, towels, and clothing is also necessary, as well as thoroughly cleaning hats, hairbrushes, combs, and anything else that comes in contact with the head. Washing items at 130° and drying them on high heat for 20 minutes is considered sufficient. Dry cleaning nonwashable items is also effective. Anything else that might harbor lice (stuffed animals, soft toys, etc.) should be tied in a dry cleaning bag and isolated for 2 weeks.

Massage?

A client who knows he or she has head lice should not receive massage. If a therapist suspects that she has been exposed, precautionary measures should be taken at once.

Body Lice

Definition: What Are They?

Body lice (*pediculus humanus*) are closely related to head lice, but they have different living and feeding patterns. Body lice tend not to live directly on their host, but in the host's clothing, especially in the seams. They are about the same size as head lice, and they also take blood meals, causing an itchy reaction.

Body lice are fairly rare except among homeless and transient populations who have limited access to laundering facilities and who spend a lot of time in unwashed clothing.

How Are They Spread?

Body lice live in clothing, so sharing unwashed clothing is the most efficient way for them to spread from one host to another. They also may crawl from infested clothing to other clothing in a laundry basket or other close proximity.

Signs and Symptoms

An itchy rash that progressively gets worse is the leading sign of body lice. They seldom live directly on the skin, and they usually lay eggs in clothing, so unless the clothing is examined, a live body louse may not be found.

Treatment

Body lice are treated most simply with good hygiene. They do not tolerate high temperatures, so frequent bathing and laundering of clothing is an effective way to eradicate an infestation.

Pubic Lice

Definition: What Are They?

Pubic lice are tiny insects that look a lot like their nickname, "crabs" (Figure 1.17). Crabs are a bit less discerning in their tastes; they like pubic hair in the groin best, but they will also live in armpit hair and coarse body hair (Figure 1.18). They also may be found in eyebrows and eyelashes.

How Are They Spread?

Pubic lice are usually spread through sexual contact, but infested massage sheets can spread them, too.

Signs and Symptoms

Pubic lice (*Pthirus pubis*) look like tiny white crabs, approximately 1 mm wide. They also leave nits, but they are so small they are just barely visible. Like all of the infestations being discussed, the primary symptom is itching.

Figure 1.17. Pubic (crab) louse.   **Figure 1.18.** Pubic louse in body hair (arrow).

Treatment

Crab lice carriers must follow the same protocols as head lice carriers. The sheets of any massage client suspected of a crab infestation should be isolated from all others and sterilized as soon as possible.

Massage?

Infestations of pubic lice, body lice, head lice, mites, and any other parasitic infestation of the skin contraindicate massage.

Parasitic infestation carries a powerful social stigma that is negatively (and inaccurately) associated with poverty and poor hygiene. Remember that *anybody* (including massage therapists) could have this problem, and people in touch professions are in a position to cause a lot more damage with it than anyone else. So be respectful, and remember that it could happen to anyone.

Warts

Definition: What Are They?

Warts are fascinating. Most of them are small, benign neoplasms caused by the ***human papillomavirus*** (HPV), which targets the keratinocytes, the same cells affected by squamous cell carcinoma. These protein-producing cells then produce a lot of extra keratin,

---

Warts in Brief

What are they?
Warts are neoplasms that arise from the keratinocytes in the epidermis; they are caused by extremely slow-acting viruses.

How are they recognized?
Typical warts (verruca vulgaris) look like hard, cauliflower-shaped growths. They usually occur on the hands. They can affect anyone, but teenagers are especially prone to them.

Is massage indicated or contraindicated?
Massage is a local contraindication for warts. The virus is contained in the blood and shedding skin cells, and it is possible to get warts from another person.

which is the material that makes our epithelial cells hard and scaly. The result: *verruca vulgaris*.

Etiology: What Happens?

Warts affect young children occasionally, adults rarely, and teenagers mercilessly. Most adults who get warts are probably somehow immune-suppressed. Warts can be contagious if the edges are roughened; the virus is contained in the blood and in the shedding skin cells. They are usually self-limiting; that is, they tend to go away on their own. In that sense they are a viral infection in slow motion: the virus slowly enters the body; it slowly takes over a few skin cells, and they slowly respond. And, slowest of all, the body finally vanquishes this not-very-threatening invader and that is the end of it. In very healthy people, they can be expected to clear within a year. For others, it can take even longer.

Signs and Symptoms

Warts look like hard, cauliflower-shaped growths on the skin (Figure 1.19). They are usually more of a nuisance than anything else, but when they occur on the bottom of the feet (*plantar warts*), they can seriously impair function. In this case (and sometimes when they occur on the palm of the hands), the warts grow *inward*, creating a sensation of always stepping on something hard that never goes away (Figure 1.20). It is important to distinguish between plantar warts and callous, to avoid the risk of making a bad situation worse.

Verruca vulgaris is the most common kind of wart; other types are worth a look as well. Sixteen different subtypes of warts have been identified; only a few are discussed here.

- *Plane warts*. These are small, brown, smooth warts that are most often seen on the faces of children.
- *Flat warts*. These are similar to verruca vulgaris, but they are much smaller and tend to occur in exposed places. Flat warts on the face can be spread by nicks and cuts with shaving.

Figure 1.19. Warts.

Figure 1.20. Plantar warts.

Compare and Contrast
PLANTAR WARTS VERSUS CALLUS

Plantar warts often look like simple callus: the thick skin that grows on areas of the feet subject to a lot of wear and tear. The problem is that although people may file or snip off their calluses with no ill effects, to do the same with a plantar wart is to risk having that wart virus spread all over the foot and lead to more growths until it becomes difficult to walk.

Massage therapists are in a unique position to observe their clients' feet and to notice the subtle differences between plantar warts and callus. As health care professionals, we may then be able to give our clients guidance about getting the right kind of care.

PLANTAR WARTS

Location
Could be anywhere on the plantar surface of the foot. Usually *not* bilateral.

Appearance
May be white, but with darker speckling under the thickened skin: this is the capillary supply for the wart.

Sensation
Very hard and unyielding: like stepping on a stone.

CALLUS

Location
Appears in areas of wear and tear, especially the back of the heels, and the lateral aspect of the feet. Callus usually grows in a similar pattern on both feet.

Appearance
Thick, white skin.

Sensation
No particular sensation.

- *Molluscum contagiosum*. This is also a children's malady, involving small white lumps. Molluscum contagiosum in adults can be a sexually transmitted disease.
- *Genital warts*. These are another sexually transmitted disease, brought about by several varieties of HPV. Some genital warts may come and go with no symptoms, but others may become cancerous. See more in *cervical cancer* (Chapter 10).

Treatment

If warts do not resolve fast enough on their own (and this can sometimes take years), medical intervention may be indicated. Any drug store carries preparations that claim to be effective, but they must be used with caution to avoid damage to surrounding tissues. The common ingredient in most of these products is salicylic acid. Recent studies have suggested that simply covering a wart with duct tape is also effective for most cases.

A standard medical approach is to freeze warts off with liquid nitrogen, but if any of the virus remains in the body, they will probably recur. Other options include electro-surgery, carbon dioxide lasers, injections, and excision. These interventions are particularly important for someone struggling with plantar warts that make it difficult to walk.

Warts seem to be especially suggestible. If a person believes that a treatment will work, it is far more likely to be successful. This has led to some interesting approaches to wart management. One of the best came from a student who said, "take a potato and cut it in six pieces. Bury each of the pieces in a different place, and *don't tell anyone where you hid them*. The wart will go away in a couple of weeks. Mine did."

Massage?

Consider warts a local contraindication. As stated above, the virus is found in the shedding skin cells around the lesion. Furthermore, warts are often caught and torn around the edges, and if the skin is not intact, the client is a walking invitation for infection.

NONCONTAGIOUS INFLAMMATORY SKIN DISORDERS

Acne Rosacea

Definition: What Is It?

Acne rosacea is an idiopathic, chronic skin condition seen mostly in fair-skinned people between 30 and 60 years of age. It primarily affects the skin of the face, centering around the nose and cheeks. Acne rosacea seldom develops elsewhere on the body.

Etiology: What Happens?

The pathophysiology of acne rosacea is not well understood. It may be inherited, but no gene has been specifically identified with this condition.

The symptoms of acne rosacea may come and go in the early stages, but ultimately may become permanent. Triggers for flare-ups are fairly predictable and may include exposure to sunlight, wind, and cold temperatures; drinking hot liquids or alcohol; eating spicy food, menopause, the use of steroidal anti-inflammatories on the face, and emotional stress.

Acne:

The root of this word is probably the result of a copyist's error. The original Greek work, *akme,* means "point of efflorescence." This describes a process in which a crystalline substance gradually changes to a powder as it dries.

Signs and Symptoms

Acne rosacea tends to progress through predicable stages. Not all patients have it severely, but it can create permanent changes in the quality of the delicate skin on the face. Four stages have been identified to mark the progression of this condition:

- *Prerosacea:* In this stage the patient may experience frequent flushing. The skin may feel hot or stinging, but it does not usually itch.
- *Vascular rosacea:* Skin is red, especially around the nose and cheeks. Small blood vessels may become permanently dilated and visible in a condition called ***telangiectasia***. Approximately half of all rosacea patients also experience chronic inflammation and irritation of the eyes and eyelids.
- *Inflammatory rosacea:* If the condition progresses to this point, papules and pustules may develop. These localized lesions respond to antibiotics, but the bacteria that cause them are not related to the bacterial infections seen with acne vulgaris.
- *Rhinophyma:* This is the damage to the skin on the nose seen with people with long-term, very severe acne rosacea. The skin becomes thickened, bumpy, distorted, and permanently reddened.

Acne Rosacea in Brief

What is it?
Acne rosacea is a chronic condition involving inflammation and damage to the skin of the face.

How is it recognized?
Acne rosacea occurs in stages of severity, starting with occasional flushing and continuing through general inflammation of the face and eyes, the formation of papules and pustules, and finally to permanent thickening and distortion of facial skin, especially around the nose.

Is massage indicated or contraindicated?
Acne rosacea has no contraindications for massage, although some clients may be sensitive to some lubricants.

Complications

Acne rosacea can lead to a number of other disorders. When it affects the eyes, it may lead to rosacea keratitis, which may eventually damage the cornea. Perhaps the greatest issue with acne rosacea is the consequences it has on self-esteem and public perception. Persons with this disorder are very likely to develop *depression* and *anxiety disorders* (Chapter 3), as they perceive being judged by the appearance of their skin. Furthermore, a traditional but incorrect association between the bulbous nose seen with advanced acne rosacea and alcoholism can lead to social stigmas that are difficult to challenge.

Treatment

This idiopathic disorder has no permanent cure and so is treated palliatively. Patients are taught to recognize their specific triggers and to avoid them when possible. Topical or oral antibiotics may be prescribed for pustules, but they are ineffective for the permanent redness seen with this condition. Laser surgery or ***dermabrasion*** may help the appearance of the skin and mask telangiectasias. Plastic surgery may be considered for a person with advanced rhinophyma.

Massage?

Acne rosacea carries no specific contraindications for massage unless the lubricant causes stinging or flushing on the face. Massage elsewhere is welcomed and appropriate.

Acne Vulgaris

Definition: What Is It?

Acne is a condition in which a person becomes susceptible to small, localized skin infections. The lesions usually appear on the face, neck, and upper back.

Acne Vulgaris in Brief

What is it?
Acne is a bacterial infection of sebaceous glands usually found on the face, neck, and upper back. It is closely associated with adolescence or liver dysfunction that results in excess testosterone in the system.

How is it recognized?
Acne vulgaris looks like raised, inflamed pustules on the skin, sometimes with white or black tips.

Is massage indicated or contraindicated?
Acne locally contraindicates massage because of the risk of spreading infection, causing pain, and exacerbating the symptoms with the application of an oily lubricant.

Demographics: Who Gets It?

Many people have painful, awkward memories of adolescence thanks to this condition. When individuals make the transition from childhood to adulthood, their bodies start to secrete the hormones (some estrogen, but mostly testosterone) that are responsible for more than sexual maturity; they also sponsor mood swings, teenage rebellion, and excess sebum production. This change in hormone levels accounts for the high incidence of acne among teenagers. Adults can get acne too, though not necessarily because of excessive testosterone production.

Up to 80% of all people experience acne at one time or another. This makes it one of the most common diseases in the world.

Etiology: What Happens?

The process of developing acne is complicated, with many contributing factors. This is a condition we often associate with puberty, but it is not exclusive to teens. A brief discussion of several of the contributing factors to acne for teens and adults follows.

Factor 1: Testosterone Production   When a person enters puberty, one of the changes that occurs is the sudden secretion of high levels of *androgens*: male hormones that are secreted by both males and females. High levels of testosterone cause sebaceous glands, the oil glands that lubricate hair shafts, to shift into high gear. At this point, it is especially important that sebaceous ducts to the surface of the skin stay clear. If any tiny particle such as a bit of duct lining or a flake of dead skin obstructs the duct, sebum rapidly accumulates behind the blockage.

Factor 2: Bacterial Activity   The pooling of oil in hair shafts is an invitation to the colonies of bacteria that grow on the skin. *Staphylococcus* may cause some acne lesions, but most of them are attributable to a special microbe: *Propionibacterium acnes*, or *P. acne*. *P. acne* produces enzymes that exacerbate inflammation and cause bacteria to clump together. This leads to more colonization of the sebaceous ducts.

Soon a localized infection leads to a pustule, a pimple, or some other type of acne lesion. These blemishes usually appear on the face, upper neck, and upper back, in the sebaceous glands that lubricate tiny, almost invisible hair shafts.

Factor 3: Stress   Stress can upset endocrine balance and slow the activity of immune system cells. ("Stress" and "adolescence" are also practically synonymous.) If the macrophages stationed in the superficial fascia are sluggish, they will not be able to fight off the bacteria that want to colonize the sebaceous glands. Furthermore, once the infection has subsided, those same suppressed macrophages will be slower to consume the residual dead bacteria and white blood cells, which means it takes longer for pimples to fade. Stress does not necessarily cause acne, but it can exacerbate it and slow the healing process.

Factor 4: Liver Congestion   When acne affects adults, it is often because liver congestion makes it difficult to neutralize the normal amounts of testosterone in the system. This leads to excess sebum production, bacterial colonization of sebaceous glands, and all the signs of acne. What causes liver congestion? It varies from person to person, but generally high-fat diets, smoking, drugs, and chemical pollutants are the most common culprits for most people. *Hepatitis* (Chapter 7) or other disorders can also severely compromise liver function.

Factor 5: Hormonal Imbalance Hormonal changes that accompany the menstrual cycle or the beginning or ending of birth control pill prescriptions will often lead to acne in mature women.

Once an infection has become established in a sebaceous gland, the resultant inflammation and destructive enzymes may destroy the walls of the structure. This causes a more extreme inflammatory response and a better chance for the bacteria to invade more skin.

Signs and Symptoms

The symptoms of acne are probably familiar to most people. It can be locally painful, but it is not generally associated with systemic infection (Figure 1.21).

Bacterial infections of the skin can cause several different types of acne lesions:

- *Pimples* are infections trapped below the surface of the skin; they involve raised, red, painful bumps or papules.

- *Cysts* are infections trapped deep in the dermis. They can protrude into the subcutaneous layer. Cysts may or may not be inflamed.

- *Open comedones* are also called "blackheads." These infections are very superficial, and the passage into the hair follicle is open to the air. This allows the trapped sebum to oxidize and turn dark. Blackheads are not, as popular belief would have it, trapped particles of dirt.

- *Closed comedones* are also called "whiteheads" or pustules. They are superficial infections that are covered with a thin layer of epithelium that traps the sebum and pus.

Figure 1.21. Acne.

Treatment

Working with diet and other life habits to cleanse the liver and make its filtering job easier often results in clearer skin, as well as a host of other benefits. Massage of the abdomen and liver may support this process, but it is erroneous to claim that massage will reliably clear up acne; there are too many other factors to consider.

For teenagers with acne, the best advice is the most difficult to follow: *do not touch the face*. Touching, scratching, and popping acne lesions does little except to spread the bacteria and open the possibility of permanent scarring.

Over-the-counter preparations usually use benzoyl peroxide or other similar substances to limit the activity of *P. acne*.

When medical help is requested for acne, interventions usually take a two-pronged attack: topical steroids are applied for their anti-inflammatory properties, and antibiotics are administered internally to go after the bacteria. The disadvantage is that being on a long-term course of antibiotics can play havoc with intestinal flora and the immune system. One alternative is a line of drugs called *retinoins*, which are effective for acne, but have a list of troubling side effects including joint pain and hair loss. Retinoins are also contraindicated if the patient may be pregnant during treatment because they are highly implicated in birth defects.

Massage?

Massage of the abdomen and liver can sometimes yield good results. But massage on the lesions themselves is out of the question. Pimples are infections, and they involve a com-

Compare and Contrast
ACNE AND BOILS

Boils and acne have a lot in common: they are both localized infections of sebaceous glands in hair follicles; they are both caused by *Staphylococcus* infections; they both have a red base with a pustule. But boils are far more serious than acne and require different precautions from massage therapists. Here are some differentiating features:

BOILS	ACNE
Pattern of Appearance One lesion at a time, or a small interconnected group of pustules	**Pattern of Appearance** Spread over large areas (the face, back, or neck)
Virulence Aggressive bacteria that attack living tissue	**Virulence** Less aggressive bacteria that simply take advantage of a hospitable growth medium
Symptoms Extremely painful	**Symptoms** Mildly painful
Communicability Highly communicable	**Communicability** Not communicable without prolonged contact
Special Precautions At least a local contraindication, but may be systemic if signs of general infection are present. Isolate and bleach sheets	**Special Precautions** Local contraindication; no other precautions necessary

promised shield: the skin is no longer intact, which means massage can make the infection worse. Also, the excellent blood supply to the skin creates at least the possibility, if not the likelihood, that the infection could spread. And finally, the lubricant can also block sebaceous glands, further aggravating an already irritable situation.

Wiping a client who is prone to acne down with alcohol after an oily treatment would seem to make some sense because it can cut right through and remove *all* of the oil from the skin. But the human body has a habit of lashing back from such extreme changes in environment: it will work overtime to replace all of the natural oils the alcohol just removed and more. If a client is concerned about the lubricant, the best options are to use a water-based lotion instead of oil or to recommend showering with an astringent soap as soon as possible after treatment.

Dermatitis/Eczema

Definition: What Is It?

Dermatitis is an umbrella term for "skin inflammation," which is about as nonspecific as a diagnosis can get. Many of the conditions in this chapter could be called dermatitis, although by convention the term *dermatitis* is reserved for disorders that are not infectious in origin. This article will focus on *eczema* and contact dermatitis, with some brief discussions of other types of skin inflammations.

Contact dermatitis is a skin inflammation caused by an *external* irritation or allergen. This separates it from other inflammatory skin conditions that arise from an *internal* source, such as bacterial infection or other internally mediated skin problems (see *cellulitis* or *psoriasis*, this chapter). Eczema is a condition connected to systemic hypersensitivity reactions expressed in the skin.

Demographics: Who Gets It?

Statistics on contact dermatitis are unavailable because this is such a general kind of problem and it can accompany many other disorders. Eczema is very common. It affects approximately one of every seven infants and young children. Most people grow out of it; its incidence is approximately 3% of adults, or roughly 15 million people in the United States.

Etiology: What Happens?

Many types of dermatitis are brought about by an overreaction in the immune system to some irritating substance. These are discussed in detail in *hypersensitivity reactions* (Chapter 5), but it is useful to look at an encapsulated version here.

The two types of hypersensitivity reactions that create skin symptoms are type I allergic reactions and type IV delayed reactions.

Eczema is an example of a type I reaction. These are systemic immune system responses to nonthreatening stimuli. In this situation, mast cells release vasodilating chemicals, including histamine, which create an inflammatory response. Someone with eczema will very likely have family members who struggle with hay fever (see *sinusitis* and *asthma*, Chapter 6).

 Eczema:

The root of this word is the Greek *ekzeo*, which means "to boil over." This is a very apt description of many types of eczema.

Dermatitis/Eczema in Brief

Pronunciation
dĕr′mă-tī′tis/ek′zĕ-mă

What is it?
Dermatitis is an umbrella term for inflammation of the skin. Eczema is a noncontagious skin rash usually brought about by an allergic reaction. Contact dermatitis is an inflammation brought about by irritation or allergic responses on the skin.

How is it recognized?
Allergic or contact dermatitis presents in various ways, depending on what type of skin reactions are elicited. Exposure to poison oak or poison ivy results in large inflamed wheals; metal allergies tend to be less inflamed and more isolated in area.
Eczema may appear as very dry and flaky skin, coin-shaped lesions, yellowish oily patches, or blistered, weepy skin.

Is massage indicated or contraindicated?
The appropriateness of massage depends completely on the source of the problem and the condition of the skin. If the skin is very inflamed or has blisters or other lesions, massage is at least locally contraindicated until the acute stage has passed. If a rash could spread (i.e., poison oak), massage is systemically contraindicated while the irritation is present. If the skin is not itchy and the affected area is highly isolated, as with a metal allergy to a watchband or earrings, massage is only locally contraindicated.

Allergic contact dermatitis is a type IV reaction, mediated by a complex organization of immune system agents. Poison oak, poison ivy, and local skin reactions to metals, soaps, dyes, or latex are examples of contact dermatitis.

Causes of Eczema

Research into the causes of eczema is proceeding, but no single factor has yet been identified. Some of the possible causes of eczema include the following:

- A deficiency in certain fatty acids has been observed in eczema patients. A lack of linoleic acid can make the skin less able to retain moisture and more susceptible to drying out.

- Certain monocytes may malfunction in persons with eczema, which causes a very extreme immune system response to minor stimuli.

- Persons with eczema tend to have elevated levels of immunoglobulin E (IgE): allergy-related antibodies that cause excessive secretion of histamine. Histamine causes many inflammatory reactions, including capillary dilation, red skin, and itching.

Although it seems clear that eczema is connected to an internal systemic immune system dysfunction, it can be exacerbated by local irritations such as rough textures, detergents, harsh chemicals, and other substances.

Causes of Contact Dermatitis

Contact dermatitis can result from simple irritation or from an allergic reaction. Irritant contact dermatitis usually arises from prolonged contact with some substance that would eventually be irritating to *anyone*; this distinguishes it from allergic contact dermatitis. Irritants that can reliably bring about a reaction include working in water, harsh cleansers, acids and alkalis, and ongoing friction. These stimuli will eventually damage even the healthiest skin, but removal from the irritation will result in a cessation of symptoms.

Allergic contact dermatitis differs from irritant contact dermatitis because the causative factors create a specific type of allergic response in the skin of the affected person. Some common allergens associated with allergic contact dermatitis include nickel (found in watchbands and earrings), preservatives used in lotions, the adhesive used in many medical bandages, some perfumes and dyes, and latex. Some substances cause an allergic reaction when the affected skin is exposed to sunlight. In this case, rashes will break out only where sun hits the skin that has been in contact with the allergen, for instance, preservatives in sunscreen.

Signs and Symptoms of Eczema

Signs and symptoms of eczema vary according to what type is present.

- *Atopic dermatitis:* This is the most common variety. It seems to be genetic in origin, and it is irritated by stress. *Atopic* dermatitis is usually red, flaky, and dry, occurring in the creases on the sides of the nose and other skin creases, such as knees, elbows, ankles, and hands (Figure 1.22). As long as the skin is dry, intact, and not puffy or itchy, atopic dermatitis does not contraindicate massage. Therapists should be cautious, though, to make sure no breaks in the skin are present, and they should use a hypoallergenic lubricant that will not exacerbate the situation.

- *Seborrheic eczema.* This form of eczema involves yellowish, oily patches, usually in the skin folds around the nose or on the scalp.

Figure 1.22. Atopic dermatitis.

Figure 1.23. Dyshidrosis.

- *Dyshidrosis.* In this condition, blisters filled with fluid appear, mostly on hands and feet. It is sometimes described as looking like a combination of *fungal infection* (this chapter) and a contact allergy (Figure 1.23). It often occurs in response to hot weather or emotional stress. Dyshydrosis can be very difficult to treat and can sometimes require systemic steroids. Like atopic dermatitis, dyshidrosis is noncontagious, but *unlike* the dry presentation of eczema, this one has the danger of blisters breaking, which exposes the client to infection. It is therefore a local contraindication for massage.

- *Nummular eczema.* This form of eczema appears in small circular lesions, often on the legs and buttocks (Figure 1.24). It can be intensely itchy.

Signs and Symptoms of Contact Dermatitis

The symptoms of contact dermatitis vary according to the causative factors. Acute situations are typically locally red, swollen, and itchy or tender, showing exactly where the irritation took place (Figure 1.25). Long-lasting low-grade reactions may not show signs of inflammation, although mild itchiness is common. Contact dermatitis locally contraindicates massage.

Figure 1.24. Nummular eczema.

Figure 1.25. Contact allergic dermatitis.

Other types of dermatitis show specific patterns but are not related to irritation or contact with allergenic substances:

- *Stasis dermatitis*: This usually appears on the lower legs, in association with poor circulation as seen with *diabetes* (Chapter 8) or *heart failure* (Chapter 4). Stasis dermatitis is very red and may occur with small ulcers where the skin has been deprived of nutrition. It often resembles *erysipelas* (this chapter). Stasis dermatitis implies severe problems with blood flow; therefore, it contraindicates circulatory massage.

- *Neurodermatitis*: This condition involves a small injury, such as a mosquito bite, that creates an enormous inflammatory response and localized scaly patches of skin. It locally contraindicates massage, until the inflammation has subsided (see *hypersensitivity reactions*, Chapter 5).

Complications

Both contact dermatitis and eczema can begin a process by which a mildly irritating skin problem can become a debilitating problem. When a person with dermatitis scratches the mildly itchy lesions, the lesions become stimulated and much itchier. This leads to more scratching, more itchiness, and a vicious circle called the "itch–scratch cycle."

Persons with dermatitis are particularly susceptible to secondary infection because their skin tends to be so irritable. *Impetigo*, *herpes simplex*, and *fungal infections* (this chapter) are all common complications for dermatitis and eczema patients.

Treatment

Self-help measures for people with contact dermatitis and eczema begin with trying to isolate the substances that irritate them and then avoiding them carefully. Persons with eczema also must try to maintain adequate hydration of the skin. This means finding a moisturizer or emollient that does not contain any irritating substances and applying it while the skin is still wet from bathing.

The medical treatment of choice for dealing with contact dermatitis and eczema is corticosteroid cream. Cortisol, among other things, is a powerful anti-inflammatory), but corticosteroid creams must be used *exactly* as prescribed because

- Steroid creams can cause their own "steroid rash," or they can quell macrophage action, making users prone to *boils* (this chapter).

- A "backlash" effect can occur: after the use of steroidal creams is stopped, the original complaint can come back in a more extreme version.

- If steroid creams are used over a long period (several months), permanent changes can be brought about by exposure to a substance that melts connective tissue: the skin can become thin, delicate, and easily damaged. (Of course massage would be inappropriate in a case like this.)

- Finally, in a worst-case scenario, the adrenal glands can suffer damage, which can be life-threatening.

Fortunately, an alternative to steroid creams has recently been developed. Called *topical immunomodulators* (TINS),

Stress, Allergies, and Cortisol

Stress can ripple through the body in a number of different chemical ways. Massage therapists study some of these effects because they too have some influence over what chemicals are being released, and that influence should be informed and intentional.

For people who are prone to allergies, long-term stress creates some special problems. Cortisol is the hormone that is specifically related to long-term stress. When it is secreted over a long time, cortisol does some things that can damage the body, such as systemically weakening the connective tissues. But cortisol does one thing that is very, *very* good: it is a powerful anti-inflammatory agent. When people undergo long-term stress, they can become depleted in their cortisol supplies. When cortisol is depleted, the body has only limited resources to quell the inflammatory reaction. And for the person subject to allergies, this means that they have a difficult time de-inflaming from immune system attacks against nonthreatening stimuli such as wheat, pollen, cat dander, or anything else. If the immune reaction takes the form of a skin rash, then it may be called dermatitis or eczema.

This is not to say stress is the only cause of allergies, or even the most important one; it is just to point out that stress can often make allergies *worse*.

these steroid-free creams have been getting excellent results without the side effects linked to steroid use.

Massage practitioners must emphasize how important it is to use medications *exactly* as they are prescribed: not less, not more. Above all, a person must make the effort to get to the *root* of the problem, rather than just patching over the symptoms. After all, if a person is allergic to her soap, what makes more sense: applying steroid cream daily for months, or changing brands?

Massage?

The appropriateness of massage depends entirely on the causes and severity of a client's dermatitis. If she has skin that is red, hot, puffy, and itchy from a morning walk through poison oak, massage is *not* appropriate. First, the inflammation will be exacerbated by extra blood in the area, and second, the irritating substance (the poison oak oils) can be distributed over more of her body, spreading the inflammation over her body, and possibly to the therapist as well. Massage for this person, and all other persons with acute dermatitis, is systematically contraindicated until the inflammation has subsided.

If, conversely, a client is displaying a small slightly reddened, flaky, circular area on the back of her left wrist (about the place where a wrist watch would usually hit), it may be possible to pursue a line of questioning that will determine that there is no danger of massage aggravating or spreading the irritation, which is probably being caused by an allergy to nickel.

The appropriateness of massage for eczema depends on the type that is present, and whether the skin has been compromised to point where there is danger of infection. For more details, see the individual descriptions above.

Hives

Definition: What Are They?

Hives, also called *urticaria*, are the result of emotional stress, an allergy, or some other stimulus. They are areas of intense heat, swelling, and itchiness on the skin.

Etiology: What Happens?

Consider someone who is allergic to shellfish. Somehow a shrimp finds its way into his Lemon Grass Soup. Within moments his immune system cells launch a full-scale attack, but they do not quite know where to go. In the confusion, specialized cells called mast cells freely distributed in the superficial fascia release histamine. This causes local capillary dilation, extra cell permeability, and *lots* of edema. Urticaria is an example of a type 1 hypersensitivity reaction (a true "allergic" reaction).

Histamine release causes a localized inflammatory response (redness), and the edema presses on nerve endings (itching). Some people need an unexpected encounter with an allergen to make this happen, but for others all it takes is an unfamiliar or threatening situation. Hives are very common; it is estimated that up to 20% of all people will experience them at some point, although they are more frequent with people who live with other allergies. Sometimes

---

Hives in Brief

What are they?
Hives are an inflammatory skin reaction to an allergen or emotional stressor.

How are they recognized?
Hives range from small red spots to large wheals, which are pink to red, warm, and itchy. Individual lesions generally subside within a few hours, but successive hives may appear; the cycle can continue for several weeks at a time.

Is massage indicated or contraindicated?
Hives systemically contraindicate massage during the acute stage and locally contraindicate it in the subacute stage. Massage would bring even more circulation to the skin, making a bad situation worse.

students break out in hives when they take a test; some may do it while reading about diseases. Exposure to cold, heat, or sunlight is a trigger for some people. Some clients who have never had massage before will get hives the first time they get on a massage table.

Signs and Symptoms

Hives begin as small, raised, reddened areas called wheals that may join to become larger irregular patches (Figure 1.26). The lesions are red around the outside and are sometimes paler in the middle. They are itchy and hot. They are not contagious but are usually brought about by a food allergy, an insect bite or sting, a reaction to medication, emotional stress, or environmental changes.

Individual hives usually clear within a few hours, but they may be replaced by other hives. It is common for a person to have ongoing hives for days or weeks at a time.

A rarer version of hives is called *chronic urticaria*. In this situation, the cycle of hives appearing, resolving, and being replaced by others lasts for 6 weeks or more. The triggers for these long-lasting episodes can be difficult or impossible to identify; evidence points toward an autoimmune component in chronic urticaria, but this condition is not well understood.

Treatment

Hives are always annoying but seldom really serious. If they require treatment, it is usually in the form of an antihistamine, to quell histamine release. Even chronic urticaria is treated this way. Antihistamines for hives are usually prescribed in heavy doses to undo all the work of the mast cells. This can be problematic because high doses of antihistamines often have a sedative effect. If antihistamines are unsuccessful, topical or systemic doses of steroidal anti-inflammatories may be recommended.

Angioedema is one variety of hives that can be a medical emergency. These hives occur in deeper layers of the skin, usually around the face and throat. The tissue can swell up to the point that breathing becomes difficult. It is rare, but angioedema can be life

Figure 1.26. Hives.

threatening, requiring an immediate injection of steroids to bring down the swelling and restore ease of breathing. (See *allergic reactions*, Chapter 5.)

Massage?

Hives systemically contraindicate massage in the acute phase, and locally contraindicate it in the subacute; there is no benefit to bringing more blood into an area that is already too congested. If a client has a history of this kind of problem, it is a good idea to take extra precautions to use an oil or lotion that will not initiate an attack.

NEOPLASTIC SKIN DISORDERS

Moles

Definition: What Are They?

Moles, or *nevi*, are benign neoplasms: areas where melanocytes replicate on site, although without threatening to invade surrounding tissues. The melanocytes produce excessive melanin, the coloring agent for skin.

Etiology: What Happens?

Most of us are genetically programmed to develop moles, and they generally appear before age 20. (If any moles appear after this time, it is recommended to consult a dermatologist to rule out melanoma.)

Moles generally begin as flat black or brown marks on the skin. They may become elevated and grow course, dark hairs (Figure 1.27). Many people find that their moles fade or may disappear as they get older.

> ### Moles in Brief
>
> **What are they?**
> Moles are isolated areas where the pigment cells in the epidermis have produced excess melanin.
>
> **How are they recognized?**
> Moles can range in color from light tan to blackish-blue. Their color is usually uniform throughout. Moles are usually circular or oval.
>
> **Are they indicated or contraindicated for massage?**
> Massage will not help or hurt moles, but massage therapists may be able to see changes in a mole that their client may be unaware of.

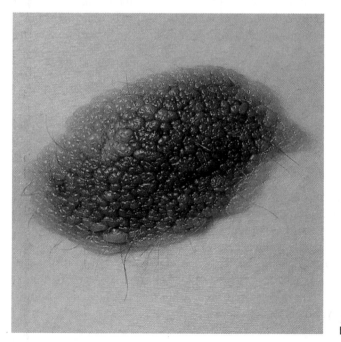

Figure 1.27. Mole.

Other Skin Pigmentations

Age and the uneven distribution of melanin in the skin can give rise to several different types of skin patches. Because massage therapists are health professionals who work closely with the skin, it is important to be familiar with the most common types of marks clients may carry.

- *Freckles.* These are simple concentrations of melanin in the skin. They can range from light tan to red, but they are always darker than the surrounding skin. Most freckles are about the size of a nail-head, although when several blend together they can seem much larger. Fair-skinned people are more susceptible to freckles than others. Freckles often darken when they are exposed to sunlight and fade when they are protected from UV radiation.

- *Lentigos.* These are similar to freckles, but they usually appear on older people, and they are often much larger than freckles. They are often mistakenly referred to as "liver spots," but they have nothing to do with liver function.

- *Seborrheic keratosis.* These are skin lesions that are very common in older people. They are benign growths on the skin that have a waxy, "pasted on" appearance. They often develop a warty appearance when they have been present for a long while. Seborrheic keratosis blemishes can appear singly or in groups. The chest, back, and face are most often affected; they rarely appear below the waist. When seborrheic keratoses are very dark, they can look like malignant melanoma, although these growths are entirely benign.

- *Port-wine stains.* These are a variety of moles that affect blood vessels near the surface of the skin. They are often quite large and are harmless.

Signs and Symptoms

Moles are usually smaller than 6 mm (the size of a pencil eraser). They generally appear in a symmetrical shape (circular or oval), and they are unicolored. These features help to distinguish moles from malignant melanoma. If an established mole begins to change, specifically if it becomes painful or itchy, if it bleeds, becomes inflamed, or suddenly changes in size, shape, or color, it should be investigated.

Treatment

A mole is not inherently dangerous, but that can change. Risk factors for moles becoming cancerous are determined by when they appear (anything that appears after age 20 is highly suspect) and how big they are (anything bigger than 6 mm bears watching). Approximately 42% of all large moles appear on the back, where clients cannot see them, but therapists can.

Two types of moles have been identified as having a higher-than-average risk for changing to melanoma: *congenital nevi* (moles that are present at birth, especially when they are quite large) and *dysplastic nevi* (moles that exhibit the ABCDE symptoms described in *skin cancer*, this chapter).

Some doctors suggest removing large moles, just as a precaution. Some doctors recommend tracing a large nevus and then comparing the tracing to the real thing a few times a year. That way, the patient can keep an accurate record of any changes.

Massage?

Massage neither hurts nor helps moles (unless they become irritated or torn), but massage practitioners are in a unique position to see what clients may not be able to; the practitioner may be the one to spot the transition from harmless nevus to life-threatening melanoma.

 Psoriasis:

Psora comes from Greek for "the itch."

Psoriasis

Definition: What Is It?

The introduction to this chapter discusses how the readiness of epithelium to repair itself is a two-edged sword. The body can heal quickly and thoroughly from most insults to the skin. However, sometimes the ease of replication in skin cells can cause problems, as with this condition. *Psoriasis* is a chronic skin disease with occasional acute episodes in which epithelial cells in isolated patches replicate too rapidly. Whereas normal skin cells replace themselves every 28 to 32 days, psoriatic skin cells divide every 2 to 4 days. The result is a pile-up of excess cells that are itchy, red or pink, and scaly. This condition comes and goes, but at present no permanent cure is available.

Demographics: Who Gets It?

Statistics on psoriasis vary. It affects approximately 5 million Americans, mostly whites. Between 150,000 and 260,000 new cases are diagnosed every year. Some psoriasis cases have a genetic link. It is most commonly diagnosed in middle years, but it has been seen on tiny babies, as well as elderly people. Psoriasis affects slightly more women than men.

Etiology: What Happens?

Psoriasis is not a well-understood disease, and research into its causes and possible cures continues. One theory is that overactive T-cells in the skin create an inflammatory response and the rapid replication of new skin cells. Vitamin D deficiencies in the skin of psoriasis patients have also been observed; vitamin D slows down the replication of skin cells. And in approximately one third of all cases, psoriasis appears within families, leading to the exploration of a genetic predisposition for the disease.

Signs and Symptoms

Psoriasis in Brief

Pronunciation
sö-rī′ă-sis

What is it?
Psoriasis is a noncontagious chronic skin disease involving the excessive production of new skin cells that pile up into isolated lesions.

How is it recognized?
The most common variety of psoriasis looks like pink or reddish patches, sometimes with a silvery scale on top. It occurs most frequently on elbows and knees, but it can develop anywhere.

Is massage indicated or contraindicated?
Psoriasis locally contraindicates massage during the acute stage because the extra stimulation and circulation massage provides can make a bad situation worse. But in subacute stages, as long as the skin is intact, massage is a good idea.

Plaque psoriasis is a very common condition; most people have at least seen it. It usually takes the form of raised red or pink patches that, if they are present for a long time, develop a white or silvery "scale" on top (Figure 1.28). They have sharply defined edges. The patches, or "plaques," may be itchy, but they are seldom really uncomfortable unless they are in an acute stage, when they can itch and burn severely. Plaques are usually on the knees or elbows, but they can be found on the scalp, trunk, palms and soles, inside the mouth, and around the genitals as well. Some patients develop psoriatic plaques over much of their skin (Figure 1.29). Psoriasis can also get under finger and toenails, where it can cause pitting, infection, and sometimes result in the loss of the nail altogether, a condition called *onycholysis*.

Figure 1.28. Psoriasis.

Figure 1.29. Severe psoriasis.

Psoriasis often occurs in cycles of acute flares followed by periods of remission; this is a pattern seen with many diseases involving immune system dysfunction. Psoriatic flares can be triggered by a number of things: physical or emotional trauma, skin damage, sunburn, hormonal changes, prescription drugs related to high blood pressure and depression, or a state of immune suppression. Psoriasis outbreaks may be more common in wintertime because of the combination of dry skin and lack of sunlight.

In its subacute or nonactive phase, a slight discoloration may remain on the skin where the lesions tend to appear. This is especially true on the trunk.

Other varieties of psoriasis are less common than plaque psoriasis but can be more serious. They include

- *Guttate psoriasis*: this version is usually triggered by a viral or bacterial infection of the respiratory tract. It looks like small circular lesions spread over large areas.
- *Pustular psoriasis*: this involves small, noninfectious pustules in the affected areas.
- *Inverse psoriasis*: this appears at skin folds under the breasts, in the armpits, and around the genitals.
- *Erythrodermic psoriasis*: this version is triggered by sunburn and steroidal anti-inflammatories. It covers large areas of skin in a bright red, hot rash.

Complications

Psoriasis is rarely a life-threatening condition, although it can be extreme and uncomfortable in the acute stages. In severe cases, profound drying and cracking of the skin can lead to infection, fluid loss, and shock. Complications due to psoriasis cause approximately 400 deaths per year in the United States.

Another complication of psoriasis is a condition called *psoriatic arthritis*. This is a type of joint inflammation that affects approximately 20% to 30% of psoriasis patients. It occurs in several subtypes but follows the typical flare–remission cycle as other autoimmune disorders. The guidelines for massage and psoriatic arthritis are the same as those for *rheumatoid arthritis* (Chapter 2).

Treatment

For such a common skin condition, psoriasis can be surprisingly difficult to treat. No single treatment is effective for a majority of patients, many of the most effective medications carry many serious side effects, and people often build up resistance to medications, making them less effective. Three main avenues are pursued with psoriasis treatments: topical applications, phototherapy, and systemic medications.

Topical medications vary from coal tar (popular because it carries a minimum of side effects, but problematic because it smells bad and stains clothing) to vitamin D ointments, to various strengths of steroid creams. The drawbacks of long-term steroid applications are spelled out in the **eczema** article. Other topical treatments include salicylic acid (which is also used to remove warts) to help dissolve and remove plaques, and oatmeal or Epsom salt baths.

Phototherapy involves limited exposure to sunshine, or carefully regulated doses of exposure to ultraviolet A or ultraviolet B lights. UV exposure stimulates vitamin D production, which in turn inhibits skin cell replication. Too much UV exposure can exacerbate symptoms, so this therapy must be used cautiously.

Systemic medications may be steroidal drugs, retinoids to limit sebaceous secretions, or cytotoxic drugs (as in chemotherapy) to limit the activity of those skin cells that have run amok. Psoriasis and cancer have a lot in common in terms of uncontrolled replication, and this option is occasionally successful.

Topical and systemic therapies are often combined with phototherapy. PUVA is a common example. It is a combination of a systemic medication (psoralen) and UV light exposure. PUVA is often successful. Unfortunately, it is also linked to increased chances of contracting basal cell or squamous cell carcinoma, as well as some other serious side effects.

Although there are many types of treatment for psoriasis, none of them has appeared to be a permanent solution. Patients with very severe cases of psoriasis must frequently change strategies as their skin builds up resistance to treatment.

Massage?

In ancient Greece, massage with olive oil was the prescribed treatment for psoriasis. It is now recognized that massage *on* the lesions during an acute outbreak will probably only aggravate the situation by stimulating circulation in an area where too much activity is already taking place. Psoriasis is a local contraindication in the acute phase, but otherwise massage is appropriate. (Of course, first it is necessary to make sure that there has not been any drying or cracking of the skin that would make the client vulnerable to infection.) Psoriasis is not spread by massage, it is not contagious, and massage may be able indirectly to help deal with some of the internal and external stress factors that can stimulate an outbreak.

Skin Cancer

Definition: What Is It?

Cancer is the uncontrolled replication of cells into tumors. These tumors can damage surrounding tissues, spread throughout the body, and can sometimes be fatal. The tissues that are most vulnerable to cancer are often those that tolerate a lot of wear and tear: skin cells, the epithelium of the lungs, and the inner layer of the colon are some good examples. These cells heal easily and rapidly, but sometimes that feature backfires and a situation develops in which cells that have endured a lifetime of abuse start "healing" in a way that could quite possibly kill.

Demographics: Who Gets It?

Some people wish that sleep could be cumulative: that a person could sleep an extra 14 hours on a weekend, and then not be tired for all of the following week. In a certain way, *sunlight* is cumulative. Picture a person playing on the monkey bars when he is 5, rollerblading when he is 10, hiking in the mountains at age 15, sailing when he is 40, and snorkeling when he is 50. His skin cells are keeping accurate records of exactly how much and how often he has insulted them with too much sun. And one day, those skin cells may respond to all that exposure by going into overactive production. This is a particular risk if a person

- has pale skin that burns but does not tan
- lives in a place with a lot of sunshine
- spends a good deal of time outside
- is in any way immune-suppressed
- is mature and has built up a lifetime of exposure to the sun in his skin cells
- has a history of exposure to coal tar, creosote, arsenic compounds, or radium.

Skin Cancer in Brief

What is it?
Skin cancer is cancer in the *stratum basale* of the epidermis (basal cell carcinoma or BCC); cancer of the keratinocytes in the epidermis (squamous cell carcinoma or SCC); or cancer of the melanocytes (pigment cells) of the epidermis (malignant melanoma).

How is it recognized?
For BCC and SCC, look for the cardinal sign: sores that never heal. These sores can resemble blisters, warts, pimples, or simple unexplained bumps and abrasions. They are usually painless but may bleed or become slightly itchy as the cells become active. For malignant melanoma, look for a mole that exhibits the ABCDEs of melanoma.

Is massage indicated or contraindicated?
For BCC, which does not metastasize, massage is a local contraindication, as long as a dermatologist has diagnosed the lesion. SCC and malignant melanoma carry the risk of metastasis. Therefore, any decisions about massage must be made according to the treatments the client is having, weighing possible benefits with possible risks.

Skin Cancer Statistics

Here is the bad news:

- By the time most people have reached 18 years of age, they will have received half or more of their lifetime's exposure to the sun.

- One serious sunburn can increase the risk of skin cancer by up to 50%.

- It is estimated that almost half of all people in the United States 65 years and older will experience some form of skin cancer at least once.

- Approximately 800,000 new cases of BCC and SCC are diagnosed each year.

- Approximately 54,200 cases of malignant melanoma were diagnosed in the United States in 2003.

- Approximately 9,800 people died of malignant melanoma in 2003; approximately 2,200 people died of other types of skin cancer.

The good news is that education and vigilance make a big difference in mortality rates for this disease. Although the exact mechanism linking sun exposure and the development of skin cancer is still being explored, it is clear that avoiding overexposure reduces the risk of developing this disease. All types of skin cancer are survivable if they are caught early enough.

Skin cancer is the most common variety of cancer that humans experience; it accounts for approximately one in three of all cancer diagnoses. It is estimated that 40% to 50% of all adults older than 65 years will experience some type of skin cancer. Non-melanoma skin cancer affects approximately 1 million Americans every year. The American Cancer Society estimates that malignant melanoma will affect 54,200 people this year and will probably kill approximately 7,600[1]. See Sidebar, "Skin Cancer Statistics."

Etiology: What Happens?

Three basic types of skin cancer and one precancerous condition are the most common forms of this disease; they are each discussed in detail.

Actinic Keratosis: Precancerous Lesions

Definition: What Is It?

Also called solar keratosis, *actinic keratosis* (AK) is a precancerous condition that can lead to squamous cell carcinoma. Other precancerous varieties of keratosis include *actinic cheilitis* (AK lesions that appear on the lips), *leukoplakia* (white patches on the tongue or inside the cheek), and *Bowen's disease*, a form of *in situ* squamous cell carcinoma.

Signs and Symptoms

Brown or red scaly lesions usually appear on the forehead, tops of ears, hands, or other areas subject to a lot of sun exposure (Figures 1.30, 1.31). These sores may form a crust, but do not heal normally. The crust falls off, and forms over again. This pattern is the

[1] Skin cancer facts. Copyright © 2003 American Cancer Society, Inc. http://www.cancer.org/docroot/PED/content/ped_7_1_What_You_Need_To_Know_About_Skin_Cancer.asp?sitearea=PED. Accessed summer 2003.

Figure 1.30. Actinic keratosis: lips.   Figure 1.31. Actinic keratosis: ear.

single most important sign of non-melanoma skin cancer. It is estimated that one person in every six will have AK lesions at some time, and up to 5% of all untreated actinic keratosis lesions can develop into squamous cell carcinoma, which is a potentially dangerous disease.

Treatment

AK lesions are usually frozen off with liquid nitrogen. They also may be injected with medication, or a topical ointment may be applied. Very large lesions may be excised.

Massage?

AK is not strictly speaking a cancerous condition and therefore does not contraindicate massage. However, if a client has AK lesions, he should consider having them removed promptly. If he has a history of AK, but nothing more serious has developed, massage is appropriate. All undiagnosed skin lesions are a caution for massage therapists, who should recommend that their clients consult their doctors as soon as possible.

Basal Cell Carcinoma

Definition: What Is It?

Basal cell carcinoma (BCC) is by far the most common type of skin cancer; it accounts for approximately 75% to 90% of all skin cancer cases. It is diagnosed roughly 800,000 times a year in this country. It is a slow-growing non-metastasizing tumor of epithelial cells in the stratum basale of the epidermis. It is not usually dangerous; although if the tumor is left untreated for years, it can become life-threatening because of the other tissues that are eroded by the tumor's growth: nearby arteries or nerves, for example.

Signs and Symptoms

Basal cell carcinoma can be tricky to describe because it looks like all sorts of different things. Typically it appears on the face, around the bridge of the nose or the eyebrow. It looks like a small, hard, pearl-colored lump, with rounded edges, and a soft, sunken middle. The borders are often hard, and they may bleed and form crusts. The middle of the lump is usually soft, with an open sore that may scab, but never permanently heals: an ulceration. BCCs are sometimes called "rodent ulcers" (Figures 1.32, 1.33, 1.34).

Figure 1.32. Basal cell carcinoma.

Figure 1.33. Basal cell carcinoma.

Figure 1.34. Basal cell carcinoma.

Another type of BCC is particularly common for elderly fair-skinned people who have spent a lot of time in the sun. This variety looks like flat sores, not on the face, but on the back and trunk. Like the typical facial BCCs, these sores do not heal, but simply crust, shed the scab, and crust again. This variety of BCC is easily mistaken for *seborrheic keratosis*, a noncancerous condition, which is why it is essential that massage therapists refer any client with suspicious lesions for further diagnosis. (See sidebar, "Other Skin Pigmentations.")

Treatment

Basal cell carcinoma, because it grows so very slowly, and does not metastasize, responds very well to simply being excised: cut out with a knife or a laser. The tumor-producing cells can also be killed off with liquid nitrogen or with radiation. Occasionally BCC recurs, so it is wise to keep a close watch for any nonhealing sores after an episode.

Massage?

The tumor itself is a local contraindication, of course. This is not something that spreads through the body or that massage makes worse in any way. And if a client fits the profile for the flat sore on the trunk, the practitioner may be the one to spot it in the first place.

Squamous Cell Carcinoma

Definition: What Is It?

Squamous cell carcinoma (SCC) is a malignancy of keratinocytes in the epidermis. Keratinocytes produce keratin, the protein that fills up the epithelial cells that are migrating toward the surface of the skin. SCC accounts for approximately 22% of all skin cancers. It is diagnosed about 200,000 times a year in this country.

Signs and Symptoms

SCC can occur anywhere epidermis tissue grows—on the skin, usually, but occasionally on mucous membranes too. It is especially common on ears, hands, and lower lips, but it can also happen *inside* the mouth, often as a response to pipe-smoking or chewing to-bacco and the constant irritation that those habits incur. It is significantly more danger-ous than BCC because it *can* metastasize through the lymph system and the tumors can infiltrate deep tissues far more quickly than BCC.

SCC tumors often happen on preexisting lesions on sun-exposed skin. In other words, they happen where the skin has had to repair itself before. Some, but not all SCC lesions begin as actinic keratosis. They generally start as hard, firm lumps that may look like a wart. The sores appear, and *do not heal*. The borders of SCCs are of-ten less distinct than the more self-contained basal cell tumors (Figures 1.35, 1.36).

AK, BCC, and SCC bear one key feature in common: an open sore that never completely heals. Often a pattern occurs: a crust forms, but it does not hold on; in-evitably it falls off and starts to form again. All the while, the sore is ulcerating, and the cancer cells are getting a deeper and deeper grip on the underlying tissues. A person who is experiencing this cycle with a sore *anywhere* on the body should *run, not walk* to the nearest dermatologist.

Treatment

As with BCC, SCCs are frozen or excised. With SCC, however, it is especially important to be sure that *all* of the affected tissue is removed, because if any "hot" cells should find their way into the lymph system, the cancer could spread to elsewhere in the body. Therefore, excess tissue is often also taken, which may require postoperative skin grafts. The area may also then be radiated, to make doubly sure that all of the cancer-causing cells are dead.

Massage?

Squamous cell carcinoma is not always an aggressive form of cancer, but it can be. People undergoing treatment for it may face surgery, skin grafts, radiation, chemotherapy, or any combination of the above. These treatments carry specific cautions for massage that are outlined in the article on *cancer* (Chapter 11). Massage can be appropriate for persons

Figure 1.35. Squamous cell carcinoma.   Figure 1.36. Squamous cell carcinoma.

who are fighting cancer, but the therapist must make sure the client and his health care team are fully informed and design a treatment that delivers maximum benefit with a minimum of risk.

Malignant Melanoma

Definition: What Is It?

Melanocytes are the pigment cells that give skin its color. They are located deep in the epidermis. Melanin protects us, as much as it can, from harmful UV radiation from the sun. As in the other cancers discussed here, if melanocytes get *too much* stimulation, they can start replicating without control. This is malignant melanoma.

Melanoma is the leading cause of death from skin diseases, and the cause of more than 75% of all deaths from skin cancer. Fortunately, it is also the least common variety of skin cancer, accounting for approximately 3% to 5% of skin cancer cases.

It is important to note that although a long history of exposure to sunlight is a leading risk factor for malignant melanoma, it can develop in areas that are not usually exposed to the sun. It can even grow in epithelial cells that are internal: mucous membranes of the respiratory, digestive, reproductive, and urinary tract may all develop malignant melanoma.

Signs and Symptoms

Melanoma often starts from a preexisting *mole* (this chapter) that, later in life, begins to change; it lightens, darkens, thickens, and may become elevated (Figure 1.37). Sometimes it is itchy or bleeds around the edges. Melanoma does not always start from a mole, however, nor does it always begin in areas that have been exposed to the sun.

Here is a simple mnemonic to remember the key diagnostic features for melanoma:

- *A: Asymmetrical*: most benign moles are circular or oval. A melanoma has an indeterminate shape.
- *B: Border*: The borders of melanomas are irregular and may be indistinct as it goes into the skin.

Figure 1.37. Superficial spreading melanoma.

- *C: Color*: The colors of most moles are consistent: they are brown or black, but not both. Melanomas are typically multicolored, with brown, black and even purple all mixed together.
- *D: Diameter*: melanomas are large. Any mole that is bigger than 6 mm across should be examined by a dermatologist.
- *E: Elevated*: melanomas are usually at least partly elevated from the skin. They may even be big enough to snag on things and bleed.

Because melanoma is a disease of cumulative sun exposure, it rarely happens in young people. Large moles that develop *after* adolescence, however, are highly suspect. Moles in areas that are subject to a lot of irritation are at especially high risk of becoming cancerous.

Men most often get melanoma on the trunk, neck or head. Women tend to get it on the arms or legs.

Four specific types of malignant melanoma have been identified:

- *Superficial spreading melanoma* is the most common variety. It spreads along the surface before invading the deeper tissues. It may be multicolored and slightly elevated (see Figure 1.37).
- *Lentigo melanoma* also begins as a superficial discoloration, usually very flat, in varying shades of brown (Figure 1.38).
- *Acral lentiginous melanoma* is the most common variety of melanoma to affect non-white people. It usually appears on the hands or feet, between the fingers or toes, or under the nails (Figure 1.39).
- *Nodular melanoma* is the most aggressive and dangerous type of skin cancer; it involves significant elevation from the skin, and the lesions often invade deeper tissues early in development (Figure 1.40).

Treatment

Treatment for melanoma is generally aggressive because this cancer spreads very rapidly, there is literally no time to lose. Once a lesion has been positively identified and staged (evaluated for how far it has progressed), it is usually attacked with every weapon available. Surgical excision involves shaving the tumor layer by layer and examining the surrounding tissues for signs of involvement. A margin of healthy tissue is usually taken along with the cancerous areas, to be sure all of the mutated cells have been removed. Radiation

Figure 1.38. Lentigo melanoma.

Figure 1.39. Acral lentiginous melanoma.

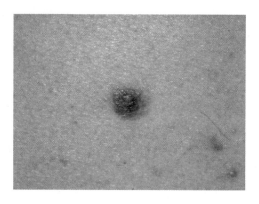

Figure 1.40. Nodular melanoma.

and examination of nearby lymph nodes follows. Perfusion chemotherapy may be employed: the affected limb is tied off with a tourniquet, then high doses of chemotherapeutic drugs are then injected and isolated just to the affected area. Another treatment intervention is called "biological therapy": man-made doses of interferon and interleukin-2 are injected to help support the body's natural cancer-fighting mechanisms.

Prognosis

The prognosis for malignant melanoma is determined largely by how far the cancerous cells have invaded the skin. Melanoma usually begins by spreading shallowly across the epidermis before invading deeper tissues. If it is caught and removed before it is approx-

Compare and Contrast
MOLES OR MELANOMA?

As public awareness about skin cancer grows, everyone is becoming more cautious about his or her moles. Although most moles are harmless, a small percentage of them become cancerous. This is why it is especially important for massage therapists, who work so intimately with the skin, to be able to recognize some of the key features that distinguish moles from melanoma. For more details about melanoma, see the article in this chapter.

MOLES	SKIN CANCER
Size	**Size**
Under 6 mm (the circumference of a pencil eraser)	Over 6 mm
Color	**Color**
Unicolored: could be brown, black, purple, or reddish, but usually not mixed	Multicolored
Shape	**Shape**
Symmetrical: round or oval	Asymmetrical, with an uneven border
Time it appears	**Time it appears**
Before puberty	After puberty

imately 0.7 mm deep, the prognosis is generally hopeful. If it gets up to 4 mm deep, it will probably have already invaded nearby lymph nodes and metastasized through the body. In this case, the prognosis is generally poor.

Massage?

Melanoma is an aggressive form of cancer that spreads through the lymph system. Persons undergoing treatment for melanoma may be on high doses of chemotherapy, radiation, or dealing with surgery and skin grafts. Cautions for massage revolve around circulatory impact and the side effects of cancer treatments. These are outlined in the article on *cancer* (Chapter 11).

In situations in which a cancer patient is terminal, massage can be a valuable part of patient care. In hospice situations, in which the patient is aware of the risks and is more interested in the quality of life than quantity, massage may be taught to family members and friends who are caring for the dying person.

SKIN INJURIES

Burns

Definition: What Are They?

Many people think about burns in the context of touching a hot iron or brushing a hand across a broiler rack. But the world of burns goes beyond household appliances. A person can sustain burn damage from dry heat such as irons and broilers, wet heat such as hot liquids or steam, electricity, friction (i.e., "rug burn"), radiation, and corrosive chemicals. Any one of these can destroy the proteins in the exposed skin cells, which causes the cells to die. If a significant amount of skin is affected, it will be unable to accomplish its protective tasks: it *will not* provide a shield from microbial invasion, it *will not* help to maintain a stable temperature, and it *will not* provide protection from fluid loss. The massive loss of water, plasma, and plasma proteins that seep out of capillaries around the injury may lead to shock.

Etiology: What Happens?

The severity of burns is determined by how deep they go, how much surface area they cover, and what part of the body has been affected. Losing more than 15% of skin function can put a person at risk for infection, shock, and circulatory collapse. Burns to the face and neck are more serious than those to other areas because the resulting inflammation can block breathing passages.

Skin is composed of three layers of tissue. Burns are graded in three levels of severity. It is not entirely coincidence.

First-Degree Burns This is a sometimes quite painful but relatively mild irritation of the superficial epidermis, characterized by redness, but no blistering. Diaper rash is an example of a burn caused by a chemical irritation. Mild sunburn is perhaps the most common example of 1st-degree burns. Overexposure to the sun damages cells in the epithelium, setting up an inflammatory response. This leads to pain, heat, redness and swelling

---

Burns in Brief

What are they?
Burns are caused by damage to the skin that causes the cells to die. They can be caused by fire, overexposure to the sun, dry heat, wet heat, electricity, radiation, extreme cold, and toxic chemicals.

How are they recognized?
First-degree burns involve mild inflammation. Second-degree burns also involve blistering and damage at the deeper levels of the epidermis. Third-degree burns go down into the dermis itself and will often show white or black charred edges. In the post-acute stage, serious burns will often involve shrunken, contracted scar tissue over the area of skin that has been affected.

Is massage indicated or contraindicated?
All burns (except, perhaps, mild sunburns) contraindicate massage in the acute stage. In the subacute and post-acute stages, massage may be performed around the damaged area within the pain tolerance of the client.

Figure 1.41. First-degree burn.

Figure 1.42. Second-degree burn.

(Figure 1.41). Sunburns generally heal in 2 to 3 days, sometimes with flaking and peeling. If the sunburn is more severe, it may blister, which is a sign of

Second-Degree Burns This is damage that involves all layers of the epidermis, and possibly some of the dermis too. Symptoms include redness, blisters, edema, and a lot of pain (Figure 1.42). Still, if the burn area is fairly small, it will heal in a week (or maybe a month if it involves the dermis). Usually the hair shafts and glands do not sustain permanent damage, although there may be some superficial scarring. Second-degree burns can come from the sun, but from lots of other things too, such as steam under pressure, toxic chemicals, or hot glue guns.

Third-Degree Burns These go right through the dermis or beyond, destroying hair shafts, sebaceous glands, erector pilae muscles, sweat glands, and even nerve endings, which paradoxically makes third-degree burns less painful than second-degree burns. Symptoms include whiteness or charring, and a leathery texture of the skin in the affected area (Figure 1.43). Third-degree burns are dangerous for all of the reasons mentioned above: risk of infection, fluid loss, and shock, especially if a significant percentage of the

Figure 1.43. Third-degree burn.

body surface has been affected. In addition, one of the special problems with 3rd-degree burns is that they tend to contract rapidly, forming a confining web of scar tissue, even with quickly applied skin grafts.

Signs and Symptoms

The symptoms of burn damage depend on what level of skin has been affected. Details on symptoms by degree of damage are listed above.

Treatment

First- and second-degree burns are seldom treated with anything more than soothing lotion and possibly antibiotic cream if the skin has been damaged to the point of not providing protection from infectious agents. Third-degree burns, however, must be treated with more care to minimize the accumulation of binding scar tissue. This often means wound cleansing and *debridement*: skin brushing to remove debris, as well as skin grafts and plastic surgery.

Massage?

The *only* kind of burn that is appropriate for circulatory massage in the acute stage is a very mild sunburn, and of course even then one must work within pain tolerance. By sloughing off dead cells, massage can speed the healing process along, but it is not something to do without a client's permission.

Other burns may be approached in the subacute stage as a local contraindication; it is all right to work around the edges within pain tolerance to improve elasticity and minimize scar tissue, without running the risk of exposing the client to infection. In this situation, it is important to be working with a doctor to establish when the burn is in a subacute stage and to rule out any other tissue trauma that may contraindicate massage. Lymph drainage techniques that specialize in working reflexively to stimulate lymph flow also may be used with recent burn victims.

Massage has been used successfully to reduce the stress associated with treatment for 3rd-degree burns. The pain of debriding damaged skin tissue is often described as worse than the burn itself. When patients receive massage before their wound care sessions, they report lower levels of anxiety, pain, and depression, and their levels of stress-related hormones and pulse rates are appreciably decreased. These benefits set the stage for a less painful, more efficient healing process.[2]

Finally, if burns are obviously long past the acute and subacute stages, that is, no pain remains and all that is left is residual scar tissue, massage is safe. The only caution here is that in serious cases permanent nerve damage might have occurred. If that is the case, the client will not be able to feel it if the massage is doing any damage.

Decubitus Ulcers

Definition: What Are They?

This condition, which is also known as *bedsores, pressure sores,* and *trophic ulcers,* is one massage therapists would most likely see when working in a hospital, a hospice, or some other setting with bed-ridden patients. It is a problem stemming from chronic inadequate blood flow to the skin that stretches over bony or otherwise prominent areas. It al-

[2] Field T. Touch Therapy. London: Churchill Livingstone 2000:53–58.

Decubitus Ulcers in Brief

Pronunciation
dē-kyū′bi-tŭs ŭl′sĕr

What are they?
Bedsores are ulcers caused by impaired circulation to the skin. Lack of blood supply leads to irreplaceable tissue death.

How are they recognized?
Unlike other sores, ulcers do not crust over; they remain open wounds that are highly vulnerable to infection.

Is massage indicated or contraindicated?
Bedsores are indicated for massage only *before* they happen. Once the tissue has been damaged it is too late, and they locally contraindicate massage until they have completely healed.

most always occurs in some area that has had constant contact with a surface: usually a bed, sometimes a cast or a splint.

Demographics: Who Gets Them?

The persons most at risk for developing *decubitus* ulcers are elderly, underweight, male, nonambulatory, and incontinent. This does not preclude other people from developing them, however; anyone who is immobile even for just a few hours can develop pressure sores.

Etiology: What Happens?

Imagine looking microscopically into the skin of an immobilized person. Nothing stimulates his circulation. Capillaries are squeezed between bone and bed, and new epithelial cells are starving for nutrition. The cells close to the surface of the skin died long ago, but now the cells in the deeper layers of the epidermis are dying too. Although the damage to deep layers of the skin may be extensive, only small lesions appear at the surface. Bacteria take advantage of the opportunity, and they begin to attack the weakened skin cells, exposing more of the damaged tissues. Capillaries are too narrow to let anything through, including the white blood cells that would otherwise limit the intruders. Gradually the surface tissue dies, and along with it the possibility of regeneration. Left unchecked, the ulcer can destroy the epidermis, the dermis, the superficial fascia, and erode tissues down to the bone (Figure 1.44). Secondary infection of the open wound can lead to blood poisoning and death.

Signs and Symptoms

The first stage of decubitus ulcers shows a marked change in skin temperature. (It can become cooler or warmer than the surrounding area.) Localized reddening becomes visible on pale skin, whereas on dark skin the discoloration may appear to be red, purple, or bluish. Pain and itching accompany these changes.

In later stages the lesions turn purple, and then necrosis, or tissue death, begins. Bacteria may invade the damaged tissue, which results in local or systemic infection.

Figure 1.44. Decubitus ulcer.

Ulcers on the skin (and anywhere else on the body) differ from other types of sores because they do not go through a normal healing process. Where most injuries stimulate the production of new epithelial cells and connective tissue fibers to replace the damaged tissues, the damage incurred by decubitus ulcers prevents this from happening. Ulcers do not even form a crust to cover regenerating epithelium. Of course, eventually, they *can* heal, but not in a normal way; when circulation to the affected area is finally restored, the lesion will close up by having scar tissue grow over the area, but there will be a permanent dip where the dead tissue will never grow back.

Bedsores can start in a surprisingly short amount of time. They can be a real danger for people with spinal injuries who may have to travel for hours strapped to a backboard or for people undergoing long surgeries. Bedsores and joint and muscle degeneration are the primary reasons comatose people are moved and turned frequently. Heels, buttocks, the sacrum, and elbows are the most common places for bedsores to appear.

Treatment

Treatment for pressure sores depends on their stage and location. Topical antibiotics and dressings can be effective for some lesions, whereas bigger, more advanced sores may require debridement and plastic surgery.

The biggest danger for someone with bedsores is the possibility of infection, which can be life-threatening for someone who is bedridden and immune-suppressed already. The treatment protocols outlined by the Agency for Health Care Policy and Research include good nutrition (extra high protein calories and minerals), avoiding pressure of any kind, and proper cleaning and dressing of the wound.[3]

Massage?

Bedsores happen because circulation is interrupted long enough that cells literally starve to death. It would make sense that massage, with its wonderful influence over circulatory flow, would be an appropriate way to deal with this problem. However, because of the peculiar open sore nature of ulcers and because it is virtually impossible to sterilize hands, massage is *not* appropriate for bedsores. If a client is at risk for developing bedsores (and does not have other conditions that contraindicate bodywork), the improved skin nutrition massage can provide could be an excellent preventive measure. But if the sore has already begun to fester, there is a significant danger of infection. The latest research shows that even working around the edges of bedsores is risky, so decubitus ulcers are considered a local contraindication.

Open Wounds and Sores

Definition: What Are They?

Many different technical names are used for all the different ways skin can be damaged. Any damaged tissue can be referred to as a *lesion*. Here is a list of common skin lesions:

- lacerations (rips and tears)
- incisions (cuts)
- excoriations (scratches)
- fissures (cracks)
- papules (firm raised areas, such as pimples)

Open Wounds and Sores in Brief

What are they?
Open wounds and sores are skin injuries that have not completely healed.

How are they recognized?
Unhealed lesions may be marked by bleeding, crusts, exuding pus, or other signs of regenerative activity.

Are they indicated or contraindicated for massage?
Any opening in the skin is an open invitation for infection. At the very least, open wounds and sores locally contraindicate massage. They may systemically contraindicate massage if they appear as a sign of serious systemic disease.

---

[3] Rovner S. Treating bedsores with a new approach. Washington Post Health, January 31, 1995.

- vesicles (blisters)
- pustules (vesicles filled with pus, such as whiteheads)
- punctures (any kind of hole)
- avulsions (something has been ripped off, such as a finger or an ear)
- abrasions (scrapes)
- ulcers (sores with dead tissue that do not go through a normal healing process)

Knowing these technical terms is important, but not as important as knowing that massage is inappropriate for any condition in which skin is not entirely intact.

Massage?

Usually these injuries are simply local contraindications for massage; it is not necessary to reschedule an appointment if a client has a scraped knee. The exception would be if the open wounds or sores were caused by some other systemically contraindicated condition such as advanced *diabetes* (Chapter 8), or *mites* (this chapter).

Scar Tissue

Definition: What Is It?

The body's ability to heal itself after injury is one of the wonders of nature. The new material generated to literally "knit" damaged tissue back together is scar tissue.

This discussion is limited to the regenerative capacities of the skin. For information on scar tissue associated with musculoskeletal injuries, see *tendinitis* (Chapter 2).

Etiology: What Happens?

The skin, because it is subject to such a lot of wear and tear, has cells with special properties not found anywhere else in the body. If a scrape or abrasion occurs, basal cells detach themselves from the basement membrane and begin to migrate in a single-layered sheet across the wound. When they reach the other side and touch other epithelial cells, an internal code makes them stop moving. (It is the absence of this internal code, called *contact inhibition*, that makes cancer cells so dangerous; nothing ever tells them to **stop**.)

Meanwhile, back at the original site, stationary basal cells duplicate to build up the ranks of migrating cells. When the whole wound has been covered, the new sheet of basal cells begin dividing to form new strata. After enough bulk has accumulated, the crust, or scab, will fall off, and the cells on the surface will become keratinized. Then the wound is healed; access to the blood supply is cut off from the outside world, and it is no longer vulnerable to infection. The whole process can take place within 24 hours to several days, depending on the size and location of the lesion.

If the injury goes deeper than the dermis, the healing process is more complicated. Fibroblasts in the area are summoned to the site, so beneath all that basal cell activity a lot of fibroblastic activity is also taking place. This "fill-in" connective tissue is called *granulation tissue*. Eventually it changes to become an accumulation of collagenous scar tissue, meant to knit up the fascia, but which may intrude on the superficial layers as well. If the scar tissue does not stay within the boundaries of the original injury, it is called *hypertrophic* scar. Sometimes the fibroblasts get much too active and produce much more collagen than is necessary. The scar overflows the injury, resulting in a permanently raised mass of tissue.

Scar Tissue in Brief

What is it?
Scar tissue is the growth of new tissue: skin or fascia, after injury.

How is it recognized?
Scar tissue on the skin often lacks pigmentation and hair follicles.

Is massage indicated or contraindicated?
Massage is contraindicated during the acute stage of any injury in which the skin has been damaged. In the subacute stage, massage may improve the quality of the healing process.

Figure 1.45. Keloid scar.

This is called *keloid* scar (Figure 1.45). Keloid scar can be a very annoying complication of surgery or any kind of deep wound healing, but it is seldom a debilitating problem.

Collagenous scar tissue differs from normal skin in some important ways: the collagen fibers are much denser, they do not lay down in the same patterns as uninjured tissue, no epidermis covers it, it has fewer blood vessels, and it is usually missing hair follicles, normal skin glands, and possibly even sensory neurons.

Treatment

Several treatment options have been developed to minimize the appearance of scar tissue on the skin, but none of them can eradicate the scars themselves. Hypertrophic scar tissue may be injected with cortisone, which dissolves the excess collagen. Keloids are frozen with liquid nitrogen and then treated with cortisone, but they may still recur. Scarred areas that dip into underlying tissues may be injected with collagen to help them "fill out" their normal area. Other options to improve the look and texture of scar tissue include dermabrasion (the skin is mechanically "buffed" to remove excess epithelium), chemical peels (the top layers of epithelium are chemically treated and removed to create more even texture and coloring), punch grafts (small pieces of normal skin are surgically implanted to replace localized scars such as old acne lesions), and laser resurfacing.

When a large surface area of skin has been damaged, it is important to control the amount of scar tissue that accumulates because large masses of scar can contract into uncomfortable and unsightly areas (see *burns*, this chapter). Skin grafts and some specialized types of gene therapy can control the accumulation of new scar tissue for the best possible long-term results.

Massage?

Obviously, massage is only appropriate in the subacute stage of healing. Why? If the skin is not intact, the client is a walking invitation for infection. If someone is healing from a deep wound such as a surgery, they will often benefit from work *around* the area, which will keep the skin supple, and may inhibit the build-up of hypertrophic scar (see *postoperative conditions*, Chapter 11). If a client has old, deep scar tissue on the skin, sensation in those areas may be reduced. In such a case, massage therapists should be extra solicitous of client feedback.

OTHER

 Ichthyosis:

Ichthys is Greek for "fish." Ichthyosis means, literally, "fish condition." Other terms for this condition are equally descriptive: "alligator skin," *"sauriasis"* (*sauros* is from the Greek for "lizard," as in *dinosaur*), *"sauroderma"* and *"sauriosis."*

Ichthyosis
Definition: What Is It?

Ichthyosis is a rare disorder in which the skin is pathologically dry. Although it can happen alone, it can also be a symptom of a variety of diseases.

Etiology: What Happens?

Ichthyosis is often linked to a problem with turnover of epithelial cells. Whereas in a normal cycle dead cells are sloughed off the skin every month or so, in ichthyosis they tend to pile up into dry, diamond-shaped plaques.

Several types of ichthyosis have been identified. It can occur alone, usually on the legs of elderly people, especially in cold weather when the air is very dry; in this kind of situation it is sometimes called *xeroderma*. Ichthyosis in infants can also be a symptom of congenital problems associated with birth defects or certain rare neurologic diseases. Other cases are indicators of a variety of other diseases, including *Hodgkin's disease* or *HIV/AIDS* (Chapter 5), *hypothyroidism* (Chapter 8), or Hansen's disease (leprosy).

Signs and Symptoms

Ichthyosis creates distinctive diamond-shaped plates on the skin that resemble fish scales, hence its name, which means "fish condition." Sometimes the affected area may become darker than the surrounding areas (Figure 1.46).

Ichthyosis in Brief

Pronunciation
ik-thē-ō′sis

What is it?
Ichthyosis is pathologically dry skin: much more severe than average dry skin.

How is it recognized?
Ichthyosis creates distinctive diamond-shaped "scales" on the skin, usually on the lower legs.

Is massage indicated or contraindicated?
When ichthyosis appears independently of other conditions, it certainly indicates massage. It probably will not be a permanent solution to this problem, but massage can certainly make it better in the short run. Take care to avoid areas where deep cracking may expose blood supply.

Figure 1.46. Ichthyosis.

Treatment

The first recourse for persons living with pathologically dry skin is to change their bathing habits. People with ichthyosis need to take special care to preserve the protective coating of sebum on their skin. This is accomplished by bathing less frequently and by applying emollients to the skin while it is still wet. A variety of preparations may be applied to help soften and remove the scales that develop with ichthyosis; these depend on the age of the patient and the cause and severity of the disorder.

Massage?

This is one of the few skin conditions that, in the absence of underlying contraindications, massage can substantially improve. It does so by adding nonirritating oil to the skin and by stimulating the sebaceous glands become active too. Be cautious, however, of skin that is *so* dry it cracks down to the capillary level, whereupon it becomes, like all compromised skin, an invitation to infection.

CHAPTER REVIEW QUESTIONS

1. What is the cardinal rule for massage and skin conditions?
2. A client has eczema on her hands that is extremely dry and flaky. Does this condition indicate or contraindicate massage? Why?
3. A client has severe ichthyosis that is cracked and oozing. Does this condition indicate or contraindicate massage? Why?
4. What does psoriasis have in common with cancer?
5. When working with a client who is prone to acne, is it a good idea to follow the treatment with an alcohol rinse to remove the oil? Why?
6. A client has white flakes that cling to hair shafts and do not brush out. What condition is probably present?
7. A client has a raised red ring on the back of his upper thigh. What condition may be present?
8. What should be done with this client's massage sheets?
9. In what stage of the development of a decubitus ulcer is massage appropriate?
10. In what situation would an open sore be a systemic rather than just a local contraindication?
11. Your client reports a small lesion that never seems to get better. What do you think is present?
12. What makes acral lentiginous melanoma different from other types?

 Answers to these questions can be found on the Student Recource CD-ROM that accompanies this book.

Bibliography

General Resources, Integumentary System

1. de Dominico G, Wood E. Beard's Massage. Philadelphia: WB Saunders, 1997.
2. Damjanou I. Pathology for the Health-Related Professions. Philadelphia: WB Saunders, 1996.
3. Travell J, Simons DG. Myofascial Pain and Dysfunction: The Trigger Point Manual. Baltimore: Williams & Wilkins, 1983.
4. Clemente CD. Anatomy: A Regional Atlas of the Human Body. 3rd Ed. Baltimore: Urban & Schwarzenburg, 1987.
5. Tortora GJ, Anagnostakos NP. Principles of Anatomy and Physiology. 6th Ed. New York: Harper & Row, 1990.
6. Taber's Cyclopedic Dictionary. 14th Ed. Philadelphia: FA Davis, 1981.
7. Stedman's Medical Dictionary. 26th Ed. Baltimore: Williams & Wilkins, 1995.

8. Memmler RL, Wood DL. The Human Body in Health and Disease. 5th Ed. Philadelphia: JB Lippincott, 1983.
9. Juhan D. Job's Body: A Handbook for Bodywork. Barrytown, NY: Station Hill Press, 1987.
10. Kunz JRM, Finkel AJ, eds. The American Medical Association Family Medical Guide. New York: Random House, 1987.
11. Marieb EM. Human Anatomy and Physiology. Redwood City, CA: Benjamin/Cummings, 1989.
12. Field T. Touch Therapy. London: Churchill Livingstone, 2000.

Boils

1. Boils (Skin Abscesses). © 1996-2003 MedicineNet, Inc. Available at: http://www.medicinenet.com/Boils/article.htm. Accessed summer 2003.
2. Boils and Carbuncles. © 1998-2003 Mayo Foundation for Medical Education and Research (MFMER). Available at: http://www.mayoclinic.com/invoke.cfm?id=DS00466. Accessed summer 2003.
3. Elizabeth P Baorto, MD, MPH, David Baorto, MD, PhD. Staphylococcus aureus infection. Copyright © 2003, eMedicine.com, Inc. Available at: http://www.emedicine.com/ped/topic2704.htm. Accessed summer 2003.

Cellulitis

1. Cellulitis. Copyright © 1995-2003 Merck & Co., Inc. Available at: http://www.merck.com/pubs/mmanual/section10/chapter112/112b.htm. Accessed summer 2003.
2. Group A Streptococcal Infections. National Institute of Allergy and Infectious Diseases. Available at: http://www.niaid.nih.gov/factsheets/strep.htm. Accessed summer 2003.

Fungal Infections

1. Rhett J. Drugge, MD. Common Dermatologic Diseases. © 1995-2000 The Internet Dermatology Society, Inc. Available at: http://telemedicine.org/common/Fungus. Accessed summer 2003.
2. Ringworm (Tinea). © 1996-2003 MedicineNet, Inc. Available at: http://www.medicinenet.com/Ringworm/article.htm. Accessed summer 2003.
3. Dermatophyte Infections (Ringworm). Copyright © 1995-2003 Merck & Co., Inc. Available at: http://www.merck.com/pubs/mmanual/section10/chapter113/113a.htm. Accessed summer 2003.
4. Nelly Rubeiz, MD, Zeina Tannous, MD. Tinea. Copyright © 2003, eMedicine.com, Inc. Available at: http://www.emedicine.com/emerg/topic592.htm. Accessed summer 2003.

Herpes Simplex

1. Genital Herpes in Women. © 1996-2003 MedicineNet, Inc. Available at: http://www.medicinenet.com/Genital_Herpes_In_Women/article.htm. Accessed summer 2003.
2. Torres G, Schinstine M. Herpes Simplex. Copyright © 2003, eMedicine.com, Inc. Available at: http://www.emedicine.com/derm/topic179.htm. Accessed summer 2003.
3. Herpes Simplex Infections (Non-Genital). © 1996-2003 MedicineNet, Inc. Available at: http://www.medicinenet.com/Herpes_Simplex_Infections_Non-Genital/article.htm. Accessed summer 2003.

Impetigo

1. Impetigo. © 1996-2003 MedicineNet, Inc. Available at: http://www.medicinenet.com/Impetigo/article.htm. Accessed summer 2003.
2. Impetigo. © 1995-2003 The Nemours Foundation. Available at: http://kidshealth.org/PageManager.jsp?dn=KidsHealth&lic=1&ps=107&cat_id=20028&article_set=22786. Accessed summer 2003.

Mites and Lice

1. Body Lice (Pediculosis). Centers for Disease Control and Prevention. Available at: http://www.cdc.gov/ncidod/dpd/parasites/lice/factsht_body_lice.htm. Accessed summer 2003.
2. Caron DM. Human Lice. Available at: http://ag.udel.edu/extension/Information/hyg/hyg-42.html. Accessed summer 2003.
3. Malerba A, Kaufman CL. Scabies. Copyright © 2003, eMedicine.com, Inc. Available at: http://emedicine.com/derm/topic382.htm. Accessed summer 2003.
4. Head Lice Infestation (Pediculosis). Centers for Disease Control and Prevention. Available at: http://www.cdc.gov/ncidod/dpd/parasites/headlice/factsht_head_lice.htm. Accessed summer 2003.
5. Pubic Lice or "Crabs" Pthirus Pubis (THEER-us pu-bis). Centers for Disease Control and Prevention. Available at: http://www.cdc.gov/ncidod/dpd/parasites/lice/factsht_pubic_lice.htm. Accessed summer 2003.
6. Scabies. © 1997-2003 New Zealand Dermatological Society. Available at: http://www.dermnetnz.org/. Accessed summer 2003.

Warts

1. Warts (Common Warts). © 1996-2003 MedicineNet, Inc. Available at: http://www.medicinenet.com/Warts_Common_Warts/article.htm. Accessed summer 2003.
2. Warts. Copyright © 2000 American Academy of Dermatology. Available at: http://www.aad.org/pamphlets/warts.html. Accessed summer 2003.
3. Your Podiatric Physician Talks About Warts. American Podiatric Medical Association. Available at: http://www.apma.org/topics/wartstxt.htm. Accessed summer 2003.
4. Focht DR 3rd, Spicer C, Fairchok MP. The Efficacy of Duct Tape vs Cryotherapy in the Treatment of Verruca Vulgaris (the Common Wart). Available at: http://ncbi.nlm.nih.gov/entrez/query.fcgi?CMD=Display&DB=PubMed. Accessed summer 2003.

Acne rosacea

1. Health Topics: Questions and Answers About Rosacea. National Institute of Arthritis and Musculoskeletal and Skin Diseases. NIH Publication No. 02–5038 Available at: http://www.niams.nih.gov/hi/topics/rosacea/rosacea.htm Accessed summer 2003.
2. Blount BW, Pelletier AL. Rosacea: A Common, Yet Commonly Overlooked, Condition. Copyright © 2002 by the American Academy of Family Physicians. Available at: http://www.aafp.org/afp/20020801/435.html. Accessed summer 2003.
3. Rosacea. Copyright © 1987 American Academy of Dermatology Revised 1991, 1993, 1995, 1999. Available at: http://www.aad.org/pamphlets/rosacea.html. Accessed summer 2003.
4. What Is Rosacea? © 1996-2003 MedicineNet, Inc. Available at: http://www.medicinenet.com/Rosacea/article.htm. Accessed summer 2003.

Acne Vulgaris

1. Acne. Copyright © 1987 American Academy of Dermatology. Available at: http://www.aad.org/pamphlets/acnepamp.html. Accessed summer 2003.
2. Questions and Answers About Acne. National Institute of Arthritis and Musculoskeletal and Skin Diseases (NIAMS). Available at: http://www.niams.nih.gov/hi/topics/acne/acne.htm. Accessed summer 2003.
3. Acne Vulgaris. Copyright © 2003, eMedicine.com, Inc. Available at: http://www.emedicine.com/derm/topic2.htm. Accessed summer 2003.

Dermatitis/Eczema

1. Atopic Dermatitis. © 1997–2003 New Zealand Dermatological Society. Available at: http://www.dermnetnz.org/. Accessed summer 2003.
2. Handout on Health: Atopic Dermatitis. National Institute of Arthritis and Musculoskeletal and Skin Diseases (NIAMS). Available at: http://www.niams.nih.gov/hi/topics/dermatitis/index.html. Accessed summer 2003.
3. Itching for a Little Relief? New Therapies Proving Effective for Millions of Adults and Children with Eczema. © American Academy of Dermatology, 2000. Available at: http://www.aad.org/PressReleases/itchingRelief.html. Accessed summer 2003.
4. What Is Eczema? © American Academy of Dermatology, 2000. Available at: http://www.skincarephysicians.com/eczemanet/whatIs.html. Accessed summer 2003.
5. Atopic Dermatitis (Atopic Eczema). © National Jewish Medical and Research Center. Available at: http://www.nationaljewish.org/medfacts/atopic.html. Accessed summer 2003.

6. Eczema/Atopic Dermatitis. © 1995-2003 The Nemours Foundation. Available at: http://kidshealth.org/PageManager.jsp?dn=KidsHealth&lic=1&ps=107&cat_id=20047&article_set=21940. Accessed summer 2003.

7. Nummular Eczema. © 2001 by A.O.C.D. American Osteopathic College of Dermatology. Available at: http://www.aocd.org/skin/dermatologic_diseases/nummular_eczema.html. Accessed summer 2003.

8. Shaberman B. Dermatology Insights: Patient Perspective: Coping with Skin Disease. © American Academy of Dermatology, 2000. Available at: http://www.aad.org/DermInsights/Fall2000/COPING.html. Accessed summer 2003.

Hives

1. Chronic Hives (Urticaria): A Guide for Sufferers. Copyright © 1997-2003 Asthma & Allergy Associates of Florida, P.A. Available at: http://www.allergyweb.com/hives_pt.asp. Accessed summer 2003.

2. Crawford MB. Urticaria. Copyright © 2003, eMedicine.com, Inc. Available at: http://www.emedicine.com/emerg/topic628.htm. Accessed summer 2003.

3. Urticaria. Copyright © 1996 - 2002; The American College of Allergy, Asthma & Immunology. Available at: http://www.allergy.mcg.edu/advice/urtic.html. Accessed summer 2003.

Moles

1. Freckles. © 1996-2003 MedicineNet, Inc. Available at: http://www.medicinenet.com/Freckles/article.htm. Accessed summer 2003.

2. What You Need to Know About Moles and Dysplastic Nevi. National Cancer Institute. Available at: http://www.cancer.gov/templates/doc_wyntk.aspx?viewid=c350807 2-3797-40c7-848b-7bbbe9ce16d4. Accessed summer 2003.

3. Moles. © 1998-2003 Mayo Foundation for Medical Education and Research (MFMER). Available at: http://www.mayoclinic.com/invoke.cfm?id=DS00121. Accessed summer 2003.

Psoriasis

1. Facts About Psoriasis. Copyright © 2003, The National Psoriasis Foundation. Available at: http://www.psoriasis.org/home/. Accessed summer 2003.

2. Psoriasis. Copyright © 1994 American Academy of Dermatology. Available at: http://www.aad.org/pamphlets/Psoriasis.html. Accessed summer 2003.

3. Birks K. What Is Psoriatic Arthritis? Copyright © 2001, Missouri Arthritis Rehabilitation Research and Training Center. Available at: http://www.muhealth.org/;arthritis/psorarth.html. Accessed summer 2003.

4. Health Topics: Questions and Answers About Psoriasis. The National Institute of Arthritis and Musculoskeletal and Skin Diseases (NIAMS). Available at: http://www.niams.nih.gov/hi/topics/psoriasis/psoriafs.htm. Accessed summer 2003.

5. Psoriasis. © 1996-2003 MedicineNet, Inc. Available at: http://www.medicinenet.com/Psoriasis/article.htm. Accessed summer 2003.

Skin Cancer

1. Skin Cancer. © American Academy of Dermatology, 2003. Available at: http://www.aad.org/pamphlets/skincan.html. Accessed summer 2003.

2. What You Need to Know About Skin Cancer. National Cancer Institute. Available at: http://www.cancer.gov/templates/page_print.aspx?viewid=22204600-fa54-4efe-8edf-7e6390b5fe6d. Accessed summer 2003.

3. Skin Cancer Facts. Copyright 2003 © American Cancer Society, Inc. http://www.cancer.org/docroot/PED/content/ped_7_1_What_You_Need_To_Know_About_Skin_Cancer.asp?sitearea=PED. Accessed summer 2003.

4. Actinic Keratosis: What You Should Know About This Common Precancer. © Skin Cancer Foundation. Available at: http://www.skincancer.org/ak/index.php?printable=1. Accessed summer 2003.

5. What Are Actinic Keratoses? © American Academy of Dermatology, 2001. Available at: http://www.skincarephysicians.com/actinickeratosesnet/whatAre.htm. Accessed summer 2003.

6. About Basal Cell Carcinoma. © Skin Cancer Foundation. Available at: http://www.skincancer.org/basal/index.php?printable=1. Accessed summer 2003.

7. Basal Cell Carcinoma. © 1997-2003 New Zealand Dermatological Society. Available at: http://www.dermnetnz.org/index.html. Accessed summer 2003.

8. About Squamous Cell. © Skin Cancer Foundation. Available at: http://www.skincancer.org/squamous/index.php?printable=1. Accessed summer 2003.

9. Squamous Cell Carcinoma. © 1997-2003 New Zealand Dermatological Society. Available at: http://www.dermnetnz.org/index.html. Accessed summer 2003.

10. About Melanoma. © Skin Cancer Foundation. Available at: http://www.skincancer.org/melanoma/index.php?printable=1. Accessed summer 2003.

11. Melanoma. © 1997-2003 New Zealand Dermatological Society. Available at: http://www.dermnetnz.org/index.html. Accessed summer 2003.

12. Information About Detection, Symptoms, Diagnosis, and Treatment of Melanoma. National Cancer Institute. Available at: http://www.cancer.gov/cancerinfo/wyntk/melanoma. Accessed summer 2003.

13. MelanomaNet Update. © American Academy of Dermatology, 2002. Available at: http://www.skincarephysicians.com/melanomanet/MelanomaRisk_november.htm. Accessed summer 2003.

Burns

1. Burns. © 1996-2003 MedicineNet, Inc. http://www.medicinenet.com/Burns/article.htm. Accessed summer 2003.

2. Burns. Copyright © 1995-2003 Merck & Co., Inc. Available at: http://www.merck.com/mrkshared/mmanual_home/sec24/277.jsp. Accessed summer 2003.

Decubitus Ulcers

1. Pershall LD. Decubitus Ulcer Information and Stages of Wounds. Available at: http://expertpages.com/news/decubitus_ulcer.htm. Accessed summer 2003.

2. Revus DR, Jr. Decubitus Ulcers. Copyright © 2003, eMedicine.com, Inc. Available at: http://www.emedicine.com/med/topic2709.htm. Accessed summer 2003.

3. Pressure Sores. Copyright © 1996, 1997, 1998, 1999, 2000 by the American Academy of Family Physicians. Available at: http://familydoctor.org/handouts/039.html. Accessed summer 2003.

4. Pressure Sores. Copyright © 1995-2003 Merck & Co., Inc. Available at: http://www.merck.com/pubs/mmanual/section10/chapter122/122a.htm. Accessed summer 2003.

5. Rovner S. Treating Bedsores With a New Approach. Washington Post Health, January 31, 1995.

Scar Tissue

1. What Is a Scar? © American Academy of Dermatology, 2003. Available at: http://www.aad.org/pamphlets/whatsina.html. Accessed summer 2003.

2. Medical Encyclopedia: Keloids. National Library of Medicine. Available at: http://www.nlm.nih.gov/medlineplus/ency/article/000849.htm. Accessed summer 2003.

3. Keloid. © 1996-2003 MedicineNet, Inc. Available at: http://www.medicinenet.com/Keloid/article.htm. Accessed summer 2003.

Ichthyosis

1. Ichthyosis Information. Copyright © 2001 Ichthyosis Information Available at: http://www.ichthyosis.com/. Accessed summer 2003.

2. Ichthyosis Support Group. Available at: http://buildingsite.igentics.com/site55/pages/ichthyosis.html. Accessed summer 2003.

Musculoskeletal System Conditions

2

Chapter Objectives

After reading this chapter, you should be able to . . .

- Name three differences between a tender point and a trigger point
- Explain the role of dystrophin in normal muscle function
- State three causative factors in muscle spasm
- Describe the feature that Paget's disease and osteoporosis have in common
- Describe the early signs of Lyme disease
- Explain the difference(s) between tendinitis and sprains
- Name three differences between osteoarthritis and rheumatoid arthritis
- Identify three structures that can be injured in whiplash
- Explain the difference(s) between specific muscle weakness and general muscle weakness
- Name three muscles and bones that can help to pin or trap the structures damaged with thoracic outlet syndrome

INTRODUCTION

This chapter discusses disorders and injuries involving muscles, bones, and joint structures: ligaments, tendons, tendinous sheaths, and bursae. Together these structures are the tools that provide humans with shape, strength and movement. They are composed almost entirely of the material that binds people together and permeates every part of the body: connective tissue.

Injury to any of the connective tissue structures (except bone and sometimes cartilage) can be tricky for many medical professionals to identify. Magnetic resonance imaging (MRIs) can be useful, but at present the ability to identify soft tissue damage is extremely limited. A thorough clinical examination still yields the most comprehensive information about injury to muscles, tendons, ligaments and other connective tissues. Massage therapists, with their in-depth understanding of the musculoskeletal system, particularly with the formation of adhesions and scar tissue, are in a unique position to be able to help persons with these types of injuries.

Bones

Bone Structure

The arrangement of living and nonliving material in bone is quite fascinating. The collagen matrix on which solid bone is built is arranged as circles within circles. Calcium and phosphorus deposits accumulate on this scaffolding in a similarly circular pattern, leaving holes for a generous blood supply. In addition, most long bones in the body grow in a gently spiraled direction, much like tree trunks. And the shaft, or *diaphysis*, of long bones is hollow, filled with red marrow in youth, yellow marrow in adulthood. All of these design features give bone some remarkable properties: terrific resilience, support, and strength combined with a relatively lightweight construction.

The commands to move the rock-like calcium and phosphorus salts around the collagen matrix are carried out by specialized cells. *Osteoblasts*, or "bone builders," help to lay new deposits, whereas *osteoclasts*, or "bone clearers" break them down. These cells are located both in the periosteum around the outside of the bone and the endosteum on the inside of the shafts. They can alter the shape of the bones from interior and exterior aspects.

Osteoblasts and osteoclasts perform their duties under the orders of two hormones. *Calcitonin*, from the thyroid, *lowers* blood calcium by telling osteoblasts to pull calcium out of the blood and put it wherever the bones need it most. Parathyroid hormone, or PTH, *raises* blood calcium by telling the osteoclasts to dismantle calcium deposits and put the valuable mineral back into the bloodstream. There it is available to help with muscle contractions, nervous transmission, blood clotting, and many other functions. The health and shape of the bones therefore depends not only on a person's physical activity, but also on whatever other chemical demands the body may be making on its calcium banks. This is, in essence, Wolff's law, which states, "Every change in the form and the function of a bone, or in its function alone, is followed by certain definite changes in its internal architecture and secondary alterations in its external conformation."[1] In other words, bone is living tissue, and remodels according to the stresses that are placed on it.

Bone Function

The skeleton provides a bony framework, protection for vulnerable organs, and leverage for movement. It also produces

new red blood cells and stores calcium and phosphorus for future use. For young people, bone is definitely not a mass of stonelike inert material; in fact, osteoblasts and osteoclasts quickly remodel bone to accommodate whatever stresses are put on it. The younger the body, the higher a percentage of living material exists within bones. Gradually, over years, however, the ratio of inert material to living material shifts; in elderly people bone has little remaining living tissue, and the density of its mineral stores has decreased; hence its brittleness and slowness to heal.

Muscles

Muscle Structure

Muscles are composed of specialized threadlike cells that, with electrical and chemical stimulation, have the power to contract while bearing weight. These cells, or *myofibers*, run the full length of the muscle, and they are encased in a connective tissue envelope, the *endomysium*. Packets of wrapped myofibers are encased in another connective tissue envelope, the *perimysium*. These bundles are called *fascicles*. Fascicles are bound together by yet another connective tissue membrane, the *epimysium* (Figure 2.1). Finally, some large muscle groups are further bound by an external connective tissue membrane, which then blends into the subcutaneous layer of the skin, the deep fascia (which is—surprise!—another connective tissue membrane).

Muscle Function

When muscles work, they consume fuel and produce both energy (the pulling together of their bony attachments) and wastes. What kinds of wastes are produced depends on how much work is done, how fast and how long it is being done, and what kind of fuel is available to do it. Muscles that work when adequate supplies of oxygen are easily accessible burn very cleanly (*aerobic metabolism*): the waste products they produce are carbon dioxide and water. But when they work without adequate oxygen (*anaerobic metabolism*), a variety of other wastes are produced. Among these is lactic acid, a byproduct of anaerobic combustion that is also a nerve irritant.

This begs the next question: what causes muscle soreness? This issue is the subject of ongoing debate. One factor is probably the accumulation of lactic acid, which irritates nerve endings in overused muscles. Another theory is that some calcium leakage from *sarcomeres* (segments of myofibrils in which chemical reactions take place) occurs. This leakage can then cause micro-spasms. Soreness also may involve tiny microscopic tears of myofibers. Even with microscopic injuries such as these, tiny pockets of inflammation accompany them. Swelling and tearing stimulate *nociceptors* (specialized nerve endings designed to transmit messages about tissue damage), which give the brain information

---

[1] Stedman's Medical Dictionary. 26th Ed. Baltimore: Williams & Wilkins, 1995:943.

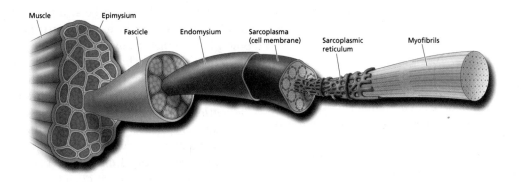

Figure 2.1. Muscles are composed of bundles within bundles, all enveloped by connective tissue membranes.

about pain and injury. Massage can influence the processing of chemical residues and minor inflammations by moving fresh, highly oxygenated blood into sore areas, while flushing old, toxic, stagnant interstitial fluid out. Imagine a person rinsing an old, dirty, smelly sponge in a stream of clean running water. Every time she squeezes, dirty, discolored liquid flows out of the sponge. Each time she releases, clean fresh water fills it up again. This is what vigorous, well-applied circulatory massage does for muscles that are sore, tired and suffused with waste products.

Joints

The joints in the body have been organized into three different classes: *synarthroses* ("immovable" joints, such as those between the cranial bones—although even these joints are not *completely* immovable); *amphiarthroses* ("slightly movable" joints, such as those between the bodies of the ver-

tebrae), and *diarthroses* ("freely movable" joints). Of these classes of joints, the diarthrotic or *synovial* joints are by far the most vulnerable to injury. For this reason, it is worth briefly reviewing synovial joints in preparation for a discussion of what happens when they are injured.

Joint Structure

As shown in Figure 2.2, synovial joints are constructed so that no rough surfaces ever have to touch, even in joints that bear an enormous amount of weight, such as knees and ankles. Articular cartilage, made of densely formed collagen fibers around *chondroitin sulfate* (very slippery material) and water, cap the ends of bones where they meet. Maintaining the slickness of that cartilage is key to maintaining the health of the joint. Fortunately, each synovial joint has a synovial membrane, which produces synovial fluid, creating a generally synovial ("egg-like") environment. As long as the

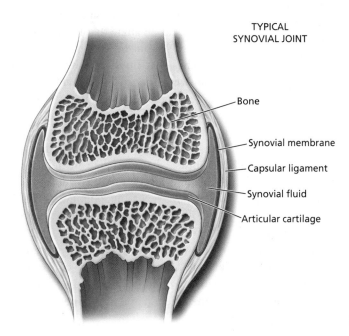

TYPICAL
SYNOVIAL JOINT

Bone

Synovial membrane

Capsular ligament

Synovial fluid

Articular cartilage

Figure 2.2. Synovial joint.

membrane and cartilage stay moist and smooth, the joint stays healthy. It takes only a very small amount of synovial fluid to lubricate the inside of a joint space.

Joint Function

Discussing joint function here is a bit redundant; this is not a kinesiology text that will define flexion as opposed to extension, or rotation versus circumduction. Suffice it to say that the function of synovial joints is to allow movement between bones, providing the fulcrum that bones can use for leverage.

Joints, like most other structures in the body, are designed for use. With healthy use, the joint structures stay smooth, slick, and well lubricated. Movement of the joint capsule stimulates the production of synovial fluid, which then circulates through the joint space for the health of all joint components. Lack of movement results in a shortage of synovial fluid; too much movement, especially too much *irritating* movement, can damage articular cartilage, or cause the bones of the joint to change shape in such a way that smooth surfaces are made rough, thus opening the door to irreversible arthritis. Other factors that can influence joint health are trauma, calcium metabolism, and nutrition.

Other Connective Tissues

Structures outside of the joint capsule (tendons, tendinous sheaths, ligaments, bursae) are also susceptible to damage. Tendons connect muscle to bone, and they are an early line of defense when a joint undergoes traumatic stress. Depending on the force of the trauma, ligaments are also quick to accrue injury: the medial and lateral stabilizers outside the joint capsule and the internal stabilizers are generally damaged before the specialized capsular ligament that constitutes the joint capsule itself. Bursae, little fluid-filled sacks that cushion areas where two bones might otherwise knock heads, or allow tendons to slide over sharp corners, tend to get irritated with repetitive stress. The body grows new bursae anywhere it needs a little extra protection, and these new bursae can also become irritated and painful.

Connective Tissue Problems in General

Every part of the body is supported by connective tissue. It wraps around muscle cells and neurons, it supports blood vessels and the tubes of the digestive tract. It is the framework on which bones grow. Connective tissue provides the structure for the functioning cells of most organs. It gives strength and elasticity to most of the body's membranes. Indeed, connective tissue is such a large proportion of the entire human body, it can be said that a person's general health can be determined by the strength, resiliency, and power held in their connective tissues.

What happens when a person's connective tissues become systemically weak? Most people know someone who seems to get injured at the drop of a hat. She twists her ankle getting out of the car; he wrenches his back when he picks up a chair. It seems that pain and injury follow them wherever they go. Very often the culprit in situations such as this is a complicated interconnected problem involving long-term stress, poor nutrition, high levels of chronic muscle contraction, elevated cortisol levels in the blood, sleep disorders, and incomplete healing.

The hormone most closely linked to long-term stress is cortisol. This is an important and beneficial chemical that helps to limit inflammation and redirects metabolism away from fast-burning glucose and toward slower-burning proteins. This is a fine mechanism for dealing with the threat of long-term hunger or famine, but what this means for people with elevated cortisol who are *not* suffering from life-threatening food shortages is that cortisol systemically weakens all types of connective tissue, increasing the chances for injury and ongoing pain.

When injury occurs, long-term stress, coupled with pain, interferes with sleep cycles to the point that secretions of somatotropin (growth hormone) are significantly inhibited, as well as the neurotransmitters that moderate pain sensation. This makes it difficult to heal from simple injuries, and reinforces a pain-stress-sleeplessness cycle that is similar to the pain-spasm-ischemia cycle seen with many muscular problems.

The point of all this is that, contrary to how many people view the body, it is not made of a series of interchangeable parts. When a car has a tire that keeps going flat, the owner replaces the tire, and the problem is solved. But when a person has an ankle that keeps getting sprained, or a back that is so fragile he cannot pick up a laundry basket, or headaches that interfere with her day-to-day functioning, the answer is not just in the ankle, or the back, or the neck muscles: it is in the totality of how mental and emotional states are echoed in the physical body; it is in how eating habits support or do not support healing; it is in whether a person gets adequate amounts of high-quality sleep. Massage therapists who specialize in helping people with musculoskeletal problems need to address all of these issues when clients have recurring, ongoing, or stubborn injuries that do not follow what is usually considered a normal healing process.

The convenient feature in musculoskeletal problems, as far as massage therapists are concerned, is that most are *not* related to an infectious agent; a person cannot catch or distribute an epidemic of sprained ankles. Nor do they usually lead to permanent damage that massage can make worse: increasing circulation does *not* spread tendinitis throughout the body. However, skillful, careful, knowledgeably applied massage administered in the appropriate stage of healing can help many musculoskeletal conditions to improve.

Sometimes that improvement is just a temporary cessation of pain (which is a noble purpose in itself), but often this work can bring about the lasting changes that make structurally based massage an important factor in the healing process.

Connective Tissue Fibers

Connective tissue comes in all shapes and forms in the body. It is difficult to accept that the loose, jiggly deposits of fat in the subcutaneous layer of the skin are technically in the same class of tissues as bones, but it is true. The unifying feature in all types of connective tissue (except blood and lymph) is the presence of particular types of protein fibers. The two that will be examined here are collagen and elastin.

Elastin is a protein fiber that lives up to its name. It is stretchy and has good potential for rebound; in other words, it snaps back to its original size after being stretched out. However, elastin is low in tensile strength; it is relatively easy to break fibers to pieces.

Collagen is another protein fiber, but it is quite different in most qualities from elastin. It has little ability to stretch and poor rebound potential; once collagen has been stretched out, it tends to stay loose rather than go back to its original length. Collagen does have tremendous tensile strength: it takes a great deal of force to stretch collagen, and even more force to physically tear or fray the fibers.

One other property of collagen is that under certain circumstances it can tend to bind things together. If general circulation to an area is impaired, the collagen-based connective tissue membranes that are intended to be slick and slippery for freedom of movement instead become thick and gluey. Collagen fibers from one structure may even fuse with fibers from a neighboring structure. This can happen at any level within muscle groups or individual muscles. Muscle sheaths can stick to each other, so that individual muscle can no longer contract independently. Fascicles can stick together within muscle bellies. Even individual myofibers can stick together. These sticky places, or *adhesions*, can greatly reduce mobility and flexibility while increasing the chances for injury when they are stretched to the point of tearing.

MUSCULOSKELETAL SYSTEM CONDITIONS

Muscular Disorders

Fibromyalgia Syndrome
Myofascial Pain Syndrome
Muscular Dystrophy
Myositis Ossificans
Shin Splints
Spasms, Cramps
Strains

Bone Disorders

Avascular Osteonecrosis
Fractures
Osteoporosis
Paget's Disease
Postural Deviations

Joint Disorders

Ankylosing Spondylitis
Dislocations

Gout
Lyme Disease
Osteoarthritis
Patellofemoral Syndrome
Rheumatoid Arthritis
Septic Arthritis
Spondylosis
Sprains
Temporomandibular Joint Disorders

Other Connective Tissue Disorders

Baker Cyst
Bunions
Bursitis
Dupuytren's Contracture
Ganglion Cysts
Hernia
Marfan Syndrome

Osgood-Schlatter Disease
Pes Planus, Pes Cavus
Plantar Fasciitis
Scleroderma
Tendinitis
Tenosynovitis
Torticollis
Whiplash

Neuromuscular Disorders

Carpal Tunnel Syndrome
Disc Disease
Myasthenia Gravis
Thoracic Outlet Syndrome

MUSCULAR DISORDERS

Fibromyalgia in Brief

Pronunciation
fī′brö-mī-al′jia

What is it?
Fibromyalgia syndrome (FMS) is a chronic pain syndrome involving sleep disorders and the development of a pre-dictable pattern of tender points in muscles and other soft tissues.

How is it recognized?
FMS is diagnosed when other diseases have been ruled out, and when 11 active tender points are found distributed among all quadrants of the body.

Is massage indicated or contraindicated?
FMS indicates massage. Care must be taken not to overtreat, however, because clients are extremely sensitive to pain and may have accumulations of waste products in the tissues that are difficult to flush out adequately.

Fibromyalgia Syndrome

Definition: What Is It?

Fibromyalgia syndrome (FMS) is a group of signs and symptoms that involve chronic pain in muscles, tendons, ligaments, and other soft tissues. It is one among a collection of chronic disorders that often go hand-in-hand. FMS is frequently seen with *chronic fatigue syndrome* (Chapter 5), *irritable bowel syndrome* (Chapter 7), *sleep disorders* (Chapter 3), and several other chronic conditions.

Demographics: Who Gets It?

FMS affects up to 3% of the US population. Women account for approximately 85% of all diagnoses, but that number may be misleading, because men may be less likely to seek medical intervention for the symptoms that fibromyalgia produces. Fibromyalgia has been seen in all ages and economic groups, but its incidence seems to increase with age.

Etiology: What Happens?

This is a very different disorder from most other muscle problems. It is not a viral or bacterial or fungal infection that causes the problem; it is not an autoimmune mistake, nor is it often a direct result of injury. Rather, some suggest it is a complicated combination of related sleep disorders, endocrine and neurotransmitter imbalances, and emotional state.

Sleep Disorder   Sleep studies of persons with fibromyalgia indicate that they seldom or never enter the deepest level of sleep, Stage IV sleep. It is in this stage that adults secrete growth hormone: the hormone that stimulates the production of new cells and collagen for healing and recovery. Furthermore, not getting adequate, high-quality sleep reduces serotonin levels. Among other things, serotonin helps to modulate pain sensation. Without adequate secretion of this important neurotransmitter, everything hurts *more*. So here is a particularly vicious circle: a person is in stress or chronic pain. This makes it difficult for her to sleep. Sleeplessness exacerbates her pain, which further limits her ability to sleep, and so on.

Fibromyalgia patients often report getting 8 hours of sleep per night or more, but they also reliably report waking up feeling unrefreshed, as though they had been working all night long. Studies in which volunteers who were deprived of Stage IV sleep rapidly developed symptoms of fibromyalgia indicate that this is a significant issue in this disorder.[2]

Fatigue   The fatigue FMS patients report may be caused by more than poor sleep. Some researchers suggest that FMS involves a problem in mitochondrial function: phos-

---

[2] Nye D. A Physician's Guide to Fibromyalgia Syndrome. Copyright © 1998, Missouri Arthritis Rehabilitation Research and Training Center. Available at: http://www.hsc.missouri.edu/~fibro /fm-md.html. Accessed summer 2003.

phates accumulate in muscle cells rather than attaching to adenosine to form adenosine triphosphate (ATP). This leads to problems with energy production and with calcium reabsorption. The result is inefficient muscle contractions and debilitating fatigue.

Pain The origin of the debilitating pain experienced by fibromyalgia patients is one of the most mysterious aspects of this problem. Current studies suggest that the pain is *not* in fact generated in the muscles, as the name implies. Instead, examinations of the cerebrospinal fluid of FMS patients show pathologically high levels of two neurotransmitters: *substance P* and *nerve growth factor*. These substances are believed to initiate nerve activity, cause vasodilation, and increase pain sensation. If the excessive secretion of substance P and nerve growth factor are found to be at the center of how fibromyalgia develops, this "muscle-fiber-pain" syndrome may eventually be reclassified as a central nervous system disorder.

Tender Points Fibromyalgia patients eventually develop tender points that are distributed all over the body (Figure 2.3) but concentrate around the neck and shoulders, and around the low back. Tender points themselves are not well understood. Histologic studies of affected tissue have yielded no useful information about how these areas develop.

History of a Disease

The history of the documentation of fibromyalgia syndrome (FMS) is a fascinating study of how information that stretches across the globe and over nearly 200 years has been gathered together to create a picture of what is still a very mysterious disorder, but one that is the second most common musculoskeletal diagnosis in the United States today.

1816: Dr. James Balfour first documents a chronic pain syndrome involving sore muscles, stiffness, and fatigue.
1904: Dr. William Gowers of Britain first uses the word *fibrositis* in relation to this disorder. This name implies an inflammatory reaction in muscle or connective tissue fibers.
1940: The word *fibrositis* first finds usage in North American medical texts.
1979: A Canadian group of physicians matches the symptoms of muscle achiness to chronic fatigue and sleep disorders.
1981: Research on this condition reveals that it does *not*, after all, involve inflammation of muscle or other tissues. Dr. Muhummad Yunus, an Illinois rheumatologist, coined the term *fibromyalgia* to refer to connective tissue, muscle tissue, and the pain that plagues them both.
1987: The American Medical Association officially recognizes that this disorder, which affects up to 3% of the American population, does indeed exist.
1990: The American College of Rheumatology creates a set of standardized diagnostic criteria for FMS.
1993: The World Health Organization officially recognizes FMS as a disorder.

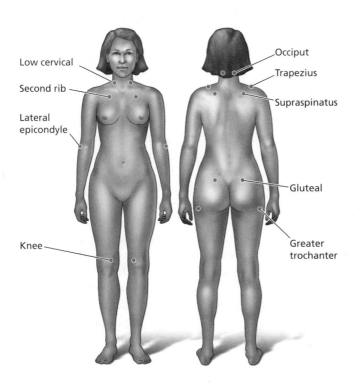

Figure 2.3. Fibromyalgia tender points map.

Signs and Symptoms

Some of the signs and symptoms of FMS include the following:

- Tender points. Nine pairs of these are distributed among all quadrants of the body. When FMS is triggered by a specific trauma, extra tender points may develop in the area around the injury.

- Widespread pain in shifting locations that is extremely difficult to pin down. The intensity of the pain may vary widely. (In other words, patients have good days and bad days.) The pain can range from a deep ache to burning and tingling.

- Stiffness after rest

- Low stamina

- Sensitivity amplification and low pain tolerance: all kinds of sensation become more likely to cause pain. This includes light and sound, but is especially true of cold and pressure.

Diagnosis

No definitive diagnostic test has been developed for FMS. It is often diagnosed when all other diseases with similar signs and symptoms have been ruled out, including Lyme disease, multiple sclerosis, rheumatoid arthritis, lupus, and several others. Obviously, this can be a long and frustrating process.

In 1990, the American College of Rheumatology officially defined a set of diagnostic criteria for FMS[3]:

- The patient must report chronic pain for a minimum of 3 months.

- The patient must show at least 11 out of 18 mapped tender points to be currently active (that is, they must elicit significant diffuse pain with digital pressure of approximately 4 kg—enough to blanch a thumbnail).

- The active tender points must be widely distributed, with some from each quadrant of the body.

In the palpation of active tender points, many practitioners also look for "control points": areas known *not* to develop tender points. If the patient reports that they, too, are painful, the diagnosis may shift away from fibromyalgia to some other chronic pain problem.

One of the challenges with diagnosing fibromyalgia is in the overlap this condition shows with other disorders. Up to 70% of the patients diagnosed with fibromyalgia meet the criteria for a diagnosis of chronic fatigue syndrome (CFS). Conversely, approximately 70% of patients diagnosed with CFS meet the criteria for fibromyalgia. Eventually it may be found that these two disorders are simply different manifestations of the same problem. For the present, however, they are approached as two closely related, yet etiologically separate, problems.

Other conditions that frequently overlap with fibromyalgia include irritable bowel syndrome, hypothyroidism, sleep disorders, *myofascial pain syndrome*, and *temporomandibular joint disorders* (this chapter). So much overlap occurs, in fact, that the diagnostic process probably depends on which conditions show up first. In other words, if a person starts with jaw pain, he may end up with a diagnosis of temporomandibular joint (TMJ) dysfunction, although his disorder may be systemic. Similarly, if another person first experiences chronic intestinal distress, she might never get past a diagnosis of irritable bowel syndrome.

[3] Gremillion, RB. Fibromyalgia. The Physician and Sportsmedicine 1998;26(4). Copyright © 1998. The McGraw-Hill Companies. Available at: http://www.physsportsmed.com/issues/1998/04apr/grem.htm. Accessed fall 2000.

The average fibromyalgia patient spends approximately 5 years and consults at least five different health care specialists before arriving at a diagnosis. This is a remarkable statistic, considering that this problem is the second most commonly diagnosed musculoskeletal problem in the United States (the first is osteoarthritis).

Complications

Although fibromyalgia is not a life-threatening disease, it is often partially or completely debilitating. The pain it causes is "invisible" pain; that is, no recognizable outward signs of a problem are perceptible. Nothing shows up on imaging tests; no signs or symptoms of this disorder are readily visible. No blood test reveals specific markers for this problem. A person with this syndrome is often discounted as a "faker" or "malingerer" by her doctors, her employers, even her friends and family. By the time a patient has reached a definitive diagnosis, her experience with the medical community has often been frustrating and overwhelmingly negative.

Consider what it would be like to live in chronic pain: pain all the time, pain that never stops, pain that no one else can see or understand. When a person lives in pain, and especially when that pain makes it difficult to sleep, she may tend to lose perspective about many things. Time ceases to have any real meaning. She hurts now; she has been hurting for a long time; she will always, *always*, **always** hurt. And ultimately, that pain begins to define what she can do, what she can eat, where she can go, and in a fundamental way, *who she is.* In other words, a person can become dependent on her experience of pain to tell her that she is alive. Take away that pain, and what is left?

It is not surprising, then, that *depression* (Chapter 3) is a common and dependable complication of FMS. Depression can exacerbate symptoms because it tends to cause people to isolate themselves from support givers, and it disrupts sleep.

Treatment

The prognosis for FMS is that for most people it is a lifelong situation. Treatment then focuses on finding ways to *manage* the disorder so that the patient may lead as normal a life as possible.

What seems to work best is a course of therapy that gives the patient control of her own healing process. The first priority is to educate her as completely as possible about her condition, emphasizing that though she may feel incapacitated, this is not a progressive or life-threatening disease.

Case History 2.1

Fibromyalgia Syndrome

Kim, Age 48: 'I'm NOT a Hypochondriac, I'm Not, I'm NOT!"

Kim, was a graphic artist, writer, and creative developer at a children's museum. She was working with the museum at its opening, after just having left an extremely stressful job in another city. It was at this time that she first began to experience new physical symptoms: powerful tingling sensations in her left arm. The sensations felt like an electrical current running up and down her arm. Eventually they spread into her right arm as well. In the beginning, the sensations came and went quickly, but eventually the episodes came in waves, leaving her arms numb and useless for hours at a time.

Fibromyalgia Syndrome, *continued*

At first she thought she was having a mini-stroke or even a heart attack because the initial symptoms were in her left arm. She went to a general practitioner who began to look for signs of stroke or heart attack with an electrocardiogram (EKG), computed tomography (CT) scan, and magnetic resonance imaging (MRI) of her neck and head. When none of these tests was positive, her doctor suggested that she had herniated a disc and recommended that she consult a neurosurgeon.

The neurosurgeon found no signs of a herniated disc and recommended that Kim consult a neurologist to look for signs of multiple sclerosis.

The neurologist found no signs of multiple sclerosis, but felt strongly that Kim was dealing with fibromyalgia syndrome (FMS), and referred her to a rheumatologist.

The rheumatologist confirmed this finding. Kim reported that when her tender points were palpated, "It felt like somebody hit me with a baseball bat."

Kim, like so many other fibromyalgia patients, endured many tests, examinations, and doctor visits before a final diagnosis was made. Because fibromyalgia is an "invisible" condition, she suffered many remarks from friends and co-workers about it all being in her head.

Kim's other symptoms are less dramatic but in many ways just as debilitating as the numbness and tingling in her arms. She has difficulty sleeping and takes a sleeping aid. She wakes up feeling foggy and extremely stiff. She reports that her pain is worst in the morning, but her neck, shoulders, and sternum hurt "all the time." Her hands and feet are constantly tingling, although this is not as extreme as her initial symptoms.

She has recently developed irritable bowel syndrome with bloating, cramping, gas, and alternating diarrhea and constipation. These symptoms are progressively becoming worse, and although she can control some of them with diet, they still interfere significantly with her life.

Kim also deals with chronic headaches that are probably a result of her fibromyalgia in combination with arthritis in her neck and ongoing sinus problems. Her vision has been affected; she reports seeing "specky things." Her balance is inconsistent. She has to keep a finger on the wall as she walks along a hall or she veers off course. Mentally Kim is frustrated (and often amused) by new problems with language. She "flips words" when she is speaking or writing and frequently accidentally substitutes one word for another when she is typing or even listening to other people. For example, she was once attempting to type "try your hand at bartering for products from Nepal," and she typed "try your hand at bartending . . ."

Kim's fibromyalgia is part of a complicated health picture. She is a recovering alcohol and drug abuser and has dealt with depression intermittently for 30 years. She has been treated for post-traumatic stress disorder since leaving her previous job. She has arthritis in her neck, bursitis in her hip, and plantar fasciitis. Her job involves a great deal of sitting, and she feels stiff and painful whenever she stands and moves. Her knees and hips make popping, crackling noises. All of these disorders together exacerbate her sleeping problems, which may then exacerbate her fibromyalgia.

Management of Kim's condition is challenging. She takes a course of vitamin and mineral supplements recommended by a fibromyalgia specialist. She recently began taking yoga classes and is excited that they seem to be providing significant relief. She also still spends plenty of time on a full-length massage mat that her mother sent her immediately after finally getting a diagnosis for her problems. She receives chiropractic care for her neck and lots of pet therapy from her two cats. Despite her many obstacles, Kim keeps a positive attitude toward life. She says that although the physical aspects of her condition are taxing, the mental twists and turns it provides are vastly entertaining.

Second, the responsibility for managing the condition must be put entirely in the patient's hands, through nutrition, sleep, exercise, stretching, and reducing emotional stress. Daily exercise is an important therapy for many fibromyalgia patients. Some specialists recommend supplementing guaifenesin, a substance that helps to flush phosphate deposits out of cells to promote more efficient ATP production. Mild tricyclic antidepressants are often prescribed both to reduce levels of depression and to improve the quality of sleep. Pain-killing drugs are generally avoided because they interfere with sleep and can be habit-forming.

Massage?

Fibromyalgia patients *live* in pain. Some moments are more severe than others, but a constant, ongoing, uninterrupted body-wide ache is a hallmark of this condition. Their tissues are drowning in irritating chemicals, and they lack the neurotransmitters that block some of the pain transmission. In other words, these people are extremely hypersensitive, and very easy to overtreat.

With that consideration, gentle massage is very appropriate for clients with fibromyalgia. Research on massage and fibromyalgia patients shows that massage is effective for reducing reported levels of pain, anxiety, and depression.[4] Massage may be used best to create relaxation and aid with toxic flushing, a little with each session. Fibromyalgia contraindicates the use of ice or ice massage; any kind of cold can exacerbate symptoms.

It usually takes a long time to become incapacitated by fibromyalgia; it also can take a long time to find ways to cope with this condition. However, if a client can experience being pain-free, even for just a short time after each massage, she will feel more able to take control of her own healing process, which is the most important step toward recovery.

Myofascial Pain Syndrome

Definition: What Is It?

Myofascial pain syndrome (MPS) is a situation that develops when muscles undergo injury or trauma, sometimes on a microscopic level, that never goes through a standard healing process. Instead, the injured area gets locked into a repeating pain–spasm cycle.

Demographics: Who Gets It?

Myofascial pain syndrome affects men and women more or less equally; this is one of the features that distinguish it from another chronic pain syndrome, *fibromyalgia* (this chapter). MPS affects people of all ages, although its prevalence seems to taper off with advancing age. Sedentary people are vulnerable to this condition as well as physically active people.

The incidence of MPS is difficult to estimate. Among one group of patients with chronic pain, 35% of them had active trigger points.[5] Even people with no symptoms can show signs of latent trigger points, however, which may develop into active myofascial pain syndrome with little provocation.

Myofascial Pain Syndrome in Brief

What is it?
Myofascial pain syndrome (MPS) is a collection of signs and symptoms that indicate trauma to muscles that leads to a cycle of chronic spasm, ischemia, and pain.

How is it recognized?
MPS is recognized mainly through the development of trigger points in predictable locations in affected muscles. Trigger points are highly painful both locally and in specific patterns of referred pain.

Is massage indicated or contraindicated?
MPS indicates massage, which can "break through" the pain–spasm cycle and help to eradicate the irritating metabolic wastes that accumulate around trigger points.

---

[4] Field T. Touch Therapy. London: Churchill, Livingstone, 2000:73.
[5] Fomby EW, Mellion MB. Identifying and Treating Myofascial Pain Syndrome. The Physician and Sportsmedicine 1997;25(2). Copyright © 1997. The McGraw-Hill Companies. Available at: http://www.physsportsmed.com/issues/1997/02feb/fomby2.htm. Accessed summer 2003.

Compare and Contrast
FIBROMYALGIA VERSUS MYOFASCIAL PAIN SYNDROME

Chronic pain disorders are identified more and more frequently as our understanding of them improves. Two such disorders that share many qualities are fibromyalgia syndrome and myofascial pain syndrome. It is certainly possible for these two conditions to occur simultaneously, but they have some differing characteristics that require some different treatment choices.

FIBROMYALGIA SYNDROME

Prevalence
Up to 3% of US population.

Demographics
85% of diagnosed patients. are women

Prognosis
This is a lifelong problem that can be managed but may never be eradicated.

Primary Symptom
"Tender points": These are predictable areas where a small amount of pressure will yield intense, diffuse pain. Tender points are often hypotonic and do not always occur in muscle tissue.

Implications for Massage
Fibromyalgia patients can benefit from massage, but manual pressure will not "melt" tender points; it will only exacerbate them.

MYOFASCIAL PAIN SYNDROME

Prevalence
Unknown

Demographics
Women and men are equally affected.

Prognosis
This can be a short-term problem that can be permanently resolved.

Primary Symptom
"Trigger points": These are predictable areas within individual muscles where microtrauma has caused an area of hypertonicity. This area may be nodular or appear as a taut band that generates a twitch response. Manual pressure on an active trigger point elicits pain locally and also in predictable patterns of referral.

Implications for Massage
Myofascial pain syndrome responds well to massage, and sustained static pressure can be an effective way to break through the "pain–spasm cycle" to eradicate trigger points.

Etiology: What Happens?

This syndrome is marked primarily by the development of trigger points. These are small, sometimes microscopic areas where chronic stress has caused a few muscle fibers to fray. Under normal circumstances, microtrauma would be followed by an inflammatory response, fibroblastic activity, the accumulation of new scar tissue, and the whole incident would be resolved. Instead, however, a trigger point forms.

A Trigger Point Is Born Consider a stereotypical postal worker. He puts in 8 long hours every day reading illegible zip codes and routing pieces of mail to the correct destinations. He *hates* his job. By 9:30 every morning, his shoulders are beginning their day-long journey up to his ears, and his trapezius is doing all the work. Furthermore, his head juts forward and downward to read the envelopes. No other muscles can keep it from slumping down onto his chest, so it falls to the trapezius, again, to do the work. It is no great surprise that a few myofibers are traumatized. They do not get the opportunity to relax and exchange waste products for nutrients, and because every myofiber in the area is similarly stressed, the blood flow to the area is severely limited.

The combination of mechanical stressors and emotional state has now created an injury. Blood components such as histamine and prostaglandins may leak into the area and cause more pain. Any normal muscle's response to injury is to *tighten up*, both as a reaction to pain, and as a splinting mechanism against even further injury. The trapezius gets stuck in a pattern of pain, which leads to spasm, which leads to local ischemia, which reinforces the pain, which creates more spasm, ad infinitum. And the tiny area where those myofibers first frayed has now become a trigger point.

Histologic studies of trigger points show some profound changes in local neuromuscular functioning. Sensory neurons in the area often permanently change into pain sensors. The neuromuscular junction between the motor neurons and their corresponding motor end plates are frequently distorted and suffused in excessive secretions of acetylcholine, the neurotransmitter involved in stimulating muscle contractions.

Satellite Points   Manual pressure on the postal worker's trigger point creates a surprising amount of pain, both locally, and, mysteriously, up over the back of his head, causing headaches. If this situation has been ongoing for a matter of weeks or months, movement patterns to compensate for the sore shoulder redistributes stress throughout the back and neck muscles. The splenius cervicis may experience more stress than it can handle, and *another* trigger point, a *satellite* trigger point, is formed. That satellite point can refer pain to yet another area, around the pectoralis major or minor, for instance. Now a new spot is constantly being told, erroneously, that it is in *pain*. What is the body's reaction to pain? *Tighten up!* That chest muscle may form its own trigger point simply because it has been told that it is hurting, even though no mechanical force is being exerted on it. And the cycle goes on, and on, and on.

Trigger points that have not been irritated will sometimes go into a latent state, during which they are not painful, nor do they refer pain. But it takes very little stimulus to turn a latent trigger point into an active one. These sore spots have palpable "knots" or taut bands that send pain shooting in predictable directions.

It is clear that trigger points form at areas that undergo microscopic amounts of trauma caused by postural habits, poor ergonomics, and repetitive motion. These tiny injuries may never be consciously felt, although the trigger points they initiate can be acutely painful. But trigger points can also be a complication of more standard types of injuries, when a person accommodates to the pain or limited range of motion that might be the result of an automobile accident, a sports injury, or any other kind of damage.

Unanswered Questions   Myofascial pain syndrome and trigger points have been documented and closely studied since the early 1950s. Still, questions about this condition outnumber answers. Why do trigger points form? Why does the whole inflammatory process not turn the affected area to scar tissue? Why does the referred pain pattern from specific trigger points not follow nerve pathways, energy meridians, or any other pattern ever observed (Figure 2.4)? Finally, why is the location of various trigger points so predictable from one person to the next?

Signs and Symptoms

Myofascial pain syndrome is recognized by the accumulation of active trigger points. These trigger points have some qualities that make them unique among muscle disorders.

- *Taut bands or nodules.* Trigger points can be palpated in muscle tissue as taut, hypertonic bands of fibers within a mass of muscle that is less tight (Figure 2.5), or as

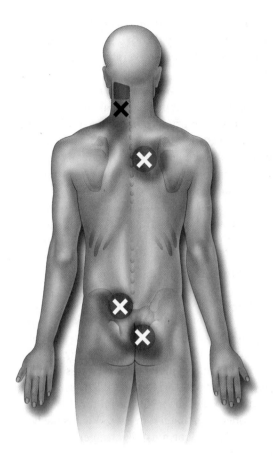

Figure 2.4. Myofascial pain syndrome: trigger points and referred pain pathways.

small nodules that dissipate under static pressure. A muscle flicker or "twitch response" is often seen when a trigger point is palpated.

- *Predictable trigger point map.* Each skeletal muscle in the body has an area or group of areas where trigger points are most likely to form. These areas have been extensively mapped.[6]

- *Referred pain pattern.* Active trigger points are always locally painful under digital pressure, but they often refer pain to other areas in the body as well. Their referred pain patterns are consistent from person to person. However, they do not follow patterns understood in the context of nerve pathways, energy meridians, or other pathways of flow through the body. Referred pain patterns of trigger points have been documented along with the maps of where they occur.

- *Regional pain.* Myofascial pain syndrome is seldom a whole-body dysfunction (another feature that distinguishes it from fibromyalgia). More often, trigger points flare up in specific regions, often around the neck and shoulders. Jaw muscles are notorious for developing trigger points, which then refer pain all over the face and head. This variety of MPS is often discussed in the context of *temporomandibular joint disorders* (this chapter).

Other symptoms of MPS are less predictable than trigger point development. Sleep disorders occur occasionally but not consistently. Depression and anxiety are also

6 Travell J, Simons DG. Myofascial Pain and Dysfunction: The Trigger Point Manual. Baltimore: Williams & Wilkins, 1983.

Figure 2.5. Myofascial pain syndrome: twitch response.

possible, especially when a person has little success in getting an accurate diagnosis and effective treatment.

Diagnosis

At this point no specific criteria have been agreed on for a definitive diagnosis of MPS. A diagnosis is usually arrived at after a thorough pain history, physical examination, movement and postural analysis, and palpation of active trigger points.

One complicating factor that interferes with getting a clear picture of this disorder is that *most* people have trigger points. They may be latent, that is, not actively causing pain, but only moderate stimulus may cause them to become active. The line between a person with some active trigger points and a person with MPS is vague indeed.

Treatment

Perhaps the best news about MPS is that this is a chronic pain disorder with an excellent prognosis. If it is treated correctly, MPS does not have to be a long-term problem. Finding the correct treatment, of course, is the challenge. Although MPS has a lot in common with fibromyalgia, the treatment protocols for the two disorders are quite different. Fibromyalgia will not improve if it is treated as MPS and MPS will not improve if it is treated as fibromyalgia.

A top priority for MPS treatment is to eradicate trigger points. This is accomplished in a number of different ways, including the use of spray and stretch (a topical application of an aerosol vapocoolant that temporarily numbs the pain of trigger points while the muscle and fascia are stretched), local injections of anesthetics, dry needling, and massage in the form of static pressure. Injections of **botulinum** toxin type A have been explored to block acetylcholine release at trigger point sites. All of these approaches work to interrupt the pain–spasm cycle, allowing the tight fibers to relax while the muscle is stretched.

Because MPS often develops out of chronic overuse or poor ergonomics, the patient's movement and work habits are often examined and adjusted so that perpetuating factors may be eliminated.

Muscle relaxants and nonsteroidal anti-inflammatory drugs (NSAIDs) have not been found to be effective at reducing the pain caused by trigger points.

Massage?

MPS indicates massage, both for its effectiveness at interrupting the pain–spasm cycle and for its ability to help clean up the debris left behind from chronic muscle tightness. Remember that when muscle cells are working, they cannot exchange nutrients for waste products. Irritating metabolic wastes accumulate in the tissues, perpetuating soreness and fatigue. Massage is an excellent mechanism to help flush the waste away, with the precaution that someone in this condition is easy to overtreat.

Muscular Dystrophy

Muscular Dystrophy in Brief

What is it?
Muscular dystrophy (MD) is a group of related inherited disorders, all of which involve the degeneration and wasting of muscle tissue.

How is it recognized?
Different varieties of muscular dystrophy destroy different areas of skeletal muscles. The age of onset, initial symptoms, and long-term prognosis depend on what kind of genetic problem is present.

Is massage indicated or contraindicated?
The early signs of MD often involve muscles that become tight and constrictive. Physical therapy is often used to prevent or minimize contractures as long as possible; massage can fit in this context as well, as long as the massage therapist is working as part of a health care team.

Definition: What Is It?

Muscular dystrophy (MD) is a group of several closely related diseases involving genetic anomalies. These mutated genes lead to the degeneration and wasting away of muscle tissue. It usually begins in skeletal muscles of the extremities but ultimately can affect the breathing muscles and the heart.

Demographics: Who Gets It?

The two most common varieties of muscular dystrophy are X-linked inherited diseases. This means the affected gene is carried by the mother, but only passed on to her sons. Other types of MD may affect females as often as males.

Etiology: What Happens?

Normal muscles convert fat or *glycogen* into fuel to do their work of pulling bony attachments together. They do this with the assistance of a special protein, recently identified and named *dystrophin*. Dystrophin is produced by specific genes located close to the periphery of muscle cells, just under the sarcolemma. The most common versions of MD involve a genetic mutation that either prevents the production of dystrophin altogether or allows its production in only subnormal levels.

In the absence of dystrophin to help create energy, muscle cells atrophy and die, to be replaced by fat and connective tissue. Antagonists to affected muscles have no resistance, and eventually their connective tissue shrinks, pulling bony attachments closer together in a permanent contracture.

Several varieties of MD have been identified, but two are more common than others, and one specifically affects adults; these are discussed in some detail. Other types of MD are much more rare, and are listed merely for identification.

- *Duchenne Muscular Dystrophy*: This is the most common and most severe variety of the disease. It affects approximately 13 to 33 boys out of every 100,000. The genetic anomaly with this condition prevents the production of any dystrophin at all.

- *Becker Muscular Dystrophy*: This variety of the disease is less common, affecting only 1 to 3 boys out of every 100,000. It is also less severe because, although the production of dystrophin will be less than normal, some of this important protein will be available to help muscles do their work.

- *Myotonic muscular dystrophy*: This type of MD affects adults more often than children. Its primary symptom is *myotonia*: stiffness or spasm after muscular contraction. This is a progressive disorder, however, that affects many systems. It can cause cataracts, gastrointestinal dysfunction, and heart problems.

- *Other varieties*: Other varieties of MD include *congenital muscular dystrophy* (several rare varieties that are diagnosed at birth or in early infancy); *facioscapulohumeral dystrophy* (a variety that primarily affects the muscles of the face, shoulder, and upper arm); *limb-girdle dystrophy* (this type begins in the shoulders, upper arms, and pelvic area); *Emery-Dreifuss muscular dystrophy* (this shows contractures of the Achilles tendon, elbow, and spine); *oculopharyngeal muscular dystrophy* (this affects the eyes and pharynx muscles first).

Signs and Symptoms

Signs and symptoms of MD vary according to what type is present, but the two most common varieties (Duchenne and Becker) are very similar in presentation. A toddler might begin to have difficulty in walking or climbing stairs. He may complain of leg pain. He develops a waddling gait with an accentuated lumbar curve to compensate for the weakness in his legs. Eventually he may not put his whole foot down at all, but he will walk on tiptoes all the time. His calves may seem to become disproportionately large, in a condition called *pseudohypertrophy*, but in actuality, the muscle mass is being replaced with fat and connective tissue.

This condition can progress to affect the spine, joints, the heart, and the lungs. Most MD patients die at a young age of cardiac or respiratory failure.

Duchenne muscular dystrophy is usually diagnosed between 3 and 5 years of age, and an affected child will probably be in a wheelchair by his 12th birthday. Its progression is fairly dependable, and its prognosis is that most patients will not live into their middle 20s.

Becker muscular dystrophy has a similar progression, but it is usually diagnosed later, it has a less severe impact, and the outlook may be a great deal brighter, depending on how much dystrophin an individual patient produces.

MD is occasionally but not always accompanied by mental retardation. Other conditions that accompany these diseases include contractures and *postural deviations* (this chapter) that develop as the skeletal muscles tighten and pull on the spine and rib cage.

Diagnosis

The ability to identify various kinds of MD has taken some giant steps forward in the past two decades. It was just in 1987 that the protein dystrophin was isolated and named. This discovery has made it possible to categorize the different types of muscular dystrophy much more accurately than ever before.

If a child shows signs of some muscular problems, he will probably be given a blood test to look for signs of creatine kinase: an enzyme produced by damaged muscles. This will probably be followed by other tests to rule out neurologic problems. Finally, a tissue biopsy may be performed to look for signs of decreased or missing dystrophin.

Treatment

If a positive diagnosis for some variety of MD is made, the family may be encouraged to meet with a genetic counselor to discuss the implications for future children. However, no treatment for a child who already has MD currently exists. Some interventions have been developed to prolong the use of muscles and limbs (massage and physical therapy may be used to minimize the progression of contractures, for instance), and surgery is sometimes recommended to release tight tendons or straighten a distorted spine. *Prednisone* is a steroidal anti-inflammatory that can preserve function temporarily, but the side effects of long-term use are very serious.

Outside of these interventions, a child with MD is aided to be as comfortable and as functional as possible. This usually means learning to use leg braces, a standing walker, and ultimately a wheelchair.

Massage?

This is a disorder of muscle function, but sensation is intact. This makes it a relatively safe condition for massage, as long as the circulatory system is strong and healthy. Massage can be used along with physical therapy to slow the progression of contractures, but it is recommended that massage therapists work as part of a health care team if they have an opportunity to work with a client who has muscular dystrophy.

Myositis Ossificans

Definition: What Is It?

Myositis ossificans means "muscle inflammation with ossification." This is a bit of a misnomer because it can happen in any type of soft tissue, and it does not always involve inflammation. Its synonym, *"heterotopic ossification,"* is closer to the mark; this describes a malpositioning of some part of the body, specifically, bone tissue.

Etiology: What Happens?

In the most common variety of myositis ossificans, an injury occurs that leads to bleeding, usually between fascial sheets where the capillary supply is practically nonexistent. The blood pools between layers of muscles, where it quickly coagulates, becoming thick and jelly-like. If the blood is never broken up and reabsorbed into the body, the liquid disperses, leaving behind a calcium/iron formation that looks and feels like a bone (Figure 2.6).

Theories about the calcification process of myositis ossificans vary. Some propose that it is an attempt by the body to "wall off" or separate the injured area. Others suggest that in the original trauma some osteoblasts are released from the damaged periosteum, and they stimulate the depositing of calcium in the soft tissues.

Myositis Ossificans in Brief

Pronunciation
mī-ö-sī′tis os′sif′ĭ-kanz

What is it?
This is the growth of a bony deposit in soft tissues. It usually follows trauma that involves significant leakage of blood between fascial sheaths.

How is it recognized?
An x-ray is the best way to see this problem, but it is palpable as a dense mass where, anatomically, no such thing should be.

Is massage indicated or contraindicated?
Massage is always a local contraindication for myositis ossificans, but work around the edges of the area may stimulate the reabsorption of the bone tissue without doing further damage.

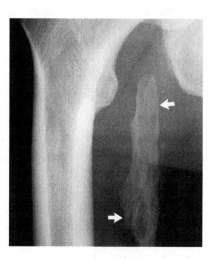

Figure 2.6. Myositis ossificans (arrows).

In the long run, the body eventually recognizes that the calcium deposits of myositis ossificans do not belong there, and it will finally begin to break down and reabsorb this bony growth. This can take months or years, but most people experience the lesion finally just going away.

Signs and Symptoms

Myositis ossificans is identified by a specific bony pattern: within weeks of the injury, an outside border of mature bone forms around an inside area of cellular material. This condition most often affects adolescents and young adults. The muscles most frequently involved are the quadriceps and the brachialis.

Myositis ossificans comes in all shapes and sizes. Usually x-rays show a clearly visible growth adjacent to a long bone. It may or may not be connected to the nearest bone. In the acute stage, the area feels bruised; later it starts to feel harder, crusty, and locally very tender. Eventually little or no local pain may be present, but a dense, unyielding mass will develop where nothing hard should be.

Treatment

Treatment for myositis ossificans tends to be conservative. Patients are recommended to rest and isolate the injured area in the acute stage, to limit further bleeding. In the subacute stage, passive stretching is employed to restore range of motion, followed by resistive exercises to restore normal muscle strength.

If a fully mature and calcified mass interferes with muscle or tendon function, it can be surgically removed. This kind of surgery is avoided when possible, however, because eventually the body will finally get around to reabsorbing this deposit of calcium.

Massage?

Myositis ossificans is always a local contraindication. If the injury is acute, it is unwise to increase the bleeding or impair the healing process by stimulating and stretching the affected tissue. If the leakage has begun to coagulate but has not yet calcified, massage can be instrumental in stimulating reabsorption, but it is still important to work just around the edges of the injury because working in the middle can aggravate it and lead to more bleeding. If the injury is old it is *still* a local contraindication; massage may impale soft tissues on the bony growth and cause more internal bleeding. Working within tolerance around the edges, however, can have the benefit of stimulating the body's own mechanisms to reabsorb this old, useless deposit.

Shin Splints

Definition: What Is It?

"Shin splints" is an umbrella term used to describe a variety of lower leg problems. The more technical terms for the injuries that often appear under this heading include acute and chronic exertional compartment syndrome, *periostitis*, tibial fractures, and medial tibial stress syndrome.

Etiology: What Happens?

Several features make the lower leg susceptible to certain injuries. Before discussing what goes wrong here, it is worthwhile to take a brief look at the construction of the lower leg and foot.

Shin Splints in Brief

What are they?
"Shin splints" refers to a collection of lower leg injuries including compartment syndromes, muscle tears, periostitis, hairline fractures, and other problems. They are usually brought about by overuse or misalignment in the ankle.

How are they recognized?
Pain along the tibia may be superficial or deep, mild or severe. The pattern of pain differs with the specific structures that are injured.

Is massage indicated or contraindicated?
Muscle injuries indicate massage, but it must be used with caution for periostitis or stress fractures. Acute exertional compartment syndrome contraindicates massage.

Anatomy Review   Many muscles in the body are almost entirely separate from their at-taching bones, touching only at the ends of their tendons. Tibialis anterior and posterior, however, attach to the tibia from beginning to end, and almost along the entire length of the muscle bellies. The tibialis anterior fascia actually blends directly into the periosteum along the whole bone (Figure 2.7). The tibialis posterior attaches to the posterior aspect of the tibia in a similar way; the endomysial sheaths blend directly into the periosteum and interosseus ligament of the tibia and fibula. The soleus muscle also has a long attachment on the medial tibial periosteum.

The musculature of the lower leg is contained in four tough fascial compartments (Figure 2.8). Each compartment has its own motor nerve supply. The fascia that wraps around these compartments is so tough and inelastic that if fluid accumulates beyond a certain point, it can interfere with normal lymph and venous drainage. This traps the excess fluid inside the fascial sheath. The pressure this causes can be very painful and can damage muscle tissue and nerves.

The other key piece to lower leg function is the shock-absorbing capacity of the feet. Feet are designed to spread out and rebound with each step. If the foot has inadequate

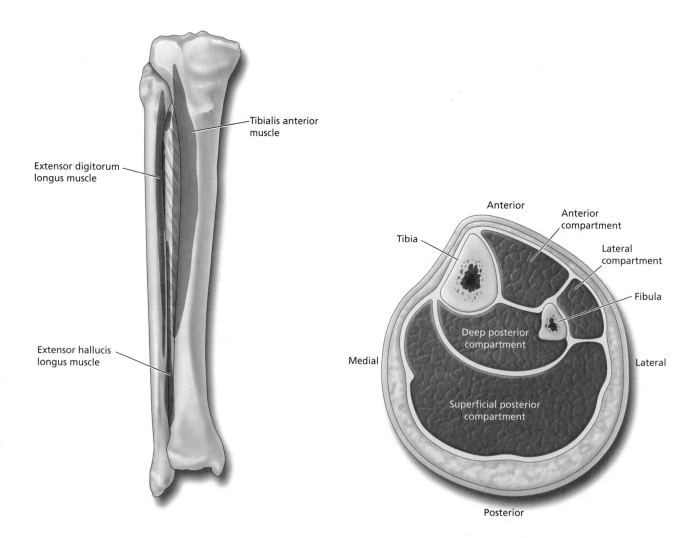

Figure 2.7. Shin splints: the anterior compartment muscles blend into the tibial periosteum.

Figure 2.8. Four fascial compartments in the lower leg.

shock absorption—from flat feet (see *pes planus*, *pes cavus*, this chapter), bad shoes, bad surfaces to walk, run, or jump on, or any combination of the above, the tibia and the muscles in the lower leg, especially soleus, tibialis anterior, and tibialis posterior, will absorb a disproportionate amount of the shock. They are not designed for this job, however, and ongoing stress causes the periosteum to become irritated, the bone to crack, and the muscles to fray and become inflamed.

Chronic overuse or misalignment may cause the lower leg muscles to accrue some internal micro-tearing along with general inflammation. The periosteum of the injured tibia may do the same. The difficulty with inflammation in this area is that there simply is not room within those fascial sheaths to allow for excess fluid retention. Even a small amount of edema puts pressure on nerve endings and limits blood flow, which, in a typical vicious circle, makes it hard for excess fluid to leave the area.

Causes for inflammation in the lower leg include exercising with inadequate foot support or on bad surfaces; unusual amounts of exercise followed by a period of rest (continued gentle movement would help the fluid to keep moving out of the area); suddenly changing an exercise routine, or running mostly uphill, downhill, or on uneven surfaces.

Signs and Symptoms

Pain from shin splints can be mild or severe, and the location varies according to which of the structures has been damaged. It gets worse with whatever actions the affected muscles do: dorsiflexion, inversion, or plantarflexion. Simple muscle injuries are rarely visibly or palpably inflamed. If the tibia is red, hot, and puffy, suspect a more severe injury than muscle damage to the lower leg.

Lower Leg Injuries

Muscle strains are the first step in a series of lower leg injuries, all of which may be referred to as "shin splints." The following lists other conditions that may fall under this heading, and the serious complications that may follow if they are not treated.

- *Tibialis anterior, tibialis posterior injury*: The pain associated with these injuries may be familiar to many people. The ache often runs most of the length of the tibia on the lateral side (for tibialis anterior) or deep in the back of the calf (for tibialis posterior).

- *Medial tibial stress syndrome*: This term refers to a muscular injury on the medial side of the tibia, usually involving the soleus and tibialis anterior.

- *Periostitis*: This is an inflammation of the periosteum, which may happen with damage to the soleus, the anterior tibialis, or posterior tibialis muscles. That seamless connection of membranes begins to rip apart, and the fibers of the muscles pull away from the bone. This condition may sometimes leave the bone feeling bumpy or pitted; that is where scar tissue has knit the connective tissue membranes back together.

- *Stress fractures*: These are small hairline fractures of the tibia. They are extremely painful, and nothing heals them except time. They are frequently the result of "running through the pain." They are best diagnosed by bone scan, which looks for areas of increased circulatory activity. Stress fractures of the tibia do not usually show up well on x-rays.

- *Chronic exertional compartment syndrome*: This situation involves the production of excessive fluid in any of the four compartments of the lower leg. The fluid, which is normally increased by up to 20% with exercise, puts mechanical pressure on local nerves, causing pain and inflammation. These symptoms are relieved by rest but recur in a predictable pattern with activity.

- *Acute exertional compartment syndrome*: This is a culmination of that vicious circle of edema that limits blood flow, which limits the exit of excess fluid mentioned previously. Because the fascia on the lower leg is such a tough container, the swelling can actually cause tissue death if it is not resolved naturally or with surgical intervention. Acute exertional compartment syndrome is an emergency situation and should be treated as quickly as possible.

Treatment

The typical approach to mild shin splints is to reduce activity and to alternate applications of heat and cold. If the situation complicates to become chronic or acute exertional compartment syndrome, steroid injections may be suggested, or surgery may be performed to split the fascia and allow room for those compressed blood vessels that were unable to do their jobs. This surgery is followed by physical therapy to limit the accumulation of scar tissue that could bind up the compartments even more tightly than before.

Massage?

As long as the problem is not too advanced, shin splints indicate massage. The lower leg muscles are impossible to thoroughly stretch out and clean up with exercise alone, but massage can give them a luxurious inch-by-inch stretching and broadening that cleanses the tissues more efficiently than anything else. In fact, massage is an excellent way to *prevent* shin splints and periostitis from complicating into exertional compartment syndrome.

For palpably hot, inflamed, painful cases, however, it is necessary to wait until the pain and inflammation have subsided. Obviously, if someone has too much fluid in a closed area, the last thing needed is massage to exacerbate it. What this person really needs, if the pain is not *much* better in 2 or 3 days, is to see a doctor. Stress fractures and exertional compartment syndrome are serious problems that require medical attention.

Spasms, Cramps

Definition: What Are They?

A spasm is an involuntary contraction of a muscle. *Clonic* spasms are marked by alternating cycles of contraction and relaxation, whereas tonic spasms are sustained periods of hypertonicity. (*Spasm* is different from *spasticity*, which is covered in the nervous system conditions, Chapter 3.) The difference between *spasms* and *cramps* is somewhat arbitrary; cramps are strong, painful, usually short-lived spasms. One could say that tight, painful paraspinals are in *spasm*, whereas a gastrocnemius with a charley horse is a *cramp*. The severity of these episodes depends on how much of the muscle is involved.

"Spasms" and "cramps" are sometimes used in reference to visceral muscle as well (i.e., *spastic constipation*), but this discussion is restricted to the involuntary contraction of skeletal, or, so-called voluntary muscle.

Spasms, Cramps in Brief

What are they?
Spasms and cramps are involuntary contractions of skeletal muscle. Spasms are considered to be low-grade, long-lasting contractions, and cramps are short-lived, very acute contractions.

How are they recognized?
Cramps are extremely painful, with visible shortening of muscle fibers. Long-term spasms are painful and may cause inefficient movement but may not have acute symptoms.

Is massage indicated or contraindicated?
Acutely cramping muscle bellies do not invite massage, although stretching and origin/insertion work can trick the proprioceptors into letting go. Muscles that have been cramping respond well to massage, which can reduce residual pain and clean up chemical wastes. Underlying cramp-causing pathologic conditions must be ruled out before massage is applied.

Long-term spasm indicates massage because it can break through the ischemia-spasm-pain cycle to reintroduce circulation to the area, as well as reduce muscle tone and flush out toxins.

Etiology: What Happens?

Four of the most common situations are addressed here.

- *Nutrition*. Calcium and magnesium deficiencies, in addition to causing all sorts of problems later in life, can also make one prone to cramping, especially in the feet.

- *Ischemia*. When a muscle, or part of a muscle, is suddenly or gradually deprived of oxygen, it cannot function properly. Rather than becoming loose and weak, it becomes tighter and tighter. Often this is a gradual process, but sometimes it is a sudden and violent reaction to oxygen shortage.

  What causes this oxygen deprivation? It can be anything that impedes blood flow into the affected areas. Consider a typical tight, painful iliocostalis: one of the paraspinal group of muscles that holds the back erect. Here is a muscle that is tight, hard, a little achy, but most of all, *overworked*. The fibers are shortened and thickened with the effort of keeping the spine upright, and this makes it harder for the supplying capillaries to deliver the goods, namely, oxygen. In protest, the iliocostalis draws up even tighter, which further inhibits the influx of oxygen: a vicious circle of ischemia causing spasm, causing pain, which leads to spasm, and so on. Furthermore, muscles that are forced to work without oxygen accumulate the chemical by-products of anaerobic combustion. These metabolic wastes are irritating to nerve fibers and further reinforce the spasm. The whole picture is complicated by the fact that as postural habits develop, the brain comes to interpret these sensations as being *normal*. The proprioceptors eventually reinforce the patterns that cause the problem. This situation can go on for years at a time without any real relief, until the circle of ischemia-spasm-pain is interrupted (Figure 2.9).

  Pregnancy can be another cause of ischemic cramping. As the fetus lays on the femoral artery (just where it splits off from the abdominal branch), it can interfere with blood flow into the leg, prompting a violent contraction of the gastrocnemius. This is a classic example of an acute cramp or charley horse. Other kinds of circulatory interruptions or nervous system problems can cause them too, so when making a decision about whether massage is appropriate it is important to be sure that no underlying pathologic condition, such as cardiac weakness for example, is creating an oxygen deficiency.

- *Exercise-Associated Muscle Cramping*. Amateur and professional athletes often report problems with muscles cramping at or near the end of vigorous workouts.

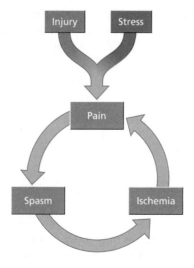

Figure 2.9. Pain-spasm-ischemia cycle.

Dehydration, electrolyte imbalance, and hyperthermia may all be contributing factors, but these cramps may be primarily due to a neurologic abnormality that over-excites muscle spindles (the proprioceptors involved in tightening) while inhibiting the activity of Golgi tendon organs (the proprioceptors that allow muscles to let go). The target muscles usually cross two joints, and they cramp when they are contracted from a shortened position. Stretching the muscles and manipulating the tendons limits these cramps, but they tend to recur if the athlete is inadequately warmed up or stretched out before beginning to exercise.

- *Splinting.* The last variety of cramps and spasms discussed here is a reflexive reaction against injury. Consider an acute *whiplash* (this chapter). The supraspinous and intertransverse ligaments have been severely wrenched, and the body senses a potentially dangerous instability in the cervical spine. Of *course* the postural neck muscles contract; as far as they are concerned, they are literally keeping the head from falling off. This kind of spasm is an important protective mechanism. It keeps the injured person from making the kind of movements that could cause further injury. The muscles create an effective splint; the range of motion of affected joints is generally very small. The proprioceptors say, "You can move this far; no further."

Massage?

Ischemic or exercise-related cramps indicate massage, as long as the ischemia is not related to a contraindicating condition. But even when the underlying pathologic condition has been ruled out, massage must be used with caution. If a therapist tries to "fluff up" a cramping gastrocnemius, the fibers may be damaged. A better strategy is to stretch the tendons and antagonists of the affected muscle to gently but quickly persuade the proprioceptors that they may safely allow the muscle to let go. When the problem has moved out of the acute stage, it is possible to go back and clean up some of the toxic waste left behind, always at the tolerance of the client.

When tight muscles splint an injured area, massage therapists should not interfere with this protective mechanism. If they do, the client will probably get up off the table with his newly loosened scalenes, but those muscles will clamp right back down, possibly even more tightly than before.

In time, the ligaments will be ready to take on some weight-bearing stress, but the muscles may no longer be able to let go spontaneously. *Now* massage can do some real good. By working to soften the hardened muscle tissue, massage can reduce toxicity, improve blood flow, and speed healing. Spasm as a splinting mechanism is to be highly respected. When the injury moves into a subacute stage, massage is indicated and will contribute to a healing process with a minimum of scar tissue, fibrosis, and permanent shortening.

Strains

Definition: What Are They?

Strains are a subject of semantic debate. Some people say that the word *strain* refers only to tendon tears; others insist it refers only to muscle tears. In this text, *strain* will refer to an injury to the muscle–tendon unit, with an emphasis on muscles.

Strains in Brief

What are they?
Strains are injuries to muscles.

How are they recognized?
Pain, stiffness, and occasionally palpable heat and swelling are all signs of muscle strain. Pain may be exacerbated by passive stretching or resisted contraction of the affected muscle.

Is massage indicated or contraindicated?
Muscle strains indicate massage, which can powerfully influence the production of useful scar tissue, reduce adhesions and edema, and reestablish range of motion.

Etiology: What Happens?

Muscle strains and other soft tissue injuries occur from specific trauma, but they appear more often in the context of chronic, cumulative overuse patterns with no specific onset.

When a muscle is injured, the process is essentially similar to tendon and ligament injuries: fibers are torn, the inflammatory process begins, and fibroblasts flood the area with collagen to knit the injury back together. For more details about this process, see *tendinitis*, this chapter. Like ligament injuries, strains are graded by severity. First-degree strains are mildly painful but do not seriously impede function, whereas third-degree strains involve ruptured muscles, and possibly avulsed bony attachment sites.

Signs and Symptoms

Symptoms of muscle strain are mild or intense local pain, stiffness, and pain on resisted movement or passive stretching. Unless it is a *very* bad tear, no palpable heat or swelling will be present. Muscles, unlike tendons and ligaments, are *not* made exclusively of connective tissue, and although this is a good thing in terms of blood supply, an accumulation of excess scar tissue in muscles has different implications than it does in tendons and ligaments:

- *Impaired contractility*. Scar tissue can seriously impede the contractility of uninjured muscle fibers. When the muscle tries to contract, it will be bearing the weight not only of its bony insertion, but also of the fibers that are disabled by the mass of collagen that binds them up. This significantly increases the chance for repeated injury, more scar tissue, and further weakening of the muscle.

- *Adhesions*. Collagen that is manufactured around an injury does not immediately lay down in alignment with the muscle fibers; it is deposited in haphazard form. Randomly arranged collagen fibers tend to bind up different layers of tissue that are designed to be separate. These areas in which one thing gets *stuck* to another are called adhesions. Adhesions can occur wherever layers of connective tissue come in contact with each other. Adhesions may be *within* the muscle, as is frequently seen with the paraspinals, or *between* muscles, when muscle sheaths stick to other muscle

Stages of Musculoskeletal Injury

Acute Injuries

The general rule for massage and soft tissue injuries is that massage therapists must *respect the acute stage of injury*. Important things are happening during this time, and therapists ought not to interfere. It is during this stage that the inflammatory reaction begins with the release of chemicals that:

1. Set up edema that limits movement
2. Call in white blood cells to eat up the debris
3. Irritate nerve endings so that the person feels pain and takes the injury seriously

Some types of massage are appropriate with some types of acute injuries, but they are highly specialized and not appropriate for casual experimentation.

How long is an acute injury acute? It depends on the injury, but the most commonly accepted guideline is 48 hours.

Subacute Injuries

This is where massage therapists can be most effective. As they strum over the newly formed scar tissue in an injured tendon or ligament, they are creating an internal environment that is conducive to the best possible healing. The tension and stretch massage creates will help determine the orientation of new collagen fibers. Massage will flush out the irritating chemicals that interfere with the inflow of fresh blood. Massage therapists are instrumental in the rehabilitation of an injured structure so that it will end up looking and behaving as though it never was hurt at all.

Chronic Injuries

In this stage, massage therapists can still be major contributors to the healing process, but their effectiveness will be determined by how big, how old, and how accessible the injury is, as well as other variables such as the diet and lifestyle of the client. These are the situations in which therapists have to use their most powerful tools: cross-fiber friction, ice, stretching, movement recommendations, everything that is at their disposal to rework that gnarled up old scar tissue inside and out.

Injured structure

Scar tissue accumulates

Scar tissue contracts: Structural weak spot

New injury at site of scar tissue

Figure 2.10. Strains, sprains, tendinitis: the injury–reinjury cycle.

sheaths. Hamstrings are a common place to see this phenomenon. Wherever they occur, adhesions limit mobility and increase the chance of injury (Figure 2.10).

Treatment

The management of muscle injuries has taken some giant steps forward in recent years. Whereas at one time an injured person would be given a prescription for anti-inflammatories and painkillers, it is now recognized that early intervention in the healing process can powerfully impact the long-term quality of the healed tissue.

Although individual specialists will approach musculoskeletal injuries with different tactics, some features are consistent:

- *Get an accurate diagnosis.* Evaluating muscular injuries requires a thorough patient history and a skilled clinical examination. Other diagnostic procedures (x-rays, bone scans, MRIs, etc.) may be recommended if the doctor suspects more than a soft tissue injury.

- *Control inflammation.* Inflammation is a valuable tool in dealing with acute injuries, but it can outlive its usefulness and end up causing more harm than good. (See more in *inflammation*, Chapter 5.) Inflammation can often be controlled by RICE (rest, ice, compression, elevation), but some physicians now use the "PRICES" protocol, which adds "protection" and "support" to the list.

- *Rehabilitate damaged tissues.* This part of the treatment involves exercises that add incremental amounts of weight-bearing stress to the injured muscle to help the scar tissue realign with the original fibers, and to gradually increase strength and fitness. This may be the most vulnerable time in the process, because athletes who are eager to resume training may try to go too fast and get injured again, and other people may neglect the need to exercise and allow scar tissue to accumulate to inefficient levels.

- *Prevent further injury.* Most chronic muscle injuries are related to controllable factors that can be adjusted to help prevent future problems. These include dealing with muscle imbalances that make one area weaker while another may be tighter; improving technique within specific sports; making sure that equipment is appropriate and in good repair; adjusting training schedules so that changes are incorporated slowly; and taping or bracing vulnerable areas.

Massage?

Skillful, knowledgeable massage can make the difference between a one-time muscle strain that takes a few weeks to resolve and a painful, limiting, chronically recurring condition that makes it impossible to do some activity a client used to love.

Once a therapist has a clear picture of what structure or structures have been injured, various kinds of lymphatic drainage techniques can help to limit edema. Cross-fiber and linear friction can influence the way old scar tissue matures and new scar tissue lays down. Passive stretches of healing muscles can also influence the correct alignment of collagen. When massage therapists apply their skills to the proper formation of scar tissue, the reduction of edema, the limiting of adhesions, and the improvement of circulation and mobility, they can help turn an irritating muscle tear into a trivial event.

BONE DISORDERS

Avascular Osteonecrosis

Definition: What Is It?

Avascular necrosis (AVN) is a condition in which blood supply to a bone is impeded by some combination of factors. Bone tissue and blood vessels disintegrate and are never fully replaced. The resulting weakness leads to a high risk of fractures, arthritis, and joint collapse.

Avascular Osteonecrosis in Brief

Pronunciation
ă-vas′kū-ler os′tē-ö-ne-krö′sis

What is it?
Avascular osteonecrosis (AVN) is a situation in which blood supply to an area of bone is interrupted and the bone tissue consequently dies. It occurs most frequently at the head of the femur.

How is it recognized?
Depending on the cause of the disorder, AVN may be silent in early stages. Later stages show pain at the affected area, along with signs of arthritis and the risk of total joint collapse if the damage is near an articulation.

Is massage indicated or contraindicated?
AVN can be brought about by several underlying disorders. Decisions about the appropriateness of massage must be made according to contributing factors. Generally speaking, massage may exacerbate pain and damage local to the affected area, but it may be appropriate elsewhere.

Demographics: Who Gets It?

AVN is diagnosed most frequently in people between 30 and 50 years old. It is rare in elderly people because of changes in the construction of bone tissue that occur with age. AVN is diagnosed approximately 10,000 to 20,000 times a year in the United States and is the reason for about 50,000 total hip replacement surgeries per year.

One version of this disease, *Legg-Calve-Perthes* disease, is almost exclusive to boys between 3 and 12 years old.

Etiology: What Happens?

Several factors may work together to interrupt blood flow to a bone. The head of the femur, because of its peculiar shape and the concentration of weight that it bears, is particularly vulnerable. The presence of tiny emboli of blood clots, fat cells, or nitrogen bubbles may block arterial capillaries in the femoral head, leading to the death of bone tissue (Figure 2.11). Congestion on the venous side of circulatory turnover also may lead to damage.

Avascular necrosis is frequently a complication of some underlying disorder. Decompression sickness ("the bends") can allow nitrogen bubbles in the blood to block flow to bony tissue. AVN frequently accompanies *lupus* (Chapter 6) because of the tendency for vascular spasm, and *Raynaud's disease* (Chapter 4) seen with this autoimmune disorder. *Pancreatitis* (Chapter 7) can lead to AVN because fat-dissolving enzymes from the pancreas may affect fatty bone marrow to form tiny plugs of fat globules in the bloodstream. *Hemophilia* and sickle cell *anemia* (Chapter 4) can lead to blockages in blood supply. Alcoholism (see *chemical dependency*, Chapter 3) and long-term use of steroidal anti-inflammatories are also associated with this disorder.

Signs and Symptoms

Early AVN is often silent and difficult to detect without intrusive tests. It often begins with joint pain just during movement, but the pain worsens and becomes prevalent even

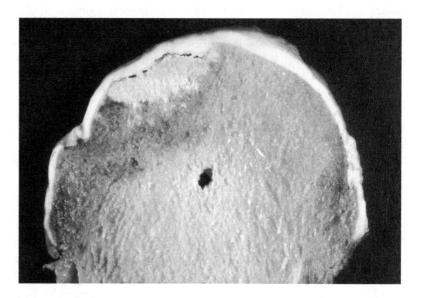

Figure 2.11. Avascular necrosis: the death of tissue in the femoral head.

during rest. In later stages it shows all of the signs of *osteoarthritis* (this chapter). Eventually it may lead to the total collapse of the joint.

Diagnosis

AVN is difficult to diagnose in early stages. X-rays, bone scans, and computed tomography (CT) scans are most useful in later stages of the disease. MRIs may show pathologic changes early, but the most definitive diagnosis involves biopsies and a bone stress test that must be conducted surgically.

Treatment

Treatment options for AVN are determined by the age of the patient, the stage of the disorder, the underlying causes, and the severity of the damage. Nonsurgical treatments are most successful if the condition is caught early, but even with early intervention the disorder is frequently progressive and difficult to control, and braces or crutches to temporarily relieve weight-bearing stress are frequently used. Electrical stimulation of the bone is recommended to stimulate healthy new growth.

Most AVN patients eventually undergo some kind of surgery to remove dead tissue, to reshape the bone for better strength, or to completely rebuild a ruined joint.

Massage?

AVN is a condition involving problems with blood flow and fragile, damaged bones. It locally contraindicates massage where symptoms could be exacerbated, but bodywork could be useful in coping with postural and movement problems that may arise because of damage to the hip joint.

Underlying conditions that may contribute to AVN must be accommodated in any decisions about bodywork.

Fractures

Definition: What Are They?

Fractures are any variety of broken bone, from a hairline crack to a complete break with protrusion through the skin.

Fractures come in all shapes and sizes. The three basic classes are *simple*, wherein the bone is completely broken but little or no damage has occurred to the surrounding soft tissues; *incomplete*, in which the bone is cracked but not completely broken; and *compound*, wherein the bone is completely broken and a great deal of soft tissue damage has occurred—in fact, the bone protrudes through the skin and is susceptible to infection. Several variations on these themes are possible, including *stress* fractures and *compression* fractures; a variety called a *march* fracture occurs in the metatarsals. *Greenstick* fractures involve bending and partial breakage of the bone; *comminuted* fractures involve shattering of the broken bone; an *impacted* fracture is a broken bone with one end wedged into the other (Figure 2.12). *Mal-union* fractures heal in a nonanatomic position. Many other types of fractures have been named for the doctors who first described them or the special joints they affect, but they are not discussed here.

Fractures in Brief

What are they?
A fracture is any kind of broken or cracked bone.

How are they recognized?
Most fractures are painful and involve loss of function at the nearest joints, but some may be difficult to diagnose without an x-ray or other imaging techniques.

Is massage indicated or contraindicated?
Acute fractures locally contraindicate massage, but work done on the rest of the body can yield reflexive benefits. Massage is indicated for people in later stages of recovery from fractures.

Comminuted   Greenstick   Oblique   Spiral   Transverse

Figure 2.12. Varieties of fractures.

Demographics: Who Gets Them?

Approximately 5.6 million people in the United States will experience a broken bone this year. It happens to children often because they engage in the risky behaviors that invite that sort of accident. Children's bones, however, have a much higher proportion of living cells and flexible cartilage to inert mass than adults' bones do. Children also have more growth hormone, which allows them a faster and more complete recovery than most adults can hope for. Elderly people, although not doing much tree climbing and skateboarding, have bones that are more brittle and less resilient than those of young people, and it takes much less stress to cause a fracture for them.

Diagnosis

Big bone breaks are usually obvious: they are painful, they usually follow a specific traumatic event, and they severely limit the function of the affected joints. However, some fractures can be difficult to identify without an x-ray or bone scan, particularly if they are accompanied by a lot of soft-tissue trauma. Sprained ankles (see *sprains*) and *shin splints* (this chapter) are two conditions that frequently hide bone fractures.

Treatment

Most fractures heal well if they are casted to immobilize the bones. Fibroblasts immediately infiltrate the area and build a framework of collagen. These are followed by osteoblasts laying down the framework for bone tissue, which will later become dense and hard.

Some fractures need more support than a standard cast can offer, especially if the break involves a joint, as in the wrist or ankle. Pins or plates may be introduced to further stabilize the joint, but these carry the risk of introducing infection to the site.

Other fractures, especially those involving the femoral neck or head, may require joint replacement surgery before they heal satisfactorily.

Several grafting procedures have been developed to speed the healing for broken bones. *Autologous* grafts are insertions of the patient's own bone tissue to provide the scaffolding on which new material may grow. Cadaverous bone has also been used with success, although the replacement process is slower than with an autologous graft. Two other substances are in current use: one is derived from coral, which has a similar growth pattern to human bone; the other is a paste made of cow collagen. All of these grafts help bone to heal faster than it would on its own, but none of them is usually strong enough to support the lesion without some kind of fixative device: pins, plates, or screws.

A variety of substances are under investigation that could take the place of various types of bone grafts. These include gels, pastes, and other compounds that may be applied to fractures to provide the framework for the growth of new tissue. Many of these compounds harden quickly to provide strong support for the new growth, and then gradually dissolve and are reabsorbed by the body when the repair is complete.

Massage?

The rules for working with fractures are guided by common sense: acute or unset broken bones obviously contraindicate massage. Casted fractures may result in stasis and edema that can be very much improved by massage, if access is available. Even if access to a broken leg is limited, for instance, reflexive benefits may be gained by working on the other limb. In addition, massage can minimize how movement compensation patterns may affect the rest of the body.

Osteoporosis

Definition: What Is It?

Osteoporosis means, literally, "porous bones." In this condition, calcium is pulled off the bones faster than it is replaced, leaving them thinned, brittle, chalky, and prone to injury.

Demographics: Who Gets It?

This disease affects an estimated 10 million Americans, although it is estimated that up to 18 million more have significant bone thinning but are unaware of their risk. It affects women approximately five times more often than men, for several reasons: women have lower bone density to begin with; they bear children—an enormous drain on calcium reserves; and changes in hormone levels have great influence on how well calcium is added to bone mass. Small-boned, thin women get osteoporosis more often than others. Women who are post-menopausal or have a history of anorexia are at especially high risk (see *eating disorders*, Chapter 3). Caucasian and Oriental women are most likely to develop this condition, but African American and Hispanic women can also have it.

Although a genetic marker for osteoporosis has been identified, other risk factors are major contributors to this disease. Therefore, bone density is determined only approximately 60% by heredity, and 40% by controllable factors such as diet, smoking, exercise, and stress levels: chronic secretions of cortisol have been shown to be extremely destructive to bone density.[7]

Osteoporosis in Brief

What is it?
Osteoporosis is loss of bone mass and density brought about by endocrine imbalances and poor metabolism of calcium.

How is it recognized?
Osteoporosis in the early stages is identifiable only by x-ray and bone-density tests. In later stages, compression or spontaneous fractures of the vertebrae, wrists, or hips may be present. Kyphosis brought about by compression fractures of the vertebrae is a frequent indicator of osteoporosis.

Is massage indicated or contraindicated?
Gentle massage is appropriate for persons with osteoporosis, with extra caution for the comfort and safety of the client. Massage will not affect the progression of the disease once it is present, but it may significantly reduce associated pain. Acute fractures, however, contraindicate massage.

[7] Depression, Bone Mass, and Osteoporosis. NIMH, 6/29/01. Available at: http://www.nimh.nih.gov/events/prosteo.cfm. Accessed winter 2004.

Etiology: What Happens?

Before discussing the bones, it is worthwhile to point out a few things about calcium.

Calcium Absorption Calcium requires an acidic environment in the stomach to be absorbed into the body. If calcium enters the body in a form that impedes its contact with hydrochloric acid (i.e., in dairy products or "calcium-rich" antacids), the body does not have access to much of the calcium that is available. Similarly, if natural secretions of hydrochloric acid are reduced, as in older women and men, it becomes even harder to absorb whatever calcium is consumed. Calcium also competes, usually unsuccessfully, with other substances for uptake. Perhaps the most notorious of these is the phosphorus found in carbonated drinks. When a person drinks a lot of soda, the phosphorus blocks out her ability to absorb calcium.

Vitamin D controls how efficiently the body absorbs and retains calcium. The body synthesizes adequate amounts of vitamin D in response to direct sunlight (it takes approximately 15 minutes of exposure per day), but vitamin D can also be easily supplemented.

Calcium Loss Calcium is constantly lost through sweat and urine. Some substances, specifically meat-based proteins, cause higher levels of calcium to be excreted in urine. Therefore, although a person may take in ample supplies of calcium, she also tends to lose a lot if she eats a lot of meat. This may help to explain why vegetarians have a statistically lower rate of osteoporosis than the general population and why, although the United States is a leading consumer of milk, it also has higher numbers of spontaneous fractures than other countries with diets that are lower in both calcium and animal proteins.

Another major cause of calcium loss is chemotherapy. Cancer patients often deal with osteoporosis as a complication of their treatment.

Maintaining Bone Density The shape and density of bones are determined by the activity of osteoclasts and osteoblasts. These cells work to remodel bones according to the commands of calcitonin and parathyroid hormone. If hormones tell the osteoclasts to work faster than the osteoblasts, bone density declines. Osteoclasts pull calcium off bones to respond to immediate needs as they arise.

Bones are *not* the only part of the body that needs calcium. Bones happen to be a convenient storage medium, but calcium is consumed in nearly every chemical reaction that results in muscle contraction and nerve transmission. Calcium is essential to blood clotting and to maintaining the proper pH balance in the blood. These are very important functions, and the body has a strict prioritizing system: chemical reactions that are crucial to moment-to-moment survival are more important than maintaining the density of the vertebrae.

Consequently, when a person develops osteoporosis, it is usually because she is using the calcium stored in her bones faster than she can replace it (Figures 2.13, 2.14). Her

Figure 2.13. Demonstrable bone loss with osteoporosis (compare to Figure 2.15).

Figure 2.14. Compare normal bone density (left) to osteoporotic bone (right).

bones, especially in the spine and pelvis, get progressively thinner, leaving her vulnerable to the primary complications of osteoporosis: spinal or hip fractures.

Complications

Complications of osteoporosis center around pathologically weak bones. Thinned vertebrae lead to a loss of height and the characteristic rounded "widow's hump" of kyphosis (see *postural deviations*, this chapter). Chronic or acute back pain appears in this stage as the vertebrae continue to degenerate. People with osteoporosis are also prone to other fractures with little or no cause; these are called spontaneous or pathologic *fractures* (this chapter). Hips (usually the femoral head rather than the ilium), vertebrae, and wrists are particularly vulnerable to breakage. And because in advanced age people are naturally low on both living osteocytes and growth hormone to induce the healing process, it is particularly difficult to recover from any injury of this severity.

Diagnosis

Osteoporosis is a virtually silent disease until it is too late to do anything about it. Even x-rays and bone density tests yield conclusive information only after density loss is between 30% and 40%. In the later stages, however, the disease is often identified by compression fractures in the vertebrae.

One important feature in the diagnosis of osteoporosis, especially in premenopausal women, is to rule out *hyperthyroidism* (Chapter 8). This condition can cause the release of too much parathyroid hormone, which consequently overstimulates osteoclasts. Hyperthyroidism may be the only type of truly reversible osteoporosis.

Treatment

Once osteoporosis has been identified, a number of treatment options are available to keep it from getting worse. Among these is hormone replacement therapy (HRT). Estrogen influences calcium absorption. Postmenopausal women secrete this hormone only in small amounts, so replacing it should improve calcium uptake. Unfortunately, estrogen supplements are also associated with breast and uterine cancers, and an increased risk of some cardiovascular diseases. Furthermore, it has been found that estrogen supplementation promotes bone density maintenance in the short run, but benefits are lost if a person ever stops taking the hormones (see *menopause*, Chapter 10). Calcitonin, a manmade version of the hormone that stimulates osteoblasts, is another treatment option, as are *biphosphates*, which inhibit bone breakdown and increase bone density.

Exercise is almost always a part of the osteoporosis treatment strategy. Because bone remodels according to the stresses placed on it, weight-bearing stress ensures that maintaining healthy mass is a high priority. For someone with this condition, gentle weight training or walking is more beneficial than cardiovascular exercises such as swimming or cycling.

Diet also plays an important part in dealing with osteoporosis. Specific vitamins and other substances may improve calcium uptake, even for postmenopausal women, but this book is not the place to discuss them.

Prevention

This is a disease that is easy to prevent, feasible to slow down or halt, and difficult or impossible to reverse. The causes are many and varied, but center around one main theme: the time to build up calcium reserves is in youth and early adulthood. The skeleton grows in height until approximately age 20, but it continues to accumulate density until about age 35. After that, it tends to progressively demineralize. Studies show that today many Americans get only half or less of the recommended daily allowance (RDA) of calcium; this, combined with our dismal rates of getting exercise, does not bode well for future osteoporosis statistics.

Four main steps have been recommended to achieve and maintain optimal bone density and avoid osteoporosis:

1. Get dietary calcium from easily accessible sources. These do *not* include dairy products, which interfere with the ability of gastric juice to absorb this important nutrient. Recommended calcium sources include "beans and greens": legumes and green leafy vegetables.
2. Exercise. Weight-bearing stress makes it necessary for the body to maintain healthy bone density.
3. Get vitamin D. The RDA for vitamin D is 200 units, or 5 μg, per day. This can be ingested in supplement form, or it can be naturally synthesized by exposure to sunlight.
4. Avoid substances and behaviors that pull calcium off bones. Salt, animal proteins, and alcohol all require calcium to be processed by the body. Cigarette smoking has also been associated with low bone density.

Massage?

In the treatment of clients with osteoporosis, the appropriateness of massage differs from person to person. The only way massage could worsen the situation would be to exert undue mechanical force, which could lead to the possibility of fractures. Conversely, consider the condition of the muscles of someone with osteoporosis; massage can offer a lot of symptomatic relief, even if it cannot reverse the degeneration of the bone tissue. In any case, caution is the key with this condition. Do not look for miracles; taking someone out of their pain for a few hours is miracle enough.

Paget's Disease

Definition: What Is It?

Paget's disease is a condition in which normal bone is reabsorbed up to 50 times faster than normal. It is replaced with disorganized fibrous connective tissue, which never completely hardens. This leaves the affected bones weakened and distorted.

Demographics: Who Gets It?

This is one of the most common metabolic bone diseases, second only to *osteoporosis* (this chapter). It affects approximately 3% of people over age 40 and 10% of people over 80 in the United States. Men have Paget's disease more often then women, and though African Americans can have it, it is especially prevalent in Caucasians from Northwestern Europe. It is very rare in Asians.

Etiology: What Happens?

Every day, on a microscopic level, small amounts of calcium in the bones are dissolved into the bloodstream, to be replaced by new supplies. The osteoclasts, which break down bone, and osteoblasts, which build it up, keep each other in balance. In Paget's disease, the osteoclasts become huge and hyperactive. Osteoblasts also increase activity, although they do not change in size or form. The result is that bony tissue is broken down and replaced at an accelerated pace.

Typically this disease occurs in two stages. In the vascular stage, bone is broken down and replaced—not with high-quality, carefully organized calcium deposits, but with jumbled, chaotic fibrous tissue, supplied by vast numbers of new blood vessels. In the sclerotic stage, the new material becomes brittle, but not strong. This shows in a characteristic mosaic pattern on x-rays. The bones most often affected by this disease are spine (Figure 2.16), skull, pelvis, femur, and lower leg.

Most people with Paget's disease have it in only one bone, but some have it in two or more. It does not seem to spread from one bone to another, however.

Cause

The cause of Paget's disease is unknown at present, but research is leaning toward the idea of a very slow-acting virus, which may live in the system for years before causing any damage. A genetic component is probable because Paget's disease often runs in families, but this may simply indicate a susceptibility to the particular virus involved.

Signs and Symptoms

Paget's disease usually has no symptoms until it has become advanced enough to cause visible changes to the affected bones. When it is found early, it is often because a person has an x-ray taken for some other reason and Paget's disease is identified by chance.

Paget's Disease in Brief

What is it?
Paget's disease is a chronic bone disorder in which healthy bone is rapidly reabsorbed and replaced with fibrous connective tissue that never fully calcifies.

How is it recognized?
Paget's disease is often silent. When it does cause symptoms, they usually include deep bone pain, local heat, and sometimes visible deformation of the affected bones. The risk of fractures is high.

Is massage indicated or contraindicated?
Paget's disease is often treated with exercise and physical therapy to maintain flexibility. Massage may fit into this context as well, with caution for the extreme fragility of the affected bones.

Figure 2.15. Normal spine.

Figure 2.16. Overgrowth of the vertebral body at L₃ in this patient with Paget's disease (compare to Figure 2.15).

Later signs and symptoms of Paget's disease include deep bone pain, palpable heat where the bones are affected, and problems related to a change in bone shape in the affected areas. These can include a loss of hearing and chronic headaches if the skull is affected, pinched nerves and vertebral fractures if the disease is in the spine, and a visible change in bone shape. The long bones of the femur and lower leg may become bowed and distorted.

Complications

Paget's disease has several serious complications brought about by changes in bone size and strength. The most common complication is *fractures* (this chapter) in the affected bones. If the cranial bones press on parts of the central nervous system, deafness or brain damage could result. *Congestive heart failure* (Chapter 4) may occur because the heart must pump blood not only through healthy, normal vessels, but also through whole new networks of vessels in the new, useless fibrous tissue.

Rare cases of Paget's disease may involve a loss of vision as the skull bones interfere with nerves from the eyes, or dental problems involving the size of the mandible or maxilla change in relation to the teeth. Approximately 1% of Paget's disease patients develop a rare form of bone cancer.

Diagnosis

This condition is diagnosed primarily by x-ray or bone scan. A blood test to look for alkaline phosphatase (an enzyme produced by overactive osteoblasts) may confirm the diagnosis.

Because this disease has a clear genetic link, family members of Paget's disease patients may be recommended to have blood tests for heightened levels of alkaline phosphatase every few years after they turn 40. This could allow for early diagnosis and more effective treatment of the disease.

Treatment

Treatment for Paget's disease is surprisingly similar to that for osteoporosis; the unwanted breakdown of healthy bone tissue is a feature common to both disorders. Exercise is the first recommendation for Paget's disease, to maintain function and healthy bone mass as long as possible. Aspirin and anti-inflammatories may be suggested for pain relief. And finally, calcitonin or biphosphates may be prescribed to inhibit osteoclast activity.

Massage?

This is a disease involving inflammation, impaired circulation, and weakened bones. All of these issues require caution from massage therapists. But if a Paget's disease patient is engaging in exercise and physical therapy to maintain bone health, massage could be a useful adjunct to this effort, as long as the client's health care team is informed.

Postural Deviations

Definition: What Is It?

Although it is tempting to think about the spine in terms of a ship's mast, a column, or a tent pole held erect by muscular tension, it is actually much stronger than any of those. The curves in the cervical, thoracic, and lumbar regions give the spine 10 times the resistance it would have if it were perfectly straight. Sometimes, though, these natural curves are overdeveloped, which *reduces* resiliency and strength, rather than enhancing it. *Kyphosis* ("humpback"), *lordosis* ("swayback"), and *scoliosis* ("S", "C" or "Reverse- C" curve) are the specific postural deviations to be addressed here (Figure 2.17).

Etiology: What Happens?

It is sometimes convenient to think about the spine in only two dimensions at a time. In other words, scoliosis would be simply an S-shaped curve from left to right, and lordosis and kyphosis would be exaggerated forward and backward curves. The truth is not nearly so simple. With any imbalance in the stacking of the vertebrae, rotations in one direction or another complicate the issue. Thus, scoliosis is not merely a left–right aberration, but involves a spiral twisting of the vertebral column as well. Similar lateral imbalances are observable with most cases of lordosis and kyphosis.

One important thing to remember with postural deviations is the difference between a *functional* problem and a *structural* one. In the early stages of either of these conditions, soft tissues may be pulling the spine out of alignment: a *functional* problem. At this point, the condition is most treatable: muscles, tendons, and ligaments can be exercised, stretched, and manipulated into new holding and movement patterns. Functional deviations also can be brought about by structural problems elsewhere in the body: unequal leg length, for instance. But if the soft tissues are left untreated and the bones are constantly pulled in one direction or another, they will eventually change shape to

---

Postural Deviations in Brief

What are they?
Postural deviations are overdeveloped thoracic or lumbar curves (kyphosis and lordosis) or an S-curve in the spine (scoliosis).

How are they recognized?
Extreme curvatures are easily visible, although x-rays are used to pinpoint exactly where the problems begin and end.

Is massage indicated or contraindicated?
All postural deviations indicate massage as long as other underlying pathologic conditions have been ruled out. Bodywork may or may not be able to reverse any damage, but it can certainly provide relief for the muscular stress that accompanies spinal changes.

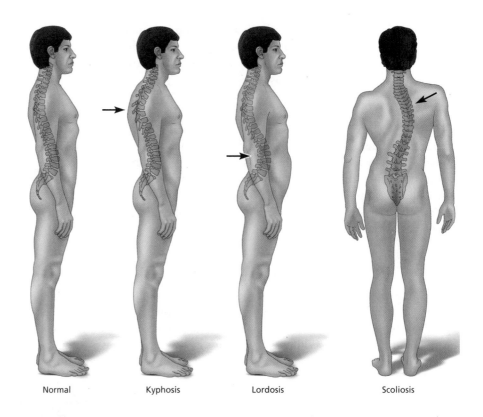

| Normal | Kyphosis | Lordosis | Scoliosis |

Figure 2.17. Postural deviations.

adapt to those stressors. At this point, the condition becomes a *structural* dysfunction and is much harder to reverse.

Most cases of postural deviations are idiopathic, that is, of unknown origin. However, a small percentage of structural problems in the spine can be related to congenital or neuromuscular problems such as *cerebral palsy*, *polio*, or *spina bifida* (all in Chapter 3). These contributing factors must be addressed before any attempt is made to correct the postural deviations they produce.

Signs and Symptoms

Postural deviations range from being painfully obvious to quite subtle. A visual examination yields a lot of information about kyphosis and lordosis, and even mild scoliosis may be visible with a forward-bending test. Patients' complaints often include muscular tension and sometimes nerve impairment along with chronic ache and loss of range of motion. If the condition is very advanced, movement of the ribs may be impaired, leaving the patient vulnerable to breathing problems and lung infections.

- *Scoliosis* is a problem for approximately 2% of all teenagers. It affects girls 7 times more frequently than boys, and almost always involves a bend to the right. It usually appears during the rapid-growth years of late childhood and early adolescence. Mild scoliosis, which is any curve less than 30° to 40° is treated, if at all, with exercise, chiropractic, a corrective brace, or electromuscular stimulation to strengthen the muscles of the stretched side of the spine. If the scoliosis appears at over 40° in childhood, the chances that it will worsen are very great. It typically progresses at 1° every year.

  Complications of scoliosis include nerve irritation as misshaped bones press on nerve roots, *spondylosis* (this chapter), and serious heart and lung problems arising from a severely restricted rib cage.

Surgery for scoliosis involves inserting rods that straighten and fuse the affected vertebrae. This limits spinal mobility, but it can definitely improve the quality of life for people with an advanced and debilitating situation.

- **Kyphosis** is an overdeveloped thoracic curve. In young people it is very often a result of muscular imbalance and may be treated with physical therapy. **Scheuermann's disease** is a type of idiopathic kyphosis that affects young men. It is usually painless and is treated with physical therapy or braces. Kyphosis in older people may be due to muscular imbalance, but it could also be a complication of *osteoporosis* or *ankylosing spondylitis* (this chapter). A kyphotic curve of 20° to 40° is considered normal. Surgical intervention is not usually suggested for anything under a 75° curvature.

- **Lordosis** or swayback is an overpronounced lumbar curve. The architecture and musculature of the low back makes it particularly vulnerable to this kind of imbalance. It can often be much improved by exercise and physical therapy (including massage). Lordosis, although not dangerous in itself, can lead to more serious low back pain (see *disc disease*, this chapter).

Treatment

Treatment options for different kinds of postural deviations are outlined in the descriptions above.

Massage?

As long as no underlying pathologic condition is contributing to spinal problems, all kinds of postural deviations indicate massage. In the early stages of these diseases, chronic soft-tissue (that is, muscular, tendinous, and ligamentous) stresses pull on the bones and change the architecture of the spine. Caught early enough, many inefficient postural habits can be reversed without permanent damage. However, bone is living, adaptable tissue, and left untreated, the vertebrae will eventually remold themselves to permanently imprint a postural pattern.

Massage certainly will not make any of these conditions any worse, and could quite possibly offer a lot of relief by simply reducing some of the tension that both causes and accompanies spinal imbalance. If a therapist is very skilled and the circumstances are just right, massage may set the stage for a permanent change in bony alignment.

JOINT DISORDERS

Ankylosing Spondylitis

Definition: What Is It?

Ankylosing spondylitis (AS) is spinal inflammation (*spondylitis*) leading to stiff joints (*ankylosis*). This means really stiff—the joints between and around vertebrae can become permanently fused. AS is a progressive inflammatory arthritis of the spine caused by an autoimmune reaction. It is sometimes called *rheumatoid spondylitis*.

Demographics: Who Gets It?

Ankylosing spondylitis is an inherited disorder that most often affects men between the ages of 16 and 35 years. A genetic marker (HLA-

Ankylosing Spondylitis in Brief

Pronunciation
ang-ki-lö'zing spon-di-li'tis

What is it?
Ankylosing spondylitis (AS) is a progressive inflammatory arthritis of the spine.

How is it recognized?
It generally begins as stiffness and pain around the sacrum, with occasional referred pain down the back of the buttocks and into the legs. It has acute and subacute episodes. In advanced AS, the vertebrae fuse together in flexion or lateral flexion.

Is massage indicated or contraindicated?
The subacute stage of AS indicates massage; along with exercise and physical therapy, it may be useful in maintaining flexibility.

B27) has been identified that seems to increase the tendency to develop this disease, but it is not a definitive factor; the incidence of AS among people with this marker is approximately 20%. Roughly 1%, or 2.5 million people, in the United States have some degree of AS; males outnumber females by approximately three to one.

Etiology: What Happens?

AS typically begins at the sacroiliac joint on one or both sides. Though it is usually limited to intervertebral and costal joints, the hips, shoulders, toes, and sternoclavicular joints may be affected too. The affected joints become inflamed in the acute or "flare" stage. When the inflammation subsides, the bony surfaces inside the joint have become damaged. Articular cartilage thickens, cartilaginous discs ossify, and bony deformation leads to the "squaring" of vertebral bodies. Surrounding ligaments and tendons may also become inflamed and ossified.

The pattern of inflammation and damage proceeds up the spine, leaving in its wake a trail of injured vertebrae that may eventually fuse (Figure 2.18) in slight or sometimes extreme flexion (Figure 2.19). If the progression reaches all the way up to the neck, the cervical vertebrae may fuse with the head in a permanently flexed position as well. Fusions also may occur at the vertebral–costal joints, resulting in a locked ribcage and difficulty with breathing.

Signs and Symptoms

Ankylosing spondylitis usually starts as chronic low back pain. Often pain is felt in the buttocks, and sometimes all the way down into the heels. This can sometimes lead to a

Figure 2.18. Ankylosing spondylitis: spinal fusions.

Figure 2.19. Ankylosing spondylitis.

misdiagnosis of herniated disc. The spine and hips feel stiff and immobile; this is usually much worse in the morning or after prolonged immobility.

As with most autoimmune diseases, this condition has acute and subacute stages. During acute episodes, a general feeling of illness and a slight fever may be present. The eyes may become dry, red, and uncomfortable. Pain and stiffness gradually spread higher and higher up the spine. Usually the disease will be limited to the low back, but occasionally it proceeds up into the neck or other joints in the body.

Complications

This condition carries a high risk for vertebral fracture. As the spine fuses and loses mobility, it becomes more vulnerable to shearing forces. Poor support from damaged ligaments means a greater chance of nerve damage and cauda equina syndrome (loss of bowel and bladder control due to pressure on the cauda equina).

Loss of lung capacity is another complication of this disease. If a person's ribs cannot expand, it is difficult to get an adequate supply of oxygen into the body, or to get carbon dioxide and air contaminants out. This results in constant shortness of breath, low stamina, and reduced resistance to chest infections such as *pneumonia* (Chapter 6) from which, depending on posture, it can be very difficult to recover.

The inflammatory nature of AS is not restricted to joints around the spine. Many patients report pain at the temporomandibular joint (see *temporomandibular joint disorders*, this chapter). The inflammation may spread to other organs, including the eyes, lungs, heart, and kidneys.

Diagnosis

Ankylosing spondylitis is diagnosed through observable symptoms, blood tests, and x-rays. It can be difficult to identify in the early stages because many disorders can cause diffuse back pain and stiffness. It sometimes takes years to confirm a diagnosis of AS. This is especially true when the condition is present in women for whom the initial symptoms tend to be less predictable.

One feature that can assist in a diagnosis of AS is that it often appears along with other disorders. Particular red flags are chronic *prostatitis* (Chapter 10), iritis (inflammation of the iris of the eyes), *Crohn disease* and *ulcerative colitis* (Chapter 7), and *psoriasis* (Chapter 1). Also, people in the immediate family of an AS patient show statistically higher rates of psoriatic arthritis, Crohn disease, and ulcerative colitis.

Treatment

The first, best option for dealing with AS (which has no known cause, and therefore no cure) is exercise. Physical therapy is recommended to develop a series of exercises that will, as much as possible, preserve the suppleness of the spine and the strength of the paraspinals, without aggravating the condition. Maintaining correct posture for as long as possible is the primary goal because the vertebrae tend to fuse in a flexed position.

If exercise alone does not help, painkillers and anti-inflammatories may be prescribed. In very extreme cases, surgery may be suggested: an ***osteotomy*** is a procedure that re-fuses joints in a straightened position. If the knees, shoulders, or hips have been impaired, joint replacement surgery also may be suggested.

Massage?

Little is well understood about this disease, and even less is known about how massage might affect it. However, because it is an inflammatory condition and because it does spread, massage practitioners must proceed with caution. Always work with this condition in conjunction with a health care team, and only work when the inflammation is subacute; reschedule an appointment rather than working on someone whose spinal joints are inflamed. If a client is in the early stages of this disease, massage may help to preserve precious mobility of the spine. If a client is in a more advanced stage, massage will probably have little effect except pain relief because the muscles are stretched over immobile joints.

Dislocations

Definition: What Are They?

When the bones in a joint are separated so that they no longer articulate, the joint is said to be dislocated. It is hard to imagine that happening without damage to most of the surrounding tissues as well: muscles, tendons, blood vessels, and nerves are generally also injured in a traumatic dislocation (Figure 2.20). Nearby bursae usually also become inflamed. Dislocations are most often caused by trauma, but some are brought about by congenital weakness of the ligaments, and others by diseases such as rheumatoid arthritis, which may involve degenerated tissue inside joints, raising the risk of having the joint literally fall apart.

Signs and Symptoms

Most of the joints in the body do not dislocate without significant force. The shoulder, because of the shallowness of the glenoid fossa, and the fingers are the joints most at risk for dislocation (Figure 2.21). The TMJ, or temporomandibular joint, is another common site. (See *temporomandibular joint disorders*, this chapter.) Symptoms of a newly dislocated joint include swelling, discoloration, loss of function, and, most obviously, a lot of pain.

Dislocations in Brief

What are they?
Dislocations are traumatic injuries to joints in which the articulating bones are forcefully separated.

How are they recognized?
Acute (new) dislocations are extremely painful. The bones may be visibly separated, and total loss of function at the joint will occur.

Is massage indicated or contraindicated?
Dislocations indicate massage in the subacute stage, as long as work is conducted within pain tolerance. As the area heals, massage may be useful for managing scar tissue accumulation and muscle spasm around the affected joint.

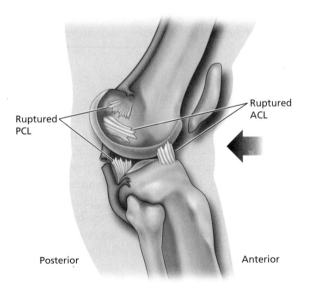

Ruptured
PCL

Ruptured
ACL

Posterior   Anterior

Figure 2.20. Dislocations often involve extensive soft tissue damage.

Figure 2.21. Fingers are common sites for dislocations.

Complications

Uncomplicated traumatic dislocations are painful and take a long time to heal, but they are not usually serious. Fibrosis and excessive scar tissue of the surrounding soft tissues may develop after prolonged splinting. Occasionally a nerve is severely damaged by the trauma, but this is the exception rather than the rule.

If, however, the ligaments supporting the damaged joint become stretched, they may lose some of their ability to do their job. The ligaments may even rupture and detach from the bone altogether. When ligaments are permanently damaged, the joint may become unstable and prone to reinjury: *"subluxation"* if the bones move out of alignment, "spontaneous dislocation" if the bones completely separate. These mishaps are especially common in the shoulder and jaw. The muscles that cross over these unstable joints are likely to be much tighter than is ideal, because the ligaments are not doing their job. This can lead to *myofascial pain syndrome* or *tendinitis* (this chapter). The most serious long-term consequence of ligament laxity is the possibility of developing *osteoarthritis* (this chapter).

Treatment

Acute dislocations require immediate attention. If large joints are not reduced within approximately 15 minutes, the tissues may swell up so much and the muscles will contract so tightly that it is difficult to move the joint without a general anesthetic. After the joint is reduced, an x-ray is usually taken to rule out the possibility of a *fracture* (this chapter). The joint is then typically be splinted for 2 or 3 weeks until the capsular ligament and other supportive ligaments are ready to carry their weight again. Physical therapy is prescribed to strengthen and retrain the muscles surrounding the joint.

If the ligaments have ruptured or are simply too lax to properly support the joint capsule, surgery may be recommended. Typically this involves shortening or reattaching the damaged ligaments to the bone by using stitches or staples. Arthroscopic surgery for dislocated shoulders is a technique that may be able to improve joint function without the complications of major surgery. *Thermal capsulorraphy* is a type of arthroscopic surgery designed to improve ligament stability. A thermal probe heats up specific areas of the joint capsule. This causes the collagen fibers to shrink, tightening the capsular ligament. This technique is currently used only for shoulders, but it may eventually be applicable to other joints.

An alternative to surgery for chronically lax ligaments is a specialized series of injections of substances called proliferants. Proliferant therapy is designed to stimulate the growth of new collagen fibers that, with appropriate stretching and exercise, lay down in alignment with the original fibers. This procedure can tighten stretched-out ligaments, thus reducing the chance of future injury.

Massage?

Obviously, massage is out of the question for an acute dislocation. In the subacute stage, massage may help untangle the muscular and tendinous scar tissue that is likely to develop as a result of dislocations, as long as basic rules about working within tolerance, following with ice, and monitoring results are followed.

If a client has an old dislocation that occasionally subluxates or even entirely dislocates without trauma, massage will do no harm as long as care is taken to be sure that he or she is positioned in a way that feels safe and comfortable.

Gout in Brief

What is it?
Gout is an inflammatory arthritis caused by deposits of sodium urate (uric acid) in and around joints, especially in the feet.

How is it recognized?
Acute gout causes joints to become red, hot, swollen, shiny, and extremely painful. It usually has a sudden onset.

Is massage indicated or contraindicated?
Gout systemically contraindicates massage when it is acute. Gouty joints locally contraindicate massage at all times.

Gout

Definition What Is It?

Gout is one of the oldest diseases in recorded medical history. In 580 A.D., Alexander of Tralles wrote,

Gout sufferers should eat little meat, drink no alcohol and eat the underground stems of calchium (autumn crocus).[9]

One of the drugs in use today for the treatment of gout is *colchicine*, a synthetic version of autumn crocus.

Gout has been known as the "disease of kings," associated with rich diets and decadent living. This is witnessed by a list of some of gout's most famous victims: Alexander the Great, Henry VIII of England, Charles V of Spain and his son Phillip II, Dr. Samuel Johnson, Wolfgang von Goethe, and Benjamin Franklin.

Gout is a type of inflammatory arthritis. This one has a chemical cause, rather than arising from wear and tear or immune system mistakes.

Demographics: Who Gets It?

Gout affects men more than women, by a wide margin: 90% of gout patients are men, for whom the prime age to develop the disease is 75 years; 10% are women, and most of those are postmenopausal. The United States has approximately 1 million gout patients.

[9] DiBacco TV. The pain of gout: Baffling condition left doctors guessing. *Washington Post.* October 11, 1994: Z19.

Etiology: What Happens?

Uric acid is a naturally occurring by-product of protein digestion. Under normal circumstances, it is extracted from the blood by the kidneys. If the kidneys are unable to perform this function, either because too much uric acid is present or because they are otherwise impaired, *hyperuricemia* will develop: this is the state of having higher than normal levels of uric acid in the blood. Hyperuricemia is the primary risk factor for gout.

The transition from hyperuricemia to an acute gouty attack is often precipitated by some specific event: binge eating or drinking, surgery, or a systemic infection. All of these things alter fluid levels in the body. When uric acid consolidates, it forms sharp, needle-like crystals that accumulate in and around the foot, grinding on and irritating synovial capsules, bursae, tendons, and other tissues (Figure 2.22). The crystals attract neutrophils, and these white blood cells initiate an extreme inflammatory response.

The foot may be the primary target because of gravity, but it also may have to do with the lower temperature found in extremities that aids in the crystallization process. Typically a person goes to bed feeling fine, and then wakes in the night with a foot that is red, throbbing, and painful.

In later stages of the disease, deposits of sodium urate called *tophi* will develop inside joints. These tophi will progressively erode all of the joint structures, leading to a complete loss of function. Tophi also grow along tendons and in subcutaneous tissues. They have been found in myocardium, pericardium, aortic valves, and even the pinna of the ear!

Risk Factors

Uric acid is a waste product from the metabolism of a component of nucleic acids called *purines*. A diet that is high in purines tends to produce more uric acid in the body than a diet that is not. Foods that are particularly high in purines include red meat, organ meats, fish, foul, lentils, alcohol, mushrooms, and some vegetables: peas, asparagus, and spinach.

Under normal circumstances, the kidneys should excrete uric acid. This is where the problems may start.

- *Metabolic gout*: In this situation the kidneys may be functioning normally, but the body is producing too much uric acid for them to keep up. This is the case for someone with a particularly high protein/alcohol intake.

- *Renal gout*: In this case, the uric acid load may be normal, but the kidneys are not functioning well. They cannot handle the job of excreting all the uric acid, and so it ends up in the bloodstream, and eventually, in the feet. This kind of kidney insufficiency may be hereditary, or related to other problems, such as *diabetes* (Chapter 8) or lead poisoning.

Figure 2.22. Gout: crystals erode joint capsules.

Figure 2.23. Gout: note the "punched out" pattern of erosion in
the first metatarsal.

- *Both*: Here the kidneys are compromised *and* the purine intake is high. This is gout, waiting to happen.

Hyperuricemia is clearly connected to gout, but the two are not always identical. Many people have hyperuricemia without ever having gout. Conversely, some people with gout show normal or even below normal levels of uric acid in the blood.

Other risk factors for gout besides a high-purine diet include obesity, sudden weight gain, moderate to high alcohol consumption, high blood pressure, and certain blood disorders that can raise uric acid levels.

Sometimes a person has just one attack of gout and then is never bothered by it again. Usually the second attack comes several years later. The third attack happens after a shorter interval, and the fourth one, shorter still. Each event resolves itself in a few days or weeks. After 10 to 20 years, a patient may end up with almost constant acute attacks of this disease, but often by that time the associated problems of this condition may make toe pain the least of his worries.

Signs and Symptoms

Acute gouty arthritis (AGA) has some very predictable patterns. It has a sudden onset and almost always happens in the feet first, especially at the joints of the great toe. Cumulative damage creates a characteristic "punched out" pattern of bony erosion (Figure 2.23). Gout may also appear in the instep, around the Achilles tendon, and in later stages in the knees and elbows.

An acute gouty joint shows all the signs of extreme inflammation. The joint may swell so much that the skin is hot, red, dry, shiny, and exquisitely painful. This phase of inflammation is often accompanied by a moderate fever (up to 101°F or so) and chills.

Complications

The complications of gout are complications of having too much uric acid in the bloodstream, which indicates kidneys that are not functioning at adequate levels. Uric acid crystals do not simply cause gout; they can also cause *kidney stones* (Chapter 9). If the kidneys become sufficiently clogged by kidney stones, the result is *renal failure* (Chapter 9). Impaired kidneys cannot process adequate fluid. This stresses the rest of the circulatory system, causing *high blood pressure* the end result of which can be *atherosclerosis* (both Chapter 4) or *stroke* (Chapter 3). All of these problems—hyperuricemia, kidney insufficiency, gout, high blood pressure, and cardiovascular disease—are closely related.

Diagnosis

Gout is usually easily recognized by its specific pain profile: sudden onset in the feet with long intervals between attacks. However, it sometimes mimics a few other conditions, including *rheumatoid arthritis*, *septic arthritis* (this chapter), psoriatic arthritis, or pseudogout: another chemically based arthritis in which crystals of an entirely different type are deposited in and around joints. The only conclusive diagnosis for gout is an examination of aspirated fluid from an affected joint to look for uric acid crystals.

Compare and Contrast
GOUT AND "PSEUDOGOUT"

Gout is a variety of arthritis brought about by the accumulation of uric acid crystals in and around joint capsules, especially in the feet. It is a manageable disorder, as long as the person keeps a close watch on his uric acid levels. *Calcium pyrophosphate dihydrate* deposition (CPDD) or *pseudogout* has a very similar presentation, but because it does not involve uric acid or hyperuricemia, it requires a different treatment plan. Massage therapists are not required to be able to tell the difference between gout and pseudogout, but we can certainly counsel our clients to explore options if the treatment they receive does not seem to meet their needs.

GOUT

Prevalence
100:100,000

Demographics
90% are men over 40; women with gout are usually postmenopausal.

Primary Symptom
Exquisitely painful inflammation, usually around the great toe, but also in the instep and heel.

Gout occasionally appears in other joints in later stages, but the foot is usually affected first.

Implications for Massage
Gout patients usually have some level of hyperuricemia and carry the risk of kidney stones or other urinary system disorders. These need to be ruled out for circulatory massage.

CPDD (PSEUDOGOUT)

Prevalence
Unknown

Demographics
Women and men are equally affected. Most patients are over 60 years old.

Primary Symptom
Exquisitely painful inflammation, usually at the knee or wrist.

Implications for Massage
CPDD is an idiopathic disease that may or may not be related to other underlying problems. Clients with CPDD need to be screened for other contributing factors, but none may be present.

Treatment
_____

A standard medical approach to gout takes three paths: pain relief (with analgesics *other* than aspirin, which inhibits uric acid excretion), anti-inflammatory drugs, and drugs that modify metabolism and uric acid management. Preventive measures include increasing fluid intake (other than caffeine or alcohol, which act as diuretics), losing weight, and limiting purine-rich foods.

Massage?
_____

Gout is at the very least a local contraindication for painful gouty joints at all times. The last thing this client needs is to have someone grind those little crystals any deeper into his flesh.

In the acute stage, gout is a systemic contraindication, but it is unlikely that anyone in a full-blown attack would try to keep a massage appointment. Ice is likewise contraindicated because lowering the temperature of the area simply helps in crystal formation. Any client who is prone to gout is a good candidate for other circulatory or excretory problems; he or she should consult a physician about these issues before receiving massage.

Lyme Disease in Brief

What is it?
Lyme disease is a bacterial infection spread by the bites of specific species of ticks. The immune response to the bacteria causes inflammation of large joints, along with neurologic and cardiovascular symptoms.

How is it recognized?
The hallmark early symptom of Lyme disease is a circular "bull's eye" rash at the site of the tick bite. The skin is red, itchy, and hot, but not usually raised. The rash may be accompanied by fever, fatigue, and joint pain. Later symptoms may include acute intermittent inflammation of one or more large joints, numbness, poor coordination, Bell's palsy, and irregular heartbeat.

Is massage indicated or contraindicated?
The inflammation associated with Lyme disease runs in acute and subacute phases. During subacute phases, massage may be appropriate to maintain joint function and relieve pain. In this situation, it is important to be working as part of a health care team for the maximum benefit and minimum risk to the infected person.

Lyme Disease

Definition: What Is It?
_____

Lyme disease is an infection with the spirochetal bacterium ***Borrelia burgdorferi***. This pathogen is spread through the bite of two species of ticks: deer ticks (*Ixodes scapularis*) and Western black-legged ticks (*Ixodes pacificus*). These ticks are very small, especially in the nymph stage, when they most frequently affect humans, which can make it difficult to find them on the skin. An unfed deer tick nymph is slightly larger than the period at the end of this sentence (Figure 2.24).

Demographics: Who Gets It?
_____

Lyme disease has been reported in 48 states and the District of Columbia, but 90% of all cases have been found in the Northeast and Mid-Atlantic states, along with Wisconsin and Minnesota.

Figure 2.24. Lyme disease: deer tick.

Smaller concentrations of the disease have been noted in Northwestern California. The nationwide statistics for Lyme disease show an infection rate of 5 of every 100,000 people, but in areas where the disease is endemic, incidence can be as high as 1% to 3% of the population.

Persons most at risk for Lyme disease are those who work or play outside in grassy or wooded areas.

Etiology: What Happens?

The life cycle of the deer tick and Western black-legged tick lasts about 2 years. Adult ticks spend fall and winter mating and taking blood meals from warm-blooded hosts. In the spring, females detach from their hosts and fall onto the ground to lay eggs. The eggs hatch and the larvae spend summer and fall taking meals from mice, birds, and large mammals, especially white-tailed deer. Dormant in the winter, the larvae molt into the nymph stage the following spring. They climb onto grass or bush stems and wait for a warm-blooded host to brush close by. This is the stage of development during which the animals most often find their way to human hosts. The final molt to the adult tick occurs in the insect's second summer, and the cycle begins again.

Ticks pick up the spiral-shaped bacterium *Borrelia burgdorferi* from the blood of their animal hosts, especially mice. If an infected tick then bites a human, that bacterium may be transmitted to the human host. The bacterial invasion can cause several different reactions, depending on the severity and the stage of the infection.

History of Lyme Disease

Although this disease was only definitively identified and named in 1982, it has probably been present for much longer.

In the early 20th century, doctors made note of red, target-shaped rashes, which were named *Erythema Migrans*. It was noted that people who developed these rashes seemed to have a high incidence of arthritis, but if they were treated with penicillin, their chances of developing arthritis were significantly lessened.

In 1974, a group of children in Lyme, Connecticut, were diagnosed with juvenile rheumatoid arthritis. Parents became suspicious of having such a high concentration of a disease that was not supposed to be in any way communicable. This led to intensive research, during which a scientist named Burgdorfer isolated the spirochete now called *Borrelia burgdorferi*. He found it in highest concentrations in the midgut of deer ticks.

Burgdorfer's discovery in 1982 began a process of surveillance that continues today. The incidence of Lyme disease rises yearly; it currently causes approximately 12,500 new infections annually.

B. burgdorferi did not make its first appearance with human infections; it probably has been around for ages. As the human population expanded into undeveloped areas, this bacterium suddenly had access to human hosts. It remains to be seen what other kinds of illnesses may be encountered as we continue to expand into previously undeveloped areas.

Signs and Symptoms

Lyme disease moves in stages, with signs and symptoms particular to each.

- *Early localized disease.* This is the first stage of a Lyme disease infection. Ticks are slow feeders, so it may take several days for the bacteria to enter the body and some days after that for symptoms to appear. Early symptoms generally appear between 7 and 30 days after an initial tick bite. They include a circular red rash (a "bull's eye" rash) that is hot and itchy, but not raised from the skin (Figure 2.25), accompanied by high fever, fatigue, night sweats, headache, stiff neck, and swollen lymph nodes.

  If no rash appears, these early symptoms may be mistaken for flu, mononucleosis, or meningitis.

- *Early disseminated disease.* In this stage, the infected person develops systemic symptoms of infection with *Borrelia burgdorferi*. These will include cardiovascular symptoms (especially irregular heartbeat), neurologic symptoms (chronic headaches, *Bell's palsy* [Chapter 3], numbness, tingling, forgetfulness, and poor coordination), along with more general problems including debilitating fatigue.

- *Late disease.* The final outcome of a Lyme disease infection is extreme inflammation of one or more large joints. The knees are the most commonly affected area, but elbows and shoulders are often inflamed as well. Most patients do not have the infection in more than three joints at a time. The inflammation can be extreme enough to damage the joint permanently, especially if it is left untreated.

Figure 2.25. Lyme disease: bull's-eye rash.

Is It Just Lyme Disease?

Lyme disease is caused by tick-borne bacteria that infect joints and cause debilitating arthritis. Some Lyme disease patients live with pain and progressive inflammation for years, in spite of antibiotics that should provide relief. Some of these patients may have more than Lyme disease alone: deer ticks can carry two other pathogens that affect humans:

- *Ehrlichiosis* is a tick-borne bacterial infection that can easily coexist with Lyme disease. Consequences of an ehrlichiosis infection include low white blood cell and platelet counts. This infection can be cleared with antibiotics from the tetracycline family, but this is a different class of antibiotics than is usually used for Lyme disease alone. Ehrlichiosis is less common than Lyme disease, so some patients may live with this infection for a long time before it is discovered.

- *Babesiosis* is a parasite similar to the protozoan that causes malaria. It can also coexist with Lyme disease. Babesiosis can cause anemia and enlarged spleen, as well as other serious problems, especially for immune-suppressed people. It responds well to quinine, *if* it is identified as an infection separate from Lyme disease.

To complicate matters further, two other tick-borne illnesses also may be confused for Lyme disease:

- *Southern tick-associated rash illness (STARI)* is a condition endemic to Southeast and South Central states. It is spread by the lone star tick, which carries a spirochete called *Borrelia lonestari*. STARI also causes a bull's-eye rash and is treatable with antibiotics.

- *Rocky Mountain spotted fever (RMSF)* is an infection with the bacterium *Rickettsia rickettsii*, spread by hard ticks all over the Western United States. Early symptoms include fever, headache, muscle pain, and malaise, followed by a spotty rash (as opposed to a bull's-eye rash). Although RMSF is treatable with antibiotics, it is a potentially life-threatening infection that can affect blood and blood vessels all over the body, leading to serious long-term consequences.

The tendency for Lyme disease to affect joints is what classifies it as an arthritic condition. In fact, the first cases of Lyme disease ever identified were among a group of children who were all initially misdiagnosed with juvenile rheumatoid arthritis.

Diagnosis

The accurate diagnosis of Lyme disease is one of the most contentious issues surrounding this condition. Blood tests that identify antibodies are unreliable—they frequently miss the presence of bacteria, leading to a "false negative" test, or they show the presence of antibodies but cannot distinguish whether the infection is currently active or part of a person's immune system history, leading to "false positive" tests.

This leaves the description of symptoms and the observation of signs as the primary means to achieve a Lyme disease diagnosis. Unfortunately, up to two thirds of all patients have no memory of a tick bite, and close to one half never develop a rash, so doctors must depend on the signs of fever, fatigue, swollen lymph nodes, and headache to make an early diagnosis. All of these symptoms can be associated with several other diseases, including mononucleosis, flu, meningitis, and several others.

At this point, whether Lyme disease is over-diagnosed or under-diagnosed is unclear. What is clear is that more accurate diagnostic tests are needed to identify this infection.

Treatment

Borrelia burgdorferi bacteria do respond to antibiotics, so the outlook for someone who is diagnosed with Lyme disease in the early stages is often hopeful. Lyme disease requires a much longer course of antibiotics than most other bacterial infections, however. It is not unusual for a person to take medication for 6 weeks or more; relapse rates for those who try shorter courses of medication are relatively high.

Lyme disease occasionally becomes a chronic ongoing problem. Patients in this situation may take high doses of antibiotics for 6 to 12 months. Some Lyme disease patients develop chronic symptoms that may last for years and that do not respond to typical antibiotics. Their disease process is much harder to explain or predict. For some of these patients, their disease may not be Lyme disease alone, but a combination of tick-borne infections (see sidebar, "Is It Just Lyme Disease?").

Prevention

The best protection against Lyme disease is protection from disease-bearing ticks. This means wearing long sleeves and long pants when working or playing in areas where tick infestation is high. Tucking pants into socks or boots may make it harder for ticks to gain access to skin. Wearing light-colored clothing is recommended, to make it easier to find and remove ticks. Using insect repellants can also reduce the risk of tick bites.

Examining the skin after being in a high-risk area is another important preventive measure. Ticks prefer to occupy warm, protected areas such as the groin, axilla, backs of knees, and insides of elbows. If a tick is found, it should be carefully removed to keep the mouth parts intact, and then the person should report being bitten and take the tick with him or her to the doctor.

Vaccines have been developed against Lyme disease, but so far they are not recommended for the general public. Persons between 14 and 70 years of age, especially those who spend a good deal of time outdoors, are the target group for these vaccines. They require a series of injections, and they do not reach full potential for a year after exposure, but at that point they are approximately 90% effective at protecting a person from Lyme disease.

Massage?

The arthritic phase of Lyme disease involves intermittently severe inflammation of joints that is acutely painful. This contraindicates massage when inflammation is acute. At other times, as long as sensation is present and the client is comfortable, a person with Lyme disease may derive significant benefits from massage. However, because this disease can affect the nervous and circulatory systems and because treatment for the disease can take a long time to take effect, it is important for massage therapists to operate as part of a client's health care team in this situation, rather than working alone.

Massage therapists who live and work in areas where Lyme disease is especially common should be aware of what deer ticks and Western black-legged ticks look like so that if they should find these parasites during a session they can counsel clients to receive appropriate medical care.

Osteoarthritis

Definition: What Is It?

Also called *degenerative joint disease*, osteoarthritis is a condition in which synovial joints, especially weight-bearing joints, are irritated and inflamed. This condition is distinguished from other types of arthritis by being directly related to wear and tear of the joint structures.

Osteoarthritis in Brief

What is it?
Osteoarthritis is joint inflammation brought about by wear-and-tear causing cumulative damage to articular cartilage.

How is it recognized?
Affected joints are stiff, painful, and occasionally palpably inflamed. Osteoarthritis most often affects knees, hips, and distal joints of the fingers.

Is massage indicated or contraindicated?
Arthritis contraindicates massage if it is acutely inflamed. It indicates massage in the subacute stage, when bodywork can contribute to muscular relaxation and mobility of the affected joint.

Arthritis Statistics

Arthritis is a term that refers to more than 100 disorders that can cause joints to become swollen, hot, and painful. Some disorders begin and end with joint trouble. Many varieties affect other body systems as well, causing skin problems, vascular inflammation, kidney dysfunction, or other difficulties.

The implications of bodywork for clients who have arthritis are many and far-reaching, especially for varieties that affect more than the musculoskeletal system. Conditions discussed in this text that can involve arthritis as primary or secondary symptoms include

Ankylosing spondylitis	Osteoporosis
Carpal tunnel syndrome	Paget's disease
Crohn disease	Pseudogout
Fibromyalgia syndrome	Psoriatic arthritis
Gout	Raynaud's syndrome
Lupus	Rheumatoid arthritis
Lyme disease	Scleroderma
Myofascial pain syndrome	Septic arthritis
Osteoarthritis	Tendinitis
	Ulcerative colitis

Approximately 42 million Americans (close to 16%) live with some version of chronic joint inflammation. Arthritis disables more people every year than heart disease and strokes combined. Arthritis treatments cost the US economy approximately $65 billion every year.

The Federal Drug Administration estimates that by 2020 approximately 60 million Americans will live with chronic arthritis, and 11 million of them will be permanently disabled by it.[10]

Demographics: Who Gets It?

This is by far the most common type of arthritis in the world. Osteoarthritis affects close to 20 million Americans, and is responsible for 7 million doctor visits each year. It is also an occupational hazard for massage therapists, who may get it at the saddle joint of the thumb because it is easy put too much pressure on this joint if good body mechanics are not employed.

Etiology: What Happens?

Joints, especially knees and hips, put up with tremendous weight-bearing stress and repetitive movements; their design is a marvel of efficiency and durability. However, the environment inside a joint capsule is precarious. Any imbalance can have cumulative destructive impact. Once the path toward arthritis has begun, it may be possible to stop it, but capacity for regeneration is limited at best.

All synovial joints have five features in common: the articulating bones, the cartilage that covers them, a ligamentous joint capsule, a synovial membrane that lines it, and the synovial fluid that serves to lubricate the cartilage. In weight-bearing joints, it is important to remember that the articulating layers of cartilage are almost always in contact; one layer of cartilage rests directly on top of the other.

Progression of Osteoarthritis

Step One: Cartilage Damage   After years of use or repetitive injury, the cartilage in a knee or hip may begin to flake, just the tiniest bit. If the cartilage on one side of the joint is even slightly roughened, it acts like sandpaper to the cartilage of the opposite side, instead of being smooth for easy, gliding movement. Then the *other* cartilage gets rough and further damages the first side. Once any cartilage damage inside the joint develops, the downhill slide has begun. The only question is, how far will it go? (Figure 2.26.)

Step Two: Bony Adaptation   The cartilaginous surfaces of two articulating bones are now rough instead of smooth. Each time one side moves, the other gets irritated. An inflammatory reaction ensues, releasing enzymes that further damage the cartilage. Because the cartilage is no longer doing its job, the bones (which are living tissue and respond to stresses put on them) begin to adapt. Bones cannot replace damaged cartilage, however. Instead of making a new, smooth surface inside the joint capsules, bones have a tendency to thicken at the condyles, and make small spurs on the ends, where they sense the most stress. This further limits freedom of movement and increases pain.

Step Three: The Muscles React   Any muscles that cross a stiff, painful, and constantly aggravated join will tend to tighten up. That is what muscles do when they are in areas

[10] Lewis C. Arthritis: Timely Treatments for an Ageless Disease. FDA Consumer Magazine. Publication No. (FDA) 00-1313. Available at: http://www.fda.gov/fdac/features/2000/300_arth.html. Accessed summer 2003.

Articular
cartilage

Bone

Extensive
cartilage damage
with bony
remodeling

Figure 2.26. Osteoarthritis.

of constant pain (see *spasms, cramps,* this chapter). They also may develop some trigger points in the process, because they cannot relax as long as that joint is in pain. The tension they cause compresses the joint, making it even more painful, which reinforces the spasm, and so on (see *myofascial pain syndrome,* this chapter).

Step Four: Atrophy   Eventually the person with arthritis wants to *stop* using the injured joint, because it hurts so much. Lack of use leads to atrophy, the wasting away of the joint structure and the tissues that surround it. The nearby muscles weaken, the synovial membranes stop functioning, and the joint fluid dries up. It could get to the point where even if the person *wanted* to move again, she would not be able to because the muscles and the joint structures will have degenerated too far.

Causes

Many changes in the body begin the process of joint degeneration. If the ligaments that surround joints are chronically lax, the joint can become unstable, raising the risk of arthritis (see *dislocations,* this chapter). Repetitive pounding stress, such as running or jumping with inadequate support, also can open the door to problems. Hormonal imbalances and nutritional deficiencies, including dehydration, inadequate calcium metabolism, and foods that trigger inflammatory responses, may compromise the health of joint structures. Being overweight adds stress to knees and hips. Age itself changes the quality of articular cartilage, making it drier and more prone to injury.

Signs and Symptoms

The symptoms of osteoarthritis all revolve around inflammation of the joint capsule. In the acute stage, the joints may be hot, painful, and swollen. More often, arthritis lingers in a chronic stage in which the joints experience ongoing pain and stiffness, especially when they are not warmed up, or when they have been overused. Osteoarthritis can be completely debilitating when it occurs at the hip or knee, because the pain and limitation are badly exacerbated by walking.

Diagnosis

Osteoarthritis is identified by physical examination and patient history. Tests may be conducted to rule out other conditions, but no blood test will absolutely confirm the presence of osteoarthritis. Even x-rays can be misleading. They may be used to confirm a diagnosis, but a surprisingly high percentage of people who show osteoarthritis-like bony deformations on x-ray experience no pain at all. Furthermore, different people are blessed with different thicknesses of cartilage. A person with thin cartilage is more likely to feel pain from arthritis than a person with thicker cartilage. (See *patellofemoral syndrome*, this chapter.)

Treatment

Treatment options for osteoarthritis have improved considerably in recent years. The goals of treatment are to reduce pain and inflammation, and to limit or reverse the damage incurred to the joint structures. These goals are accomplished in a number of different ways, depending on how advanced the condition is.

- *Nonsteroidal anti-inflammatory drugs*: These are the usually the first recourse to deal with arthritis pain. Although some patients do not tolerate them well (they can cause stomach irritation), a recently developed variety of painkillers is getting good results. Called *cox-2 inhibitors*, these drugs work to limit the action of the prostaglandin-related enzyme (*cyclooxygenase-2*) associated with pain and inflammatory response.

- *Exercise*: Arthritis patients are advised to exercise within pain tolerance to achieve three goals: to improve and maintain healthy range of motion, to increase stamina and lose weight, and to improve the strength of muscles surrounding affected joints.

- *Nutritional supplements*: **Glucosamine** and **chondroitin sulfate** are two substances that may not only limit the progression of arthritis damage, but may be able to reverse it. Research on how (or whether) taking supplements of these naturally occurring connective tissue building blocks helps to repair damaged cartilage is still ongoing. Although public interest in these supplements is high, they are unregulated by the Food and Drug Administration (FDA), and so potency and dosages may vary widely from one brand to another.

- *Injections of lubricating fluid*: Another recent development in arthritis treatment has been the injection of lubricants made essentially of **hyaluronic acid** (the liquid matrix of much of the body's connective tissue) directly into damaged joints. Although the patient often will have temporary swelling and irritation of the joint after this procedure, this is usually followed by an improvement in the quality and quantity of synovial fluid secreted into the joint capsule.

- *Joint replacement surgery*: A last resort for debilitating osteoarthritis is to replace the surfaces of the affected joint with artificial cartilage. Joint replacement surgery for knees and hips has become a commonplace intervention, and the expected recovery time from such surgery is a matter of weeks.

Massage?

Acute arthritis, like other acute inflammatory conditions, contraindicates massage. However, most osteoarthritis patients seldom experience acute swelling with pain, heat, and redness. Chronic osteoarthritis indicates massage, when goals would be to reduce pain through release of the muscles surrounding the affected joints, and to maintain range of motion through gentle stretching and passive gymnastics.

Patellofemoral Syndrome

Definition: What Is It?

Patellofemoral syndrome (PFS) is a condition in which the patellar cartilage becomes damaged as it contacts the femoral cartilage. This situation can be a precursor of *osteoarthritis* at the knee (this chapter).

PFS is almost always associated with overuse, although it may be precipitated by a specific injury or trauma. For a long while, the term *patellofemoral syndrome* was used interchangeably with ***chondromalacia patellae***; it is now recognized that these terms refer to significantly different types of knee problems. More current synonyms for PFS include *jumper's knee, movie-goer's knee, anterior knee pain syndrome,* and *over-utilization syndrome.*

Etiology: What Happens?

If the patellar cartilage is going to wear out, it usually happens in one of two ways. First is by simple overuse. Unfortunately, one person's "I've overused it" is another person's "I barely got started." This is because everyone is born with a different amount of cartilage on the patella. People with "thick cartilage" genes may never get PFS, but for people with "thin cartilage" genes, it takes much less use to wear it out and land with a textbook example of overuse PFS.

The other way to wear down patellar cartilage is something that, unlike genetic structure, people have some control over: the alignment of the knee. If the patella is pulled slightly to one side or the other, the wear on the cartilage is uneven, and leaves a person vulnerable to cartilage damage. The uneven tracking seen with PFS usually occurs toward the lateral aspect of the knee. It is especially prevalent in women athletes, because they tend to have an exaggerated "Q-angle": the line of traction as the quadriceps pull on the patella and tibial tuberosity.

Signs and Symptoms

Symptoms of PFS include pain that is usually felt on the anterior aspect of the knee, stiffness after long immobility, difficulty walking down stairs, and a characteristic crackling, grinding noise on movement, called *crepitus.*

Diagnosis

PFS can be difficult to diagnose, especially in the early stages before visible damage to the bones has occurred. The problem is that what is often called PFS may actually be another condition, *patellar tendinitis.* This is significant because, although PFS is largely unaffected by massage, patellar tendinitis responds beautifully and can have a virtually pain-free resolution. Consequently, it is important to have a clear idea of what a client really has. One clue that is sometimes useful is that patellar tendinitis often hurts going *up* stairs (resisted extension of the leg) whereas PFS may hurt more going *down*

Patellofemoral Syndrome in Brief

What is it?
Patellofemoral syndrome (PFS) is an overuse disorder that can lead to damage of the patellar cartilage.

How is it recognized?
PFS causes pain at the knee, stiffness after immobility, and discomfort in walking down stairs.

Is massage indicated or contraindicated?
PFS indicates massage, as long as the knee is not acutely inflamed. Massage may or may not be useful to correct this problem, but it certainly will do no harm and can address issues of muscle tightness and imbalance.

stairs—the weight of the femur pushing on the patella. However, these two conditions can certainly be present simultaneously. Ultimately only a doctor with imaging techniques can give an absolutely definitive diagnosis.

Treatment

The long-term prognosis for a person with PFS depends entirely on what he or she does with it. Although damage to the patellar cartilage may set the stage for osteoarthritis in the knee, PFS does not always get to the point of requiring a joint replacement. However, this condition is badly irritated by jarring, jouncing, bouncing kinds of exercise. If one kind of activity becomes prohibitive (running and aerobics are not great choices for someone with PFS), it can probably be replaced it with something else, such as swimming, walking, cycling, or skating. Patients may have to experiment, under a doctor's supervision, to find the exercise activities that work best.

Physical therapy for PFS often includes exercises to strengthen and balance tension in the muscles that cross the knee and that influence knee alignment. The quadriceps, hamstrings, tensor fascia latae, and deep lateral rotators are often addressed in the challenge to improve alignment and stop the progression of damage that PFS can cause.

Massage?

If the knee is inflamed and painful, it locally contraindicates massage. But PFS is more often a chronic, low-level irritation that interferes with normal activity, and massage certainly will not make it any worse. Whether massage can be instrumental in *improving* the situation depends on the situation. Massage can address the stiffness and chronic pain experienced in muscle–tendon units that cross the knee joint. If a treatment strategy is developed to retrain the knee extensors to track the patella appropriately over the joint, massage may be a useful part of an effort to slow down or stop permanent cartilage damage.

Rheumatoid Arthritis

Rheumatoid Arthritis in Brief

What is it?
Rheumatoid arthritis (RA) is an autoimmune disease in which immune system agents attack synovial membranes, particularly of the joints in the hands and feet. Other structures, such as muscles, tendons, blood vessels, and serous membranes, also may be affected.

How is it recognized?
In the acute phase, affected joints are red, swollen, hot, and painful. They often become gnarled and distorted. It tends to affect the body symmetrically, and it is not determined by age.

Is massage indicated or contraindicated?
Massage is indicated in the subacute stages of RA only. At that point, it may be used to reestablish mobility and to reduce the stresses that can trigger another flare.

Definition: What Is It?

Rheumatoid arthritis (RA) is an autoimmune condition in which the synovial membranes of various joints are attacked by immune system cells. Unlike many forms of arthritis, RA also can involve inflammation of tissues outside the musculoskeletal system.

Demographics: Who Gets It?

This disease affects 2.1 million people, or approximately 1% of all Americans. Women are affected roughly three times more frequently than men. Statistics indicate that it is most common among 20- to 40-year-olds, but it can strike anyone, including children and adolescents.

Etiology: What Happens?

Autoimmune diseases are brought about by a mistake in the vastly complex and usually very effective immune system: normal, healthy tissues are mistakenly identified as threatening invaders and attacked by immune system agents. Some autoimmune diseases are triggered by pathogens that closely resemble some part of the body's own proteins. A pathogen's protein coat needs to have only five amino acids in the same order as some normal, healthy part of the body to trigger an autoimmune disease response.

In RA, an immune system attack is targeted for a specific protein, but that protein *is not* on an invading microbe; it is in the synovial membranes. This leads to all of the cardinal signs of inflammation: heat, pain, redness, swelling, and loss of function. In later stages, the antibodies also may attack the pericardium, blood vessels, lungs, and fascia.

Several pathogens have been identified that may initiate RA. They include a variety of streptococcus bacterium, *B. burgdorferi* (the same bacterium that causes Lyme disease), and some retroviruses. Contracting and sustaining damage from RA begins with exposure to one of these pathogens. RA typically progresses in this pattern:

- A person has a bout with a pathogen. She goes through the usual process of producing T-cells, B-cells, and antibodies. She wins the fight, and the bacterium or virus is vanquished, but now she has a regiment of memory cells and antibodies in circulation, looking for any remnants of the invading microorganisms.

- Her antibodies get confused. The proteins in her synovial membranes look so much like the proteins in the pathogen's molecules that her immune system raises the alarm and launches a full-scale attack. This is where genetics may play a role; this person's antibodies may actually programmed to be "auto-antibodies."

- The synovial membrane thickens and swells. Fluid inside the joint capsule begins to accumulate, which causes pressure and pain.

- The inflamed tissues release enzymes that erode cartilage, eventually right down to the bone. This is the process that causes the tell-tale deformation of the joint capsules, and gnarled appearance of RA (Figure 2.27).

- Fibrous scar tissue develops to connect the raw ends of the bones.

- The scar tissue ossifies, and the joint is permanently fused.

Actually, the disease seldom progresses all the way to the final two steps. As serious as RA could be, it rarely fulfills the worst of its promises. After coping with the disease for 10 to 15 years, approximately 20% of affected people are in remission. Most are able to retain full-time employment. After 15 to 20 years of living with RA, approximately 10% of affected people are permanently disabled.

Signs and Symptoms

Symptoms of RA vary considerably at the onset of the disease. Many people experience a period of weeks or months with a general feeling of illness: lack of energy, lack of appetite, low-grade fever, and vague muscle pain, which gradually becomes sharp, specific joint pain. Approximately 10% experience a sudden onset with joint pain alone.

Figure 2.27. Rheumatoid arthritis.

Rheumatic nodules, small, painless bumps that appear around fingers, elbows, and other pressure-bearing areas, are also common indicators of the disease.

In the acute stage, the affected joints are red, hot, painful, and stiff, although they improve considerably with moderate amounts of movement and stretching. The joints RA most often attacks are the proximal knuckles in hands and toes. It also can appear in ankles and wrists; knees are less common, and one of the most serious places to get it is in the neck. It generally affects the body bilaterally, although it is sometimes worse on one side than the other.

Like many autoimmune diseases, RA appears in cycles of flare followed by periods of remission. Some patients have only a few flares in their life and are never affected again. Moderate cases involve cycles of flare and remission up to several times a year. Severe RA involves chronic inflammation that never fully subsides.

Complications

If someone has rheumatoid arthritis, it means that her immune system is confused about what it should be fighting off. Synovial membranes are just one of the types of tissue that may be attacked. Other possibilities include:

- Rheumatic nodules on the sclera ("whites") of the eyes
- *Sjögren's* syndrome (pathologically dry eyes and mouth).
- Pleuritis, which makes breathing painful and increases vulnerability to lung infection.
- Pericarditis, or inflammation of the pericardial sac around the heart.
- Vasculitis, or inflammation of blood vessels. This complication carries another set of risks: *Raynaud's syndrome* (Chapter 4), *decubitus ulcers* (Chapter 1), bleeding intestinal *ulcers* (Chapter 7), and internal hemorrhaging.

Bursitis (this chapter) and *anemia* (Chapter 4) are also common complications of RA, especially when onset of the disease occurs in childhood.

Advanced structural damage also brings a set of complications. Deformed and bone-damaged joints may dislocate or even collapse, rendering them useless. The tendons that cross over distorted joints sometimes become so stretched that they snap. If the disease is at the C_1–C_2 joint and the joint collapses, the resultant injury to the spinal column may even result in paralysis.

Diagnosis

Rheumatoid arthritis can be difficult to diagnose because its early symptoms are often subtle, they vary greatly from one person to another, and a long list of diseases with similar symptoms must be ruled out before a diagnosis can be conclusive. A sense of urgency exists around a conclusive diagnosis, however, because it has been found that cartilage and bone damage may occur as early as the first or second year of the disease process, and if treatment can be administered earlier, this damage can be averted.

RA is typically diagnosed through a description of symptoms, x-rays, and a blood test to check for rheumatoid factor, a substance that is present in most, but not all, cases. An erythrocyte sedimentation test may be conducted to look for signs of general inflammation, and the blood is also examined for signs of anemia. Even when all signs are positive, the diagnosis is sometimes not considered conclusive until the patient has been under observation for a long while.

Treatment

Once the presence of rheumatoid arthritis has been confirmed, the goals of treatment are to reduce pain, limit inflammation, halt joint damage, and improve function. Medications that help to achieve these goals are divided into "first-line" and "second-line" drugs.

Compare and Contrast
OSTEOARTHRITIS AND RHEUMATOID ARTHRITIS

Of the 100 conditions that cause painful inflammation of joints, the two most common varieties are osteoarthritis and rheumatoid arthritis. Osteoarthritis (OA) is a wear-and-tear disorder that could possibly be exacerbated by over-enthusiastic bodywork, but cannot be spread through the body. Rheumatoid arthritis (RA) is an autoimmune disorder that *can* spread from joint to joint, and must be avoided by bodyworkers in the acute or "flare" stage.

It is important for clients to know what the source of their joint pain is. Massage therapists are not equipped to tell the difference between the two conditions—and of course it is a perfectly reasonable possibility that a client could have both simultaneously. Still, it can be difficult to come to a conclusive diagnosis for joint pain. The following is a brief list of the most common patterns seen with osteoarthritis compared with rheumatoid arthritis.

OSTEOARTHRITIS

Prevalence
X-rays show bony deformation in 33%–90% of people over 65.

Demographics
Most common in people over 40. Men and women are affected equally.

Pain Patterns
Spine, knees, and hip joints are most frequently affected. Distal joints of the fingers and the saddle joint (trapezium—1st metacarpal) are also at risk.

Other Symptoms
None

Implications for Massage
Massage can be useful to maintain range of motion and to relieve pain in muscles that cross over affected joints, as long as inflammation is not acute.

RHEUMATOID ARTHRITIS

Prevalence
Up to 1.5% of the population

Demographics
Women are affected twice to three times as often as men, although men will be more likely to have systemic symptoms. RA may affect children as well as adults.

Pain Patterns
Proximal joints in hands and feet, ankles, and wrists are usually affected. Extreme distortion of the joint capsules can cause the joints to become visibly misshapen.

The pain appears in "flare" and "remission" stages.

Other Symptoms
In early stages and during acute episodes fever, malaise, lack of appetite, and muscle pain may be present.

Implications for Massage
During remission, massage can be useful to help maintain joint function. During acute stages, however, circulatory massage should be avoided.

First-line drugs include NSAIDs and cox-2 inhibitors to limit inflammation and pain. These are often used along with exercise, hydrotherapy, physical therapy, and occupational therapy in the hopes that progression can be limited without further intervention.

Second-line drugs attempt to interfere with the disease process. These include steroidal anti-inflammatories and immune suppressant drugs. They often give significant relief, but they also carry a long list of serious side effects and cannot be used for long-term care.

Until recently, RA was treated as conservatively as possible, but new research indicates that joint damage occurs much earlier than had been suspected, so many rheumatologists and other specialists now recommend an aggressive course of treatment as soon as the diagnosis is confirmed, to limit cumulative joint damage.

Surgery can be a successful option for RA patients, if their disease has affected joints that can be easily treated. Joint replacement is sometimes an option, along with surgery to rebuild damaged or ruptured tendons, and to remove portions of affected synovial membranes. The synovial membranes grow back, however, so this surgery is a temporary measure.

Massage?

In its acute (flare) phase, RA is an inflammatory condition caused by agents in the circulatory system. Anything that increases circulation also increases the risk that the disease may spread to other joints in the body.

In its subacute phase, RA leaves the joints stiff but not inflamed, and the muscles and tendons around them stressed and tight from chronic pain. Rheumatoid arthritis indicates massage in the subacute stage. Massage can improve mobility and the health of the soft tissues surrounding the joints. In addition to the structural benefits it offers, massage also can be an important part of the keep-healthy-and-stress-free part of prevention strategy. If massage can help to balance the autonomic nervous system, it may also help to reduce the incidence of attack.

Septic Arthritis in Brief

What is it?
Septic arthritis is joint inflammation caused by infection inside the joint capsule.

How is it recognized?
This condition shows the cardinal signs of inflammation: pain, heat, redness, and swelling, although these symptoms may be mild. It is often accompanied by fever.

Is massage indicated or contraindicated?
Massage is contraindicated for septic arthritis until the infection is completely gone from the joint. At that time, massage may be useful to help restore function.

Septic Arthritis

Definition: What Is It?

Septic arthritis is a form of arthritis brought about by a bacterial infection. *Neisseria gonorrhea* or *Staphylococcus aureus* are the most common infectious agents.

Demographics: Who Gets It?

Septic arthritis is most common among very young, very old, or immune-suppressed persons. It is more common among people with other immune system dysfunctions; it is sometimes a complication of *rheumatoid arthritis* (this chapter) or *lupus* (Chapter 6). It is unusual for a healthy mid-range adult to have this kind of infection.

Etiology: What Happens?

Because no direct blood supply nourishes joints structures, it is difficult for bacteria to get inside a joint. The most common ways for infections to be introduced into a joint capsule are through puncture wounds, contaminated needles (used for IV drugs or for steroid injections), or susceptibility brought about by underlying illness, especially gonorrhea (see *sexually transmitted diseases*, Chapter 10), rheumatoid arthritis, or *diabetes* (Chapter 8).

Once a bacterial colony is established, it can thrive in the warm, dark, moist growth medium supplied by synovial capsules. Septic arthritis can become very serious as the bacteria feast on the tissues, filling the joint space with fluid and pus. Permanent damage to the joint will occur if the infection is not treated promptly.

Signs and Symptoms

Symptoms of joint infections include redness, pain, heat, swelling, and mild to high fever, sometimes reaching 104°F, which is quite extreme for adults. Usually just one joint is affected; knees and hips are the most common sites. Surprisingly, the pain generated by septic arthritis is often mild and indistinct when the infection is just getting started. This is a problem because studies show that if a person does not receive care within 7 days of contacting an infection, the chance of permanent joint damage is much higher.

Septic arthritis due to gonorrhea has a slightly different pattern: It starts around the sacroiliac joint and progressively moves up the spine much in the manner of *ankylosing spondylitis* (this chapter), but it shares the same inflammatory symptoms as standard septic arthritis.

Diagnosis

Septic arthritis is diagnosed when aspirated fluid from an affected joint is examined for signs of bacterial infection. This test may be followed by blood cultures to look for signs of inflammation and an increased white blood cell count. Finally, x-rays or ultrasounds may be used to determine the extent of the infection and the amount of damage that has occurred.

Treatment

Infected joints are repeatedly aspirated, either with needles or with open shunts. Arthroscopic surgery may be performed to débride or scrape the insides of the synovial capsule, to be sure all bacteria are removed. Antibiotic drugs are administered orally, as an injection into the joint, or both. After the infection has subsided, the patient is recommended for physical therapy to prevent, or at least limit, permanent loss of function.

Prognosis

The expected outcome for such limited infections is surprisingly grave. Up to 10% of all people with septic arthritis die of complications from their infections. Thirty percent of all patients sustain some lasting damage in the affected joints. Only 60% of all septic arthritis patients can expect to achieve full recovery.

Massage?

Absolutely not, under any conditions, should vigorous massage be given to someone with septic arthritis. Think about what a full range-of-motion gymnastic would do to the bacteria hiding in a corner of an ankle joint: not only could the infection spread more thoroughly through the joint capsule, the infection could get into another part of the body altogether. And because this condition often goes hand-in-hand with a high fever, it strictly and systemically contraindicates massage, until the infection is gone.

Once the possibility of infection is past, however, massage can be beneficial to help restore range of motion and suppleness to the joint and surrounding structures.

Spondylosis

Definition: *What Is It?*

Spondylosis is the term used to describe osteoarthritis as it happens specifically in the spine. Another term for the same condition is *degenerative joint disease*. In addition to referring to arthritis joints, the term *spondylosis* is often used in the context of a narrowing or *stenosis* of the spinal canal.

Etiology: *What Happens?*

Spondylosis usually occurs in the most mobile parts of the spine: the lumbar and cervical regions. Bony remodeling of the vertebral bodies and joints leads to inflammation and restricted range of motion. Several factors may contribute to the process:

- *Thinning discs*: One contributor to spondylosis is thinned discs that are no longer elastic or resilient. The soft part of the disc calcifies with the aging process, reducing the shock-absorbing capacity between vertebrae.

- *Damaged discs*: Spondylosis is also a frequent complication of *disc disease* (this chapter). Damaged discs, like thinning ones, cannot easily absorb shock and bear weight. This puts extra stress on the vertebrae, which, according to Wolff's law, adapt by becoming thickened and distorted.

- *Chronic misalignment*: This situation signals misaligned bones to thicken in a peculiar pattern that is exclusive to spondylosis. The bony growths, called *osteophytes*, can also grow inside joint capsules or in the intervertebral foramen, where they put pressure on the nerve roots there (Figure 2.28). Eventually, arthritic vertebrae may fuse together completely (Figure 2.29).

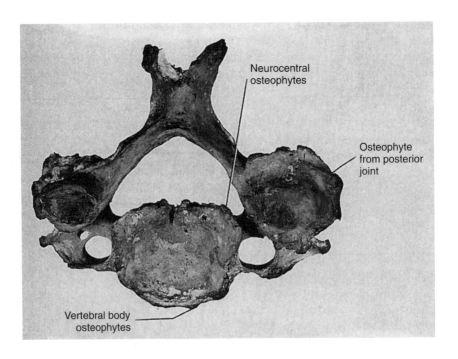

Figure 2.28. Osteophytic growths with spondylosis.

Figure 2.29. Fusion of vertebral bodies with spondylosis.

Signs and Symptoms

Often spondylosis has no symptoms whatever. If the bony changes do *not* press on nerve roots, but grow somewhere that impedes movement, the main symptom is a slow, painless, but irreversible stiffening of the spine.

When the osteophytes *do* press on nerve roots, the symptoms include shooting pain, tingling, pins and needles, numbness, and muscle weakness only in those muscles supplied by the affected nerve. One distinguishing feature of nerve pressure from osteophytes is that the pain is absolutely consistent; if the bone spurs are in a place to create pain when a person is in a certain position or posture, that pain is predictable, and it will probably get worse over time instead of better.

Pain from lumbar spondylosis has a pattern all its own. Patients with arthritis in the low back often feel pain in the low back and legs that is consistently aggravated by standing and walking, and usually relieved by sitting or forward bending. This pattern helps to distinguish lumbar spondylosis from disc or other problems that can cause pain that radiates from the back into the legs.

Complications

Spondylosis is a slowly progressing arthritis that mostly affects middle-aged and elderly people who have accumulated the kind of wear-and-tear in their spine that would make them vulnerable to this kind of condition. What makes spondylosis more dangerous is the seriousness of the complications that can arise from it:

- *Spreading problems in the spine.* This is not a progressive disease that travels through the blood, but if two vertebrae become fused through bony remodeling, that puts much more stress on the joints above and below the fusion to provide mobility. Those joints can then become unstable, develop arthritis, and experience the same bony remodeling that created the first problem. Or the stress of hypermobility may cause disc problems. Disc disease can be both a predisposing factor and a complication of spondylosis.

- *Nerve pain.* This is the consequence of having osteophytes grow where they can put pressure on nerve roots in the foramina.

- *Secondary spasm.* This accompanies nerve pain. Muscle spasm may be confined to the paraspinals, where it exacerbates the problem by compressing the affected joints, or it may follow the path of referred pain. Muscles also may go into spasm to protect the spine from movement that would otherwise be excruciatingly painful.

- *Blood vessel pressure.* Osteophytes in the neck are sometimes situated to press on the vertebral arteries as they go up the transverse foramina. If the head is turned or extended in a certain position, the patient may feel dizzy or may have headaches or double vision from impaired blood flow into the head.

- *Spinal cord pressure.* This is an extremely serious complication of spondylosis in the neck. In 5% to 10% of patients with spondylosis symptoms, osteophytes may grow in a place to put pressure not on the nerve roots, but in the spinal cord itself, a condition called **cervical spondylitic myelopathy.** This is felt as progressive weakening down the body, possible loss of bladder and bowel control, and even eventual paralysis. The surgery for this condition involves creating a larger foramen for the spinal cord to pass through and permanently fusing the involved vertebrae.

Diagnosis

The characteristic thickening or hypertrophy of the vertebral bodies that accompanies spondylosis is easily identified by x-ray. The facet joints in the lumbar spine tend to become distorted in a predictable pattern, and the ligamentum flava—the ligament that lines the spinal canal—often visibly thickens and buckles with spondylosis.

A random sampling of x-rays of people over 50 years old show signs of spondylosis 25% to 50% of the time. X-rays of 75% of people over 75 years old are positive for spondylosis—and most people never experience arthritic pain![11] Therefore, if a mature person complains of low back or neck pain, an x-ray is likely to point toward spondylosis, although the pain may actually be from something completely different, such as an injured disc or inflamed spinal ligaments.

Spondylo-Tongue Twisters

The terminology used in the discussion of arthritis and stenosis in the spine can be puzzling. Here is a brief look of some of the most confusing terms:

- *Spondylosis:* a general term for any degenerative condition of the vertebrae. This comes from the Greek root *spondylo-,* for "vertebra."

- *Spondylolysis:* a specific defect in vertebrae, usually in the lumbar spine, which impairs the weight-bearing capacity of the bone. The word roots are *spondylo-* and *lysis,* or "loosening."

- *Spondylolisthesis:* an anterior displacement of the body of a lumbar vertebra onto its inferior vertebra or onto the sacrum. This is a combination of *spondylo-* and *olisthesis,* Greek for "a slipping and falling."

All three of these conditions can contribute to *stenosis* or a narrowing of the spinal canal.

Treatment

Treatment for spondylosis depends on which (if any) complications are present. Anti-inflammatories are the usual first recourse. Movement and exercise can limit progression once the damage has begun.

If symptoms get worse, a variety of surgeries can create more space for nerve roots or the spinal cord. These often involve spinal fusions, however, and they work best for younger patients who have not been having arthritic symptoms for a long time or in more than one joint.

[11] Cervical Spondylosis. © All rights reserved by NYU Dept. of Neurosurgery. Available at: http://www.publishedresearch.com/AAAca/cervical_spondylosis.htm. Accessed summer 2003.

Massage?

Massage for spondylosis is appropriate with caution. If the joints are acutely inflamed, the surrounding muscles tend to splint them against painful movement. This splinting mechanism is important and must be respected by massage therapists. For this reason, and because of the other serious complications of spondylosis, in this situation it is highly recommended to work with a primary caregiver who has a complete set of x-rays.

Sprains

Definition: What Are They?

Sprains are tears to ligaments: the connective tissue strapping tape that links bone to bone throughout the body.

Etiology: What Happens?

Sprains, strains, and tendinitis are all injuries to structures that are composed largely of connective tissue fibers arranged in linear patterns. They have a lot in common in the way of symptoms, healing mechanisms, and treatment protocols. Thus, much of the information in this segment is applicable to all three conditions. Their differences will be emphasized here, as well as guidelines for how they may be seen in the same light.

Anatomy Review   Linearly arranged structures such as muscles, tendons, and ligaments are injured when some of their fibers are ripped. The severity of the injury depends on what percentage of the fibers is affected. First-degree injuries involve just a few fibers; second-degree injuries are much worse, and third-degree injuries are ruptures: the entire structure has been ripped through and no longer attaches to the bone.

Sprains in Brief

What are they?
Sprains are injured ligaments. Injuries can range from a few traumatized fibers to a complete rupture.

How are they recognized?
In the acute stage pain, redness, heat, swelling, and loss of joint function are evident. In the subacute stage, these symptoms are less extreme, although perhaps not entirely absent. Passive stretching of the affected ligament is painful until all inflammation has subsided.

Is massage indicated or contraindicated?
Subacute sprains indicate massage. Bodywork can influence the healthy development of scar tissue and reduce swelling and damage caused by edematous ischemia. Therapists must take care to rule out bone fractures or other injuries that sprains may temporarily mask.

Common Orthopedic Injuries

Injuries of muscles, tendons, and ligaments are among the most common complaints clients may carry, and they are among the most satisfying things massage therapists can work with. Cross-fiber friction, linear friction, PNF, lymph drainage, and dozens of other modalities have been developed to help create a healing process that is efficient and long-lasting.

The purpose of this text is to provide information about the appropriateness of massage in the context of many diseases and disorders, but *not* to give specific guidelines about exactly what modalities to use when and in what circumstances; that judgment must be made by the individual therapist, depending on his or her own bodywork skills and the needs of the client. For this reason, many orthopedic injuries are not specifically addressed in the body of the text, because they fit into the broader headings of *strains*, *sprains*, and *tendinitis* (all this chapter).

Nonetheless, it is useful to make a list of some of the most common orthopedic injuries, and some reference to where they may fit in the context of massage.

Soft tissue injuries can often be identified with carefully isolated resisted contractions or passive stretches, but it must be remembered that injuries seldom happen in a vacuum: they often appear in combination with other damage. This is why it is important to accompany a massage therapist's informed opinion with a thorough diagnosis conducted by a medical professional.

Common tendon injuries
Rotator cuff tears
These can affect any combination of the rotator cuff muscles of the shoulder. One of the trickiest things about rotator cuff tears is that they can refer pain down the arm or even into the wrist and hand. This can make it difficult to get a clear diagnosis. Rotator cuff injuries can involve chronic tendinosis (damage to tissues without acute inflammation) or acute tendinitis. They often respond well to friction and rehabilitative exercise.
Patellar tendinitis
This is obviously an injury to the quadriceps attachment somewhere around the patella or distally in the patellar tendon on the way to the tibia. Several things make patellar tendinitis difficult to

(continues)

Common Orthopedic Injuries, *continued*

pin down: the quadriceps are so strong that they often will not be painful with resisted contractions unless they are already fatigued; the patellar tendon is large and thick, and it can be difficult to pin down exactly where the lesion has developed; and this injury is frequently misdiagnosed as *patellofemoral syndrome* (this chapter), which can be problematic because patellofemoral syndrome implies damage *inside* the joint capsule, whereas this condition involves irritation *outside* the joint.

Patellar tendinitis often arises in conjunction with muscular imbalances and overuse. It responds well to massage, both at the site of injury and generally around the lower extremity as the injured person works to create better balance.

Epicondylitis

This is a term that has been used to refer to irritation of either the extensors or flexors of the forearm. "Golfer's elbow" refers to flexor problems, whereas "tennis elbow" refers to extensor injuries. These injuries respond very well to friction and carefully gauged exercise, but they *will not* improve if the massage is applied to the wrong area. The greatest challenge with both flexor and extensor injuries is isolating the damaged structure and the exact site of injury.

Common Ligament Injuries

Ankle Sprains

Most ankle injuries involve rolling outward and stressing structures on the lateral side of the foot. The most commonly injured ligament in the body is the anterior talofibular ligament, which is almost always a part of lateral ankle sprains.

Ligaments are not contractile structures, so they are not isolated by muscle contractions, and they are not rehabilitated by exercise. Rather, friction, stretching, and gradually increasing weight-bearing stress are the interventions that work best for most ankle sprains.

If a ligament ruptures, it will be unable to stabilize its joint. This situation may require surgery to reattach the ligament and restore its ability to function.

Cruciate ligament sprains or ruptures

The anterior and posterior cruciate ligaments (ACL and PCL) inside the knee joint capsule are responsible for most of the anterior–posterior stability of this massive weight-bearing joint. When they are injured, the whole joint becomes unstable and susceptible to further injury.

Cruciate ligament sprains break the pattern of most orthopedic injuries: they do not benefit from immediate mobilization, and they are not accessible for friction or other hands-on therapies. Instead, these injuries often require arthroscopic surgery to repair the damage, followed by physical therapy to limit scar tissue and restore function. Massage can be useful in the postsurgical recovery period, but has no access to an untreated cruciate ligament injury.

Common joint injuries

Meniscus Tears

The menisci are mobile pieces of cartilage that help track the femur on top of the tibia. Occasionally they can crack, tear, fragment, or otherwise sustain damage. This situation requires surgery to remove loose bits of cartilage before joint surfaces become rough and arthritic. Because they are inside the joint capsule, massage therapists have no access to meniscus injuries. Massage can be a beneficial part of the postsurgical recovery period, however.

Acromial clavicular (AC) joint

The gliding joint where the clavicle meets the acromion of the scapula is a vulnerable spot because it is subject to bumps, falls, and other trauma. When the joint is inflamed, movement at the shoulder is limited and painful. AC joint problems often respond well to friction followed by ice to limit inflammation.

Frozen shoulder (adhesive capsulitis)

This disorder involves the synovial joint capsule at the glenohumeral joint. Often precipitated by some other inflammatory problem (bursitis or tendinitis), the joint capsule gradually adheres to the articulating bones, causing pain, inflammation, and loss of range of motion. The onset is usually gradual, and without intervention it will often spontaneously resolve, although it may leave a permanent loss of range of motion at the joint. Physical therapy is often recommended for persons with frozen shoulder, to minimize and reverse the adhesive process; massage can fit into this context as well.

The process of repairing from muscle, tendon, or ligament tears involves the laying down of new collagen fibers, *not* in alignment with the injured structure, but whichever way the fibroblasts happen to deposit them (see *inflammation*, Chapter 5). The perfect combination of movement, stretching, and weight-bearing stress in the subacute phase of recovery helps to reorient the fibers in alignment with the uninjured structure. If this happens in the best possible way, the new scar tissue actually becomes part of the muscle fascia, tendon, or ligament. However, if a new injury is immobilized, the scar tissue becomes dense and contracted, pulling on all of the uninjured fibers nearby, and significantly hampering the weight-bearing capacity of the ligament (see Figure 2.10).

Distinguishing Features

What makes sprains unique? A few things distinguish sprains from strains and tendinitis, which are discussed in other sections.

- *Sprains are injured ligaments, not muscles or tendons*. Ligaments are the connectors that hold the bones together. Structurally they are a little different from tendons; the dense linear arrangement of collagen fibers affords little stretch and almost no rebound. If a ligament is stressed enough to become injured, it tends to tear before it stretches. And if it *does* get stretched, it will not rebound to its original length, and it will not stabilize the joint as well as it did before the injury. This ligament laxity is also seen with chronic injury–reinjury situations.

- *Sprains are more serious than strains and tendinitis.* Because tendons and muscles tend to be more elastic and less densely arranged than ligaments, they will stretch before a ligament does. The "lines of defense" in joint injuries are: muscles, tendons, ligaments, joint capsule—so a sprain is one step away from a *dislocation* (this chapter). Furthermore, ligaments do not have the same rich blood supply as muscles, and they are denser than tendons. Consequently, they do not have the same access to circulation, which makes them slower to heal than muscles or tendons.

- *Sprains tend to swell.* With a few exceptions, acute sprains swell much more than muscle strains or tendinitis; this is one way to differentiate between injuries. Swelling is a protective measure that recruits the body's healing resources and limits movement, which prevents further injury. Ligaments are sometimes contiguous with the joint capsules of the joints they cross over, so an injury to them will sometimes signal the joint to swell as well. Ligaments that are *not* attached to joint capsules swell much less than those that are.

Signs and Symptoms: Acute Stage

Acute sprains show the usual signs of inflammation: pain, heat, redness, and swelling, with the added bonus of loss of function because the rapid swelling splints the unstable joint and makes it extremely painful to move. Inflamed ligaments are especially painful with passive stretches of the structure.

Sprains can happen at almost any synovial joint, but the anterior talo-fibular ligament of the ankle is the most commonly sprained ligament in the body. Ligaments overlying the sacroiliac joint are also very commonly injured, as are various ligaments around the knees and fingers.

Signs and Symptoms: Subacute Stage

In the subacute stage, signs of inflammation may still be present, but they will have subsided and the joint will have begun to regain some function. The physiologic processes are no longer geared toward blood clotting and damage control; they have shifted toward clearing out debris and rebuilding torn fibers. The amount of time that passes between acute and subacute stages varies with the severity of the injury, but the 24- to 48-hour rule is usually dependable. It is important to remember, though, that some injuries can waver back and forth between acute and subacute, especially in response to certain kinds of activity or massage.

Complications

Injured ligaments can occasionally lead to more serious problems. Sprains are such a common injury that it is important for massage therapists to be familiar with all of their repercussions.

- *Masking symptoms.* An acute sprain may mask the symptoms of a bone fracture, especially in the foot. It is important to have clients get an x-ray to rule out fractures before beginning to work with a sprained ankle.

- *Repeated injury.* Internal scar tissue (scar tissue that accumulates within a specific structure) that never remodels just lies there in a big, gummy mass. It can interfere with the function of undamaged fibers. It can weaken the integrity of the whole structure, which, along with the increase in ligament laxity (see below), makes repeated injury a very common complication of sprains. This pattern is present with strains and tendinitis also.

- *Ligament laxity.* A ligament that has been injured, in addition to having torn some fibers, is often looser than uninjured ligaments. This is because it has been asked to stretch further than it could go, and ligaments have almost no rebound capability. When a joint becomes unstable because of loose, lax ligaments, excessive movement of the bones becomes possible. The bones may rock around and knock together, causing *osteoarthritis* (this chapter) and a host of other problems.

Treatment

A long time ago, the recommendations for sprains included hot soaks and total immobilization. Clearly both of these strategies were counter-productive: heat increases edema and the accumulation of scar tissue, whereas immobilization prevents the fibers from becoming aligned with the injured structure.

These days *RICE* therapy (rest, ice, compression, elevation) is considered the norm, with an emphasis on moving the joint within range of pain tolerance absolutely as soon as possible. The potential benefits are clear: ice keeps edema at bay, limiting further tissue damage from ischemia; compression does the same; elevation also encourages lymph flow *out* of an already impacted area.

Introducing movement is exactly what bodies are designed to do to help form scar tissue that strengthens, rather than weakens, an injured ligament. If exercise is overdone, more tearing accumulates, and more scar tissue is produced. If it is done too little, the scar tissue glues itself in its original random arrangement, and binds up the undamaged ligament fibers as well, increasing the risk of future injury. But if it is done *just right*, exercise and stretching "teach" the new collagen fibers which way to lie, and they will remodel themselves according to the stresses put on them. Interestingly, the issue of when exactly to introduce movement and weight-bearing stress is still not settled; different ligaments seem to have different needs. However, most evidence points toward early mobilization as an important part of the rehabilitation of most ligament sprains.

Massage?

Massage is *great* for sprains. It can reduce adhesions and influence the direction of new collagen fibers in the healing process. It can address edema and toxic accumulations from secondary muscle spasm. Massage will also help with stiffness from the temporary loss of joint function. But most massage must be done *after* the acute stage has subsided. Modalities in lymph drainage for dealing with acute sprains are effective, but it is a highly technical field and not for casual experimentation.

Temporomandibular Joint Disorders

Definition: What Are They?

The term *temporomandibular joint (TMJ) disorders* can mean a multitude of problems in and around the jaw. This collection of signs and symptoms is usually associated with *malocclusion* (a dysfunctional bite), *bruxism* (teeth grinding), and loose ligaments surrounding the

Temporomandibular Joint Disorders in Brief

What are they?
Temporomandibular Joint (TMJ) disorders arise when constant strain, stress, and malocclusion of the jaw lead to pain and loss of function of the temporomandibular joint.

How are they recognized?
Symptoms of TMD include head, neck, and shoulder pain, ear pain, mouth pain, clicking or locking in the jaw, and loss of range of motion in the jaw.

Is massage indicated or contraindicated?
Massage can be useful for TMJ problems, if intervention is begun before bony deformation begins. However, this condition can be difficult to diagnose, so it is important to be working with other medical professionals in these situations.

jaw that cause excessive movement between the bones, damage to the internal cartilage, and possible dislocation of the joint. (See *dislocations*, this chapter.) TMJ disorders are also referred to as *TMD*, for **t**emporo**m**andibular joint **d**isorders.

Demographics: Who Gets It?

It is difficult to pin down exact numbers of people who live with distortions in the jaw. Some estimates suggest that up to 20% of the US population has some degree of TMJ disorders, but only a small fraction may ever seek help. Of those who do, women outnumber men by approximately three to one.

Etiology: What Happens?

When chronic misalignment, trauma, or muscle tension affect the highly specialized joints at the jaw, a person may find it difficult to open or close her mouth without pain. Chewing and swallowing become problematic, and pain in the jaw can reverberate systemically throughout the body. The construction of the jaw is so intricate, it is easy for structures to become injured or improperly balanced.

Anatomy Review The temporomandibular joint is like no other in the body. Far from being a simple hinge joint, the TMJ moves up, down, forward, back, and side to side. The jaw is unusually mobile, as the shape of the joint actually stretches with the position of the mouth (Figure 2.30). A fibrocartilage disc cushions the two bones (the temporal bone

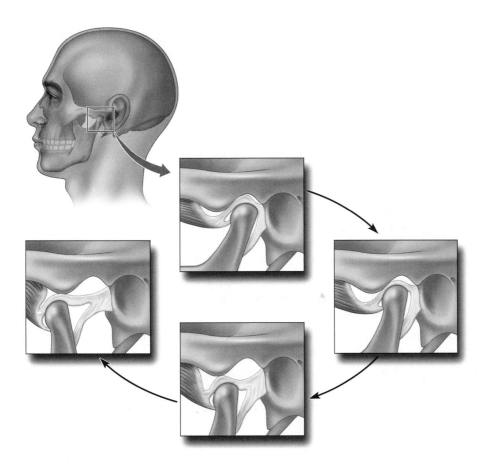

Figure 2.30. The temporomandibular joint allows great mobility as the jaw protracts.

and the condyle of the mandible) but, like the menisci in the knee, this disc is sometimes pulled awry or injured, which can lead to problems in the joint. And lastly, a muscle involved in this joint, the lateral pterygoid that attaches directly to the fibrocartilage disc, is an unusual structure: it does not relax by order of the central nervous system. Instead, it constantly pulls on the disc, acting as a kind of spring. This constant tension makes the lateral pterygoid especially prone to trigger points, which can both mimic and precipitate TMJ disorders.

Causes

The American Dental Association estimates that 44% to 99% of TMJ problems are precipitated by some kind of trauma. This may be direct impact to the face or head, or indirect repercussions of trauma elsewhere in the body. For instance, a childhood fall could set up imbalances in the spine, which would culminate in neck and jaw problems.

TMJ disorders also may be a frequent consequence of car wrecks. A whole scenario of the progression of "jaw-lash" has been developed to explain the whiplash-like results seen after this kind of acceleration–deceleration accident (see *whiplash*, this chapter).

Precipitating trauma aside, this is often a "circular" disorder. That is, the things that cause TMJ disorders can also be the symptoms. This is true of teeth grinding, muscle tightness, and *osteoarthritis* (this chapter). *Rheumatoid arthritis* (this chapter) occasionally strikes here, but osteoarthritis is a far more frequent cause for TMJ problems. Other factors include misalignment of the bite and congenital malformations of the bones. Some sources suggest that TMJ disorders are entirely muscular in nature, but this is contradicted when the problems progress to arthritis and bony adaptation. Travell points out that when the jaw flexors, especially the lateral pterygoid, are over-engaged, the constant pulling mechanically displaces the internal disc, thus starting the downward slide toward arthritis. In other words, *myofascial pain syndrome* (this chapter) that is linked to painful trigger points is both a cause and a complication of this disorder. According to her findings, approximately 70% of the people who complain of TMJ disorder symptoms show some disc displacement.[12]

It is impossible to ignore the emotional component of TMJ disorders. If one looks at the body as a physical expression of the emotional state, it is clear that chronic emotional stress and chronic jaw stress are linked. Regardless of whether a precipitating injury occurred, people who persistently clench their teeth are setting themselves up for jaw problems in the future.

Signs and Symptoms

The signs and symptoms of TMJ disorders are as follows:

• *Jaw, neck, and shoulder pain.* This can be from actual deterioration of bony structures inside the capsule (arthritis), or it can be local and referred pain generated by tight, trigger-point–laden muscles.

• *Limited range of motion.* Deformation or displacement of the cartilage inside the joint can make it difficult or impossible to open the mouth all the way.

• *Popping in the jaw.* This is usually attributed to having the disc or bone out of alignment, which then interferes in jaw opening. A similar "clicking" sensation is sometimes felt by people with knee problems involving the discs there.

[12] Travell J, Simons DG. Myofascial Pain and Dysfunction: The Trigger Point Manual. Baltimore: Williams & Wilkins 1983, p. 176.

- *Locking of the joint.* Again, this is a result of having the fibrocartilage disc interfere with normal joint movement.

- *Grinding teeth (bruxism).* Like many things about this disorder, this symptom is also a possible cause of the problem. A chronically shortened set of jaw flexors contributes to clenching and grinding of teeth, especially during sleep, when the joint should be as relaxed as possible.

- *Ear pain.* Because of the location of the joint, pressure may be exerted directly on the eustachian tubes. Symptoms in this case would include a feeling of stuffiness in the ears, and loss of hearing.

- *Headaches.* Two thousand pounds per square inch of pressure are exerted at the second molar when the teeth are clenched. It is no surprise that the cranial bones would be affected if this happened all night long. Headaches can also be related to trigger points of muscles in spasm and to cervical subluxation.

- *Chronic misalignment of cervical vertebrae.* This is probably a result of the muscular hypertonicity that is generated by this problem. As pain refers from the jaw to the neck and shoulders, the muscles there tighten up and pull asymmetrically on the neck bones. No matter how often the neck is adjusted, or how brilliantly the neck muscles are massaged, this pain–spasm cycle will not abate until the jaw situation is addressed.

Diagnosis

Many conditions present signs and symptoms similar to TMJ disorder, but they do not respond at all to the most advanced kinds of interventions. Therefore, it is important to differentiate between true TMJ disorder, which involves bony or cartilaginous deformation inside the joint capsule, and the other diseases and conditions that can cause head, neck, and shoulder pain.

First among these differential diagnoses is myofascial pain syndrome. More than any other condition, this one is both a precursor and a complication of TMJ disorder. Jaw surgery will not resolve trigger points, but resolving trigger points could eliminate the need for future jaw surgery. It is important to remember, however, that true TMJ disorder can (and probably will) be present simultaneously with myofascial pain syndrome. Other conditions that cause head, neck, and shoulder pain include:

- *Sprain* of the ligament that attaches the stylomandibular joint to the base of the skull can cause pain in the jaw and head. This is also called *Ernest syndrome.*

- *Trigeminal neuralgia,* also called *tic douloureux,* is an extremely painful result of damage to the trigeminal nerve (see *trigeminal neuralgia* Chapter 3).

- *Occipital neuralgia* is damage to the greater or lesser occipital nerves.

- *Osteomyelitis* is a complication of dental surgery in which tissue death occurs at the site of extracted teeth, which causes pain in the face.

Some diagnostic tools that identify TMJ disorder include MRIs, which can show whether the internal cartilage is chipped or subluxated; x-rays of the jaw and head; and electromyography, which will show muscle function around the joint. A trained clinician also can feel a subluxation when fingers are inserted in the ear of the patient during chewing.

Treatment

Treatment for TMJ disorder is divided into surgical and nonsurgical options. In most cases, nonsurgical options are tried first. These include applying heat to painful areas, physical therapy, ultrasound and massage for jaw muscles, anti-inflammatory medicine, and local anesthetics. Special splints that reduce bone-to-bone pressure may be prescribed, although some specialists feel that ill-fitting splints will make matters worse rather than better. Proliferant injections to tighten the ligaments that surround the jaw also may be effective. If these noninvasive techniques are successful, the TMJ disorder may be averted before permanent bony distortion or cartilage damage inside the joint occurs.

In some situations, the onset of symptoms may be very fast, for instance, with a car wreck or a fall. If such a patient has been severely debilitated, or if noninvasive techniques have been unsuccessful and other problems have been ruled out, surgery may be considered. Several different surgeries have been developed. These range from an outpatient procedure in which scar tissue and adhesions are dissolved by injecting special substances into the joint, to arthroscopic surgery to manipulate the cartilage, to full prosthetic joint replacement.

Massage?

Massage can be especially useful in the early teeth-clenching stages of TMJ problems, not only by addressing the jaw flexors, but also by helping to increase the client's awareness of this habit. It is surprising how often people grit their teeth without realizing it; the proprioceptors can adapt to assume that this is *normal*, even if it is not *optimal*. And of course, in addition to helping reduce excessive muscle tone, massage can also deal with some of the referred pain patterns that can be such a problem with this condition.

OTHER CONNECTIVE TISSUE DISORDERS

Baker Cysts

Baker Cysts in Brief

What are they?
Baker cysts are fluid-filled extensions of the synovial membrane at the knee. They protrude into the popliteal fossa, usually on the medial side.

How are they recognized?
Baker cysts are usually painless sacs that are palpable deep to the superficial fascia in the popliteal fossa. They may cause pain or a feeling of tightness in the knee in flexion.

Is massage indicated or contraindicated?
Massage is locally contraindicated in the popliteal fossa anyway, especially if a Baker cyst is present. In addition, if any signs of circulatory disruption (coldness, clamminess, edema) are visible distal to the cyst, the client needs to be cleared of the possibility of thrombosis.

Definition: What Are They?

Baker cysts are posterior extensions of the joint capsule of the knee.

Etiology: What Happens?

Baker cysts form when the joint capsule at the knee develops a pouch at the posterior aspect. A structural weak spot of the joint capsule, called the *popliteal* recess, is the most common site for these extensions. Although Baker cysts are relatively common in children, in whom they usually spontaneously resolve within a few months, when they occur in adults it is usually connected to general joint inflammation: *osteoarthritis, rheumatoid arthritis* (this chapter), or meniscus tears.

Baker cysts are not usually dangerous. The only risk they pose is that a cyst could become big enough to press on nerves or impair blood flow through the lesser saphenous vein in the back of the leg. If that is the case, clients may experience some numbness, which contraindicates massage, or they could be at risk for forming blood clots, another contraindication (see *thrombophlebitis/deep vein thrombosis*, Chapter 4).

Signs and Symptoms

Baker cysts themselves are generally asymptomatic, but the affected knee is often painful from the underlying cause of inflammation. The cysts usually extend into the medial side

Figure 2.31. Baker cyst: the mass posterior to the femoral condyle is probably the original cyst; the mass in the gastrocnemius is leaked fluid.

of the popliteal fossa and may protrude down the leg, deep to the gastrocnemius (Figure 2.31). Patients with Baker cysts often report a feeling of tightness or fullness when the knee is in flexion.

Baker cysts occasionally spontaneously rupture, the symptoms of which mimic thrombophlebitis: deep acute pain in the calf with temporary edema from the leaking fluid.

Treatment

Most Baker cysts are first treated with ice and NSAIDs, in the hopes that they will spontaneously resolve. If this is unsuccessful, they may be aspirated, followed by cortisone shots to resolve joint inflammation. This is often an impermanent solution, however, because they may easily come back.

Surgery to remove the cyst is another possibility, although even in this case if the area is irritated again, another cyst may form. Baker cysts are resolved most successfully when the underlying cause for joint inflammation is effectively identified and treated.

Massage?

It is possible, though unlikely, that massage could rupture a Baker cyst, but a therapist would have to be working much deeper in the popliteal fossa than good sense allows. Baker cysts are considered local contraindications for massage, however, because of their proximity to the lesser saphenous vein. Therapists should watch for signs of fluid accumulation and poor blood return below the knee: coldness, clamminess, and edema that is more pronounced on the cyst side than the non-cyst side (Figure 2.32). These are all signs that the cyst is big enough to cause a problem. If this is the case, the client should visit a doctor to rule out the possibility of thrombophlebitis.

Figure 2.32. Baker cyst: note the disparity in size and color between the two calves.

Bunions

Definition: What Are They?

Bunions are also known as ***hallux valgus***, which means, "laterally deviated big toe." The first phalanx of the great toe is distorted toward the lateral aspect of the foot. The joint capsule stretches, and callus grows over the protrusion. A smaller version of the same problem sometimes appears at the base of the little toe; this is called "tailor's bunion," or "bunionette."

Demographics: Who Gets Them?

Bunions occur approximately 10 times more often in women than in men. The condition is linked to a habit of wearing high-heeled, narrow toed shoes. A genetic weakness in the toe joints may predispose some people to bunions regardless of footwear, but anyone can develop bunions.

Etiology: What Happens?

Bunions begin with a bony misalignment in which the proximal phalanx of the great toe is laterally deviated. This misalignment may be the result of an overarched foot, which places excessive pressure on the medial aspect of the foot. Bunions also arise when feet are forced into pointed-toe shoes, shoes that are too small, and shoes with high heels. A history of other joint problems in the feet, i.e., osteoarthritis or rheumatoid arthritis, also may precipitate bunions.

The distortion of the metacarpal–phalangeal joint in itself can cause erosion and irritation, but the acute pain of bunions is more often related to a variety of *bursitis* (this

---

Bunions in Brief

What are they?
A bunion is a protrusion at the metatarsal–phalangeal joint of the great toe that occurs when the toe is laterally deviated.

How are they recognized?
Bunions are recognizable by the large bump on the medial aspect of the foot. When they are inflamed, they are red, hot, and possibly edematous.

Is massage indicated or contraindicated?
Massage is locally contraindicated at the point of a bunion regardless, and especially when or if it is inflamed. Massage elsewhere on the foot or body is very much indicated within pain tolerance to help with compensation patterns that occur when it is difficult to walk.

chapter). Bursae spontaneously generate in places subject to a lot of wear and tear. The bump formed by a bunion is a natural spot for that protective impulse. If that new bursa should get irritated and inflamed, it becomes a case of friction bursitis, which can be extremely painful, even debilitating. Ultimately if this badly misaligned weight-bearing joint is not somehow corrected or supported in a way that limits erosion of the joint structures, the bunion patient also can develop bone spurs or degenerative joint disease (see *osteoarthritis*, this chapter), which can make it debilitatingly painful to do anything with the foot, including walking.

Signs and Symptoms

Bunions look like an enormous lump on the medial side of the metatarsal–phalangeal joint of the great toe. If the bunion is not irritated, a simple protrusion, often covered with a thick layer of callus, is obvious (Figure 2.33). If the bursa happens to be inflamed, the area will be red, hot, and painful.

Treatment

The first steps in treating a bunion are to remove whatever irritants are making it happen, or making it worse. This usually means switching footgear, or even cutting holes in shoes to make room for the protrusion. Other noninvasive techniques include the use of massage and ultrasound to reduce internal adhesions and inflammation. Elevating the heel to an appropriate height can diminish pain, and a corticosteroid injection can reduce inflammation. However, if damage has developed inside the joint, and if the bunion is painful enough to limit the patient's activity, surgery may be recommended to realign and fuse the joint. This eradicates the bunion, but it also can eradicate any movement at the joint, so surgery is considered a "last ditch" option.

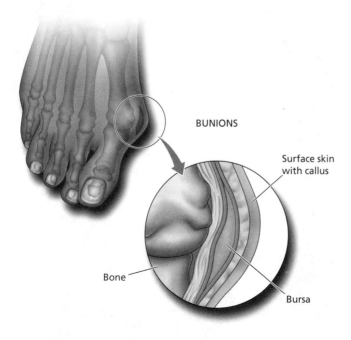

Figure 2.33. Bunion.

Massage?

Acutely inflamed bunions locally contraindicate massage; massage elsewhere on the body is perfectly safe. If no acute inflammation is present, massage is appropriate, although the bump itself is still a local contraindication because of the risk of irritating a bursa or osteophyte. Massage does not make bunions go away. Therapists do not have access to genetic patterning, nor to the inner workings of the affected joint. The best massage can do is work with the compensation patterns that will ripple through a body that is forced to move differently because of foot pain. This can mean concentrating on the intrinsic muscles of the affected foot, and it can mean working with the extrinsic muscles for gross movement everywhere else on the body.

Bursitis in Brief

What is it?
A bursa is a fluid filled-sack that acts as a protective cushion at points of recurring pressure, eases the movement of tendons and ligaments moving over bones, and cushions points of contact between bones. Bursitis is the inflammation of a bursa.

How is it recognized?
Acute bursitis is painful and is aggravated by both passive and active motion. Muscles surrounding the affected joint often severely limit range of motion. It may be hot or edematous if the bursa is superficial enough to be palpated.

Is massage indicated or contraindicated?
Acute noninfectious bursitis locally contraindicates massage. Massage elsewhere on the body during an acute phase, and directly on the muscles of the affected joint (within pain limits) in a subacute phase is perfectly appropriate.

Bursitis

Definition: What Is It?

Bursae are small closed sacks made of connective tissue. They are lined with synovial membrane, and they are filled with synovial fluid. Bursitis is inflammation of the bursae: these fluid-filled sacks, when irritated, generate excess fluid, which causes pain and limits mobility (Figure 2.34). Most bursae are very small, but the ones that protect the knee and shoulder can be quite large.

Bursitis comes in all shapes and forms, some of which have descriptive names, such as *housemaid's knee* and *student's elbow*, which occurs on the point of the olecranon. *Weaver's bottom* is bursitis on

Figure 2.34. Calcaneal bursitis.

the ischial tuberosity. Trochanteric or hip bursitis is another common variety. The most common type of bursitis, at the pad between the humerus and the acromion, is called subacromial bursitis, but could be labeled *"jackhammerer's shoulder."*

Etiology: What Happens?

Imagine stretching a rubber band over the sharp edge of a table. Now imagine moving it back and forth for several minutes. Before long that rubber band would fray and then break. But if a small water balloon is inserted between the rubber band and the edge of the table, the rubber band (i.e., tendon) has freedom to move without the friction from the table (i.e., bone). The water balloon (i.e., bursa) has protected it from damage. Bursae are the water balloons; they serve to ease the movement of tendons over bony angles (Figure 2.35). They also cushion the bones where they would otherwise bang against each other. Bursae pad people's sharpest corners: they are on elbows, knees, heels, ischial tuberosities, and between layers of fascia. Bursae can grow anywhere the body experiences extra wear and tear around a joint.

Without bursae to protect them, several tendons would fray and rupture in shor order. Some bones that are not meant to touch *would* touch, with great force. Sharp corners, such as elbows or hallux valgus (*bunions*, this chapter) would have no protection.

Causes

Repetitive stress is usually the culprit behind bursitis. Performing the same movement or rubbing the same spot over and over, day after day, sooner or later irritates that fluid-filled sack. Then the inflammatory process will try to pack a tangerine's worth of fluid into a sack the size of a grape, which *hurts*. In response to the pain, the muscles that surround the joint go into spasm, splinting the injury. This drastically limits the range of motion of the affected joint. Sometimes the muscles can actually aggravate and prolong an attack of bursitis by compressing the joint and the bursa at the same time.

Bursitis often occurs in concert with other inflammatory conditions. It tends to accompany general area inflammation, so if a person has shoulder tendinitis, bursitis will

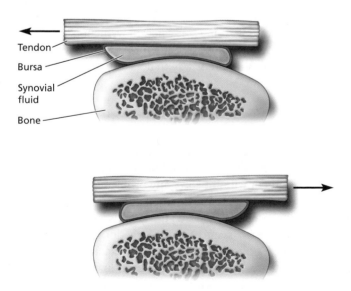

Figure 2.35. Bursae allow tendons to move freely over bony prominences.

often be present as well. (Unfortunately, it is hard to treat the tendinitis if the bursitis is in the way.) It will also attend *gout*, *rheumatoid arthritis* (this chapter), and *tuberculosis*, (Chapter 6).

Signs and Symptoms

The symptoms of bursitis include pain on *any* kind of movement, passive or active, along with heat, edema, and extremely limited range of motion because of the muscular splinting reaction to pain. If the affected bursae are deep, no heat or edema may be palpable, but the pain and limitation of movement are still present.

Diagnosis

Bursitis is not usually caused by an infectious agent, and bursae do not show up on x-rays. Therefore, its diagnosis largely depends on ruling out anything else it could be, which includes tendinitis, arthritis, ligament sprains, and any other problems specific to the joint or area being affected.

Treatment

Opinions vary about the duration of the average bursitis episode. Some orthopedists predict several weeks; others suggest it will usually clear up in about 2 weeks. For some people, bursitis can last much longer: untreated bursitis can become a chronic situation that lasts several months or even years. Obviously, a lot depends on which bursae are inflamed, and what the precipitating factors are. Treatment strategies range from NSAIDs to warm moist applications (cold is too intense for this inflammation; the muscles seize up and make it worse), to aspiration of excess fluid, to corticosteroid injections. One or two injections generally clear away even chronic inflammation, and because the chemical is being injected into a closed cavity, one does not have to deal with the same side effects that a systemic dose of steroids involves.

As a last resort, some doctors suggest the possibility of a *bursectomy* to simply remove a badly inflamed bursa. But the only way to be sure that the bursitis is permanently cured is to get rid of the aggravating factors that caused it. No matter how often or how effectively bursitis is treated, if the stimulus that irritated the bursa to begin with is not removed, no treatment will be permanently successful. Even removing the bursa may eventually backfire, because the body can grow new ones! What does removing the irritating stimulus mean? It means learning some new movement patterns that do not put so much stress in just one spot. It means strengthening the muscles that surround the affected joint. It means finding a different way to do a job, or possibly even finding a new line of work.

Massage?

This is a local contraindication, especially in an acute phase. It is tempting to try to release the muscles around an inflamed bursa, but although the muscles are likely to be tight, working to loosen them will not solve any problems until the inflammation itself has subsided. Bursitis usually does not involve a pathogen that can spread, so massage is certainly indicated for the rest of the body. (If the bursitis *is* caused by an infectious agent, it systemically contraindicates massage until the infection has subsided.)

In the subacute stage, a skilled massage therapist can address the muscles that cross over the affected joint and may well have some success at decompressing the bones that are re-irritating the affected bursa. As with any condition that involves prolonged pain and immobility, it is a good idea to look for compensation patterns that may contribute to pain.

Dupuytren Contracture

Definition: What Is It?

Dupuytren contracture, also called *palmar fasciitis*, is an idiopathic thickening and shrinking of the palmar fascia that limits the movement of the fingers. Usually the ring and little fingers are most severely affected, although the index and middle fingers also may be bent (Figure 2.36).

Demographics: Who Gets It?

This condition strikes mostly middle-aged white men. It shows some statistical links to alcoholism and epilepsy, but no direct connections have been established. It affects 5% to 15% of men over 50 years old. It is rarer among women. Approximately 10% of Dupuytren contracture patients have other family members with the same condition.

Etiology: What Happens?

No one knows exactly *why* the palmar fascia shrinks in this condition, although some think it may have to do with repetitive trauma. The development of Dupuytren contracture resembles the growth of scar tissue in response to trauma, but to an excessive degree. Specialized fibroblasts and other cells contribute to proliferations of type III collagen fibers, both in the fascia on the palm and in the fingers. As the condition progresses, the collagen thickens and toughens, but the active cells recede, leaving tight, thick bands of connective tissue that interfere with the use of the hand.

Signs and Symptoms

Dupuytren contracture may be mildly painful in early stages, but then usually becomes painless. It is sometimes progressive. The pattern is unpredictable, and varies greatly from person to person. Some people experience only the growth of tough, fibrous bumps on their hands, whereas others will end up with severely bent, strangulated, unusable fingers. Dupuytren contracture is bilateral in almost half of all cases.

Treatment

If this condition is left untreated, the connective tissue may simply strangle the muscles and nerves until the affected fingers eventually lose all function. If it is caught before too much atrophy occurs, corticosteroid injections to reduce fascial build-up can be an effective treatment. Injections of collagenase, an enzyme that dissolves collagen, is another treatment option.

> ### Dupuytren Contracture in Brief
>
> **Pronunciation**
> doo-pwē-trah′
>
> **What is it?**
> Dupuytren contracture is an idiopathic shrinking and thickening of the fascia on the palm of the hand.
>
> **How is it recognized?**
> This is a painless condition that usually affects the ring and little fingers, pulling them into permanent flexion.
>
> **Is massage indicated or contraindicated?**
> Massage is indicated for Dupuytren contracture as long as sensation is present, although it may do little to reverse the process if it has progressed too far.

Figure 2.36. Dupuytren's contracture.

Surgical intervention is generally not recommended until fingers become bent and too stiff to move. At that point, the surgery involves making several zig-zag cuts in the palm to release the fascia, followed by skin grafts, physical therapy, and massage to limit the growth of scar tissue. Even when surgery is successful, Dupuytren's contracture recurs in approximately one third of all cases.

Massage?

Dupuytren's contracture does not stem from nerve injury, and sensation is present in the hand, at least before the progression has damaged nerves. Therefore, massage is appropriate. But the connective tissue involved with Dupuytren's contracture is particularly tough and strong. Although massage will certainly not make the condition any worse, it may not make it better either. Massage is a good preventive measure for contractures, but if this condition is already present, it may not be possible to reverse it.

Massage is sometimes recommended along with physical therapy and exercise to help minimize the growth of scar tissue in postsurgical situations.

Ganglion Cysts in Brief

What are they?
Ganglion cysts are small fluid-filled synovial sacks that are attached to tendinous sheaths, or joint capsules.

How are they recognized?
Ganglion cysts form small bumps that usually appear on the hand, wrist, or ankle. They are not usually painful, unless they are in a place to be injured by normal wear and tear.

Is massage indicated or contraindicated?
Ganglion cysts locally contraindicate massage. Friction or direct pressure will not make them go away and may irritate them by stimulating excessive fluid flow.

Ganglion Cysts

Definition: What Are They?

Ganglion cysts are small connective tissue pouches filled with fluid. They grow on joint capsules or tendinous sheaths. They usually appear on the wrist, the hand, or the top of the foot.

Etiology: What Happens?

Although some ganglion cysts seem to be a response to a direct trauma, the vast majority of them simply appear without an identifiable reason. A ganglion cyst is essentially a synovial pouch that forms as an extension of a joint capsule or tenosynovial sheath; in this sense they are very similar to *Baker cysts* (this chapter).

Ganglion cysts are not inherently dangerous, but when they appear on the distal phalanges of the fingers, they can interfere with normal fingernail growth. They also may interfere with joint capsule function at the distal interphalangeal joint.

Signs and Symptoms

Ganglion cysts may be too small to notice, or they may grow to the size of a tennis ball, obstructing joint function and getting in the way of a normal range of motion. Most ganglion cysts are not usually painful, except that they have a habit of growing in places where they can be easily irritated: on the fingers and around the wrists (Figure 2.37). This can put them in a state of chronic irritation, and it can make it difficult for them to heal and subside.

When a cyst grows on the flexor tendon of a finger, movement of that finger may become limited and painful. Some cysts around the wrist or ankle joints may become large enough to limit the normal range of motion for those joints. Most ganglion cysts are not acutely painful.

Figure 2.37. Ganglion cyst.

Treatment

Generally the treatment for ganglion cysts is to leave them alone. It may take a while, but they usually resolve themselves without interference. They may be injected with cortisone, or aspirated to relieve internal pressure, but they grow back approximately half the time. The traditional "home remedy" for ganglion cysts used to be to smash them with a bible. Patients are not recommended to use this option, however, as smashing a ganglion cyst with a book or any other heavy object may rupture the cyst but will probably cause a lot of other soft tissue damage as well.

Cysts may be surgically excised if they are big enough to be a significant problem. They often grow back, but usually they are not as large as the original cyst.

Massage?

Ganglion cysts are a local contraindication. Massage certainly will not make ganglion cysts bigger, worse, or more painful, *unless* they are overstimulated. Massage cannot make them go away, either, so massage therapists should leave them alone. If, however, a client has a mysterious bump on her wrist, foot, or anywhere else, it is important to get a diagnosis before working anywhere in the area.

Hernia

Definition: What Is It?

"Hernia" means hole. Specifically, in this case, it means "hole through which contents that are supposed to be contained are protruding." Muscles may herniate through fascial walls; vertebral discs may herniate; the brain may even herniate through the cranium. But this article discusses the most common types of hernias, which occur in various places around the abdomen.

Etiology: What Happens?

Hernias can be caused by a number of different factors, from congenital weakness of the muscular wall, to childbirth, to abnormal straining, which increases internal abdominal pressure. They can

---

Hernia in Brief

What is it?
A hernia is a hole or rip in the abdominal wall or the inguinal ring through which the small intestines may protrude.

How is it recognized?
Abdominal hernias usually show some bulging and mild to severe pain, depending on whether a portion of the small intestine is trapped.

Is massage indicated or contraindicated?
Untreated hernias locally contraindicate massage. If the hernia is accompanied by fever or other signs of infection, it systemically contraindicates massage. Recent hernia surgeries fall under the category of postsurgical situations. Old hernia surgeries with no complications are fine for massage.

go undetected for a long time if they have a slow onset and the hole is large enough that the intestine is not impaired in any way. Most hernias are *reducible*, which means that the contents can easily be put back where they belong manually. Generally, though, they get worse and worse, bulging more and more often, and perhaps a bigger and bigger hole may develop. Therefore, once a hernia has been identified, surgery to tighten up or close the hole is recommended sooner rather than later. Where a hernia happens and what it will feel like depends mainly on gender and what forces push the abdominal contents against their walls.

Signs and Symptoms

The signs and symptoms of hernias depend on what part of the abdominal wall has been compromised.

- *Epigastric hernia.* This is a bulging superior to the umbilicus. In this condition, the linea alba is split, and a portion of the omentum pushes through. The symptoms, besides a visible lump protruding above the navel, may include a feeling of tenderness or heaviness in the area, but seldom extreme pain. This hernia happens with women and men, but it is more common in men.

- *Paraumbilical hernia.* This is another split of the linea alba, this time right at the navel. It is sometimes a complication of childbirth. The symptoms are the same as the epigastric type, but the bulge is lower. This type of hernia is almost always experienced by women.

- *Femoral hernia.* This is the female equivalent to the inguinal hernia. In this case, the abdominal contents protrude through the femoral ring just below the inguinal ligament. Femoral hernias usually happen only in women, and they can be hard to detect. They can be very dangerous, however, because the hole around the intestine is usually quite small, which increases the chance of strangulation or obstruction of the intestine.

- *Inguinal hernia.* This is the most common variety of hernia. Inguinal hernias are holes in the abdominal wall at the inguinal ring. This opening for the spermatic cord to enter the abdomen is a structurally weak spot. A sudden change in internal abdominal pressure, such as coughing, sneezing, or heavy lifting (especially with simultaneous twisting), may force a section of small intestine right through the hole at this point (Figure 2.38). Inguinal hernias are especially common in infant boys, whose peri-

Small intestine

Figure 2.38. Inguinal hernia.

toneum may not be fully formed. Approximately 700,000 surgeries to correct inguinal hernias are performed every year.

Complications

The seriousness of a hernia is determined by how big it is. Paradoxically, the bigger the hernia, the safer it is, at least for the short term. Small holes, as seen with femoral hernias, have a much greater danger of trapping the intestine in such a way that it cannot function. Either it becomes obstructed, in which case the patient experiences abdominal pain, nausea, and vomiting, or it becomes strangulated, cut off from its blood supply. In this case, the area rapidly becomes red, enlarged, and extremely painful. If no medical intervention is taken, the strangulated loop of intestine may become infected, and possibly gangrenous.

Treatment

Surgery is frequently recommended even for mild hernias because they will tend to get worse and worse as time goes on. Sewing up a small stretch of abdominal fascia is a lot easier than repairing a big rip. The standard surgical technique involves inserting a small piece of mesh at the site of the tear. This helps to distribute the force of abdominal pressure more evenly than do stitches or staples alone, reducing the risk of subsequent hernias at the site of the surgery.

If a person does not need immediate surgery, a special corset or truss may be recommended to prevent sudden changes in abdominal pressure, but trusses are considered only temporary measures, not a solution to the problem.

Massage?

If a client has been diagnosed with a hernia but has not had surgery, that part of the body locally contraindicates any kind of deep massage. Vigorously stretching the fascia around an already weakened area could have disastrous results. If, however, a client has had surgery, follow the guidelines for postoperative cautions. If his or her hernia surgery is ancient history and no pain is present, massage does not pose a danger in any way.

Marfan Syndrome

Definition: What Is It?

Marfan syndrome is the result of a genetic mutation that leads to the production of dysfunctional *fibrillin*, a key connective tissue fiber. The responsible gene, FBN1, is located on chromosome 15. This is an autosomal defect, which means it is not gender specific.

Demographics: Who Gets It?

Marfan syndrome is relatively rare, affecting approximately 1 out of every 5,000 to 10,000 people. It is estimated to affect more than 20,000 people in the United States today. Although it is usually passed from parent to child, approximately 25% of all cases are suspected to be spontaneous mutations of otherwise healthy genes.

Marfan Syndrome in Brief

What is it?
Marfan syndrome is a genetic defect leading to problems in the construction of fibrillin, a connective tissue fiber. Consequently, connective tissues are systemically affected, with the most serious problems occurring in the skeleton, cardiovascular system, and the eyes.

How is it recognized?
Marfan syndrome patients are often taller than average, with very long fingers. Joints tend to be hypermobile. Listening to the heart may show signs of valve problems. Many Marfan syndrome patients are myopic, and up to half experience a dislocated lens in the eye.

Is massage indicated or contraindicated?
Marfan syndrome patients must adjust their daily activities to accommodate for fragility in their connective tissues. Massage must likewise be adjusted to meet the reduced capacity to adjust to changes in their environment.

Marfan Syndrome: History of a Genetic Disorder

Antoine Bernard Marfan was a pioneering specialist in pediatric medicine in Paris at the end of the Nineteenth Century. At a meeting in 1896, he presented a case involving a 5-year-old girl who was abnormally tall, and whose fingers, arms, and legs were disproportionately long. Later studies of this patient showed other anomalies that were eventually classified and named after Dr. Marfan.

As the ability to recognize specific genetic defects developed, Marfan syndrome continued to be a condition that generated a lot of interest. In 1991, the specific chromosome, gene, and component of connective tissue affected by this mutation were finally identified. Future studies of fibrillin and its role in the creation of healthy connective tissue may result in new treatment options for people affected by Marfan syndrome.

Etiology: What Happens?

Marfan syndrome is a result of the production of faulty protein fibers with the consequence that certain connective tissues throughout the body may be weak or otherwise dysfunctional. The musculoskeletal system, the heart and aorta, and the eyes are most at risk for problems related to Marfan syndrome.

Signs and Symptoms

Marfan syndrome is a multisystem disorder, but it manifests most often as problems with the musculoskeletal system, heart and aorta, or eyes.

- *Musculoskeletal system anomalies*: People with Marfan syndrome frequently have unusually long fingers and toes (Figure 2.39), and disproportionately long arms and legs. One test for this disorder is the wrist test: persons with Marfan syndrome can overlap the thumb and fifth digit (little finger) of one hand while encircling the other wrist. Ligament laxity is another common sign, which opens the door to joint injuries and *osteoarthritis* (this chapter).

Other skeletal signs include chest deformities: a flat chest with a protruding sternum, or with a sunken sternum, is common. This anomaly can contribute to pulmonary problems and a high risk of congestive *heart failure* (Chapter 4). Early-onset and rapidly progressive *scoliosis* (this chapter) is another common sign of Marfan syndrome.

- *Cardiovascular system anomalies*: The aortic and mitral valves are particularly vulnerable to problems with connective tissue stability. Prolapsed valves lead to regurgitation of blood and irregular heartbeat. Furthermore, people with Marfan syndrome develop a progressively stiff, inelastic aorta, especially at the ascending section. A ruptured *aneurysm* (Chapter 5) or aortic dissection is a common cause of death for this population.

Figure 2.39. Marfan syndrome: abnormally long fingers.

- *Eye disorders*: *Myopia* (nearsightedness) is very common with Marfan syndrome. Up to 50% of all patients have a dislocated lens. A high risk of detached retina, a medical emergency that could lead to blindness, is also present.

Diagnosis

No easily accessible blood or genetic test is available to identify Marfan syndrome, and this disorder closely resembles some other rare cardiovascular problems, so it is usually diagnosed through clinical examination, family history, and careful observation.

Treatment

Marfan syndrome can only be treated by symptom; no therapy can reverse the action of mutated genes. Beta-blockers are frequently prescribed to reduce the load on the aorta. Prophylactic antibiotics are recommended when even distant procedures are performed, because heart valves are highly susceptible to infection.

Surgical interventions are not always necessary, but when the curve of scoliosis or the shape of the thorax interferes with normal breathing, this may be corrected. Similarly, if early-stage aneurysm or mitral valve prolapse is identified, these situations can be surgically addressed.

Massage?

Marfan syndrome weakens connective tissue and interferes with some activities of daily living. Patients are recommended not to engage in contact sports, or activities that put undue stress on the heart and aorta. With these cautions in mind, careful massage that respects the fragility of connective tissues may be appropriate for clients with Marfan syndrome, as long as their cardiovascular health can keep up with the changes massage may bring about. This is a good situation in which to work as part of a well-informed health care team.

Osgood-Schlatter Disease

Definition: What Is It?

Osgood-Schlatter disease (OSD) is a condition involving irritation and inflammation at the site of the quadriceps insertion on the tibial tuberosity. It occurs when the quadriceps muscles are vigorously used in combination with rapid growth of the leg bones.

Demographics: Who Gets It?

OSD is a condition that is practically exclusive to adolescent athletes. It is especially common among people who participate in sports that involve running, jumping, and making fast, tight turns. Soccer, basketball, figure skating, and dancing are all sports with a high incidence of athletes who develop OSD.

OSD occurs in both boys and girls, although it is more common in boys. The average age of onset for boys is 11 to 18 years old; for girls it can occur a little earlier, between 10 and 16 years of age.

Incidence of OSD in the United States is unknown. Some experts estimate that it affects between 16% and 20% of young athletes to some extent.

Osgood-Schlatter Disease in Brief

Pronunciation
oz'good shlaht'ere dĭ-zēz'

What is it?
Osgood-Schlatter disease is the result of chronic or traumatic irritation at the insertion of the quadriceps tendon, in combination with adolescent growth spurts.

How is it recognized?
When Osgood-Schlatter disease is acute, the tibial tuberosity is hot, swollen, and painful. The bone may grow a large protuberance at the site of the tendinous insertion.

Is massage indicated or contraindicated?
An acute flair of Osgood-Schlatter disease locally contraindicates circulatory massage, which could exacerbate inflammation. Techniques for reducing lymphatic retention and work elsewhere on the body are certainly appropriate. A client with a history of Osgood-Schlatter disease but no current inflammation at the knee may benefit from the pain relief and balance in quadriceps muscle tone that massage can supply.

Figure 2.40. Osgood Schlatter disease: a protuberance at the tibial tuberosity is visible, and the blurry area indicated by the arrow shows where inflammatory edema has accumulated.

Etiology: What Happens?

When children enter their teen years, they begin a time of rapid bone growth, especially in their femurs and tibias: the bones that eventually determine how tall a person will be. Most of the time the muscles, fascia, and other connective tissues in the legs can easily keep up with the accelerated growth rate during this time, but when the quadriceps muscles are particularly taxed through demanding athletics, the combination of stresses can cause the insertion of this powerful muscle group to become irritated and inflamed.

OSD involves acute inflammation of the quadriceps insertion at the tibial tuberosity. The tendon can pull away from the bone, causing a variety of *tendinitis* (this chapter), or in extreme cases the tibia itself can become damaged and even develop an avulsion: a forceful separation of a part of the bone from chronic tendinous tension. Even if the tibia does not break, it is common for OSD patients to develop a large, permanent bump at the tibial tuberosity; this is where the bone adapts to the constant pull of the quadriceps insertion (Figure 2.40). OSD is usually unilateral, but a small number of athletes may develop inflammation at both knees.

The severity of OSD varies greatly from one person to the next; one person may have to be careful about not over-stressing her knee, whereas another athlete may have to quit the team altogether. It is generally a self-limiting condition, which means that when the connective tissue growth "catches up" to the bone growth, the pain and irritation subsides. Unfortunately, this can take anywhere from several months to 2 years.

Signs and Symptoms

OSD is easy to identify because the people susceptible to it are such an unambiguous group: athletic teens. In acute stages of OSD, the knee is hot, swollen, and painful, just distal to the patella at the tibial tuberosity. Any activity that stresses or stretches the quadriceps will aggravate symptoms.

When OSD is not acute, pain and inflammation are resolved, but the characteristic bump of the remodeled tibia will be permanent. A person who had OSD as a child may never be comfortable kneeling, because of tibial distortion.

Treatment

Treatment for OSD focuses on reducing pain and limiting damage to the quadriceps attachment at the tibia. Mild cases can be managed by heating the knee with hot packs before athletic events, and icing them afterward. NSAIDs may be suggested to help with pain and inflammation, and doctors or physical therapists may recommend that stretches designed to reduce tension in the quadriceps be performed several times a day.

More severe cases may require that the athlete suspend his or her activity until the pain and inflammation have been gone for several weeks. In the meantime, the knee may be supported with a brace or cast. This period is followed by aggressive quadriceps exercise to strengthen the muscles and reduce the chance of a recurrence when the athlete becomes active again.

In rare cases, the knee may require surgery to remove bits of the tibia that may have been pulled off and suspended in the tibial tendon.

Massage?

In its acute stages, OSD locally contraindicates circulatory massage, which only exacerbates inflammation. Other techniques that may reduce edema can be appropriate, as is work anywhere other than the affected knee.

When the knee is not acutely painful, massage may be useful in reducing quadriceps tension that pulls on the tibial tendon. Massage is unlikely to resolve or reverse a case of OSD, but it may help to deal with the pain it causes, and speed up recovery so that a teen athlete may more quickly and safely resume activity.

Pes Planus, Pes Cavus

Definition: What Are They?

Pes planus ("flat feet") is the medical term for feet that lack the medial arch between the calcaneus and the great toe, the lateral arch between the calcaneus and the little toe, and the transverse arch that stretches across the ball of the foot.

Pes cavus ("caved feet") is the term for feet with jammed arches: a hyperaccentuated arch that does not flatten out with each step, but instead stays high and immobile.

Etiology: What Happens?

Pes planus and pes cavus may develop because of a congenital problem in the shape of the foot bones, or the strength of the foot ligaments. They may arise from the unending battle between the deep flexors and everters, combined with footwear that offers little or no support to the intertarsal ligaments that are supposed to hold up the arches (Figure 2.41).

Pes planus in particular has been studied in relation to a poorly functioning tibialis posterior tendon. This leads to hypertonicity and imbalanced pulling, especially at the peroneus muscles on the lateral aspect of the foot.

Pes cavus, when it is serious enough to interfere with function, is often examined as a complication of an underlying or preexisting disorder. Malunion *fractures* and *shin splints* (this chapter) are often considered. Other neuromuscular disorders such as Charcot-Marie-Tooth syndrome, *muscular dystrophy* (this chapter), *polio*, or *cerebral palsy* (Chapter 3) are other factors that may contribute to jammed arches.

Complications

Whichever direction the tarsal bones go—to the floor or to the roof—if they lack mobility, a critical feature of foot architecture is missing: shock absorption. Each time the foot hits the ground, thousands of pounds of downward pressure should be softly

---

Pes Planus, Pes Cavus in Brief

Pronunciation
pes plăˈnŭs, pes kăˈvŭs

What are they?
These are the medical terms for flat feet or jammed arches.

How is it recognized?
In pes planus, the feet lack any arches. Pronation of the ankle also may be present. Persons with pes cavus have extremely high arches with little or no mobility between the tarsal bones.

Is massage indicated or contraindicated?
Pes planus and pes cavus indicate massage. In some cases, the health of intrinsic foot muscles and ligaments can be improved to the point where alignment in the foot is also improved. In cases in which the ligaments are lax through genetic or other problems, massage may not correct the situation, but neither will it make it worse.

Figure 2.41. Pes planus: the "stirrup" of lower leg muscles that support
the medial arch of the foot.

distributed through the tarsal bones, which flatten out and then rebound in preparation
for the next step. If the arches are somehow compromised and the bones lose their
rebound capacity, all that force reverberates through the rest of the skeleton. This is how
flat feet or jammed arches can lead to arthritis in the feet, heel spurs, *plantar fasciitis* (this
chapter), **neuromas**, knee problems, hip problems, back problems, even headaches and
TMJ disorders. Furthermore, foot problems can be especially dangerous for people with
poor peripheral circulation, such as *diabetes* patients (Chapter 8) because chronic friction
and irritation at isolated spots can lead to sores on the feet.

     All of these processes point back to the central idea that should echo throughout
good anatomy training: *everything in the body is connected to everything else*. Pes planus and
pes cavus are excellent examples of how an "insignificant" problem in one place can
create *very* significant problems elsewhere. These problems can be difficult to track down
and correct unless a therapist knows where to look.

Treatment

Unless they lead to serious arthritis or plantar fasciitis, flat feet or jammed arches often do not hurt in the feet as much as causing dysfunction in other places in the body. When this is the case, they may never be treated at all. If a person is aware that the alignment in his feet is a problem, he may be recommended to switch to highly supportive shoes, perhaps with orthotic inserts. Physical therapy to strengthen the peroneus longus and tibialis posterior muscles may be suggested. Rarely, surgery may be performed to repair injured tendons that can contribute to flat feet, or to reshape foot bones, or to fuse foot joints for reduced pain and improved stability.

When pes cavus is related to an underlying condition and function could be restored by surgically releasing tight tissues, this may be considered a viable choice.

Massage?

Pes planus and pes cavus indicate massage. If the problems are congenital, massage will not have much lasting effect, but even temporary relief from pain is better than nothing. Furthermore, massage can ameliorate some of the distant effects of foot problems: knee strain, hip rotation, etc.

If flat feet or jammed arches are related to muscular or ligamentous stresses, massage may have some success at equalizing the tensions between antagonistic muscles and stimulating circulation to the ligaments. Deep, specific massage tips the scales, drawing lots of fresh nutrition to ligaments that otherwise would not get it.

Plantar Fasciitis

Definition: What Is It?

This is a condition involving pain and inflammation of the plantar fascia, which stretches from the calcaneus to the metatarsals on the plantar surface of the foot.

Demographics: Who Gets It?

This is a common problem; 95% of all heel pain is diagnosed as plantar fasciitis. Up to two million cases are reported a year, and that includes only people who seek treatment. It affects men and women equally, and though children *can* get it, adults are far more susceptible because their plantar fascia has generally lost some of its youthful elasticity.

Two populations seem to be at highest risk for developing plantar fasciitis: runners (some estimates suggest that up to 10% of all runners experience plantar fasciitis at some time), and non-athletes who may be overweight, especially if a sudden change is made that puts unusual stress on the foot.

Etiology: What Happens?

When the plantar fascia is overused or stressed by misalignment, its fibers tend to fray or become disorganized (Figure 2.42). Some controversy is developing over whether plantar fasciitis is actually an inflammatory condition or whether it has more to do with the degeneration of the collagen matrix of the *plantar aponeurosis*, putting it more in

---

Plantar Fasciitis in Brief

What is it?
Plantar fasciitis is the pain and inflammation caused by injury to the plantar fascia of the foot.

How is it recognized?
Plantar fasciitis is acutely painful after prolonged immobility. Then the pain recedes, but it comes back with extended use. It feels sharp and bruise-like, usually at the anterior calcaneus or deep in the arch, but the pain can appear almost anywhere the plantar fascia goes.

Is massage indicated or contraindicated?
Massage is indicated for plantar fasciitis. It can help release tension in deep calf muscles that put strain on the plantar fascia; it also can help to affect the development of scar tissue at the site of the tear.

Area of
involvement

Figure 2.42. Plantar fasciitis.

the category of tendinosis, rather than tendinitis. This has some implications for determining the best treatment options, so it is an important point to consider.

X-rays of people with plantar fasciitis often show that a bone spur has developed at the attachment to the calcaneus. It was once assumed that these bone spurs caused the pain of plantar fasciitis. It is now clear that the chronic irritation of injured fascia stimulates the growth of bone spurs; bone spurs do not cause the fascial irritation.

The pain that accompanies plantar fasciitis occurs when the foot has been immobile for several hours, and then used. The fibers of the fascia begin to knit together during rest, and are re-irritated each time the foot goes into even gentle weight-bearing dorsiflexion.

Causes

Causes of plantar fasciitis vary, but most boil down to overuse or alignment stresses. Being overweight can predispose someone to plantar fasciitis, as can wearing shoes without good arch and lateral support. Flat or pronated feet are associated with this problem, as are jammed arches (see *pes planus, pes cavus*, this chapter). Very tight calf muscles are also contributing factors, especially for runners. Plantar fasciitis may occur as a secondary complication to an underlying disorder such as *gout* or *rheumatoid arthritis* (this chapter).

Signs and Symptoms

Plantar fasciitis follows a distinctive pattern that makes it easy to identify: it is acutely painful for the first few steps every morning. Then the pain subsides or disappears altogether, but becomes a problem again with prolonged standing, walking, or running. A sharp "bruised" feeling either just anterior to the calcaneus on the plantar surface or deep in the arch of the foot often marks this disorder.

Treatment

The most important thing to do for plantar fasciitis is to remove the tensions that cause the plantar fascia to be reinjured every morning when the foot first hits the floor. This can be accomplished in a number of ways: warming and massaging the foot and lower leg before getting out of bed can make the tissue more flexible. Shoe inserts can be helpful to keep the foot from going into deep dorsiflexion; these should be in *all* shoes, including bedroom slippers. Someone with plantar fasciitis should *never* go barefoot until the fascia can stretch without tearing. Another helpful device is a night splint that holds the foot in a slightly dorsiflexed position. This allows the plantar fascia fibers to knit back together in a way that will not be stressed and re-torn so easily.

NSAIDs and topical anti-inflammatories, ice, stretching, and deep massage to the calf muscles and at the site of the tear are frequently prescribed for plantar fasciitis. Corticosteroid injections are sometime given to reduce inflammation if other interventions are unsuccessful, but steroids leak into the fat pads on the heels, and may weaken the collagen fibers and increase the risk of plantar fascia rupture, so they are used only sparingly. As a last-ditch option, surgery may be performed to sever the plantar fascia altogether. This may eradicate pain, but it also creates more instability in the foot, which can lead to problems in the rest of the body. Shockwave lithotripsy, similar to that used to break up kidney stones, is being used with some success as an alternative to surgery for plantar fasciitis. Long-term success rates for this modality are not yet available.

No single treatment is universally effective; each patient must experiment with the treatments that meet his or her own needs. It takes patience to overcome this stubborn injury; even the most successful treatment options often take up to 12 weeks to completely resolve injuries.

Massage?

Plantar fasciitis responds well to bodywork. Massage is often suggested both to decrease tension in the deep calf muscles and to have an organizing influence on collagen fibers within the plantar fascia itself.

Scleroderma

Definition: What Is It?

Scleroderma is a chronic autoimmune dysfunction in which abnormal proteins called *autoantibodies* attack and damage small arteries. This stimulates the production of excessive amounts of collagen in the skin, hence the name: *sclero* (from Greek for "hard")–*derma* (from Greek for "skin").

Demographics: Who Gets It?

Like many autoimmune diseases, scleroderma affects women more often than men; in this case the ratio is about four to one. It is a relatively rare disease, affecting approximately 300,000 people in the United States. Most scleroderma patients are women between 35 and 54 years of age. It is rare in children and elderly people.

Etiology: What Happens?

Scleroderma is the result of an overactive immune system that launches attacks against normal tissue. In this case, the tissue under

---

Scleroderma in Brief

Pronunciation
sklēr-ö-der'mă

W hat is it?
Scleroderma is a chronic autoimmune disorder involving damage to small blood vessels that leads to abnormal accumulations of scar tissue in the skin. Internal organs also may be affected.

How is it recognized?
Scleroderma can have many varied symptoms, depending on which tissues are involved. The most common outward signs are edema followed by hardening and thickening of the skin, usually of the hands and face.

Is massage indicated or contraindicated?
Scleroderma may indicate massage if circulatory and kidney damage is not advanced. Clients whose systems are not capable of keeping up with the changes circulatory massage brings about may benefit from bodywork with less mechanical impact.

attack is the lining of arterioles. Damage to these small blood vessels causes local edema and the stimulation of nearby fibroblasts to spin out huge amounts of collagen: the basis for scar tissue. Eventually the edema subsides, but the scar tissue deposits remain hard and unyielding for years at a time. Scleroderma takes two forms: localized or systemic.

- *Localized scleroderma.* When scleroderma is a localized situation, the areas of blood vessel damage are usually limited to the skin. The initial edema may last for several weeks or months, the thickening of the skin may accumulate over a course of about 3 years, and then the symptoms gradually stabilize or even reverse.

   Localized scleroderma is often discussed in two forms: *morphea*, in which it affects disconnected patches of skin, and *linear*, in which it appears as a discolored line or band on a leg, arm, or over a forehead.

- *Systemic scleroderma.* When scleroderma is a systemic problem, blood vessel damage occurs in the skin as with localized scleroderma, but also in other organs and systems. Tissues most at risk are in the digestive tract, the heart and circulatory systems, the kidneys, lungs, and various parts of the musculoskeletal system, especially synovial membranes in joints and around tendons. When systemic scleroderma attacks the lungs, kidneys, or heart, the prognosis becomes much more serious. This disease can be fatal.

   Systemic scleroderma is also called "systemic sclerosis," and it is recognized in three forms.

- *Limited systemic scleroderma* has a slow onset and begins as CREST syndrome (see *signs and symptoms* below) but may eventually infiltrate internal organs

- *Diffuse scleroderma* has a more sudden onset and earlier involvement of internal organs.

- *Sine scleroderma* does not involve the skin at all; it only involves internal organs. (*"Sine"* means "without.")

Causes

The cause of scleroderma is unknown, but several contributing factors have been identified. One of the most interesting features of this disease is that a large number of patients have accumulated *"chimeric* cells" in their sclerotic deposits. These are cells that contain genes not only of the patient, but of someone else as well: usually they are leftover fetal cells, from pregnancies that may date from many years previously. Somehow these fetal cells, which traveled from child to mother during gestation, manage to survive in the mother, stimulating an autoimmune attack many years later. When scleroderma occurs in children, men, or in women who have never had a child, it is postulated that the chimeric cells may be maternal cells that traveled into the patient during gestation.

The presence of chimeric cells alone does not seem to be the only stimulus for the autoimmune activity associated with scleroderma. But when these cells are present and a person experiences other kinds of triggers, the chance for the disease to develop is much higher. Other triggers for scleroderma involve exposure to specific chemicals, including vinyl chloride, epoxy resins, uranium, and aromatic hydrocarbons.

Signs and Symptoms

Scleroderma can produce a huge variety of symptoms, depending on which blood vessels are under attack. The term "CREST syndrome" has been coined as a mnemonic for the most common scleroderma symptoms:

   C: *Calcinosis* refers to the accumulation of calcium deposits in the skin.

   R: *Raynaud's phenomenon* is a result of impaired circulation and vascular spasm in the hands (see Chapter 4).

Figure 2.43. Scleroderma.

E: *Esophageal dysmotility* refers to sluggishness of the digestive tract and chronic gastric reflux.

S: *Sclerodactyly* is "hardening of the fingers," a result of the accumulation of scar tissue in the hands (Figure 2.43).

T: *Telangiectasia* is a discoloration of the skin caused by permanently stretched and damaged capillaries. It is a synonym for "spider veins."

Other symptoms of systemic scleroderma include skin ulcers where circulation prevents normal nutrition for healthy cells, changes in pigmentation, and hair loss. Muscles may become weak, whereas tendons and tendinous sheaths become swollen. Lungs may accumulate edema where blood vessels are under attack. Heart pain, arrhythmia, and *heart failure* (Chapter 4) may develop as the heart tries to push blood through a system that cannot accommodate it. And kidneys, working under high blood pressure and damaged arterioles, may go into *renal failure* (Chapter 9). *Trigeminal neuralgia* (Chapter 3) and Sjögren syndrome (pathologically dry mucous membranes) also may be a part of the scleroderma picture.

Treatment

Scleroderma is typically treated by symptom. Calcium channel blockers may be recommended for Raynaud's phenomenon; diuretics for kidney function; antacids for gastric reflux, NSAIDs for muscle and joint pain. Physical or occupational therapies are often employed to maintain flexibility in the hands. Patients are usually advised to avoid smoking, cold conditions, and spicy foods to minimize symptoms.

As more research is conducted on the presence of chimeric cells in many scleroderma patients, medications may be developed that will help the body recognize these "nonself" entities more efficiently, and eradicate them before they can trigger significant damage.

Massage?

Scleroderma is a disease that presents very differently in each client. One person may have some stiffness and coldness in her hands, and another may be undergoing dialysis because her kidneys are failing. The decision about massage in the context of scleroderma must be made based on the client's circulatory health and resiliency. It is inappropriate to try to mechanically push fluid through a system in which the blood vessels are either inflamed or severely scarred. Bodywork that does not challenge fluid flow, however, can be beneficial.

Tendinitis

Definition: What Is It?

Tendinitis involves injury and inflammation in tendinous tissues. The injury process has a lot in common with strains and sprains, and in fact these injuries may sometimes be difficult to delineate from each other.

Etiology: What Happens?

Tendinitis can occur anywhere in the tendon, but tears happen most frequently at the tenoperiosteal junction or the musculotendinous junction. These areas mark the shift of one tissue type into another. Though the transition may be gradual, this is still a weak point in the structure that is vulnerable to injury.

Signs and Symptoms

The symptoms of tendinitis are very similar to those of muscle strains, though they may be more intense. The acute stage may show some heat and swelling, depending on which tendons are affected. Most tendon swelling is not visible, with a few exceptions, particularly in the Achilles tendon and the posterior tibialis tendon at the medial ankle, both of which may swell significantly with injury.

In all stages of tendinitis, stiffness and pain are present on resistive movements and in stretching. It is easier to sustain a serious tendon tear than a serious muscle tear; muscles are a lot more elastic than tendons are. This condition has a more distinct acute and subacute stage than muscle strains.

Treatment

The quality of the healing of a torn tendon depends largely on what happens between the subacute and maturation phase of scar tissue development. Although the initial collagen fibers generated by the inflammatory response lie down randomly during the subacute phase of healing, weight-bearing stress and stretching cause them to rearrange in alignment with the direction of force once the initial inflammation has subsided. A more in-depth discussion of the stages of injury is covered in *inflammation*, Chapter 5.

If an injured tendon gets too little weight-bearing stress during its maturation phase, the scar tissue fibers do not realign, the collagen is of poor quality, and the tendon is permanently weakened and prone to developing adhesions to nearby structures. This condition is often referred to as *tendinosis*. If the injured tendon gets *too much* use during this time it can rip again, go back into an acutely inflamed state, and accumulate excessive scar tissue. The challenge for the injured person and his health care team is to figure out how much is just the right amount of weight-bearing stress for the maximum benefit to injured tendons.

As with muscle and ligament tears, standard medical approaches to this kind of injury often focus on symptom abatement rather than scar tissue management. Unfortunately, this can create a stubborn, serious problem out of a potentially very minor one, as the unresolved scar tissue weakens rather than strengthens the tendon

---

Tendinitis in Brief

What is it?
Tendinitis is inflammation of a tendon, usually attributable to injury at the tenoperiosteal or musculotendinous junction.

How is it recognized?
Pain and stiffness are usually present, and in acute stages palpable heat and swelling will occur. Pain is exacerbated by resisted exercise of the injured muscle–tendon unit.

Is massage indicated or contraindicated?
Tendinitis indicates massage. In the acute stage, lymph drainage techniques may help to limit and resolve inflammation. In the subacute stage, massage may influence the production of useful scar tissue, reduce adhesions and edema, and reestablish range of motion.

Tendinitis? Tendinosis? Is There a Difference?

Inflammation is not the only cause of tendon pain and weakness. Another term, *tendinosis*, has been used to describe tendons that have sustained significant damage but are no longer inflamed. Tendons with tendinosis may have significant accumulations of disorganized scar tissue, poorly formed collagen, and a reduction is weight-bearing strength, but the inflammatory process is no longer at work—that is, until the structure is re-injured.

Massage is frequently suggested for athletes and other persons with tendinosis to stimulate circulation and improve nutrition in the avascular connective tissue structures, as well as to help stretch and mobilize the damaged tissues.

(see sidebar, "Tendinitis? Tendinosis? Is There a Difference?"). Fortunately, recent advancements in the understanding of how scar tissue develops have begun spreading into more mainstream applications, so the "take painkillers and do not move it for 2 weeks" kinds of treatment strategies for soft tissue injuries are becoming less and less common.

Massage?

Tendinitis definitely indicates massage. Again, however, this condition is more serious than a simple muscle tear, and the acute phase must be respected to allow the body to begin the process of cleaning up debris and laying down new fibers in peace. Practitioners familiar with lymph drainage techniques may be able to limit the accumulation of edema and minimize scar tissue. In the subacute stage, massage will be valuable not only for the mechanical action it can have on badly placed collagen fibers, but for the circulatory turnover it will stimulate in the area of nonvascularized tendons.

Sprains, strains, and tendinitis all respond best to mechanical types of massage in a subacute phase, as soon as the acute symptoms have passed. This is when direct manipulation can have the most profound influence over the quality of healing. The sooner an injury is treated, the more complete resolution a client is likely to have. However, even years-old injuries respond well to massage if the circumstances are right. It may not be possible to completely reverse a 10-year-old tendinitis or tendinosis, but any amount of improvement is significant. For a client who has been living with pain and limitation, any improvement is a lot better than nothing.

Tenosynovitis

Definition: What Is It?

Tenosynovitis is a situation in which tendons that pass through a synovial sheath become irritated and inflamed.

Etiology: What Happens?

Some tendons have to pass through very narrow, crowded passageways or around sharp corners to get to their bony attachments. Without any lubrication, those tendons and their neighbors would soon be worn and frayed. But they *do* have lubrication, provided by special sheaths made of connective tissue and lined with synovial membrane: tenosynovial sheaths. As the tendon or group of tendons pass through the sheath, synovial fluid is secreted to provide lubrication and ease of movement (Figure 2.44).

Repetitive stress, percussive movement, or constant twisting can cause the tendons inside tenosynovial sheaths to become irritated. The sheath may become inflamed and then shrink around the tendons in such a way that it inhibits freedom of movement. A cycle of stiffness followed by irritating movement, which creates more stiffness, pain, and inflammation, may develop.

Causes

Tenosynovitis is usually caused by trauma, repetitive movement, or excessive exercise. It can happen anywhere synovial sheaths protect tendons: the wrist, the ankle, the long head of the biceps, or near the thumb, where it has a special name: *De Quervain's*

Tenosynovitis in Brief

What is it?
Tenosynovitis is the inflammation of a tendon or its surrounding tenosynovial sheath. It can happen wherever a tendon passes through a sheath, but is especially common in the wrist and hand.

How is it recognized?
Pain, heat, and stiffness mark the acute stage of tenosynovitis. In the subacute stage, only stiffness and pain may be present. The tendon may feel or sound gritty as it moves through the sheath. It is difficult to bend fingers with tenosynovitis but even harder to straighten them.

Is massage indicated or contraindicated?
Tenosynovitis contraindicates massage in the acute stage of inflammation and indicates massage when the swelling has subsided.

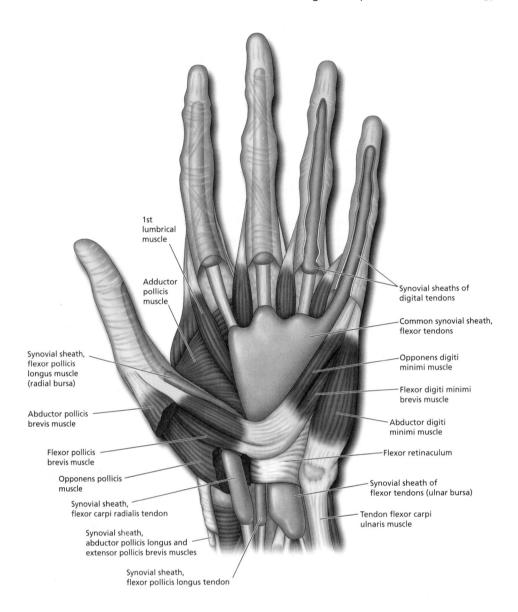

1st
lumbrical
muscle

Adductor
pollicis
muscle

Synovial sheaths of
digital tendons

Common synovial sheath,
flexor tendons

Synovial sheath,
flexor pollicis
longus muscle
(radial bursa)

Opponens digiti
minimi muscle

Flexor digiti minimi
brevis muscle

Abductor pollicis
brevis muscle

Abductor digiti
minimi muscle

Flexor pollicis
brevis muscle

Flexor retinaculum

Opponens pollicis
muscle

Synovial sheath of
flexor tendons (ulnar bursa)

Synovial sheath,
flexor carpi radialis tendon

Tendon flexor carpi
ulnaris muscle

Synovial sheath,
abductor pollicis longus and
extensor pollicis brevis muscles

Synovial sheath,
flexor pollicis longus tendon

Figure 2.44. Synovial sheaths allow groups of tendons to slide easily over each other.

tenosynovitis. Occasionally it can be caused by a local infection that inflames the synovium, but it is usually brought about by mechanical stress. Tenosynovitis also occurs as a complication of other inflammatory wrist problems such as *rheumatoid arthritis* or *fractures* (this chapter).

Signs and Symptoms

Symptoms of tenosynovitis are predictable: local pain, sometimes with swelling and heat. In the case of "trigger finger," it maybe difficult bend the joint, and *unbending* it is even harder; excessive force must be applied to slide the tendon through its sheath, and the joint usually extends with a sudden "pop." A grinding noise or gritty feeling called crepitus occurs when the affected joint is moved. Movement of the tendon through the sheath tends to exacerbate the problem, but lack of movement decreases the production of synovial fluid. It can be a very frustrating condition, because nothing seems to make it better.

Treatment

If the synovium is inflamed because of infection, the obvious course is to treat it with antibiotics. Noninfectious tenosynovitis is typically treated with anti-inflammatory drugs, then injected with steroids, and if that is unsuccessful, the synovium is surgically split.

Massage?

This is an inflammatory condition, and even worse, the inflammation is confined to a very small, crowded space. This makes it counterproductive to work when the condition is hot and painful, because massage will make it hotter and more swollen. During the acute phase, tenosynovitis locally contraindicates massage.

When inflammation is not acute, however, massage can help to reduce inflammation, flush out toxins, and create very specific movements of structures against each other to prevent the accumulation of scar tissue or adhesions. Massage may or may not be able to actually solve the problem of irritation inside the synovial sheath, but it can improve the nutrition and freedom of movement available to the affected structures.

Torticollis

Definition: What Is It?

Torticollis ("wryneck") is an umbrella term for any condition that causes the head to be pulled to one side. A unilateral spasm of a neck muscle or muscles causes the head to become stuck in flexion and rotation.

Etiology: What Happens?

Torticollis can be a simple matter of having "slept funny" so that the neck is stiff and painful all day, or it could be a symptom of a more serious underlying problem.

- *Congenital Torticollis*: In this situation, a genetic abnormality results in the development of only one sternocleidomastoid muscle. Because so many other muscles can rotate and flex the head, this problem may be overcome by physical therapy.

- *Infant Torticollis*: In the late stages of pregnancy, the fetus may lie with the head twisted to one side. This can create a shortened or weakened sternocleidomastoid, as well as cranial bone distortion. This condition is usually successfully treated with exercise and special helmets designed to reshape the cranial bones.

- *Spasmodic Torticollis*: This idiopathic condition is the most common type of *focal dystonia*: abnormal muscle contraction related to a central nervous system disturbance. The spasms may be tonic (sustained contractions), clonic (tremors), or both. Spasmodic torticollis affects approximately 90,000 adults in the United States, creating chronic pain in the neck, back, and shoulder. It has a slow onset that peaks within 2 to 5 years. Occasionally it spontaneously resolves, but it may occur again in later years. Spasmodic torticollis is a life-long condition.

- *Wryneck*: This is a simple stiff neck, often caused by irritation of the intertransverse ligament at C_7. A cervical misalignment also may create the problem, which will not be relieved until both the muscles and the bony alignment have been addressed.

Torticollis in Brief

What is it?
Torticollis is a unilateral spasm of neck muscles. It can be caused by a variety of factors, including mild musculoskeletal injury, congenital abnormalities, or central nervous system problems.

How is it recognized?
Flexion and rotation of the head are the main symptoms. The spasm may be constant or intermittent. Torticollis may also cause pain in the neck, shoulders, and back.

Is massage indicated or contraindicated?
This depends on the cause of the problem. Simple wryneck from trigger points, cervical misalignment, ligament sprain, or trauma may be appropriate for massage if no acute inflammation is present. Spasmodic torticollis patients may benefit from pain relief offered by massage, but work should be done in cooperation with the patient's health care team. If symptoms do not improve, or if signs of systemic infection are present, a more thorough diagnosis should be sought.

Figure 2.45. Torticollis.

Trigger points and spasm in the splenius cervicis are another possible cause. Short-lived cases of wryneck may be brought about by sleeping in a bad position, or some other event or trauma that might cause irritation in the neck muscles (Figure 2.45).

- *Other*: Torticollis can, on rare occasions, be the earliest presenting sign of a more serious condition. Cases have been documented in which it was the first symptom of bone cancer in the spine (the tumor may affect the motor or sensory neurons); bone infections, and even a bad infection of the adenoids: lymph nodes in the neck, which can get so filled with pus that they irritate and cause spasm in the nearby muscles.

Signs and Symptoms

Symptoms of torticollis vary according to the predisposing causes. For specific information, refer to the types of torticollis described above.

Treatment

Treatment for torticollis depends on the underlying cause. Congenital or infantile situations call for exercise and physical therapy to strengthen the auxiliary muscles. For spasmodic torticollis, anticholinergic drugs, injections of botulinum toxin, or surgery to sever the motor nerves in the affected muscles may be recommended. Wryneck from subluxated vertebrae can be addressed by bony manipulation. Specific frictions to the lesion may resolve wryneck caused by ligament irritation; if the scar tissue is very old and difficult to access, corticosteroid injections to limit inflammation and reduce scar tissue may be helpful. Torticollis related only to muscle spasm and trigger points responds well to massage.

Massage?

Chiropractic or manipulation *with* massage for uncomplicated wryneck is a powerful combination, because both the hard and soft tissues receive the attention they need. It is important to remember, however, that torticollis can be an early symptom of some other more serious problems, so if the client's condition does not improve, or if he or she is showing any other signs of infection, a more complete diagnosis is necessary.

Whiplash

Definition: What Is It?

Whiplash, or CAD (cervical acceleration–deceleration) is a broad term used to refer to a mixture of injuries, including sprains, strains, and joint trauma. Bone fractures, herniated discs, and concussion are commonly seen along with these soft tissue injuries, and so are often addressed simultaneously. Whiplash injuries are usually, but not always, associated with car accidents in which the head "whips" backward and forward in rapid succession (Figure 2.46).

Etiology: What Happens?

The nature of damage incurred by whiplash accidents depends on many variables, including the direction of impact, the speed with which the vehicles were moving, the relative weight of the vehicles involved, whether the individual was wearing a seatbelt, the position of the individual's head, and whether the person was aware of the impending impact and had time to brace. Analysis of rear-impact accidents shows that the initial movement of the head is into extension, as the momentum of the car seat forces the thorax forward while the head initially stays stable. Then energy is magnified by the leverage of the neck to increase the forward-moving acceleration of the head. At an impact of 20 miles per hour, the maximum acceleration of the head has been measured at 12 Gs![13]

Accidents of this nature put the cervical muscles (especially the sternocleidomastoid, scalenes, and splenius cervicis) at risk (see *strains*, this chapter). Spinal ligaments also may be damaged (see *sprains*, this chapter). Two ligaments that massage cannot touch are also frequently traumatized: the anterior and the posterior longitudinal ligaments. However, the supraspinous and the intertransverse ligaments *are* accessible, and they are highly vulnerable to injury.

[13] Mahar R. Musculotendinous Injuries of the Neck. Available at: http://www.theberries.ns.ca/Archives/Whiplash.html. Accessed summer 2003.

Whiplash in Brief

What is it?
Whiplash is an umbrella term referring to a collection of soft tissue injuries that may occur with cervical acceleration/deceleration. These injuries include sprained ligaments, strained muscles, damaged cartilage and joint capsules, and TMJ problems. Although whiplash technically refers to soft-tissue injury, damage to other structures including vertebrae, discs, and the central nervous system frequently occurs at the same time.

How is it recognized?
Symptoms of whiplash vary according to the nature of the injuries. Pain at the neck and referring into the shoulders and arms along with chronic headaches are the primary indicators.

Is massage indicated or contraindicated?
An acute whiplash injury contraindicates circulatory or mechanically based massage. In the subacute and maturation phases of scar tissue formation, however, massage along with chiropractic or manipulation can be important contributors to a positive resolution to the problem.

Figure 2.46. Cervical acceleration–deceleration: whiplash.

Other structures that may be injured with CAD include the joint capsules of the facet joints, the esophagus and larynx, spinal discs that may herniate or rupture (see *disc disease*, this chapter); vertebrae that can come out of alignment or fracture (see *fractures*, this chapter); the temporomandibular joint (see *temporomandibular joint disorders*, this chapter); and the spinal cord, which may get stretched and then become edematous, and the brain, which can become bruised and damaged in concussion (see *traumatic brain injury*, Chapter 3).

Signs and Symptoms

A lot of crossover exists between what may be considered a symptom of whiplash, and what is a complication, or resulting disorder; the following is a list of both. Basic signs and symptoms include head and neck pain, which may radiate into the trunk or arms; loss of range of motion, and paresthesia. One of the curious aspects of whiplash is that it is common for symptoms to be delayed for days, weeks, and occasionally months before coming to full intensity. This phenomenon is not well understood.

- *Ligament sprains.* The supraspinous and intertransverse ligaments that connect the vertebrae to each other are at risk of injury in a whiplash-type accident. These ligaments can refer pain up over the head, into the chest, and down the arms. It is important to know about these structures because referred pain from ligaments can easily be misdiagnosed as pain from nerve damage.

  Ligament sprains often take a long time to heal, and they tend to accumulate excess scar tissue. They may be the most common cause of lasting pain and dysfunction when a whiplash injury occurs.

- *Misaligned cervical vertebrae.* This generally shows clearly on an x-ray. Vertebrae may be displaced to the front, back, side, or rotated one way or another. In some very extreme cases, fractures may occur. Left untreated or incompletely treated, misaligned vertebrae with lax ligaments and lack of structural support may develop *spondylosis* (this chapter).

- *Damaged disc.* This is not inevitable, but it frequently happens that the neck ligaments are so stressed in a trauma of this force that the annulus cracks too, allowing the nucleus pulposus to seep into spaces where it does not belong. Car wrecks and other major traumas of this type are the easiest way to cause a herniation in the cervical region.

- *Spasm.* When a neck injury is acute, the paraspinals and other neck muscles go into spasm to "splint" or give extra support to the stretched neck ligaments. However, this reaction has a tendency to outlive its usefulness. Spasm of neck muscles also significantly limits range of motion and blood flow to nearby connective tissues.

- *Trigger points.* Traumatized muscles often develop trigger points: localized tight areas that refer pain, often into the head, causing chronic headaches (see *myofascial pain syndrome*, this chapter).

- *Neurologic symptoms.* These can include dizziness, blurred vision, abnormal smell or taste, *tinnitus* (ringing in the ears), or loss of hearing. These signs indicate cranial trauma: the brain has been bruised and may have some internal bleeding. This is usually the result of a specific blow, hitting the head on the steering wheel, for instance, but postconcussion syndrome can also happen without direct impact.

- *TMJ disorders.* Again, direct impact of the jaw on a steering wheel or dashboard can obviously damage the TMJ, but some research suggests that the joint can be traumatized just by the rapid acceleration/deceleration that accompanies whiplash injuries. TMJ disorders often go unaddressed until the more critical, acute aspects of whiplash have passed.

- *Headaches* (Chapter 3). These arise for a variety of reasons, including but not limited to referred pain and trigger points from spasming muscles in the neck; sprained ligaments that refer pain up over the head; cranial bones that may be out of alignment; stress and its autonomic action on blood flow, and muscle tightness in the neck and head, TMJ problems, and concussion.

Diagnosis

Some assumptions can be made about which precise structures have been injured based on whether the car wreck was a direct head-on or a rear-end collision. These assumptions will not hold true if the impact occurred at an angle, however, or if the person's head was turned in any direction at the moment of contact.

The techniques that are currently available to measure the extent of injury (MRIs, x-rays, CT scans, nerve conduction velocity tests) are extremely valuable for evaluating one particular type of whiplash damage: direct, mechanical nerve pressure. Pressure on a nerve causes "radicular pain": pain that radiates directly along the distribution of the affected nerve. Care must be taken, however, to delineate between what these tests show and what patients report: very frequently MRI or x-ray pictures show anomalies that actually do not create symptoms for the patient.

Unfortunately, much of the pain associated with whiplash injuries is *not radicular* pain, but referred pain brought about by trauma to connective tissue and muscle tissue that feed into the same nerve root as the associated spinal nerve. This type of damage is much harder to quantify. It is best evaluated with good palpation skills that show information about localized tenderness, muscle spasm, and trigger point activity.

Treatment

Neck collars are used for acute whiplash patients to take the stress off their wrenched ligaments, and to try to reduce muscle spasm. But the sooner the injured structures are put back to use, the less scar tissue accumulates. Therefore, collars are strictly for short-term use, because this kind of immobilization can create more long-term problems than benefits.

Medical intervention typically focuses on pain relievers, anti-inflammatories, and muscle relaxants. These substances can change the quality of the tissues, so massage therapists should be aware when clients use them. Physical therapy to strengthen injured neck muscles is usually recommended later in the treatment process.

Other treatments for whiplash depend on the type and severity of specific injuries that have occurred. It has been noticed that most whiplash patients recover completely within a year, but anywhere from 5% to 20% may have long-lasting pain. Whether this disability is from unresolved injury, psychological stress associated with long-term injury, or other factors is difficult to assess. The fact that much of the pain generated by whiplash injuries is difficult to measure makes this a condition that is easy to take advantage of by patients willing to "work the system" for financial gain, and easy to discount by health care professionals and insurers who become frustrated with patients' slow recovery.

Massage?

The acute stage of this injury contraindicates mechanical massage. This is an important phase of healing that massage therapists must not disrupt. Gentle reflexive work with the intention of balancing the autonomic nervous system rather than making changes in the tissue may ameliorate the emotional trauma and shock such an injury often incurs. As long as it does not disrupt the cellular activity at the site of the injury, this type of work is a fine idea.

If it has been established that no other serious disorder is present, such as a herniated disc or spinal fracture, chiropractic or manipulation alone can be sufficient to undo the damage done to the cervical vertebrae in a whiplash injury. However, if muscle spasm is not addressed, bony adjustments are difficult to perform and often do not hold for long

Case History 2.2
Whiplash

Client X: "The Sneezer"
A massage therapist met with a first-time client approximately 1 year after the client had been involved in a car accident. The client was still in considerable pain. He was diagnosed with whiplash and was seeking massage under prescription from his doctor.

The therapist worked slowly and carefully and was encouraged by the client to go deeper into his neck muscles, all the way down to the transverse processes of the neck vertebrae. He felt better after the massage; his muscles were looser and he had an improved range of motion.

Several hours later, the client sneezed. The force of the motion wrenched his neck and re-injured the tissues so that he was in greater pain, more spasm, and had much less range of motion than he had *before* his massage. He returned for another session, but it was ineffective at reducing his pain and dysfunction. He never sought massage again.

What is the moral here? It is utterly unclear whether the first massage put the client at risk of re-injuring himself just by sneezing. The therapist followed all the rules of good sense, worked under medical supervision, and let the client guide her into how much pressure felt comfortable to receive. However, it is necessary to entertain the possibility that the massage somehow *did* put the client at risk, even though the therapist was well-informed and made what seemed to be the right decisions. The point is that no two people will go through the same kind of healing process, and no two people will respond to massage the same way. Massage therapists must weigh the benefits and risks of their work on a case-by-case basis. It is impossible to rely only on books and rules to make decisions about whether to give massage.

because the muscles will simply pull the bones out of alignment again. Furthermore, in the absence of the circulation that can be stimulated by massage, the injured ligaments have little access to nutrition. They tend to accumulate masses of scar tissue that bind to other ligaments and other muscle sheaths, thus turning a temporary loss of range of motion into a permanent one.

Chiropractic or manipulative therapy *with* massage can yield good results, blending the best of soft tissue work (to prevent or reduce muscle spasm, scar tissue accumulation, adhesions, fibrosis, and ischemia) with the best of bony alignment. It is not unusual for someone to emerge from a whiplash recovery with this kind of care in better shape than before they began.

NEUROMUSCULAR DISORDERS

Carpal Tunnel Syndrome

Definition: What Is It?

Carpal tunnel syndrome (CTS) is a set of signs and symptoms brought about by the entrapment of the median nerve between the carpal bones of the wrist and the transverse carpal ligament that holds down the flexor tendons (Figure 2.47). The median nerve supplies sensation to the thumb, forefinger, middle finger, and half of the ring finger (Figure 2.48). If it is caught or squeezed in any way, it creates symptoms in the part of the hand the nerve supplies.

Demographics: Who Gets It?

It is estimated that carpal tunnel syndrome affects up to 1% of the United States population, and up to 10% of people over 40 years old. Up to one million surgeries for this condition are performed every year.

As the physical demands of many occupations have changed over the past few decades, many jobs have become more specialized. Fewer movements are needed to accomplish assigned tasks, but those movements may be performed several thousand times a day. This is true for manufacturing jobs, as well as for people working on

Carpal Tunnel Syndrome in Brief

What is it?
Carpal tunnel syndrome (CTS) is irritation of the median nerve as it passes under the transverse carpal ligament into the wrist. It can have several different causes.

How is it recognized?
CTS can cause pain, tingling, numbness, and weakness in the part of the hand supplied by the median nerve.

Is massage indicated or contraindicated?
Depending on the underlying factors, some CTS cases may respond well to massage. Work on or around the wrist must stop immediately if any symptoms are elicited. It is necessary to get a medical diagnosis to know which type of CTS is present.

Figure 2.47. The carpal tunnel is formed by the transverse ligament (flexor retinaculum) and the carpal bones.

Figure 2.48. Carpal tunnel syndrome affects the thumb, index finger, middle finger, and half of the ring finger.

computers, cash registers, and assembly lines. The National Institute for Occupational Safety and Health reports that the incidence of carpal tunnel syndrome in job-related settings increased by 300% between 1982 and 1992.[14]

CTS is an occupational hazard for massage practitioners and anyone else who performs repetitive movements for several hours every day: people who work with keyboards, string musicians, bakers, check-out clerks. Women with CTS outnumber men by approximately three to one; this may be because their carpal tunnels are smaller to begin with, and so less irritation may lead to symptoms.

Etiology: What Happens?

Pressure on the median nerve may arise from several sources. To develop a treatment strategy (and to assess the appropriateness of massage), the aggravating factors must be determined. The following are some possible causes, with basic medical treatment strategies included:

- *Edema.* Fluid retention, which is common for overweight people as well as menopausal and pregnant women, will create extra pressure in an area where there is no room to spare. The wrist is particularly susceptible because of its normal gravitational position; it is easy for fluid to pool here. CTS caused by edema is usually bilateral and is quite common. It is most often treated with diuretics or other methods designed to help get rid of excess fluid.

- *Subluxation.* Sometimes the carpal bones, especially the capitate bone in the center of the distal row of carpal bones, subluxate toward the palmar side. This can put mechanical pressure on the median nerve that is *not* relieved by diuretics, anti-inflammatories, or any other drugs. This type of CTS is almost always unilateral. Manipulation is the treatment of choice, although the bones often move back into place without intervention. Waiting for that to happen can be something of a gamble; however, because the longer the irritation goes on, the higher the chances of sustaining nerve damage, and the less likely it is that the problem will spontaneously resolve.

- *Fibrotic build-up.* This is the most common variety of carpal tunnel syndrome. The human body simply was not designed to perform the same movements for 8 hours a day, 5 days a week. In an attempt to keep up with demands, the body will tend to

[14] NIOSH Facts: Carpal Tunnel Syndrome. National Institute of Occupational Safety and Health. Available at: http://www.cdc.gov/niosh/muskdsfs.html. Accessed winter 2004.

hypertrophy, or grow bigger and thicker wherever we use it most. This is true of muscles and bones, and it also happens with the tendons and synovial sheaths at the wrist. When they thicken because of overuse, they press on anything soft trying to get through tiny "tunnel" formed by the carpal bones, namely, the median nerve. The transverse carpal ligament also may swell with chronic irritation, adding to the pressure on the median nerve.

Treatment for this situation often begins with a wrist splint: the goal is to keep the carpal tunnel in a neutral position (in which it is as open as possible), and to require less work from the supportive tissues. Steroidal or nonsteroidal anti-inflammatories may be prescribed. Corticosteroid injections into the wrist also may be recommended to reduce inflammation and melt excess connective tissue. If the ligaments surrounding the wrist have become loose enough to allow nearby structures to become irritated, proliferant injections may be recommended to tighten them up.

CTS treatment culminates with surgery: the transverse carpal ligament is split, and some of the accumulated connective tissue is scraped away. Innovations in endoscopic surgery techniques allow surgeons to use tiny incisions and pencil-thin cameras to cut through the transverse ligament from the inside of the carpal tunnel without opening the rest of the tissues of the hand. This allows for a much shorter recovery time and a reduced risk of fresh scar tissue accumulation that would lead to a recurrence of symptoms.

It is important to point out that CTS is one of several conditions, brought about by repetitive stress, called RSIs, or "repetitive stress injuries." The physical stress of repeating the same movements hour after hour, day after day, is one part of this picture, but nutritional deficiencies, poor alignment, fatigue, and the resulting risk for trauma and accidents are also contributing factors.

Signs and Symptoms

Depending on the source and severity of the problem, CTS can manifest as tingling, pins and needles, burning, shooting pains, intermittent numbness, and weakness as innervation to the hand muscles is interrupted. The *thenar* pad may flatten out as the thumb muscles atrophy from lack of nerve stimulation. It is often worse at night, when people may sleep on their arm or turn their wrist into awkward positions. It can be painful enough to wake someone out of a deep sleep. If pressure is taken off the nerve promptly, symptoms tend to disappear. But the worst-case scenario involves permanent damage to the median nerve, resulting in some loss of muscle function and sensation in the hand.

Diagnosis

Carpal tunnel syndrome is generally diagnosed by the description of symptoms and two simple tests: *Tinel test* involves tapping on the wrist while the hand is extended; *Phalen maneuver* involves holding the wrist in flexion for 2 minutes or more to see whether symptoms occur in this position. These are often followed by a nerve conduction test or *electromyogram* that measure nerve impulses passing through the wrist into the hand. Unfortunately, these tests are not conclusive.

Doctors also look for underlying conditions that can contribute to nerve pain in the hands, specifically hypothyroidism, diabetes, gout, rheumatoid arthritis, Lyme disease, pregnancy, and obesity. Any of these factors may cause pain and irritation of the median nerve, but they will not be relieved with standard CTS interventions. It is important to get a very solid diagnosis before attempting to treat this problem, because many other disorders can cause similar problems.

Many factors can contribute to pain or reduced sensation in the wrist and hand. The possibilities include but are not limited to the following:

- *Neck injuries*: Herniated discs and irritated neck ligaments refer pain distally. The worse the irritation, the further the pain refers.

- *Shoulder injuries*: Some rotator cuff tendons also refer pain down the arm. The worse the injury, the further it refers. So again, really bad shoulder injuries can actually cause pain in the wrist.

- *Thoracic outlet syndrome*: Nerve and vascular entrapment at the pectoralis minor or scalenes can create pain in the wrist.

- *Nerve entrapment elsewhere in the arm*: The pronator teres is especially likely to trap a piece of the median nerve between its attachments on the forearm. This can lead to symptoms in the wrist and hand, but they also tend to radiate up the forearm, whereas the symptoms of true CTS only radiate distally.

- *Nerve elongation elsewhere in the arm*: when nerves are inappropriately stretched along bones or around joints, they sustain damage and transmit pain signals.

- *Other wrist injuries*: These can include osteoarthritis, rheumatoid arthritis, tendinitis, and ligament sprains, all of which can cause pain in the wrist and hand, and none of which are affected by any of the standard treatments for CTS.

One difficult thing about CTS is that injuries often run in combinations; this may be referred to as "double crush syndrome." In other words, wrist and hand pain can be caused by any blending of real CTS factors and factors that mimic CTS, but that do not fully respond to typical CTS remedies or interventions.

Treatment

The treatment options for CTS depend entirely on what the causes are. Treatments may range from vitamin therapy, to bony manipulation, to surgery. For more details, review the *causes* section of this article.

Various kinds of carpal tunnel syndrome and other nerve impairment problems often respond well to acupuncture. The National Institute of Health has conducted studies that come to the conclusion that acupuncture is a useful adjunct treatment for this and other nerve conduction disorders.[15] If a client is not getting relief through other non-invasive methods and is reluctant to consider surgery, acupuncture may be a viable alternative.

Massage?

The appropriateness of massage absolutely depends on which kind of CTS the client has, and that determination is not a massage therapist's job. So what can a responsible therapist do? Be sensible: work conservatively, check with the client's health care team, monitor results. Edematous CTS responds well to massage that focuses on draining the forearm. Fibrotic CTS may or may not improve with massage, depending on how thick and where the fibrosis is. CTS due to a subluxation *may* respond to massage and traction, but wrist adjustments are *not* in the scope of practice of massage.

If work on or around the wrist creates any symptoms, stop immediately! If, however, a client experiences some improvement, the therapist may be on the right track. Bodyworkers should proceed slowly, have a clear image of what needs to be accomplished, and work with a doctor for a definitive diagnosis.

[15] Packer-Tursman J. Treatment of Choice. Special to The Washington Post. Tuesday, October 17, 2000; Page Z35 . Copyright © 2000 The Washington Post. Available at: http://www.washingtonpost.com/wp-dyn/articles/A21028-2000Oct17.html. Accessed summer 2003.

Disc Disease

Definition: What Is It?

Disc disease is a situation in which the *soft nucleus* pulposus or the *annulus fibrosis* extend beyond their normal borders. If the disc puts pressure on the spinal cord or spinal nerve roots, pain will be present. If the bulge does not happen to interfere with nerve tissue, no symptoms may be present at all.

Etiology: What Happens?

A typical intervertebral disc is quite a complex package. It has an outer wrapping of very tough, hard material called the *annulus fibrosis*, which envelopes a soft, gelatinous center called the *nucleus pulposus*. Ideally, the shape of the nucleus should be roughly spherical, with the harder annulus layers forming flat surfaces above and below the ball. This combination of textures gives the disc the advantages of strength and resiliency, which it needs to do its job of separating and cushioning the vertebrae (Figure 2.49). The spine is capable of bearing a great deal of weight, partly thanks to this arrangement of the discs.

The outer ring of annulus fibrosis is an arrangement of concentric circles of collagen fibers. These fibers are arranged in such a way that the tighter they are pulled, the stronger they become. Conversely, the closer the vertebrae are, the looser (and weaker) the collagen fibers are. This has great implications for the nucleus pulposus, which relies on a very tight, solid exterior wall for support.

The annulus fibrosis is very strong, but studies show that it starts to degenerate at approximately 25 years. It can sustain multitudes of micro-traumas, but they all contribute to setting the stage for future trouble. At the same time, the nucleus pulposus tends to shrink and dry with age. By the time most people are in their 50s, the nuclei of their discs are no longer soft and gelatinous; they have hardened and thinned. This process begins in the neck where the discs are thinner, but eventually also affects the more massive lumbar discs.

Disc Disease in Brief

What is it?
Disc disease is a situation in which the nucleus pulposus or the surrounding annulus fibrosis of an intervertebral disc protrudes in such a way that it puts pressure on nerve roots, the cauda equina, or on the spinal cord.

How is it recognized?
The symptoms of nerve pressure include back or neck pain, radiculopathy (pain along the dermatome), specific muscle weakness, paresthesia, and numbness.

Is massage indicated or contraindicated?
Back or neck pain that is not acutely inflamed or undiagnosed indicates massage.

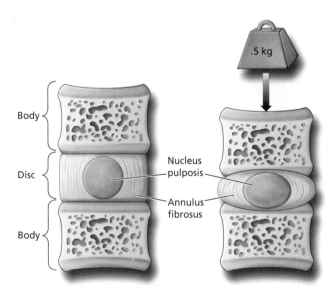

Figure 2.49. Intervertebral discs increase the weight-bearing capacity of the spine.

Causes

Causes of disc injury may vary according to the general health of the connective tissues of the person involved. For some people it takes a major trauma such as a car accident to damage the tissues enough to cause pain. For people with weak, loose intervertebral ligaments, the spine is less stable, and the risk of disc damage from ordinary everyday activity is higher. The classic scenario for this kind of disc damage is an incident that involves simultaneous lifting and twisting.

When the nucleus pulposus protrudes through a hole or crack in the annulus, it can press on nerve tissue and cause very severe problems. This scenario is generally the case for people under 45 or 50 years of age. For older people, the annulus itself may crack and exert pressure on nerve tissue. Of course, if these protrusions do not happen to press on nerve roots or the spinal cord, no symptoms may develop at all.

Progression

When an intervertebral disc is injured and puts pressure on nerve tissue, it is often because of a certain sequence of events on top of a lifetime of normal wear and tear. Here is a typical example of how a lumbar disc may herniate:

- A person bends over to pick up something heavy, a basket full of laundry, for example. Going into trunk flexion flattens the anterior portion of the nucleus, and opens up a posterior space while stretching the posterior fibers of the annulus.

- The person jerks into an erect posture, possibly twisting at the same time, while carrying a heavy load. Suddenly coming back into extension, especially while carrying something heavy, quickly redistributes the nucleus, and shoots it into that posterior space with great force.

- The protruding section of nucleus presses against the weakest part of the posterior annulus and breaks through, which then puts pressure on nerve roots. Or the force

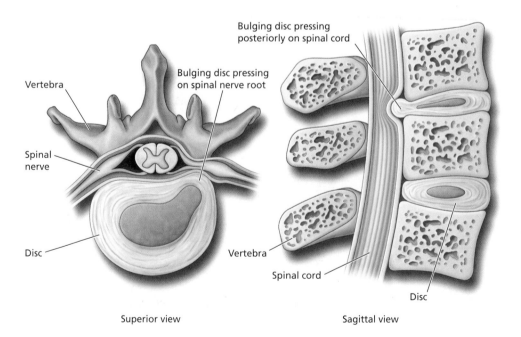

Superior view   Sagittal view

Figure 2.50. Herniated nucleus pulposus.

of the motion, combined with the brittleness of the annulus, causes the annulus to crack and put pressure on nerve tissue. The chemical substance of the nucleus pulposus creates a very extreme inflammatory response that can be a major contributor to the nerve pain that accompanies these injuries.

Many variations may develop on this theme. Discs that cause pain usually bulge posterolaterally, because that is the path of least resistance in the tight space they inhabit, but they also can go to the left or the right side (Figure 2.50). A "mushroom" disc may bulge in both directions. Occasionally a disc bulges directly posteriorly, which puts pressure on the spinal cord or *cauda equina* rather than nerve roots. This is a very serious situation that can lead to permanent damage. However, usually the protrusion is on nerve roots rather than the spinal cord, and the amount of herniated material is very small. It dries up and takes pressure off the nerve roots within a few days or weeks. This leaves the disc permanently thinned, but does not necessarily lead to long-lasting problems.

L_4 and L_5 injuries are the most common with the kind of lifting or lifting-and-twisting injury described here. Cervical disc lesions are an occasional problem for car crash survivors; the action of a *whiplash* (this chapter) can be similar to the injury described above. Thoracic injuries are possible, but rarer, because the ribs make the thoracic spine much more stable than its cervical and lumbar counterparts.

Types of Disc Problems

It does not make a great deal of difference to the applicability of massage to specific cases, but it is useful to be able to recognize the terminology for different types of disc problems that may turn up in a diagnosis.

- *Herniated nucleus pulposus*: In this case, the nucleus pulposus extends beyond the posterior margin of the vertebral body.
- *Degenerative disc disease*: This refers to mild tears of the annulus, along with decreased disc height and dehydration of the nucleus. Degenerative disc disease is often considered a normal part of the aging process, although it is accelerated by smoking, obesity, and sedentary lifestyle.
- *Internal disc disruption*: This condition is often related to trauma in addition to cumulative degenerative disc disease. In this case, the nucleus protrudes through the annulus.
- *Bulge*: This refers to a situation in which the entire disc protrudes beyond the normal boundaries of the vertebral body.
- *Protrusion*: In this, the nucleus pulposus extends out of the annulus at a specific location. If it protrudes posterolaterally it may put pressure on nerve roots. If it protrudes straight back, it could put pressure on the spinal cord or cauda equina.
- *Extrusion*: This is a protrusion of a small piece of the nucleus with a narrow connection back to the body of the nucleus. In some cases, the protrusion can separate from the nucleus altogether.
- *Rupture*: The nucleus pulposus has burst and leaked its entire contents into the surrounding area. Ruptures are less painful than other disc problems, because the pressure has been removed from the nerve tissue.

Signs and Symptoms

Discs have no direct nerve or blood supply, so the only symptoms they elicit are from the pressure that they put on surrounding ligaments and nerve fibers. The pressure can come and go as the patient's position and alignment shifts, and so the symptoms may be intermittent. This is very important: it is appropriate to work with a herniated disc client when their symptoms are abated; it is *not* appropriate to work when the affected disc is irritated and painful. Symptoms of an acute situation include:

- *Local and radicular pain.* Pain is felt locally from inflammation and ligament irritation, as well as along the dermatome for the affected nerve roots. A dermatome chart is a critical piece of equipment for a massage therapist working with this population.

- *Specific muscle weakness.* It is important to clarify the difference between general weakness, which will occur after a length of time of disuse or injury to whole muscle areas, and specific weakness, which will occur fairly quickly, and only in the muscles supplied by the affected nerve.

- *Paresthesia.* "Pins and needles." It happens along the affected dermatomes.

- *Numb-likeness.* Numb-likeness is a feeling of reduced sensation, but not completely absent sensation. It is a common symptom of ligament damage (which may frequently accompany disc damage).

- *Numbness.* Total numbness is one distinguishing factor between disc problems and ligament injuries. A disc protrusion can completely cut off sensation to areas within a particular dermatome, whereas a ligament injury cannot. When a person experiences numbness in a "saddle distribution," i.e., the low back, groin, and medial thigh, this is an indication of pressure on the cauda equina, or "cauda equina syndrome." This is a medical emergency, and requires immediate attention.

Diagnosis

It is important to get a solid diagnosis for disc injuries because many of the signs and symptoms listed above may be caused by other disorders entirely. Many neurologists agree that disc pressure accounts for less than 2% of all neck and back pain.

Discs are generally examined by a combination of x-rays, CAT scans, myelograms, and MRIs. Similar symptoms may be exhibited by two other conditions that require vastly different treatment. *Spondylosis* (this chapter) may lead to osteophytes, and bone cancer may cause tumors. Both may lead to the same kind of nerve pressure that creates the signs of a herniated disc.

One situation that mimics a disc problem but is actually much less serious is a ligament sprain. Irritated spinal ligaments running between spinous or transverse processes can refer pain along the same dermatomes as the nearby discs. Ligament injuries do *not* cause total numbness or specific muscle weakness, however, and they respond well to specific types of massage (see *sprains*, this chapter).

Treatment

The best of all possible resolutions for a herniated disc is for the bulging nucleus pulposus to be reabsorbed into the center of the disc, and for the annulus to close down behind it. Chiropractors and osteopaths will work to correct bony alignment to create a maximum of space for the nucleus to retreat. Medical doctors recommend strict bed rest or traction for the same reason. Physical therapy and special classes on correct posture and body mechanics are often recommended to people recovering from disc problems. Drugs that are prescribed for herniated discs are aimed at the tendency for muscles to seize up in response to this kind of trauma: muscle relaxants and painkillers. If nothing else works, cortisone is sometimes injected into the area. This powerful anti-inflammatory helps only approximately half of the time, and is often considered the last resort before surgery.

If bed rest does not help and the protrusion does not run its course of drying up and disintegrating, it may be necessary to consider other kinds of intervention. One option is called *chemonucleolysis*. This procedure involves injecting a preparation of papain, an enzyme from papayas that dissolves proteins (it is also used in meat tenderizer) into the

Compare and Contrast
IS IT REALLY DISC DISEASE?

Injured discs are generally diagnosed through a combination of x-rays, CT scans, myelograms, and MRIs. It is important to arrive at a clear diagnosis, because similar symptoms may be exhibited by three other conditions that require vastly different treatment: *spondylosis* (this chapter), ligament *sprains* (this chapter), and, infrequently, bone tumors.

Spondylosis may lead to osteophytes that can put direct pressure on nerve tissue.

Irritated spinal ligaments running between spinous or transverse processes can refer pain along the same dermatomes as the nearby discs. Ligament sprains do *not* cause total numbness or specific muscle weakness, however, and they respond well to specific types of massage (see *sprains*, this chapter).

Bone tumors, by far the least common of these options, may involve growths in the spine that put mechanical pressure on nerve roots in much the same way that bulging discs may do.

Individuals seeking a definitive diagnosis for their back, neck, arm, or leg pain may be frustrated by the fact that spondylosis, herniated discs, and irritated spinal ligaments may all exist simultaneously and in any combination. Here are some basic guidelines in trying to sort out the most common sources of pain.

DISC DISEASE

Best diagnostic tool . . .
MRI to see soft tissue distortion

When the person coughs or sneezes . . .
Symptoms are elicited.

Things that make it worse . . .
Sitting for long periods, flexion of the spine

Pattern of weakness:
Specific muscle weakness in the muscles supplied by the affected nerve root.

Pattern of pain:
Shooting electrical pain along dermatome, numbness, reduced sensation, paresthesia. May be intermittent as the disc changes shape and size.

SPONDYLOSIS

Best diagnostic tool . . .
X-ray or CT scan for bony definition

When the person coughs or sneezes . . .
Symptoms do not change.

Things that make it worse . . .
Extension of the spine

Pattern of weakness:
Specific muscle weakness in the muscles supplied by the affected nerve root.

Pattern of pain:
Same symptoms as with disc disease are dependably elicited when the spine is in a position that lets osteophytes press on nerve tissue.

LIGAMENT IRRITATION

Best diagnostic tool . . .
A skilled clinical examination to identify areas of injury

When the person coughs or sneezes . . .
Symptoms do not change.

Things that make it worse . . .
Standing, twisting movements

Pattern of weakness:
General muscle weakness may gradually appear if the situation is present for a prolonged period.

Pattern of pain:
Pain (usually not electrical) along dermatome, reduced sensation, paresthesia.

disc. This material reduces the size of the protrusion, takes pressure off the nerve tissue, and so restores the patient to a pain-free state, all without major surgery. *Transcutaneous diskectomies*, the removal of disc material through a tiny incision, are sometimes also possible. Laser discectomy is a newer procedure that is having good results but is not yet widely available.

Open surgery is generally recommended, however, when the disc puts pressure directly on the spinal cord. In this procedure, a portion of the posterior arch of the vertebra is cut, and the protruding part of the disc is removed, along with the rest of the nucleus pulposus. Another surgical option is to fuse the affected vertebrae together. This certainly increases stability at the spot but may lead to hypermobility at the joints above and below the fusion as they compensate for the loss of motion at the fused joint. Hypermobility then increases the risk of future disc problems at the joints above and below the site of the original problem.

Massage?

Most people with disc disease have good days and bad days. Massage therapists should avoid mechanical techniques on the bad days, and on the good days, work with the intention of creating space for the retreat of the bulging tissue. Referred pain and muscle spasms always accompany this condition. Compensation patterns that develop with chronic back pain also demand attention.

It is especially important not to work alone with a disc injury. Muscle spasm can serve an important protective function for newly damaged discs, and releasing it too soon may put a client in danger (See *spasms, cramps*, this chapter). Working with another professional who can handle the bony or medical end of the injury helps the client recover faster and more completely than he or she would have with either professional alone.

Myasthenia Gravis in Brief

Pronunciation
mī-as-thē′nē-ă gra′vis

What is it?
Myasthenia gravis (MG) is a neuromuscular disorder in which an autoimmune attack is launched against acetylcholine receptors at the neuromuscular junction. This makes it difficult to stimulate a muscle to contract, leading to fatigue and weakness.

What does it look like?
Myasthenia gravis can develop at any age, but it is most common in women in their 20s, and in men in their 50s. It often begins with weakness in facial muscles and in the muscles used in speech, eating, and swallowing. MG is a progressive disease, but it is usually treatable with medical intervention.

Massage?
Massage can be appropriate for persons with MG, because this disease does not affect sensation. Massage may not impact acetylcholine uptake in any positive way, but it will not make it worse either. Care must be taken to respect the side effects that accompany medications used to treat MG.

Myasthenia Gravis

Definition: What Is It?

In 1890, a German doctor named Wilhelm Erb documented several patients with a "grave muscular weakness." This was the first written reference to what is now called *myasthenia gravis* (MG). MG is an autoimmune disease that involves the degeneration or destruction of specific receptor sites at neuromuscular junctions. It is a progressive disease, but it is usually manageable with the right kinds of intervention.

Demographics: Who Gets It?

Although MG has been diagnosed in babies as young as 1 and in adults as old as 80, it is seen most often in women in their 20s and men in their 50s. It affects approximately 14 out of every 100,000 people, and anywhere from 24,000 to 36,000 Americans live with this condition.

Etiology

MG is one of the best-understood autoimmune diseases. In learning about this condition, we have come to a much clearer understanding of the chemistry of muscular contractions. Before we examine the disease process, however, it will be worthwhile to review how nerves normally work with muscles.

Anatomy Review: The Neuromuscular Junction Every motor neuron contacts its muscle cell at a specialized area on the cell membrane called the motor end plate. At this junction, a chemical called *acetylcholine* is released from the motor neuron. Acetylcholine moves across the synaptic cleft onto specialized receptor sites within the motor end plate. This stimulates the opening of channels into the membrane of the muscle cell. Sodium ions that have traveled the length of the motor neuron then flow through the channels, stimulating the release of positively charged calcium ions from the sarcolemma, or muscle cell membrane. The release of these calcium ions initiates muscular contraction. Acetylcholine, a neurotransmitter associated with increased excitability, is a key player in the lightning-fast cascade of events that translates electrical stimulation into chemical reactions.

Two theories have developed about the origins of the autoimmune reactions that lead to MG. One states that B-cells trained in the thymus are inappropriately sensitized against acetylcholine receptor sites on motor end plates. This causes the production of antibodies that attack the sites, reducing their efficiency or blocking them altogether. The fact that the thymus gland of people with MG is abnormal up to 90% of the time points to this possibility. Thymic abnormalities usually involve hypertrophic thymuses or the growth of benign tumors (thymomas) that are easily removed.

Another theory behind the development of MG is that the immune system simply misinterprets the target tissue, in this case, acetylcholine receptor sites, as "nonself." This kind of autoimmune mistake is usually made after exposure to some pathogen with a protein coat pattern similar to the target tissue. Some evidence indicates that exposure to the *herpes simplex* (Chapter 1) virus can lead to MG.

In either case, molecular studies of affected motor endplates indicates that acetylcholine receptors are impaired or completely disabled in MG patients. This means that the muscle cell cannot be stimulated by its motor neuron.

Signs and Symptoms

Most people with MG report weakness and fatigability in affected muscles. The process begins most often around the eyes or lower face. Early signs include a flattened smile; droopy eyelids *(ptosis)*; and difficulty with eating, swallowing, and speech.

Symptoms tend to fluctuate during the day, being worse early in the morning and late at night. Repetitive activity, emotional stress, overexertion, exposure to heat, and some medications can make symptoms much worse.

The typical MG patient experiences degeneration of muscle function for 2 or 3 years after diagnosis, and then symptoms tend to level off, sometimes even going into complete remission. However, MG is a progressive disease, and without intervention it can move from the muscles of the face and head to the muscles of the arms and legs, and ultimately to the muscles that control respiration. This is the final stage of the disease, although it is rarely seen now that effective treatments for this condition have been developed.

Treatment

Before the 1970s the prognosis for MG was indeterminate at best. Approximately one third of people died of the disease; approximately one third experienced permanent damage and loss of motor function; and approximately one third experienced spontaneous remission with no lasting effects. When the relationship between acetylcholine and muscle contractions was finally unraveled, it opened new possibilities for treating this disease.

Treatment of MG usually has a double intention: to boost nerve transmission and to suppress immune system activity at neuromuscular junctions. Medications include drugs that limit the normal destruction of acetylcholine by local enzymes (this allows the acetylcholine more time and opportunities to bind with whatever receptor sites are functioning), and steroids that suppress immune system activity. Surgery is occasionally recommended to remove an abnormal thymus gland. In the event of a MG crisis (a sudden onset that threatens the patient's ability to breathe), *plasmapheresis* may be used to remove antibodies from the blood. This is an invasive procedure with only short-term benefits, so it is usually saved for extreme circumstances.

Massage?

MG is a disorder that involves motor loss but no sensory loss. It is exacerbated by stress, repetitive motion, and overexertion. Massage could be appropriate for MG patients, bearing in mind that excessive heat also can aggravate symptoms, and that these clients may be taking immunosuppressive medications that put them at increased risk for picking up other people's infections.

Thoracic Outlet Syndrome in Brief

What is it?
Thoracic outlet syndrome (TOS) is a collection of signs and symptoms brought about by occlusion of nerve and blood supply to the arm.

How is it recognized?
Depending on what structures are compressed, TOS shows shooting pains, weakness, numbness, and paresthesia ("pins and needles") along with a feeling of fullness and possible discoloration of the affected arm from impaired circulation.

Is massage indicated or contraindicated?
This depends on the source of the problem. If it is related to muscle tightness, it indicates massage. TOS symptoms due to muscle atrophy or some other disorder such as spondylosis or disc disease may not respond well to massage.

Thoracic Outlet Syndrome

Definition: What Is It?

Thoracic outlet syndrome (TOS) is a neurovascular entrapment. The nerves of the brachial plexus or the blood vessels running to or from the arm (or some combination of both) are impinged or impaired at the thoracic outlet: the area behind the clavicle between the insertions of the trapezius and sternocleidomastoid.

Etiology: What Happens?

The brachial plexus, that tangled network of spinal nerves that supplies the arm with sensation and motor control, is composed of spinal nerves C_5 to T_1. These nerves interconnect as they travel a complicated path to get to their final destinations in the arm: they go from intervertebral foramina through the anterior and medial scalenes, between the clavicle and the first rib, under the pectoralis minor, and around the humerus. If some part of the plexus is somehow compressed along the way, a person feels it somewhere along the distance of that nerve. The nerve roots C_8 and T_1, both of which contribute to the ulnar and median nerves, are most at risk for compression with TOS.

Pinched nerves are only one part of TOS. This is a neuro*vascular* entrapment, and the vessels at risk are the subclavian vein and the axillary artery, which is the distal portion of the subclavian artery. These vessels, while not being vulnerable to osteophytes and disc disease like the nerves, are equally at the mercy of the compression that can happen when muscles in small spaces get too tight (Figure 2.51).

TOS has become a somewhat controversial topic in orthopedic medicine, because it has so many possible configurations. It is often discussed as three varieties:

- *True neurogenic TOS*: This is a situation with nerve impingement that is established by electromyogram or nerve conduction studies.

- *True vascular TOS*: In this case, TOS is identified by venogram or arteriogram that shows where exactly an obstruction has developed.

- *Nonspecific or disputed TOS*: In this situation, symptoms are present, but standard tests do not reveal any specific obstruction. This is the most common presentation of TOS.

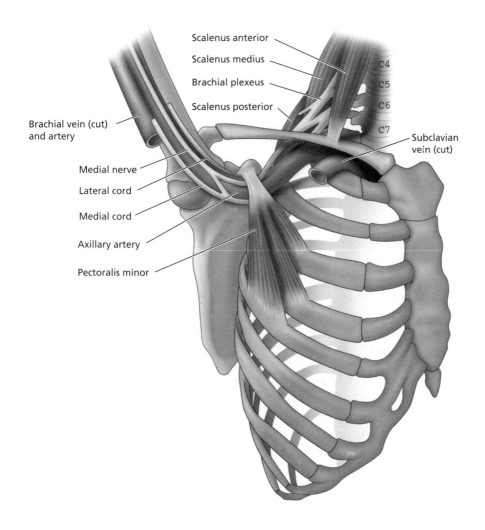

Scalenus anterior
Scalenus medius
Brachial plexeus
Scalenus posterior
C4
C5
C6
C7
Brachial vein (cut) and artery
Subclavian vein (cut)
Medial nerve
Lateral cord
Medial cord
Axillary artery
Pectoralis minor

Figure 2.51. Thoracic outlet syndrome.

Contributing Factors

Symptoms of TOS can be caused by any factor that impinges on brachial plexus nerves or blood vessels to and from the arm, anywhere from the neck to the shoulder. Although postural habits and bony growth patterns can make a person susceptible to TOS, it often seems to be precipitated by a specific traumatic event: a hyperextension injury (see *whiplash*, this chapter) or a repetitive stress situation similar to the factors seen with *carpal tunnel syndrome* (this chapter).

Although TOS is only diagnosed when the impingement occurs at the thoracic outlet, other factors can contribute to identical symptoms. Treating this condition successfully means finding out exactly where that interference is happening. Some possibilities include the following:

- *Cervical misalignment.* This could be a subluxation, but would more likely be a rotation *with* subluxation of any combination of lower cervical vertebrae. Which nerves are affected (and therefore the location of the symptoms) depends on what level or levels of spinal nerves are being compressed.

- *Cervical ribs.* In approximately 1% of the population, the transverse processes of the cervical vertebrae grow longer than normal, extending into territory where they do not belong. On an x-ray, they actually look like little ribs sticking out into the soft tissues of the neck. They are usually unilateral, and C_7 is the vertebra that grows them most frequently.

- *Spondylosis.* If a bone spur intrudes right into the nerve root at C_6 (or any other cervical nerve root), symptoms are identical to those of classical TOS (see *spondylosis*, this chapter.)

- *Rib misalignment.* The joints that join the ribs to the spine are full synovial joints, called **zygapophyseal joints.** Like the intervertebral joints, the rib joints sometimes subluxate. When this happens to the first rib, two different spots could cause problems: right under the anterior scalene, and between the coracoid process and the ribs. In both of those locations, the brachial plexus nerves can easily be caught between a bone (the first rib) and a hard place (a tight muscle or another bone).

- *Tight muscles.* The anterior and medial scalenes and the pectoralis minor are the muscles most immediately involved with TOS. Microscopic studies of the scalenes of TOS patients show that the muscles are often bound up with large amounts of scar tissue. This can make the muscles tight and unyielding, putting mechanical pressure on the nerve roots.

- *Atrophied muscles.* Many cases of TOS may be related to muscle atrophy as an outcome of chronic muscle tightness. The pectoralis minor, in a constant battle with the rhomboids and levator scapulae, is especially prone to this phenomenon, particularly for people with a "caved in" posture. Eventually the pectoralis minor becomes shrunken and fibrotic, whereas its antagonists on the back, especially the rhomboids, become stretched out and hypotonic. If muscles that support the shoulder girdle are abnormally underdeveloped, the clavicle and scapula may collapse onto the ribs, compressing and irritating brachial plexus nerves and the subclavian vein.

- *Other factors.* Other, more serious developments can put direct or indirect pressure on brachial plexus nerves or local blood vessels. *Lung cancer* (Chapter 6) with tumors in the apex of the lung, *aneurysm* or *thrombus* (Chapter 5), or nerve damage to the spinal accessory nerve during a cervical lymph node biopsy can all lead to the collapse of the shoulder girdle and pressure on delicate structures.

Signs and Symptoms

Symptoms of TOS include all signs of nerve irritation: shooting pains; numbness, numblikeness; weakness; tingling; pins and needles. Add to these the vascular symptoms: a feeling of "fullness" when blood return from a vein is blocked, or coldness and weakness when blood flow to the axillary artery is impaired. A difference in coloration or temperature of the affected arm also may be noticeable. Symptoms tend to be worse at night, when the patient lifts the affected arm over her head, or when the person is tired from other activities.

Diagnosis

Several tests to look for the presence of TOS have been developed. Unfortunately, none of them is always accurate for every patient, so a diagnosis is usually based on a physical examination combined with a description of symptoms from the patient. The challenge then is to locate exactly where the impingement is taking place.

In the Wright hyperabduction test, the hand is placed over the head and the head is turned toward the affected side. If this exacerbates symptoms or reduces the strength of the pulse of the affected side, impingement to the axillary artery and lower brachial plexus nerves is suspected.

For Adson's test, the head is extended and rotated toward the affected side. The client takes a deep breath, and the radial pulse on the affected side diminishes or even completely disappears. TOS that is due to muscle atrophy may show best when a client lies on his affected side and the pulse is diminished from axillary artery compression.

Nerve velocity conduction tests and electromyograms (tests that measure electrical activity during muscle action) are sometimes used, but they are often inconclusive. X-rays, MRIs, and other imaging techniques may be used to look for bone spurs, cervical ribs, or other mechanical obstructions, but they yield little information about chronic muscle tightness or atrophy.

Confusing Signs

Many, many factors cause pain in the shoulders, arms, wrists, and hands. Some of these problems are often missed by standard diagnosis, simply because most soft tissue injuries do not show up on most medical tests. This is unfortunate because it makes it difficult for people to get an accurate diagnosis for their most common and treatable problems. The following list includes just a few of the things that will cause pain in the shoulder, arm, wrist, or hand and that can be hard to pin down in an accurate diagnosis.

Spondylosis
Vertebral misalignment
Cervical rib pressing on the brachial plexus
Tight scalenes, pectoralis minor
Carpal tunnel syndrome
Wrist tendinitis or sprain
Shoulder bursitis
Disc disease
Costal misalignment
Injured cervical ligaments
Rotator cuff tendinitis
Elbow tendinitis
Arthritis in shoulders, elbows, or wrists

Treatment

The treatment for thoracic outlet syndrome depends entirely on its causes, which is why it is important to get an accurate diagnosis of the cause of this problem. Different strategies are more appropriate for spondylosis than for tight scalenes, for instance. TOS due to muscle atrophy or tightness responds best to strengthening exercises and stretching. A small percentage of TOS patients are good candidates for surgery, which has the goal of releasing pressure on the affected nerves. This can mean the removal of a cervical rib, or the resectioning of the first rib, or both.

Massage?

If the TOS is not from a muscular spasm or weakness, massage will not make much lasting difference. However, if it *is* related to muscular problems, it can respond very well to massage. The client should also learn some specific stretches and exercises for pectoralis minor, its antagonists, and the scalenes to make the massage have lasting impact.

 # CHAPTER REVIEW QUESTIONS

1. What is the relationship between fibromyalgia and sleep disorders?
2. What does *hernia* mean? Name three kinds of abdominal hernias.
3. Describe the differences between tender points and trigger points.
4. Where do massage therapists often get osteoarthritis?

5. Why are women more prone than men to osteoporosis?

6. Describe how pes planus can lead to headaches.

7. What kind of muscle spasm serves an important function in the healing process?

8. Describe several factors that may influence bone density and risk of osteoporosis.

9. In which stage of healing do soft tissue injuries generally contraindicate circulatory massage? Why?

10. What does RICE stand for?

11. List the lines of defense against a joint injury.

12. Define "specific muscle weakness."

13. Describe the pain-spasm-ischemia cycle.

14. Describe the differences between strains, sprains, tendinitis, and tendinosis.

15. Describe the relationship between stress and chronic injury.

Answers to these questions can be found on the Student Recource CD-ROM that accompanies this book.

Bibliography

General Resources, Musculoskeletal System

1. de Dominico G, Wood E. Beard's Massage. Philadelphia: WB Saunders, 1997.
2. Damjanou I. Pathology for the Health-Related Professions. Philadelphia: WB Saunders, 1996.
3. Travell J, Simons DG. Myofascial Pain and Dysfunction: The Trigger Point Manual. Baltimore: Williams & Wilkins, 1983.
4. Clemente CD. Anatomy: A Regional Atlas of the Human Body. 3rd Ed. Baltimore: Urban & Schwarzenburg, 1987.
5. Tortora GJ, Anagnostakos NP. Principles of Anatomy and Physiology. 6th Ed. New York: Harper & Row, 1990.
6. Taber's Cyclopedic Dictionary. 14th Ed. Philadelphia: FA Davis, 1981.
7. Stedman's Medical Dictionary. 26th Ed. Baltimore: Williams & Wilkins, 1995.
8. Memmler RL, Wood DL. The Human Body in Health and Disease. 5th Ed. Philadelphia: JB Lippincott, 1983.
9. Juhan D. Job's Body: A Handbook for Bodywork. Barrytown, NY: Station Hill Press, 1987.
10. Kunz JRM, Finkel AJ, eds. The American Medical Association Family Medical Guide. New York, NY: Random House, 1987.
11. Marieb EM. Human Anatomy and Physiology. Redwood City, CA: Benjamin/Cummings, 1989.
12. Field T. Touch Therapy. London: Churchill Livingstone, 2000.

Fibromyalgia Syndrome

1. Nye D. A Physician's Guide to Fibromyalgia Syndrome. Copyright © 1998, Missouri Arthritis Rehabilitation Research and Training Center. Available at: http://www.hsc.missouri.edu/~fibro/fm-md.html. Accessed summer 2003.

2. Winfield J. Fibromyalgia. Copyright © 2003, eMedicine.com, Inc. Available at: http://www.emedicine.com/med/topic790.htm. Accessed summer 2003.
3. Fibromyalgia & Chronic Myofascial Pain Information: A Frequently Missed Diagnosis. Copyright © 1995-2002 Devin J. Starlanyl & Mary Ellen Copeland. Available at: http://www.sover.net/~devstar/phdefine.htm. Accessed summer 2003.
4. Guaifenesin. Copyright © 1995-2002 Devin J. Starlanyl & Mary Ellen Copeland. Available at: http://www.sover.net/~devstar/phguai.htm. Accessed summer 2003.
5. Questions and Answers About Fibromyalgia. NIAMS (National Institute of Arthritis and Musculoskeletal and Skin Diseases.) Available at: http://www.niams.nih.gov/hi/topics/fibromyalgia/fibrofs.htm. Accessed summer 2003.
6. Gremillion RB. Fibromyalgia. The Physician and Sportsmedicine, vol 26, no. 4; April 98. Copyright © 1998. The McGraw-Hill Companies. Available at: http://www.physsportsmed.com/issues/1998/04apr/grem.htm. Accessed summer 2003.
7. FM Online Newsletter, A publication of National Fibromyalgia Association. Hellerwork: Using Deep Tissue Bodywork, Movement Education and Dialogue to Treat FM. Vol. 3, No. 16, September 3, 2003. Copyright © 2003 National Fibromyalgia Association. Available at: http://www.fmaware.org/fmOnlineNewsletter/vol3_no16/hellerwork.htm. Accessed summer 2003.
8. Davis JL. WebMD Medical News. Massage Helps Fibromyalgia. Copyright © 2002 WebMD Inc. URL http://my.webmd.com/content/article/16/1673_50941. Accessed summer 2003.

9. What Is Fibromyalgia Syndrome? copyrighted by Fibromyalgia Network. Available at: http://www.fmnetnews.com/pages/basics.html. Accessed summer 2003.

Myofascial Pain Syndrome

1. Fibromyalgia & Chronic Myofascial Pain Information: A Frequently Missed Diagnosis. Copyright © 1995-2002 Devin J. Starlanyl & Mary Ellen Copeland. Available at: http://www.sover.net/~devstar/phdefine.htm. Accessed summer 2003.
2. Filner BE. Fibromyalgia or Myofascial Pain Syndrome? Understanding and Treating, the Differences. National Fibromyalgia Partnership. Available at: http://www.immunesupport.com/library/showarticle.cfm/ID/3390/e/1/T/CFIDS_FM/. Accessed summer 2003.
3. Myofascial Pain—a Neuromuscular Disease. Copyright © 1995-2002. Devin J. Starlanyl & Mary Ellen Copeland. Available at: http://www.sover.net/~devstar/myopain.htm. Accessed summer 2003.
4. Treatment of Myofascial Pain Syndrome Requires Team Effort. Copyright © 2003 Specialty Physicians Alliance. Available at: http://www.spa-ortho.com/library/gen2.htm. Accessed summer 2003.
5. Fomby EW, Mellion MB. Identifying and Treating Myofascial Pain Syndrome. The Physician and Sportsmedicine 1997; 25(2). Copyright © 1997. The McGraw-Hill Companies. Available at: http://www.physsportsmed.com/issues/1997/02feb/fomby2.htm. Accessed summer 2003.
6. Bruno AA. Myofascial Pain in Athletes. Copyright © 2003, eMedicine.com, Inc. Available at: http://www.emedicine.com/sports/topic158.htm. Accessed summer 2003.

Muscular Dystrophy

1. What Are Duchenne and Becker Muscular Dystrophies? Copyright © 2003 The Muscular Dystrophy Association. Available at: http://www.mdausa.org/publications/fa-dmdbmd-what.html. Accessed summer 2003.
2. Carol Sowell. Marvelous Massage: Pain Relief, Relaxation and Comfort Can Result When You Get Rubbed the Right Way. Quest 2000;7(6). Copyright © 2003 The Muscular Dystrophy Association. Available at: http://www.mdausa.org/publications/Quest/q76massage2.html. Accessed summer 2003.
3. Robinson R. Fight Against Contractures . . . An Ongoing Battle. Quest 1996;3(4). Copyright © 2003 The Muscular Dystrophy Association. Available at: http://www.mdausa.org/publications/Quest/q34contrc.html. Accessed summer 2003.
4. What Can Be Done to Treat DMD or BMD? Copyright © 2003 The Muscular Dystrophy Association. Available at: http://www.mdausa.org/publications/fa-dmdbmd-treat.html. Accessed summer 2003.
5. Welcome to the Internet Home of the FSH Society. Fascioscapulohumeral Muscular Dystrophy Society. Available at: http://www.fshsociety.org/fsh/fshd.html. Accessed summer 2003.

Myositis Ossificans

1. Larson CM, Almekinders LC, Karas SG, et al. Evaluating and Managing Muscle Contusions and Myositis Ossificans. The Physician and Sportsmedicine 2002;30(2). Copyright © 2002 The McGraw-Hill Companies. Available at: http://www.physsportsmed.com/issues/2002/02_02/larson.htm. Accessed summer 2003.
2. Moore DS, Cho G. Heterotopic Ossification. Copyright © 2003, eMedicine.com, Inc. Available at: http://www.emedicine.com/radio/topic336.htm. Accessed summer 2003.
3. D'Alessandro DM, Takle TE. Virtual Pediatric Patients: Case 3—An Adolescent With Leg Pain. Copyright © 1992-2003 the Author(s) and The University of Iowa. Available at: http://www.vh.org/pediatric/provider/pediatrics/VirtualPedsPatients/Case03/Case03.html . Accessed summer 2003.
4. Myositis Ossificans. Bonetumor.org. Available at: http://www.bonetumor.org/tumors/pages/page177.html. Accessed summer 2003.

Shin Splints

1. Hutchinson MR, Cahoon S, Atkins T. Chronic Leg Pain: Putting the Diagnostic Pieces Together. The Physician and Sportsmedicine 1998;26(7). Copyright © 1998. The McGraw-Hill Companies. Available at: http://www.physsportsmed.com/issues/1998/07jul/hutch.htm. Accessed summer 2003.
2. Couture CJ, Karlson KA. Tibial Stress Injuries: Decisive Diagnosis and Treatment of 'Shin Splints.' The Physician and Sportsmedicine 2002;30(6). Copyright © 1998. The McGraw-Hill Companies. Available at: http://www.physsportsmed.com/issues/2002/06_02/couture.htm. Accessed summer 2003.
3. Wallace SB. Compartment Syndrome, Lower Extremity. Copyright © 2003, eMedicine.com, Inc. Available at: http://www.emedicine.com/orthoped/topic596.htm. Accessed summer 2003.

Spasms, Cramps

1. Schwellnus MP. Skeletal Muscle Cramps During Exercise. The Physician and Sportsmedicine 1999;27(12). Copyright © 1998. The McGraw-Hill Companies. Available at: http://www.physsportsmed.com/issues/1999/11_99/schwellnus.htm. Accessed summer 2003.
2. Mayers LB, Noakes TD. A Guide to Treating Ironman Triathletes at the Finish Line. The Physician and Sportsmedicine 2000;28(8). Copyright © 1998. The McGraw-Hill Companies. Available at: http://www.physsportsmed.com/issues/2000/08_00/mayers.htm. Accessed summer 2003.

Strains

1. Ahh . . . Ice Massage for Pain Relief. Copyright © 1999-2003 Spine-health.com. Available at: http://www.spine-health.com/topics/conserv/ice/ice001.html. Accessed summer 2003.
2. Reeves RK, Laskowski ER, Smith J. Weight Training Injuries: Part 1: Diagnosing and Managing Acute Conditions. The Physician and Sportsmedicine 1998;26(2). Copyright © 1998. The McGraw-Hill Companies. Available at: http://www.physsportsmed.com/issues/1998/02feb/laskow.htm. Accessed summer 2003.
3. Best TM, Garrett WE Jr. Hamstring Strains: Expediting Return to Play. The Physician and Sportsmedicine 1996;24(8). Copyright © 1998. The McGraw-Hill Companies. Available at: http://www.physsportsmed.com/issues/1996/08_96/best.htm. Accessed summer 2003.

Avascular Osteonecrosis

1. Questions and Answers About Avascular Necrosis. National Institute of Arthritis and Musculoskeletal and Skin Diseases (NIAMS). Available at: http://www.niams.nih.gov/hi/topics/avascular_necrosis/. Accessed summer 2003.
2. Legg Calve Perthes Disease. Copyright © 1996, C.R. Wheeless MD. Available at: http://www.ortho-u.net/orthoo/242.htm. Accessed summer 2003.
3. Nochimson G. Legg-Calve-Perthes Disease. Copyright © 2003, eMedicine.com, Inc. Available at: http://www.emedicine.com/emerg/topic294.htm. Accessed summer 2003.
4. Aiello MR. Avascular Necrosis, Femoral Head. Copyright © 2003, eMedicine.com, Inc. Available at: http://www.emedicine.com/radio/topic70.htm. Accessed summer 2003.

Fractures

1. Bone Fracture Repair. National Library of Medicine. Available at: http://www.nlm.nih.gov/medlineplus/ency/article/002966.htm. Accessed summer 2003.
2. Farley D. New Ways to Heal Broken Bones. FDA Consumer Magazine (April 1996). Available at: http://www.fda.gov/fdac/features/396_bone.html. Accessed summer 2003.
3. Brukner P, Bradshaw C, Bennell K. Managing Common Stress Fractures: Let Risk Level Guide Treatment. The Physician and Sportsmedicine 1998;26(8). Copyright © 1998. The McGraw-Hill Companies. Available at: http://www.physsportsmed.com/issues/1998/08aug/brukner.htm. Accessed summer 2003.

Osteoporosis

1. McCormick CC. Calcium & Osteoporosis—A Weak Link. Copyright © 1998-99 Cornell University. Available at: http://www.cce.cornell.edu/food/expfiles/topics/mccormick/mccormickoverview.html Accessed summer 2003.
2. Beck BR, Shoemaker MR. Osteoporosis: Understanding Key Risk Factors and Therapeutic Options. The Physician and Sportsmedicine 2000;28(2). Copyright © 1998. The McGraw-Hill Companies. Available at: http://www.physsportsmed.com/issues/2000/02_00/beck.htm. Accessed summer 2003
3. Protecting Your Bones. Physicians Committee for Responsible Medicine. Available at: http://www.pcrm.org/health/Preventive_Medicine/strong_bones.html. Accessed summer 2003.
5. Which Drugs Are Used for Osteoporosis? Copyright © 2003, Arthritis Foundation. Available at: http://www.arthritis.org/resources/arthritistoday/2001_archives/2001_11_12_yourmedicine_q6.asp. Accessed summer 2003.
6. Preventing and Reversing Osteoporosis. Physicians Committee for Responsible Medicine. Available at: http://www.pcrm.org/issues/Nutrition_Curriculum/nutr_curr_7.html. Accessed summer 2003.
7. Depression, Bone Mass, and Osteoporosis. National Institute of Mental Health (NIMH). Available at: http://www.nimh.nih.gov/events/prosteo.cfm. Accessed winter 2004.
8. Fast Facts on Osteoporosis. National Institute of Health Osteoporosis and Related Bone Diseases—National Resource Center. Available at: http://www.osteo.org/newfile.asp?doc=fast&doctitle=Fast+Facts+on+Osteoporosis&doctype=HTML+Fact+Sheet. Accessed summer 2003.

9. Matsen F III. Osteoporosis. Copyright © 2003 University of Washington. Available at: http://www.orthop.washington.edu/arthritis/types/osteoporosis/01. Accessed summer 2003.

Paget's Disease

1. The Management of Paget's Disease of Bone. National Institute of Health Osteoporosis and Related Bone Diseases-National Resource Center. Available at: http://www.osteo.org/newfile.asp?doc=p132i&doctitle=The+Management+of+Paget%27s+Disease+of+Bone&doctype=HTML+Fact+Sheet. Accessed summer 2003.
2. Kurtzweil P. Help for People with Paget's Disease. FDA Consumer magazine (October 1996). Available at: http://www.fda.gov/fdac/features/896_pag.html. Accessed summer 2003.
3. Information for Patients About Paget's Disease of Bone. National Institute of Health Osteoporosis and Related Bone Diseases-National Resource Center. Available at: http://www.osteo.org/newfile.asp?doc=p110i&doctitle=Information+for+Patients+about+Paget%27s+Disease+of+Bone&doctype=HTML+Fact+Sheet. Accessed summer 2003.
4. Matsen F III. About Paget's disease. Copyright © 2003 University of Washington. Available at: http://www.orthop.washington.edu/arthritis/types/pagets/01. Accessed summer 2003.

Postural Deviations

1. Scoliosis / Kyphosis. Copyright © 1998, 99 Intermedx . Available at: http://www.orthospine.com/ask_doctor/faq_scoliosis_kyphosis.html. Accessed summer 2003.
2. Scoliosis: Information & Treatment. Copyright © 1996–2001 by James H. Clay. Available at: http://danke.com/Orthodoc/scoliosis.html. Accessed summer 2003.
3. Richardson ML. Scoliosis. Copyright © 2000 University of Washington Department of Radiology Available at: http://www.rad.washington.edu/mskbook/scoliosis.html. Accessed summer 2003.
4. Lordosis. Copyright © 2003, *University of Utah* Health Sciences Center. Available at: http://www.uuhsc.utah.edu/healthinfo/pediatric/orthopaedics/lordosis.htm. Accessed summer 2003.
5. Dalton E. Scoliosis: A Case Study of Deep Tissue Massage Therapy. Rolf Lines, Fall 2000. Copyright © 2000 Rolf Institute. Available at: http://www.erikdalton.com/massagearticles.htm. Accessed summer 2003.
6. Odom JA Jr. Spinal Deformities: Benefits of Early Screening and Treatment. Copyright © June 1, 1995, Joel R. Cooper, All rights reserved. Available at: http://medicalreporter.health.org/tmr0795/scoliosis0795.html. Accessed summer 2003.

Ankylosing Spondylitis

1. Humphreys SC. Ankylosing Spondylitis. Copyright © 2003, eMedicine.com, Inc. Available at: http://www.emedicine.com/orthoped/topic13.htm.
2. Matsen FA III. Ankylosing Spondylitis. Copyright © 2003 University of Washington. Available at: http://www.orthop.washington.edu/arthritis/types/ankylosingspondylitis/01. Accessed summer 2003.
3. Ankylosing Spondylitis. Copyright © 1995-2003 Merck & Co., Inc. Available at: http://www.merck.com/pubs/mmanual/section5/chapter51/51a.htm. Accessed summer 2003.
4. Ankylosing Spondylitis. Copyright © 1996-2003 MedicineNet, Inc. Available at: http://www.medicinenet.com/Ankylosing_Spondylitis/article.htm. Accessed summer 2003.

Dislocations

1. Bach AW. Finger Joint Injuries in Active Patients: Pointers for Acute and Late-Phase Management. The Physician and Sportsmedicine 1999;27(3). Copyright © 1999. The McGraw-Hill Companies. Available at: http://www.physsportsmed.com/issues/1999/03_99/bach.htm. Accessed summer 2003.
2. Welsh S. Shoulder Dislocations. Copyright © 2003, eMedicine.com, Inc. Available at: http://www.emedicine.com/orthoped/topic440.htm. Accessed summer 2003.
3. Joy EA. Self-Reduction of Anterior Shoulder Dislocation. The Physician and Sportsmedicine 2000;28(11). Copyright © 1999. The McGraw-Hill Companies. Available at: http://www.physsportsmed.com/issues/2000/11_00/joy.htm. Accessed summer 2003.
4. Arthroscopic Shoulder Surgery: Thermal Capsulorrhaphy. American Academy of Orthopaedic Surgeons. Available at: http://orthoinfo.aaos.org/fact/thr_report.cfm?Thread_ID=228&topcategory=Shoulder. Accessed summer 2003.

Gout

1. Rothschild BM. Gout. Copyright © 2003, eMedicine.com, Inc. Available at: http://www.emedicine.com/orthoped/topic124.htm. Accessed summer 2003.
2. Gout and Hyperuricemia. Copyright © 1996-2003 MedicineNet, Inc. Available at: http://www.medicinenet.com/Gout/article.htm. Accessed summer 2003.
3. DeGroot H III. Gout. bonetumor.org. Available at: http://www.bonetumor.org/tumors/pages/page184.html. Accessed summer 2003
4. CPPD Deposition Disease. Copyright © 2003 University of Washington. Available at: http://www.orthop.washington.edu/arthritis/types/cppd. Accessed summer 2003.

5. DiBacco TV. The Pain of Gout: Baffling Condition Left Doctors Guessing. Washington Post, October 11, 1994: Z 19.

Lyme Disease

1. CDC Lyme Disease Home Page. Centers for Disease Control and Prevention. Available at: http://www.cdc.gov/ncidod/dvbid/lyme/index.htm. Accessed summer 2003.
2. NINDS Neurological Sequelae of Lyme Disease Information Page. National Institute of Allergy and Infectious Diseases. Available at: http://www.ninds.nih.gov/health_and_medical/disorders/lyme_doc.htm. Accessed summer 2003.
3. Lyme Disease Basic Information. The International Lyme and Associated Diseases Society (ILADS). Available at: http://www.ilads.org/axioms.htm. Accessed summer 2003.
4. Vector Ecology. Centers for Disease Control and Prevention. Available at: http://www.cdc.gov/ncidod/dvbid/lyme/history.htm. Accessed summer 2003.
5. Prevention and Control. Centers for Disease Control and Prevention. Available at: http://www.cdc.gov/ncidod/dvbid/lyme/prevent.htm. Accessed summer 2003.
6. Epidemiology. Centers for Disease Control and Prevention. Available at: http://www.cdc.gov/ncidod/dvbid/lyme/epi.htm. Accessed summer 2003.
7. Diagnosis. Centers for Disease Control and Prevention. Available at: http://www.cdc.gov/ncidod/dvbid/lyme/diagnosis.htm. Accessed summer 2003.
8. Lyme Disease: The Facts The Challenge. NIH Publication no. 03-7045. April 2003. Available at: www.niaid.nih.gov. Accessed summer 2003.
9. Southern Tick-Associated Rash Illness. Centers for Disease Control and Prevention. Available at: http://www.cdc.gov/ncidod/dvbid/stari/index.htm. Accessed summer 2003.
10. Human Ehrlichiosis in the United States. Centers for Disease Control and Prevention. Available at: http://www.cdc.gov/ncidod/dvrd/ehrlichia/Signs/Signs.htm. Accessed summer 2003.
11. Herwaldt BL, McGovern PC, Gerwel MP, et al. Endemic Babesiosis in Another Eastern State: New Jersey. Emerg Infect Dis [serial online] Available at: http://www.cdc.gov/ncidod/EID/vol9no2/02-0271.htm. Accessed summer 2003.
12. Rocky Mountain Spotted Fever. Centers for Disease Control and Prevention. Available at: http://www.cdc.gov/ncidod/dvrd/rmsf/index.htm. Accessed summer 2003.

Osteoarthritis

1. Lewis C. Arthritis: Timely Treatments for an Ageless Disease. FDA/Office of Public Affairs. Publication No. (FDA) 01-1313.

Available at: http://www.fda.gov/fdac/features/2000/300_arth.html. Accessed summer 2003.

2. Kelly GS. The Role of Glucosamine Sulfate and Chondroitin Sulfates in the Treatment of Degenerative Joint Disease. © THORNE Research, Inc. Available at: http://www.thorne.com/altmedrev/.fulltext/3/1/27.htm. Accessed summer 2003.

3. What Is Hip Replacement? A Review of Total Hip Arthroplasty, Hip Resurfacing, and Minimally-Invasive Hip Surgery. Copyright © 2003 University of Washington. Available at: http://www.orthop.washington.edu/faculty/Leopold/hipreplacement/01. Accessed summer 2003.

4. Handout on Health: Osteoarthritis. National Institute of Arthritis and Musculoskeletal and Skin Diseases. Available at: http://www.niams.nih.gov/hi/topics/arthritis/oahandout.htm. Accessed summer 2003.

5. Thumb Arthritis. Southeastern Hand Center. Available at: http://www.handsurgery.com/arthritis.html. Accessed summer 2003.

6. Osteoarthritis: What Is It? Copyright © 2003, Arthritis Foundation. Available at: http://www.arthritis.org/conditions/Disease Center/oa.asp. Accessed summer 2003.

Patellofemoral Syndrome

1. Post WR. Patellofemoral Pain: Let the Physical Exam Define Treatment. The Physician and Sportsmedicine 1998;26(1). Copyright © 1998. The McGraw-Hill Companies. Available at: http://www.physsportsmed.com/issues/1998/01jan/post.htm. Accessed summer 2003.

2. Patellofemoral Syndrome. Copyright © 1996-2003 MedicineNet, Inc. Available at: http://www.medicinenet.com/Patellofemoral_Syndrome/article.htm. Accessed summer 2003.

3. Potter PJ. Patellofemoral Syndrome. Copyright © 2003, eMedicine.com, Inc. Available at: http://www.emedicine.com/pmr/topic101.htm. Accessed summer 2003.

4. Liss H, Liss D. Patellofemoral syndrome. The Physical Medicine and Rehabilitation Center, PA. Available at: http://www.rehabmed.net/documents/patelloff.htm. Accessed summer 2003.

Rheumatoid Arthritis

1. Handout on Health: Rheumatoid Arthritis. National Institute of Arthritis and Musculoskeletal and Skin Diseases. Available at: http://www.niams.nih.gov/hi/topics/arthritis/rahandout.htm. Accessed summer 2003.

2. Krupp DC, Graber MA. Rheumatology: Rheumatoid Arthritis. Copyright © 1992-2003 the Author(s) and The University of Iowa. Available at: http://www.vh.org/adult/provider/familymedicine/FPHan

dbook/Chapter07/02-7.html Accessed summer 2003.

3. Gupta K. Rheumatoid Arthritis. Copyright © 2003, eMedicine.com, Inc. Available at: http://www.emedicine.com/pmr/topic124.htm. Accessed summer 2003.

4. Rheumatoid Arthritis Fact Sheet. Copyright © 2003, Arthritis Foundation. Available at: http://www.arthritis.org/conditions/af_statements/af_state_ra.asp. Accessed summer 2003.

Septic Arthritis

1. Munoz G. Septic Arthritis. Copyright © 2003, eMedicine.com, Inc. Available at: http://www.emedicine.com/orthoped/topic437.htm. Accessed summer 2003.

2. Krupp DC, Graber MA. Rheumatology: Septic Arthritis. Copyright © 1992-2003 the Author(s) and The University of Iowa. Available at: http://www.vh.org/adult/provider/familymedicine/FPHandbook/Chapter07/06-7.html. Accessed summer 2003.

Spondylosis

1. Oró J. What Is Cervical Spondylosis? Copyright © Department of Surgery University of Missouri-Columbia. Available at: http://www.surgery.missouri.edu/ns/neurospine/disorders_spondylosis.html. Accessed summer 2003.

2. Cervical Spondylosis. Copyright © All rights reserved by NYU Dept. of Neurosurgery. Available at: http://www.publishedresearch.com/AAAca/cervical_spondylosis.htm. Accessed summer 2003.

3. Lumbar Stenosis (Spondylosis). Copyright © 2003 New York University. Available at: http://www.med.nyu.edu/neurosurgery/articles/spine_1.html. Accessed summer 2003.

4. Baron EM. Cervical Spondylosis: Diagnosis and Management. Copyright © 2003, eMedicine.com, Inc. Available at: http://www.emedicine.com/neuro/topic564.htm. Accessed summer 2003.

Sprains

1. Trojian TH, McKeag DB. Ankle Sprains: Expedient Assessment and Management. The Physician and Sportsmedicine 1998;26(10). Copyright © 1998. The McGraw-Hill Companies. Available at: http://www.physsportsmed.com/issues/1998/10Oct/mckeag.htm. Accessed summer 2003.

2. Meislin RJ. Managing Collateral Ligament Tears of the Knee. The Physician and Sportsmedicine 1996;24(3). Copyright © 1998. The McGraw-Hill Companies. Available at: http://www.physsportsmed.com/issues/1996/03_96/meislin.htm. Accessed summer 2003.

3. Stamford B. Giving Injuries the Cold Treatment. The Physician and Sportsmedicine 1996;24(3). Copyright © 1998. The McGraw-Hill Companies. Available at: http://www.physsportsmed.

com/issues/1996/03_96/cold.htm. Accessed summer 2003.

Temporomandibular Joint Disorders

1. Temporomandibular Disorders (TMD). National Institute of Dental and Craniofacial Research. Available at: http://www.nidcr.nih.gov/health/pubs/tmd/text.htm. Accessed summer 2003.

2. Temporomandibular Joint Disorder (TMJ). Copyright © 1996-2003 MedicineNet, Inc. Available at: http://www.medicinenet.com/Temporomandibular_Joint__Disorder/article.htm. Accessed summer 2003.

3. Shankland W. The Effects of Glucosamine and Chondroitin Sulfate on Osteoarthritis: A Preliminary Report of 50 Patients. The American Academy of Head, Neck & Facial Pain. Available at: http://www.drshankland.com/glucos.html. Accessed summer 2003.

4. Temporomandibular Disorders. Copyright © 1998-2003 Mayo Foundation for Medical Education and Research (MFMER). Available at: http://www.mayoclinic.com/invoke.cfm?id=DS00355. Accessed summer 2003.

5. Shankland W. Pain Disorders That Are Confused with TMJ. The American Academy of Head, Neck & Facial Pain. Available at: http://www.drshankland.com/disorders.html. Accessed summer 2003.

6. TMJ Function. Copyright © 1998, 1999, 2000 Dr. Brendan C. Stack. Available at: http://www.tmjstack.com/Animation/animation.html. Accessed summer 2003.

Baker Cysts

1. Baker Cyst (Popliteal Cyst). Copyright © 1996-2003 MedicineNet, Inc. Available at: http://www.medicinenet.com/Baker_Cyst/article.htm. Accessed summer 2003.

2. Langsfeld M, Matteson B, Johnson W, et al. Baker's Cysts Mimicking the Symptoms of Deep Vein Thrombosis: Diagnosis with Venous Duplex Scanning. J Vasc Surg 1997 Apr;25(4):658–662. Available at: http://www.ncbi.nlm.nih.gov/entrez/query.fcgi?cmd=Retrieve&db=PubMed&dopt=Abstract&list_uids=97275860. Accessed summer 2003.

3. Yu WD, Shapiro MS. Cysts and Other Masses About the Knee: Identifying and Treating Common and Rare Lesions. The Physician and Sportsmedicine 1999;27(7). Copyright © 1999. Available at: http://www.physsportsmed.com/issues/1999/07_99/yu.htm. Accessed summer 2003.

4. Bui-Mansfield LT. Baker Cyst. Copyright © 2003, eMedicine.com, Inc. Available at: http://www.emedicine.com/radio/topic72.htm. Accessed summer 2003.

Bunions

1. Bunions. Copyright © 1998-2003 Mayo Foundation for Medical Education and Research (MFMER). Available at:

http://www.mayoclinic.com/invoke.cfm?
id=DS00309. Accessed summer 2003.
2. Richardson ML. Radiographic Evaluation
   of Hallux Valgus. Copyright © 1997
   Michael L. Richardson, M.D. Available at:
   http://www.rad.washington.edu/anatomy/
   modules/HalluxValgus/HalluxValgus.html.
   Accessed summer 2003.
3. Bunions. Copyright © 1996-2003
   MedicineNet, Inc. Available at:
   http://www.medicinenet.com/Bunions/
   article.htm. Accessed summer 2003.

Bursitis

1. Bursitis. Copyright © 1998-2003 Mayo
   Foundation for Medical Education and
   Research (MFMER). Available at:
   http://www.mayoclinic.com/invoke.cfm?
   id=DS00032. Accessed summer 2003.
2. Bursitis. Copyright © 1996-2003
   MedicineNet, Inc. Available at:
   http://www.medicinenet.com/Bursitis/
   article.htm. Accessed summer 2003.
3. Bursitis. Copyright © 1995-2003 Merck &
   Co., Inc. Available at: http://www.merck.
   com/pubs/mmanual/section5/
   chapter59/59c.htm. Accessed summer 2003.

Dupuytren Contracture

1. Dupuytren Contracture. Copyright ©
   1996-2003 MedicineNet, Inc. Available at:
   http://www.medicinenet.com/Dupuytren_
   Contracture/article.htm. Accessed summer
   2003.
2. Revis DR Jr. Duypuytren Contracture.
   Copyright © 2003, eMedicine.com, Inc.
   Available at: http://www.emedicine.com/
   med/topic592.htm. Accessed summer 2003.

Ganglion Cyst

1. Honing EW. Wrist Injuries. Part 2:
   Spotting and Treating Troublemakers. The
   Physician and Sportsmedicine 1998;26(10).
   Copyright © 1998. The McGraw-Hill
   Companies. Available at: http://www.
   physsportsmed.com/issues/1998/10Oct/
   honing.htm. Accessed summer 2003.
2. What is a Ganglion Cyst? Copyright ©
   Manus 2000. Available at: http://www.
   indianahandcenter.com/med_gang.html.
   Accessed summer 2003.
3. Ganglion Cyst. Copyright © 1996-2003
   MedicineNet, Inc. Available at: http://www.
   medicinenet.com/Ganglion/article.htm.
   Accessed summer 2003.

Hernia

1. Hernia. Copyright © 1996-2003
   MedicineNet, Inc. Available at:
   http://www.medicinenet.com/Hernia/
   article.htm. Accessed summer 2003.
2. Inguinal hernia. Copyright © 1998-2003
   Mayo Foundation for Medical Education
   and Research (MFMER). Available at:
   http://www.mayoclinic.com/invoke.cfm?
   id=DS00364. Accessed summer 2003.

Marfan Syndrome

1. Channell K. Marfan Syndrome. Copyright
   © 2003, eMedicine.com, Inc. Available at:
   http://www.emedicine.com/orthoped/topic
   414.htm. Accessed summer 2003.
2. Marfan Syndrome. Copyright © 2003
   University of Washington. Available at:
   http://www.orthop.washington.edu/
   arthritis/types/marfan/01. Accessed
   summer 2003.
3. National Marfan Foundation Fact Sheet.
   National Marfan Foundation (NMF).
   Available at: http://www.marfan.org/
   pub/factsheet.html. Accessed summer 2003.
4. Salim MA, Alpert BS. Sports and Marfan
   Syndrome: Awareness and Early Diagnosis
   Can Prevent Sudden Death. The Physician
   and Sportsmedicine 2001;29(5). Copyright
   © 1998. The McGraw-Hill Companies.
   Available at: http://www.physsportsmed.
   com/issues/2001/05_01/salim.htm.
   Accessed summer 2003.
5. Marfan Syndrome. Copyright © 2003,
   Arthritis Foundation. Available at:
   http://www.arthritis.org/conditions/Disease
   Center/marfan_syndrome.asp. Accessed
   summer 2003.

Osgood-Schlatter Disease

1. Meisterling RC, Wall EJ, Meisterling MR.
   Coping With Osgood-Schlatter Disease.
   The Physician and Sportsmedicine
   1998;26(3). Copyright © 1998. The
   McGraw-Hill Companies. Available at:
   http://www.physsportsmed.com/
   issues/1998/03mar/wall_pa.htm. Accessed
   summer 2003.
2. Chang AK. Osgood Schlatter Disease.
   Copyright © 2003, eMedicine.com, Inc.
   Available at: http://www.emedicine.com/
   EMERG/topic347.htm. Accessed summer
   2003.
3. Osgood-Schlatter Disease: A Cause of Knee
   Pain in Children. Copyright © 2000 by the
   American Academy of Family Physicians.
   Available at: http://familydoctor.org/
   handouts/135.html. Accessed summer 2003.
4. Osgood-Schlatter disease. Copyright ©
   1998-2003 Mayo Foundation for Medical
   Education and Research (MFMER).
   Available at: http://www.mayoclinic.
   com/invoke.cfm?id=DS00392. Accessed
   summer 2003.

Pes Planus, Pes Cavus

1. Pediatric Orthopaedics. Copyright © The
   Cleveland Clinic 2003. Available at:
   http://www.clevelandclinic.org/ortho/peds/
   flatFoot.htm. Accessed summer 2003.
2. Coady CM, Gow N, Stanish W. Foot
   Problems in Middle-Aged Patients:
   Keeping Active People Up to Speed. The
   Physician and Sportsmedicine 1998;26(5).
   Copyright © 1998. The McGraw-Hill
   Companies. Available at: http://www.
   physsportsmed.com/issues/1998/05may/sta
   nish.htm. Accessed summer 2003.

3. Berlet G. Pes Planus. Copyright © 2003,
   eMedicine.com, Inc. Available at:
   http://www.emedicine.com/orthoped/topic
   540.htm. Accessed summer 2003.
4. Turner N. Pes Cavus. Copyright © 2003,
   eMedicine.com, Inc. Available at:
   http://www.emedicine.com/orthoped/topic
   539.htm. Accessed summer 2003.

Plantar Fasciitis

1. Petrizzi MJ, Petrizzi MG, Roos RJ. Making
   a Tension Night Splint for Plantar Fasciitis.
   The Physician and Sportsmedicine
   1998;26(6). Copyright © 1998. The
   McGraw-Hill Companies. Available at:
   http://www.physsportsmed.com/
   issues/1998/06jun/petrizzi.htm. Accessed
   summer 2003.
2. Plantar Fasciitis, Heel Spur, Heel Pain.
   Copyright © 2001 heelspurs.com LLC.
   Available at: http://heelspurs.com/
   index.html. Accessed summer 2003.
3. Shea M, Fields KB. Plantar Fasciitis:
   Prescribing Effective Treatments. The
   Physician and Sportsmedicine 1998;30(7).
   Copyright © 1998. The McGraw-Hill
   Companies. Available at: http://www.
   physsportsmed.com/issues/2002/07_02/
   fields.htm. Accessed summer 2003.
4. Roberts WO. Plantar Fascia Injection. The
   Physician and Sportsmedicine 1999;27(9).
   Copyright © 1998. The McGraw-Hill
   Companies. Available at: http://www.
   physsportsmed.com/issues/1999/09_99/
   roberts.htm. Accessed summer 2003.
5. Lowe W. Plantar Fasciitis. Copyright 2003
   Massage Magazine, Inc. Available at:
   http://www.massagemag.com/2003/
   issue105/assess105.htm. Accessed summer
   2003.

Scleroderma

1. About Scleroderma. Copyright © 2002
   Scleroderma Research Foundation.
   Available at: http://www.srfcure.org/
   sclerod/index.html. Accessed summer 2003.
2. Fetal Cells Found in Skin Lesions of
   Women with Scleroderma. The National
   Institute of Arthritis and Musculoskeletal
   and Skin Diseases. Available at:
   http://www.niams.nih.gov/ne/press/1998/
   04_22.htm. Accessed summer 2003.
3. Handout on Health: Scleroderma. National
   Institute of Arthritis and Musculoskeletal
   and Skin Diseases (NIAMS). Available at:
   http://www.niams.nih.gov/hi/topics/
   scleroderma/scleroderma.htm. Accessed
   summer 2003.
4. Scleroderma is . . . Copyright © 2003
   Scleroderma Foundation. Available at:
   http://www.scleroderma.org/medical/
   overview.htm. Accessed summer 2003.
5. CREST Syndrome. Copyright © 1998-
   2003 Mayo Foundation for Medical
   Education and Research (MFMER).
   Available at: http://www.mayoclinic.com/
   printinvoker.cfm?objectid=7DAEE064-

FFE0-4465-BF7D9482CE73940D. Accessed summer 2003.

6. Scleroderma. Copyright © 1998-2003 Mayo Foundation for Medical Education and Research (MFMER). Available at: http://www.mayoclinic.com/printinvoker.cfm?objectid=3830E935-0B28-4EE9-85E99C261470826D. Accessed summer 2003.

7. Scleroderma. Copyright © 2003, Arthritis Foundation. Available at: http://www.arthritis.org/conditions/DiseaseCenter/scleroderma.asp. Accessed summer 2003.

8. Dziankowska-Bartkowiak B. Systemic Sclerosis. Copyright © 2003, eMedicine.com, Inc. Available at: http://www.emedicine.com/derm/topic677.htm Accessed summer 2003.

Tendinitis

1. The Tendinosis Injury. Copyright © 2002, Laurie Erickson. Available at: http://www.tendinosis.org/injury.html. Accessed summer 2003.

2. Khan KM, Cook JL, Taunton JE, et al. Overuse Tendinosis, Not Tendinitis. Part 1: A New Paradigm for a Difficult Clinical Problem. The Physician and Sportsmedicine 2000;28(5). Available at: http://www.physsportsmed.com/issues/2000/05_00/khan.htm. Accessed summer 2003.

3. Cook JL, Khan KM, Maffulli N. Overuse Tendinosis, Not Tendinitis: Part 2: Applying the New Approach to Patellar Tendinopathy. The Physician and Sportsmedicine 2000;28(6). Copyright © 1998. The McGraw-Hill Companies. Available at: http://www.physsportsmed.com/issues/2000/06_00/khan.htm. Accessed summer 2003.

4. Wolf WB III. Calcific Tendinitis of the Shoulder: Diagnosis and Simple, Effective Treatment The Physician and Sportsmedicine 1999;27(9). Copyright © 1998. The McGraw-Hill Companies. Available at: http://www.physsportsmed.com/issues/1999/09_99/wolf.htm. Accessed summer 2003.

5. Tendinitis. Copyright © 1998-2003 Mayo Foundation for Medical Education and Research (MFMER). Available at: http://www.mayoclinic.com/invoke.cfm?id=DS00153. Accessed summer 2003.

Tenosynovitis

1. Medical Encyclopedia: Tenosynovitis. Copyright © 2002 A.D.A.M., Inc. Available at: http://www.nlm.nih.gov/medlineplus/ency/article/001242.htm. Accessed summer 2003.

2. Steele M. Tenosynovitis. Copyright © 2003, eMedicine.com, Inc. Available at: http://www.emedicine.com/emerg/topic571.htm. Accessed summer 2003.

Torticollis

1. Understanding Spasmodic Torticollis. National Spasmodic Torticollis Association. Available at: http://www.torticollis.org/. Accessed summer 2003.

2. Medical Encyclopedia: Torticollis. Copyright © 2002 A.D.A.M., Inc. Available at: http://www.nlm.nih.gov/medlineplus/ency/article/000749.htm. Accessed summer 2003.

3. Dystonia. Copyright © 1996-2003 MedicineNet, Inc. Available at: http://www.medicinenet.com/Dystonia/article.htm. Accessed summer 2003.

4. Vangelova L. Botulinum Toxin: A Poison That Can Heal. FDA Consumer magazine (December 1995). Available at: http://www.fda.gov/fdac/features/095_bot.html. Accessed summer 2003.

5. NINDS Dystonias Information Page. The National Institute of Neurological Disorders and Stroke. Available at: http://www.ninds.nih.gov/health_and_medical/disorders/the_dystonias.htm?format=printable. Accessed summer 2003.

6. Ross M. Torticollis. Copyright © 2003, eMedicine.com, Inc. Available at: http://www.emedicine.com/emerg/topic597.htm Accessed summer 2003.

Whiplash

1. Lowe W. Whiplash. Copyright © 2003 Massage Magazine, Inc. Available at: http://www.massagemag.com/2003/issue104/assess104.htm. Accessed summer 2003.

2. Hunter OK Jr. Whiplash. Copyright © 2003, eMedicine.com, Inc. Available at: http://www.emedicine.com/pmr/topic28.htm. Accessed summer 2003.

3. NINDS Whiplash Information Page. The National Institute of Neurological Disorders and Stroke. Available at: http://www.ninds.nih.gov/health_and_medical/disorders/whiplash.htm. Accessed summer 2003.

4. Verhagen AP, Peeters GGM, de Bie RA, et al. Conservative Treatment for Whiplash. Copyright © 2003 The Cochrane Collaboration. Available at: http://www.medscape.com/viewarticle/455163. Accessed summer 2003.

5. Mahar R. Musculotendinous Injuries of the Neck. Available at: http://www.theberries.ns.ca/Archives/Whiplash.html. Accessed summer 2003.

Carpal Tunnel Syndrome

1. Carpal Tunnel Syndrome Fact Sheet. National Institute of Neurological Disorders and Stroke. Available at: http://www.ninds.nih.gov/health_and_medical/pubs/carpal_tunnel.htm. Accessed summer 2003.

2. Viera AJ. Management of Carpal Tunnel Syndrome. Copyright © 2003 by the American Academy of Family Physicians. Available at: http://aafp.org/afp/20030715/265.html. Accessed summer 2003.

3. Carpal tunnel syndrome. Copyright © 1998-2003 Mayo Foundation for Medical Education and Research (MFMER). Available at: http://www.mayoclinic.com/invoke.cfm?id=DS00326. Accessed summer 2003.

4. Carpal Tunnel and Tarsal Tunnel Syndrome. Copyright © 1996-2003 MedicineNet, Inc. Available at: http://www.medicinenet.com/Carpal_Tunnel_Syndrome/article.htm. Accessed summer 2003.

5. Fuller DA. Carpal Tunnel Syndrome. Copyright © 2003, eMedicine.com, Inc. Available at: http://www.emedicine.com/orthoped/topic455.htm. Accessed summer 2003.

6. NIOSH Facts: Carpal Tunnel Syndrome. National Institute of Occupational Safety and Health. Available at: http://www.cdc.gov/niosh/muskdsfs.html. Accessed winter 2004.

7. Packer-Tursman J. Treatment of Choice. Special to The Washington Post. Tuesday, October 17, 2000; Page Z35. Copyright © 2000 The Washington Post. Available at: http://www.washingtonpost.com/wp-dyn/articles/A21028-2000Oct17.html. Accessed summer 2003.

Disc Disease

1. Furman MB. Cervical Disc Disease. Copyright © 2003, eMedicine.com, Inc. Available at: http://www.emedicine.com/pmr/topic25.htm. Accessed summer 2003.

2. El-Khoury GY. Diagnosis of Disk Disease. All contents copyright © 1992-2003 the Author(s) and The University of Iowa. Available at: http://www.vh.org/adult/provider/radiology/DiagnosisDiskDisease/DiagnosisDiskDisease.html. Accessed summer 2003.

3. Patel J. Laser Discectomy. Copyright © 2003, eMedicine.com, Inc. Available at: http://www.emedicine.com/neuro/topic683.htm. Accessed summer 2003.

4. Lumbar Degenerative Disc Disease. Copyright © 1999-2003 Spine-health.com. http://www.spine-health.com/topics/cd/overview/lumbar/young/degen01.html. Accessed summer 2003.

5. Lumbar Disc Herniation. Copyright © 1999-2003 Spine-health.com. Available at: http://www.spine-health.com/topics/cd/overview/lumbar/young/lum01.html. Accessed summer 2003.

6. Aptaker RL. Neck Pain: Part 1: Narrowing the Differential. The Physician and Sportsmedicine 1996;24(10). Copyright © 1996. The McGraw-Hill Companies. http://www.physsportsmed.com/issues/1996/10_96/aptaker.htm. Accessed summer 2003.

7. Aptaker RL. Neck Pain: Part 2: Optimizing Treatment and Rehabilitation. The Physician and Sportsmedicine 1996;24(11). Copyright © 1996. The McGraw-Hill

Companies. Available at: http://www.
physsportsmed.com/issues/1996/11_96/
aptaker2.htm. Accessed summer 2003.

8. Chen AL, Spivak JM. Degenerative Lumbar
Spinal Stenosis: Options for Aging Backs.
The Physician and Sportsmedicine
2003;31(8). Copyright © 1996. The
McGraw-Hill Companies. Available at:
http://www.physsportsmed.com/
issues/2003/0803/chen.htm. Accessed
summer 2003.

9. Foster MR. Herniated Nucleus Pulposus.
Copyright © 2003, eMedicine.com, Inc.
Available at: http://www.emedicine.com/
orthoped/topic138.htm. Accessed summer
2003.

10. Patel RK. Lumbar Degenerative Disc
Disease. Copyright © 2003, eMedicine.com,
Inc. Available at:
http://www.emedicine.com/
pmr/topic67.htm. Accessed summer 2003.

Myasthenia Gravis

1. Myasthenia Gravis. Copyright © 1996-2003
MedicineNet, Inc. Available at:
http://www.medicinenet.com/Myasthenia_
Gravis/article.htm. Accessed summer 2003.

2. Shaw AK. Myasthenia Gravis. Copyright ©
2003, eMedicine.com, Inc. Available at:
http://www.emedicine.com/neuro/topic232.
htm. Accessed summer 2003.

3. Myasthenia Gravis. Copyright © 1998-2003
Mayo Foundation for Medical Education
and Research (MFMER). Available
at:http://www.mayoclinic.com/invoke.cfm?i
d=DS00375. Accessed summer 2003.

4. NINDS Myasthenia Gravis Information
Page. The National Institute of
Neurological Disorders and Stroke.
Available at: http://www.ninds.nih.gov/
health_and_medical/disorders/myasthe-
nia_gravis.htm Accessed summer 2003.

Thoracic Outlet Syndrome

1. NINDS Thoracic Outlet Syndrome
Information Page. National Institute
of Neurological Disorders and Stroke.
Available at: http://www.ninds.nih.
gov/health_and_medical/disorders/
thoracic_doc.htm. Accessed summer
2003.

2. Sucher BM. Thoracic Outlet Syndrome.
Copyright © 2003, eMedicine.com, Inc.
Available at: http://www.emedicine.com/
pmr/topic136.htm. Accessed summer
2003.

3. Dubuisson AS. The Thoracic Outlet
Syndrome. Louisiana State University
Health Sciences Centers Department of
Neurosurgery. Available at: http://www.
medschool.lsumc.edu/Nsurgery/TOS.html.
Accessed summer 2003.

NERVOUS SYSTEM CONDITIONS

3

Chapter Objectives

After reading this chapter, you should be able to . . .

- Name three diseases that can be confused with multiple sclerosis.
- Identify the neurotransmitter that is in short supply in Parkinson's disease.
- State the causative agent of herpes zoster.
- Describe three types of depression.
- Describe three types of anxiety disorders.
- Describe two types of stroke.
- Identify the nerve that is involved in Bell's palsy.
- Name three complications of spinal cord injury.
- Identify two signs that indicate that a headache could be a medical emergency.
- Describe the feature that multiple sclerosis and Guillain-Barré syndrome have in common.

INTRODUCTION

By the time most massage therapists finish their training, they probably know more about the nervous system than they ever suspected even existed, and they will probably still feel like rank amateurs on the subject. That feeling is common to most people who study this topic. Fortunately, only a passing familiarity with the structure and function of this system is needed to make educated decisions about massage and most nervous system disorders. Most of the conditions considered here affect the peripheral nerves rather than the central nervous system (CNS), so this introductory discussion focuses mainly on the structure and function of the parts of the nervous system massage therapists can touch—which, not coincidentally, are also the parts of the system that are most vulnerable to injury.

Function

What are nerves? Nerves are bundles of individual neurons: fibrous cells capable of transmitting electrical impulses from one place to another. At their most basic level, their function is to transmit information from the body to the brain (sensation) and responses from the brain back to the body (motor control). Interconnected neurons in the brain also provide the potential for consciousness, creativity, memory, and other fascinating abilities, but they are beyond the scope of what massage therapists are qualified to deal with, and so are not discussed in any detail here.

Structure

Peripheral nerves are composed of bundles of long filaments (neurons) that run from the spinal cord to wherever in the body they supply sensation or motor control. Each neuron is a single living cell. It is a bit boggling to realize that the neuron running from the low back to the skin of the great toe is all one unbroken microscopic fiber, but that is how we are built.

Neurons have three parts: the **dendrite** (which carries impulses *toward* the cell body), the cell body with a nucleus, and the **axon** (which carries impulses *away* from the cell body). Sensory neurons therefore have exceptionally long dendrites to carry information from the periphery toward the cell body in the dorsal root ganglia; they have short little axons to continue carrying their impulses into the spinal cord. Motor neurons have tiny axons and cell bodies inside the spinal canal and very long axons to carry messages out to their terminating sites in the muscles and glands. Motor and sensory neurons communicate via synapses in the spinal cord, usually by way of some combinations of central, or association, neurons. At the same time that an immediate response is generated at the spinal cord level, the information also travels up the spine into the brain. This immediate reaction is called the reflex arc (Figure 3.1).

🔘 *The animation "Nerve Synapse" can be found on the Student Resource CD-ROM that accompanies this book.*

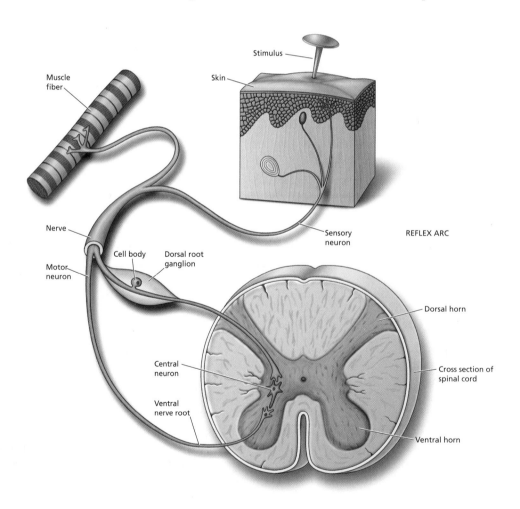

Figure 3.1. The reflex arc connects sensation to motor response.

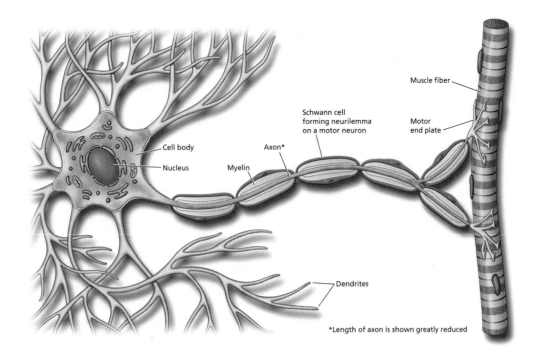

Figure 3.2. Neurons in the peripheral nervous system are covered with Schwann cells, forming myelin and neurilemma.

Most neurons in the peripheral and central nervous system have a waxy insulating coating called myelin. This layer of material speeds nerve conduction along the fiber, and also prevents the jumping of electrical impulses from one fiber to another. In the peripheral nervous system, neurons have another protective feature in *neurilemma*: an out covering of special cells that can help to regenerate damaged tissue (Figure 3.2).

Peripheral nerves typically run close to the bone, where they are protected from most injuries. In a few places they are vulnerable, however. These spots are *endangerments* for massage therapists, who could potentially cause injury to delicate tissues at these points; self-defense classes call them *targets*. For specific information on nerve endangerment sites, refer to Appendix 3.

It is a convenient analogy to think about nerves as bundles of electrical wires. The similarities are obvious: here are thousands of filaments carrying electrical impulses, each one wrapped by an insulating layer of myelin, and they are bundled together for efficiency. The analogy stops, however, when one considers the effect of external pressure on nerve fiber transmission. In *Job's Body*, Deane Juhan points out that a piece of electrical cable with a truck parked on it continues to carry its electrical messages, but a sciatic nerve squeezed by a tight piriformis has a drastically reduced flow of energy through it.[1] Nerves function with a combination of electrical and fluid flow; fluid flow may be severely limited by external pressure. Consider the implications of that pressure on a femoral nerve that is hugged by a psoas in spasm or the brachial plexus nerves running through a tangled maze of scalenes and pectoralis minor muscles.

General Neurologic Problems

Most of the nervous system disorders that massage can affect involve some kind of mechanical pinching or distortion of peripheral nerves as they wend their ways from the spinal cord to their destinations in the body. Peripheral nerve damage has a generally good prognosis because of the regenerative properties provided by the neurilemma.

[1] Juhan D. Job's Body: A Handbook for Bodywork. Barrytown, NY: Station Hill Press, Inc., 1987:158.

The Stress Response System

The *stress response system* is the link between the central nervous system and the endocrine system that allows humans to respond to both short-term and long-term stressors. It is controlled by the hypothalamus-pituitary-adrenal axis (HPA): the communication between the hypothalamus, the pituitary gland, and the adrenals. A healthy stress response system allows immediate reactions that are appropriately gauged to the circumstances: big reactions to big threats, small reactions to small threats. And when the stress response system works well, the chemical changes it brings about are transitory and quickly neutralized once the threat has passed.

Some people have a stress-response system that does not work well. The chemical messages issued first from the hypothalamus, then by the pituitary gland, are slow to leave the brain and reach the adrenals. This takes longer to have an effect on the body, decreasing the ability to respond quickly to threat. However, the stress reaction, once it takes hold, is tenacious. Its after-effects linger much longer than for someone who has a healthy stress response system. Furthermore, people who have a sluggish stress response system also tend to have *more* stress responses, *more* often, to *less threatening* stimuli, and those responses will have longer-lasting effects on the body. This is a person who fumes in a long checkout line, who frets in heavy traffic, and who blows her top when the kids leave their bikes in the driveway. This is someone who may have a sluggish but over-reactive stress response, and this person has a high propensity to develop, among other things, depression.

What determines the health of the stress response system? Studies with animals reveal one reliable predictor for a sluggish stress response: lack of tactile stimulation, or touch. Under-stimulated animals have consistently slower, longer lasting, and more frequent stress responses than animals that had been regularly petted and fondled. Consider what this means for the average under-touched person in our society: most of us have low-functioning, but longer-lasting, stress reactions, and they occur with unnecessary and unhealthy frequency. The good news is, the health of the stress response system can be improved with an abundance of healthy, nurturing touch.

Other neurologic problems involve the brain or spinal cord, which have very limited ability to regenerate and which massage obviously cannot directly access. But even when the spinal cord has been injured, overlapping patterns of innervation created by the twists and turns of the plexuses often allow at least partial use of what would otherwise be a totally lost limb. This is a remarkable advantage that begins to explain the benefits of the confusing routes that nerves take through the plexuses. The best plan, when faced with a client who has sustained CNS damage, is to address the *symptoms* of these disorders as well as possible, looking for sensation where it is present, and to create as hospitable an internal environment as possible.

Survivors of various kinds of CNS damage often experience loss of motor function that becomes progressively worse. This traditionally has been viewed as an inevitable consequence, but this idea may prove to be a myth. In many cases, loss of motor function may be an issue of proprioceptive adaptation more than true nerve loss. In other words, a stroke or traumatic brain injury survivor may experience some loss of strength in an arm or a leg, and their compensatory movement patterns allow for further degeneration of affected muscle fibers. This type of progressive loss may be possible to interrupt and even reverse with massage, stretching, and careful exercise.

Organic and mechanical problems with the central and peripheral nervous systems are one class of neurologic problem massage therapists will encounter. Psychiatric disorders, which also can be classified as neurologic problems, are another situation altogether. Many people have a bewildering array of mental or psychological qualities that set them apart from the arbitrary standards called "normal." Some of these people seek massage as a way to deal with some of the difficulties that their "abnormalities" create. This is often a good impulse; touch is an integral part of physical and psychological health—in fact, it could be said that touch is the primary link between physical and psychological health (see sidebar, "The Stress Response System").

Massage therapists can thus be put in the precarious position of deciding whether their work is an appropriate part of someone's healing (or even just coping) process. Sometimes the answer will clearly be "no" (for instance, with someone who obviously is in need of psychological counseling instead of or in addition to massage). At other times it will be less clear, and it will be necessary to seek out the opinion of other professionals. Mental health patients who are on heavy, long-term doses of medication are in a particularly vulnerable position with regard to massage. Though massage is usually a good thing, it can change the internal chemistry of the body and brain significantly. When massage elicits a parasympathetic response, the types of neurotransmitters and hormones circulating in the body may shift radically away from "flight or fight" chemicals to substances that allow for relaxation and even sleepiness. If a client is on medication to achieve equilibrium, it is inappropriate for a well-meaning but ignorant massage therapist to throw him off balance. It is important to consult with the client's medical and health care team before proceeding.

Disorders of the nervous system can produce a bewildering variety of startling and sometimes intimidating symptoms. In working with these patients, as with all others, massage therapists must remember that their prime objective must always be to "do no harm."

NERVOUS SYSTEM CONDITIONS

Chronic Degenerative Disorders

Alzheimer's Disease
Amyotrophic Lateral Sclerosis
Multiple Sclerosis
Parkinson's Disease
Peripheral Neuropathy
Tremor

Infectious Disorders

Encephalitis
Herpes Zoster
Meningitis
Polio, Postpolio Syndrome

Psychiatric Disorders

Anxiety Disorders
Attention Deficit Hyperactivity
Disorder
Chemical Dependency
Depression
Eating Disorders

Nervous System Injuries

Bell's Palsy
Cerebral Palsy
Reflex Sympathetic Dystrophy
Spina Bifida
Spinal Cord Injury
Stroke
Traumatic Brain Injury
Trigeminal Neuralgia

Other

Guillain-Barré Syndrome
Headaches
Seizure Disorders
Sleep Disorders

CHRONIC DEGENERATIVE DISORDERS

Alzheimer's Disease

Definition: What Is It?

Alzheimer's disease is a progressive degenerative disorder of the brain causing memory loss, personality changes, and eventually death. The precise causes of the disorder are not fully understood, but it is now known that although most people can expect a certain degree of memory loss as they age, the severe dementia associated with Alzheimer's is not normal and not an inevitable fate for every person.

Demographics: Who Gets It?

Alzheimer's disease affects approximately 5% of the US population, or roughly 4.5 million people. It affects approximately half of all people living in nursing homes and costs some $110 billion per year in direct medical expenses, and an estimated $61 billion per year in lost productivity from primary caregivers.

   The incidence of Alzheimer's disease increases with age. Approximately 14% of people older than 65 are diagnosed with the disease and close to half of those older than 85 have severe dementia.

Alzheimer's Disease in Brief

Pronunciation
awlz′-hī-měrz

What is it?
Alzheimer's disease is a degenerative disorder of the brain involving shrinkage and death of neural tissue.

How is it recognized?
Alzheimer's disease is difficult to definitively diagnose in a living person, but signs and symptoms include progressive memory loss, deterioration of language and cognitive skills, disorientation, and lack of ability to care for oneself.

Is massage indicated or contraindicated?
If an Alzheimer's disease patient feels comfortable and nurtured while receiving touch, then massage is very much indicated. However, if the patient feels disoriented and threatened, the therapist must change tactics. Alzheimer's patients may not be able to communicate verbally, so therapists must be sensitive to nonverbal cues.

Most cases of Alzheimer's disease are diagnosed around age 80. Because baby boomers will soon be entering the at-risk age group, it is estimated that by 2050 this disease will disable some 16 million people.[2]

Alzheimer's disease affects more women than men, but this may be related to the fact the women generally live longer than men, rather than a gender-based predisposition.

Etiology: What Happens?

Alzheimer's disease is named for a German doctor, Alois Alzheimer, who in 1906 first documented the trademark lesions in the brain seen with this disease. He performed an autopsy on a female patient who died in a mental institution in her mid-50s and noticed two specific changes in her brain tissue: plaques and tangles. These observations have become the primary postmortem diagnostic features of this disease, and they have become the focus of the leading edge of research today.

Features of Alzheimer's Disease

Plaques   Sticky deposits of a certain type of naturally occurring cellular protein called *beta amyloid* have been noted on brain tissue of people with Alzheimer's disease. Beta amyloid is a protein produced by many cells throughout the body, and it occurs in different lengths and qualities, depending on where it is found. In the brain, it seems to be particularly adhesive. When it accumulates in sufficient amounts, the deposits appear to stimulate an inflammatory response in the brain that kills off not only the cells affected by beta amyloid plaques, but nearby unaffected cells as well.

Neurofibrillary Tangles   Another Alzheimer-related protein is called *tau*. This substance helps to physically support long fibers in the CNS that allow cells to communicate. The tau proteins in Alzheimer's patients degenerate, and the long fibers collapse and become twisted and tangled together. Eventually the cells, which are incapable of transmitting messages to each other, shrink and die. This results in significant atrophy of the entire structure of the brain (Figures 3.3a, 3.3b).

Low Neurotransmitters   The presence of beta amyloid plaques and tau-related tangles means that fewer brain cells function at normal levels. With the loss of neural tissue, levels of neurotransmitters in the brains of Alzheimer's patients become pathologically low. This makes it difficult for the functioning nerve cells that remain to communicate with each other. Consequently, the Alzheimer's patient loses access to memories and loses the ability to process new information.

Genetics   Although having Alzheimer's disease in the family only marginally increases a person's chance of developing it, some specific genetic markers have been found that can identify a higher-risk population. The genes involved probably determine how effectively a person can clear off beta amyloid plaques. Genetic research has yielded especially clear markers for people susceptible to an early onset of the disease.

Most of the information we have about how Alzheimer's develops has been gathered in the last 10 years and is still in rapid development. Just recently it has been found that other issues, including genetics, chronic inflammation, a history of head injury, exposure to environmental toxins, high cholesterol levels, low estrogen levels (in women), and many other variables are also contributing factors for many patients.

[2] What Is Alzheimer's Disease? Copyright © 2003 Alzheimer's Disease and Related Disorders Association, Inc. Available at: http://www.alz.org/AboutAD/overview.htm. Accessed fall 2003.

Figure 3.3a. Normal brain.   **Figure 3.3b.** Visible atrophy of cerebrum associated with Alzheimer's disease.

Signs and Symptoms

The protocol for staging Alzheimer's disease is somewhat variable, but the Global Deterioration Scale outlines seven distinct phases of the disease.[3]

Stage 1   No impairment

Stage 2   Very mild decline. No impairment is obvious to observers, but the person may be aware of some brief memory lapses. This stage may also be called "mild cognitive impairment," a pre-Alzheimer's condition.

Stage 3   Mild dementia. Some memory loss or loss of function is objectively observable by friends or family, but coping skills remain intact. Word loss becomes apparent at this stage.

Stage 4   Moderate dementia. The person experiences a loss of knowledge of current events, reduced ability to do complex math problems, short-term memory loss, and a tendency to withdraw from social situations.

Stage 5   Moderately severe dementia. The person experiences major gaps in the ability to perform activities of daily living. Assistance is necessary for complex tasks such as cooking, shopping, and maintaining finances.

Stage 6   Severe dementia. In this stage, profound memory loss is evident, personality changes may develop, and the person may become easily disoriented even in familiar surroundings. Wandering becomes a danger. Some loss of bowel or bladder control may occur.

---

[3] What Is Alzheimer's Disease? Copyright © 2003 Alzheimer's Disease and Related Disorders Association, Inc. Available at: http://www.alz.org/AboutAD/overview.htm. Accessed fall 2003.

Stage 7 Very severe dementia. The patient is completely incapacitated. Language is mostly lost. Muscular problems in the form of weakness, rigidity, and *dysphagia* develop.

Most people with Alzheimer's disease live about 8 years after their diagnosis, but this number can range from 3 to 20 years.

Diagnosis

Diagnosis of Alzheimer's disease has always been problematic because the presence of plaques and tangles can only be confirmed posthumously. This disease is diagnosed through a variety of tests to rule out other causes of dementia, in combination with mental status examinations. It is important to try to come to an accurate diagnosis of Alzheimer's for two reasons. First, the earlier treatment is introduced, the longer memory may be preserved. Second, dementia and loss of memory can sometimes be indicators of diseases *other* than Alzheimer's, some of which can be reversible.

As our ability to gather information about living brains develops, it may become easier to diagnose Alzheimer's disease. New technologies allow doctors to observe interactions of brain chemicals at a molecular level in living patients. Nonetheless, a diagnosis of Alzheimer's is based on a physical examination, a mental examination, and ruling out other dementing diseases.

Differential Diagnosis

Alzheimer's disease is only one of several diseases that can cause dementia and memory loss. Some conditions involve permanent brain damage, but others may be only temporary problems, if they are treated appropriately.

Causes of permanent memory loss other than Alzheimer's include

- *Vascular dementia*: this is caused by a narrowing of the arteries to the brain, usually associated with advanced cardiovascular disease.
- *Stroke and transient ischemic accident (TIA)*: these events cause brain tissue to die because of an interruption in blood supply. These issues are more fully discussed elsewhere in this chapter.
- *Parkinson's disease*: this disease involves the degeneration of certain motor centers in the brain, but it also often involves dementia. Parkinson's disease is discussed in a separate article in this chapter.
- *Lewy body dementia*: Lewy bodies are protein deposits similar to beta amyloid plaques that lead to dementia. This disease has features in common with both Alzheimer's disease and Parkinson's disease.
- *Huntington's disease*: this is another progressive degenerative central nervous system disease, involving the destruction of nerve cells and resulting changes in personality and intellect. Huntington's is a genetic disease.
- *Creutzfeldt-Jakob disease* is a type of dementia that affects young and middle-aged people. It is associated with eating meat that is contaminated with *bovine spongiform encephalitis* (mad cow disease).

Other conditions can cause memory loss that is recoverable. Naturally, it is important to consider these possibilities before deciding that a patient has irreversible Alzheimer's disease. Some examples of things important to test for include

- Chronic high blood pressure
- Depression
- Diabetes
- Hypothyroidism

- Side effects to medication
- Vitamin B$_{12}$ deficiency

Treatment

Current treatment options often revolve around the deficit of neurotransmitters in the brain that make it difficult for nerves to communicate. ***Cholinesterase*** inhibitors are often prescribed to prevent the reuptake of acetylcholine, an essential neurotransmitter that is often in short supply for Alzheimer's patients. These drugs effectively improve memory, at least in the short term. Other medications may be prescribed to address some of the behavioral and mood distortions seen with Alzheimer's.

Other promising options include the use of some nonsteroidal anti-inflammatory drugs (NSAIDs) (specifically, ibuprofen, naproxen sodium, and ***indomethacin***—*not* aspirin or acetaminophen) that seem to limit the reaction to plaques that causes cell damage. Observations that postmenopausal women who supplement estrogen have a lower risk of Alzheimer's disease, and that some antioxidants seem to limit the progression of the disease also may point the way to effective treatments or preventive measures in the future.

Massage?

Alzheimer's disease patients, even in advanced stages of the disease when language is difficult or impossible, still respond positively to touch. Research done on the effects of massage with Alzheimer's patients shows that although bodywork does not slow or reverse the disease, it improves the quality of life for patients to the extent that they become measurably less disruptive, show better sense of orientation, and have more positive social interactions in nursing home settings.

Two cautions must be kept in mind when working with Alzheimer's patients. One is that most of these clients are elderly, and consequently may have a number of other complicated disorders that may or may not contraindicate various kinds of bodywork. The other is that when a client cannot communicate clearly, it becomes the responsibility of the massage therapist to interpret nonverbal signals about how the bodywork is being accepted. Alzheimer's clients generally respond well to massage, but if they become anxious and frightened for unknowable reasons, the therapist must be sensitive to the client's mental and emotional state.

Amyotrophic Lateral Sclerosis

Definition: What Is It?

Also known as *Lou Gehrig's disease,* ***amyotrophic lateral sclerosis*** (ALS) is a progressive condition that destroys motor neurons in the central and peripheral nervous systems, leading to the atrophy of voluntary muscles.

Demographics: Who Gets It?

Three types of ALS have been identified: sporadic, which accounts for 90% to 95% of the cases in the United States; familial, which shows a genetic link for 5% to 10% of US cases; and the Mariana Island variety, which is endemic to a specific population in the Western Pacific islands.

Amyotrophic Lateral Sclerosis in Brief

Pronunciation
ă-mī-ö-trö′fik lat′ĕr-ăl sklĕ-rö′sis

What is it?
Amyotrophic lateral sclerosis (ALS) is a progressive disease that begins in the central nervous system. It involves the degeneration of motor neurons and the subsequent atrophy of voluntary muscles.

How is it recognized?
Symptoms of ALS include weakness, fatigue, and muscle spasms. It appears most frequently in patients between 40 and 70 years old.

Is massage indicated or contraindicated?
ALS indicates massage, with caution, when a massage therapist works as part of a health care team.

ALS usually affects people between 40 and 70 years old; the average age at diagnosis is 55. Familial ALS tends to have a younger onset than the sporadic type. Between 4,000 and 5,000 new cases of ALS are diagnosed in the United States every year; approximately 30,000 people in this country are living with this disease right now. Men get it only slightly more often than women do. One of the most interesting features about this disease is that it has a virtually identical incidence among all nations and races. Two populations carry a higher-than-normal risk in the United States, however: electrical utility workers and airline pilots.

Etiology: What Happens?

The cause or causes of ALS is unknown. When the disease develops, it leads to the degeneration of motor neurons in the spinal cord, which leads to the progressive and irreversible atrophy of voluntary muscle.

Several possible causative factors have been identified, including some features that are strikingly similar to *Alzheimer's disease* (this chapter): tangled neural fibers and deposits of abnormal proteins on clumps of cells. This leads to the degeneration of the neuron's cytoskeleton, and the "strangulation" of the presynaptic axons. ALS interrupts only motor function, however, and does not affect intellect or memory.

One well-established feature in ALS is the accumulation of a neurotransmitter called *glutamate* in the synapses. This excitatory neurotransmitter is not neutralized or reabsorbed by the presynaptic neuron, and it eventually damages and even kills the motor neuron it is meant to stimulate.

Other possible causes of ALS include a genetic susceptibility to damage from free radicals (this has been reliably established in the case of familial ALS), and exposure to environmental toxins such as lead, agricultural chemicals, and selenium. It is important to point out, however, that these associations are simply observations; causative factors for ALS have not been defined.

Signs and Symptoms

ALS presents different early symptoms in different people. The most common pattern is stiffness, weakness, and awkwardness in one body part, which slowly spreads to other parts of the body. Approximately one third of ALS patients have their first symptoms in the legs; another third begin with changes in hand and arm function; and the final third begin with "thick speech" and difficulty with swallowing. Fasciculations, or visible muscle twitching, may be present. One side is typically worse than the other, but the stiffness eventually spreads and moves proximally up the limbs, eventually to affect the trunk muscles for breathing.

The nerve damage seen with ALS is to motor neurons; sensory neurons are not attacked. This can be a painful disease, however, as the body gradually collapses and gravity puts musculoskeletal stresses on muscles that have no power to respond. Immobility also leads to a high risk of *decubitus ulcers* (Chapter 1) and constipation.

ALS does not affect intellectual capacity at all.

Diagnosis

No single test can identify ALS. It is typically diagnosed through history, physical examination, nerve conduction studies, and electromyographs, all of which show loss of muscle function caused by lack of nerve stimulation. Tests are also conducted to differentiate ALS from other conditions that have some similar symptoms, for instance *muscular dystrophy* (see Chapter 2), *hyperthyroidism* (Chapter 8), *multiple sclerosis, postpolio syndrome,* and *peripheral neuropathy* (all in this chapter).

Treatment

Until very recently, treatment for ALS has been strictly palliative, that is, aimed at managing the severity of the symptoms only. Some of these options include moderate exercise and physical and occupational therapy to maintain muscle strength as long as possible. Heat and whirlpools are used to control muscle spasms, and speech therapy helps with difficulties in swallowing and speech. Assistive devices such as leg braces, arm braces, or wheelchairs can improve a patient's ability to function. In advanced cases, swallowing may be so difficult that the insertion of a stomach tube (*gastrostomy*) may be recommended. Because this disease does not impede cognitive or emotional processes at all, psychological therapy for ALS patients and their families is an important part of the treatment plan.

Drug treatment for ALS traditionally has been used only to help combat general fatigue or secondary infections, but drugs have now been developed that limit the amount of glutamate in the CNS, so motor nerves live longer. They are not a cure for ALS, but they may significantly prolong the lives of people affected by this disease.

Prognosis

Once diagnosed, this disease, which has no known cure, usually results in death within 2 to 10 years. Usually death comes about by complications of paralysis, particularly systemic infections such as *pneumonia* (Chapter 6) or *kidney infection* (Chapter 9). One half of all ALS patients succumb within 3 years of diagnosis. Ninety percent die within 6 years. Some ALS patients, however, have survived for decades. How? No one knows.

Massage?

This disease is not blood or lymph-borne, it does not involve sensory paralysis, and it is not contagious. It is treated with heat, exercise, and physical therapy. Therefore, *within limits*, and in the absence of other contraindicated circumstances, massage also may be appropriate. Massage therapists who get a chance to work with ALS patients should do it as part of a health care team.

Multiple Sclerosis

Definition: *What Is It?*

This is a condition characterized by the inflammation and then gradual degeneration of myelin sheaths in the spinal cord and brain. It is thought to be an autoimmune disease, but the triggering pathogen or other stimulus has not yet been identified.

Demographics: *Who Gets It?*

Multiple sclerosis (MS) affects whites approximately twice as often as any other ethnic group. Its highest incidence is among people who live far from the equator (either north or south) or who did so before they were 15 years old.

MS is generally diagnosed in patients somewhere between 20 and 40 years of age. Young women are diagnosed up to twice as often as young men, but when it is diagnosed among older patients, the female–male distribution is about the same.

Multiple Sclerosis in Brief

What is it?
Multiple sclerosis (MS) is an idiopathic disease that involves the destruction of myelin sheaths around both motor and sensory neurons in the CNS.

How is it recognized?
MS has many symptoms, depending on the nature of the damage. These can include fatigue, eye pain, spasticity, tremors, and a progressive loss of vision, sensation, and motor control.

Is massage indicated or contraindicated?
Massage is indicated in subacute stages of MS, when the client is in remission rather than during acute periods in which function is diminishing.

Between 300,000 and 350,000 Americans live with MS; approximately 9,000 new cases are diagnosed every year.

Etiology: What Happens?

The word *sclerosis* means hardened scar or plaque. In MS, myelin is attacked and destroyed. Early in the process, research indicates that **oligodendrocytes**, the myelin-producing cells in the CNS, multiply and attempt to repair the damage, but eventually they fail.

As attacks progress, normal myelin is replaced with scar tissue. As the disease advances, the electrical impulses meant to tie the whole system together literally short circuit. This results in motor and sensory paralysis, instead of coordinated movement and feeling. The signs and symptoms of the disease, like so many disorders of the CNS, depend entirely on where and how much nerve tissue has been damaged.

MS, like many autoimmune diseases, often works in cycles of inflammatory "flares" followed by periods of remission. During flares, the myelin is under attack and is replaced by scar tissue. During remission, inflammation subsides, and some myelin regenerates. In this way MS patients may lose some neurologic function during flares but regain some or all of it during remission.

If flares are persistent and repetitive, the damage may affect the neuron itself. In this case, lost function is more likely to be permanent.

Causes

The leading theories behind MS point to immune system attacks against some component of myelin sheaths in the central nervous system. This leads to an inflammatory response that destroys the protective myelin sheath and may eventually attack the nerve tissue itself. Most autoimmune diseases have some specific pathogenic trigger that begins the immune system mistake leading to tissue damage, but no specific trigger has yet been identified for MS.

It also seems clear that a genetic predisposition raises the risk of developing MS, but this seems to be a relatively small factor. The population-wide risk of developing MS is less than 1%; people with a first-degree relative who has the disease carry a risk of only 1% to 3%. Identical twins carry a 30% risk of developing the disease if their twin has it.

This collection of information indicates that MS is probably an autoimmune disease to which some people are genetically predisposed, but that requires some combination of environmental triggers to initiate the disease process. The fact that in a few isolated cases the incidence of MS among a local population ("MS clusters") is much higher than the statistical norm supports the influence of environmental factors that are not yet understood.

Signs and Symptoms

This disease is sometimes called *The Great Imitator* because its initial symptoms can look like a variety of other diseases, depending on what area of nerve tissue has been affected. The order with which symptoms appear also varies greatly from one person to the next. Some of the most dependable signs and symptoms include

- *Weakness*: The onset of this problem may be gradual or sudden. It comes about because the loss of myelin makes nerve transmission slow.
- *Spasm*: This can take the form of chronic muscle stiffness or of active acute cramping (see *spasms, cramps* Chapter 2).

- *Changes in sensation*: MS patients often report numbness or paresthesia ("pins and nee- dles") in various parts of the body. These sensations may last for hours or days at a time.
- *Optic neuritis*: Attacks on the myelin of the optic nerve results in extreme eye pain, coupled with progressive loss of function. Vision may be minimally impaired (for in- stance, red/green color distortions), or it may be fully lost until the episode has past. Most MS patients recover full or close to full vision when they go into remission.
- *Urologic dysfunction*: MS patients may find it difficult to urinate, or they may experi- ence incontinence.
- *Sexual dysfunction*: For men, difficulty in maintaining an erection, or for women, in having an orgasm, are sometimes early signs of this disease.
- *Difficulty walking*: This problem can be a product of several different factors, includ- ing muscle stiffness, numbness, and loss of coordination.
- *Loss of cognitive function*: A frequently overlooked issue for many MS patients is a change in mental ability: short-term memory and the ability to learn and perform complex tasks is often challenged. Most MS patients have limited loss of cognitive function, but they can compensate. A smaller percentage experience severe changes in cognitive skills.
- *Depression*: This is a complication of many chronic progressive diseases, especially in situations as unpredictable as those created by multiple sclerosis. Up to 70% of MS patients live with depression, which can exacerbate symptoms.
- *Lhermitte's sign*: In this neurologic test, electrical sensations run down the spine when the neck is in flexion.
- *Digestive disturbances*: Many MS patients experience severe digestive disturbances (nausea, diarrhea, constipation) that vary greatly from day to day.
- *Fatigue*: Perhaps the most common symptom for all MS patients is debilitating fa- tigue, which is particularly exacerbated by heat. The fatigue may be a result of slower or impaired nerve transmission (this requires fewer muscle fibers to work harder), muscle spasm, and other factors.

Progression

The progression of this disease is highly unpredictable. It has a few characteristic pat- terns, but some patients move from one pattern type to others within their disease process. Some of the basic patterns are these:

- *Benign MS:* The patient has only one flare in her lifetime.
- *Relapse/remitting (RRMS):* Definite periods of flare are followed by long periods of re- mission. It may be years between episodes.
- *Secondary progressive MS (SPMS):* Cycles of flare and remission occur, but recovery during remission is only partial.
- *Primary progressive (PPMS):* Patients show a steady decline in function; episodes of flare are low-grade but constant.
- *Malignant MS:* This is a rapidly progressive form of the disease, with little respite (if any) between flares.

Diagnosis

No single test can definitively diagnose MS. The disease is identified through a descrip- tion of symptoms, a family health history, a spinal tap to look for raised antibody levels and myelin fragments, and MRIs that can reveal central nervous system lesions. (The lesions shown in MRIs may be from sources other than MS, however, so they are not considered a definitive diagnosis.) Nerve conduction tests to measure the speed of electrical impulses through nerves also may be conducted.

An official list of criteria has been developed to identify MS that incorporates the use of MRI imaging. To achieve a positive diagnosis, a patient must have

- Objective evidence of at least two episodes (this can be achieved through MRIs, examinations of cerebrospinal fluid, or evoked potential tests that show the speed of nerve transmission in the brain)
- Episodes of flare are separated by at least 1 month and by location of affected function;
- No other explanation for symptoms can be found

Several conditions can produce MS-like symptoms. Part of a thorough diagnosis is ruling these out:

Lyme disease	Herniated or ruptured disc
HIV/AIDS	Lupus
Scleroderma	CNS tumors
Vascular problems in the brain	Fibromyalgia
Complications of encephalitis	Vitamin B_{12} or folic acid deficiency

The process of coming to a conclusive diagnosis of MS is so challenging that patients are often labeled before their tests are conclusive as "possible MS," and "probable MS."

Treatment

Until recently, standard treatment options for MS included symptomatic treatment (for fatigue, muscle pain, etc.) with doses of steroidal anti-inflammatories to quell the severity of flares. Steroids can reduce symptoms in the short run, but have not been shown to have long-lasting benefits, and their side effects can be severe. Therefore they are usually used only as a temporary measure.

A class of drugs called *interferon betas* works specifically to limit immune system activity. These drugs can shorten the duration of periods of flare, as well as prolong periods between episodes. They are cumulatively toxic to the heart and liver, however, and must be used extremely carefully.

Research into MS treatment is now examining the possibility of transplanting myelin-producing cells into MS patients. This may become the standard treatment option until the understanding of the exact causes of the disease yield enough information to stop the myelin damage before it starts.

Other interventions for people living with MS include mild exercise and physical or occupational therapy designed to maintain strength and function as long as possible. Eating well and getting adequate amounts of high-quality sleep are important for maintaining health and prolonging remissions. Stress management techniques, including massage, are often recommended for the same reasons.

Prognosis

Even though not much is understood about the cause of this disease, many statistics have been collected about how it affects the people who have it. Until recently, up to 50% of all MS patients have had some level of disability within 10 years of the onset of their disease. Sixty-six percent of all MS patients could expect to be in a wheelchair at 30 years after their diagnosis. Those statistics may change as interferon beta–based medicines slow the progression of the disease.

MS is not a terminal disease in itself. People who have MS generally have a lifespan approximately 6 years shorter than average. People who die prematurely of this disease are usually immobile, and they fall prey to an opportunistic disease such as a *kidney infection, urinary tract infection,* (Chapter 9) or *pneumonia* (Chapter 6).

Massage?

This disease usually has acute and subacute periods; massage is indicated in the subacute stages. However, care must be taken not to overstimulate the client, which can result in painful and uncontrolled muscle spasms. Symptoms also may be exacerbated by heat, so therapists must avoid allowing their clients' core temperature to rise by working in an overly warm environment.

Every client with MS presents her symptoms and problems differently. If sensation is present, massage can be useful as an agent against stress (which has been shown to exacerbate symptoms for some patients), depression, and spasticity, and it helps to maintain the health and mobility of the tissues. In areas in which sensation is not present, non-mechanical types of work (i.e., very light effleurage and energy work) is more appropriate.

Case History 3.1

Multiple Sclerosis

Tricia, Age 36: "It Takes All the Courage I Can Muster Just to Stand Up in the Morning."

Everyone has problems. Everyone gets in their own world so much. Now I look at someone with a disability and I wonder if they have it. You start to watch people walk and wonder if they've got it.

One and a half years ago, we had just moved into a new house and my youngest child had just started school. For the first time in 15 years I was looking forward to having some time, to getting on with my life.

Then there was a pain in my left heel that felt like a stone bruise. We were just back from a long vacation, so I thought it was from too much walking. Two weeks later, there was a lack of sensation in my foot and it traveled up my leg to my knee. It began affecting my right leg too. Then there was numbness and tingling in my left hand. It felt like I had just had a shot of Novocain; it was that kind of tingling.

Try walking on the balls of your feet for a whole day. Then you'll get an idea of how hard it was. I couldn't put my heels down because there would be a sharp tingling "funny bone" feeling. My walking was so labored, I got to the point where I would rather shimmy on my chest like an army guy to get from room to room. I wasn't crying, I wasn't upset; it was just easier to crawl.

Although I felt stressed about not knowing what was happening to me, I put off going to the doctor. I finally went to my OB for my headaches. He gave me migraine medication, but it didn't work.

He sent me to a neurologist, who checked me out and watched me walk. Then while I was sitting there, he went out into the hall with another doctor and they started speaking in medical jargon that I couldn't understand; it made me really nervous. When he came back he asked me, "Will you come in for a spinal tap?"

"Why?"

"There are some things we want to check out."

"What do you think I have?"

"I think you have MS."

"Excuse me?"

I never *dreamed* it would be something like this.

Multiple Sclerosis, *continued*

They started me on IV steroids. The next morning I got up after a bad night, and for the first time in 2 months I could walk normally. I was so excited, I woke my family and called my mom on the phone. But by the end of that morning I was already beginning to feel tired. My condition deteriorated in spite of the steroids. By the end of the week, I couldn't even get up off the couch to let the home care nurse in.

My neurologist finally sent me to the University Hospital. There they did lots of other tests, more spinal taps, and an MRI. The MRI showed tiny spots in my brain, but nothing like what they were expecting. The spinal taps all came back negative.

They had me talking to teams of doctors. I talked to neurologists, immune specialists, nutritionists, and psychiatrists. The head of the department was prepared to tell my family I had chronic progressive MS, which meant I could be dead in a matter of weeks. I finally decided that I needed to be home, I needed to be with my family, so I checked out even though they didn't want me to.

I continued physical therapy at a local clinic. At first they would have me sit in a warm pool with jets of water after I exercised, and I would go home feeling so drained and worn out, it was awful. Finally they adjusted that part of it and I did better.

Today I still don't have much sensation below my knees. It takes all the courage I can muster to just to stand up in the morning. I never know what kind of day I'll have, whether I'll be able to walk without a cane, whether I'll be tied to the house because my digestive system is unpredictable. I have terrible headaches that begin on the lower half of one side of my face and go up into my ear. I have days when I can't eat at all. I've had episodes of dizziness and double vision. I'm not on steroids now, but I take an antidepressant for the headaches. We're still struggling to find the right dose. My greatest fear, even more than being in a wheelchair, is that I will loose bladder or bowel control, or go blind.

But my doctor says my scenario is good. It's been a year and a half without any exacerbations, and he says that I'm in remission. The only thing that's worse is my headaches, which are more painful and happen more often.

I think everything depends on your attitude. A major thing for me is to feel needed. If I have a purpose, I feel better. My aunt has MS, and she practically runs her family business. It's just amazing to see her get up and go. She says there are some days that if she didn't have that business to go to, she wouldn't be able to get out of bed. I have a chance now to see what other people have to deal with, and some of them are so much worse off than I am, because of physical problems, but other kinds of problems too. I have five wonderful children and a husband who loves me. My doctor thought I was going to die, and here I am in remission. I just feel so lucky to be here.

Parkinson's Disease:

Dr. James Parkinson (1755–1824) was a British physician who first documented this chronic degenerative nervous system disorder.

Parkinson's Disease

Definition: What Is It?

Parkinson's disease, first discussed by the British physician James Parkinson in 1817 as the "shaking palsy," is a movement disorder involving the progressive degeneration of nerve tissue and a reduction in neurotransmitter production in the CNS.

Demographics: Who Gets It?

Parkinson's disease affects approximately one person out of every thousand of the population overall, but its incidence rises considerably with age. It occurs at a rate of about 1–2:100 in people older than 50 years. Men with Parkinson's disease outnumber women by approximately 3:2.

Roughly 500,000 people with Parkinson's live in the United States today; approximately 50,000 new cases are diagnosed each year.

Etiology: What Happens?

Parkinson's disease is one of a variety of conditions classified as "movement disorders." It involves changes in CNS structures that cause them to work inefficiently. To discuss this condition thoroughly, it is necessary to review some of the inner workings of the brain.

Parkinson's Disease in Brief

What is it?
Parkinson's disease is a degenerative disease of the substantia nigra cells in the brain. These cells produce the neurotransmitter dopamine, which helps the basal ganglia to maintain balance, posture, and coordination.

How is it recognized?
Early symptoms of Parkinson's include general stiffness and fatigue; resting tremor of the hand, foot, or head; stiffness; and poor balance. Later symptoms include a shuffling gait, a "mask-like" appearance to the face, and a monotone voice.

Is massage indicated or contraindicated?
Parkinson's disease indicates massage, with caution. Care must be taken for the physical safety of these clients, who cannot move freely or smoothly.

Anatomy Review

Voluntary muscle control is managed in two areas in the brain: the *basal ganglia* and the cerebellum. The basal ganglia are found at the lower edges of the cerebrum. They are pockets of gray matter embedded in white matter that work with the cerebellum to provide learned reflexes, motor control, and coordination. ("Coordination" here means the balance in action between prime movers and their antagonistic muscles.)

Healthy basal ganglia cells are supplied with a vital neurotransmitter, *dopamine*, by another nearby structure, the *substantia nigra* (a.k.a. "black stuff"). In Parkinson's disease, the substantia nigra cells die off, depriving the basal ganglia of dopamine. Without dopamine, the basal ganglia cannot maintain the careful balance between agonists and antagonists in the body, and so coordination degenerates, and controlled movement becomes very difficult.

For Parkinson's symptoms to appear, the substantia nigra must be approximately 60% lost. This loss of tissue results in an 80% loss of dopamine production in the area of the basal ganglia. New imaging techniques that can track chemical reactions in the brain may allow diagnoses of Parkinson's disease before the damage has reached this advanced stage.

Causes

No one really knows what causes the substantia nigra to degenerate in most Parkinson's disease cases. Environmental agents may be found to be one cause; a statistical rise in patients younger than 50 years of age substantiates that theory. In some families, a genetic connection is clear, and research has identified specific sites of genetic abnormality for those individuals with familial Parkinson's. A small percentage of cases can be traced to specific other issues: carbon monoxide poisoning may be one factor, as is heavy metal poisoning, and exposure to pesticides or specific combinations of agricultural chemicals. It also can follow repeated head trauma (*pugilistic parkinsonism* is a diagnosis given to affected boxers), neurovascular disease, and exposure to certain drugs. The drug-induced form is reversible.

Whatever the root cause, research is focusing on the process of *apoptosis* (cellular "suicide") that occurs in the substantia nigra. One theory holds that immune system agents create a surplus of chemical messengers in the substantia nigra that carry instructions for cells to self-destruct. A similar problem with apoptosis of specific nervous system cells has been seen in other neurodegenerative diseases such as *amyotrophic lateral sclerosis* and *Alzheimer's disease* (this chapter).

Signs and Symptoms

Symptoms of Parkinson's disease can be divided into primary and secondary problems. Primary symptoms arise from the disease itself, and secondary symptoms are results of primary symptoms.

Primary Symptoms

- *Nonspecific achiness, weakness, and fatigue.* Parkinson's disease has a slow onset and is most common in elderly people. Therefore, these early symptoms are often missed, either because they are too subtle to be seen or because of an assumption that a certain amount of fatigue and stiffness is just a natural part of growing older.

- *Resting tremor.* This phenomenon is present in approximately 75% of all Parkinson's patients, and is often one of the first noticeable symptoms. A rhythmic shaking or "pill rolling" action of the hand is often seen. Tremor also may affect the foot, head, and neck. This tremor is most noticeable when the patient is at rest but not sleeping. It often disappears entirely when the patient is engaged in some other activity.

- *Bradykinesia.* This means difficulty in initiating or sustaining movement. It can take a long time to begin a voluntary movement of the arm or leg, and the limb's movement may be halting and interrupted midstream. Parkinson's patients sometimes report feeling "rooted to the floor" when they can visualize moving a leg, but it does not happen without sustained effort.

- *Rigidity.* Gradually the muscles, particularly the flexor muscles, of Parkinson's patients become permanently hypertonic. This can give rise to a characteristically stooped posture as the trunk flexors contract more strongly than the paraspinals. This will be particularly visible when Parkinson's accompanies *osteoporosis* (Chapter 2), as it often does. Rigidity also makes it difficult to bend or straighten arms and legs, and can cause a particular "mask-like" appearance to the face as the facial muscles lose flexibility and ease of movement (Figure 3.4). This also accounts for a reduced rate of eye blinking and increased drooling and difficulty with eating and swallowing.

  The rigidity that accompanies Parkinson's is *not* the same thing as spasticity, which implies a different kind of nerve damage. (See *spinal cord injury*, this chapter.) Rigidity indicates massage (with caution), whereas spasticity, which often accompanies numbness, must be more carefully approached.

- *Poor postural reflexes.* Disruption in the activity of basal ganglia cells results in uncoordinated movement and poor balance. Parkinson's patients are particularly susceptible to falling.

Secondary Symptoms

- *Shuffling gait.* Difficulty in bending arms and legs make walking a special challenge for Parkinson's patients. Often the ability to swing the arm is noticeably diminished on one side. The patient takes small steps and may then have to stumble forward to avoid falling. This chasing after the center of gravity is called a *festinating gait.*

- *Changes in speech.* Parkinson's patients experience progressive rigidity of the muscles in the larynx that control vocalization. Their speech gradually becomes monotone and expressionless, and progresses toward constant whispering. Muscular changes in the mouth and throat also create problems with swallowing and drooling, particularly while laying down.

CLINICAL FEATURES

- Tremors of the head
- Head bent forward
- Masklike facial expression
- Drooling
- Rigidity
- Stooped posture
- Weight loss
- Tremor
- Bradykinesia
- Loss of postural reflexes
- Bone demineralization
- Festinating gait

Figure 3.4. Clinical features of Parkinson's disease.

- *Changes in handwriting.* The loss of coordination in fine motor muscles will change the ability of a Parkinson's patient to write by hand. *Micrographia* or progressively shrinking, cramped handwriting is one of the later symptoms of this disease.
- *Sleep disorders.* Parkinson's patients experience a variety of sleep disorders, from a complete reversal of normal sleeping schedules to sleeplessness because it is difficult or impossible for them to move in bed.
- *Depression.* The progressive nature of this condition makes anxiety and depression a very predictable part of the disease process. Depression also can be related to insomnia, or it can be a side effect of medication. Sometimes the symptoms of depression can outweigh the symptoms of the disease, and treatment for depression can lessen Parkinson's symptoms as well.
- *Mental degeneration.* This is a subject of some controversy. Some sources suggest that advanced Parkinson's patients experience memory loss and deterioration of thought processes. Others suggest that mental problems are side effects of Parkinson's medication and not necessarily a part of the disease itself.

Treatment

In Parkinson's disease, a dopamine deficiency develops in the basal ganglia of the brain. A manmade precursor of dopamine called *levodopa (L-dopa)* can cross the blood-brain barrier, but it is usually a temporary solution. Patients seem to build up a resistance to the drug, and it has a number of troubling side effects, including hallucinations and dementia. Some dopamine agonists can be substituted when it becomes necessary, or L-dopa can be prescribed with other drugs that serve to mediate side effects.

Other drug therapies include substances that slow the metabolism of dopamine, so that whatever is available stays for a longer time, and substances that stimulate dopamine receptors in the basal ganglia so that uptake of the neurotransmitter happens more easily. *Anticholinergic* agents that work to limit muscle contraction and antivirals are also employed. None of these is a permanent solution, however. Doctors working with Parkinson's patients must monitor their medications carefully and make frequent adjustments.

New discoveries about the pathology of neural tissue have yielded several other treatment options for Parkinson's patients who do not respond to medication. One of them is deep brain stimulation, in which an electrode is inserted in the thalamus. The patient can activate the thalamus by passing a magnet over a pacemaker-like device that is implanted in the chest. Stimulating the thalamus in this way causes an immediate cessation in tremors. Other surgical options include alterations to the thalamus and other midbrain structures to try to modulate motor dysfunction. As neurosurgery advances, these surgeries are becoming safer and more dependable, but they are still considered a viable option only when medications are no longer effective. Stem cell implantation: the insertion of cellular "blanks" that will grow into healthy substantia nigra cells, holds some promise for the future of Parkinson's disease treatment.

Physical, speech, and occupational therapies are often employed to maintain the health and general functioning levels of Parkinson's patients for as long as possible. Psychotherapy and support groups are recommended to cope with the effects of depression.

Massage?

Parkinson's patients experience progressive stiffness and rigidity of voluntary muscles. Massage, as part of a health care team, can be a valuable tool not only to maintain flexibility and range of motion, but also to reduce anxiety and depression. It is important to work in cooperation with a client's primary physician, because massage may impact the need for antidepressive medication. Be aware, however, that clients with Parkinson's disease do not have the freedom of movement that most other people do, and they may have great difficulty in getting on and off tables safely. Some massage therapists solve this by doing their work with these clients on mats on the floor.

Peripheral Neuropathy in Brief

What is it?
Peripheral neuropathy is damage to peripheral nerves, usually of the hands and feet, often as a result of some other underlying condition such as alcoholism, diabetes, or lupus.

How is it recognized?
Sensory damage, motor damage, or both may be present. Symptoms include burning or tingling pain beginning distally and slowly moving proximally, loss of movement or control of movement, hyperesthesia, and eventual numbness.

Is massage indicated or contraindicated?
Peripheral neuropathy contraindicates massage when numbness interferes with the client's ability to give accurate feedback. In other cases, therapists will need to make case-by-case judgments about whether massage fits in the context of the underlying factors.

Peripheral Neuropathy

Definition: What Is It?

Peripheral neuropathy is not a disease in itself, but a symptom or a complication of other underlying conditions. Peripheral nerves, either singly or in groups, are damaged through lack of circulation, chemical imbalance, trauma, or other factors.

Etiology: What Happens?

Peripheral neuropathy can affect one nerve at a time (*mononeuropathy*) or multiple nerves (*polyneuropathy*.) Most cases of polyneuropathy are complications of long-standing bouts with *diabetes* Chapter 8) or alcoholism (see *chemical dependency*, this chapter). More rarely this condition develops because of certain vitamin deficiencies (especially B_1 or B_{12}), or exposure to toxic substances. The toxins in question include arsenic, mercury, lead, and the organophosphates in insecticides.

Peripheral neuropathy can be associated with various cancers, human immunodeficiency virus/acquired immune deficiency syndrome *(HIV/AIDS)*, *lupus*, (Chapter 5), *rheumatoid arthritis*, *scleroderma* (Chapter 2), and other diseases that cause *vasculitis*, or inflammation of blood vessels.

Mechanical pressure on nerves from injury or overuse situations generally leads to mononeuropathy. Examples of this kind of problem include *carpal tunnel syndrome* and disc disease (Chapter 2), *trigeminal neuralgia* (this chapter), and any kind of trauma or tumors that might result in nerve pressure.

Signs and Symptoms

Most cases of peripheral neuropathy begin subtly and slowly. Damage to sensory neurons produces burning pain or tingling in the hands and feet, which gradually spreads proximally into the limbs and finally the trunk. Extreme sensitivity to touch can follow, but that will eventually be replaced by a far more dangerous symptom: numbness. Numbness is dangerous because if a person cannot feel something—her toe, for instance—she cannot tell if it is injured or infected. Secondary ulcers and infections are common complications of numbness with any disease.

Damage to motor neurons causes weakness and possibly limited or uncontrolled movement. Specific muscle weakening and atrophy are also a part of advanced peripheral neuropathy.

Treatment

Treatment for peripheral neuropathy depends entirely on the underlying pathologic condition that is causing the nerve damage. Chronic pain is often treated with tricyclic antidepressants or anti-seizure medications. Topical ointments with pepper sometimes offer some relief. Other therapies include TENS units (electrical stimulators that interrupt pain transmission), biofeedback, acupuncture, relaxation techniques, and massage to improve circulation in the affected extremities.

The good news is, if the disease is interrupted early, the peripheral nerves may be able to regenerate, and the patient may regain full function. However, if it is left untended, peripheral neuropathy can progress to become a chronically painful long-term condition.

Massage?

If a client has undiagnosed tingling or numbness, he or she needs to see a doctor; it could be any number of things, peripheral neuropathy included. If a client is numb or has reduced sensation, these are contraindications too because he is unable to give informed feedback about his comfort. Clients with nerve damage are likely to be hypersensitive; massage may exacerbate or soothe this symptom.

Massage therapists must make case-by case decisions for clients with peripheral neuropathy to balance the possible benefits (soothing irritable nerves, improving circulation) with the possible risks (further irritating irritable nerves, damaging numb tissue).

Tremor

Definition: What Is It?

This condition refers to involuntary movements, which can be a symptom of a number of different types of CNS problems. The key characteristics of tremor disorders are that the movements are *rhythmic oscillations* of antagonistic muscle groups, and the movement occurs in a fixed plane. Tremor varies by frequency and amplitude.

Tremor in Brief

What is it?
Tremor is rhythmic, involuntary muscle movement. It can be a primary disorder (unrelated to other problems), or it can be a symptom of other neurologic diseases.

How is it recognized?
Tremor is identified through uncontrolled fine or gross motor movements.

Is massage indicated or contraindicated?
Tremor may indicate massage, as long as no contraindicating conditions are contributing factors.

Chorea:

This word, which is a synonym for tremor, comes from the Greek *choreia*, a "choral dance." It has the same root as the word "chorus," which gives some insight into what those Greek choruses were doing during all those tragedies.

Etiology: What Happens?

Tremors can occur in a variety of ways. The most common versions are discussed below. They are generally classified as *resting tremor* (the oscillations occur when the patient is at rest), *postural tremor* (the oscillations occur when the patient attempts to hold a limb against gravity, i.e., holding an arm out in front of him), and *kinetic* (the tremor occurs with simple movement), *task-specific tremor* (the oscillations occur when the patient attempts to use his hands for fine or complex tasks), and *psychogenic* (this type is often stress-related and disappears when a person is distracted).

Tremors may be further classified by whether they are *physiologic* (exacerbated by stress, fear, or underlying problems such as alcohol withdrawal, hypoglycemia, hyperthyroidism, or drug reactions) or *pathologic* (either idiopathic, or caused by some other disease).

Understanding why a person may be experiencing tremors is important because treatment options for this disorder vary according to cause and classification. Some of the most common tremor types are listed here:

- *Essential tremor* is an idiopathic chronic tremor that is not secondary to any other pathologic condition. Up to 10 million people in the United States have essential tremor (20 times more than have Parkinson's disease). This condition is slowly progressive but not usually debilitating. Onset can occur as early as adolescence, but essential tremor most often shows up at about 45 years of age. It is often an inherited disorder.

  Neurologic studies show that the cerebellum, thalamus, red nucleus, and **globus pallidus** are all more active than normal in persons with essential tremor.

- *Huntington's disease* is a hereditary degeneration of nerve tissue in the cerebrum. Symptoms do not usually show until adulthood, when tremors and progressive dementia become irreversible. The average age of onset is between 35 and 50 years. It affects approximately 5 out of every million people in the United States.

  Huntington's disease is diagnosed by CT scan, MRI, and DNA marker studies.

- *St. Vitus' dance*, or chorea minor, is a rare disorder. This is a problem that begins in childhood, or occasionally during pregnancy. Again, there is no known cure, but the prognosis is not so bleak; it usually passes without serious incident, although sedation during convulsive episodes may be recommended.

- *Parkinson's disease* is another CNS disorder involving involuntary movement, but it is discussed elsewhere in this chapter.

- *Other factors* that can cause tremor include alcohol withdrawal, *peripheral neuropathy*, and damage to the cerebellum from *stroke*, *multiple sclerosis* (all this chapter), or tumors.

Treatment

Tremor is treated according to underlying causes. Dopamine precursors, beta blockers, tranquilizers, antiseizure medications, botulinum toxin (if it affects muscles of the voice or head), and small doses of alcohol may be suggested. Surgical interventions may be used if the tremor is debilitating and unresponsive to medication; these include surgical interruptions at the thalamus or globus pallidus.

Massage?

If a client has episodes of uncontrolled muscular contraction and he has not been diagnosed, it is important to get medical clearance before performing massage. It may be that massage can help to reconnect these patients with their bodies in a way that is beneficial, but it is vital to work as part of a health care team.

INFECTIOUS DISORDERS

Encephalitis

Definition: What Is It?

Encephalitis is a central nervous system infection, usually caused by a variety of different viruses.

Demographics: Who Gets It?

Until recently, many different types of encephalitis were considered to be *endemic* to certain areas, that is, specifically limited to geographical regions. However, as the potential for international travel has essentially made the world smaller, strains of virus that had previously been restricted to certain areas are being found all over the globe.

Encephalitis infections are relatively rare. Even with a recent introduction of a previously unknown strain in the United States, national incidence stays between 150 and 5,000 cases per year.

Etiology: What Happens?

Most cases of encephalitis are transmitted by mosquitoes, although some rare varieties can be transmitted by ticks. The virus usually affects other animals first; wild and domestic birds and horses are common hosts. Parasites bite an infected animal and pick up the virus, and then bite a human being, introducing the virus into the bloodstream.

Encephalitis infections affect the brain and sometimes the spinal cord. Very often infections are mild and do not lead to long-lasting damage. Occasionally, and especially if the patient is very young or very old, encephalitis infections can cause permanent neurologic damage or even death.

Encephalitis is usually brought about by a viral infection, but occasionally it is from something more exotic such as a paramecium carried by the tsetse fly (see sidebar, "West Nile Encephalitis"). Inflammation of the brain also can be a complication of other diseases, notably *HIV/AIDS* (Chapter 5).

Signs and Symptoms

Symptoms of encephalitis can range from being so mild that they are never even identified to very, very severe. How the disease presents depends on the virus involved and the age and general health of the patient. Infants, elderly, and AIDS patients are most vulnerable to the very extreme forms of the disease, whereas others will only rarely experience any lasting damage from the inflammation.

The mild end of the symptomatic scale includes a sudden onset of fever with headaches, drowsiness, irritability, and disordered thought processes. In more severe cases, drowsiness can progress to stupor and then coma. The patient also may experience double vision, confused sensation, impaired speech or hearing, convulsions, and partial or full paralysis. Changes in personality, intellect, and memory may develop, depending on which parts of the brain are affected.

Diagnosis

The presenting symptoms for any CNS disturbance are so varied and individualized it is difficult to make a conclusive diagnosis without a full range of intrusive testing. For en-

---

Encephalitis in Brief

Pronunciation
en-sef-ă-lī'tis

What is it?
Encephalitis is inflammation of the brain usually brought about by a viral infection.

How is it recognized?
Signs and symptoms of encephalitis include fever, headache, confusion, and personality and memory changes. In rare cases, encephalitis may cause permanent neurologic damage or even death.

Is massage indicated or contraindicated?
Acute encephalitis contraindicates massage, but if a client has had it in his history with no signs of present infection or neurologic damage, massage is perfectly acceptable.

cephalitis, this means a spinal tap to look for signs of inflammation in the cerebral spinal fluid, along with a CT scan or MRI to look for signs of inflammation. Newly designed blood tests are becoming more accurate at identifying signs of infection as well. This is a lot better than how it was done long ago, when a biopsy of brain tissue was required to make a diagnosis!

Treatment

Viruses do not respond to antibiotic therapy, which is designed to disable bacteria only. Encephalitis is treated with anti-viral medications to slow viral activity, along with steroids to limit inflammation, sedatives to moderate convulsions, and "supportive therapy," which is to say, tender loving care.

Prognosis

The prognosis for encephalitis depends on the vulnerability of the patient, the virulence of the pathogen, and how early treatment is administered. Very often healthy people can emerge from a short-term infection with no lasting damage. However, prolonged inflammation in the central nervous system may cause permanent damage to structures that have little or no capacity to heal. Thus, permanent paralysis or cognitive changes may be the result of a serious bout with this disease.

Massage?

If a client exhibits the major signs of an encephalitis infection, especially headache, fever, and irritability, *it systemically contraindicates massage*. If, however, it shows up on her medical history as a long-ago infection and she has no permanent damage, massage should be just fine.

West Nile Encephalitis: Watching a Virus Take Hold

In August 1999, six residents of Queens, New York, checked into local hospitals with high fevers in combination with debilitating headaches. Five of them also developed alarming neurologic symptoms: weakness, paralysis, and even coma.

Initial tests suggested an outbreak of Saint Louis encephalitis (SLE), a mosquito-borne viral infection. However, patients showed a different pattern than usually seen with SLE; several of them were much sicker than medical professionals expected. Within days, several more people in the area were reporting similar symptoms.

At the same time, a few miles to the north of where most of the encephalitis patients were, birds in the Bronx Zoo were dying at a startling rate. Crows all over the city were showing an alarming mortality rate. Horses in nearby suburbs were also falling to a mysterious brain fever.

It took some time, but epidemiologists finally put the phenomena together and realized that the viruses attacking humans were the same as those attacking the birds and horses. It was firmly established that the infectious agent was one never before seen in the United States. West Nile encephalitis virus was being transmitted from horses and birds to humans by common mosquitoes.

By the time the first frost killed the mosquito population, a total of 56 confirmed cases were identified among humans, with 7 deaths. The people who died of encephalitis were all older than 68 years of age.

It has never been firmly established exactly how the West Nile Virus (WNV) got to New York. One of the patients had been to Africa the previous June and might have been infected then, or it is possible that one of the birds in the Bronx zoo carried the virus into the United States. Aggressive mosquito abatement programs limited the spread of the disease.

The appearance of the WNV in the United States provides an unprecedented opportunity to observe how an infectious agent spreads through a new environment. In 2002, more than 4,000 people were diagnosed with WNV (this does not reflect how many were infected and never sought treatment), and 284 people died of the infection. Since then, it has spread rapidly westward.

Exposure to WNV does not guarantee illness: although many people develop nonspecific flu-like symptoms, only approximately 1 in every 150 develop severe neurologic symptoms.

What does this bode for the future? It is difficult to say. This virus carries several challenges, including how to develop ways of predicting high-risk areas for outbreaks of the disease, creating measurably useful mosquito abatement programs, screening for infected blood and organ transplants, and setting up a wide-ranging surveillance program to carefully monitor the geographic progress of the disease.

Herpes Zoster

Definition: What Is It?

Also known as *shingles*, this condition is a viral infection of the nervous system. In this case, the targeted tissues are the dendrites at the end of sensory neurons. Imagine growing painful, fluid-filled blisters on all of the nerve endings of a specific dermatome: this is fair idea of what a bad case of shingles feels like. Shingles affects approximately 300,000 people in the United States every year. It seldom affects the same person twice, unless that person is severely immunocompromised.

Etiology: What Happens?

The virus at fault here is the chickenpox virus, also called *varicella zoster virus*. When a person is exposed to chickenpox in childhood, the normal course of events is to go through the disease process, have painful itchy blisters, let them fade away, and then go back to business as usual. The difference with chicken pox is that although after the infection a full complement of anti–chickenpox antibodies is present, the virus is never fully expelled from the body. Instead, it goes into a dormant state in the dorsal root ganglia (the meeting point for all the sensory neurons in each dermatome). Later in life the virus may reactivate.

Sometimes the immune response quells future attacks before any symptoms appear. But if the virus awakens when the immune system is below par for some other reason—stress, old age, or other diseases—a person might get chicken pox again, but adults are much more likely get shingles.

Causes

It is hard to predict what might cause a reactivation of the herpes zoster virus. Contributing factors include the ones listed above: stress, old age, impaired immunity because of other diseases (shingles is notorious for accompanying *HIV/AIDS* (Chapter 5) advanced *tuberculosis*, or *pneumonia*, Chapter 6), chemotherapy, or having had an initial infection before 18 months of age. Shingles occasionally occurs after severe trauma or as a drug reaction. And of course if an adult has never been exposed to chicken pox, that person is vulnerable if they have contact with the varicella zoster virus.

Although the fluid in zoster blisters is filled with virus, shingles is not particularly contagious, unless a person has never been exposed to the virus in the first place. In this case, an adult may develop either shingles or chickenpox, but shingles is more likely.

Signs and Symptoms

Pain is the primary symptom of this disease. Pain is present for 1 to 3 days before the blisters break out. Pain is present for the 2 to 3 weeks in which blisters develop, erupt, and scab over. Pain is often present for months even after the lesions have healed and the skin is intact again.

Shingles' name derives not from its appearance, but from the Latin *cingulum*, which means girdle or belt. This describes the typical distribution of blisters around the chest or abdomen on a single dermatomal line.

Herpes Zoster in Brief

What is it?
Herpes Zoster, or shingles, is a viral infection of sensory neurons from the same virus that causes chicken pox.

How is it recognized?
Shingles creates rashes and extremely painful blisters unilaterally along the affected dermatomes. The trunk or buttocks are the most common areas, but it occasionally affects the trigeminal nerve.

Is massage indicated or contraindicated?
This is an extraordinarily painful condition, and it contraindicates massage in the acute stage. After the blisters have healed and the pain has subsided, massage is appropriate.

A Chickenpox Vaccine?

A controversy exists over the need for a chickenpox vaccine. It is usually such a benign childhood rite of passage that some doctors and parents argue that such a vaccine is really unnecessary. (The parents of children who die of complications due to chickenpox might argue this point.)

A chickenpox vaccine was licensed in the United States in 1995, and is currently available through state health departments. Many schools require that children entering kindergarten be vaccinated against chickenpox. No statistics are available on how the vaccine affects the chances of contracting shingles later in life.

From the perspective of economic impact, a chickenpox vaccine might well become popular, simply for the amount of money to be saved by employers who pay for sick days while parents stay home with infected children.

Figure 3.5. Herpes zoster: shingles.

The blisters may grow along the entire dermatome of the host dorsal root ganglion, but more often they appear along an isolated stretch. It is nearly always a unilateral attack (Figure 3.5). Sensory nerves that supply the trunk and buttocks are the most frequently affected, although the trigeminal nerve also may be attacked.

Complications

The most common complication of herpes zoster is secondary bacterial infection of the blisters. Other complications involve a viral attack on the trigeminal nerve, which can lead to eye damage, hearing loss, and temporary or permanent facial paralysis. This is sometimes referred to as ***Ramsey-Hunt syndrome Type 1. Postherpetic neuralgia*** is a complication in which the pain generated by the viral attack outlives the infection by weeks or months.

Herpes zoster occasionally leads to secondary viral and bacterial infections. Pneumonia, *encephalitis*, and *meningitis* (this chapter) are all possible complications of this disease.

Treatment

Herpes zoster is treated mainly palliatively. *Acyclovir*, an anti-viral medication, has some success with herpes zoster; it is believed to shorten any possible bouts with postherpetic neuralgia. Beyond that, soothing lotion, steroids for anti-inflammatory action, and painkillers are the interventions used most often. If postherpetic neuralgia develops, more aggressive pain interventions may be recommended, including antidepressants, antiseizure medications, topical lidocaine patches, and nerve blocks.

Massage?

Herpes zoster is the kind of disease that is very kind to massage practitioners: during an acute outbreak of this condition the *last* thing a client will go looking for is someone to *touch* her. Occasionally very mild outbreaks may occur, for which massage may be only locally contraindicated, according to the tolerance of the client. After the infection has passed and the lesions have completely healed, massage is perfectly appropriate.

Meningitis

Definition: What Is It?

Meningitis is "meninges" + "itis": an inflammation of the meninges, specifically the pia mater and arachnoid layers of the connective tissue membranes that surround the brain and spinal cord.

Demographics: Who Gets It?

Approximately 300 people die of meningitis every year in this country. More than 70% of meningitis infections are in children younger than 5 years of age, although in recent years a second high-risk group has been identified: college students living in dormitories. Most dangerous cases of meningitis are among people whose resistance is low: immunosuppressed people, babies, and the elderly.

Etiology: What Happens?

Meningitis is usually caused by bacterial or viral infection. It is important to know the causative factor for this condition because the severity and best treatment options vary according to the pathogen.

- *Bacterial meningitis*: This infection is usually due to an invasion of *Streptococcus pneumoniae* or *Neisseria meningitides* bacteria. Bacterial meningitis tends to be more severe than viral infections, and the risk of long-term CNS damage, specifically hearing loss or mental retardation, is much higher. It does respond to antibiotics, as long as the correct ones are administered early in the disease process.
- *Viral meningitis*: The viruses that can cause meningitis are many and varied, and include a number of enteroviruses (usually associated with intestinal infections), herpes, coxsackievirus, and others. Viral meningitis tends to be less severe than bacterial meningitis, and seldom causes permanent damage.

Signs and Symptoms

The symptoms of an acute meningitis infection include very high fever and chills, a deep red or purple rash, extreme headache, irritability, aversion to bright light, and a stiff, rigid neck. The neck is held tightly because any movement or stretching of the swollen meninges is excruciatingly painful. Drowsiness and slurred speech may be present. More extreme infections cause nausea, vomiting, delirium, and possibly convulsions or coma.

A bacterial meningitis infection incubates from 2 to 10 days. It takes up to 3 weeks for viral infections to develop. Symptoms generally peak and then recede over a period of 2 to 3 weeks.

Diagnosis

Meningitis is diagnosed through a spinal tap that examines the cerebrospinal fluid for pus, fragments of pathogens, and reduced glucose levels. (The infectious agents consume the glucose that would normally be available to the CNS.)

Meningitis in Brief

Pronunciation
men-in-jī'tis

What is it?
Meningitis is an infection of the meninges, specifically the pia mater and the arachnoid layers.

How is it recognized?
Symptoms of acute meningitis include very high fever, rash, photophobia, headache, and stiff neck. Symptoms are not always consistent, however; they may appear in different combinations for different people.

Is massage indicated or contraindicated?
Meningitis, a contagious and inflammatory disease, strictly contraindicates massage in the acute phase. People who have recovered from meningitis with no lasting damage are perfectly fine to receive massage.

Treatment

If the pathogen is identified as a bacterium, large doses of antibiotics are administered immediately to forestall the possibility of central nervous system damage. Steroids also may be prescribed to limit inflammation in the brain. Viral meningitis is generally treated with supportive therapy: rest, fluids, and good nutrition while the patient's immune system fights back.

Most people emerge from meningitis infections with no lasting damage if the correct treatment is administered early in the infection.

Communicability

Meningitis can be contagious. Its mode of transmission is much like that of the common cold: an infected person sneezes or coughs, and then touches some surface such as a doorknob or light switch. An uninfected person contaminates her hand, then touches her eye or mouth. Meningitis brought about by the intestinal enterovirus family can also be spread by oral–fecal contact, which is an issue when it occurs in young children or in day-care settings.

Some parts of the world experience epidemics of meningitis. The "meningeal belt" of sub-Saharan Africa has seasonal outbreaks of the severe bacterial version of this disease.

Not all of the people exposed to meningitis-causing pathogens contract the disease. A high percentage of exposed people experience no symptoms, or symptoms of a cold or mild flu. Only about one out of every thousand people exposed to meningitis develop the disease.

Prevention

In the United States, the HiB (*Haemophilus influenzae*) vaccine is probably the most effective prevention against children getting meningitis; before this vaccine was available, this was the most common causative agent of bacterial meningitis infections. Vaccines against two of the three types of meningococcus bacteria have been developed, but they are generally recommended only for people planning to travel to places where epidemics are in progress, or college students who plan to live in a high-density dormitory setting.

Massage?

Meningitis contraindicates massage in the acute stage. These people do not just need bed rest; they may need hospital care. Clients who have recovered from meningitis with no lasting effects are perfectly appropriate candidates for massage.

Polio:

This is from the Greek word for "gray." Polio denotes damage to the gray matter of the central nervous system. Poliomyelitis indicates damage and inflammation in the gray matter, specifically in the spinal cord (*myelos* means "marrow").

Polio, Postpolio Syndrome

Definition: What Is It?

Poliomyelitis or *infantile paralysis*, as it used to be known, is a viral disease. Most viruses have a target tissue, or a "favorite food," so to speak. Herpes zoster targets sensory neuron dendrites; most cold viruses attack mucous membranes. AIDS goes after helper T cells. The poliovirus targets intestinal mucosa first, and anterior horn nerve cells later.

Postpolio syndrome (PPS) is a progressive muscular weakness that develops anywhere from 10 to 40 years after an initial infection with the poliovirus.

Demographics: Who Gets It?

It is estimated that some 300,000 polio survivors live in the United States. Of them, approximately 25% have some symptoms of PPS, although polio survivors are also more than usually prone to arthritis, tendinitis, and other orthopedic problems that mimic PPS.

Etiology: What Happens?

The poliovirus usually enters the body through the mouth; contaminated water is the usual medium. It gets past the acidic environment of the stomach and sets up an infection in the intestine. New virus is released in fecal matter, possibly to contaminate water elsewhere.

For 99% of people exposed to the poliovirus, this is the end of the story. Symptoms resemble a severe flu: headache, deep muscular ache, and high fever. These are followed by an intestinal infection, a bout with diarrhea, and then the infection is over. However, in approximately 1% of people who are infected, the virus travels into the central nervous system, where it targets and destroys nerve cells in the anterior horns of the spinal cord. This impedes motor messages leaving the spinal cord, which in turn leads to rapid deterioration and atrophy of muscles and motor paralysis.

The paralysis caused by polio is motor only; sensation is still present. Because the motor nerves overlap muscle groups in the extremities, some muscle fibers may still function, even though a whole level of motor neurons may have been damaged. In other words, consider the dermatomes for the quadriceps. Even if all the impulses to the motor neurons in L_2 have been eliminated, L_3 supplies other motor neurons to the same muscle group (Figure 3.6). Furthermore, anterior horn cells that survive the initial attack can create new nerve connections to help reestablish motor control during recovery. Unfortunately, these cells can become overtaxed later in life, giving rise to PPS.

PPS is *not* a resurgence of the original polio infection. Instead, it seems to be the result of normal aging combined with the loss of some percentage of anterior horn cells from the initial polio attack. The surviving cells, in spite of or because of whatever new synapses they were able to make in the recovery process, are severely overtaxed. PPS may be the result of over-stressed motor neurons.

Signs and Symptoms

Polio is little more than a memory for most people in this country, but some people who had polio as children, especially those who experienced significant loss of function, have found as they reach middle age that they have a sudden and sometimes extreme onset of fatigue, achiness, and weakness, not always in just the muscles originally affected. Breathing difficulties, sleep disturbances, and trouble swallowing also may develop. These symptoms usually begin many years after the original infection. They tend to run in cycles in which function is progressively lost, followed by periods of stability, and then more loss of function.

Diagnosis

PPS is diagnosed by looking for a confirmed prior episode of paralytic polio, along with an electromyogram to look for changes to anterior horn nerves. Other diseases, such as *amyotrophic lateral sclerosis* (this chapter), must also be ruled out.

Polio, Postpolio Syndrome in Brief

What is it?
Polio is a viral infection, first of the intestines, and then (for approximately 1% of exposed people) the anterior horn cells of the spinal cord. Postpolio syndrome (PPS) is a group of signs and symptoms common to polio survivors, particularly those who experienced significant loss of function in the acute stage of the disease.

How is it recognized?
The destruction of motor neurons leads to degeneration, atrophy, and finally paralysis of skeletal muscles in polio patients. Later in life they may develop a sudden onset of fatigue, achiness, and weakness. Breathing and sleeping difficulties also may occur.

Is massage indicated or contraindicated?
The polio virus does not affect sensation or cognition. Therefore, massage is appropriate for polio survivors, as long as acute phase of the infection has passed. PPS also indicates massage.

Figure 3.6. Dermatome patterns in the leg muscles allow multiple nerves to supply muscle.

Treatment

Moist heat applications, physical therapy, and massage have been used to treat polio survivors once the initial infection has subsided. Together hydrotherapy and massage can help to limit contractures and to keep functioning muscle fibers healthy and well nourished.

PPS is treated as a problem that may be fixed by reducing muscular and neurologic stress: adjusted braces, a change in activity levels, and exercise programs that encourage the use of muscles *not* supplied by the damaged nerves. People with PPS need to avoid excessive use of their affected muscles, because exercise to these compromised tissues can cause permanent damage to the working fibers.

Prevention

Polio is stunningly easy to prevent. Two inexpensive, stable, easy-to-administer vaccines are effective against this disease. The Salk vaccine injects inactivated poliovirus into the bloodstream, causing the recipient to create a set of antibodies against it. This vaccine, although protecting the patient, does not eliminate the possibility of that person's transmitting the disease to someone else. People who handle the diapers of infants who have received the oral vaccine need to be aware that live virus may be in the fecal matter. Immune-suppressed persons should avoid contact with infants who are undergoing this treatment.

The Sabin vaccine, an oral medication, introduces weakened viruses into the digestive system, where they attract antibodies exactly where the virus first tends to reside. The advantages of the Sabin vaccine are that this approach prevents the patient from being a carrier of the disease, as well as creating an internal immune response, and because it is given orally rather than hypodermically, it can be administered by anyone.

In the United States, the injected form of vaccine is now the only one recommended; the oral version is still in use in worldwide vaccination programs.

Massage?

Massage therapists in the United States are *extremely* unlikely to encounter an acute case of polio in their practice (see sidebar, "Polio: It Is Almost Extinct"). Polio survivors experience only a motor paralysis; sensation is still intact. Massage can be performed for these clients with good possibility of benefit and little risk of danger.

PPS indicates massage: it will reduce muscle tone, improve local nutrition, and generally decrease strain on the nervous system.

Polio: It Is Almost Extinct

The statistics on polio are extremely promising. In 1988, The Global Poliomyelitis Eradication Initiative combined efforts by the World Health Organization (WHO), UNICEF, Rotary International, and the Centers for Disease Control in the largest public health effort for the eradication of a disease. As a result of this effort, the last new case of wild poliovirus in the entire Western hemisphere was diagnosed in Peru in August of 1991. The Western Pacific Region was certified polio free in October of 2000. The last reported case in Europe was in 1998.

Outbreaks of vaccine-derived virus occurred in the Dominican Republic, Haiti, and the Philippines in 2000 and 2001, but better distribution programs to follow up on incompletely administered vaccine series can limit this threat.

As of 2002, wild poliovirus is endemic to only seven countries on the planet, and outbreaks occurred in tightly restricted areas. Approximately 99% of all the new cases of polio were in small areas of India, Pakistan, and Nigeria.

Countries with little or no incidence of polio infection are still vulnerable to invasion with the virus, especially along borders with countries in which the virus is still active. Therefore, it is recommended that even "safe" countries maintain their vaccination schedules until the globe is free of the poliovirus.

PSYCHIATRIC DISORDERS

Attention Deficit Hyperactivity Disorder

Definition: What Is It?

Attention deficit hyperactivity disorder (ADHD) is a neurobiochemical disorder resulting in difficulties with attention, movement, and impulse control. Recognized in children since the 1900s, it has had several names, including "minimal brain dysfunction." It was not discussed as an issue for adults in medical literature until 1976.

Demographics: Who Gets It?

Most estimates suggest that approximately 3% to 5% of school-age children could have ADHD. Many unofficial surveys, however, show that up to 17% of school-age children within certain areas are medicated for ADHD, and the numbers are disproportionately high among upper middle class white boys. Many authorities recognize that non-white children, and children with limited access to health care, are probably an underserved population with regard to this disorder. This gives ADHD the distinction of being both over- and under-diagnosed.

Boys with ADHD are diagnosed approximately three times as often as girls. This may be because the way boys often manifest this disorder is with hyperactivity and

Attention Deficit Hyperactivity Disorder in Brief

What is it?
Attention deficit hyperactivity disorder (ADHD) is a neuro-biochemical imbalance in the brain resulting in problems with focus, impulse control, and motor activity. It occurs among children and adults.

How is it recognized?
ADHD is recognized by the behavior changes it brings about: inattention, inappropriate impulsivity, and when hyperactivity is present, difficulty with controlling movement. The diagnostic criteria for ADHD depend on the observations of people close to the patient, along with ruling out other possible sources for the problems.

Is massage indicated or contraindicated?
ADHD indicates massage, although the preference for the type of bodywork and the length of time it can be administered, may vary greatly from one client to another.

inappropriate, attention-getting behaviors, whereas girls with the disorder are more often simply inattentive, but not disruptive.

Studies suggest that approximately 4% of all adults may have ADHD. Symptoms, especially the inability to control movement, are often less severe, but many complicating factors contribute to difficulties in the life of an adult with ADHD, including the high probability that he or she is also raising a child with ADHD; approximately half of all patients have another first-degree relative with this disorder.

Etiology: What Happens?

The etiology of this disorder remains a mystery, although new technologies that allow researchers to watch chemical pathways in living brains are beginning to offer some new ideas about how ADHD works.

This disorder is clearly a neurochemically mediated issue. It has been traced to problems with dopamine production, transportation, and reabsorption, and with *noradrenaline* disruption in various areas in the brain that have to do with decision-making and movement.

Although its causes are still unclear, some contributing factors have been identified: genetics are certainly an issue, because up to 50% of all ADHD patients have a first-degree relative with the same disorder; altered brain function is observable because motor control and planning centers in the brain are affected by disturbed chemical levels; and maternal behaviors (smoking and alcohol consumption) and exposure to toxins (dioxins and polychlorinated biphenyls [PCBs]) have been seen to increase the risk of ADHD in children.

Signs and Symptoms

Three specific patterns of behavior indicate ADHD: inattentiveness, hyperactivity, and impulsivity. A person with ADHD may only be inattentive or have a combination of these patterns, but they are consistent in multiple settings, i.e., at school or work, at home, and in social situations.

Signs of inattention include becoming easily distracted by irrelevant sights and sounds; failing to pay attention to details and making careless mistakes; rarely following instructions carefully and completely; and losing or forgetting things such as toys, or pencils, books, and tools needed for a task

Some signs of hyperactivity and impulsivity include feeling restless, fidgeting with hands or feet, or squirming; running, climbing, or leaving a seat in situations in which sitting or quiet behavior is expected; blurting out answers before hearing the whole question; and having difficulty waiting for others to complete a task.

Diagnosis

No conclusive test reliably and definitively identifies ADHD. In children it is usually diagnosed through ruling out other possibilities, and then gathering observations from teachers and parents. In adults, the same procedure includes feedback from family members and work associates. Perhaps the most important part of an ADHD diagnosis is the process of ruling out other disorders that can lead to the same symptoms, and recognizing how other psychiatric conditions often coexist and influence the behavior of a person with ADHD.

- *Differential diagnosis:* a number of things can cause children to become easily distractible and disruptive. It is important to rule these out before assuming that ADHD is the primary cause of their trouble. Depression, anxiety disorders, learning disabilities, sleep disorders (specifically sleep apnea or snoring), fetal alcohol syndrome, vision or hearing problems, Tourette's syndrome, mood disturbances, and seizure disorders could all be considered, along with the possibility that the child is simply demonstrating age-appropriate behavior.

• *Coexisting conditions:* the issue of ADHD diagnosis is made more difficult by several disorders that commonly occur concurrently. These include oppositional defiant disorder, *depression*, and *anxiety disorders* both this chapter.

Complications

Untreated ADHD carries the risk of several serious consequences. Children with this disorder have difficulty with self-esteem, maintaining relationships, and performing well with schoolwork or other jobs. Later in life, untreated or unsuccessfully treated ADHD patients have a high rate of automobile accidents, and an elevated risk of developing substance abuse or other addictive behaviors (i.e., gambling, shopping, engaging in sexual encounters) in attempts to "self-medicate" to manage their disease.

Treatment

At this moment, the most successful treatment options for ADHD involve the use of psychostimulants, usually from classes of drugs called *methylphenidates* or *dextroamphetamines*. Studies of children treated with medication alone, medication in addition to counseling and training in coping skills, and just counseling, show that the best results occur with medication. A new option has recently been released with good results; this medication is not a psychostimulant, but a norepinephrine reuptake inhibitor.

Side effects of ADHD medications are a concern, especially if the patient is a young child. They can include appetite suppression, increased blood pressure and heart rate, sleep problems, and sometimes the development of facial or vocal tics. These signs indicate that a medication is being poorly tolerated, or the dosage needs to be adjusted. Some ADHD medications cannot be combined with some asthma medications. Perhaps the issue of most concern for many parents is that the long-term effects of ADHD medications are not well known.

Non-drug approaches for ADHD include the use of nutritional supplements and adjusting the diet to avoid sugar, caffeine, and other stimulants. Although these are recognized as good options, the research indicates that they are not as successful at dealing with the symptoms of ADHD as pharmacologic intervention.

Massage?

Massage holds no risks for children or adults with ADHD. Bodywork has been seen to improve classroom behavior and interpersonal relationships in children with this disorder.[4] It is important to have realistic expectations about what a child or adult with ADHD can tolerate within a bodywork session. Although some love the stimulation of a rigorous, fast-paced sports massage–type of modality, others prefer the chance to achieve the stillness found with subtler energy techniques. Regardless of preference, however, many ADHD patients cannot expect to be able to receive massage for a full hour or more.

---

[4] Ewart H III. Attention-Deficit/Hyperactivity Disorder: Why Massage Works. Copyright © 2002, American Massage Therapy Association. Available at: http://www.amtamassage.org/infocenter/adhd.html. Accessed fall 2003.

Anxiety Disorders in Brief

What are they?
Anxiety disorders are a group of mental disorders that have to do with exaggerated, irrational fears and the attempts to control those fears. Some anxiety disorders come and go, some are chronic progressive problems, and others reach a peak and then sometimes recede or remain stable. All anxiety disorders begin as emotional responses that create inappropriate sympathetic reactions.

How are they recognized?
Although triggers for individual cases may vary, many anxiety disorders involve sympathetic reactions in the body, including fast heart rate, sweating, dizziness, faintness, nausea, and other symptoms. In addition, some disorders bring about feelings of impending death, a sense of physical detachment, unwelcome or frightening thoughts, and other reactions.

Is massage indicated or contraindicated?
If the stimulus of bodywork is perceived as something safe and welcome, then massage can have a useful place in dealing with a variety of anxiety disorders.

Anxiety Disorders

Definition: What Are They?

Anxiety disorders are a collection of distinct psychiatric disorders that all have to do with irrational fears and extensive efforts to avoid or control them. Anxiety disorders range from being mild to being completely debilitating.

Demographics: Who Gets Them?

Statistics for specific types of anxiety disorders are discussed individually, but overall it is estimated that up to 19 million people in the United States have some type of anxiety disorder. Many anxiety disorders are more common in women than in men, but men are more likely to seek treatment for disorders that make it hard to function in public settings. These disorders take a huge toll on a person's ability to complete school or hold a job. Consequently, a disproportionately high percentage of people with anxiety disorders never earn a high school diploma and are in the lowest end of socioeconomic ranking.

Etiology: What Happens?

"Am I safe?" At this moment, every person who is alive and awake is asking this question at some level of consciousness. The answer for people with anxiety disorders is, *"Probably not."*

Each type of anxiety disorder has its own etiology, but some group generalizations can be made. These disorders involve neurotransmitter imbalances in the brain, although which parts of the brain vary by individual problem. The areas most frequently affected are parts of the limbic system: the area of the brain that stores memory and compares it to current experience to gauge an appropriate sympathetic or parasympathetic response. Many people with anxiety disorders tend to interpret incoming stimuli as potentially threatening and consequently live in a constant hypervigilant, sympathetic state. Other parts of the brain that are frequently affected are the basal ganglia (the site that initiates much muscular activity) and the frontal lobes (the area associated with judgment and decision-making).

The neurotransmitters that are most frequently disturbed by anxiety disorders include *norepinephrine* (chemically related to adrenaline), *gamma-aminobutyric acid* (GABA), and *serotonin*.

Some types of anxiety disorders can always be linked to a specific trigger. Posttraumatic stress disorder, for instance, is initiated by some traumatic incident. Other types can be occasionally but not always traced to an initial event. A genetic link appears to be a factor in some types of anxiety disorders, but the specific genetic mutation has not been found. This blend of genetics, life-changing events, and neurotransmitter imbalances produces emotions and behaviors that can completely debilitate a person, making it impossible to go to school, to maintain relationships, or to hold a job. The risk of *depression* (this chapter) and suicide with several anxiety disorders is many times higher than it is with the general population.

Types of Anxiety Disorders

Dozens of distinct anxiety disorders have been documented, each with a specific list of criteria for diagnosis. This list includes of some of the most common versions, along with brief descriptions.

- *General anxiety disorder (GAD)*

  This disorder affects some 4 million people in this country. Women with GAD outnumber men by approximately two to one. This disorder involves chronic, exaggerated, consuming worry and the constant anticipation of disaster. It does not cause the person to avoid stressful situations, but she lives in a constant state of anxiety that makes it difficult to accomplish many tasks. It appears earlier and develops more slowly than other anxiety disorders.

  GAD is diagnosed when symptoms persist for 6 months or longer. Physical symptoms include insomnia, fatigue, muscle tension, and headaches. Over half of all GAD patients also deal with depression, substance abuse, and other anxiety disorders.

- *Panic disorder*

  Panic disorder is characterized by the sudden onset (often with no identifiable trigger) of very extreme sympathetic symptoms: a pounding heart, chest pain, sweatiness, dizziness, faintness, alternating flushing and chilling. Hyperventilation causes numbness and tingling in the lips and extremities. A feeling of being smothered, of impending doom, and the nearness of death usually lasts for approximately 10 minutes, but it may persist for many hours.

  Panic disorder affects approximately 2.4 million Americans, with women again outnumbering men by roughly two to one. It is complicated by worrying about having another attack: fear of fear. When it causes a person to avoid situations in which panic attacks have happened before or may happen in the future, it can cause another anxiety disorder, *agoraphobia*, or fear of open places. Gradually a person's perceived "safety zone" shrinks to the point where she becomes reluctant to leave her immediate environment. Approximately one third of all panic disorder patients develop agoraphobia.

  People with panic disorder are four times more likely than the general population to abuse alcohol or drugs, and 18 times more likely to commit suicide, although this rarely happens *during* a panic attack. Panic disorder patients also have high rates of depression, migraine *headache* (this chapter), and *irritable bowel syndrome* (see Chapter 7).

  Panic disorder is one of the most successfully treated of all anxiety disorders, but treatment is most successful if it is initiated before the onset of agoraphobia.

- *Posttraumatic stress disorder (PTSD)*

  Traditionally associated with soldiers returning from the horrors of war, PTSD has also been known as "shell shock." It affects approximately 5.2 million Americans, most of them men.

  PTSD is a disorder involving persistent visceral memories of a specific ordeal, which could be combat, physical or sexual abuse, rape, assault, torture, natural disaster, terrorist attack, or any other life-threatening event. Sometimes a PTSD patient was a witness to an attack or threat to someone else. Memories of the event are relived in nightmares and waking flashbacks. The patient often becomes withdrawn, irritable, and occasionally aggressive as these memories intrude more and more frequently into his life. Some PTSD patients find that their symptoms subside with time and eventually no longer affect them, but others find that without treatment this is a lifelong problem.

  Symptoms of PTSD usually appear within 3 months of the triggering event, but some patients are not affected until many years later. People with PTSD tend to be hypervigilant, always on the lookout against the possibility of a repeated attack or trauma. Studies of the brain activity of PTSD patients show some differences in brain chemicals, depending on whether the trauma was impersonal, such as a hurricane or flood, or a personal attack, such as a rape or kidnapping.

Generally, survivors of impersonal experiences have less severe symptoms, although the severity of the stressor does not necessarily correspond to the severity of the symptoms.

- *Obsessive-compulsive disorder (OCD)*

  Obsessive-compulsive disorder is a combination of intrusive, uncontrollable, unwelcome thoughts (*obsessions*) along with highly developed rituals designed to try to quell or control those thoughts (*compulsions*). Approximately 3.3 million Americans have it, and the ratio of men to women is about even. Unlike many other anxiety disorders, OCD can come and go throughout a lifetime, and it is not always progressive.

  Some of the most common obsessions experienced by OCD patients include fear of contamination by dirt, germs, or sexual activity; fear of violence or catastrophic accidents; fear of committing violent or sexual acts; and fears surrounding disorder or asymmetry. The rituals used to battle these fears include repeated hand washing (often to the point of damaging the skin); refusing to touch other people or contaminated surfaces; repeatedly checking locks, stoves, irons, or other appliances; counting telephone poles; carefully and symmetrically arranging clothes, food, or other items; and persistently repeating words, phrases, or prayers. Although many people occasionally engage in some of these behaviors, OCD patients often devote hours every day to the rituals that are designed to keep them safe.

- *Phobias: social and specific*

  - *Social phobia*

    Social phobia is also called *social anxiety disorder*. It involves intense, irrational fears of being judged negatively by others or of being publicly embarrassed. It can involve specific situations, such as speaking or performing in public, or it can involve any social setting at all. Physical symptoms include blushing, sweating, trembling, and nausea, but many social phobia patients display no outward signs of their disorder.

    Whereas many people may feel shy or nervous among strangers, patients with social phobia are significantly distressed and even disabled by their fear, which can interfere with work, school, or relationships.

    Social phobia affects some 5.3 million people in the United States. Women with social phobia outnumber men, but men are generally more likely to seek treatment. Approximately 16% of all social phobia patients are alcoholic. They are four times more likely to have depression, and they have a higher than normal risk for suicide.

  - *Specific phobias*

    A phobia is an intense, irrational fear of something that poses little or no real danger. Some common phobias include fear of closed-in places, heights, flying, elevators, tunnels, and bridges. Untreated phobias can severely restrict a person's ability to hold a certain kind of job, live in a certain kind of building, or perform mundane tasks, such as grocery shopping.

    Approximately 6.3 million people have specific phobias. Women outnumber men. Persons with this disorder often respond better to controlled desensitization and relaxation techniques than they do to medication.

Signs and Symptoms

Signs and symptoms of anxiety disorders vary according to type. Although they usually involve irrational fears and inappropriate sympathetic nervous system responses, they present differently by each variety and in each patient. The *Diagnostic and Statistical Manual of Mental Disorders*[5] has extensively documented signs, symptoms, and diagnostic criteria for each of the individual anxiety disorders, but brief descriptions of their signs and symptoms have been included in the descriptions above.

Treatment

Most anxiety disorders are treated with a combination of medication and psychotherapy. Some varieties respond better to psychotherapy and the development of coping skills alone, whereas others also require chemical intervention to reestablish neurotransmitter balance in the central nervous system. Most patients with anxiety disorders can find some combination of therapies that successfully treats their problem—if they seek treatment. Sadly, many patients are incorrectly diagnosed, or never seek treatment at all.

Medications to treat anxiety disorders fall in three classes: antidepressants, antianxiety drugs, and beta-blockers. Antidepressants include *selective serotonin reuptake inhibitors* (SSRIs), *tricyclics*, and *monoamine oxidase inhibitors* (MAOIs). These drugs often take several weeks to become effective, and they cause unpleasant side effects in the initial stages. Anti-anxiety medications include *benzodiazepines*: tranquilizers that influence levels of the neurotransmitter GABA. These can be effective drugs, especially because they can produce results in a short period. Unfortunately, they also can be highly addictive, and they react dangerously with alcohol. Therefore, they are not appropriate for long-term treatment, or for anxiety patients who are also chemically dependent on alcohol or other drugs (which is a high percentage of this population). Beta-blockers are usually prescribed for high blood pressure patients to decrease the force of heart contractions. They can also help to ameliorate some of the heart-pounding discomfort of panic attacks and social phobias, but they are strictly palliative; they do nothing to fix the problem, they simply quell some of the symptoms.

Psychotherapeutic techniques used for anxiety disorders vary from supported resistance to compulsive behaviors for OCD patients, to controlled exposure to frightening stimuli for people with specific phobias, to various forms of behavioral–cognitive therapies to help patients learn ways to address and often overcome the irrational fears that limit their lives.

Massage?

Relaxation techniques, breathing exercises, and biofeedback are often taught to anxiety disorder patients as coping mechanisms; it seems reasonable that massage and bodywork would fit under this heading as well. It is important to remember, however, that massage therapy is a fine choice for an anxiety disorder patient *as long as the stimulus is perceived as safe and nurturing*. Although a therapist's intent may be completely benign and supportive, the survivor of touch abuse or other types of trauma may not be able to interpret it as such.

Some people with issues and phobias about touch may specifically seek out massage as a way to experience positive touch in their lives. It is a privilege to work with these clients, but massage therapists must be especially vigilant about maintaining clear and careful boundaries around these relationships, so that no one—neither the therapist nor the client—feels abused or taken advantage of.

---

[5] Diagnostic and Statistical Manual of Mental Disorders—IV TR 2000. Copyright © 2000, American Psychiatric Press, Inc.

Chemical Dependency

Definition: What Is It?

Here is a controversial topic! Although definitions for chemical use, abuse, and dependence are relatively clear, the whole issue is clouded by value judgments imposed on whether a substance is legal. A person may become addicted to nasal decongestants or to cocaine, but decongestants are not generally considered a substance abuse problem, whereas cocaine certainly is.

Alcoholism is form of chemical dependency that, because of its prevalence in the culture, and the profound effects it has on virtually every system of the body, is discussed as a specific subset of chemical dependency within this article.

- *Use:* The issue of chemical dependence falls into three categories: use, abuse, and dependence, or addiction. "Use" is easy to identify; if a person ingests a substance specifically to change mood or physical experience, that could be called substance use.

- *Abuse:* "Abuse" is harder to define, especially when the substances under question are examined without the qualifiers of "legal" and "illegal." After all, are caffeine or sugar inherently less damaging than an illegal substance such as cannabis? What is more "abusive": smoking a cigarette or eating a cheese Danish?

The official definition of substance abuse is simply "the use of a substance in a way that is potentially harmful to the user or to other people." Abuse is identified when use of the product interferes with a person's ability to function normally, when the user's behavior becomes unacceptable to those around her, and when she continues to use the substance in spite of recurring problems that it causes.

- *Dependence:* The line between substance *abuse* and chemical *dependency* is sometimes blurry. Most experts agree that abuse becomes dependency when the user develops a progressive tolerance, and so must use more of the substance to achieve the same effects, and when signs of physical and psychological addiction develop. Some substances can be abused without developing dependency.

Demographics: Who Becomes Chemically Dependent or Alcoholic?

Statistics on chemical dependency are difficult to gather, especially because many people never get medical treatment, and they may move back and forth between being a substance user and being free from use.

The Department of Health and Human Services estimates that in 2002 19.5 million Americans over 12 years of age were ongoing users of illicit drugs, although not all of them become dependent.[6] Dependency is more common in men than in women. The peak years for dependency among adults are 18 to 29. The lowest rates of chemical dependency are found among adults older than 65 years.

Statistics on alcoholism are similarly alarming. Approximately 18% of all Americans have lived in a house with an alcoholic. An estimated 14 million Americans regularly abuse alcohol, leading to a yearly average of 100,000 alcohol-related deaths, and over $150 billion in health care costs.[7]

---

[6] Overview of Findings from the 2002 National Survey on Drug Use and Health. Available at: http://www.samhsa.gov/oas/nhsda/2k2nsduh/Overview/2k2Overview.htm#toc. Accessed fall 2003.

[7] Alcoholism. Copyright © 1998-2003 Mayo Foundation for Medical Education and Research (MFMER). Available at: http://www.mayoclinic.com/invoke.cfm?id=DS00340 Accessed fall 2003.

Etiology: What Happens with Chemical Dependency?

The process of developing dependence on a particular substance depends on the chemical makeup of that product and the susceptibility of the user. Many of the most common addictive stimulants available today (cocaine, amphetamines, nicotine) work in the central nervous system by slowing the rate at which dopamine is reabsorbed at key synapses. Dopamine in certain parts of the brain can trigger pleasure responses, but if it lingers too long, the receptors become desensitized. In other words, it takes more dopamine—and more drug—to produce the same pleasurable results.

Etiology: What Happens with Alcoholism?

Alcohol and sedatives such as tranquilizers and barbiturates work by depressing central nervous system arousal, enhancing the activity of the inhibitory neurotransmitter GABA. Alcohol slows activity of the brain and nervous system. Although it is technically a depressant, the loss of inhibitions felt by the drinker can give the impression that alcohol is a stimulant. Although some people bear a genetic susceptibility to alcohol addiction, many alcoholics develop the disease over many months or years of repeated use that finally changes the chemistry in the brain. Consequently, a physical addiction develops: the person is incapable of functioning normally without the substance. The affect of alcohol on specific organ systems is discussed in more detail in the *complications* section of this article.

Risk factors

Several risk factors contribute to a person's susceptibility to chemical dependency.

- *Genetic predisposition*. The rate of drug abuse and alcoholism is demonstrably greater in the families of other addicts than in the general population. This is partly an environmental and availability issue, but studies have shown that even children who are not raised with their chemically dependent parents have a higher than normal incidence of addiction themselves.

- *Other mental illness*. The presence of *depression* or *anxiety disorders* (this chapter) raises the risk of a person becoming a substance abuser because the person may attempt to self-medicate to cope with problems.

- *Environmental factors*. These include availability of the substance in question, peer pressure, self-esteem, a history of physical or sexual abuse, being a child in the household of a substance abuser, and other stressors that may make drug use look like a reasonable choice to the person at risk.

- *Age*. The younger a person is when she begins to use an addictive substance, the more likely she is to develop a long-term dependency on it.

- *Medical reasons*. A patient's need for medication sometimes outlives the problem that required the initial prescription. Addiction to painkillers and sleeping pills are examples of this phenomenon.

Types of Addiction

Once a person becomes dependent on a substance, two things happen: it takes more and more of the substance to achieve the desired effects, and to *stop* using the substance can create physical responses that are daunting to contemplate. Addiction is defined in two categories: psychological addiction and physical addiction. Most addicts have a combination of these two phenomena.

- *Psychological addiction*. This is a dependency on the pleasurable or satisfying sensations that some substance provides—in other words, the addict likes the way she feels when she is using.

- *Physical addiction.* This is a dependency arising from the need to avoid withdrawal symptoms, which can involve hallucinations, nausea and vomiting, seizures, and general physical pain.

Two issues are especially important to bear in mind in any discussion of chemical dependency. One is that even easy-to-get, over-the-counter drugs can change body chemistry and make it very hard to cope without them. Nasal decongestants are an excellent example: why should a body's antihistamines do any work if some externally supplied nasal decongestant will do it for them? The difficulty lies in how long it takes to convince the body that no more decongestants will be consumed. The same kinds of dependency can develop with the use of sleeping pills, muscle relaxants, and some kinds of painkillers.

The body builds up chemical tolerances to most kinds of drugs. That is, it takes more and more decongestant to clear up that stuffy nose, more sleeping pills, more painkillers, more caffeine, and so on. The higher the doses a person needs to feel satisfied, the harder it is to shake off the dependency.

Signs and Symptoms of Chemical Dependency and Alcoholism

Symptoms of chemical dependency vary according to the substance, but four main features are consistent:

- The person feels a persistent craving for the substance
- The person is unable to voluntarily control her own use of the substance
- The person develops an increasing tolerance to the effects of the substance and so must consume more to achieve the same results
- Cessation of use creates unpleasant, alarming, and even physically dangerous withdrawal symptoms

In addition to these signs, the addict or alcoholic also may devote a significant amount of time to the process of using and then recovering from her substance use. He or she may neglect responsibilities to family, job, friends, and other relationships because of being distracted by substance use. The addict often denies that substance use seriously impedes or endangers his or her life: "I'm not dead yet, so that proves I'm okay."

Complications of Chemical Dependency

Complications depend on the substance in question. They can range from paranoid delusions to coma, or even death. Some of the worst effects of drug use are not limited to the users, however. People close to substance abusers also suffer tremendously. Drug-related violent crime, car accidents, industrial accidents, impaired judgment leading to the spread of AIDS, and high rates of child abuse are other complications of chemical dependency that affect many people beyond the user.

Complications of Alcoholism

Alcohol use affects virtually every system of the body. Here is a brief synopsis:

The Digestive System Alcohol irritates the stomach lining, and high levels of consumption are responsible for a specific type of *gastritis*. It is also very rapidly absorbed through the gastric mucosa into the portal system. The portal vein dumps the alcohol directly into the liver, where it then enters the rest of the bloodstream. The effects of alcohol are felt until the liver has finished neutralizing the poison.

People who have preexisting gastrointestinal problems are especially vulnerable to the worst effects of alcohol. It is implicated in the development of cancer in the upper gastrointestinal tract, especially in the esophagus (*esophageal cancer*), pharynx, larynx, and mouth. Alcoholism can cause *ulcers*, internal hemorrhaging, and *pancreatitis*. Approximately 20% of long-term drinkers go on to develop *cirrhosis* (see all of these articles in Chapter 7).

The Cardiovascular System   Alcohol use decreases the force of cardiac contractions and can lead to irregular heartbeats, or arrhythmia. Alcohol is also toxic to myocardial tissue and can lead to *alcoholic cardiomyopathy*. Alcohol tends to agglutinate red blood cells, making them stick together. This leads to the possibility of *thrombi* (see Chapter 4) not only in the brain (see *stroke*, this chapter), but in the coronary arteries as well (see *atherosclerosis*, Chapter 4). Alcohol use also can have the opposite effect: liver damage can lead to suppressed clotting factors and poor Vitamin K synthesis, which may result in uncontrollable bleeding.

Moderate alcohol consumption may actually help prevent cardiovascular disease by increasing high-density lipoprotein (HDL) levels (the "good" cholesterol) in the blood.

The Nervous System   Memory loss frequently occurs for biochemical reasons as well as from *agglutinated* red blood cells getting stuck in the cerebral capillaries, causing brain cells to starve to death. Even some "social drinkers" sustain measurable brain damage from repeated agglutination. In the short term, alcohol slows reflexes, slurs speech, impairs judgment, and compromises motor control. In the long term, the same effects can happen on a permanent basis, in a condition known as *organic brain syndrome*. In advanced stages of cirrhosis, the blood accumulates toxic levels of metabolic wastes that can cause brain damage.

The Immune System   Prolonged alcohol use severely impedes resistance, especially to respiratory infections. Alcoholics are especially vulnerable to *pneumonia* (see Chapter 6).

The Reproductive system   Alcoholism can cause reduced sex drive, erectile dysfunction, menstrual irregularities, and infertility. Babies of alcoholic women are susceptible to fetal alcohol syndrome (FAS): the most common type of environmentally caused mental retardation in the United States. FAS affects 4,000 to 12,000 babies every year.

Alcoholic Families   Children raised in homes with one or more alcoholic adults show a threefold increase in the risk of becoming substance abusers themselves; their chances of developing depression, general anxiety disorders, and phobias are higher than those of the general population; their health costs average 32% higher than other children.

Other Complications   Alcohol is a factor in almost half of all automobile fatalities. It is involved in 40% of all industrial accidents, and up to 65% of adult drownings. It costs approximately $86 billion per year in lost productivity, health care, and death costs. It contributes to approximately 100,000 deaths every year.

Treatment

The first and most important step in treating any kind of chemical dependency is recognizing that a problem exists. Once a person has reached that point, most treatment programs have good success rates. It often seems to be a matter of finding which program best fits the personality of the patient. Treatment goals for chemical dependency are threefold: abstinence, rehabilitation, and prevention of relapses.

Most programs begin with a detoxification process, during which the drugs are expelled from the body. This may be ameliorated with sedatives, tranquilizers, or even less potent versions of the drug in question, until all chemical remnants have been processed out of the body. The length of time this requires varies according to the substance in question.

Detoxification is then followed by a process of rehabilitation, during which the patient is educated about the effects of chemical use and often is trained in avoidance behaviors to give them some ammunition against the temptation to fall back into old habits.

Aftercare has been shown to be the most important part of treatment for chemical dependency: this sets up the patient with a support system that will carry her throughout a lifetime choice of total drug abstinence.

Some medications have been developed that can help to suppress the craving for alcohol, or that can cause violent physical illness when alcohol is consumed. The potential for relapse into substance abuse lasts indefinitely, so this is a condition that is treated most successfully with long-term coping skills rather than short-term patches. Total abstinence is essentially the only successful conclusion to treatment for most chemical dependency.

Massage?

Massage has a useful place in the treatment of chemical dependency. Some rehabilitation facilities employ massage therapists to help ameliorate withdrawal symptoms and reduce the need for tranquilizers and other drugs. However, a client with a history of alcohol or drug abuse is at high risk for secondary health problems. For this reason, it is important to work as part of a health care team and to beware of complications that are associated with "hard" drug use: staphylococcus or streptococcus infections, hepatitis B and C, AIDS, and heart problems.

Clients who are in long-term recovery with no lasting contraindications are good candidates for massage.

Current alcohol or other drug use at the time of an appointment contraindicates massage, mainly because of the risk of overtaxing a liver that is already occupied. This guideline can be a judgment call, based on the level of intoxication (one glass of wine poses less stress on the liver than a fifth of vodka), the setting of the massage session, the behavior of the client, and the safety boundaries set by the therapist.

Depression in Brief

What is it?
Depression is an umbrella term covering a number of mood disorders that can result in persistent feelings of sadness, guilt, or hopelessness.

How is it recognized?
Symptoms vary according to the type of depression and the individual, but they usually include a loss of enjoyment derived from usual hobbies and activities, disappointment with oneself, hopelessness, irritability, and a change in sleeping habits.

Is massage indicated or contraindicated?
Most types of depression indicate massage, which can work in several ways to alleviate symptoms both temporarily and in the long run.

Depression

Definition: What Is It?

Depression is a group of disorders that involve changes in emotional state. One of the best descriptions of this disease is: "a genetic-neurochemical disorder requiring a strong environmental trigger whose characteristic manifestation is an inability to appreciate sunsets."[8]

In other words, depression is a central nervous system disorder involving a genetic predisposition, chemical changes, and often a triggering event, that results in a person losing the ability to enjoy life. Depression is more than a temporary spell of "the blues"; it can be a long-lasting, self-propagating, and ultimately debilitating disease.

Demographics: Who Gets It?

Statistics on the incidence of depression in all of its forms are hard to gather, because many affected people never seek help. Most estimates suggest that somewhere between

[8] Salpolsky RM. Why Zebras Don't Get Ulcers: An Updated Guide to Stress, Stress-Related Diseases, and Coping. Copyright © 1994 and 1998 by W.H. Freeman and Company, New York. p. 230.

10% and 20% of the US population experiences an episode of depression every year; this amounts to 11 to19 million people.

Women seem to be either more susceptible to depression, more likely to seek help, or both. The incidence of depression among women is approximately twice as frequent as it is among men.

Depression can affect people of any age. It has been observed in young children, up through senior adults, in whom its symptoms can mimic other specifically geriatric diseases. Depression in seniors can be misdiagnosed as early *Alzheimer's disease, Parkinson's disease* (this chapter), or other problems.

Etiology: What Happens?

What a great question. No one really knows how depression comes about. Several distinctive features have been noted in the brains and endocrine systems of depressive individuals, but whether these features *cause* the problem or are *caused by* the problem is still a mystery. Nonetheless, as we learn more about the chemical changes associated with depression, we also learn new ways to attempt to treat it.

- *Neurotransmitter imbalance.* Three main neurotransmitters have been associated with depression: serotonin, norepinephrine, and dopamine. The assumption is that these neurotransmitters are in short supply, and if medical interventions make them more readily available, the patient will improve. Some research, however, points in a slightly different direction: that these neurotransmitters are actually present in *too much* concentration, and the brain builds up resistance to receiving them. Regardless, the drugs most often prescribed for depression change brain chemistry by increasing the accessibility of these important neurotransmitters.

- *Hormonal imbalance.* Neurotransmitter disruption leads to disruption in hormonal secretions, especially progesterone, estrogen, endorphins (which increase the sensation of pleasure), and cortisol: the hormone most closely related to long-term stress. It is also possible that this is a two-way street, in other words, that the hormonal shifts associated with long-term stress can disrupt neurotransmitter secretion.

- *Pituitary–adrenal axis.* This is the tight connection between the central nervous system and the endocrine system. The pituitary gland, under the control of the hypothalamus, controls the adrenal glands (which secrete adrenaline and cortisol, among other things) by way of a specific chemical: corticotrophin-releasing factor (CRF). Depressive people tend to secrete excessive amounts of CRF, meaning that they create stress responses to minimal stimuli, and those responses tend to have a longer-lasting effect on the body.

- *Atrophy in the hippocampus.* The hippocampus is a structure deep in the brain that is involved with learning and memory. The hippocampus in persons with major depressive disorder is often smaller than normal, showing up to 20% atrophy. The factors in hippocampus atrophy vary, but they may be linked to long-term stress and the hypersecretion of cortisol.

Causes

Many contributing factors collide to initiate a depressive episode. Some of them are controllable, but many are not. Whether someone ends up in a depression depends on her own personal chemistry, genetics, and something much harder to quantify: her personality.

- *Genetics.* The rates of various kinds of depression show higher-than-normal incidence among family members, pointing to a distinct genetic predisposition to this disorder. Because this is such a common and widely distributed disease, many different sites of genetic abnormality may be responsible.

- *Environmental triggers*. Most episodes of depression can be related to specific life events that initiate a slide into a depressed state. Sometimes the triggers are less clear, or they could be not recent. Triggers can range in severity from losing a loved one to losing a telephone number. The more depressive episodes a person has had, the smaller the trigger that may send her into another.

- *Personality traits*. Some people, through their childhood experiences and family history, are simply more prone to depression than others. Psychological testing can identify people with a basically passive, "things in my life happen to me; I don't make things in my life happen," kind of attitude. These people carry an increased risk for developing depression.

- *Chronic illness*. People who live with chronic illness show a much higher rate of depression than the general population. This is easy to understand because chronic pain or the prospect of sliding into inevitable disability would naturally deprive a person of a sense of hopefulness or investment in life. Often the symptoms of depression can outweigh the symptoms of the chronic illness. If the depression can be resolved, then coping skills for the illness also may improve.

- *Other issues*. Several other issues can contribute to depression, but these are often much more easily controlled than those so far discussed. *Hypothyroidism* (Chapter 8), smoking, alcohol, drug use, or side effects of medication all can create depressive symptoms. Also, certain nutritional deficiencies, notably vitamin B_{12} and folate, can contribute to depressive symptoms.

Signs and Symptoms

The signs and symptoms of depression depend partly on what type is present. The leading symptoms include a persistent sad or "empty" feeling, experiencing less enjoyment from usual activities (including sex) and hobbies; a deep sense of guilt or disappointment with oneself, a feeling of hopelessness—that things will never get better, irritability, and a change in sleeping habits: either the person sleeps very little, or he sleeps much more than usual.

Other signs and symptoms can include a decreasing ability to concentrate, weight changes (the person either eats much more than usual or loses all interest in food), a loss of energy, a feeling of helplessness, persistent physical pain that is unresponsive to treatment (headaches, digestive discomfort), and suicidal thoughts or even suicidal attempts. A person is typically diagnosed with depression when five or more of these symptoms are present or in a new pattern for a minimum of 2 weeks.

Types of Depression

The Diagnostic and Statistical Manual of Mental Disorders (DSM) has officially recognized at least eight etiologically distinct types of depression. Five of them are relatively common and are discussed here:

- *Major depressive disorder*. This is the classic, debilitating "clinical depression." It involves the major symptoms listed above, in very severe form, for periods longer than 2 weeks. Left untreated, episodes of major depression may last anywhere from 6 to 18 months, and on the average they may reoccur anywhere from four to six times over a lifetime. Someone who does not treat her major depressive disorder can expect to spend up to 10 years of her life feeling hopeless, helpless, and worthless.

- *Dysthymia*. This is a less extreme version of depression, involving fewer symptoms in less extreme forms, but it can last for years at a time. Someone who has dysthymia can function, but she will not ever feel normal or at her best.

- *Bipolar disease*. This is also called *manic depression*. It is marked by mood swings from major depression to mania: a state defined by heightened energy, elation, irritability, racing thoughts, increased sex drive, decreased inhibitions, and unrealistic or grandiose notions that lead to decisions made with extremely poor judgment. Someone in a manic state might spontaneously quit her job, buy a car, or make some other major life change without realizing the long-term implications—which will of course be waiting for her when her manic episode subsides.

- *Seasonal affective disorder*, or *SAD*. This is a depression that seems to be related to absence of sunlight. Incidence of it in the general population goes up according to distance from the equator. SAD is thought to be related to low levels of melatonin, a neurotransmitter stimulated by exposure to sunlight. SAD is most prevalent during December, January, and February.

- *Postpartum depression*. The depression experienced by new mothers is different from other types. It is related to several factors, including sleep deprivation, vast hormonal shifts, and the challenge of matching expectations of parenthood with reality. A woman with postpartum depression has all of the symptoms of major depression, along with the deep-rooted fear of having harm come, or of actually doing harm, to her baby. In the most extreme version of postpartum depression, a woman can become psychotic and have hallucinations that may put her or her baby in danger. A woman with a history of postpartum depression with one infant is at increased risk for repeated episodes with other children.

Diagnosis

Depression is diagnosed with a combination of physical tests to rule out factors such as hypothyroidism, vitamin deficiencies, or underlying disease, and psychological tests designed to identify exactly which type of depression might be present.

Treatment

Most types of depression are treatable; up to 90% of all depression patients eventually find some treatment option that significantly improves their quality of life. A combination of medical intervention and various types of psychotherapy seems to be the most effective way to treat most types of depression.

Antidepressant Drugs   Medications used for depression usually fall into one of three categories: SSRIs, MAOIs, or tricyclics. All of these classes of medication aim to make neurotransmitters more easily accessible in the mood-determining areas of the brain.

SSRI stands for *selective serotonin reuptake inhibitors*. These drugs, which include Prozac and Zoloft, work by preventing the recycling of secreted serotonin into axon terminals. In other words, serotonin lingers in synapses for longer than it normally would, which reinforces its power to work. Tricyclic antidepressants, including amitriptyline (Elavil), do essentially the same thing, although they do not focus specifically on serotonin. Monoamine oxidase inhibitors (MAOIs) limit the action of an enzyme that would normally break down and clear away secretions of neurotransmitters. Phenelzine (Nardil) and tranylcypromine (Parnate) are examples of MAO inhibitors.

Antidepressants are effective drugs for most people, but they have two major disadvantages: they take several weeks to establish any noticeable mood changes, and they tend to produce unpleasant side effects during that initial adjustment period. Side effects usually include dry mouth, dizziness, constipation, skin rashes, sleepiness or sleeplessness, sexual dysfunction, and restlessness. Side effects generally subside within 4 to 6 weeks, which is about when the benefits of the medication begin to be felt.

Lithium is another drug used specifically with bipolar depression. Rather than altering levels of neurotransmitter reuptake or recycling, lithium works simply to "smooth out" mood swings.

Psychotherapy   Psychologists and psychiatrists may employ various types of talk therapy to help patients improve coping skills and reduce both the effects and the recurrence of depressive episodes. Three major approaches have been found to be most useful, depending on the personality and needs of the affected individual. *Cognitive–behavioral therapy* focuses on the patient's skills at managing her life and making choices that benefit her. *Interpersonal therapy* focuses on how relationships color a person's life for better or worse. *Psychodynamic* therapy looks at how unresolved inner conflicts can affect the way a person makes choices and lives with those choices.

Psychotherapy in addition to medication often works better than medication alone, because it can help the patient take some control of her situation: a feeling many depressive people do not often have.

Other Therapies

Light therapy   Persons living with SAD may not need medication or talk therapy; they need sunlight. Exposure to broad-spectrum lights can help to reduce symptoms.

Electroconvulsive therapy (ECT)   Some major depressive disorder patients do not respond to medication, and they are at high risk for suicide. Electroconvulsive (ECT) or "shock" therapy may be the best choice for these patients. Although this may bring up disturbing memories of *One Flew Over a Cuckoo's Nest*, modern ECT is conducted under light anesthesia, and with muscle relaxants to limit uncontrolled contractions. It is not entirely clear why it works, but it can be a highly effective intervention for people who do not get relief from other options.

St. John's Wort   This herbal extract has received a lot of attention as a mood enhancer without the side effects that other antidepressants carry. Although some studies indicate that it can be effective for mild dysthymia, it has been shown to be ineffective as a treatment for major depressive disorder. St. John's wort is not without its risks; if a person takes medication to control HIV or any cytotoxic drugs (to reduce the risk of organ rejection, for instance), St. John's wort has been seen to make these medications less effective.

Others   A number of other interventions for depression continue to be explored. A dietary supplement called SAM-e (*S-adenosyl-methionine*), omega-3 fish oil, and others are under investigation as possible alternatives to standard antidepressant medications.

Complications

The most obvious, and most serious, complication of depression is suicide. Up to 15% of all major depression patients successfully commit suicide. Numbers on how many depression patients attempt suicide are unavailable.

In addition to suicide risk, a history of depression is now being found to have a statistical correlation to several other conditions, notably *heart attack* and other forms of cardiovascular disease (see Chapter 4). Although the cause-and-effect relationship between depression and cardiovascular disease has not yet been established, an obvious connection can be made between depression and heart disease in terms of physical manifestations of long-term stress.

Massage?

The ways massage can help a depressed person are varied and many. Although some cautions must be borne in mind, most people with depression can reap several benefits from bodywork.

Touch improves the efficiency of the pituitary–adrenal axis. Receiving nonsexual, nurturing, nonthreatening touch is one of the most important ways humans and other mammals have of keeping a healthy stress response.

Massage moves people from a sympathetic into a parasympathetic state. This brings about several physiologic and chemical changes in the body, including an increase in serotonin secretion, and a decrease in cortisol.

Research about how massage affects mood indicates a shift in EEG (electroencephalogram) activation from the right frontal lobe (usually associated with sad affect) to the left frontal lobe (usually associated with happy affect), or at least to a symmetric reading.[9]

Receiving massage is one of the few distinctively pleasurable things people can do that is also really good for them. The act of scheduling and receiving this gift is a step toward self-determination that depressive people can take with little risk of having it backfire on them.

Some cautions about working with depression patients remain, however. Some clients who receive massage and enjoy its benefits may wish to stop taking their medication. Well-meaning massage therapists may view this as a successful outcome and encourage their clients to try it, but balancing medication for depressive people is a difficult business. The only people who should get involved in changing doses are the depressed person and her doctor.

Depression often accompanies complex emotional issues that a client may have trouble sorting out on her own. Client–therapist relationships run the risk, in some cases, of becoming distorted when boundaries are not carefully respected. If a massage therapist has a client who is depressive in connection with other problems (for instance, recovering from emotional or physical or sexual abuse), that relationship can be precarious, especially if the client is not getting adequate support outside the massage clinic. Therapists in cases such as these have the obligation to refer clients for other kinds of help, and to prevent the client–therapist relationship from becoming more central to the client's life than it should be.

[9] Field T. Touch Therapy. London: Churchill Livingstone; 2000:165.

Case History 3.2

Depression

Dave, Age 50: "Everybody Wants to See the Evidence!"

I don't know for sure when I first started to notice any symptoms of depression. Maybe when I was around 45. I remember I spent about a year trying to figure out what was wrong. I thought I had an infection or something, maybe a sinus infection that was making me feel tired all the time.

One day I went to get a physical, and my doctor asked me a couple of questions about things, about my life. I didn't think anything of it; I thought he was just making conversation. Then he said, "You know, Dave, you have depression." I laughed at him because there wasn't anything to be depressed about. My life was wonderful, I had no real problems; everything was good.

When I was first diagnosed, my problem was nowhere near its peak. After that, though, it got really bad. I couldn't concentrate on anything, and I spent weeks in bed. I couldn't respond to any questions, I didn't even know what was going on. When I did tune in, I had this indescribable horrible feeling. The only way I made it through that time was by asking Jesus to hold me. I just pulled the covers up over my head and asked God to just hold me. That gets me through the bad times.

Depression, *continued*

I took short-term disability, for 6 months, from my job as a safety engineer. When it was over, I tried to go back to work, but it wasn't any good. I used up all my sick leave, and one day the personnel officer came and told me I was through. I haven't worked since then. I got 18 months of disability, and they shut the door. If I'd broken my back, they would have paid disability for the rest of my life. But this kind of illness gets no respect. With mental illness, people think you're either slothful or you're insane. Slothful people are expected to get up and pull their own weight. Insane people are just ignored.

My illness is not the result of any outside situation; it is a chemical thing, an imbalance. I tried antidepressant drugs. They're hard, though, because when you try one you have to give it a good 2 months before you know if it'll do any good. For about 90% of all people with depression, those drugs help them out. I'm in the 10% they don't help.

I've taken lots of tests in the past 2 years. My latest diagnosis is that I have schizoid-affective disorder along with depression. It's hard to categorize. Now I'm taking anti-psychotic drugs. I had a really bad episode about a month ago. I was in tears, tearing out my hair, just crawling out of my skin. I ended up in the hospital. I thought it was a reaction to the medication, but apparently the medication wasn't working yet. It was just my disease, hitting a big crest.

That's how it goes, in cycles. From day to day, hour to hour, week to week. It's impossible to predict, but it's always wave-like, never steady. Medications are a crap shoot. You take your meds and hope something happens. By now I've taken so many, and the combinations are so complicated, it's really hard to make any changes. I think I developed tolerance to all the antidepressants. The anti-psychotics are new, and there are times when I feel pretty good.

The worst part of all this for me is that on my bad days I have no energy to do anything. I just lie there and sleep. I'm completely unreliable. I can't be sure I'll show up for church or for choir practice. It's a real bummer.

I get lots of support at home. My wife has an incredible burden, but she's been behind me 100% all the way. She knows that when I'm in bad shape there's nothing to do but wait until I'm feeling better. Then we just go on with life without dwelling on what we've missed—that's a good approach for me.

I know I'm in lots of people's prayers. I feel that's a powerful tool. I know the prayers being lifted up for me are helping, without a doubt. But when I'm feeling bad, you can't come over and cheer me up, because that's not what I need. When people come visit me in the middle of the day and I've been in bed, I'm not showered or shaved, then I get so embarrassed, almost paranoid. It's not an atmosphere I like to see people in.

I don't think I'm at risk for suicide, although since I've had this disease I know more about why people do it. You get to a point where you say, " This. Is. Intolerable. This. Cannot. Go on." But it does. For now I don't see suicide being a danger for me.

At this point, the only people who really understand depression are people in the medical profession, people who *have* it, or people who have someone in their family who has it. No one else really gets it. They all want to see the proof: where's the blood test, where's the x-ray, where's the *evidence*? I see a lot of the attitude that if you don't have the evidence, you must be faking it. I would like for everyone to understand that mental illness can be as debilitating as any other disease, and it deserves the same respect and concern that any other kind of disease gets.

Eating Disorders

Definition: What Are They?

Eating disorders include a variety of poor eating habits that may begin slowly but over time become difficult or even impossible to break. Eating disorders usually arise in response to specific kinds of emotional or physical stressors. They often begin as a coping mechanism but become a serious impairment to health.

- *Anorexia nervosa* is the use of fasting, severely restricted eating, or compensatory activities to drastically reduce the number of calories that enter the digestive system. It is, essentially, self-starvation.

- *Bulimia nervosa* involves normal or higher-than-normal calorie consumption, followed by compensatory activities to prevent the absorption of those calories.

- *Compulsive overeating* involves the consumption of food for reasons other than hunger. Those reasons may vary according to the individual. Eating is then *not* followed by compensatory activity, leading to rapid weight gain. Compulsive overeating has not been studied as a specific subset of eating disorders, but it happens so frequently and affects so many people, it is worth including in this discussion.

Demographics: Who Gets Them?

> ### Eating Disorders in Brief
>
> **What are they?**
> Eating disorders are a group of psychological problems involving compulsions around food and weight gain or loss. Anorexia, bulimia, and compulsive overeating are each distinct problems, although overlap between them frequently occurs.
>
> **How are they recognized?**
> Signs and symptoms of anorexia and bulimia may be hard to recognize in early stages because these behaviors are usually done in private. Long-term consequences include esophageal and colon damage, tooth damage, arrhythmia and low cardiac stroke volume, electrolyte imbalance, hormonal disturbance, osteoporosis, and many other problems. Compulsive overeating is recognizable by eating habits, in combination with significant weight gain, often in a short period.
>
> **Is massage indicated or contraindicated?**
> Massage may be very supportive and appropriate for all types of eating disorders, as long as the body's chemistry can keep up with the changes bodywork brings about. If a client is in an advanced stage of anorexia or bulimia, bodywork choices may need to change to respect the delicacy of her system.

The typical anorexia or bulimia patient is a girl somewhere between adolescence and college age. Some estimates predict that up to 1% of all girls in this age range may experience anorexia, and 2% to 5% of all girls may have bouts of bulimia. Although men also may have this problem, more than 90% of all eating disorder patients are female.

Eating disorders are found in all economic and social groups. The incidence among Hispanics and whites is about even, but rates are slightly higher among Native Americans. Black women are more likely to be bulimic than anorexic.

Statistics on compulsive overeating are difficult to gather, but given the fact that 100 million people in the United States are overweight or obese and that obesity accounts for $100 billion dollars per year in health costs, it is reasonable to suggest that many people have a dysfunctional relationship with food.

Etiology: What Happens?

Anorexia and Bulimia The personality profiles of anorexia and bulimia patients point toward people with high expectations of themselves. They are often eager-to-please overachievers who do well in school and in athletics. Anorexia and bulimia are often control issues for a population that often feels powerless: adolescent girls in a culture that bombards them with impossible standards with which to compare themselves. A young woman may not be able to control how people treat her, but she can at least control what goes into her mouth—for many, that feels like a major victory, at least in the short run.

Most people in this society are exposed to essentially the same cultural pressures, but not all young women develop eating disorders. This has led some researchers to look for organic causes in the chemistry of the brain. Not surprisingly, serotonin levels are found to be generally lower in eating disorder patients than in the general population. Whether this is a cause or a result of anorexia and bulimia is debatable, but it does open the door to some extra treatment options.

When a person begins to change the way she eats, ultimately it does not matter whether it is because of a neurotransmitter imbalance or because she is desperate to get on the track team. The impact her choices have on her body will eventually change the way it functions. If her problems go on long enough, she may even reach the point where it is impossible to go back; she can lose the ability to break down nutrients, absorb nutrition, or process waste. Anorexia and bulimia can be terminal illnesses.

Compulsive Overeating   The etiology of overeating is a complex mixture of physical and psychological issues. It has significance for massage therapists for several reasons.

- *Touch:* Recall that the experience of *touch* is a basic human need. Touch deprivation in infancy has been shown to lead to sluggish stress response systems and all manner of severe psychological dysfunction. When adults are deprived of touch, they have weaker immune systems, they have higher incidence of chronic diseases, and they have shorter life spans. What does this mean for this under-touched society? It means that if a person does not get touch on the *outside*, she can at least get touch on the *inside*. Think of the digestive tract is a seamless continuation of the external skin. Eating to the point of satiation causes a specific snug, comforting feeling that may be in short supply for some people.

  Eating for comfort can become a vicious circle because this culture places a high premium on physical attractiveness (i.e., being slender), which means that overweight people may have a harder time making and keeping supportive touch-rich relationships. Massage therapists are in a position to provide nurturing, restorative, educated, and *nonjudgmental* touch to a population of people who may have little or no other access to this important sensory "food."

- *Protection:* Weight gain creates a physical barrier between a person and the world around her. This protective device may be a person's conscious or subconscious attempt to protect and distance herself from experiences she wants to avoid. It is common to see overeating and weight gain, for instance, in people who experience physical, verbal, or sexual abuse. Survivors may use overeating as a strategy to discourage their abusers. If they can make themselves unattractive by gaining weight, they can hope to lose the sexual interest of the person who abuses them.

  Many survivors of touch abuse are compulsive overeaters. Many survivors also eventually explore massage as a way to experience touch that is positive and nurturing. Massage therapists who work with this population must be very aware of how closely these clients' emotional state may be reflected in their physical state.

Signs and Symptoms: What Do They Look Like?

Anorexia   As a person moves toward being anorexic, she may begin to avoid social eating situations, where people may notice her new habits. Anorexics often do not see themselves accurately. Seeing herself as fat, a pathologically thin woman may dress herself in large, shapeless, baggy clothes. These serve to hide her weight loss, as well as they would to hide her perceived weight gain.

Anorexia has been divided into two varieties: *restrictive*, in which a person simply does not take in enough calories to sustain her, and *purge-type*, in which calorie intake may be adequate for sustenance, but it is negated by compensatory activities, including vomiting, laxative use, diuretics, enemas, and excessive exercise.

Advanced anorexics, in addition to being extraordinarily thin, sometimes experience the growth of *lanugo*: fine, downy hair usually seen only in early infancy. This grows all over the body, possibly as an effort to compensate for the absence of any insulating fat in the superficial fascia.

Bulimia Bulimia patients may appear to eat normally but then binge in private. Bingeing episodes are often triggered by emotionally stressful experiences: a fight with a loved one, a failed test, or some other disappointment.

The bingeing food is usually chosen to be self-indulgent. Bulimics do not binge on celery; they binge on candy bars. These episodes of drastic overeating are then followed by some kind of compensatory activity. *Purge-type* bulimics will attempt to prevent calorie uptake by removing the food they have just eaten through vomiting, laxatives, diuretics, or enemas. In *non–purge-type* bulimia, eating episodes are followed by excessive exercise, or periods of fasting.

Bulimia patients do not experience the same weight loss that anorexics do; this can make it harder to recognize the disease in early stages. The complications they develop, however, can be more visible than those seen with anorexics.

Compulsive Overeating Compulsive overeating may be done in public or in private, or both. The reasons behind it often have the same roots as the triggers for anorexia and bulimia: stress and a feeling that the person has little or no control over what happens to her. Because the overeating is not followed by excessive exercise, fasting, or purging, compulsive overeaters tend to gain a lot of weight. If the behavior is related to a specific trauma or emotional problem, this can take place over a relatively short period. The good news is, the long-term physical damage and dangers to the body that arise from compulsive overeating are much easier to undo than those associated with anorexia and bulimia.

Complications

The complications associated with eating disorders can be divided into mental/emotional issues and physical issues. Many eating disorder patients struggle with *depression*, irritability, *sleep disorders*, and *anxiety disorders*, especially obsessive-compulsive disorder (all in this chapter). Physical disorders vary according to eating behaviors.

Anorexia Physical problems related to self-starvation include a slow heart rate (*bradycardia*), low blood pressure, and *arrhythmia*. Severely reduced caloric intake interferes with hormone secretion and leads to infertility and *osteoporosis* (see Chapter 2). Overuse of laxatives can cause colon dysfunction, and self-induced vomiting can lead to tooth damage, esophageal erosion, and dangerously upset electrolyte imbalances.

Bulimia The physical complications seen with bulimia are all related to repeated self-induced vomiting or the use of laxatives or enemas to empty the bowel. Advanced erosion of the enamel of molars is a hallmark of bulimia. The esophagus may develop ulcers, strictures (scar tissue that restricts movement), or it may rupture altogether. The colon may progressively lose function when its work is replaced by laxative or enema use. Electrolyte imbalances brought about by vomiting and diarrhea may reach life-threatening levels. Eventually a bulimic person may find it difficult to keep food down even if she wants to.

Compulsive Overeating Compulsive overeaters put themselves at risk for cardiovascular disease, *osteoarthritis* (Chapter 2), *diabetes mellitus* (Chapter 8), and other physical problems associated with being overweight, if their eating habits are never modified. However, these patients do not accrue the same life-threatening chemical imbalances that anorexic or bulimic patients do. If eating behaviors are changed, compulsive overeaters may sustain few if any long-term problems.

Diagnosis

The *Diagnostic and Statistical Manual of Mental Disorders* has identified four main criteria for the diagnosis of anorexia, and five for the diagnosis of bulimia.[10] (Compulsive overeating has not been examined as an official eating disorder in this document.)

The four criteria for a diagnosis of anorexia are:

• Refusal to maintain weight at or above a normal level; weight is below 85% of normal for height

• Intense fear of gaining weight

• Distorted self-perception; the patient sees herself as heavier than she is

• Menstrual periods stop (*amenorrhea*) for at least 3 months in a row

The five criteria for bulimia are:

• Recurrent episodes of binge eating

• A sense of lack of control; the patient could not stop eating, even if she wanted to

• Inappropriate compensatory behaviors, including self-induced vomiting, laxative or enema use, or excessive exercise (persisting in exercise when exhaustion or injury are present)

• A binge/compensation pattern occurs at least twice a week for at least 3 months in a row

• Behaviors are influenced by body image

Treatment

Treatment for eating disorders is most successful when the emphasis is *not* on gaining or losing weight, but on resolving the issues that led to the behaviors in the first place. Although it is important to stabilize weight and educate patients about good eating habits, these interventions are generally unsuccessful until the patient's psychological and emotional issues have been addressed.

New research revealing neurotransmitter imbalances in the brains of many eating disorder patients has opened the door to medications that may help. Addressing some of the emotional and psychological complications of eating disorders also can help to stabilize a patient's emotional state so that she can begin to understand more clearly the consequences of her actions.

Massage?

If a client with eating disorders is stable and her circulatory system is not overly taxed (as might be seen with an advanced anorexic client, for instance), massage can be a wonderful experience for a person who has a generally negative perception of her body. One study showed that anorexia patients who received massage over time self-reported fewer eating disorder symptoms than other patients who were treated only with traditional interventions.[11]

Overeaters, undereaters, and people who interfere with the absorption of food can all benefit from time spent focused on how *good* they can feel. The main cautions for bodywork concern the possibility of cardiovascular weakness, and these can be circumvented by choosing modalities that do not focus on increasing circulation.

[10] Pritts SD, Susman J. Diagnosis of Eating Disorders in Primary Care. Copyright © 2003 by the American Academy of Family Physicians. Available at: http://www.aafp.org/afp/20030115/297.html. Accessed fall 2003.

[11] Anorexia Nervosa Symptoms Reduced by Massage. Copyright © 2003 Massage Magazine, Inc. Available at: http://www.massagemag.com/2002/issue95/research95.htm. Accessed fall 2003

Case History 3.3

Eating Disorders

Jessica, Age 19: "Food Was the One Thing I Thought I Could Control Completely."

I think my eating problems began when I was around 12 years old. I was an only child and a gymnast, and working hard in my program. All my coaches wanted muscle, muscle, muscle—no flab. At that time I got in the mindset that the more I worked out, the more muscle I'd have, so I started skipping meals to have more body-building time. Having muscles and doing my routines perfectly were the only things on my mind.

I went on a pretty much just-rice diet. Rice doesn't have any fat, but lots of carbs to burn for energy. I'd have a bowl of rice and some water, which would make me feel really full. I think due to that my stomach shrank; just eating regular foods became really hard. Since I was always by myself, my parents didn't realize my problem. I always wore baggy clothes because I was constantly cold, and if I wore something tighter, my mother would say I looked fat; but in truth I was barely 5 feet tall and about 70 to 75 pounds. When I was in 7th grade I also got food poisoning from a school lunch. I ended up in the hospital. After that I couldn't eat lunch anymore until I was 18.

When I was 15, my grandfather, who had been the center of my life, died. I went into a deep depression. I had already lost gymnastics because of an injury. So I'd just go to school, home, go to sleep, get up for a little bit to eat, and go back to sleep to do it all over again. When I slept I had terrible dreams, and I heard voices when I was awake. I started to lose a lot of hair and have irregular menstrual cycles.

At this time, and up until I turned 18, I felt like my parents controlled everything: what I wore, who I spent time with, where I was, every minute of the day. Food was one thing I thought I could control completely. Sometimes I'd get up in the middle of the night and eat and eat like I was about to die. I would feel awful later, but I would never make myself throw up. I saw a movie on bulimia once, and saw how much damage it caused, so instead, I would not eat for a day or two after I binged. I still do that sometimes, but not as severely as I used to.

I had always been a straight-A student in school until my senior year in high school. That is when I learned of my eating problem. Several of my friends noticed how I never seemed to eat and started to help me break out of my cycle. The best thing I did was to go to Europe by myself. That gave me a chance to "break out of my box," which opened a whole new world of options to me. I'd say that was when I began to heal from both my depression and my eating problems.

Now I'm in massage school. I eat about 2 ½ meals every day. I was kind of surprised that getting massage was so easy for me. I did have some fears about laying supine on the table, but I'm over it. I have chronic back pain, and I enjoy deep massage. I still have some fears about long-term problems from anorexia. My periods were irregular then, and they're painful now. I lose a lot of blood every month; I'm definitely anemic.

Still, I know I was lucky. I was able to control my eating before it got so bad that I needed to be admitted to the hospital. My whole sense of who I am and what makes me feel good is different now. I still really like getting compliments. If I hear, "You look great," or "That shirt looks good on you," then I feel like I can eat a chicken sandwich or a bowl of ice cream without feeling guilty later. But for the most part, for stuff like the grades I get in school, or what courses I take, no one decides what I need now. I am my own person, and I am in control of my life once again. It feels really good.

Bell's Palsy:

Sir Charles Bell (1774–1842) was a Scottish surgeon, anatomist, and physiologist. He pioneered neurologic research in several areas, including damage to the facial nerve and the structure of the spinal cord (Bell's law states that the ventral horns of the spinal cord are for motor function, whereas the dorsal horns are for sensory function).

NERVOUS SYSTEM INJURIES

Bell's Palsy

Definition: What Is It?

This disorder is the result of damage to or impairment of cranial nerve VII, the facial nerve. This nerve is composed almost entirely of motor neurons and is responsible for providing facial expression, blinking the eyes, and providing some taste sensation (Figure 3.7). It exits the cranium through a small foramen just behind the earlobe. This spot is palpable by *gently* putting the index finger just behind the earlobe and slightly opening the mouth.

Demographics: Who Gets It?

Bell's palsy is a fairly common condition that affects approximately 40,000 people per year in the United States. It is most common among young and middle-aged adults, although it has been seen in children. Men and women are affected equally, although pregnant women are more at risk than the rest of the population.

Etiology: What Happens?

When a peripheral nerve is irritated or damaged, it cannot function efficiently. Because the facial nerve provides most of the motor control for muscles of facial expression, damage to this nerve results in weakness or total paralysis of the face on the affected side. The good news is that because the facial nerve is a peripheral nerve, it has a protective layer of neurilemma that allows it to regenerate. The facial nerve regenerates at a speed of approximately 2 mm/day.

Causes

Bell's palsy is a type of *peripheral neuritis* (this chapter), that is, inflammation of a nerve, usually from some mechanical interference. Several contributing factors have been identified, but most cases are evidently stimulated by a reactivation of the herpes simplex virus. The virus, which lays dormant in the nervous system until it becomes active again, stimulates the production of antibodies and elicits an inflammatory response. Usually the virus attacks nerves on the face (see *herpes*, Chapter 1). However, when an inflammatory response focuses specifically around where the facial nerve must pass through a narrow bony canal near the ear, the swelling damages the nerve, and function is temporarily lost. Another common trigger for Bell's palsy, especially in the northeastern part of the country, is *Lyme disease* (Chapter 2).

The stimulus for a bout of Bell's palsy varies from one person to another. Depressed immunity, lack of sleep, stress, and flares of autoimmune diseases are often identified as triggers. Up to 75% of all recorded cases are preceded by an upper respiratory infection.

Herpes and Lyme disease are the leading factors in Bell's palsy episodes, but other problems also can put pressure on the facial nerve. Some possibilities include tumors, bone spurs at the foramen, severe middle ear infections, upper cervical subluxation, and

---

Bell's Palsy in Brief

What is it?
Bell's palsy is a flaccid paralysis of one side of the face caused by inflammation or damage to cranial nerve VII, the facial nerve.

How is it recognized?
Symptoms of Bell's palsy include drooping of the muscles on the affected side, difficulty with drinking and eating, and difficulty in closing the eye on one side. Pain, headaches, hypersensitivity to sound, and drooling also may occur.

Is massage indicated or contraindicated?
Bell's palsy indicates massage to maintain flexibility and good circulation in the affected muscles. It is important, however, to rule out causes for the nerve damage that may contraindicate massage.

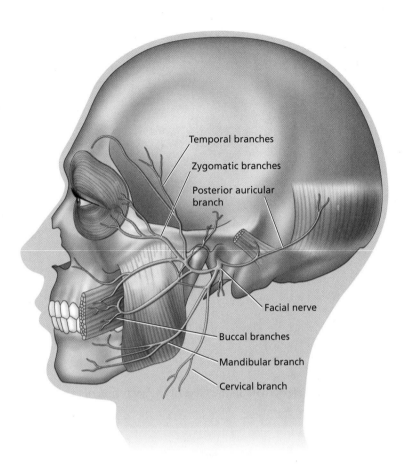

Figure 3.7. The facial nerve.

TMJ disorder (see Chapter 2), all of which can increase surrounding pressure on an already crowded area.

This condition is also associated with *diabetes* (see Chapter 8); diabetes can cause peripheral neuritis. *Guillain-Barré syndrome* (see Chapter 5), exposure to certain toxins, and facial infections are also seen hand-in-hand with facial nerve damage.

Signs and Symptoms

Symptoms of Bell's palsy are brought about by the sudden loss of enervation to the muscles on one side of the face: flaccid paralysis, drooping, and distortion of the affected side of the face (Figure 3.8). It is difficult to eat, drink, and close the eye of the affected side. Sometimes the ear on that side becomes hypersensitive, because a muscle connected to the eardrum is paralyzed. The affected side may have pain, but it is not the sharp, electrical pain seen with *trigeminal neuralgia* (this chapter). This is a motor paralysis, not a sensory one (except for the facial nerve taste buds that may be affected), so sensation throughout the face stays intact.

Complications

Bell's palsy is usually a short-lived disorder with few serious complications. One serious problem to consider is corneal ulcers. These can occur if the lubrication and cleaning of the eyeball provided by blinking is impaired. Another, rarer complication occurs when, as the facial nerve heals, it forges some new and inappropriate connections. The result

Figure 3.8. Bell's palsy.

may be unpredictable muscle activity in the face, or the secretion of excessive tears during salivation.

Treatment

Treatment for Bell's palsy is usually conservative because most cases are self-limiting, that is, they resolve without interference. A combination of steroidal anti-inflammatories and acyclovir to slow down herpes activity are effective for up to 85% of Bell's palsy patients. Patients are counseled to tape the affected eye closed at night, and to protect it from drying and dust during the day. Massage may be recommended to stretch and mobilize facial muscles until the nerve is repaired.

A small number of patients do not experience full or close to full recovery, however. These patients, who can be identified early by nerve conduction studies to measure the extent of nerve damage, may benefit from a surgical intervention to release bony pressure on the nerve.

Prognosis

This condition almost always has a sudden onset (the textbook Bell's palsy patient will simply wake up with it one morning), and it also nearly always has a rapid recovery rate. Improvement is usually seen within 2 to 3 days, and complete restoration of function can be expected within weeks or months. Some cases take longer, however, and they often see a less complete recovery without some intervention to remove mechanical pressure on the facial nerve.

Massage?

Bell's palsy is a flaccid paralysis with sensation left intact. If the underlying cause of the neuritis has been diagnosed to be safe for massage (i.e., not a tumor, Lyme disease, etc.), then massage is a very appropriate treatment choice. Massage keeps the facial muscles elastic and the local circulation strong. This sets the stage for a more complete recovery when nerve supply is eventually restored.

Case History 3.4
Bell's Palsy

Jim S.: "No Dimple for a Year!"

When I think about what may have precipitated my bout with Bell's palsy, I remember one of the most stressful years of my life. I had recently moved to the Pacific Northwest and had to go back to school to receive Washington State licensure as a massage practitioner. I was working three jobs and going to school. I had also spent some days plunging into the cold water of a tributary of the Breitenbush river. I was over-cooked!

When the paralysis started, I thought it was a temporary effect of some bodywork I had received. I was told to take Advil and ice my neck. I was given massage to help with the pain. But nobody recognized the seriousness of the symptoms. Within a day I had full-on Bell's palsy complete with hyperacusis (abnormal acuteness of hearing), full facial muscle paralysis, an eyelid that would not blink (with the inherent rolling of the eye up and out of danger when the lid would normally blink), and a distorted soapy beer taste on the affected side of my tongue.

It was clear in my subsequent research that these symptoms could not have been caused by a massage. With Bell's, the location of impediment on the facial nerve is described by the symptoms. In other words, if I had only had facial paralysis, I would know that the nerve was impaired at a point above the jaw line. As you add symptoms (*hyperacoustic* sensitivity, taste impairment), you trace further up proximal to the *geniculate ganglion*, located inside the area near the ear.

Because I neglected to see a neurologist for over a week, my facial nerve degenerated, and it took almost a year for near full function to resume. I couldn't use my dimple for a year! I'm adamant about people seeing a neurologist immediately these days when I hear of a case of Bell's palsy.

The whole experience was generally frustrating because there's a lot of poor information out there, but it was a great emotional process; when you've used your face for a calling card all your life and suddenly it's not available to you anymore, you have to really deal with what's underneath.

Cerebral Palsy

Definition: What Is It?

Cerebral palsy (CP) is a term that refers to many possible injuries to the brain during gestational development, birth, and early infancy. Several different types of CP have been identified, each involving damage to different parts of the brain, at different moments in development.

Demographics: Who Gets It?

The incidence of CP in the United States is every 2 to 4 out of 1,000 live births. Approximately 500,000 to 1 million CP patients live in the United States today, and approximately 1,500 are born every year. In spite of improved prenatal care, the rate of CP has remained unchanged for many years. The persons most likely to develop CP are infants who experience intracranial bleeding. Other high-risk

---

Cerebral Palsy in Brief

What is it?
Cerebral palsy (CP) is an umbrella term used to refer to a variety of central nervous system injuries that may occur prenatally, at birth, or in early infancy. These injuries usually result in motor impairment, but they may also lead to sensory and cognitive problems as well.

How is it recognized?
Cerebral palsy is usually diagnosed early in infancy, when voluntary motor skills are expected to begin to develop. CP patients may have hypertonic or hypotonic muscles, suppressed or extreme reflexes, poor coordination, and they may show random, involuntary movement.

Is massage indicated or contraindicated?
As long as sensation is intact and the patient is able to communicate with the therapist in some way, massage is appropriate and potentially very useful for persons with CP, as they work to maintain muscular elasticity and improve motor skills.

populations are hard to identify, but statistics are highest among children of mothers who smoke, who live in poverty, who do not receive prenatal care, and who have previously had preterm babies.

Etiology: What Happens?

Cerebral palsy is the result of brain damage, usually to motor areas of the brain, specifically the basal ganglia and the cerebrum. The damage can be brought about in a number of ways. For a long time it was believed that most cases of CP happened when a baby was deprived of oxygen for a dangerously long time during the process of childbirth. That myth has been dispelled by studies that show that most babies who experience *anoxia*, or oxygen depletion during childbirth, never develop brain damage, and most CP patients had uncomplicated, uneventful births. The causes of most cases of CP are now being recognized to be multifactorial situations that occur much earlier in pregnancy.

Causes

Causes of CP can fall into three groups, according to when they occur.

- *Prenatal causes.* Most cases of CP can be traced to problems during pregnancy, often attributable to maternal illness. Contributing factors include infections with *herpes* (see Chapter 1) or toxoplasmosis, *hyperthyroidism*, *diabetes* (see Chapter 8), Rh sensitization (the mother essentially has an allergic reaction to the blood type of her unborn child), or abdominal trauma.

- *Birth trauma.* CP can result if the child experiences anoxia or *asphyxia* (lack of air from a mechanical blockage) during birth. Respiratory distress and head trauma (often from a difficult presentation or the use of forceps in delivery) also may increase the risk of brain damage.

- *Acquired CP.* This is CP that is acquired in early infancy. Causes include head trauma (often from car accidents or child abuse: "shaken baby syndrome"), infection with *meningitis* or *encephalitis* (this chapter), vascular problems (brain hemorrhages), or neoplasms in the brain that may lead to brain damage.

Regardless of the cause of the brain damage, the child with cerebral palsy has some impairment of function. The problem could be so subtle that only people who know what to look for may see it, or it may be completely debilitating both physically and mentally; it all depends on what part and how much of the brain has been affected.

Types of Cerebral Palsy

CP is classified into four types: spastic, athetoid, ataxic, and mixed.

- *Spastic cerebral palsy.* This is the most common form of the disorder, accounting for 50% to 80% of all CP patients. Spastic CP means that in some areas of the body muscle tone is so high that the tight muscle's antagonists have completely let go. This is called the "clasp knife" effect. (See more details on spasticity in the sidebar "Nerve Damage Terminology" with *spinal cord injury*, this chapter.)

- *Athetoid cerebral palsy.* This variety is less common than spastic CP, accounting for up to 30% of all patients. It involves very weak muscles and frequent involuntary writhing movements.

- *Ataxic cerebral palsy.* This rare variety of the disorder involves chronic shaking and tremors and very poor balance. Fewer than 10% of all CP patients live with ataxic CP.

- *Mixed cerebral palsy.* Many CP patients live with combinations of the CP forms.

CP may also be classified by what part of the body is affected. These terms are consistent with those used for other CNS disorders: *hemiplegic CP* means the left or right side is affected; *diplegic CP* means either two arms or two legs are affected; and *quadriplegic CP* means all the extremities are affected to some extent.

Types of CP may come and go, or change entirely from one kind to another, as the child grows. CP is not a progressive disorder, however, and if symptoms seem to be getting significantly worse over time, a different kind of CNS dysfunction must be considered.

Complications

Damage to the motor systems of the body is only the beginning for many CP patients. Complications of this disorder include several other serious challenges. Many CP patients have changes in sensation, including partial or total hearing loss. Up to 75% of all CP patients have some amount of *strabismus* (eyes that do not focus on the same axis). This condition can be corrected to prevent further sight loss. Although CP does not necessarily imply cognitive problems, up to 50% of CP patients experience some level of mental retardation. Approximately 25% of all CP patients have *seizure disorders* (this chapter), which can require very powerful medication to control. And finally, the muscles of CP patients can become so chronically tight that they are replaced with tight, restrictive connective tissue; these are called contractures. Contractures can pull on the skeleton so constantly and so powerfully that the patient is at risk for developing pathologic levels of *scoliosis* (see Chapter 2) that can make it painful to sit or stand and difficult to breathe.

Signs and Symptoms

Signs and symptoms of CP vary according to the location and extent of brain injury. Some of the most common features of CP include hypotonicity, hypertonicity, poor coordination and voluntary muscle control, unusually weak muscles, random movements, and early hearing or vision problems.

Because infants do not develop voluntary motor skills until they are approximately 6 months old, CP may be difficult to diagnose earlier than this point.

Treatment

The central nervous system damage that occurs with CP is incurable and irreversible. CP is therefore managed, rather than treated, by providing skills and equipment to live as fully and functionally as possible. For some CP patients, this means braces for one foot that is slightly weaker than the other; for others, it could mean intensive occupational, physical, and speech therapy for many years.

Interestingly, many CP patients who undergo extensive and aggressive physical therapy and massage experience a surprising recovery or maintenance of function. This indicates that the proprioceptive response to the motor loss in the CNS reinforces and exacerbates the process in the musculature. Therapies that work to maintain peripheral function may be able to interrupt this self-fulfilling prophecy.

Medication for CP is prescribed to help manage seizures and to reduce muscle spasm; this may include injections of botulinum toxin. Some surgical interventions have been developed to lengthen contracted muscles, to realign vertebrae that have become distorted by scoliosis, and to alter nerve pathways in the brain to reduce the severity of tremors.

Massage?

Massage therapy can have a valuable role in improving the quality of life of a person with CP. As stated above, if physical therapy is used to stretch and strengthen skeletal muscles, massage will also be a safe choice. The only caution is that people with very severe CP may not be able to communicate their wants or concerns clearly. If a massage therapist works with a client who cannot speak, other modes of communication, including nonverbal signals, become especially important. It is the responsibility of the massage therapist to make sure that his or her work is welcome and freely accepted at all times.

Reflex Sympathetic Dystrophy Syndrome

Definition: What Is It?

Reflex sympathetic dystrophy syndrome (RSDS) is a collection of signs and symptoms that involve changes to the skin, muscles, joints, nerves, and blood vessels of the affected areas. It usually (but not always) begins after some trauma or injury that initiates a reflex response (*reflex*). A problem in the sympathetic response leads to a chronic reinforcement of the initial pain (*sympathetic*). The chronic pain and resulting changes in blood flow lead to problems in tissue nutrition and growth (*dystrophy*). RSDS is classified as a variant of a broader phenomenon, *causalgia* (see sidebar "Pain by Any Other Name").

Demographics: Who Gets It?

Statistics on RSDS have been difficult to gather, and different agencies quote contradictory numbers. Some estimates say that chronic pain follows after 2% to 5% of all peripheral nerve injuries, and up to 21% of all hemiplegic injuries (see *stroke*, this chapter).

Although it has been observed in all ages from babies to elderly adults, the largest number of RSDS patients are diagnosed when they are 40 to 60 years old. Estimates of the numbers of RSDS patients in the United States range from 5 to 7 million people. Some resources say that men are affected as often or more often than women; other resources suggest that women are diagnosed three or four times more often than men.

What these conflicting pieces of information reveal is that this condition is not well understood, that many people are not sure whether it is a real phenomenon, and that reliable standards for diagnosis have not yet been developed.

Etiology: What Happens?

When a person experiences a stimulus, a sensory neuron carries that information to the spinal cord, where a reflex response begins. At the same time, that impulse travels up the spinal cord to the brain, where the stimulus is interpreted at a conscious or subconscious level. The response might be regulated by the parasympathetic nervous system, for instance, if the stimulus was a soothing, confident effleurage stroke. The response is regulated by the sympathetic nervous system if the stimulus is interpreted as something threatening or painful.

Reflex Sympathetic Dystrophy Syndrome in Brief

What is it?
Reflex sympathetic dystrophy syndrome (RSDS) is a chronic pain condition in which an initial trauma causes pain that is more severe and longer lasting than is reasonable to expect. The pain can become a self-sustaining phenomenon that becomes a lifelong affliction.

How is it recognized?
RSDS moves in stages, although symptoms may overlap. In early stages, it involves redness, heat, sweating, and severe burning pain. In later stages, the skin may turn bluish, and the nearby joints and muscles may atrophy. Bones in the area thin and become vulnerable to breakage. Late-stage RSDS can involve irreversible changes to the affected area and symptoms that spread to other parts of the body.

Is massage indicated or contraindicated?
Most RSDS patients have little or no tolerance for touch of any kind, at least in the area where the pain syndrome began. Physical therapy is often recommended to keep the affected joints moveable and functioning; massage may help to relieve some of the pain associated with this therapy. Massage within tolerance in other parts of the body may be welcome and supportive.

Pain by Any Other Name . . .

In October of 1864, a group of doctors compared their observations of Civil War soldiers recovering from gunshot wounds. Their comments were remarkably astute, and constitute a vivid picture of the experience of the condition eventually termed "*causalgia*," from the Greek *kausis* (burning) and *algia* (pain).

"In our early experience of nerve wounds, we met with a small number of men who were suffering from a pain which they described as 'burning' or as 'mustard red-hot' or as 'red-hot file rasping the skin' . . . Its intensity varies from the most trivial burning to a state of torture, which can hardly be credited, but which reacts on the whole economy, until the general health is seriously affected . . . "[12]

Over the years this condition has come to be known by many names. Sympathetic maintained pain syndrome is another name, as is complex regional pain syndrome, types 1 and 2. Shoulder–hand syndrome and Sudeck's atrophy are other terms used to describe this phenomenon. Causalgia itself is now considered the umbrella term for other chronic pain syndromes, and reflex sympathetic dystrophy is a subtype under this heading.

---

[12] Reflex Sympathetic Dystrophy. Copyright © RSDHope.org. Available at: http://rsdhope.org. Accessed winter 2001.

In RSDS, the nervous system makes a mistake. An initial trauma, (often to a hand or foot, but anywhere on the body can be affected), begins a pain sensation that is moderated by the sympathetic nervous system. RSDS is often associated with high-velocity traumas such as bullet or shrapnel wounds, but it has also been seen with minor strains and sprains, as a postsurgical complication, along with cerebrovascular accidents, and sometimes with no identified causative trauma at all.

The pain, whatever its source, initiates a sympathetic response, which then reinforces the pain sensation. In other words, the pain becomes a self-fulfilling prophecy: a person hurts, which makes her feel anxious, which makes her hurt worse, and the normal healing processes that would interrupt this sequence are unable to overcome the power of the vicious circle.

Eventually the physiologic changes that occur when a specific part of the body is stuck in a sympathetic loop cause their own kinds of damage—damage that can be irreversible. This pain cycle also has the potential to spread proximally on the affected limb, to the eyes, internal organs, and even to the *contralateral* limb.

Signs and Symptoms

Four main symptoms have been observed in most RSDS patients: constant burning pain with little or no stimulus; local inflammation and sweating; spasm of both skeletal and smooth muscle in nearby blood vessels; and chronic insomnia, which gives rise to a number of other mental disorders, including *depression* (this chapter)

RSDS has been broken into three or four loosely defined stages. Overlap of these stages often occurs, so they are useful mainly as a time reference for how long a person has been affected by this condition, and what treatment options have the best chance of interfering with its progression.

- *Stage I:* Stage I signs and symptoms are prevalent during the first 1 to 3 months of pain. They include severe burning pain at the site of the injury, muscle spasm, reduced range of motion, excessive hair and nail growth if the injury is on a hand or foot, and hot, red, sweaty skin (Figure 3.9). Stage I is sometimes called the acute stage.

Figure 3.9. Reflex sympathetic dystrophy syndrome.

- *Stage II:* In this stage, changes in the growth pattern of the affected tissues can be observed. The swelling spreads proximally from the initial site, the hair stops growing, and the nails become brittle and easily cracked. Skin that was red in stage I takes on a bluish caste in stage II. In this intensely painful stage, the muscles begin to atrophy from underuse, and the nearby joints may thicken and become stiffer. Stage II usually lasts from 3 to 6 months. It is also called the *dystrophic* stage.

- *Stage III:* Stage III RSDS shows signs of irreversible changes to the affected structures. The bones become thin and brittle, the joints become immobile, and the muscles tighten into permanent contracture. The condition may spread proximally up the limb, to the contralateral limb, or anywhere else in the body. At this point, the pain sensation is a self-sustaining phenomenon in the brain. In other words, the neurotransmitter balance and pain sensation centers in the brain are essentially incapable of letting go of this sensation. This is known as the *atrophic* stage.

Diagnosis

It is not difficult to identify RSDS, but this disease is not well recognized or understood, so it is probably under-diagnosed. This is a problem, because the long-term outlook for someone with this problem is significantly better if he can begin treatment in stage I than if he tries to intervene in stage III.

Visible signs and patients' descriptions of symptoms are usually straightforward with this condition. Diagnosis can be confirmed with *thermography*: a test that measures blood flow and localized heat in the body. X-rays or bone scans may be used to look for signs of *osteoporosis* at the site of injury.

Treatment

Treatment options for RSDS vary according to which stage the patient is in when he is diagnosed. The earlier in the process treatment begins, the better the chance for a full or nearly full recovery.

Stage I RSDS may be treated with simple analgesics: NSAIDs or short-term steroids if necessary. Patients get good benefit from heat, especially moist heat applications such as paraffin baths or hot packs. Although cool packs may be useful, ice is absolutely out of the question for RSDS patients in any stage.

Stage II and III RSDS patients need to be more aggressive with their pain management. *Intrathecal* pumps that introduce morphine directly into the spinal canal are used with mixed results. TENS machines are successful for some people but not all. Calcium channel blockers may improve blood flow and relieve pain. Eventually a patient may consider a *sympathectomy*: the surgical severing of parts of the sympathetic nervous system to stop the endless cycle of repeating pain signals. This intervention can be successful, but many patients report that the benefits are short-lived and the pain comes back postsurgically.

Massage?

RSDS locally contraindicates massage in acutely affected areas, where any stimulus is painful and unwelcome. Some cases of RSDS are treated with physical therapy to limit bone and joint atrophy. Massage that is well tolerated may be appropriate and important in this context as well. If massage is perceived as pleasant anywhere else on the body, it could certainly add to the quality of life of a person who has some extreme physical challenges.

Spina Bifida

Definition: What Is It?

Spina bifida (literally, "cleft spine") is a neural tube defect in which the vertebral arch fails to close completely over the spinal cord. This defect can be so subtle that it is only found through incidental radiographs, or it can be so severe that the spinal canal is open at birth, or the baby may not survive the birth process.

Demographics: Who Gets It?

Spina bifida statistics in the United States have recently been declining, but it still occurs about once out of every 1,000 live births, or 1,500 to 2,000 times per year. It clearly has a genetic component, because having this disorder in the family raises the risk of having a child with SB; however, approximately 95% of all cases occur in families with no history of the disease.

Etiology: What Happens?

Several types of neural tube defects may occur between day 14 and day 28 after conception. At this time, the woman may not know she is pregnant, and the fetus is approximately the size of a grain of rice, but all of the cells that eventually differentiate into connective, muscle, and epithelial tissue at various levels of the spinal cord are in place. If something interrupts their development, spina bifida may occur.

Some risk factors for spina bifida have been identified: folic acid deficiency raises the risk for neural tube defect significantly, as does *diabetes* (Chapter 8). If the mother takes certain anti-seizure medications, spina bifida may develop. And if a family history of spina bifida exists, the chances of having another child with this disease are much higher. However, as previously stated, 95% of all cases occur in families with no previous spina bifida history.

Spina bifida can be classified as occulta (invisible without looking for it) and cystic.

- *Spina bifida occulta (SBO):* In this situation, the vertebral arch, usually in a lumbar vertebra, may not completely fuse, but no signs or symptoms are obvious. Indeed, a person with SBO may never be aware of it, unless a low back x-ray is taken at some point for another reason. It is difficult to estimate how common SBO is; some sources suggest that 10% or more of the population may be affected. Some people with SBO have a small dimple, birthmark, or tuft of hair on the spine at the location of the abnormality, but they do not experience any change in function because of it.

- *Spina bifida meningocele:* This is the rarest version of cystic spina bifida. In this case, only the dura mater and arachnoid layers of the meninges press through at the site of the vertebral cleft, forming a cyst that is visible at birth. It is easily repairable with surgery, and generally has little or no long-term consequences for the baby.

- *Spina bifida myelomeningocele:* This is the most common and most severe version of cystic spina bifida, accounting for approximately 94% of all cases. In this case, the spinal cord or extensions of the cauda equina protrude along with the meninges through several incompletely formed vertebral arches. Occasionally the skin does not cover the protrusion, raising a serious risk of CNS infection without immediate intervention.

Spina Bifida in Brief

Pronunciation
spī'nă bī'fi-dă

What is it?
Spina bifida is a neural tube defect resulting in an incompletely formed vertebral arch, damage to the meninges or spinal cord, and a high risk of distal paralysis and infection.

How is it recognized?
Spina bifida can be detected through prenatal testing, but the most obvious sign is a protrusion, sometimes covered by skin, of a cyst containing the dural and arachnoid layers of the meninges, and, usually, the spinal cord as well.

Is massage indicated or contraindicated?
Infants recovering from spina bifida surgery are given rigorous physical therapy to establish and maintain function, especially in the abdomen and legs. Massage is appropriate in this context as well. For adults with spina bifida, the judgment about massage depends on the extent of the damage, complicating factors, and the presence or absence of sensation.

Signs and Symptoms

Spina bifida occulta is not obvious at birth, although it sometimes causes a birthmark, patch of hair, or a dimple at the site of the abnormality. Cystic spina bifida is obvious, because a sac containing meninges or spinal cord material protrudes on the back of the newborn infant. It usually occurs in the lumbar spine, and the sac is often red and raw-looking (Figures 3.10, 3.11, 3.12).

Complications

Spina bifida is a complex disorder with several possible complications. *Hydrocephalus*, or "water on the brain," is a common issue after a cyst has been reduced. This is usually dealt with by the insertion of a shunt that drains cerebrospinal fluid from the brain, down the neck, and into the abdominal cavity.

Although most children with spina bifida have normal intelligence, many experience mild to severe learning disabilities that may make it difficult to function in a mainstream classroom situation. Many spina bifida patients develop very severe latex hypersensitivity, possibly from having multiple intrusive surgeries and other medical procedures early in life. This allergy may create a dangerous anaphylactic reaction later in life (see *allergic reactions*, Chapter 5).

Other common complications include *decubitus ulcers* (Chapter 1), digestive tract problems, obesity, and severe muscle imbalances that can lead to flaccidity on one side, contractures on the other, scoliosis, and kyphosis (see *postural deviations*, Chapter 2).

Diagnosis

Spina bifida is detectable prenatally. Testing begins with a blood sample; if that comes up positive for a substance called *alfa-fetoprotein*, a follow-up ultrasound or *amniocentesis* may be scheduled. If a woman is found to be carrying a child with spina bifida, a number of options might be considered. Some research indicates that having a Cesarean section is a safer birth process for a baby with spina bifida; this can obviously be planned in advance. Furthermore, a few facilities have begun to try in utero corrective surgery. This approach is very new, and it is too early to gauge long-term success.

Spina bifida occulta: Vertebrae are incompletely fused; no external sac is present

Meningocele: External sac contains meninges and cerebrospinal fluid

Myelomeningocele: External sac contains meninges and cerebrospinal fluid, peripheral nerves, and spinal cord tissue

Figure 3.10. Spina bifida occulta.

Figure 3.11. Spina bifida: meningocele.

Figure 3.12. Spina bifida: myelomeningocele.

Case History 3.5

Spina Bifida

Observations from the 2000 Paralympic Games by Jan Fields, LMT

With an effortless motion, he pulled himself onto the table. He grasped his lifeless legs and twisted his whole body until he was lying in a prone position. To gaze on his body was to grasp two opposing realities at once. His legs, clad in a loose-fitting pair of sweatpants, were shriveled and limp. Even his hips and buttocks were hollowed out and gaunt after years of frustrated growth and nearly useless service to the greater whole.

Yet, beginning with his lower back, and especially with the lower border of his rib cage, a transformation of epic proportions occurred. The sides of his torso tapered out dramatically to accommodate his thickly muscled back. Indeed, his entire upper body resembled that of a professional bodybuilder. Thus, while the lower half of his body revealed a life of disease, death, and despair, his upper body reflected a life filled with drive, determination, ambition, and hope.

At the end of the session, after my client had gotten off my table and had dressed and left the building, I reflected on the meaning of wholeness. It dawned on me that wholeness is not a disease-free condition, at least in this life, in this reality.

Instead, wholeness is a realized and utilized connection between the human will and a greater purpose, a greater goal. This athlete thrives because his sights are set on goals that diminish the significance of his lower body and magnify the significance of his upper body, including especially his mind. Similarly, I thrive when my sights are set on goals that are adorned in truth and immersed in love—on my best days, and even on my worst days.

Treatment

A baby born with cystic spina bifida needs to undergo surgery within a few days to reduce the cyst and preserve as much spinal cord function as possible. Afterwards, even tiny babies are supported with rigorous physical therapy and exercises to maintain function in the leg muscles as much as possible. As children mature and their functional level becomes clear, they may be trained to use crutches, braces, wheelchairs, or other equipment as necessary.

Many spina bifida patients undergo multiple surgeries, not only to reduce the protruding cyst, but also to correct a "tethered cord" in which the spinal cord does not slide freely within the spinal canal, to deal with the complications of hydrocephalus as discussed above, and to address whatever complications may be brought about by severe scoliosis or kyphosis.

Massage?

The guidelines for massage and spina bifida are the same as for most CNS disorders. Judgments must be based on the presence of sensation, the level of function, and other contraindications that may accompany this complex and serious CNS dysfunction. Many patients engage in physical therapy and exercise to preserve function, and massage can certainly be appropriate in this context.

Spinal Cord Injury in Brief

What is it?
Spinal cord injury (SCI) is a situation in which some or all of the fibers in the spinal cord have been damaged, usually by trauma, but occasionally from other problems such as tumors or bony growths in the spinal canal.

How is it recognized?
The signs and symptoms of SCI vary with the nature of the injury. Loss of motor function follows destruction of motor neurons, but that paralysis may be flaccid or spastic, depending on the injured area. Loss of sensation follows the destruction of sensory pathways. If the injury is not complete, some motor or sensory function may remain in the affected tissues.

Is massage indicated or contraindicated?
Mechanical types of massage are appropriate only where sensation is present and no underlying pathologic conditions may be exacerbated by the work. Areas without sensation contraindicate massage that intends to manipulate and influence the elasticity of tissue.

Spinal Cord Injury

Definition: What Is It?

The definition of spinal cord injury (SCI) is self-evident: damage to some percentage of nerve tissue in the spinal canal has occurred. How that damage is reflected in the body depends on where and how much of the tissue has been affected.

Spinal cord injuries fall into one of five categories: *concussions*, in which tissue is jarred and irritated but not structurally damaged; *contusions*, in which bleeding in the spinal cord damages tissue; *compression*, in which a damaged disc (see *disc disease*, Chapter 2), a bone spur, or a tumor puts mechanical pressure on the cord; *laceration*, in which the spinal cord is partially cut, as with a gunshot wound; and *transection*, in which the spinal cord is completely severed.

An injury that affects the lower abdomen and extremities, but leaves the chest and arms intact, is called paraplegia. An injury that impacts the body from the neck down is called tetraplegia or quadriplegia. For more terminology in the context of CNS injuries, see sidebar, "Nerve Damage Terminology."

Demographics: Who Gets It?

Frequency of SCIs in the United States is estimated at approximately 10,000 to 11,000 per year, excluding those persons who die at the scene of the accident. Approximately 250,000 people in this country currently live with permanent spinal cord injuries. The average age at the time of injury is 32 years. Male patients outnumber females by more than 4 to 1.

Nerve Damage Terminology

Nerve damage can manifest in several different ways. Familiarity with some of the vocabulary of nervous system damage can make it much easier to "talk shop" with clients and doctors dealing with these problems.

- *Paresthesia*: This is a technical term for any abnormal sensation, particularly the tingling, burning, and prickling feelings associated with "pins and needles."

- *Hyperkinesia*: This is excessive muscular activity.

- *Hypokinesia*: This is a condition involving diminished or slowed movement.

- *Hypertonia*: This is a general term for extreme tension, or *tone* in the muscles.

- *Hypotonia*: This is the opposite of hypertonia; it means an abnormally low level of muscle tone, as seen with flaccid paralysis.

- *Spasticity*: This is a type of hypertonia. It is a condition in which the stretch reflex is overactive. The flexors want to flex, but the extensors do not want to give way. Finally the extensors are stretched too far, and then they release altogether. This phenomenon is called the "clasp-knife effect."

- *Paralysis*: This comes from the Greek for "loosening." It means the loss of any function controlled by the nervous system.

- *Paresis*: This is partial or incomplete paralysis.

- *Flaccid paralysis*: This is typically a sign of *peripheral nerve damage*. It accompanies conditions such as *Bell's palsy* (this chapter). Flaccid paralysis involves muscles in a state of *hypo*tonicity.

- *Spastic paralysis*: This indicates *central nervous system* damage. Spastic paralysis combines aspects of hypertonia, hypokinesia, and hyperreflexia. This situation is never resolved, which distinguishes it from mere *spasm* (see Chapter 2).

Types of spastic paralysis:

- *Hemi*plegia means one vertical half (or **hemi**sphere) of the body has been affected. This is the variation that most often accompanies *stroke* (this chapter).

- *Para*plegia means the bottom half of the body, or some part of it, has been affected. These patients still have at least partial use of their arms and hands.

- *Di*plegia is a symmetric paralysis of upper or lower extremities resulting from injuries to the cerebrum.

- *Tetra*plegia, or quadriplegia, means that the body has been affected from the neck down. Tetraplegics can eat, breathe, talk, and move their heads because these functions are controlled by the cranial nerves, which are usually protected from injury.

Motor vehicle accidents cause approximately 50% of all SCIs, and sports-related injuries contribute to 14% of all spinal cord injuries.

The neck is the most vulnerable part of the spine; approximately half of all injuries occur here. The levels most often injured, by order of frequency, are C_5, C_4, C_6, T_{12}, and L_1. Roughly 51.6% of SCI survivors are tetraplegic, and 46.3% are paraplegic.

Etiology: What Happens?

A primary injury to the spinal cord is usually a crushing blow (Figure 3.13), but the cord also can be injured through direct compression exerted by tumors, bone spurs, or cysts, or by stretching the spinal column (this is most frequently seen in children). Gunshot wounds may lacerate the cord. Spinal cords are rarely completely transected, and when they are, the mortality rate is very high.

As researchers learn more about spinal cord injuries, some very exciting information has emerged: a large part of the damage to delicate central nervous system tissue is incurred not by the trauma itself, but by post-traumatic reactions in the body. These secondary reactions, which include excessive bleeding, localized edema, free radical activity, an overabundance of scar tissue formation, white blood cell attacks on healthy tissue, and gradual demyelination of healthy cells, can be controlled and limited with appropriate early intervention.

A newly injured spinal cord goes through a period called "spinal cord shock." During this time, which may last 3 months or more, many body functions are severely impaired: blood pressure is dangerously low, the heart beats slowly, peripheral blood vessels dilate, and the patient is susceptible to *hypothermia*. Any or all of the secondary reactions discussed above may set in at this time. These secondary responses can interrupt function up to two full levels above the primary injury, so it is vital that an injury patient get aggressive care during this window of opportunity.

Figure 3.13. Spinal cord injury.

During this acute phase of injury, the affected muscles may be flaccid, or hypotonic. When the inflammatory process begins to subside, the muscles supplied by damaged axons begin to tighten, and their reflexes become hyperreactive. *Spasticity* along with *hyperreflexia* is a hallmark of SCI. If muscles stay flaccid and reflexes are dull or nonexistent, the damage is probably to the nerve roots rather than to the spinal cord itself. Injuries to the low back often show this pattern, as the spinal canal is occupied by the cauda equina nerve extensions from T_{12} down to the sacrum. Depending on the nature of the accident, injury to both the spinal cord and the nerve roots simultaneously is possible.

Signs and Symptoms

The motor and sensory impairment caused by SCI is entirely determined by what parts of the cord are damaged, and at what levels. Obviously, the higher the damage, the more of the body is affected. Injuries to the anterior cord affect motor function, whereas damage to the posterior aspect affects the senses of touch, proprioception, and vibration. Damage to the lateral parts of the cord interrupts sensations of pain and temperature.

Complications

Spinal cord injuries can lead to many serious long-term complications. An SCI patient will spend a lot of time and energy in working to prevent, manage, or recover from these secondary problems.

- *Decubitus ulcers.* Also known as bedsores or pressure sores, *decubitus ulcers* (see Chapter 1) can arise anywhere circulation is limited by mechanical compression of the skin. Because these wounds do not heal quickly or easily, they are highly susceptible to infection.

- *Heterotopic ossification.* This is the formation of calcium deposits in soft tissues. It is very similar to *myositis ossificans* (see Chapter 2), but this particular process is seen only in SCI patients. It typically occurs around the hips or knees, where it can be acutely painful. Heterotopic ossification can only be corrected with surgery.

- *Deep vein thrombosis, pulmonary embolism.* The formation of blood clots in the venous system is a high risk for new SCI patients, but the risk decreases only slightly with time. Blood that goes into the legs, but that lacks the muscular support to get back up the leg veins, can pool and thicken, causing *deep vein thrombosis*. If a fragment of a clot breaks loose, it will inevitably go to the lungs, causing a life-threatening *pulmonary embolism* (see Chapter 4); this is the second leading cause of death for SCI patients.

- *Respiratory infection.* SCI patients are at high risk for respiratory infection, especially if the damage is higher than T_{12}. When the chest cannot fully expand and contract and the cough reflex is limited, it is difficult to expel pathogens from the body. The leading cause of death for SCI patients is *pneumonia* (see Chapter 6).

- *Urinary tract infection.* SCI patients who must use a catheter to urinate are at high risk for contamination and infection of the urinary tract. Left untended, the risk of these infections invading the kidneys is significant. (See *urinary tract infection, pyelonephritis,* Chapter 9).

- *Autonomic hyperreflexia.* Damage to the spinal cord above T_6 raises the risk of developing autonomic *hyperreflexia*: a condition in which a minor stimulus (a full bladder or bowel, a ridge of cloth caught under the skin, menstrual cramps, etc.) creates an uncontrollable sympathetic reaction. It causes a pounding headache, increased heart rate, sweating, and other flight or fight symptoms, including dangerously high blood pressure. Autonomic hyperreflexia can be a medical emergency.

- *Cardiovascular disease.* Suddenly changing from being ambulatory to being confined to a wheelchair means a significant reduction in physical activity for most SCI patients. The risk of developing *hypertension, atherosclerosis,* and other cardiovascular problems (see Chapter 4) is high for this sedentary population.

- *Numbness.* Most SCI patients experience some numbness or reduction in sensation, depending on which part of the spinal cord has been damaged. The absence of pain is a dangerous feature, because it allows for damage to occur without warning. Small cuts or abrasions can become infected and an SCI patient may never know.

- *Pain.* Some SCI patients experience various kinds of pain along with numbness and lack of sensation. Some chronic pain problems are generated in the spine itself but refer sensation to the damaged limbs; nerve root pressure may refer pain along the associated dermatome; pain may be generated by the development of calcium deposits (see *heterotopic ossification,* above); or pain may be related to musculoskeletal injury as a person must learn to use his arms and shoulders in new ways to propel his wheelchair, and lift himself into and out of it.

- *Spasticity, contractures.* As the muscles supplied by damaged motor axons begin to tighten, an SCI patient loses range of motion. Some spasticity may become a permanent feature of the injury. Chronically tight muscle fibers eventually atrophy, to be replaced by thick, tough layers of connective tissue; this is called a contracture. If any sensory or motor function is left in the limb, temporary episodes of spasticity also may be a problem. These may be caused by any kind of stimulus; the reflexes of active muscle fibers in SCI patients are very extreme and sensitive.

Treatment

If something presses directly on the spinal cord or cauda equina, emergency surgery to remove it is indicated. The other very important early intervention with these traumas is to limit inflammation and other secondary body reactions that may damage uninjured tissue, so anti-inflammatories and other medications that limit this kind of activity are usually administered as quickly as possible.

Some later treatments for SCI include the implantation of electrodes in muscles that are controlled from an external computer. These implants can provide pinching and gripping capabilities for people who otherwise would not have the use of their hands. Surgical transfer of healthy tendons also can be helpful. For some people, the triceps muscle may be paralyzed, whereas the deltoid is not. Surgically extending the posterior deltoid tendon and attaching it to the olecranon can provide these people with the power it takes to use a wheelchair.

Treatment for SCI survivors is targeted at providing them with the skills to live as fully as possible. Physical and occupational therapists specialize in helping these patients gain the skills they need to function; mental/emotional therapists are also critical, especially for those who are adapting to their paralysis as a new way of life. Ultimately approximately 90% of all SCI patients are able to live independently with these new skills.

The focus of current research in SCI treatment is on influencing the growth of CNS neurons. It has been found that some proteins in cerebrospinal fluid inhibit neuronal growth, whereas others stimulate it. Furthermore, it may be that different types of neurons require different chemical environments for repair. Eventually, through a combination of stem cell implantation, genetic manipulation, and the creation of highly conducive chemical environments, it may be possible for someone with extensive spinal cord damage to regenerate damaged tissue and emerge with full or nearly full function.

Massage?

Massage can be an important part of the life of people with SCIs, as long as the complications listed above are considered and respected.

One aspect of living with an SCI that may be frequently missed is that in incomplete injuries where part of the spinal cord still functions, sensation and some motor control are still present. Some of the proprioceptors in these muscles still send messages about tightness and movement. If those messages consistently relay information about limitation, that limitation can become a self-fulfilling prophecy: a muscle that is partially limited can become completely unusable. It is vital that the proprioceptors in affected muscles be stimulated to allow the *most* use possible, rather than the least. When physical therapy and massage for SCI survivors focus on this goal, the long-term prognosis for maintaining function is much better.

SCI patients have very different physical and emotional stressors than the rest of the population, but they are prone to the same kinds of injuries as anyone else. Imagine being in a wheelchair and having shoulder tendinitis; would it not be a relief to get rolling, pain-free, again?

It takes a lot of courage to work with SCI survivors; massage therapists may have fears of accidentally hurting them, physically or emotionally, by saying or doing the wrong thing. But within this group is a population of people waiting eagerly for the chance to receive bodywork.

Stroke

Definition: What Is It?

Stroke, also called brain attack or cerebrovascular accident (CVA), is damage to the brain caused by oxygen deprivation.

⊙ *The animation "Stroke" can be found on the Student Resource CD-ROM that accompanies this book.*

Demographics: Who Gets It?

Stroke is the single most common type of CNS disorder. It is the third leading cause of death in the United States, coming in behind heart disease and cancer. It is the leading cause of adult disability.

Approximately 700,000 people will have a stroke this year (that is one every 45 seconds). Of them, 500,000 will experience their first attack, whereas 200,000 will have a repeat stroke. Close to 170,000 Americans will die of stroke this year (one every 3.1 minutes). Of the survivors, 15% to 30% will be permanently disabled, and 20% will require institutionalized care. Approximately 4.7 million stroke survivors are alive in this country today.

More men have strokes than women, but more women tend to die of strokes than men do. The chance of having a stroke before age 70 is approximately 1 in 20. After age 70, however, the risk rises significantly each year, especially if risk factors are present.

Etiology: What Happens?

Oxygen deprivation in the brain can be caused by ischemia or bleeding in the cranium (Figure 3.14). Ischemic strokes are related to oxygen deprivation because of blocked arteries. They typically occur in one of two forms:

- *Cerebral thrombosis*: A clot becomes lodged in a cerebral artery and starves off nerve cells. These strokes account for up to 88% of all CVAs. They are closely related to

Stroke in Brief

What is it?
A stroke is damage to brain tissue caused either by a blockage in blood flow or by an internal hemorrhage.

How is it recognized?
The symptoms of stroke include paralysis, weakness, or numbness on one side; blurry or diminished vision on one side with asymmetrically dilated pupils; dizziness and confusion; difficulty in speaking or understanding simple sentences; sudden extreme headache; and possibly loss of consciousness.

Is massage indicated or contraindicated?
Most people who survive strokes are at high risk for other cardiovascular problems. Rigorous circulatory massage should probably be avoided with this group, although they may certainly benefit from other types of bodywork to augment their rehabilitative physical therapy.

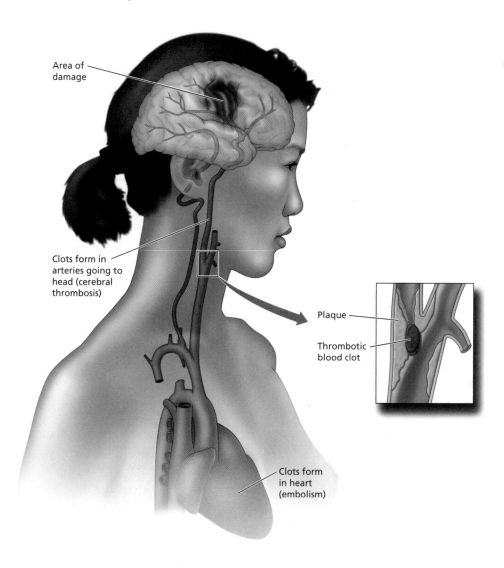

Area of damage

Clots form in arteries going to head (cerebral thrombosis)

Plaque

Thrombotic blood clot

Clots form in heart (embolism)

Figure 3.14. Ischemic stroke.

Carotid Artery Disease: Nowhere to Go But Up

The discussion of *atherosclerosis* (see Chapter 4) points out that because of chronically high blood pressure, both the aorta and coronary arteries are particularly prone to the development of atherosclerotic plaque. The carotid arteries, which emerge from the aortic arch, are similarly vulnerable. Although they are further from the heart, blood pressure in the arteries that supply the head is ordinarily very high to ensure adequate blood flow to the brain. This puts the carotid arteries at risk for the same endothelial damage and plaque development seen with the aorta and the coronary arteries; this is called *carotid artery disease*.

The problem with carotid artery disease is that if any fragment of plaque or blood clot should break free, it has only one direction to go: straight up into the brain. When this happens in very tiny increments, it is called transient ischemic attack, or TIA. But the presence of carotid artery disease significantly raises the risk of a major stroke—so much so that identifying this disorder often leads to aggressive treatment, in the shape of *carotid endarterectomy*: the artery is surgically opened, cleaned out, and closed up again.

Massage therapists working with clients who know they have carotid artery disease need to stay away from the neck, especially the anterior triangle, which is bordered by the sternocleidomastoid muscle, running superficially over the carotid arteries.

atherosclerosis (see Chapter 4). Cerebral thrombosis strokes usually occur during sleep or early in the morning.

• *Embolism*: This is much the same thing except that the origins of the obstruction are usually different. Emboli generally come from inefficient pumping of a heart with **atrial fibrillations**; incomplete and arrhythmic contractions allow blood in the left atrium to thicken and form clots before being forced out into the bloodstream. Emboli account for 8% to 14% of all CVAs.

   Ischemic strokes are distinct from but closely related to another phenomenon: *transient ischemic attacks*, or TIAs. In a TIA, a very tiny blood clot creates a temporary blockage in the brain, but it quickly disperses before any lasting damage can occur. Consequently, TIAs are associated with ischemic rather than hemorrhagic CVAs. Symptoms of TIA are very similar to those of stroke, except that they last only a few minutes or hours. They are, however, like the muffled rumblings of an incipient eruption; approximately one third of all people who have a stroke had a TIA beforehand.

   Another type of stroke has to do with bleeding inside the cranium (Figure 3.15). These are called hemorrhagic strokes, and they also occur in two forms:

• *Cerebral hemorrhage*: This is the rupture of a blood vessel that can cause tissue death in the brain. Cerebral hemorrhages are often associated with *aneurysms* (see Chapter 4), which may be a result of chronic hypertension, bleeding disorders, head trauma, or malformation of blood vessels.

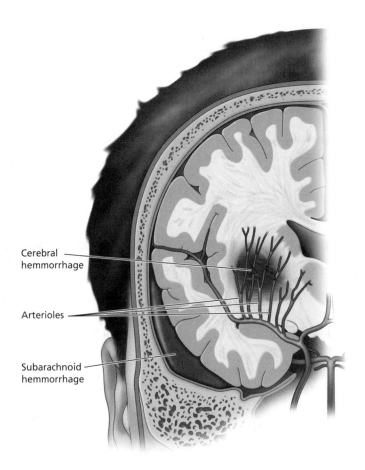

Cerebral hemmorrhage

Arterioles

Subarachnoid hemmorrhage

Figure 3.15. Hemorrhagic stroke.

- *Subarachnoid hemorrhage*: This is the rupture of a blood vessel on the surface of the brain rather than within the tissue itself. The leaking blood fills the space between the brain tissue and the arachnoid, eventually putting pressure against the cranium.

  The amount of damage a stroke causes is determined primarily by the location and numbers of neurons that are damaged by oxygen deprivation. Secondary responses to tissue damage have been seen also to contribute heavily to stroke damage. Inflammatory reactions, free radical activity, and other factors can cause tissue damage that far exceeds the oxygen deprivation brought about by the stroke itself. The good news in this discovery is that these secondary responses can be interrupted and moderated if treatment begins quickly enough.

Risk Factors

Although a person can have a genetic predisposition toward a CVA, many factors contribute to the likelihood of stroke that are well within the reach of personal control.

Risk Factors That Can Be Controlled

- *High blood pressure*: Untreated hypertension is the biggest single contributing factor to the risk of stroke. See *hypertension*, Chapter 4.
- *Smoking*: Nicotine constricts blood vessels and raises blood pressure.
- *Atherosclerosis, high cholesterol*: This situation also contributes to high blood pressure, as well as raising the risk of emboli.
- *C-reactive protein (CRP)*: This is a substance that is present with long-term low-grade inflammation. A high CRP level is a dependable predictor for both ischemic stroke and atherosclerosis.
- *Atrial fibrillation*: Left untreated, this condition can help to form the emboli responsible for some ischemic embolic strokes.
- *High alcohol consumption*: This is generally considered to be more than 2 drinks per day.
- *Obesity and sedentary lifestyle*
- *Diabetes*: Untreated, this condition can contribute to high blood pressure and atherosclerosis. (See Chapter 8.)
- *High-estrogen birth control pills*: especially when taken by a smoker
- *Hormone replacement therapy*: Some research indicates that women who supplement estrogen and progesterone as a way to manage symptoms of *menopause* (Chapter 10) have a significantly increased risk of stroke.
- *Overall stress*

Risk Factors That Cannot Be Controlled

- *Age*: Two thirds of all stroke patients are older than 65 years of age. The incidence of stroke doubles each decade after 55.
- *Gender*: Approximately 25% more men have strokes than women. However, women seem to have more severe strokes; strokes kill 100,000 women in this country each year, double the rate of death by breast cancer.
- *Race*: African Americans have a higher incidence of hypertension than whites. They are approximately twice as likely to have a stroke as whites, and they are almost twice as likely to die of a stroke.
- *Family history*: Having a family history of stroke and cardiovascular disease can be a predisposing factor. Structurally weak blood vessels can be an inherited problem. However, in cases of ischemic strokes, the question needs to be asked—what is inherited: the status of the blood vessels, or the diet and exercise habits?

- *Previous stroke*: Having one stroke usually predisposes a person to having another. Predisposition is not predestination, however; by taking control over whatever factors are within reach, a person can take big steps toward reducing the chances that he or she will have another stroke.

Signs and Symptoms

It is important to be able to recognize the signs of stroke; the sooner treatment is administered, the less damage will occur. Surprisingly, many Americans do not recognize the major symptoms of stroke, which are as follows:

- Sudden onset of unilateral weakness, numbness or paralysis on the face, arm, leg, or any combination of the three
- Suddenly blurred or decreased vision in one or both eyes; asymmetric dilation of pupils
- Difficulty in speaking or understanding simple sentences; confusion
- Sudden onset of dizziness, clumsiness, vertigo
- Sudden very extreme headache
- Possible loss of consciousness

Note that the symptoms of a TIA are very similar to those of a stroke. Whereas TIA symptoms may subside after a few minutes or hours, it is inappropriate to take a "wait and see" approach to any stroke symptoms. The effectiveness of stroke treatments depends on how soon treatment begins, so any symptoms should be immediately investigated.

After a debilitating stroke, the extent of the damage depends on what part and how much of the brain has been affected. Occasionally, progressive degeneration may continue over 1 or 2 days, but usually a stroke is complete within a few hours.

Motor damage from strokes can result in partial or full paralysis of one side of the body; this is called *hemiplegia*. *Aphasia* (loss of language), memory loss, and mild or severe personality changes also may occur. Sensory damage may result in permanent numbness or vision loss.

Diagnosis

When a person suspects that he may have had a stroke, the first priority is to determine whether it was an ischemic or hemorrhagic event, because these two phenomena require a very different treatment approach. A diagnosis may be reached through a combination of a physical examination, CT scan, MRI, ultrasound, *arteriography*, and blood tests.

Treatment

The treatment of choice for ischemic stroke survivors is anticoagulant medication to minimize the risk of more clotting. Severe brain damage may be averted if the anticoagulants are administered within a few hours of the stroke. One anticoagulant, called *tissue plasminogen activator* (tPA), has been found to be extremely effective for minimizing the blood clots involved in both stroke and *heart attack* (see Chapter 4), if it is administered within the first few hours of onset.

If the CVA was from a hemorrhage, however, anticoagulant treatment could be dangerous, or even deadly. A brain aneurysm caught before it ruptures may be treated with surgery to take the pressure off or strengthen the affected artery.

Once the dust has settled and it is clear how much function was lost during a stroke, therapy may begin to help a patient relearn how to do basic tasks such as walking, speaking, eating, and self-care. Because the brain has a vast resource of backup wiring, this is often a very successful part of the recovery process. It needs to be started very soon after the CVA, however, to prevent the fibrosis and atrophy of muscle tissue that happen so quickly when nerve signals have been interrupted. Physical, occupational, and speech therapists may be enlisted in this process; massage, with respect for the risk of cardio-vascular disease, may have a role here too.

Limiting controllable risk factors is also important: stopping smoking, improving diet and exercise habits, and reducing stress are all important actions to take. If necessary, surgery may be performed either on the blood vessels leading to the brain or inside it to widen the lumina and reduce the possibility of more clots being caught or formed inside.

Massage?

Massage can play a role in the recovery of a stroke survivor, but some cautions need to be considered. First and foremost is the client's general cardiovascular health. Most stroke patients have other circulatory problems. Therefore, it is very important to work as part of a client's health care team. Second, hemiplegia is a type of spastic paralysis, which carries specific cautions and guidelines for massage. (See sidebar "Nerve Damage Terminology").

Persons who are in physical and occupational therapy for stroke recovery may derive significant benefit from massage as well; remember that proprioceptors in affected limbs may misinterpret the amount of limitation that occurs, leading to an unnecessary degeneration of muscular function. Stretching, exercising, and improving circulation in areas that have good sensation can slow that process.

Traumatic Brain Injury

Definition: What Is It?

Traumatic brain injury (TBI) is an insult to the brain, not brought about by congenital or degenerative conditions, leading to altered states of consciousness, cognitive impairment, and disruption of physical, emotional, and behavioral function.

TBI is usually due to external force: a direct blow or a rapid acceleration/deceleration incident. Motor vehicle accidents, gunshot wounds, falls, sports, and physical violence are leading causes.

Demographics: Who Gets It?

Approximately 1.5 million TBIs are reported every year, with 1 million emergency room visits. Approximately 70,000 deaths from head injuries occur every year.

A TBI occurs approximately every 21 seconds in this country. Approximately 270,000 people experience moderate to severe TBIs; the rest are classified as mild injuries, although the risk of long-term disability even in mild cases is very high.

Between 2.5 and 6.5 million TBI survivors are living in the United States today. The direct and indirect costs of treating this injury are over $48 billion per year.

Etiology: What Happens?

Several different classifications for head injuries have been created to try to organize the vast number of ways the brain, although encased in a protective casing, can be injured.

Traumatic Brain Injury in Brief

What is it?
Traumatic brain injury (TBI) is damage to the brain brought about by trauma rather than congenital or chronic degenerative disease.

How is it recognized?
Symptoms of TBI vary according to the location and severity of the injury. Long-term effects range from mild cognitive impairment, learning problems, and motor control difficulties to varying types of coma or persistent vegetative state.

Is massage indicated or contraindicated?
Many TBI patients undergo intensive physical, occupational, and speech therapy to preserve or recover motor function. Carefully administered massage is also appropriate, as long as it is incorporated within the patient's health care plan and does not pose any risk in the presence of spasticity, numbness, or psychiatric disturbance.

- *Skull fracture:* This occurs when the bones around the skull are broken, usually from a direct blow. This can lead to a number of internal injuries, but, interestingly, the prognosis for an "open head injury" is often better than for a "closed head injury," because the risk of damage from too much pressure is somewhat less.

- *Penetrating injury:* This is usually due to a gunshot wound but also may be from a knife or other object. Penetrating injuries are the leading cause of death among TBI patients.

- *Concussion:* This is a temporary loss of consciousness (less than 20 minutes), often brought about by jarring of the cranium. Concussion is the most common type of TBI.

- *Contusion:* This is bruising inside the cranium. When a contusion happens at the point of impact and also where the brain hits the opposite wall, it is referred to as a "*coup-contrecoup.*"

- *Diffuse axonal injury:* This is internal tearing of nerve tissue throughout the brain. It is often related to acceleration/deceleration accidents as seen with *whiplash* (see Chapter 2) or shaken baby syndrome.

- *Anoxic brain injury:* This is the complete lack of oxygen in the brain. It can be brought about by airway obstruction or sudden apnea.

- *Hypoxic brain injury:* This is an inadequate supply of oxygen, often associated with ischemic *stroke* (this chapter), or toxic exposure, especially carbon monoxide poisoning.

- *Hemorrhage:* This is bleeding inside the brain, often associated with ruptured aneurysms (see hemorrhagic *stroke*, this chapter).

- *Hematoma:* This is the development of a large amount of coagulated blood, either pressing outside or within the brain.

- *Edema:* A secondary inflammatory response can follow any or all of the causes of TBI. The swelling of brain tissue and action of free radicals against healthy tissue may ultimately be responsible for more damage than the original source of the trauma.

Signs and Symptoms

Signs and symptoms of a TBI vary according to what areas of the brain are affected, and how severe the injury is. Trauma to the frontal lobes is most common and may result in language and motor dysfunction; trauma to structures closest to the brainstem is more likely to lead to massive loss of function.

Symptoms of an acute TBI include the leakage of cerebrospinal fluid from the ears or nose; dilated or asymmetric pupils; visual disturbances; dizziness and confusion; *apnea* or slowed breathing; nausea and vomiting; slow pulse and low blood pressure; loss of bowel and bladder control; possible seizures, paralysis, numbness, lethargy, or loss of consciousness. In infants, chronic crying, lethargy, or unusual sleep patterns are cause for concern. Symptoms may occur immediately or grow in severity over a course of days or even weeks.

Long-term consequences of TBI include mild to severe cognitive dysfunction, especially with memory and learning skills. Movement disorders may range from hypertonicity to spasticity. *Seizure disorders* (this chapter) are a frequent complication. Permanent changes in behavioral and emotional function are also common; many TBI survivors are emotionally volatile, and may develop new patterns of aggressiveness and hostility. More severe cases of TBI (usually those that affect the brainstem) may lead to various levels of coma or a persistent vegetative state.

Treatment

TBI is treated with surgery to remove pressure on the brain if necessary, followed by intensive physical, recreational, occupational, and speech therapy to preserve or recover function. The prognosis with children is generally better, because their brains seem to be more capable of establishing new pathways to relearn skills. Nonetheless, "brain plasticity," or the ability to tap into unused areas for motor and mental function, is a new field, and further research continues to brighten the outlook even for mature TBI survivors.

Prevention

Preventive measures to guard against the risk of TBI are self-evident, but worth repeating. Most TBIs happen as a "transport injury," that is, in an altercation involving cars, motorcycles, bicycles, scooters, skates, or skateboards. Driving only while alert and sober, using seatbelts, and wearing helmets can help to reduce the risk and severity of these accidents. Other preventive measures include making sure homes are safe for young children and elderly people to reduce the risk of falls, and the appropriate storage of firearms.

Massage?

Decisions about bodywork in the presence of a TBI must be made based on the client's ability to adapt to the changes brought about by massage. If sensation is present and the client is able to communicate clearly about his or her comfort, massage is not only appropriate but could be an important part of the rehabilitation picture to assist in the maintenance of healthy muscles and connective tissues.

If a client is comatose, massage or other stroking techniques may be performed to help preserve the health of the tissues and prevent complications such as *decubitus ulcers* (Chapter 1), but this must be conducted with caution because the risk of over-treatment cannot be managed by the client himself.

In either case, TBI is a complicated, serious problem with many long-term problems that affect many aspects of health. Any TBI survivor who receives massage as part of a rehabilitative process should do so as part of an integrated health care approach, incorporating massage with other therapies for the best result.

Trigeminal Neuralgia

Definition: What Is It?

Trigeminal neuralgia (TN) is neuro-algia ("nerve pain") along one or more of the three branches of cranial nerve V, the trigeminal nerve (Figure 3.16). It is also called *tic douloureux*, which is French for "painful spasm" or "unhappy twitch."

Demographics: Who Gets It?

Trigeminal neuralgia is a relatively rare disorder; its incidence is approximately 16 per 100,000. The average TN patient is a woman older than 50 years of age, although it has been documented among all ages.

Etiology: What Happens?

Trigeminal neuralgia is usually classified as a primary or a secondary problem. In either case, the trigeminal nerve is irritated, and the result is brief, repeating episodes of sharp, electrical, stabbing pain on one side of the face.

Trigeminal Neuralgia in Brief

What is it?
Trigeminal neuralgia (TN) is a condition involving sharp electrical or stabbing pain along one or more branches of the trigeminal nerve (cranial nerve V), usually in the lower face and jaw.

How is it recognized?
The pain of TN is very sharp and severe. Patients report stabbing, electrical, or burning sensations that occur in brief episodes, but that repeat with or without identifiable triggers. A muscular tic is often present as well.

Is massage indicated or contraindicated?
TN is intensely painful, and even very light touch may trigger an attack. It therefore contraindicates massage on the face, unless the client specifically guides the therapist into what feels safe and comfortable. Massage elsewhere on the body is appropriate, although TN clients may prefer not to be face down.

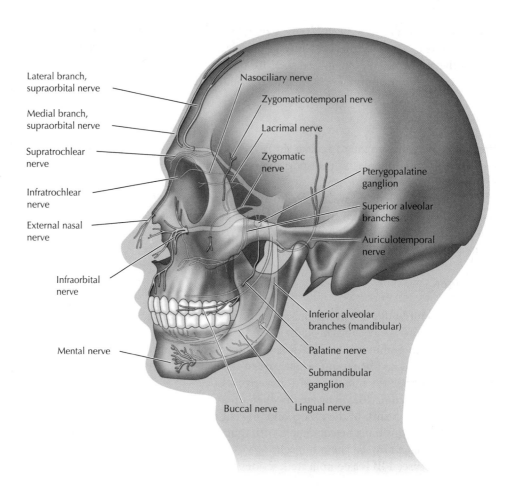

Figure 3.16. The trigeminal nerve.

Primary TN is considered to be idiopathic: the cause or source of the nerve irritation may never be identified.

Secondary TN is due to mechanical pressure on the nerve or some other structural problem. Causative factors include tumors, bone spurs, a recent infection, complications of dental surgery, or *multiple sclerosis* (this chapter). Cervical misalignment or *temporomandibular joint dysfunction* (see Chapter 2) also may contribute to symptoms. Perhaps the most common cause of TN is the growth of tiny blood vessels that may strangulate or otherwise irritate the nerve. This usually occurs just at the junction between the trigeminal nerve and the brain.

Episodes of trigeminal nerve pain can be triggered by speaking, chewing, swallowing, sitting in a draft, a light touch to the wrong spot, and sometimes by no stimulus at all. Episodes may happen several times a day for days, weeks, or months, and then suddenly disappear—only to begin again months or years later. TN can be a debilitating lifelong condition if it is not treated.

Signs and Symptoms

Some people call the pain of TN among the worst in the world. It is often described as sharp, electrical stabbing or burning sensations. The words "hot poker" appear in a lot of the literature associated with this condition. These episodes may last for 10 seconds to a minute, or several jabs may occur in rapid succession. A muscular tic sometimes develops along with the nerve pain.

Triggers of TN attacks may vary, or episodes may be completely spontaneous. The incidence of attacks also may vary: they can occur regularly, then disappear for a while, then come back with renewed vigor.

Treatment

Treatment strategies for this problem depend on the source of the pain. Sinus and tooth infections can sometimes mimic trigeminal neuralgia, so an early step is to rule those out. Cervical misalignment or TMJ problems can be sorted out by the appropriate professionals. Acupuncture often works well for trigeminal neuralgia, as it does for many problems with nerve conduction.

The mainstream medical approach to TN starts with painkillers, and then proceeds to anti-seizure drugs that inhibit nerve conduction. Many patients do not tolerate these drugs very well, however, or they build up resistance and the drugs provide less and less relief.

Several more invasive interventions have been developed to treat TN. Some of them involve the controlled destruction of part of the nerve, with lasers, radiation, or injected chemicals. These options often provide some relief, with the understanding that the patient may experience permanent numbness as a result. Microvascular surgery to relieve pressure on the trigeminal nerve is conducted through a hole in the mastoid process. This process leaves sensation intact and is successful for many patients, but carries more risks of complication than other approaches.

Massage?

Clients who currently experience TN attacks will probably feel unsafe with any pressure or work on their face; massage therapists should respect this caution. Face cradles also may be uncomfortable; it may not be possible to work with TN clients in a prone position.

Massage anywhere else on the body is certainly indicated.

OTHER NERVOUS SYSTEM DISORDERS

Guillain-Barré Syndrome

Definition: What Is It?

Guillain-Barré syndrome (GBS) is a condition involving acute inflammation and destruction of the myelin layer of peripheral nerves, specifically in the extremities. Its synonym is *acute idiopathic polyneuritis*, which is highly descriptive: it is a severe, extreme inflammation of multiple peripheral nerves, which comes about for reasons no one fully understands.

Other Cranial Nerve Disorders

Any damage or irritation to a cranial nerve may lead to symptoms in the face. Trigeminal neuralgia and Bell's palsy are two of the most common disorders that may cause facial symptoms. But a few other cranial nerve disorders deserve a passing glance as well:

- *Postherpetic neuralgia*. This is a complication of *herpes zoster* (this chapter). It may occur wherever the shingles blisters appeared but can outlast the visible lesions by several weeks or months. When the herpes infection affects the optic nerve, postherpetic neuralgia can create extremely painful facial symptoms.

- *Glossopharyngeal neuralgia*: This is etiologically identical to vascular compression on the trigeminal nerve, but this condition affects cranial nerve IX, which supplies sensation to the back of the throat.

- *Atypical face pain*. This is a condition similar to trigeminal neuralgia, and in some cases may be a predecessor to it. It is characterized by pain that is less severe than trigeminal neuralgia, but it tends to be continuous rather than intermittent. The pain also may go up over the back of the head and into the scalp, and it may involve the occipital as well as the trigeminal nerve.

- *Hemifacial spasm*. This condition creates a painless tic that is related to blood vessel compression of the facial nerve rather than the trigeminal nerve.

Guillain-Barré Syndrome in Brief

What is it?
Guillain-Barré syndrome (GBS) is a demyelinating disorder of peripheral nerves. It usually begins in the feet and moves proximally. It is probably autoimmune in nature, but the specific triggers have not been identified.

How is it recognized?
Guillain-Barré syndrome is marked by its sudden onset (symptoms usually begin quickly and peak within 2 weeks) followed by its gradual remission (most patients have full or nearly full recovery within 18 months). Furthermore, GBS affects limbs symmetrically, and moves proximally toward the trunk, which distinguishes it from other peripheral nerve problems.

Is massage indicated or contraindicated?
When a person has reached the peak of his or her GBS attack, physical and occupational therapy are often employed to speed recovery and prevent muscle atrophy. Massage may be useful at this stage as well, to improve circulation, and to reduce fatigue and anxiety.

Demographics: Who Gets It?

GBS can affect anyone at any time. Men with the syndrome slightly outnumber women, but it is seen in all ages and races. Although it is not a particularly common problem, affecting approximately 1 of every 100,000 people, it is the most frequently seen form of acute neuromuscular paralysis since the eradication of polio in the Western hemisphere.

Etiology: What Happens?

Guillain-Barré syndrome was first documented in 1916, but our understanding of how this disease comes about has not progressed a great deal since then. Many patients have an infection of the respiratory or gastrointestinal tract several days before developing GBS symptoms. It is believed that this preceding infection stimulates an immune system attack mistakenly directed against the myelin sheaths of peripheral nerves. Current research indicates that a common cause of *gastroenteritis* (Chapter 7) may be behind many cases of GBS; this is a bacterium called **Campylobacter jejuni**.

Some GBS patients do not experience a preceding infection. This disorder has also been seen in conjunction with immune system changes brought about by pregnancy, surgery, and as a reaction to certain vaccines, specifically the swine flu vaccine that was distributed in 1976.

Regardless of what initiates the disease process, the end result is that the myelin sheaths on peripheral nerves is attacked and destroyed. The damage progresses proximally, and also may affect cranial nerves. This can be a life-threatening situation if the nerves that control breathing are damaged; many GBS patients spend time on a ventilator before they recover.

Signs and Symptoms

GBS is notorious for being unpredictable, but it has a few features that distinguish it from other peripheral nerve disorders. Onset is typically fast and severe; a patient may go from being fully functional to being in a hospital within a matter of hours or a couple of days. GBS is usually symmetric, affecting both legs equally. Also, myelin damage progresses proximally, moving up toward the trunk rather than distally, which is different from most other nerve problems.

When GBS first appears, it often involves weakness or tingling in the affected limbs. Reflexes become dull or disappear altogether. Loss of sensation progresses proximally, although pain frequently develops in the hips and pelvis. If the GBS affects cranial nerves of the face, facial weakness, pain, and difficulty with speech may develop.

GBS symptoms usually peak at 2 or 3 weeks after onset, and then they may linger for several weeks before they begin to subside. The amount of damage that accrues while the nerves are inflamed depends on what treatments were introduced when, and how soon the patient can begin to use his or her muscles after the paralysis resolves.

Diagnosis

The signs and symptoms of GBS are so distinctive that it is usually not difficult to diagnose. A lumbar puncture may be performed to look for elevated proteins in cerebrospinal fluid, and a nerve conduction test may be recommended to confirm that nerve transmission to the extremities is impaired.

Treatment

Because GBS is an idiopathic disease, no specific cure has been developed. Two treatment options have been successfully used to shorten recovery time: *plasmapheresis* ("blood cleansing") and injections of high concentrations of immunoglobulin or gamma globulin (donated antibodies).

Plasmapheresis is a process by which blood cells are removed from the patient's blood, placed in fresh donated plasma, and then replaced in the body. This removes autoimmune antibodies and reduces attacks against myelin. This procedure is most effective within 2 weeks of onset.

Intravenous doses of immunoglobulin or gamma globulin are believed to inhibit the patient's antibody and cytokine activity, thus limiting the autoimmune attack against myelin sheaths on peripheral nerves.

Clinical trials of both of these treatment options show them to be approximately equally effective. They can shorten the duration of the recovery process by up to 50% compared with patients who do not receive these treatments.

Other interventions for GBS patients are dictated by their individual needs. Many patients require the use of a ventilator for a time until the respiratory nerves regain full function. Anticoagulants may be used against the danger of blood clots in immobilized legs (see *deep vein thrombosis*, Chapter 4). Once the acute inflammation has passed, occupational and physical therapy are used to help the patient regain as much muscle function as possible.

Prognosis

The good news is most people who develop GBS have a full or nearly full recovery, although the process may take 18 months or more. A small number of patients (5%–15%) have permanent disability because of the disease. Some people (roughly 5%) don't ever get better; their condition becomes a chronic inflammation that does not resolve. Approximately 10% of all GBS patients experience a relapse later in life. Approximately 3% to 4% of GBS patients die of instability of the autonomic nervous system that comes about with such rapid changes in functional levels.

Massage?

A person in the acute stage of GBS is unlikely to seek massage, and it would be wisest to avoid trying to mechanically stimulate the body while this immune system confusion is still raging.

Once the acute stage is over, physical and occupational therapy play a key role in the rehabilitation process of a person recovering from GBS. As long as sensation is present and accurate (i.e., the client can give feedback about pressure and comfort), massage could be a very useful adjunct in this long and frustrating process.

Headaches

Definition: What Are They?

Headaches are one of the most common physical problems in the range of human experience. Up to 90% of adults in the United States will experience a headache each year. Although they can herald some serious underlying problems, most of the time headaches are self-contained, temporary problems, only peripherally related to other conditions in the body.

Headaches in Brief

What are they?
Headaches are pain caused by any number of sources. Muscular tension, vascular spasm and dilation, and chemical imbalances all can contribute to headache. Headaches only rarely indicate a serious underlying disorder.

How are they recognized?
Tension-type headaches are usually bilateral and steadily painful. Vascular headaches are often unilateral and have a distinctive "throbbing" pain from blood flow into the head. Headaches brought about by central nervous system injury or disease are extreme, severe, and prolonged. They can have a sudden or gradual onset.

Is massage indicated or contraindicated?
Headaches due to infection or CNS injury contraindicate massage. Persons experiencing vascular headaches generally avoid stimuli such as massage, but massage is definitely indicated for tension-type headaches.

Types of Headaches

New advances in headache research have uncovered similarities between headache types that had never been suspected. As we learn more about the physiologic processes of these disorders, our methods for classifying them may change, but for the present, most headaches can be put into one of four categories. Headaches defy categorization, however; some headaches share qualities from more than one of these classifications.

- *Tension-type headaches.* By far the most common type of headache people experience (90%–92%), these are triggered by muscular tension, bony misalignment, *TMJ disorders*, *myofascial pain syndrome* (see Chapter 2), ligament irritation, or other musculoskeletal imbalances.
- *Vascular headaches.* These include classic and common migraines, cluster headaches, and possibly sinus headaches. They account for a total of approximately 6% to 8% of all headaches. Many vascular headaches are triggered by food sensitivities, alcohol use, or chemical shifts seen with the menstrual cycle.
- *Chemical headaches.* The triggers for these headaches can be any kind of chemical disturbance, including low blood sugar ("hunger headache"), hormone shifts, and dehydration, including the dehydration brought about by alcohol use ("hangover" headaches). "Rebound headaches" that accompany the overuse of painkillers could be classified at chemical headaches.
- *Traction-inflammatory headaches.* These are the rarest type of headache, and the most dangerous: they are indicative of severe underlying pathologic conditions such as tumors, aneurysm, hemorrhage, or infection in the central nervous system.

Etiology: What Happens?

Although headaches are fairly easy to categorize by type, it turns out that the actual pain-causing mechanisms of the various headache categories (which had always been assumed to be fundamentally different) are probably much closer than we thought. Therefore, as we learn more about this phenomenon, the perceived differences between tension-type and vascular-type headaches may fade. This is good news, as a more thorough understanding of these mechanisms may lead to more effective ways to treat and even prevent the debilitating pain headaches can cause.

The common denominator that has been observed in tension and vascular headaches (by far the two most common types) has been the activity of serotonin, a neurotransmitter that has been implicated in a number of other central nervous system disorders. Both migraine and tension headache episodes show significant drops in serotonin levels. This may cause the trigeminal nerve (the major sensory nerve for the head and face, to release *neuropeptides* that dilate blood vessels in the periphery of the brain. This vasodilation puts pressure on the meninges, the main source of sensation for the brain. The primary difference between migraine headaches and tension headaches, therefore, may simply be the triggers. Migraines are generally associated with chemical triggers such as food sensitivities or hormonal shifts, whereas tension headaches are more often associated with mechanical triggers such as tight muscles or misaligned vertebrae. However, both types of triggers evidently may lead to serotonin shifts and intracranial vasodilation.

The specific changes brought about by headache triggers are discussed below.

Tension Headaches

Definition: What Are They?

Tension headaches are headaches triggered by mechanical stresses that initiate the central nervous system changes in serotonin levels and blood vessel dilation discussed above.

Etiology: What Happens?

The average head weighs about 18 to 20 pounds. The area of bone-to-bone contact between the occipital condyles and the facets of C1 is about the same as two pairs of fingertips touching. The whole mechanism is kept in balance by tension exerted by muscles and ligaments around the neck and head. The muscles primarily responsible for the posture of the head form two inverted triangles just below the occiput (Figure 3.17). It is not surprising, then, that when this delicate balance is a little off, the resulting pain reverberates throughout the whole structure.

Similarly, when postural or movement patterns elsewhere in the body exert force on the spine, the end result can be tension at the occipital connection. In this way, a foot that strikes the ground too hard on the lateral side may pull on the knee, which may then demand compensation in the hip. The sacrum moves to adjust to the tip in the *os coxae*. This creates a slight twist in the lumbar vertebrae, which then reverberates all the way up the spine to the head. The result: headaches because the feet are not in alignment.

Triggers

These are almost too numerous to list here, precisely because staying pain-free involves such a precarious balance of muscle tension, bony alignment, and a myriad of other factors. Here are some of the major causes for tension headaches:

- Muscular, tendinous, or ligamentous injury to the head or neck structures can lead to headaches. The ligaments in the neck may be most easily injured; they are vulnerable to fraying and irritation with uncontrolled movement, and they refer pain over the back of the head. (See *whiplash*, Chapter 2.)

- Simple muscle tension in the suboccipital triangle or the jaw flexors can cause headaches. These muscles are especially vulnerable to the effects of emotional stress. When people are worried or angry, they tend to clench their jaws and tighten their necks.

- Subluxation or fixation of cervical vertebrae can irritate ligaments or cause muscle spasms, both of which lead to headaches.

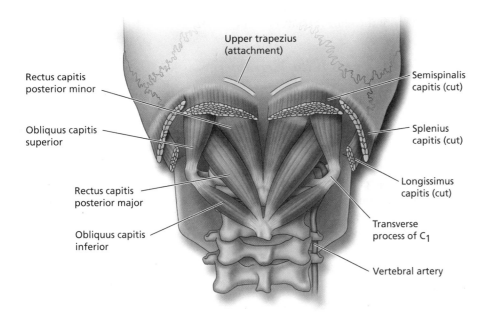

Figure 3.17. Muscular imbalance at the suboccipital triangle is a contributing factor in many headaches.

- Structural problems in the alignment of the cranial bones (which are not completely immobile) or in the temporomandibular joint can cause headaches.
- Trigger points in the muscles of the neck and head can refer pain all around the head. (See *myofascial pain syndrome*, Chapter 2.)
- Eyestrain: the chronic contraction of muscles in the eye to focus on reading material or other visual input can cause tension headaches. (These may be relieved when corrective eyewear successfully reduces eye muscle tension.)
- Any kind of ongoing mental or physical stress can change postural and movement patterns, which will lead to muscle spasm, subluxation, fixation, and so on. Poor ergonomics, especially in repetitive work situations, are frequently the culprit behind chronic tension headaches.

Vascular Headaches

Definition: What Are They?

These are headaches that are often triggered by food sensitivities, hormonal shifts, alcohol use, or other factors that are difficult to identify. The pain they cause comes from excessively dilated blood vessels in the meninges. They are characterized by a pain that "throbs" with the patient's pulse.

Migraines

Demographics: Who Gets Migraines?

Approximately 28 million people in the United States experience diagnosed migraines. This malady is responsible for an overwhelming $50 billion in lost wages and medical expenses every year.

Women get migraines more often than men do. It is estimated that up to 18% of all women will have a migraine at some time in their life; that number is closer to 6% for men. Many migraines are genetically linked; 70% to 80% of migraine patients have other family members with the same malady.

Etiology: What Happens With Migraines?

Migraine headaches begin with extreme vasoconstriction in the affected hemisphere, which one would expect to be painful, but it is not. Instead a sense of euphoria is felt, although it is mixed with dread that the worst is yet to come. The vasoconstriction is then followed by a huge vasodilation: a veritable flood of blood into the affected part of the brain. It is all still contained within the vessels, of course, but all the excess pressure presses against the vessel walls and meninges, which causes excruciating pain.

People with migraines are frequently deficient in magnesium. Supplementing this mineral sometimes decreases the frequency of migraine episodes.

Migraines are associated with increased risk of *seizure disorders* and *stroke* (this chapter).

Triggers

No one has identified an exact reason for what sets up the process for migraines to take place. Some triggers have been identified, such as the consumption of certain kinds of foods, including red wine, cheese, chocolate, coffee, tea, aspartame, MSG, and any kind of alcohol. Abnormal levels of stress can bring them on, as can hormonal shifts such as menstruation, pregnancy, and menopause. (These hormonal shifts can also make pre-existing migraines disappear.) The good news about migraines is that they usually subside by middle age. It is not unheard of, but quite uncommon, for mature people to suffer from migraines.

Signs and Symptoms

The word *migraine* comes from the French, hemi-craine, or "half-head." This is because migraine headache has a characteristic unilateral presentation. In classic migraines, the pain will be preceded by blurred vision, the perception of flashing lights or auras, and even auditory hallucinations. Classic migraines constitute only about 15% to 20% of all migraines. Then, as with the aura-less common migraines (the other 80%–85% of migraines), the patient experiences extreme throbbing pain on one side of the head, which may cause the affected eye and side of the nose to water. Hypersensitivity to light, nausea, and vomiting are all possible. Symptoms can persist for anywhere from several hours to several days.

Cluster Headaches

Definition: What Are They?

These are a fairly rare, not well-understood variety of vascular headache. Cluster headaches affect men more often than women, and they affect less than 1% of the US population. They come, one right after the other, for days or weeks at a time. Cluster headaches usually happen at night, with pain severe enough to wake a person out of a sound sleep. Like migraines, they cause the eye and nostril of the affected side to water. They also may cause facial swelling and unilateral sweating.

Reliable triggers for cluster headaches have not been identified. They may occur seasonally, once or twice in a year, or just once in a lifetime.

Sinus Headaches

Sinus headaches are worth a mention among the vascular headaches because they also have to do with too much fluid in the skull. The fluid is contained in the sinuses rather than the cranium itself. When a person has sinus-related allergies or sinusitis, the membranes can become irritated and inflamed. This is discussed further in *sinusitis*, Chapter 6.

Chemical Headaches

Definition: What Are They?

Chemical headaches are triggered by a variety of chemical imbalances in the body. They are often warning signs that the person has too much or too little of some substance vital to maintaining homeostasis. Examples of chemical headaches can include:

- Headaches caused by very low blood sugar, indicating that the person needs to eat soon (see *hypoglycemia*, Chapter 8)
- Headaches caused by hormonal shifts such as those seen with the menstrual cycle and childbirth (see *premenstrual syndrome* and *menopause*, Chapter 10).

- Headaches caused by extreme dehydration—both from physical exertion and from alcohol consumption. This is the typical "hangover" headache.
- "Rebound headaches" occur when a person takes too much headache medication, especially NSAIDs. These headaches may last for 2 weeks or more, and the only way to treat them is to stop taking pain medication.

Traction–Inflammatory Headaches

Headaches are occasionally a sign of a serious CNS injury or infection. Headaches in combination with extreme fever often have a bacterial or viral precipitator. They are usually short-lived, subsiding when the fever passes the crisis point. The time to become concerned is when headaches are severe, repeating, and have a sudden onset ("thunderclap headache"); when they appear in a new pattern after age 50; or when they have a gradual onset but no remission. In these cases, headache may be a symptom of some serious underlying condition. This is particularly true if the headache is accompanied by slurred speech, numbness anywhere in the body, and difficulties with motor control. The first things to investigate in cases such as this are *encephalitis*, *meningitis*, *stroke* (this chapter) or a tumor or an *aneurysm* (Chapter 4).

Treatment

Avoiding or managing headache triggers is the most proactive and least invasive way to deal with this problem. People who experience recurrent headaches of any type are usually encouraged to keep a "headache journal" to try to pin down their own specific triggers for headaches.

As our understanding of the most common types of headaches changes, treatment options will likewise probably also shift. For the moment, medical headache treatment falls into two categories: prophylactic treatment that works to prevent the headache from beginning, and abortive treatment that works to end the headache once it has begun. A class of medications developed for depression called selective serotonin reuptake inhibitors (SSRIs) are finding use in both categories to deal with migraine headaches. Other migraine treatments include *ergot* compounds, beta-blockers, and calcium channel blockers, all of which work to interrupt the vasoconstriction phase of the early headache process. Because migraines often involve vomiting, some medications are poorly tolerated when taken orally; nasal spray applications work well for some patients.

Tension-type headaches are still treated primarily with NSAIDs when they require medical intervention at all.

Massage?

The appropriateness of massage depends on what kind of headache the client has. If it is related to a serious underlying pathologic condition, or to a bacterial or viral infection, any massage is obviously inappropriate.

Vascular headaches are usually so extreme and painful that clients prefer to wait until the acute stage has passed. Hydrotherapy to draw fluid out of the congested cranium may be successful if the client can tolerate it.

However, for the most common tension-type headaches, massage is resoundingly indicated. These episodes are an excellent opportunity to demonstrate how many seemingly disconnected postural and movement patterns can create pain in entirely different area of the body.

Seizure Disorders

Definition: What Are They?

A seizure disorder is any kind of problem that can cause seizures as one of its symptoms. Epilepsy, one type of seizure disorder, is one of the oldest conditions recorded in medical history. It was first described about 2,000 years before Christ, but it was not studied as a specific problem other than "demonic possession" until the mid 19th century. Epilepsy is identified as a specific disorder when a person has two or more seizures that are *not* related to any identifiable cause such as head injury, stroke, infection, or fever. This rules out approximately 75% of all people who have a history of seizure.

Demographics: Who Gets Them?

Seizure disorders are the second most common type of central nervous system problem in the country; *stroke* (this chapter) is the first. Approximately 1% of the population will experience a seizure at some point. Approximately 25% of those people may eventually be diagnosed with epilepsy. In the United States, approximately 30,000 cases of epilepsy are diagnosed each year; an estimated 4 million people live with epilepsy at the present time. Epilepsy occurs in males and females about equally.

Etiology: What Happens?

When interconnecting neurons in the brain are stimulated in a certain kind of way, a tremendous burst of excess electricity may stimulate the neighboring neurons. The reaction is repeated, and soon millions of neurons in the brain are giving off electrical discharge. This is the central nervous system "lightning storm" of the epileptic seizure, and it affects the rest of the body in a number of different ways.

For the most part, no one knows what starts the storm in the first place. Triggers vary for different people. For some, sudden changes in light level, from dark to light or vice versa, will trigger a seizure. For others, flashing or strobe lights, or the strobe effect created by ceiling fans, will be the trigger. For others, certain sounds, or even particular notes of music cause a seizure. High anxiety or other sicknesses such as cold or flu also can lead to seizures.

Whatever the trigger, the result is uncoordinated neuronal activity that allows electrical signals to get progressively more extreme, sometimes to the point of collapse and loss of consciousness. Close studies of the synapses of seizure patients has revealed the possibility that these disorders may be linked to some important neurotransmitter imbalances; these patients have either underactive inhibitory neurotransmitters, overactive excitatory neurotransmitters, or both. This discovery has opened some new possibilities in seizure treatment.

Causes

In some cases, the cause of seizures can be definitively linked to a mechanical or chemical problem in the brain. Birth trauma, *traumatic brain injury* (this chapter), brain tumors, and penetrating wounds all can cause seizures, as can some types of metabolic distur-

---

Seizure Disorders in Brief

What are they?
Seizure disorders are any condition that causes seizures. They are often related to some kind of neurologic damage in the shape of tumors, head injuries, or infection, although it may be impossible to delineate exactly what that damage is. Epilepsy is a subtype of seizure disorder.

How are they recognized?
Seizures may take very different forms for different people; they range from barely noticeable to life-threatening. Seizure disorders are diagnosed through physical examination, a description of symptoms, CT scans, MRIs, and EEGs.

Is massage indicated or contraindicated?
Seizure activity itself contraindicates massage, but bodywork is certainly appropriate for patients with most kinds of seizure disorders at any other time.

bances, infections, exposure to some toxins, and extreme hypotension or hemorrhage. Rarely, seizures can be traced to a hereditary problem. However, approximately 35% of all seizure disorder patients have idiopathic seizures that are untraceable to any identifiable problem.

Signs and Symptoms

Seizures take very different forms in each person they affect. From the original oversimplified categories of "petit mal" and "grand mal" seizures, more than 30 different classes of seizures have been identified. Seizures are classified by what parts of the brain they affect, when that information can be gathered. *Generalized* seizures affect the whole brain, whereas *partial* seizures involve abnormal activity in isolated areas. The most common types of seizures are described here:

- *Partial seizures.* These are seizures that involve abnormal activity only in isolated areas. The motor cortex and the temporal lobes are the sites most often affected. Partial seizures come in two subtypes:

  - *Simple partial.* In this type of seizure, the patient has no change in consciousness. He may become weak, or numb; he may smell or taste things that are not there; he may have some changes in vision, or have temporary vertigo along with some muscular tics or twitching.

  - *Complex partial.* This type of seizure is specifically associated with temporal lobe dysfunction. The patient may exhibit repetitive behaviors such as pacing in a circle, rocking, or smacking his lips. He may laugh uncontrollably or experience fear. Hallucinations and strange odors are other symptoms of complex partial seizures.

- *Generalized seizures.* These seizures involve electrical signals that occur all over the brain. They may be very subtle or dramatic.

  - *Absence seizures.* These involve very short episodes of loss of consciousness. The patient does not fall to the floor, but he may simply "check out" for 5 to 10 seconds, and have no memory of his lapse.

  - *Tonic-clonic seizures.* These are what have traditionally been called "grand mal" seizures. They involve uncontrolled movement of the face, arms, and legs, followed by loss of consciousness and a fall to the floor. They may last for 5 to 20 minutes, and the patient is usually tired and disoriented after an episode.

  - *Myoclonic seizures.* These involve bilateral muscular jerking, which may be very pronounced or almost unnoticeable. They are usually seen among very young patients.

  - *Status epilepticus.* These are a life-threatening variation of tonic-clonic seizures; they last for a prolonged period and can put such a strain on the body that they can cause death. Status epilepticus, or "static seizures," are a medical emergency.

Diagnosis

Epilepsy is usually diagnosed by an electroencephalogram, or EEG: a test that measures electrical activity in the brain. X-rays, CT scans, or MRIs may be used to look for identifiable lesions. Tests are conducted in part to delineate seizures from other conditions that produce seizure-like symptoms: migraine headaches, stroke, fainting spells, heart arrhythmia, narcolepsy, hypoglycemia, some anxiety disorders, and reactions to some medications.

Treatment

Seizures are generally treated with anticonvulsant medication, which acts to make neurons in the brain harder to stimulate. It can be difficult to find the right dosage of these powerful medications, and although most patients can find an anticonvulsant that works for them, some patients do not tolerate them well.

Some epilepsy patients find that their seizures are less frequent and less extreme when they follow a strict high-fat, low-fiber *ketogenic* diet.

Surgical intervention for seizure disorders is reserved for when an isolated and expendable mass (i.e., a tumor or clump of scar tissue) can be determined to be the cause of the seizures. Some patients who experience tonic-clonic seizures can successfully control them when their *corpus callosum* is severed.

One device that is successful for some patients for whom medications do not work is a vagus nerve stimulator. This mechanism is implanted in the vagus nerves in the neck, and activated when the patient waves a magnet over the implant. It is believed that stimulating the vagus nerve in this way helps to activate some of the inhibitory neurotransmitters that seizure disorder patients lack.

Massage?

It is inappropriate to try to massage someone who is in the midst of a seizure of any kind. In the event of a tonic-clonic seizure, the practitioner's job is to make sure the client is safe, call 911 or the local emergency number, and then wait until the seizure has subsided. If a client has a history of seizures, it is perfectly fine to work with him at any other time, although if his seizures tend to come on fast with no warning, the therapist should be alert to the possibility of its happening during an appointment.

Someone recovering from a severe seizure will probably find that he is sore and tender, as if he had been doing a lot of unaccustomed exercise, which in fact he has. Serious injury are also very possible when these seizures happen in unprotected surroundings. Sprains, bruises, even broken bones can happen during tonic-clonic seizures.

Sleep Disorders

Definition: What Are They?

Sleep disorders are any disorders that interfere with the ability to fall asleep, to stay asleep for an adequate period, or to wake up feeling refreshed. More than 70 different sleep disorders have been defined, but this article covers the most common varieties: insomnia, sleep apnea, restless leg syndrome, *narcolepsy*, and *circadian rhythm* disruption.

Demographics: Who Gets Them?

Approximately 40 million Americans report chronic, ongoing problems with sleep every year, and another 20 million have short-term difficulties. Men tend to outnumber women with sleep problems by a small margin. The incidence of sleep disorders increases with age; elderly people are less likely to feel refreshed by sleep than younger people.

Sleep Disorders in Brief

What are they?
Sleep disorders are a collection of problems including insomnia, sleep apnea, restless leg syndrome, narcolepsy, and circadian rhythm disruption that make it difficult to get enough sleep, or to wake up feeling rested and refreshed.

How are they recognized?
The primary symptom of sleep disorders is excessive daytime sleepiness. If this continues for a prolonged period, a weakened immune system, memory and concentration loss, and an increased risk of automotive or on-the-job accidents may occur.

Is massage indicated or contraindicated?
Sleep disorders indicate massage. Bodywork may not correct a mechanical or psychological dysfunction that leads to sleep deprivation, but it can improve the quality of sleep and can reduce the mental and physical stresses that may interfere with sleep.

Etiology: What Happens?

To understand what happens when sleep is interrupted, it is useful to take a brief look at the phenomenon of sleep itself. Until recently sleep was considered to be a strictly passive, uneventful activity. As researchers have examined it more closely, they have found that sleep occurs in cycling stages, and each of those stages performs a specific function in keeping the body healthy. Although human beings can adapt to living in colder or warmer temperatures, and although they can adapt to living with more food or less, humans simply *cannot* adapt to sleep deprivation. It is such a vital process that without the proper balance of the stages of sleep people can end up with disorders that range from slowed reflexes and lower cognitive skills, to poor immune system efficiency, to *fibromyalgia syndrome* (see Chapter 2) to chronic pain, *depression* (this chapter), hallucinations, and psychosis. The circular relationship between poor health and poor sleep is another complicating factor. If a person does not feel well and consequently does not sleep well, he will probably continue *not* to feel well, *because* he does not sleep well.

The need for sleep is determined partly by the hormone **melatonin**, a secretion of the pineal gland, located deep within the brain. This hormone is secreted in the absence of full-spectrum sunlight. Melatonin contributes to a feeling of drowsiness. A standard rotation of wakefulness and sleepiness usually runs on a 24- to 25-hour cycle, called the circadian rhythm.

Sleep occurs in five distinct phases or stages:

- *Stage I*: In this light sleep, a person is easily wakened. Eye movement is slow. A phenomenon called **hypnic myoclonia** occurs in this stage: this is the feeling that a person is suddenly starting to fall.

- *Stage II*: In this stage, the eyes stop moving. Brain waves slow down but still show occasional bursts of activity called "sleep spindles."

- *Stage III*: Brain waves are much slower in stage 3. A particular "deep sleep" pattern called delta waves are intermixed with slightly faster brain waves during this stage.

- *Stage IV*: Only delta waves are emitted from the brain during this stage. Stage 4 sleep is when the body secretes the hormones that enable new growth for children and adolescents, and repair and regeneration for adults.

- *REM sleep*: In REM (rapid eye movement) sleep, breathing is rapid, shallow, and irregular. Eyes move quickly, but muscular activity in the limbs is usually absent. Heart rate and blood pressure approach waking levels. REM sleep is the stage in which dreams occur.

A person cycles through each of the five stages, and then starts over again at Stage 1. It takes about 90 to 100 minutes to complete a sleep cycle, although the amount of time spent in each stage varies according to the time of night. In other words, a person spends more time in Stages 3 and 4 at the beginning of the night, and the majority of time in Stage 1 and REM sleep toward the morning. Overall, a healthy balance of sleep stages allows an adult to spend approximately 20% of his time in REM sleep, 50% of his time in stage 2, and 30% of his time in the other stages.

Types of Sleep Disorders

This article discusses five of the more than 70 different sleep disorders that have been documented.

Insomnia   Literally, this means "lack of sleep." Insomnia can involve difficulty falling asleep, difficulty in staying asleep, or difficulty in sleeping long enough for the body to get the rest it needs. Insomnia can be described as *transient*, in which case it occurs for less than 4 weeks at a time, or *chronic*, in which a person cannot sleep most nights for a period of over a month at a time.

Transient insomnia is usually attributable to habits or environmental issues that are controllable. Caffeine taken too close to bedtime can ruin some peoples' sleep (for many people, "too close to bedtime" means any time at all). Alcohol, while being a depressant, reduces the quality of sleep. Some medications, including diet pills, antihistamines, and antidepressants, can interfere with sleep or can reduce the time spent in REM stage. Cigarette smoking can cause a person to wake up too early from nicotine withdrawal.

Environmental conditions also can contribute to insomnia: having a room that is too cold, too hot, too loud, or too light can make it hard to get to sleep or to stay asleep. Having a bed partner who snores or moves around a lot in the night can interrupt sleep. Exercising too late in the day, or not exercising at all, also can make it hard to fall asleep.

Emotional stress is of course a major contributor to sleep loss. Ironically, the longer a person lays in bed feeling the need to sleep, the less likely he is to drop off; the stress of waiting for sleep will ensure that it never comes.

Chronic insomnia is usually examined as a sign of some deeper medical or psychological problem. *Hyperthyroidism* (see Chapter 8), fibromyalgia, depression, *kidney failure* (see Chapter 9), heart problems (see Chapter 4), or *chronic fatigue syndrome* (see Chapter 5) are all possibilities when a person does not sleep well or long enough.

Sleep Apnea   "Apnea" means absence of breath. Sleep apnea is a disorder in which the air passage of a sleeping person temporarily shuts down, depriving him of oxygen for up to 60 seconds at a time. Repeated episodes may occur dozens or even hundreds of time each night, reducing the quality of sleep, but more importantly putting the person at risk for serious damage from oxygen deprivation.

Statistics on sleep apnea vary widely, with some estimates suggesting that it affects up to 18 million Americans. Obstructive sleep apnea is a mechanical problem, in which the air passage collapses when muscles relax during sleep, so that oxygen cannot enter during inhalation. When O_2 levels fall sufficiently, muscles tighten slightly, and air reenters the passageway with a loud snort or gasp; loud snoring is one sign of possible sleep apnea. Other signs are excessive daytime sleepiness and morning headache from oxygen deprivation. Obstructive sleep apnea is a possible complication of obesity; excessive body weight can increase the tendency to block air passageways.

Central sleep apnea is a neurologic problem involving decreased respiratory drive. A rise in CO_2 in the blood is the signal to waken and breathe again.

Frequent waking leads to sleep deprivation and an increased risk of motor vehicle accident or on-the-job injury. Patients with sleep apnea also have an increased risk of *stroke* (this chapter), *heart attack*, and *hypertension* (see Chapter 4). In some extreme cases, sleep apnea has caused sudden death from respiratory arrest during sleep.

Restless Leg Syndrome (RLS)   This is a disorder that often runs in families, although it also can be associated with *pregnancy* (see Chapter 10), *diabetes* (see Chapter 8), and *anemia* (see Chapter 4). It involves a constant crawling, prickling, tingling sensation in the extremities, especially the legs, that is only relieved by rubbing and movement. It is closely related to another disorder called periodic limb movement disorder (PLMD), in which a person experiences repeated jerking movements of the legs every 20 to 40 seconds.

Although RLS is present at all times, its symptoms are most pronounced when a person lies still in an effort to sleep. It is relieved by movement, massaging the affected areas, or by warm baths.

Some estimates suggest that RLS affects up to 12 million Americans, most of them elderly.

Narcolepsy This chronic neurologic dysfunction gets its name from the Greek *narco* for stupor, and *lepsis*, for seizure. It involves unpredictable "sleep attacks" at inappropriate times, often in response to intense emotional reactions such as laughing or anger.

Narcolepsy is generally diagnosed in adolescence; this is one sleep disorder that does not increase in incidence with age. It affects some 200,000 Americans.

Narcolepsy has three basic symptoms, not all of which must be experienced for a positive diagnosis. *Cataplexy* refers to a sudden loss of muscle tone, even during waking hours. These events can last anywhere from several seconds to 30 minutes. *Sleep paralysis* is a phenomenon in which a person temporarily experiences a complete inability to speak or move while dozing. *Hypnagogic hallucinations* are episodes of hallucinations that occur while drifting off to sleep. Narcolepsy patients often experience poor nighttime sleep, which adds to a general problem with drowsiness during the day.

Circadian Rhythm Disruption The Circadian rhythm is the normal cycle of drowsiness and wakefulness that all humans experience. It is regulated by exposure to ambient light and the secretion of melatonin. Most people run through this cycle every 24 to 25 hours. They feel drowsy as the sun goes down, and more awake as it rises. When people are forced to be physically or mentally active in a different cycle, their circadian rhythms are disrupted and the quality of their sleep, as well as the quality of their waking hours, is compromised.

Circadian rhythm disruption can occur in response to shift work, having to be awake all night for a graveyard shift, losing a night's sleep, or changing time zones through travel. Short-term difficulties associated with this problem are excessive sleepiness along with degenerating reflexes and mental functioning that accompanies exhaustion. Longer-term problems can include depression and other physical and psychological disorders brought about by sleep deprivation.

Some 25 million Americans do not work a "standard" daytime shift and are forced to adjust their sleep to accommodate a different schedule. Whereas numbers on how many of those people experience dysfunction are difficult to gather, these workers have been found to carry a higher than normal risk for motor vehicle accidents and on-the-job injuries. They also have more colds, flu, hypertension, weight gain, irregular menstrual cycles, and digestive discomfort than the rest of the population.

Signs and Symptoms

The primary sign of someone with a sleep disorder is excessive daytime sleepiness. Chronic sleep deprivation also can cause irritability, decreased ability to focus or concentrate, mood changes, and poor short-term memory. Other symptoms are associated with specific disorders, as described above.

Complications

The National Highway Traffic Safety Administration estimates that about 1.5% of all motor vehicle accidents have excessive fatigue as a primary cause.[13] Approximately 1,500 fatalities and 71,000 injuries occur every year because of these accidents. In addition to car crashes, fatigue and sleep deprivation also contribute dangerously to on-the-job injuries that affect not only the sleep-deprived person but many others as well.

Deprivation of specific stages of sleep also has been associated with specific disorders. Lack of REM sleep over a prolonged period can lead to hallucinations and psy-

[13] Facts About Drowsy Driving. National Sleep Foundation. Available at: http://www.sleepfoundation.org/activities/daaafacts.cfm. Accessed fall 2003.

chosis. Fibromyalgia syndrome patients do not get adequate stage IV sleep, which means they do not secrete the hormones that stimulate healing and repair in adults.

Diagnosis

If a person experiences excessive drowsiness that makes it difficult to accomplish basic tasks, it is worth pursuing with a medical professional, on the chance that sleep apnea could be interfering with his nighttime oxygen supply. Patients are often encouraged to keep a "sleep diary" in which they record activities in relation to how well they sleep. This is a useful tool to look for behavioral patterns that may interfere with a good night's rest. A physical examination is usually conducted to rule out other causes of insomnia, such as hyperthyroidism. A *polysomnograph* is a sleep study conducted in a laboratory in which a person's heart rate, respiratory rate, blood pressure, and other vital signs are measured while he sleeps. How much time a person spends in each stage also may be measured.

These tests can yield useful information about the nature of an individual's sleeping problem, along with possibilities for treatment.

Treatment

Cases of transient insomnia are treated with lifestyle changes that better support healthy sleep. This can mean changes in diet and exercise habits, quitting smoking, adjusting temperature or sound levels in the bedroom, or other simple interventions. By the time insomnia has become a chronic problem, it can be difficult to recondition the body to sleeping well, so the earlier intervention can be taken, the better.

Over-the-counter sleeping aids are generally discouraged, because they tend to create an imbalance in the time spent in each stage of sleep. Prescription sleeping aids can be helpful for short periods, but several of them can become habit-forming, and so long-term use is not a viable solution.

Sleep apnea can be treated in a variety of ways. A surgery to keep airways open may be conducted, or a nose mask to provide continuous positive airway pressure may be used. Apnea patients should not sleep on their backs, and if they are obese they should work to lose weight and reduce their risk of apnea complications. It is especially important that sleep apnea patients not drink alcohol or use sleeping aids at night; these substances may interfere with their already challenged breathing mechanisms.

Restless leg syndrome is believed to be associated with dopamine deficiencies in certain brain areas. It is managed with dopamine agents, as well as tranquilizers, and for very extreme cases, opioids and anticonvulsants. Less severe cases of RLS can be managed with mild exercise, warm baths, and massage.

Narcolepsy is treatable with some medications, as well as increasing exercise, which has been seen to reduce the number of sleep attacks.

Massage?

Most types of sleep disorders certainly indicate massage. Anyone who experiences restless nights and persistent daytime sleepiness appreciates the opportunity to "tune out" while he receives bodywork. Some studies indicate that massage increases the time spent in Stage III or IV restorative sleep[14], which decreases pain sensation and speeds healing. Massage can improve the quality of sleep for insomniac clients, and although it does not reverse sleep apnea, a massage therapist may be the first person to bring the habit of not breathing and then gasping during sleep to a client's attention.

---

[14] Field T. Touch Therapy. London: Churchill Livingstone Press; 2000:67.

CHAPTER REVIEW QUESTIONS

1. What is the difference between spastic and flaccid paralysis? Where in the nervous system does each indicate damage?

2. How can a person who has experienced spinal cord damage at C_6 still have control of his head and neck?

3. Why is massage indicated for Bell's palsy, when it is contraindicated for most other types of paralysis?

4. Is postpolio syndrome contagious? Why or why not?

5. Describe the safest course of action for a client who experiences an epileptic seizure during a massage.

6. A client who has multiple sclerosis comes for massage. The therapist performs a rigorous sports-massage–type treatment and then recommends a soak in a hot tub. Is this a good idea? Why or why not?

7. Can a person who has had chicken pox catch herpes zoster from another person? Why or why not?

8. A person with reflex sympathetic dystrophy may have poor circulation and bluish skin in the affected area. Is it appropriate to massage her here? Why or why not?

9. List five types of depression.

10. A client is recovering from a major stroke. What are some of the key criteria on which to base a judgment about the appropriateness of Swedish massage?

 Answers to these questions can be found on the Student Recource CD-ROM that accompanies this book.

Bibliography

General Resources, Nervous System

1. de Dominico G, Wood E. Beard's Massage. Philadelphia: WB Saunders, 1997.
2. Damjanou I. Pathology for the Health-Related Professions. Philadelphia: WB Saunders, 1996.
3. Travell J, Simons DG. Myofascial Pain and Dysfunction: The Trigger Point Manual. Baltimore: Williams & Wilkins, 1983.
4. Clemente CD. Anatomy: A Regional Atlas of the Human Body. 3rd Ed. Baltimore: Urban & Schwarzenburg, 1987.
5. Tortora GJ, Anagnostakos NP. Principles of Anatomy and Physiology. 6th Ed. New York: Harper & Row, 1990.
6. Taber's Cyclopedic Dictionary. 14th Ed. Philadelphia: FA Davis, 1981.
7. Stedman's Medical Dictionary. 26th Ed. Baltimore: Williams & Wilkins, 1995.
8. Memmler RL, Wood DL. The Human Body in Health and Disease. 5th Ed. Philadelphia: JB Lippincott, 1983.
9. Juhan D. Job's Body: A Handbook for Bodywork. Barrytown, NY: Station Hill Press, 1987.

10. Kunz JRM, Finkel AJ, eds. The American Medical Association Family Medical Guide. New York, NY: Random House, 1987.
11. Marieb EM. Human Anatomy and Physiology. Redwood City, CA: Benjamin/Cummings, 1989.
12. Field T. Touch Therapy. London: Churchill Livingstone, 2000.

Alzheimer's Disease

1. Alzheimer's and Lewy Body Disease: Important Similarities and Differences. Copyright © 1998, 1999, 2001, 2002 Alzheimer's Association, Northern California & Northern Nevada. Available at: http://www.alznorcal.org/research/resrchlewy.asp. Accessed fall 2003.
2. Rodrigo O. Kuljis MD. Alzheimer's Disease. Copyright © 2003, eMedicine.com, Inc. Available at: http://www.emedicine.com/neuro/topic13.htm. Accessed fall 2003.
3. Alzheimer's Disease. Copyright © 1998-2003 Mayo Foundation for Medical Education and Research (MFMER). Available at:

http://www.mayoclinic.com/invoke.cfm?id=DS00161. Accessed fall 2003.
4. Alzheimer's Disease. Copyright © 1996-2003 MedicineNet, Inc. http://www.medicinenet.com/Alzheimers_Disease/page1.htm. Accessed fall 2003.
5. NINDS Dementia With Lewy Bodies Information Page. National Institute of Neurological Disorders and Stroke. http://www.ninds.nih.gov/health_and_medical/disorders/dementiawithlewybodies_doc.htm?format=printable. Accessed fall 2003.
6. What Is Alzheimer's Disease? Copyright © 2003 Alzheimer's Disease and Related Disorders Association, Inc. Available at: http://www.alz.org/AboutAD/overview.htm. Accessed fall 2003.
7. Alzheimer's Disease Research: Slow-Stroke Massage. Source: J Gerontol Nurs 1999 Jun;25(6):22-34. Copyright Copyright © The Internet Health Library 2000. Available at: http://www.internethealthlibrary.com/Health-problems/Alzheimers_disease_research.htm. Accessed fall 2003.

8. Alzheimer's Disease. Centers for Disease Control and Prevention. Available at: http://www.cdc.gov/nchs/fastats/alzheimr.htm. Accessed fall 2003.

9. Meaningful Activities for Caregiver. Copyright © 2001 Alzheimer's Association of Greater Indiana. Available at: http://www.memorywalk2003.org/feature.cfm?docPKey=24. Accessed fall 2003.

10. NINDS Alzheimer's Disease Information Page. National Institute of Neurological Disorders and Stroke. Available at: http://www.ninds.nih.gov/health_and_medical/disorders/alzheimersdisease_doc.htm?format=printable. Accessed fall 2003.

11. What Causes AD? Alzheimer's Disease Education & Referral Center. Available at: http://www.alzheimers.org/index.html. Accessed fall 2003.

12. Brandt NJ. Pharmacotherapy for Dementias. Copyright © 1994-2003 by Medscape. Available at: http://www.medscape.com/viewprogram/560_pnt. Accessed fall 2003.

Amyotrophic Lateral Sclerosis

1. ALS and Lead: The Polymorphism Possibility. Environmental Health Perspectives Volume 111, Number 10, August 2003.

2. Mayfield E. Glimmer of Hope for People with ALS. FDA Consumer magazine (September 1996). Available at: http://www.fda.gov/fdac/features/796_als.html. Accessed fall 2003.

3. Neurology 101: Neurophysiology of ALS. ALS Survival Guide Copyright © 1998, 1999, 2000, 2001, 2002, 2003. Available at: http://www.lougehrigsdisease.net/als_pages/neurolog.htm. Accessed fall 2003.

4. NINDS Amyotrophic Lateral Sclerosis Information Page. National Institute of Neurological Disorders and Stroke. Available at: http://www.ninds.nih.gov/health_and_medical/disorders/amyotrophiclateralsclerosis_doc.htm?format=printable. Accessed fall 2003.

5. Causes of ALS. ALS Survival Guide Copyright © 1998, 1999, 2000, 2001, 2002, 2003. Available at: http://www.lougehrigs-disease.net/als_causes_of_als.htm. Accessed fall 2003.

6. Amyotrophic Lateral Sclerosis (ALS or "Lou Gehrig's Disease"). Copyright © 1996-2003 MedicineNet, Inc. Available at: http://www.medicinenet.com/Amyotrophic_Lateral_Sclerosis/article.htm. Accessed fall 2003.

7. What is ALS? and 44 other frequently asked questions about the disease. ALS Survival Guide. Copyright © 1998, 1999, 2000, 2001, 2002, 2003. Available at: http://www.lougehrigsdisease.net/als_what_is_als.htm. Accessed fall 2003.

Multiple Sclerosis

1. Massage and Multiple Sclerosis. Internet Health Library. Available at: http://www.internethealthlibrary.com/Health-problems/Multiple%20Sclerosis%20-%20research AltTherapies(incomp).htm#Massage. Accessed fall 2003.

2. Massage and Bodywork Therapy. Copyright © 2003 The National Multiple Sclerosis Society. Available at: http://www.nationalmssociety.org/Sourcebook-Massage.asp. Accessed fall 2003.

3. NINDS Multiple Sclerosis Information Page. National Institute of Neurological Disorders and Stroke. Available at: http://www.ninds.nih.gov/health_and_medical/disorders/multiple_sclerosis.htm?format=printable. Accessed fall 2003.

4. Rao SM. Medical College of Wisconsin. Cognitive Impairment in Multiple Sclerosis. Copyright © 2003 Healthology, Inc. Available at: http://www.understandingms.com/focus_article.asp?f=m_sclerosis&c=article_cogimpairms. Accessed fall 2003.

5. Viruses. Copyright © 2003 The National Multiple Sclerosis Society. http://www.nationalmssociety.org/Sourcebook-Viruses.asp. Accessed fall 2003.

6. Cause of MS (Etiology). Copyright © 2003 The National Multiple Sclerosis Society. Available at: http://www.nationalmssociety.org/Sourcebook-Etiology.asp. Accessed fall 2003.

7. Interferons. Copyright © 2003 The National Multiple Sclerosis Society. Available at: http://www.nationalmssociety.org/Sourcebook-Interferons.asp. Accessed fall 2003.

8. Prognosis. Copyright © 2003 The National Multiple Sclerosis Society. Available at: http://www.nationalmssociety.org/Sourcebook-Prognosis.asp. Accessed fall 2003.

9. Diagnosis. Copyright © 2003 The National Multiple Sclerosis Society http://www.nationalmssociety.org/Sourcebook-Diagnosis.asp. Accessed fall 2003.

10. Clusters. Copyright © 2003 The National Multiple Sclerosis Society. Available at: http://www.nationalmssociety.org/Sourcebook-Clusters.asp. Accessed fall 2003.

11. New Study Suggests Link between Increased Sun Exposure and Decreased Risk of MS. Copyright © 2003 The National Multiple Sclerosis Society. Available at: http://www.nationalmssociety.org/Research-2003Aug8.asp. Accessed fall 2003.

12. Frazin N. Brain Produces New Cells in Multiple Sclerosis. National Institute of Neurological Disorders and Stroke. Available at: http://www.ninds.nih.gov/news_and_events/news_article_ms_repair.htm. Accessed fall 2003.

13. Stress Exacerbates MS Symptoms. British Medical Journal, September 20, 2003. Copyright 2002 Reuters. Available at: http://www.nlm.nih.gov/medlineplus/news/fullstory_14037.html. Accessed fall 2003.

Parkinson's Disease

1. Massage Reduces Symptoms of Parkinson's Disease. Source: The Touch Research Institute and the Department of Neurology at the University of Miami School of Medicine; Duke University Department of Pharmacology. Copyright © 2003 Massage Magazine, Inc. Available at: http://www.massagemag.com/2003/issue101/research101.htm. Accessed fall 2003.

2. Treatment Methods. Copyright © 1996-2003 The National Parkinson Foundation, Inc. Available at: http://www.parkinson.org/treament.htm. Accessed fall 2003.

3. Parkinson's disease research shows promise. Copyright 2003 by United Press International. Available at: http://www.nlm.nih.gov/medlineplus/news/fullstory_13985.html. Accessed fall 2003.

4. Primary Symptoms. Copyright © 1999-2002 Parkinson's Disease Foundation. Available at: http://www.pdf.org/AboutPD/symptoms.cfm. Accessed fall 2003.

5. Combination of Two Widely Used Pesticides Linked to Parkinson's Disease. University of Rochester Medical Center. Available at: http://www.niehs.nih.gov/centers/2001news/ctrnews5.htm. Accessed fall 2003.

6. Barclay L. NSAIDs May Protect Against Parkinson's Disease. Medscape Medical News 2003. Copyright © 2003 Medscape. Available at: http://www.medscape.com/viewarticle/460264. Accessed fall 2003.

7. What the Patient Should Know. Copyright © 1996-2003 The National Parkinson Foundation, Inc. Available at: http://www.parkinson.org/pdedu.htm. Accessed fall 2003.

8. NINDS Parkinson's Disease Information Page. The National Institute of Neurological Disorders and Stroke. Available at: http://www.ninds.nih.gov/health_and_medical/disorders/parkinsons_disease.htm?format=printable. Accessed fall 2003.

9. Dr. David Nicholl. Parkinson's Disease. Department of Clinical Neuroscience. Available at: http://medweb.bham.ac.uk/http/depts/clin_neuro/teaching/tutorials/parkinsons/parkinsons1.html. Accessed fall 2003.

10. NIH Researchers Find First Parkinson's Disease Gene. National Human Genome Research Institute (NHGRI). Available at: http://www.nhgri.nih.gov/DIR/LGDR/PARK2/media_release.html. Accessed fall 2003.

11. Mueller JM. Elderly Parkinson's Patient—Feeling Good. Massage Therapy Journal. 1996;35(1). Accessed fall 2003.

Peripheral Neuropathy

1. Boucaud-Obali D. Overcoming Peripheral Neuropathy. Body Health Resources Corporation. Available at: http://www.thebody.com/bp/julaug02/pn.html. Accessed fall 2003.

2. NINDS Peripheral Neuropathy Information Page. The National Institute of Neurological Disorders and Stroke. Available at: http://www.ninds.nih.gov/health_and_medical/disorders/peripheral-

neuropathy_doc.htm?format=printable. Accessed fall 2003.
3. Peripheral Neuropathy. Copyright © 1998-2003 Mayo Foundation for Medical Education and Research (MFMER). Available at: http://www.mayoclinic.com/invoke.cfm?id=DS00131. Accessed fall 2003.
4. Diabetic Neuropathy. Harvard Medical School. Available at: http://www.intelihealth.com/IH/ihtPrint/WSIHW000/24479/408/233221.html?d=dmtContent&hide=t&k=basePrint. Accessed fall 2003.

Tremor

1. Classification of Tremor and Update on Treatment. Charles PD, Esper GJ, Davis TL, et al. Copyright © 1999 by the American Academy of Family Physicians. Available at: http://aafp.org/afp/990315ap/1565.html. Accessed fall 2003.
2. Essential Tremor. Copyright © 1996-2003 Aetna InteliHealth Inc. Available at: http://www.intelihealth.com/IH/ihtPrint/WSIHW000/9339/10898.html?hide=t&k=basePrint. Accessed fall 2003.
3. NINDS Tremor Information Page. The National Institute of Neurological Disorders and Stroke. Available at: http://www.ninds.nih.gov/health_and_medical/disorders/tremor_doc.htm?format=printable. Accessed fall 2003.
4. Clinical Characteristics of Essential Tremor. Copyright © WE MOVE 2003. Available at: http://www.wemove.org/et/default.htm. Accessed fall 2003.
5. Essential Tremor. Copyright © 1998-2003 Mayo Foundation for Medical Education and Research (MFMER). Available at: http://www.mayoclinic.com/invoke.cfm?id=DS00367. Accessed fall 2003.

Encephalitis

1. Information on Arboviral Encephalitides. Centers for Disease Control and Prevention. Available at: http://www.cdc.gov/ncidod/dvbid/arbor/arbdet.htm. Accessed fall 2003.
2. Pritz T. Herpes Simplex Encephalitis. Copyright © 2003, eMedicine.com, Inc. Available at: http://www.emedicine.com/emerg/topic247.htm. Accessed fall 2003.
3. West Nile Virus 2002 Case Count. Centers for Disease Control and Prevention. Available at: http://www.cdc.gov/ncidod/dvbid/westnile/surv&controlCaseCount02.htm. Accessed fall 2003.
4. Fact Sheet: West Nile Virus (WNV) Infection: Information for Clinicians. Centers for Disease Control and Prevention. Available at: http://www.cdc.gov/ncidod/dvbid/westnile/resources/fact_sheet_clinician.htm. Accessed fall 2003.
5. NINDS Encephalitis and Meningitis Information Page. The National Institute of Neurological Disorders and Stroke http://www.ninds.nih.gov/health_and_medical/disorders/encmenin_doc.htm?format=printable. Accessed fall 2003.

6. Statement of Jesse L. Goodman, M.D., M.P.H. Deputy Director, Center for Biologics Evaluation and Research, Food and Drug Administration, U.S. Department of Health and Human Services, before the Subcommittee on Criminal Justice, Drug Policy and Human Resources Committee, on Government Reform, United States House of Representatives. Food and Drug Administration. Available at: http://www.fda.gov/ola/2002/wnvresponse1003.html. Accessed fall 2003.

Herpes Zoster

1. Postherpetic Neuralgia. Copyright © 1998-2003 Mayo Foundation for Medical Education and Research (MFMER). Available at: http://www.mayoclinic.com/invoke.cfm?id=DS00277. Accessed fall 2003.
2. Herpes Zoster (Shingles) Eye Infections. Copyright ©1996-2003 Steen-Hall Eye Institute. Available at: http://www.steen-hall.com/zoster.html. Accessed fall 2003.
3. NINDS Shingles Information Page. The National Institute of Neurological Disorders and Stroke. Available at: http://www.ninds.nih.gov/health_and_medical/disorders/shingles_doc.htm?format=printable. Accessed fall 2003.
4. Shingles (Acute Herpes Zoster) and Postherpetic Neuralgia (PHN). Copyright © 2000 Continuum Health Partners, Inc. Available at: http://stoppain.org/pain_medicine/shingles.html. Accessed fall 2003.
5. Herpes Zoster. Copyright © 1988 American Academy of Dermatology. Available at: http://www.aad.org/pamphlets/herpesZoster.html. Accessed fall 2003.
6. NINDS Ramsay Hunt Syndrome Type I Information Page. The National Institute of Neurological Disorders and Stroke. Available at: http://www.ninds.nih.gov/health_and_medical/disorders/ramsay1_doc.htm?format=printable. Accessed fall 2003.
7. Zamula E. Shingles: An Unwelcome Encore. FDA/Office of Public Affairs. Available at: http://www.fda.gov/fdac/features/2001/301_pox.html. Accessed fall 2003.

Meningitis

1. Meningitis. Copyright © 1998-2003 Mayo Foundation for Medical Education and Research (MFMER). Available at: http://www.mayoclinic.com/invoke.cfm?id=DS00118. Accessed fall 2003.
2. Meningitis. Copyright © 1996-2003 Aetna InteliHealth Inc. Available at: http://www.intelihealth.com/IH/ihtIH/WSIHW000/9339/10302.html. Accessed fall 2003.
3. Meningococcal Disease. National Center for Infectious Diseases (NCID); Division of Bacterial and Mycotic Diseases (DBMD). Available at: http://www.cdc.gov/ncidod/dbmd/diseaseinfo/meningococcal_g.htm. Accessed fall 2003.
4. Viral (Aseptic) Meningitis. Available at: http://www.cdc.gov/ncidod/dvrd/virlmen.htm. Accessed fall 2003.

Polio, Postpolio Syndrome

1. Lorraine Alexander, Trudy Murphy. Poliomyelitis. Centers for Disease Control and Prevention. Available at: http://www.cdc.gov/travel/diseases/polio.htm. Accessed fall 2003.
2. Public Health Dispatch: Certification of Poliomyelitis Eradication—Western Pacific Region, October 2000. Centers for Disease Control and Prevention. Available at: http://www.cdc.gov/mmwr/preview/mmwrhtml/mm5001a1.htm. Accessed fall 2003.
3. NINDS Post-Polio Syndrome Information Page. The National Institute of Neurological Disorders and Stroke. Available at: http://www.ninds.nih.gov/health_and_medical/disorders/post_polio_short.htm?format=printable. Accessed fall 2003.
4. Progress Toward Global Eradication of Poliomyelitis, 2002. MMWR 52(16):366-369, 2003. Copyright © 2003 Centers for Disease Control and Prevention (CDC). Available at: http://www.medscape.com/viewarticle/453008. Accessed fall 2003.

Attention Deficit Hyperactivity Disorder

1. AD/HD in Adults—Fact Sheet #7. Copyright © 1996–2003 CHADD. Available at: http://www.chadd.org/fs/fs7.htm. Accessed fall 2003.
2. Ewart H. III Attention-Deficit/Hyperactivity Disorder: Why Massage Works. Copyright © 2002, American Massage Therapy Association. Available at: http://www.amtamassage.org/infocenter/adhd.html. Accessed fall 2003.
3. ADHD—Coexisting Conditions. Copyright © 2001 American Academy of Pediatrics. Available at: http://www.medem.com/MedLB/article_detaillb.cfm?article_ID=ZZZ6ZRWVYSC&sub_cat=21. Accessed fall 2003.
4. ADHD—Common Behaviors and Symptoms. Copyright © 2001 American Academy of Pediatrics. Available at: http://www.medem.com/MedLB/article_detaillb_for_printer.cfm?article_ID=ZZZCEF4MXSC&sub_cat=21. Accessed fall 2003.
5. Parental Report: Impact of Attention Deficit-Hyperactivity May Be Underestimated. The National Institute of Environmental Health Sciences. Available at: http://www.nih.gov/news/pr/feb2002/niehs-04.htm. Accessed fall 2003.
6. Dopheide JA. ADHD Part 1: Current Status, Diagnosis, Etiology/Pathophysiology. Copyright © 1994–2003 by Medscape. Available at: http://www.medscape.com/viewprogram/560_pnt. Accessed fall 2003.
7. Stoner SC. Part 2: Treatment. Copyright © 1994–2003 by Medscape. Available at: http://www.medscape.com/viewprogram/560_pnt. Accessed fall 2003.
8. Attention-Deficit Hyperactivity Disorder (ADHD). Copyright © 1996–2003 Aetna

InteliHealth Inc. Available at: http://www.intelihealth.com/IH/ihtIH/WSIHW000/9339/9505.html. Accessed fall 2003.

9. Attention Deficit Hyperactivity Disorder. National Institutes of Health (NIH). Available at: http://www.nimh.nih.gov/publicat/adhd.cfm. Accessed fall 2003.

10. ADHD—Making the Diagnosis. Copyright © 2001 American Academy of Pediatrics. Available at: http://www.medem.com/MedLB/article_detaillb_for_printer.cfm?article_ID=ZZZY612KXSC&sub_cat=21. Accessed fall 2003.

11. NIMH Research on Treatment for Attention Deficit Hyperactivity Disorder (ADHD): The Multimodal Treatment Study—Questions and Answers. National Institutes of Health (NIH). Available at: http://www.nimh.nih.gov/events/mtaqa.cfm. Accessed fall 2003.

12. Attention-deficit/hyperactivity disorder: Meeting the challenge. Copyright © 1998–2003 Mayo Foundation for Medical Education and Research (MFMER). Available at: http://www.mayoclinic.com/invoke.cfm?id=DS00275. Accessed fall 2003.

13. Rosenthal D. Atomoxetine (Strattera™) in the Treatment of ADHD. People with Attentional and Developmental Disabilities Association. Available at: http://www.padda.org/index.shtml. Accessed fall 2003.

Anxiety Disorders

1. Anxiety Disorders. National Institute of Mental Health (NIMH). Available at: http://www.nimh.nih.gov/anxiety/anx4. Accessed fall 2003.

2. Epidemiological Facts About PTSD. A National Center for PTSD Fact Sheet. Available at: http://www.ncptsd.org/facts/general/fs_epidemiological.html. Accessed fall 2003.

3. Generalized Anxiety Disorder: What Is It? Copyright © 1996-2003 Aetna InteliHealth Inc. Available at: http://www.intelihealth.com/IH/ihtIH/WSIHW000/8271/8558/187873.html?d=dmtContent. Accessed fall 2003.

4. Obsessive Compulsive Disorder. Copyright © 1993–2000 tAPir Available at: http://www.algy.com/anxiety/ocd.html. Accessed fall 2003.

5. Panic Disorder. Copyright © 1993–2000 tAPir. Available at: http://www.algy.com/anxiety/panic.html. Accessed fall 2003.

6. Let's Talk Facts About . . . Phobias. Copyright © 1999 American Psychiatric Association. Available at: http://www.psych.org/public_info/phobias.cfm. Accessed fall 2003.

7. Bruce TJ, Saeed SA. Social Anxiety Disorder: A Common, Under recognized Mental Disorder. Copyright © 1999 by the American Academy of Family Physicians. Available at: http://www.aafp.org/afp/991115ap/2311.html. Accessed fall 2003.

8. Study: Stress Takes Toll On Brain. Copyright 2002 The Associated Press. Available at: http://www.intelihealth.com/IH/ihtIH/WSIHW000/333/24603/345038.html. Accessed fall 2003.

9. Hsu K. Anxiety. Copyright © 2003, eMedicine.com, Inc. Available at: http://www.emedicine.com/emerg/topic35.htm. Accessed fall 2003.

10. Facts About Anxiety Disorders. National Institute of Mental Health (NIMH). Available at: http://www.nimh.nih.gov/anxiety/adfacts.cfm. Accessed fall 2003.

11. What Is OCD? Copyright © 1998 by The Obsessive-Compulsive Foundation (OCF). Available at: http://www.ocfoundation.org/ocf1010a.htm. Accessed fall 2003.

12. Obsessive-Compulsive Disorder. Copyright © 1998-2003 Mayo Foundation for Medical Education and Research (MFMER). Available at: http://www.mayoclinic.com/invoke.cfm?id=DS00189. Accessed fall 2003.

13. Plewa MC. Panic Disorders. Copyright © 2003, eMedicine.com, Inc. Available at: http://www.emedicine.com/emerg/topic766.htm. Accessed fall 2003.

14. Post-Traumatic Stress Disorder. Copyright © 1996-2003 Aetna InteliHealth Inc. Available at: http://www.intelihealth.com/IH/ihtPrint/WSIHW000/24479/9476.html?k=basePrint. Accessed fall 2003.

15. Social Anxiety Fact Sheet. Copyright © 1999, 2000. Available at: http://www.algy.com/anxiety/social/fact.html. Accessed fall 2003.

16. What is Posttraumatic Stress Disorder? A National Center for PTSD Fact Sheet. Available at: http://www.ncptsd.org/facts/general/fs_what_is_ptsd.html. Accessed fall 2003.

Chemical Dependency

1. Children of Alcoholics: Important Facts. National Association for Children of Alcoholics. Available at: http://www.health.org/nongovpubs/coafacts/. Accessed fall 2003.

2. Pathophysiology. The National Institute on Drug Abuse (NIDA). Available at: http://www.nida.nih.gov/Diagnosis-Treatment/Diagnosis4.html. Accessed fall 2003.

3. Substance Abuse. Copyright © 1988, 1989 American Psychiatric Association. Available at: http://www.psych.org/public_info/sub_ab_1.cfm. Accessed fall 2003.

4. Alcoholism. Copyright © 1998-2003 Mayo Foundation for Medical Education and Research (MFMER). Available at: http://www.mayoclinic.com/invoke.cfm?id=DS00340. Accessed fall 2003.

5. IV. Alcohol-Related Disorders: Treatment Principles and Alternatives. Copyright © 1988, 1989 American Psychiatric Association. Available at: http://www.psych.org/clin_res/pg_substance_4.cfm. Accessed fall 2003.

6. Marley D. Chemical Addiction, Drug Use, and Treatment. Copyright © 1994–2003 by Medscape. Available at: http://www.medscape.com/viewprogram/560_pnt. Accessed fall 2003.

7. Overview of Findings from the 2002 National Survey on Drug Use and Health. Available at: http://www.samhsa.gov/oas/nhsda/2k2nsduh/Overview/2k2Overview.htm#toc. Accessed fall 2003.

Depression

1. Bipolar I Disorder. Copyright © 1995-2003 by Phillip W. Long, M.D. Available at: http://www.mentalhealth.com/dis1/p21-md02.html#DepEp. Accessed fall 2003.

2. St. John's Wort and the Treatment of Depression. National Center for Complementary and Alternative Medicine (NCCAM); National Institutes of Health (NIH). Available at: http://nccam.nih.gov/health/stjohnswort/index.htm. Accessed fall 2003.

3. Depression and Stress. Copyright © 1999, 2000, 2001, 2002, 2003 by John McManamy. Available at: http://www.mcmanweb.com/article-44.htm. Accessed fall 2003.

4. Depression. On The Brain, Volume 2. Available at: http://www.med.harvard.edu/publications/On_The_Brain/Volume2/Special/SPDepr.html. Accessed fall 2003.

5. Sapolsky RM. Depression, antidepressants, and the shrinking hippocampus. Copyright © 2001 by the National Academy of Sciences. Available at: http://www.pnas.org/cgi/content/full/98/22/12320. Accessed fall 2003.

6. Dysthymia. Copyright © 1996–2003 Aetna InteliHealth Inc. Available at: http://www.intelihealth.com/IH/ihtIH/9339/32040.html. Accessed fall 2003.

7. Frequently Asked Questions (FAQs) for Depression. Copyright © 2002 The Depression Clinical and Research Program at Massachusetts General Hospital. Available at: http://www.mghmadi.org/depression/faqs.htm. Accessed fall 2003.

8. Manic Depression (Bipolar Disorder). Copyright © 1996–2003 Aetna InteliHealth Inc. Available at: http://www.intelihealth.com/IH/ihtPrint/WSIHW000/9339/9803.html?hide=t&k=basePrint. Accessed fall 2003.

9. Major Depression. Copyright © 1996–2003 Aetna InteliHealth Inc. Available at: http://www.intelihealth.com/IH/ihtIH/WSIHW000/9339/9805.html. Accessed fall 2003.

10. Depression. Copyright © 1998-2003 Mayo Foundation for Medical Education and Research (MFMER). Available at: http://www.mayoclinic.com/invoke.cfm?id=DS00175. Accessed fall 2003.

11. Depression Facts. National Institute of Mental Health (NIMH); National Institutes of Health (NIH). Available at: http://www.nimh.nih.gov/publicat/depheart.cfm. Accessed fall 2003.

12. Postpartum Depression. Copyright © 1996–2003 Aetna InteliHealth Inc. Available at: http://www.intelihealth.com/IH/ihtIH/WSIHW000/9339/32034.html. Accessed fall 2003.

13. Gallagher RM. The Pain-Depression Conundrum: Bridging the Body and Mind. Copyright © 1994–2003 by Medscape. Available at: http://www.medscape.com/viewprogram/2030_pnt. Accessed fall 2003.

Eating Disorders

1. Anorexia Nervosa. Copyright © 2000–2001 Support Concern and Resources for Eating Disorders. Available at: http://www.eating-disorder.org/anorexia.html. Accessed fall 2003.
2. Anorexia Nervosa. National Institute of Mental Health (NIMH); National Institutes of Health (NIH). Available at: http://www.nimh.nih.gov/publicat/eatingdisorder.cfm. Accessed fall 2003.
3. Binge Eating Disorder. Copyright 2000–2001 Support Concern and Resources for Eating Disorders. Available at: http://www.eating-disorder.org/binge_eating.html. Accessed fall 2003.
4. Bulimia Nervosa. Copyright 2000–2001 Support Concern and Resources for Eating Disorders. Available at: http://www.eating-disorder.org/bulimia.html. Accessed fall 2003.
5. Pritts SD, Susman J. Diagnosis of Eating Disorders in Primary Care. Copyright © 2003 by the American Academy of Family Physicians. Available at: http://www.aafp.org/afp/20030115/297.html. Accessed fall 2003.
6. Eating Disorders. Copyright © 2003 Society for Neuroscience. Available at: http://www.sfn.org/content/Publications/BrainBriefings/eating_disorders.html. Accessed fall 2003.
7. Uwaifo GI, Arioglu E. Obesity. Available at: http://www.emedicine.com/med/topic1653.htm. Accessed fall 2003.
8. Anorexia Nervosa Symptoms Reduced by Massage. Copyright © 2003 Massage Magazine, Inc. Available at: http://www.massagemag.com/2002/issue95/research95.htm. Accessed fall 2003.
9. Signs and Symptoms of Eating Disorders. Copyright © 2000–2001 Support Concern and Resources for Eating Disorders. Available at: http://www.eating-disorder.org/signs_and_symptoms.html. Accessed fall 2003.
10. Understanding Eating Disturbances and Disorders: A Guide for Helping Family and Friends. Available at: http://www.mckinley.uiuc.edu/health-info/nutrit/eatdisor/und-ed-d.html. Accessed fall 2003.

Bell's Palsy

1. Bell's Palsy. Copyright 1995–2003 Merck & Co., Inc. Available at: http://www.merck.com/pubs/mmanual_home2/sec06/ch096/ch096e.htm. Accessed fall 2003.
2. Lotfipour S. Bell Palsy. Copyright © 2003, eMedicine.com, Inc. Available at: http://www.emedicine.com/aaem/topic41.htm. Accessed fall 2003.
3. Bell's palsy. Copyright © 1998–2003 Mayo Foundation for Medical Education and Research (MFMER). Available at: http://www.mayoclinic.com/invoke.cfm?id=DS00168. Accessed fall 2003.
4. NINDS Bell's Palsy Information Page. National Institute of Neurological Disorders and Stroke (NINDS); National Institutes of Health (NIH). Available at: http://www.ninds.nih.gov/health_and_medical/disorders/bells_doc.htm?format=printable. Accessed fall 2003.
5. Facial Nerve Paralysis. Copyright © 2003 The University of Texas Medical Branch. Available at: http://www.utmb.edu/otoref/Grnds/face961.htm. Accessed fall 2003.
6. What is Bell's Palsy? Copyright 2000–2003 Bell's Palsy Information Site. Available at: http://www.bellspalsy.ws/. Accessed fall 2003.

Cerebral Palsy

1. Ratanawongsa B. Cerebral Palsy. Copyright © 2003, eMedicine.com, Inc. Available at: http://www.emedicine.com/neuro/topic533.htm. Accessed fall 2003.
2. Cerebral Palsy. Copyright © 1996–2003 MedicineNet, Inc. Available at: http://www.medicinenet.com/cerebral_palsy/article.htm. Accessed fall 2003.
3. Edwards D, Bruce G. For cerebral palsy patients, massage makes life better. Massage Magazine, July/Aug 2001:93–110. Accessed fall 2003.
4. Johnson VM. My healing journey. Massage Magazine, July/Aug 2001:97–101. Accessed fall 2003.
5. Bourne RA. To Onar, with love. Massage Therapy Journal, spring 1996:68–76. Accessed fall 2003.
6. Cerebral palsy. Copyright © 1998–2003 Mayo Foundation for Medical Education and Research (MFMER). Available at: http://www.mayoclinic.com/invoke.cfm?id=DS00302. Accessed fall 2003.
7. Studies Suggest Ways to Prevent Cerebral Palsy. Copyright © 2003 Reuters. Available at: http://www.nlm.nih.gov/medlineplus/news/fullstory_14825.html. Accessed fall 2003.
8. Englehaupt C. Finding the Right Combination Reiki-ssage, Chiropractic and Cerebral palsy. Copyright © 2002 Associated Bodywork & Massage Professionals. Available at: http://www.massageandbodywork.com/Articles/DecJan2003/RightCombination.htm. Accessed fall 2003.
9. NINDS Cerebral Palsy Information Page. National Institute of Neurological Disorders and Stroke (NINDS); National Institutes of Health (NIH). Available at: http://www.ninds.nih.gov/health_and_medical/disorders/cerebral_palsy.htm. Accessed fall 2003.
10. Cerebral Palsy. Copyright © 2000–2003, Pediatric Orthopedics, P.C. Available at: http://www.pediatric-orthopedics.com/Topics/CP/cp.html. Accessed fall 2003.
11. Werner R. Working with Clients Who Have Cerebral Palsy. All Rights Reserved, Massage Today, 2003. Available at: http://www.massagetoday.com/archives/2002/08/21.html. Accessed fall 2003.

Reflex Sympathetic Dystrophy Syndrome

1. Complex Regional Pain Syndrome (also called Reflex Sympathetic Dystrophy Syndrome) Fact Sheet. National Institute of Neurological Disorders and Stroke (NINDS); National Institutes of Health (NIH). Available at: http://www.ninds.nih.gov/health_and_medical/pubs/rsds_fact_sheet.htm?format=printable. Accessed fall 2003.
2. Complex regional pain syndrome. Copyright © 1998–2003 Mayo Foundation for Medical Education and Research (MFMER). Available at: http://www.mayoclinic.com/invoke.cfm?id=DS00265. Accessed fall 2003.
3. Reflex Sympathetic Dystrophy (RSDS). Copyright © 1996–2003 MedicineNet, Inc. Available at: http://www.medicinenet.com/reflex_sympathetic_dystrophy_syndrome/article.htm. Accessed fall 2003.
4. Revis DR Jr, Goldberg E. Reflex Sympathetic Dystrophy. Copyright © 2003, eMedicine.com, Inc. Available at: http://www.emedicine.com/med/topic2936.htm. Accessed fall 2003.
5. Reflex Sympathetic Dystrophy Syndrome (RSDS). Copyright © 2003 Arthritis Foundation, Available at: http://www.arthritis.org/conditions/DiseaseCenter/rsds.asp. Accessed fall 2003.
6. Reflex Sympathetic Dystrophy. Copyright © American Society for Surgery of the Hand 2001. Available at: http://www.assh.org/Content/NavigationMenu/Patients_and_Public/Hand_Problems_and_Diseases/Reflex_Sympathetic_Dystrophy/Reflex_Sympathetic_Dystrophy.htm. Accessed fall 2003.

Spina Bifida

1. Spina Bifida. Copyright © 1998–2003 Mayo Foundation for Medical Education and Research (MFMER). Available at: http://www.mayoclinic.com/invoke.cfm?id=DS00417. Accessed fall 2003.
2. Spina Bifida—Ask a Neurosurgeon. Copyright © 1998–2003 American Association of Neurological Surgeons/Congress of Neurological Surgeons. Available at: http://www.neurosurgery.org/health/patient/askaneuro.asp?disorderID=29 Accessed fall 2003.
3. Spina Bifida. Copyright © 1996–2003 Aetna InteliHealth Inc. Available at: http://www.intelihealth.com/IH/ihtIH/WSIHW000/9339/31351.html. Accessed fall 2003.
4. Spina Bifida. Copyright © 2003 March of Dimes Birth Defects Foundation. Available at: http://www.marchofdimes.com/professionals/681_1224.asp. Accessed fall 2003.
5. Spina Bifida—Fact Sheet 12—National Dissemination Center for Children with

Disabilities (NICHCY). Available at: http://www.nichcy.org/pubs/factshe/ fs12txt.htm. Accessed fall 2003.
6. Foster MR. Spina Bifida. Copyright © 2003, eMedicine.com, Inc. Available at: http://www.emedicine.com/orthoped/ topic557.htm. Accessed fall 2003.

Spinal Cord Injury

1. Carrano I. Helen Hayes Hospital. Spinal Cord Injury. Available at: http://www.spinal cord-injury.com/spinalcordinjury.html. Accessed fall 2003.
2. Spinal Cord Injury Facts and Figures at a Glance May, 2001. Copyright © 1998–2003 University of Alabama at Birmingham. Available at: http://www.spinalcord.uab. edu/show.asp?durki=21446. Accessed fall 2003.
3. Spinal Cord Injury—InfoSheet #12 "Heterotopic Ossification". Copyright © 1998–2003 University of Alabama at Birmingham. Available at: http://www. spinalcord.uab.edu/show.asp?durki=21485. Accessed fall 2003.
4. NINDS Spinal Cord Injury Information Page. National Institute of Neurological Disorders and Stroke (NINDS); National Institutes of Health (NIH). Available at: http://www.ninds.nih.gov/health_and_med ical/disorders/sci.htm?format=printable Accessed fall 2003.
5. Garcia R. Deep Venous Thrombosis and Pulmonary Embolism in Spinal Cord Injury. Available at: http://www.geocities. com/garciaronald/scidvtpe.htm. Accessed fall 2003.
6. Spinal Cord Injury. Copyright 2003. The Thomson Corporation. Available at: http://www.ahealthyme.com/topic/spinalin- jury;jsessionid=BAPPJO42AI4RICTYAIRS 4EQ?_requestid=80794. Accessed fall 2003.
7. Spinal Cord Injury: Emerging Concepts. National Institute of Neurological Disorders and Stroke (NINDS); National Institutes of Health (NIH). Available at: http://www.ninds.nih.gov/health_and_ medical/pubs/sci_report.htm?format=print- able. Accessed fall 2003.
8. Werner R. Working with Clients Who Have Spinal Cord Injuries. All Rights Reserved, Massage Today, 2003. Available at: http://www.massagetoday.com/archives/ 2002/05/13.html. Accessed fall 2003.

Stroke

1. About Stroke. Copyright © 2002 American Heart Association, Inc. Available at: http://www.strokeassociation.org/presenter. jhtml?identifier=11402. Accessed fall 2003.
2. Carotid Artery Disease. Copyright © 1996- 2003 Texas Heart Institute. Available at: http://www.tmc.edu/thi/carotida.html. Accessed fall 2003.
3. Bouchez C. HRT Linked to Increased Stroke Risk. Copyright © 2003 ScoutNews, LLC. Available at: http://www.hon.ch/News/ HSN/511784.html. Accessed fall 2003.
4. Inflammation, Heart Disease and Stroke: The Role of C-Reactive Protein. Available at: http://www.americanheart.org/ presenter.jhtml?identifier=4648. Accessed fall 2003.
5. Stroke. Copyright © 1996–2003 MedicineNet, Inc. Available at: http://www. medicinenet.com/stroke/article.htm. Accessed fall 2003.
6. NINDS Cerebral Aneurysm Information Page. The National Institute of Neurological Disorders and Stroke (NINDS); National Institutes of Health (NIH). Available at: http://www.ninds.nih. gov/health_and_medical/disorders/ ceraneur_doc.htm?format=printable. Accessed fall 2003.
7. NINDS Stroke Information Page. The National Institute of Neurological Disorders and Stroke (NINDS); National Institutes of Health (NIH). Available at: http://www.ninds.nih.gov/health_and_ medical/disorders/stroke.htm?format= printable. Accessed fall 2003.
8. NINDS Transient Ischemic Attack (TIA) Information Page. The National Institute of Neurological Disorders and Stroke (NINDS); National Institutes of Health (NIH). Available at: http://www.ninds. nih.gov/health_and_medical/disorders/ tia_doc.htm?format=printable. Accessed fall 2003.
9. Inflammation, Heart Disease and Stroke: The Role of C-Reactive Protein. Available at: http://www.americanheart.org/presen- ter.jhtml?identifier=4648. Accessed fall 2003.
10. Tissue Plasminogen Activator (tPA). Available at: http://www.americanheart.org/ presenter.jhtml?identifier=4751. Accessed fall 2003.
11. Effect of Estrogen Plus Progestin on Stroke in Postmenopausal Women. Copyright © 2003 American Medical Association. All Rights Reserved. Available at: http://jama. ama-assn.org/cgi/content/abstract/289/ 20/2673. Accessed fall 2003.

Traumatic Brain Injury

1. Brain Injury Is Unpredictable in its Consequences. Brain Injury Association of America. Available at: http://www.biausa. org/Pages/what_is_brain_injury.html. Accessed fall 2003.
2. JAMA Patient Page—Head Injury— Protecting Against Head Injuries. JAMA & Archives. Copyright © 2002–2003 Medem, Inc. Available at: http://www.medem.com/ medlb/article_detaillb.cfm?article_ID=ZZZ 8ZI10NAC&sub_cat=366. Accessed fall 2003.
3. Traumatic Brain Injury: Hope Through Research. National Institute of Neurological Disorders and Stroke Traumatic. Available at: http://www.ninds. nih.gov/health_and_medical/pubs/TBI.htm. Accessed fall 2003.
4. Traumatic Brain Injury—Fact Sheet 18— National Dissemination Center for Children with Disabilities (NICHCY). Available at: http://www.nichcy.org/pubs/ factshe/fs18txt.htm. Accessed fall 2003.
5. NINDS Traumatic Brain Injury Information Page. The National Institute of Neurological Disorders and Stroke. Available at: http://www.ninds.nih.gov/ health_and_medical/disorders/tbi_doc.htm. Accessed fall 2003.
6. Traumatic Brain Injury: No one pathway to recovery. Copyright © 1998–2003 Mayo Foundation for Medical Education and Research (MFMER). Available at: http:// www.mayoclinic.com/invoke.cfm?id=BN00 005. Accessed fall 2003.
7. Brain Injury. Brain Injury Association of America. Available at: http://www.biausa. org/word.files.to.pdf/good.pdfs/ 2002FactSheetBrainInjury.pdf. Accessed fall 2003.
8. Traumatic Brain Injury: Cognitive and Communication Disorders. National Institute on Deafness and Other Communication Disorders. National Institutes of Health. Available at: http:// www.nidcd.nih.gov/health/voice/tbrain.asp. Accessed fall 2003.

Trigeminal Neuralgia

1. Trigeminal Neuralgia. Copyright © 2003 Department of Neurosurgery, University of Pittsburgh. Available at: http://www. neurosurgery.pitt.edu/cranialnerve/ disorders/trigeminal_neuralgia.html. Accessed fall 2003.
2. Tatter SB. Microvascular Compression Syndromes: Treatment of Trigeminal Neuralgia, Glossopharyngeal Neuralgia, and Hemifacial Spasm. Copyright © 2000 MGH Neurosurgical Service. Available at: http://neurosurgery.mgh.harvard.edu/mvd.h tm#TN. Accessed fall 2003.
3. NINDS Trigeminal Neuralgia Information Page. The National Institute of Neurological Disorders and Stroke (NINDS); National Institutes of Health (NIH). Available at: http://www.ninds. nih.gov/health_and_medical/disorders/trige min_doc.htm?format=printable. Accessed fall 2003.
4. Trigeminal Neuralgia. Copyright © 1998–2003 Mayo Foundation for Medical Education and Research (MFMER). Available at: http://www.mayoclinic.com/ invoke.cfm?id=DS00446. Accessed fall 2003.
5. Lenaerts ME, Couch JR. Trigeminal Neuralgia. Copyright © 2003, eMedicine.com, Inc. Available at: http://www.emedicine.com/oph/topic512.ht m. Accessed fall 2003.
6. Makela J. Trigeminal Neuralgia. Available at: http://facial-neuralgia.org/conditions/ tn.html. Accessed fall 2003.

Guillain-Barré Syndrome

1. McGovern TV. Hard Time. Copyright The Washington Post Company. Tuesday, September 5, 2000; Page Z10. Accessed fall 2003.
2. Barclay L. AAN Offers New Guidelines for Treatment of Guillain-Barré Syndrome.

Copyright © 2003 Medscape. Available at: http://www.medscape.com/viewarticle/461780. Accessed fall 2003.

3. Sater RA. Acute Inflammatory Demyelinating Polyradiculoneuropathy. Copyright © 2003, eMedicine.com, Inc. Available at: http://www.emedicine.com/neuro/topic7.htm. Accessed fall 2003.

4. Guillain-Barré Syndrome. Copyright © 1998–2003 Mayo Foundation for Medical Education and Research (MFMER). Available at: http://www.mayoclinic.com/invoke.cfm?id=DS00413. Accessed fall 2003.

5. Development of Guillain-Barré Syndrome Following Campylobacter Infection. National Institute of Allergy and Infectious Diseases (NIAID); National Institutes of Health (NID). Available at: http://www.niaid.nih.gov/dmid/meetings/gbssumfi.htm. Accessed fall 2003.

6. Guillain-Barré Syndrome Fact Sheet. National Institutes of Neurological Disorders and Stroke (NINDS); National Institutes of Health (NIH). Available at: http://www.ninds.nih.gov/health_and_medical/pubs/guillain_barre.htm. Accessed fall 2003.

Headaches

1. Cluster Headache. Copyright © 1998–2003 Mayo Foundation for Medical Education and Research (MFMER). Available at: http://www.mayoclinic.com/invoke.cfm?id=DS00487. Accessed fall 2003.

2. What You Should Know About Headache. Copyright © 2003, American Council for Headache Education. Available at: http://www.achenet.org/understanding/. Accessed fall 2003.

3. Migraine. Copyright © 1998–2003 Mayo Foundation for Medical Education and Research (MFMER). Available at: http://www.mayoclinic.com/invoke.cfm?id=DS00120. Accessed fall 2003.

4. Coleman MJ, Burchfield TM. Migraines: Myth Vs. Reality. Copyright © 1994, 1995, 1996, 1997, 1998, 1999, 2000, 2001, 2002, 2003, and all other years Magnum, Inc. Available at: http://www.migraines.org/myth/mythreal.htm. Accessed fall 2003.

5. Martin CO. Neurology: Headache. Copyright © 1992–2003 the Author(s) and The University of Iowa. Available at: http://www.vh.org/adult/provider/familymedicine/FPHandbook/Chapter09/01-9.html. Accessed fall 2003.

6. Tension-Type Headache. Copyright © 1998–2003 Mayo Foundation for Medical Education and Research (MFMER). Available at: http://www.mayoclinic.com/invoke.cfm?id=DS00304. Accessed fall 2003.

7. Tension-Type Headache. Copyright © 2003, National Headache Foundation. Available at: http://www.headaches.org/consumer/topicsheets/tension_type.html. Accessed fall 2003.

8. Headache Definitions and What Causes Headache? Copyright © 2003, American Council for Headache Education. Available at: http://www.achenet.org/understanding/causes.php. Accessed fall 2003.

Seizure Disorders

1. Epilepsy (Seizure Disorder). Copyright © 1996–2003 MedicineNet, Inc. Available at: http://www.medicinenet.com/seizure/article.htm. Accessed fall 2003.

2. Huff JS, Huff M. Epilepsy. Copyright © 2003, eMedicine.com, Inc. Available at: http://www.emedicine.com/aaem/topic183.htm. Accessed fall 2003.

3. Information on Epilepsy: What is epilepsy? Copyright © The National Society for Epilepsy March 2002. Available at: http://www.epilepsynse.org.uk/pages/info/leaflets/explaini.cfm. Accessed fall 2003.

4. Seizures and Epilepsy: Hope Through Research. The National Institute of Neurological Disorders and Stroke (NINDS); National Institutes of Health (NIH). Available at: http://www.ninds.nih.gov/health_and_medical/pubs/seizures_and_epilepsy_htr.htm. Accessed fall 2003.

5. Epilepsy Overview. Copyright © 1998–2003 by Healthcommunities.com, Inc. Available at: http://www.neurology-channel.com/seizures/index.shtml. Accessed fall 2003.

6. Epilepsy. Copyright © 1998–2003 Mayo Foundation for Medical Education and Research (MFMER). Available at: http://www.mayoclinic.com/invoke.cfm?id=DS00342. Accessed fall 2003.

Sleep Disorders

1. Facts about Drowsy Driving. National Sleep Foundation. Available at: http://www.sleepfoundation.org/activities/daaafacts.cfm. Accessed fall 2003.

2. Excessive Daytime Sleepiness. Copyright © 1999, National Sleep Foundation. Available at: http://www.websciences.org/nsf/epworth/quizfaq.htm. Accessed fall 2003.

3. Facts about PLMS, What are Periodic Limb Movements in Sleep (PLMS)? National Sleep Foundation. Available at: http://www.websciences.org/nsf/publications/fact_plms.html. Accessed fall 2003.

4. Facts about Restless Legs. National Sleep Foundation. Available at: http://www.websciences.org/nsf/publications/fact_rls.html. Accessed fall 2003.

5. Facts about Insomnia. National Institutes of Health (NIH); National Heart, Lung, and Blood Institute (NHLBI). Available at: http://www.nhlbi.nih.gov/health/public/sleep/insomnia.txt. Accessed fall 2003.

6. Facts about Narcolepsy. National Institutes of Health (NIH); National Heart, Lung, and Blood Institute (NHLBI). Available at: http://www.nhlbi.nih.gov/health/public/sleep/narcolep.txt. Accessed fall 2003.

7. Facts about Restless Legs Syndrome (RLS). National Institutes of Health (NIH); National Heart, Lung, and Blood Institute (NHLBI). Available at: http://www.nhlbi.nih.gov/health/public/sleep/rls.txt. Accessed fall 2003.

8. Sleep apnea. Copyright © 1998–2003 Mayo Foundation for Medical Education and Research (MFMER). Available at: http://www.mayoclinic.com/invoke.cfm?id5DS00148. Accessed fall 2003.

9. Problem Sleepiness. National Institutes of Health (NIH); National Heart, Lung, and Blood Institute (NHLBI). Available at: http://www.nhlbi.nih.gov/health/public/sleep/pslp_fs.pdf. Accessed fall 2003.

10. Bonds CL. Sleeping Disorders. Copyright © 2003, eMedicine.com, Inc. Available at: http://www.emedicine.com/med/topic609.htm. Accessed fall 2003.

11. Cataletto ME, Hertz G. Sleeplessness and Circadian Rhythm Disorder. Copyright © 2003, eMedicine.com, Inc. Available at: http://www.emedicine.com/neuro/topic655.htm. Accessed fall 2003.

CIRCULATORY SYSTEM CONDITIONS

4

Chapter Objectives

After reading this chapter, you should be able to . . .

- Name two deficiencies that can cause nutritional anemia.
- Identify the only destination for loose blood clots in the venous system.
- Describe three possible destinations for loose blood clots and other debris in the arterial system.
- Describe two signs or symptoms of deep vein thrombosis.
- Name what tissue is damaged first with chronic hypertension.
- List three risk factors for the development of atherosclerosis.
- Explain the difference(s) between primary and secondary Raynaud's syndrome.
- Describe two factors that determine the severity of a heart attack.
- Identify the most common causative factor for right-sided heart failure.
- Cite the statistic for the incidence of death from cardiovascular disease in the United States.

INTRODUCTION

Most of the diseases that contraindicate massage do so because of the way the circulatory system works. This introduction gives a brief overview of how this system feeds, cleans, and protects the body, with emphasis on the aspects of the system that are relevant to the conditions listed in this chapter.

The body's cells are highly specialized and complex in their functioning and metabolism. Most of them are fixed, immobile, unable to move *toward* nutrition or *away* from toxic wastes. They depend on the circulatory system for the constant delivery of food and fuel, and the constant carrying away of garbage. Suppose a person needed someone to run to the grocery store for him *and* to flush his toilets *and* to take out his trash. How long would he last if his services were interrupted? Massage can sometimes interrupt or interfere with circulatory service. If a massage therapist is going to make wise choices about to whom and when to give massage, he or she *must* have a strong understanding of how massage affects the cardiovascular system.

General Function: The Circulatory System

The body depends on the process of *diffusion*, that random distribution of particles throughout an environment, for the exchange of nutrients and wastes. For diffusion to happen, there must be a medium, an environment that allows substances to move freely. What could be better than the combination of blood and lymph? People contain approximately 6 gallons of *liquid*. In every milliliter of it, particles are flowing this way and that, chemicals are reacting, and *life* is happening.

The circulatory system, through the medium of the blood, works to *maintain homeostasis*, that *tendency to maintain a stable internal environment*. It does this in a number of different ways.

- *Delivery of nutrients and oxygen.* The blood carries nutrients and oxygen to every cell in the body. If for some reason the blood cannot reach a specific area, cells in that area will starve and die. This is the situation with many disorders, including *stroke* (Chapter 3), *heart attack* (this chapter), and *decubitus ulcers* (Chapter 1).

- *Removal of waste products.* At the same time as dropping off nutrients, the blood, along with lymph, picks up the waste products generated by metabolism. These include carbon dioxide and other more noxious compounds that, left to stew in the tissues, can cause problems. Again, if blood and lymph supply to an area is limited, the affected cells can "drown" in their own waste products and be damaged or even die.

- *Temperature.* Superficial blood vessels dilate when it is hot, and they constrict when it is cold. Furthermore, blood prevents the hot places (the heart, the liver, working muscles) from getting too hot by flushing through and distributing the heated blood throughout the rest of the body. By keeping a steady temperature, the circulatory system helps to maintain a stable internal environment.

- *Clotting.* This is an often overlooked but truly miraculous function of the circulatory system without which people would quickly die. Every time there is a rough place in the endothelium of a blood vessel, a whole chain of chemical reactions happens that results in the spinning of tiny fibers that catch cells to plug any possible gaps. Unfortunately, under certain circumstances, this reaction is sometimes more of a curse than a blessing.

- *Protection from pathogens.* Without white blood cells (WBCs), there would be no defense against the hordes of

microorganisms that are longing to gain access to the body's precious (and precarious) internal environment. For a closer look at what actually happens to those would-be invaders, see the section in the introduction to Lymph and Immune System Conditions (Chapter 5).

- *Chemical balance.* The body has a very narrow margin of tolerance for variances in internal chemistry. A person can actually *die* if his or her blood gets even 15% too alkaline or too acidic. Happily, blood components, including red blood cells (RBCs), are supplied with enzymes and other mechanisms specifically designed to keep pH balance within the safety zone.

Structure and Function: The Blood

Red Blood Cells (Erythrocytes)

Almost all of the blood cells, red and white alike, are born in the red bone marrow. Red blood cells (erythrocytes; RBCs) are created at the command of a hormone secreted by the kidneys called **erythropoietin**. RBCs are constantly being produced and dying, at a rate of approximately 2 million per second. They constitute 98% of all blood cells. Their life span is approximately 4 months, and during that time, they do a single job: they deliver oxygen to the cells and carbon dioxide to the lungs. They are so devoted to this task that they have given up their nuclei to make more room to carry their cargo. (One indicator of disease is the presence of nuclei in RBCs; it means they are being released from the bone marrow prematurely.)

Red blood cells are tiny; 1 mL of blood holds approximately 5 million of them. They are built around an iron-based molecule called **hemoglobin**. This molecule (there are 250 million of them in each RBC) is extremely efficient at carrying oxygen, slightly less so at carrying CO_2. Much of the carbon dioxide in blood is suspended in plasma, like a carbonated drink—which once prompted a student to ask why, when we jump up and down, don't we fizz up and explode? (The answer is, we are not *that* carbonated.) Another key quality to healthy RBCs is their shape: they are discs that are thinner in the middle than around the edges. They are very smooth and should be flexible enough to bend and distort themselves to get through the tiniest capillaries. If for some reason they are not round, smooth, and flexible, big problems ensue.

White Blood Cells (Leukocytes)

Leukocytes are not really white; they are more or less clear. Unlike RBCs, which are all identical, different classes of white blood cells (WBCs) fight off different types of invaders in different stages of infection. Types of WBCs include neutrophils, basophils, eosinophils, monocytes, and

Figure 4.1. Varieties of blood cells.

lymphocytes (Figure 4.1). This is discussed in more detail in the Lymph and Immune System Conditions, Chapter 5.

Platelets (*Thrombocytes*)

These are not whole cells at all, but fragments of huge cells that are born in the red bone marrow. *Thrombo* means clot, and *cyte* means cell, so it is clear what thrombocytes do. As stated above, thrombocytes have the job of going through the system looking for leaks or rough places in the blood vessels. If they should find one, a series of chemical reactions occurs, which causes tiny threads of fibrin, a special protein, to be woven in the injured area. These act as a net to catch not only passing thrombocytes, but passing RBCs as well, forming a *crust* if on the skin, or a *clot* (*thrombus*) if internal. This is a good thing, it is very important, and it is usually not a problem because other chemicals circulate in the blood whose job is to *melt* clots; these are called *anticoagulants*. Under certain circumstances, however, this clotting mecha-

nism has cause to overwork, which ultimately can become life threatening.

Structure and Function: The Heart

The heart is divided into left and right halves. The right half pumps blood to the lungs (the pulmonary circuit), and the left half pumps to the rest of the body (the systemic circuit). Each half of the heart is further divided into top and bottom. The small top chambers, where blood returning from the lungs and body enters, are called the atria (the singular form is *atrium* from the Latin for *entrance hall*), and the larger bottom chambers are the ventricles (from the Latin for *belly*). The two-part "lub-dup" of the heartbeat is the coordinated contraction with closing valves, first in the atria, and then in the ventricles.

The cardiac muscle of the atria is much thinner and weaker than that of the ventricles. This is because the atrial contraction needs to push blood only a few centimeters downhill into the ventricles. The cardiac muscle of the ventricles, however, is much thicker and stronger than that found in the atria because the ventricular contraction pushes blood out into the circulatory system—through the pulmonary circuit to the lungs from the right ventricle, and through the systemic circuit to the rest of the body from the left ventricle. The differences in how hard various parts of the heart have to work has great implications for the seriousness of myocardial infarctions (heart attacks)—the location of the dead tissue determines how well the heart will function without it.

Structure and Function: Blood Vessels

The vessels *leaving* the heart are called *arteries* and **arterioles**; the vessels *going toward* the heart are called **venules** and *veins*; the vessels that connect them are called *capillaries*. Ideally this should be a closed system; that is, although WBCs are free to come and go through capillary walls, the RBCs should never be able to leave the 60,000 miles of continuous tubing that constitute the circulatory system. If they *do* leak out, the system has an injury, and a blood clot should be forming.

Arteries and veins share the same basic properties of most of the tubes in the body. They have an internal layer of epithelium (called *endo*thelium here because it is on the inside), a middle layer of smooth muscle, and an external layer of tough, protective connective tissue. This combination of tissues makes these tubes strong, pliable, and stretchy.

Capillaries are delicate variations of basic tube construction. As the arteries divide into smaller arterioles, their outer layers get thinner and thinner. Finally, all that is left is one layer of simple, squamous epithelium: the capillaries. This construction is ideal for the passage of substances back and forth, because most diffusion happens readily through single-cell layers. However, because capillaries lack the tougher muscle and connective tissue layers of the larger tubes, they are much more vulnerable to injury.

Blood cells leave the heart through the thick-walled arteries, crowd into arterioles, and line up one-by-one to squeeze through the capillaries. Once they have dumped their cargo of oxygen and picked up their CO_2, there is more breathing room; now they are in the venules. Again the three-ply construction design is present, but with a difference. Much of the venous system operates against gravity. Blood flows upward in the legs, the arms and the trunk partly by indirect pressure exerted by the heart on the arterial system, but also with the help of hydrostatic pressure and muscular contraction. To help the blood move along without backing up in the system, small epithelial flaps or valves line the veins. The smooth muscle layer here is present, but

thinner and weaker than in the arteries, which have to cope with much higher pressure coming directly from the heart. Veins get wider, bigger, and stronger as they approach the heart, but they are never as strong as arteries. Fortunately, the force with which blood moves through them is never as strong either.

When blood returns from the body to the heart (the systemic circuit), it then goes to the lungs to be re-oxygenated (the pulmonary circuit, Figure 4.2).

The chapter on cardiovascular conditions is the most self-referential portion of this book. Most of the conditions discussed here are caused by, are complications of, or are both caused by and complications of other conditions in this chapter.

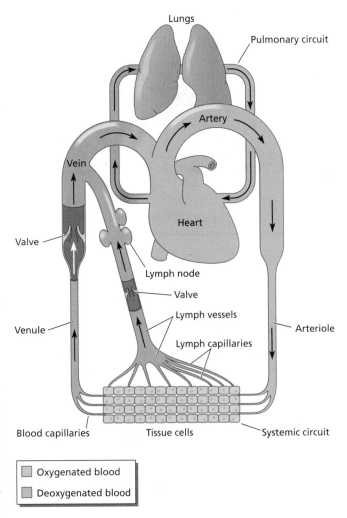

Figure 4.2. The right side of the heart pumps blood to the lungs in the pulmonary circuit; the left side of the heart pumps blood through the rest of the body in the systemic circuit.

CIRCULATORY SYSTEM CONDITIONS

Blood Disorders

Anemia
Embolism, Thrombus
Hemophilia
Hematoma
Leukemia
Thrombophlebitis, Deep Vein
thrombosis

Vascular Disorders

Aneurysm
Atherosclerosis
Hypertension
Raynaud's Syndrome
Varicose Veins

Heart Conditions

Heart Attack
Heart Failure

BLOOD DISORDERS

Anemia

Definition: What Is It?

Anemia is the condition of having either an insufficient supply of RBCs or an insufficient or somehow functionally impaired supply of *hemoglobin* within those cells, or both. In any case, "anemia" all by itself is not a diagnosis; it is a description. The diagnosis comes when one determines *why* a shortage of RBCs or hemoglobin has developed.

Etiology: What Happens?

Several different kinds of anemia are possible, each with different guidelines for treatment and the appropriateness of massage. Some of the most common varieties are examined here, with discussions of what is really happening in the body and how massage might positively or negatively affect it.

> ### Anemia in Brief
>
> **What is it?**
> Anemia is a symptom rather than a disease in itself. It indicates a shortage of red blood cells, or of hemoglobin, or both.
>
> **How is it recognized?**
> Symptoms of anemia include pallor, shortness of breath, fatigue, and poor resistance to cold. Other symptoms may accompany specific varieties of anemia.
>
> **Is massage indicated or contraindicated?**
> Anemia that is idiopathic or caused by nutritional deficiency may indicate massage, as long as no neurologic damage has occurred. Anemia related to bone marrow suppression (i.e., cancer), chronic disease or inflammation, or premature destruction of red blood cells may contraindicate rigorous bodywork, although some types of energy work may be appropriate.

Idiopathic Anemias   These conditions, which have no well-understood cause, may be caused by poor nutritional uptake because of how stress affects gastric juices, or by other, more mysterious factors. But once other pathologic conditions are ruled out, these anemias (which are usually comparatively mild) may respond well to massage.

Nutritional Anemias   These anemias occur because the body is missing something vital in its diet, and no amount of massage, no matter how brilliantly administered, will replace it. However, most of these conditions will not be negatively affected by massage. The only exception to this rule is advanced cases of pernicious anemia.

- *Iron-deficiency anemia.* Iron is at the center of the hemoglobin molecule. An insufficiency of iron in the diet leads to insufficiencies of hemoglobin, and then to pathologically small or thin RBCs and "iron-poor blood." Iron-deficiency anemia is the most common variety of anemia. It can result from diets that are poor in iron, an inability to absorb iron from digestion, chronic bleeding, or lead poisoning. Iron-deficiency anemia is estimated to affect approximately 2 in every 1,000 Americans, and up to half of all pregnant women.

- *Folic acid deficiency anemia.* Folic acid is a nutrient found in green leafy vegetables that is absolutely critical to the formation of red blood cells. If a person does not get enough, it is impossible to produce the 2 million cells per second that it takes to keep up with the cells that are dying off. Folic acid is also water-soluble. That means it cannot be stored for later use; a steady fresh supply is necessary. Folic acid anemia is usually related to dietary insufficiencies or malabsorption, often attributable to *alcoholism* (Chapter 3) or *celiac disease* (Chapter 7). It affects approximately 4 in every 100,000 Americans.

- *B_{12} deficiency anemia.* Vitamin B_{12}, or cobalamine, is another critical ingredient for the making of new RBCs. It comes *only* in animal food sources: meat and eggs. Total vegans must supplement their B_{12} supply or they could end up with the much more serious *pernicious anemia.*

- *Pernicious anemia.* Of all the nutritional anemias, this is the most serious because it can lead to irreversible damage to the central nervous system. Vitamin B_{12} is necessary for the formation of RBCs. Very few people in the United States have a B_{12} deficiency; however, pernicious anemia does happen here. This is because, to *absorb* B_{12}, a special chemical in gastric secretions called *intrinsic factor* is needed. Without it a person may take in all the B_{12} she requires, but her body has no access to it, and she will not produce enough erythrocytes to keep up with her needs.

    The causes behind reductions in intrinsic factor are not always understood. Genetic tendencies, alcoholism, tapeworms, and *Crohn disease* (Chapter 7) all may interfere with intrinsic factor activity. Most often, though, it happens when some section of the stomach is surgically removed because of another condition. Whatever the reason, once it is gone, it is gone for good, and the affected person faces a lifetime commitment to supplementing B_{12} by injection.

    This pales in comparison to the alternative, however. B_{12} is also critical to the maintenance of the central nervous system. Without it, a person will experience the slow onset of paralysis and brain damage. This is often irreversible, and it contraindicates massage, especially if any impairment in sensation has developed.

- *Other nutritional deficiencies.* Anemia can be the result of shortages of several other substances, notably copper and protein. Massage will not improve this condition, and if it is very advanced (with extreme shortness of breath, fatigue, and low stamina), massage could possibly tax the already overworking heart in a dangerous way. Anemia this advanced is relatively rare, however.

Hemorrhagic Anemias Hemorrhagic anemias are those brought about by blood loss. Usually this is from a slow leak, but occasionally it is from some trauma; this would be acute hemorrhagic anemia. The most common causes for hemorrhagic anemia are *ulcers* (Chapter 7), heavy menstruation, and large wounds. Obviously bleeding ulcers and large wounds contraindicate rigorous circulatory massage. Heavy menstruation would not be badly affected unless the therapist worked deeply in the abdomen during flow, but it is a sign that something may be wrong, and the client should consult with her health care team to rule out some other disorder such as *endometriosi* or *fibroid tumors* (Chapter 10).

Hemolytic Anemias These are a group of anemias that involve the premature destruction of healthy red blood cells. In addition to the basic symptoms of anemia, *splenomegaly* is often present. This is the abnormal growth of the spleen as it works

Figure 4.3. Sickle cell anemia

overtime to process all of those dying RBCs. Another sign of *hemolytic* anemia is the presence of *reticulocytes* in the blood. These are simply immature red blood cells that have not yet lost their nucleus, and therefore are not equipped to carry the load of a normal mature cell. Reticulocytes are released from the bone marrow when it is sensed that the supply of erythrocytes is getting dangerously low.

In hemolytic anemias, the red blood cells may die for a variety of reasons, but they all leave their membrane or "ghost" behind while their hemoglobin leaks into the blood instead of being processed in the liver as it is supposed to. One consequence of this is the additional risk of blood clotting because of extra debris in the stream (see *embolism*, *thrombus*, this chapter). Furthermore, all that extra hemoglobin in the blood breaks down into bilirubin, which may result in *jaundice*: a condition that can have a profound impact on the liver (see Chapter 7).

Causes of hemolytic anemia range from genetics (sickle cell is an example of this) to allergic reactions to certain drugs, to malaria.

Sickle cell anemia is a special type of hemolytic anemia in which the hemoglobin molecules (remember, 250 million in each red blood cell) are not normal. They are rod-shaped, and cause RBCs to develop a characteristic stiff, "sickle" shape (Figure 4.3). Symptoms and complications of sickle cell anemia include blood that is viscous and prone to clotting; joint pain; *meningitis*, *seizures*, and *stroke* (all in Chapter 3), and several varieties of organ damage from blockages caused by blood clots. The spleen, overcome by too many dying erythrocytes, is typically destroyed by age 4. Trauma or infection can bring on extremely painful sickle cell "crises" when the body may experience yet more damage from the sticky, lumpy blood flow. Sickle cell anemia has no cure; treatment is limited to addressing the symptoms alone.

An estimated 2 million Americans carry the sickle cell trait (one sickle cell gene), whereas 72,000 have sickle cell disease.

Aplastic Anemia In aplastic anemia, normal bone marrow activity is sluggish or even nonexistent. The production of every kind of blood cell is slowed or suspended. When this moment's 2 million cells report to the spleen for destruction, no new RBC replacements are available. Likewise, no new WBCs are manufactured, so resistance to infection is

Sickle Cell Anemia and Malaria: A Close Connection

A person has sickle cell anemia if he or she inherits a gene for it from *both* parents. If only one gene is present, a person has the sickle cell *trait*, but not the disease. This is a crucial distinction because the sickle cell trait usually does not create any negative impact on the body, although some people experience a mild anemia. However, the presence of this single gene *does* limit the rupturing of erythrocytes during an attack of malaria. Sickle cell genes are mostly found in populations (and descendants of populations) from the Mediterranean, subtropical Africa and Asia—otherwise called the *malarial belt*. Isn't it an amazing world?

impaired. Finally, the stream of thrombocytes dries up too, making persons with aplastic anemia prone to uncontrolled bleeding.

Aplastic anemia can be caused by an autoimmune attack against bone marrow, renal failure, folate deficiency, certain viral infections, exposure to some types of radiation, and some environmental toxins, namely benzene and some insecticides. Bone marrow transplants have proven fairly successful at solving the problem if it is caught early.

Myelodysplastic anemia is a closely related problem, but in this case, the bone marrow makes multitudes of abnormal cells rather than being suppressed altogether.

Secondary Anemias   Anemia is a frequent complication of other disorders. Sometimes a direct cause-and-effect relationship is obvious, and sometimes the association is a less clear but still present. A short list of some of the conditions that anemia frequently accompanies includes the following:

- *Ulcers.* Gastric, duodenal, and colonic ulcers all can bleed internally. This might not be very obvious, but it results in a steady draining of red blood cells, which can impair general oxygen uptake and energy levels. This is a type of *hemorrhagic anemia*, discussed above. See *ulcers*, Chapter 7.

- *Kidney disease.* The capillaries inside the kidneys have a tremendous workload. Not only do they filter toxins and maintain water balance, but they do it under tremendous mechanical pressure from the renal arteries. Sometimes the kidney capillaries are damaged and leak red blood cells into the urine. Again, it is a leak rather than a gusher, but just as that dripping faucet drives up a person's water bill, a leaking kidney slowly but surely drains away viable red blood cells.

   Furthermore, the kidneys secrete the hormone that stimulates bone marrow to produce red blood cells (**erythropoietin**, or EPO). When the kidneys are not functioning well, EPO levels drop, and red blood cell production goes down. See more in *renal failure*, Chapter 9.

- *Hepatitis.* The liver contributes vital proteins to the blood, and it is responsible, with the spleen, for breaking down and recycling the iron from dead erythrocytes. If liver function is disrupted for any reason, the quality and amount of hemoglobin available to new red blood cells may suffer. See *Hepatitis*, Chapter 7.

- *Acute infectious disease.* Anemia is sometimes a sign or indicator that the body is under attack. It is a frequent follower of pneumonia, tuberculosis, and rheumatoid arthritis. Infectious disorders often cause iron to be used elsewhere in the body, reducing the amount of hemoglobin available to new red blood cells. Anemia in these cases usually clears up spontaneously once the primary condition has been resolved.

- *Leukemia, lymphoma.* In these conditions, masses of nonfunctional white blood cells are produced in bone marrow or in lymphatic tissues. These WBCs essentially crowd out functional RBCs. See *Leukemia*, this chapter, and *Lymphoma*, Chapter 6.

Signs and Symptoms

No matter what the cause of anemia is, some signs and symptoms are consistent. These include:

- *Pallor.* Pallor is present because there is either a reduced amount of RBCs or a reduced amount of hemoglobin to carry the oxygen that gives the RBCs their color. Pallor is visible in the skin, and also in mucous membranes, gums, and nail beds. In dark-skinned people, pallor shows as an ashy-gray appearance to the skin.

- *Dyspnea.* This is shortness of breath. *Dyspnea* is a symptom of anemia because, with less oxygen-carrying capacity, a person has to breathe harder and more often just to keep up. Another sign of anemia is a higher than normal respiratory rate.

- *Palpitations.* This does not mean that the heart is beating irregularly; it is probably beating faster and harder, and a person is more *aware* of it. Another term for this is *tachycardia*.

- *Fatigue.* Often this is the first noticeable symptom of anemia. Less oxygen is available to go around, so muscles wear out sooner, and stamina is nonexistent. Unfortunately a host of other conditions may make a person feel worn out, so this is rarely enough to go on for a whole diagnosis.

- *Intolerance to cold.* Oxygen is needed for muscle contraction and for heat production (shivering). Someone who is in short supply of oxygen runs out of steam in a hurry.

Massage?

The appropriateness of massage for clients with anemia varies according to the cause. Massage has been seen to increase red blood cell count, at least temporarily, but this is probably because of the action of pushing red blood cells that were moving sluggishly back into circulation; these effects do not tend to last very long. Massage certainly will not provide missing nutrients, but the resulting parasympathetic response may improve uptake in the digestive system.

Anemia contraindicates massage when it accompanies other disorders that may be negatively affected. Specifically, if pernicious anemia has resulted in a decrease in sensation, or if the anemia were present because of acute infection, circulatory massage would be inappropriate. Similarly, sickle cell disease, which is associated with a high risk of thrombosis, contraindicates rigorous circulatory massage.

Very advanced anemia of any kind is fairly rare. However, if the blood is especially low in hemoglobin or oxygen, the heart has to work extremely hard to pump the diminished supply through the body. For this reason, very advanced anemia of any kind contraindicates rigorous circulatory massage.

Embolism, Thrombus

Definition: What Are They?

An *embolism* is a traveling clot or collection of debris, and *thrombus* is a lodged clot (Figure 4.4). Thrombi that form on the venous side of the systemic circuit are discussed in the *thrombophlebitis, deep vein thrombosis* section of this chapter. Emboli and thrombi that form on the arterial side of the systemic circuit are part and parcel of the whole interrelated cardiovascular disease picture. Having them can cause heart trouble, and heart trouble can cause them.

Etiology: What Happens?

Blood leaves the left ventricle of the heart through the aorta, and goes to its destination through smaller and smaller vessels: arteries, arterioles, and finally capillaries. Nutrient-waste exchange happens at the capillary level, and then the vessels get bigger and bigger as they zoom back toward the right atrium: venules, veins, and the vena cava. The same telescoping action happens in the pulmonary circuit: blood leaves the right ventricle through the huge pulmonary artery, and vessels going into the lungs get smaller and smaller. Oxygen and carbon dioxide are exchanged through capillaries in the lungs, and

Embolism, Thrombus in Brief
What are they? Thrombi are stationary clots; emboli are clots that travel through the circulatory system. Emboli are usually composed of blood, but they also may be fragments of plaque, fat globules, air bubbles, tumors, or bone chips. **How are they recognized?** If venous thrombi break loose or *embolize*, they can only land in the lungs, causing pulmonary embolism (PE). Symptoms of PE include shortness of breath, chest pain, and coughing up sputum that is streaked with blood. Many venous thrombi and pulmonary emboli are silent; that is, they cause no symptoms until the damage has been done. Clots that form on the arterial side of the system can lodge anywhere their artery carries them. Some of the most common (and dangerous) locations for arterial clots to land are in the coronary arteries (heart attack), the brain (transient ischemic attack or stroke), and the kidneys (renal infarction). **Is massage indicated or contraindicated?** Any disorder than involves the potential for lodged or traveling clots contraindicates circulatory massage.

Figure 4.4. A thrombus is a lodged clot; an embolus is a moving clot.

the freshly oxygenated blood goes back toward the heart through venules, veins, and finally the large pulmonary vein, as seen in Figure 4.2.

Jagged-edged platelets constantly flow through the circulatory system looking for rough spots, which indicate injury. If they find any disruption in the walls of the blood vessels, they stick to that spot. Then they release the chemicals that cause blood proteins to weave fibers, making a net to catch other blood cells, and a clot is formed. Clots can also form in places where blood does not flow quickly; the clotting factors accumulate enough to thicken the fluid even without having an injury to initiate the action. This kind of stasis thrombosis happens frequently enough that it now has a name: "coach class syndrome."

The construction of the circulatory system is such that clots cannot pass through capillaries; they either form on the arterial side of the systemic circuit, or on the venous side. The kind of damage that ensues depends on the origin of the clot, its size, and where it finally gets stuck.

Pulmonary Embolism   The lungs are the one and only destination for clots or debris anywhere on the venous side of the systemic circuit. When something, usually a sudden movement after prolonged immobility, knocks any debris in any vein loose, it jets toward the heart in increasingly bigger tubes. It goes through the right atrium and ventricle, enters the pulmonary artery, and ends up in the lungs (Figure 4.5). Most pulmonary emboli occur as small fragments in multiple places in both lungs simultaneously. The extent of damage can vary from a temporary loss of a tiny bit of lung function to total circulatory collapse when suddenly little or no blood returns to the heart from the lungs.

Every year, approximately 600,000 people in the United States have a pulmonary embolism. Many of them resolve spontaneously, but approximately 60,000 people die of PE every year. This condition is usually related to thrombophlebitis or deep vein thrombosis that develops as a complication of surgery or trauma.

Risk Factors for Pulmonary Embolism

Risk factors for pulmonary embolism include other types of cardiovascular disease, recent trauma, extended bed rest, taking oral contraceptives, and any kind of surgery, although surgeries for femur and hip fractures have a particularly high embolism rate.

Infected venous
catheter

Pulmonary
embolus without
infarction

Pulmonary
embolus with
infarction

Injection
(air, foreign
material)

Tumor emboli
(e.g., renal cell
carcinoma)

Amniotic fluid
embolism

Fracture with
fat embolism

Deep venous
thrombosis

Figure 4.5. Sources of pulmonary embolism.

Women in advanced stages of *pregnancy* (Chapter 10) or who have recently given birth are also at high risk for pulmonary embolism because the weight of the uterus on the femoral vessels can cause blood to pool and thicken in the legs, and hormonal changes associated with pregnancy and childbirth also can cause the blood to thicken.

Signs and Symptoms of Pulmonary Embolism

Some studies estimate that up to 80% of all PE cases show no discernible signs or symptoms until after lung damage has occurred. Classic symptoms of pulmonary embolism include difficulty breathing, chest pains, and coughing with bloody sputum. Other symptoms that may or may not be present are shortness of breath, lightheadedness, fainting, dizziness, rapid heartbeat, and sweating.

Complications of Pulmonary Embolism

A person with a history of PE has an increased risk of another PE episode. Furthermore, if a significant amount of lung function is lost, pulmonary hypertension and right-sided *heart failure* (this chapter) may develop as the heart tries to push blood through the damaged, restricted, pulmonary circuit.

Treatment

Treatment of non–life-threatening pulmonary embolism situations is usually an aggressive course of anticoagulants and attention to the cause of the deep vein thrombosis. If it is a major embolism, surgery may be required to vacuum it out of the lung.

Prevention

Pulmonary embolism is the leading cause of death from surgical complication. Because this condition is very difficult to diagnose early, emphasis has shifted from treatment to prophylaxis, or prevention. Preventive measures include identifying patients who are at particularly high risk for developing clots, administering low-dose anticoagulants starting shortly before surgery, tight stockings on the legs, elevation of the legs, external compression on the legs, and early ambulation after surgery.

Arterial Embolism   This is one of the many complications of *atherosclerosis* (this chapter). Emboli in the arteries also can be a complication of bacterial infection, atrial fibrillation (the uncoordinated flutter of the atrium instead of a rhythmic, strong contraction), or rheumatic heart disease, which can create clots inside the heart. Emboli can be made of some foreign object in the bloodstream such as a bit of plaque, a bone chip, an air bubble, or a knot of cancer cells.

   The main difference between arterial emboli and venous ones is the final resting place. If the clot is somewhere on the arterial side of the systemic system it could wind up virtually anywhere, *except* the lungs. Therefore, the damage it causes is very different. The brain, the heart, the kidneys, and the legs are statistically the most common sites for arterial emboli to lodge.

Signs and Symptoms

Symptoms of emboli in organs may be nonexistent until the affected tissue has significant loss of function. This is particularly dangerous in the kidneys, where many tiny clots can come to rest somewhere in the renal arteries, leading to progressive *renal failure* (see Chapter 9). If clots lodge in the legs, however, symptoms involve sharp, tingling pain, followed by numbness, weakness, coldness, and blueness. Left untreated, this tissue may become necrotic in a matter of hours; immediate medical attention is necessary.

   If the embolus lodges in the brain, it is called a *transient ischemic attack* if the symptoms are short-lived, and a *stroke* (Chapter 3) if they are more serious. And finally, if it lodges in a coronary artery, it is called a *heart attack* (this chapter).

Treatment

If a person has a tendency to form clots easily, anticoagulant medications may be prescribed to circumvent the complications of heart attack or stroke.

Massage?

The tendency to form thrombi or emboli is a situation that systemically contraindicates rigorous circulatory massage. Lodged thrombi are a medical emergency. If a person knows an embolism is present in either the venous or arterial sides of the system, he should be under treatment. Clients who take anticoagulant medications require extra care from massage therapists. These clients have two significant issues: they have a history of excessive clotting, and they are taking medication that limits their ability to clot, which means they bleed easily. Both of these require the use of techniques that do not have the intention of pushing a lot of fluid, or of challenging the tissue to the point that bruising might occur.

Hematoma

Definition: What Is It?

Technically, *hematoma* refers to extensive bleeding and pooling of blood between muscle sheaths. The simple leakage of blood from damaged capillaries that causes the familiar discoloration of the skin known as a bruise is called *ecchymosis*. Although the size and seriousness of these two conditions vary widely, their treatment guidelines are very much the same, so they are considered together here.

Signs and Symptoms

Bruises are reddish or purplish (or black and blue) in the acute stage. They fade to yellowish green in the subacute stage, when the local macrophages have migrated in to clean up the debris. The processes for cleaning up capillary leaks deeper than the skin, for instance in a gastrocnemius that has been kicked, are invisible but otherwise identical.

Larger bleeds can involve quite a bit of inflammation along with discoloration. They can occur when an arteriole between deep muscle layers is injured. It seeps blood into an area until local pressure closes it off. A large acute hematoma feels like hot, half-congealed gelatin under the muscle layers, and it is painful to the touch. They happen most often in large fleshy areas such as the calf or buttocks.

A special variety of hematomas (subdural hematomas) happen in the brain; this is covered in *strokes* (Chapter 3).

Treatment

Small bruises require no medical intervention, although they respond well to alternating hot and cold applications, which stimulate macrophages to come into the area, and flush wastes from the tissue damage away. Larger bleeds, however, can be more complicated. If they are caught relatively early they can be aspirated or drained, but if they are left too long they will have a tendency to congeal from the concentration of clotting factors in the blood. At that point, only time, hydrotherapy, and gentle movement will help to break up the pooled blood into a form that the body can reabsorb. An occasional complication of hematoma is *myositis ossificans* (see Chapter 2).

Massage?

Hematomas and bruises contraindicate local massage in the acute stage because of pain and the possibility of disturbing blood clots. In the subacute stages (at least 2 days after the injury occurs), the local blood vessels will be sealed off. Gentle massage may be appropriate around the edges of the lesions, always within the tolerance of the client.

Hematoma in Brief

Pronunciation
hē-mă-tö′mă

What is it?
A hematoma is a deep bruise (leakage of blood) between muscle sheaths.

How is it recognized?
Superficial hematomas are simple bruises. Deep bleeds may not be visible, but they will be painful, and if extensive bleeding has occurred, a characteristic "gel-like" feel will develop in the affected tissue.

Is massage indicated or contraindicated?
Massage is at least locally contraindicated for acute hematomas because of the possibility of blood clots and pain. In the subacute stage (at least 2 days later), when the surrounding blood vessels have been sealed shut and the body is in the process of breaking down and reabsorbing the debris, gentle massage around the perimeter of the area and hydrotherapy can be helpful.

Hemophilia

Definition: What Is It?

Hemophilia is a genetic disorder involving the absence of some plasma proteins that are crucial in the clot-forming process. Anyone who has studied Russian history has at least a vague idea about this disease; the last ruling family in Russia, the Romanovs, had it in their genes, and because it weakened the Royal Family, hemophilia changed the course of world history.

Hemophilia is actually a collection of different types of genetic disorders, each one of them affecting a different clotting factor in the blood. Their presentations are all much the same, however, so the only people who need to know which type of hemophilia is present are the patients themselves and the people who administer clotting factors after a bleeding episode.

Demographics: Who Gets It?

In this country, hemophilia affects approximately 18,000 men. The incidence of the most common variety is about 1 in every 5,000 males, and the disease appears equally among races and socioeconomic status. The disease is carried on the X chromosome of female genes, so female carriers pass the mutation on to their sons. It is possible that a girl could have hemophilia, if she got a positive X chromosome from both her father and mother, but this is a rare circumstance.

Etiology: What Happens?

Von Willebrand's Disease: An Equal Opportunity Mutation

The kinds of hemophilia that most of us are familiar with involve X-linked genes that affect clotting factors VII or IX. But these types of hemophilia affect a relatively small proportion of the population. It turns out that another type of genetic mutation causes another type of clotting factor deficiency, and it is *not* on the X chromosome, which means men and women can be equally affected.

The condition is called von Willebrand's disease, and it involves a deficiency or poor quality of von Willebrand factor: one of the last clotting factors to participate in the cascade of chemical reactions that cause the spinning of fibrinogen to make blood clots. Von Willebrand's disease is the most common type of genetically linked bleeding disorder in the world.

Von Willebrand's disease is usually very mild. Signs and symptoms include frequent bloody noses, bleeding from the gums, and, in women, heavy menstrual flow. A person may never be diagnosed until he or she has a tooth pulled or goes through childbirth or undergoes some other experience that can lead to prolonged bleeding.

If a client knows he or she has von Willebrand's disease, no special precautions need to be taken for massage, other than to avoid bruises and other lesions—but these are precautions for all clients.

Thrombocytes constantly cruise around the circulatory system looking for signs of damage. When they encounter any kind of rough spot inside a blood vessel, they stick to that spot and secrete a series of chemicals that cause plasma proteins to weave nets of fibers called *fibrinogen*. These nets then catch passing platelets and red blood cells, forming a plug to limit loss of blood through the damaged vessel. The plasma proteins that weave the fibrinogen have been identified as 12 distinct factors. Hemophilia occurs when a genetic mutation causes a deficiency in one or more of these clotting factors.

The most common variety of hemophilia is hemophilia A, which accounts for approximately 80% of all cases. It involves a deficiency in clotting factor VIII. Hemophilia B, also called Christmas disease, involves insufficient levels of factor IX. Hemophilia B affects approximately 15% of all hemophilia cases. Other clotting factor deficiencies are possible, but they are much more rare than hemophilia A or B.

If a person is deficient in clotting factor VIII, IX, or both, he has difficulty in forming a solid, long-lasting clot. Hemophiliacs do not bleed *faster* than normal, but they do bleed *longer*. Hemophilia is rated mild, moderate or severe, depending on what percentage of normal levels of clotting factors the patient has. Severe hemophiliacs, who account for 70% of all hemophilia patients, have lower than 1% of normal levels of clotting factors.

Signs and Symptoms

Hemophilia first appears at birth when the umbilical cord bleeds excessively, or in early childhood, as babies begin to engage in physical activities that can involve mild bruising. These babies experience extensive bruising and bleeding with very mild irritation, and small scrapes and lesions tend to bleed for a long time.

As the person matures, he finds that he is prone to subcutaneous bleeding (bruising), intramuscular hemorrhaging (see hematoma, this chapter), nosebleeds (*epistaxis*), blood in the urine (*hematuria*), and severe joint pain brought about by bleeding in joint cavities. Bleeding episodes may follow minor trauma, or they may occur spontaneously.

Complications

Bleeding into joint cavities is the main problem for people with hemophilia. Unless clotting factors are administered very soon after an episode, the blood inside the joint may collect and become very difficult for the body to reabsorb. This can lead to debilitating *arthritis* (Chapter 2).

Infected blood products have been another major worry for people with hemophilia. Before proper screening methods were used consistently, contracting HIV (see *HIV/AIDS*, Chapter 5) was a significant risk for hemophiliacs. *Hepatitis* (see Chapter 7) is another potential problem for people who use blood products. Blood and plasma screening techniques are successful at filtering out most kinds of hepatitis viruses, but hepatitis A and hepatitis G can still get through. Hemophiliacs and other people who rely on using blood products are recommended for vaccinations against hepatitis A and B.

Treatment

Treatment protocols for people with hemophilia have taken gigantic leaps forward in the past 30 years. Before 1965, the only treatment available was transfusions of whole blood: a time-consuming and inefficient means of replacing clotting factors for someone experiencing an internal hemorrhage. Consequently, most hemophiliacs were in wheelchairs by their teens, and their life expectancy was much shorter than the norm. In 1965, techniques were developed to isolate the specific missing clotting factors, allowing a much more efficient treatment. More recently, these clotting factors have been manufactured in a form that can be self-administered, which radically increases a hemophiliac's independence and ability to work and travel.

Although the plasma products that are processed into concentrated clotting factor are as free from contaminants as it is possible to make them, another option has been developed with recombinant clotting factors. These are clotting factor proteins that have been genetically engineered from human and nonhuman DNA. Because they do not involve the use of blood or blood products, the risk of contamination with infectious diseases is eliminated. Unfortunately, a significant percentage of hemophilia patients develop an antibody response against their clotting factors, which interferes with the action of the medication.

Massage?

Severe hemophilia contraindicates rigorous, mechanical, circulatory massage. People who have been diagnosed with mild or moderate cases should consult with their medical team about receiving bodywork. Although the mechanisms that cause spontaneous bleeds in hemophiliacs are largely unknown, massage therapists should not put themselves in the position of being even indirectly responsible for tissue damage to a client. Energetic and noncirculatory techniques may be appropriate and welcome.

Leukemia

Definition: What Is It?

Leukemia, or "white blood," is a cancer of white blood cells that are produced in bone marrow. This distinguishes it from lymphoma, which is a cancer involving white blood cells produced in lymph nodes. *Lymphoma* is discussed in Chapter 5.

Dozens of types of leukemia have been identified; however, the four most common varieties are the focus of this article. These types of leukemia have much in common, but each has some unique features that will be examined under individual headings.

Etiology: What Happens in all Types of Leukemia?

White blood cells   Healthy leukocytes come in several shapes and sizes, each with a specific role to play in the effort to keep us free from potential invaders.

Most white blood cells are born in bone marrow. They develop from nonspecific stem cells into whatever type of cell is needed at the moment. Two types of stem cells manufacture WBCs in bone marrow: myeloid stem cells and lymphoid stem cells. Leukocytes are classified as *myeloid cells* or *lymphocytic cells*, depending on their origin. Leukemia occurs when a mutation in the DNA of one or more stem cells in the bone marrow causes the production of multitudes of nonfunctioning leukocytes. These cells can crowd out the functioning cells in the bone marrow and in the blood. Leukemia can be aggressive and quickly progressive, involving the release of immature cells into the circulatory system ("acute"), or it can be slowly progressive, leading to the release of mature but nonfunctioning cells ("chronic"). In either case, the mutated cells are not a functioning part of the immune system, and they live far longer than normal cells, leading to dangerous accumulations. The four most common varieties of leukemia are:

- *Acute Myelogenous Leukemia* (AML). Aggressive cancer of the myeloid class of cells
- *Chronic Myelogenous Leukemia* (CML). Slowly progressive cancer of the myeloid class of cells
- *Acute Lymphocytic Leukemia* (ALL). Aggressive cancer of the lymphocytes
- *Chronic Lymphocytic Leukemia* (CLL). Slowly progressive cancer of the lymphocytes

Each one of these is discussed in detail below.

Unlike many types of cancer, leukemia spreads through the blood rather than the lymph. It can cause tumors in the lymph nodes (although not as readily as lymphoma), but it also affects the liver, spleen, and central nervous system.

Left untreated, leukemia results in death, usually from excessive bleeding or infection.

Leukemia: General Statistics

Leukemia in various forms is diagnosed in about 31,000 Americans every year. Although this is a disease many people associate with children, adult cases are far more common; about 28,000 adults are diagnosed, and just over 3,000 children are diagnosed every year. Approximately 178,000 leukemia patients are living in the United States today.

Research into new and better treatment options has drastically improved the outlook for most leukemia patients. In 1960, the survival rate for childhood cases was approximately 14%. Now it is 80% for acute lymphocytic leukemia, and 43% for acute myelogenous leukemia. Death rates from leukemia among patients older than 65 years of age have also gone down. Overall, the 5-year survival rate has tripled in the last three decades.

Nonetheless, leukemia kills approximately 22,000 Americans every year: approximately 12,000 are males, and 10,000 are female. Acute myelogenous leukemia is at the top of the list, with 7,800 deaths. It is followed by chronic lymphocytic leukemia with 4,400 deaths. Chronic myelogenous leukemia is next with 1,700 deaths, and acute lymphocytic leukemia comes in last with 1,400 deaths. The remaining 6,600 patients die of the several other less common forms of leukemia.[1]

[1] Leukemia Facts & Statistics. Copyright © 2003–2004 The Leukemia & Lymphoma Society. Available at: http://www.leukemia.org/all_page?item_id=12486. Accessed winter 2003.

Signs and Symptoms of All Types of Leukemia

Signs and symptoms of all types of leukemia point back to bone marrow dysfunction. When the marrow is sabotaged by a genetic mutation that causes the overproduction of nonfunctioning cells, then functioning cells are produced in smaller numbers, if at all. A leading sign of leukemia is fatigue and low stamina due to *anemia* (this chapter): low numbers of red blood cells are available to deliver oxygen to working tissues. A person with leukemia bruises easily, or he or she may experience bruises with no particular trauma. Small cuts and abrasions may bleed for long periods. Unusual bleeding or bruising comes about because platelet production is suppressed, and the person has limited ability to make blood clots. Finally, a person with leukemia is susceptible to chronic infections—these can be skin infections such as hangnails or pimples, or they can be respiratory infections such as colds and flu. They can even be chronic urinary tract infections. Whatever the infectious agent is, the person with leukemia has very limited resources to fight it off because functioning white blood cells are in short supply.

Other signs and symptoms of leukemia are unique to each type, and so are discussed in their individual sections.

Diagnosis

All types of leukemia are diagnosed by a combination of blood tests and bone marrow examinations. It is important to find out exactly which kinds of cells have been affected and whether the cancer is an acute or chronic variety. Furthermore, each type of leukemia has subtypes that respond differently to various treatment options.

Treatment of All Types of Leukemia

Chemotherapy   Leukemia treatment depends to a certain extent on what types of cells have been affected, how aggressive the disease is, and what kinds of treatments the patient has already had. Treatment usually begins with chemotherapy: the introduction of chemicals that are highly toxic to any cells that reproduce rapidly. Exactly which chemotherapy drugs are used depends on the type of cancer that is present. A course of chemotherapy for leukemia usually takes place in four stages:

- *Induction*. Chemotherapeutic drugs are introduced into the system, usually by IV.

- *Central nervous system (CNS) prophylaxis*. Some types of leukemia attack the central nervous system, but normal chemotherapeutic agents are blocked from these areas by the blood-brain barrier. To overcome this, chemotherapeutic drugs may be introduced directly into the CNS.

- *Consolidation*. Once the process has begun, chemotherapy is administered in high doses for several weeks or months in an effort to be sure that all cancerous cells have been killed.

- *Maintenance therapy*. Lower doses of chemotherapy are used over several years to maintain remission.

Other Treatment Options   If a person does not respond well to chemotherapy, or if his or her cancer keeps recurring (this is called "refractory leukemia"), it is necessary to explore other treatment options. This can include adding radiation therapy or surgery, especially if cancerous cells have aggressively invaded any particular organ or location.

The treatment options for leukemia (and other types of cancer) are broadening every day. Bone marrow transplants with preserved marrow of the patient (autogenic or autologous transplants) or closely matched donors (allogenic transplants) are useful for some leukemia cases, but the incidence of complications is high. It is also possible to harvest stem cells from the bloodstream, bone marrow, or umbilical cords of healthy people, and to transplant these "cellular blanks" into leukemia patients, so that they can make healthy, functioning blood cells.

New treatments for leukemia also include the use of interferon or other medication to slow the production of cancerous cells, or the use of manufactured antibodies that are designed to identify and destroy leukemic cells.

The treatment for leukemia, especially the acute varieties, can seem to take as hard a toll on the body as the disease itself. Chemotherapy introduces substances into the body whose function is to kill off any rapidly reproducing cell. Unfortunately, this does not only mean cancer cells; it also means epithelial cells in the skin and the digestive tract, and, ironically, healthy blood cells. The side effects of chemotherapy on epithelial tissues include the development of ulcers in the mouth, nausea and diarrhea from gastrointestinal irritation, and hair loss as the epithelial cells in follicles are killed. One of the difficulties with digestive system disturbances is that if the patient cannot eat well, the whole system becomes weaker and less able to cope with the stresses of both the disease and its treatment.

Chemotherapy also exacerbates symptoms of leukemia, as red and white blood cells and platelets are suppressed. Consequently, chemotherapy patients often experience anemia, blood clotting problems, and low resistance to infection—all signs of leukemia itself.

Acute Myelogenous Leukemia (AML)

Definition: What Is It?

Acute myelogenous leukemia (AML) is a rapidly progressive cancer of the myeloid group of white blood cells.

Demographics: Who Gets It?

Approximately 10,000 new cases of AML are diagnosed every year in the United States. This variety of leukemia is associated with age; most cases occur in people over 50 years old; the average age diagnosis is 65 years.

Etiology: What Happens?

Like other forms of leukemia, AML begins with genetic damage to the DNA of specific stem cells. These cells then begin producing leukemic cells in great numbers. The new nonfunctioning white blood cells are released into the circulatory system before they fully mature. These immature cells are called blast cells, which is why one synonym for AML is *acute myeloblastic leukemia*. (Other synonyms are *acute myelocytic leukemia*, and *acute granulocytic leukemia*.)

The genetic damage that causes AML has been associated with certain specific environmental factors. High doses of radiation, chemotherapy for other types of cancer, and exposure to benzene all increase the risk of contracting AML in later years.

Signs and Symptoms

Suppression of normal bone marrow activity leads to shortages of normal blood cells. The result is anemia with fatigue, shortness of breath, and low stamina; persistent bleeding and easy bruising, indicating a shortage of platelets; and low resistance to infections because of a lack of functioning white blood cells.

Treatment

A diagnosis of AML is only the first step in designing a treatment protocol. Each leukocyte type responds best to an individualized course of chemotherapy drugs. Therefore, it is necessary to identify which subtype of AML is present.

Because this variety of leukemia is aggressive and rapidly progressive, it is important to start treatment as soon as possible. The steps in administering chemotherapy are outlined in the general treatment section above.

Prognosis

The prognosis for AML has improved drastically over the past 40 years, but even with all of the treatment options available today, most people have recurrent leukemia. Children with AML tend to fare better; they have a 43% remission rate.

Chronic Myelogenous Leukemia (CML)

Definition: What Is It?

Chronic myelogenous leukemia (CML) is a slow-growing cancer of myelogenous cells in the bone marrow. It is also called *chronic granulocytic leukemia* and *chronic myeloid leukemia*. It involves the myeloid class of white blood cells: granulocytes and monocytes.

Demographics: Who Gets It?

Approximately 5,000 new cases of CML are diagnosed in the United States every year. Most patients are adults, but a small number of children contract CML as well.

Etiology: What Happens?

The genetic mutations involved in CML may be the best understood of any kind of leukemia. Specific sites on the affected chromosomes have been identified; one of these sites is now called the *Philadelphia chromosome*, for the city in which researchers nailed down the exact location of the genetic anomaly.

Chronic leukemia involves the production of nonfunctioning white blood cells, but unlike acute leukemia, these white blood cells are produced relatively slowly, and they are released into the bloodstream when they are fully mature. These leukemic cells can interfere with and slow down normal immune system activity, but they do not usually bring it to a halt, as acute leukemic cells can do.

Signs and Symptoms

All of the predictable signs and symptoms of leukemia are present in CML patients, but they tend to have a slow onset. In addition, CML patients often experience spleen enlargement and pain as leukemic cells congregate in this organ. Night sweats, unexpected weight loss, and a decreasing tolerance of warm temperatures are other signs and symptoms commonly experienced by CML patients.

Treatment

CML can often be controlled with chemotherapy. When it occurs in young patients, stem cell transplants or autologous bone marrow transplants may be able to totally eradicate the disease.

CML occasionally changes its pattern and becomes more aggressive. This is called an *accelerated phase* of the disease, and it is treated as if it were acute myelogenous leukemia.

Prognosis

Without bone marrow transplants, CML patients have a generally poor prognosis; the 5-year survival rate is 15% to 25%. With a bone marrow transplant or new medications available to slow the growth of cancer cells, the prognosis is much better. Children have higher survival rates than adults; this is probably because young leukemia patients have better success with tissue transplants than adults do.

Acute Lymphocytic Leukemia (ALL)

Definition: What Is It?

Acute lymphocytic leukemia (ALL) is a rapidly progressive, aggressive form of leukemia that involves DNA mutations in stem cells that produce bone marrow lymphocytes. Synonyms for acute lymphocytic leukemia include *acute lymphoid leukemia* and *acute lymphoblastic leukemia*.

Demographics: Who Gets It?

This variety of leukemia affects young children more often than adults—until adults become mature. The incidence of this disease peaks among 4 year olds, and then subsides among older children and young adults. It becomes more common among people over the age of 50 years.

ALL is most common in developed countries and among higher socioeconomic groups. Approximately 4,000 new cases of ALL are diagnosed each year; about half of them are in children.

Etiology: What Happens?

ALL is an acute cancer of bone marrow lymphocytes. The affected cells can be B cells, T cells, or natural killer cells. As with myelogenous leukemia, it is important to identify exactly which cells are cancerous, because different treatment options are used for the different cells.

As an acute form of leukemia, the genetic injury to a stem cell results in the proliferation of nonfunctioning white blood cells, which do not die off as normal cells do. This happens at such a rate that all other bone marrow activity is suppressed and immune system function is crippled. Leukemic lymphocytes (*lymphoblasts*) are released into the blood before they are fully mature.

Causative agents and risk factors for ALL are not clear, but this disease has been associated with high doses of radiation, and exposure to toxic substances during gestation or in early childhood.

Signs and Symptoms

ALL symptoms follow the basic leukemia pattern: anemia, loss of blood clotting, low resistance to infection. In addition to these, leukemic lymphocytes may gather in lymph nodes, or they may gain access to the central nervous system, where they accumulate and can cause seizures, severe headaches, and vomiting.

Treatment

Treatment for ALL depends on several variables, including the age of the patient, the severity of the disease, and which type of cell is involved. Aggressive treatment with chemotherapy is usually recommended. Because this disease can invade the CNS, chemotherapeutic drugs may be directly injected into the cerebrospinal fluid.

Prognosis for ALL

Among children, the remission rate for ALL is 80%. Among adults, the 5-year survival rate is 25% to 35%.

Chronic Lymphocytic Leukemia (CLL)

Definition: What Is It?

Chronic lymphocytic leukemia (CLL) is a slow-growing version of lymphocytic leukemia. Although it can involve T cells or natural killer cells, 95% of all cases involve B cell malignancies.

Demographics: Who Gets It?

CLL is a disease found primarily in elderly people. Up to 95% of all cases are among patients older than 50 years, and the incidence rises sharply with age. Approximately 8,000 cases of CLL are diagnosed every year.

Etiology: What Happens?

This a slowly developing cancer of bone marrow lymphocytes, usually B cells. As normal working B cells are replaced with cancerous cells, circulating levels of antibodies go down, making the CLL patient especially susceptible to infections.

Signs and Symptoms of CLL

This disease has a slow onset and may not be discovered until blood is tested for other problems. Signs and symptoms include many features that are automatically associated with old age: fatigue, low stamina, low immunity, and weight loss.

Treatment for CLL

Sometimes CLL is so stable and so nonthreatening that no treatment is recommended. If numbers of functioning blood cells drop to dangerous levels, chemotherapy may be recommended, along with radiation to shrink enlarged lymph nodes. Bone marrow and stem cell transplants are seldom successful for CLL.

Prognosis for CLL

CLL has the best prognosis of all the types of leukemia: 71% of all patients make it to 5 years of remission.

Massage?

The question of whether massage is appropriate for all clients with cancer may never be settled. It seems clear that the benefits massage can bring (reinforcing a parasympathetic state, improving immune system function, reducing pain perception) can be enjoyed with a minimum of risk, if simple precautions are taken.

Leukemia is a type of cancer that can spread through the circulatory system. It involves seriously impaired immunity and a tendency to bleed easily. Some types of bodywork, especially those that enlist the healing energies of the client rather than trying to impose outside forces on blood flow or tissue manipulation, may be helpful and supportive for a person going through a difficult and often painful treatment procedure. It is important in this situation to work as part of a well-informed health care team, so that the possibility of secondary infection or other complications can be carefully avoided.

For more guidelines about massage in the context of cancer and cancer treatments, see *cancer*, Chapter 11.

Thrombophlebitis, Deep Vein Thrombosis

Thrombophlebitis, Deep Vein Thrombosis in Brief

What is it?
Thrombophlebitis and deep vein thrombosis (DVT) are inflammations of veins due to blood clots.

How is it recognized?
Symptoms for thrombophlebitis may or may not include pain, heat, redness, swelling and local itchiness, and a hard cord-like feeling at the affected vein. Symptoms for DVT may be nonexistent, or they can be more extreme: possibly pitting edema distal to the site, often with discoloration, and intermittent or continuous pain that is exacerbated by activity or standing still for a long period.

Is massage indicated or contraindicated?
Thrombophlebitis and deep vein thrombosis contraindicate any kind of bodywork that may disrupt clots, which could lead to a pulmonary embolism.

Definition: What Is It?

Thrombophlebitis and deep vein thrombosis refer to inflammation of a vein caused by clots. These clots can form anywhere in the venous system (see Figure 4.5), but they develop most often in the calves, thighs, and pelvis. Thrombophlebitis is a term used for clots in superficial leg veins (lesser and greater saphenous), whereas deep vein thrombosis (DVT) is much the same problem in deeper leg veins, specifically the popliteal, femoral, and iliac veins.

Demographics: Who Gets It?

The clots of thrombophlebitis and deep vein thrombosis happen more often in women than in men, and they are especially associated with the elderly and the overweight. DVT is diagnosed anywhere from 250,000 to 2 million times each year. It progresses to pulmonary embolism approximately one third of the time.

Etiology: What Happens?

These conditions are major concerns for well-trained massage practitioners. They involve thrombi, stationary clots somewhere in the venous system. If they break loose, nothing stops them from traveling up the vena cava, through the right atrium and ventricle, straight into the pulmonary artery, causing pulmonary embolism (see *embolism*, *thrombus*, this chapter).

The causes of thrombophlebitis and DVT can be many and varied. Any circumstance involving venous stasis (slowed movement of venous blood), increased *coagulability*, or blood vessel damage increases the chances of developing this problem. Here are a few of the most common precipitators of thrombophlebitis or DVT:

- *Physical trauma* is a predisposing factor; being kicked or hit in the leg can damage the delicate venous tissue, which is then prone to clot formation. Athletes are particularly vulnerable to this problem.

- *Varicose veins* (this chapter) are another risk factor because they too involve damaged tissue and the risk of clot formation. Fortunately, the clots that form in superficial veins tend to embolize, or to break loose, much less frequently than those in deeper veins.

- *Local infection* can cause an inflammatory reaction leading to clot formation.

- *Reduced circulation*, either from physical restriction such as too-tight socks or immobility, can cause the clotting factors in the blood to accumulate in amounts that will cause coagulation even without damage to a vessel wall. People who must sit still for many hours at a time run the risk of developing DVT; this phenomenon has given rise to a layman's term for this condition: "coach class syndrome."

- *Pregnancy* (Chapter 10) and childbirth can increase the risk of blood clotting. The weight of the fetus on femoral vessels slows blood return, and hormonal changes can cause the blood to thicken and become more viscous.

- *Blood diseases* that are particularly disposed to complicate into thrombophlebitis or DVT include polycythemia and sickle cell *anemia* (this chapter). Both of these involve blood that is viscous, sticky, and not free-flowing.

- *Certain types of cancer* can lead to thrombophlebitis or DVT, either because of changes to the blood or because of irritation at the site of a catheter.

- *Surgery* is another major risk for DVT. In fact, thrombosis and subsequent pulmonary embolism is the leading cause of death for orthopedic surgery, especially for knee and hip replacements. Heart and any kind of pelvic surgery also hold high risks for thrombosis.

- *High-estrogen birth control pills or hormone replacement therapy* can increase the risk of developing blood clots.

- *Other factors* that increase the risk for DVT include cigarette smoking, *hypertension* and other cardiovascular diseases (this chapter), paralysis (see *spinal cord injury* Chapter 3), and some genetic conditions that lead to excessive coagulation in the blood.

Most blood clots causing DVT or thrombophlebitis form in the lower legs, but most clots that break off and go to the lungs originate in the thigh or pelvis. Sudden movement or change in position is often the factor that will cause part of a clot to detach and become a pulmonary embolism. Another alarming fact is that a patient who is immobile because of some leg injury is almost as likely to throw a clot from the *uninjured* leg as she is from the injured side. This is because lack of ambulation can thicken the blood systemically, even where no damage to blood vessels has occurred.

Signs and Symptoms

Thrombophlebitis can show the major signs of inflammation: pain, heat, redness, and swelling. Sometimes itchiness, a hard cord where the vein is affected, and edema with discoloration distal to the area are present (Figure 4.6). Thrombophlebitis that has become a chronic problem may result in poor blood flow to the skin, leading to flaking, discoloration, and skin ulcers. If it is caused by a local infection, fever and general illness also may be present.

Deep vein thrombosis is considered the more dangerous of these two conditions because the clots in deeper veins can be big enough to do serious damage in the lungs and because clots in superficial veins usually melt under the influence of the body's own anticoagulants before they have a chance to break off and do any damage.

If DVT shows any signs (and it often does not), it may show more swelling and edema than thrombophlebitis because the clot inhibits more blood flow back to the heart. The backup forces extra fluid out of the capillaries and into the interstitial spaces, thus adding general edema to any localized swelling of the vein. The capillary exchange may become so sluggish that the edema "pits," or leaves a little dimple wherever it is touched. Pitting edema is a huge red flag for massage therapists. It is an indication that this person's circulation is absolutely not capable of dealing with the internal changes brought about by massage.

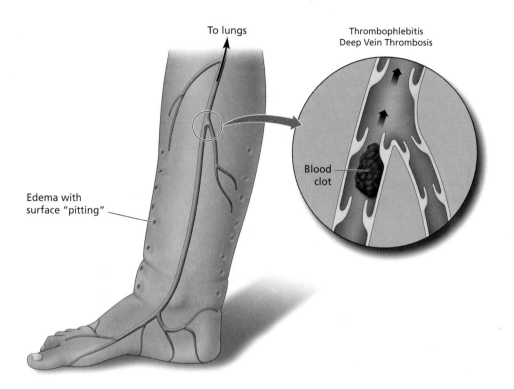

Figure 4.6. A blood clot lodged in a vein can cause distal edema.

Diagnosis

Thrombophlebitis and DVT can be diagnosed in various ways, each with inherent benefits and disadvantages. Ultrasound is a fast and noninvasive technique, but it tends to yield "false positives," leading to unnecessary prescriptions of anticoagulants, which can lead to risks of uncontrolled bleeding. *Venography*—injecting the blood vessel with dye and watching how it moves through the system—can be more accurate, but it is slow, and the injection itself can damage delicate tissue.

Treatment

The treatment for both thrombophlebitis and deep vein thrombosis is anticoagulants. The risk is that these chemicals make a person prone to excessive bleeding with minor trauma: another caution for massage. If the patient is bedridden, she may be given pneumatic compression: a machine mimics the pumping action of exercise by inflating and deflating a tubular balloon around the affected leg. Support hose to prevent the accumulation of postoperative edema are also recommended.

People with thrombophlebitis in superficial veins are at much less risk for embolism than those with DVT. Self-care measures such as hot packs, analgesics, and gentle exercise may be recommended to resolve episodes of vein inflammation.

High-risk patients who have clotting disorders that make anticoagulants prohibitive may have a special filter implanted in the vena cava to prevent clots from reaching the lungs.

Massage?

A client who is at high risk for throwing a blood clot and developing pulmonary embolism is obviously not a candidate for Swedish, circulatory, rigorous massage. The trick is that although thrombophlebitis *may* show obvious signs, it may *not* as well, or the signs could be indistinct. A client may come complaining of an ache deep in her calf that she really wants "worked out." This is a reasonable request—except that what the massage therapist may be "working out" is a blood clot that will land the client in the hospital with the other 600,000 pulmonary embolism cases this year. This is one of the rare situations in which it is wisest not to work at all, but to refer the client emphatically and immediately to a primary health care provider.

Case History 4.1

Deep Vein Thrombosis

Anne, Age 67: "It Was Just a Broken Knee!"

Anne is a retired schoolteacher who spends her winters in Arizona and summers in the mountains of Colorado. In May, 1 week after she had moved to her summer home, she took a bad fall over a curb and sustained a lateral plateau fracture to the tibia of her left leg: a leg with which she had a history of varicose veins and phlebitis.

Because her health maintenance organization was out of state (in Arizona), it was reluctant to cover any treatment for conditions not considered "life threatening." For that reason, Anne, a mildly overweight moderate smoker, spent 3 days sitting in a chair all day at 10,000 feet of altitude (which thickens the blood because there is less oxygen in the air). She was unable to move except with the use of a walker. Her broken knee was never set or seen by an orthopedist.

Eventually, the swelling in the leg became so severely painful that she sought out a general practitioner in the Colorado town. He sent her to a local hospital for an ultrasound, which showed a blood clot from her ankle to her groin. She immediately checked into the hospital and was put on anticoagulant medication.

Four days later, she was sent home. Still basically immobile, but taking anticoagulants, she returned to sitting in her chair with her leg elevated for 12 to 14 hours a day. On her second night home, she woke in the night with severe chest pains and shortness of breath. The emergency medical team took her back to the hospital, where it was revealed that she had thrown a large clot to the lung: a pulmonary embolism. At this point, her condition was too severe to be treated at a small rural hospital. After 2 days in the intensive care unit, she was transferred to a larger facility about 100 miles away, where a filter was inserted into her vena cava to prevent any further clots from reaching her lungs.

When she checked out of the second hospital, she was prescribed supplemental oxygen to compensate for the loss of lung function and the high altitude. She used an oxygen tank for several weeks and had to quit smoking in the process. Several months later, Anne has no severe pain in her knee, but there is a constant achiness. She limps when she gets tired, which happens easily; her energy level never quite returned to what it used to be.

VASCULAR DISORDERS

Aortic Aneurysm

Aneurysm in Brief

Pronunciation
an′ū-rizm

What is it?
An aneurysm is a bulge or outpouching in a vein, artery, or the heart. They usually occur in the thoracic or abdominal aorta or in the arteries at the base of the brain.

How is it recognized?
Symptoms of aneurysms are determined by their location. Thoracic aneurysms may cause chronic hoarseness; abdominal aneurysms may cause local discomfort, reduced urine output, or severe backache. Cerebral aneurysms may be silent or may cause extreme headache when they are at very high risk for rupture.

Is massage indicated or contraindicated?
If a client has been diagnosed with an aneurysm, circulatory massage is contraindicated. Massage is also strongly cautioned for clients who fit the profile for aneurysms, but who have not been diagnosed.

Definition: What Is It?

An *aneurysm* is a permanent bulge in the wall of a blood vessel or the heart. The damage may be brought about by any combination of injury, congenitally weak smooth muscle tissue, high blood pressure, atherosclerosis, and compromised connective tissue. If an aneurysm ruptures, the person can bleed to death in a very short time.

Demographics: Who Gets It?

Most aortic aneurysm patients are men older than 55 years of age. The risk of aneurysm rises with age; up to 5% of all men over 80 have had an aortic aneurysm. Approximately 15,000 aneurysm patients die every year. Statistics show that the rate of aortic aneurysm in the United States has tripled in the last 40 years. This is probably because of an increase in the number of people who smoke, combined with longer life spans and better survival rates for other types of heart disease.

Etiology: What Happens?

The three-ply construction of the arteries includes the endothelial inside layer, the smooth muscle middle layer, and the tough connective tissue outer layer. Blood pressure in the aorta, the largest artery, is very high. If the walls of the aorta lose their elasticity, they can bulge wide with blood. This bulge is an aneurysm. As the aneurysm grows, the walls stretch and become weaker, increasing the risk of rupture and death.

Aneurysms happen most often in the abdominal aorta and at the base of the brain. Thoracic aneurysms are usually associated with specific diseases such as *Marfan's syndrome* (Chapter 2), which frequently exhibits a congenital weakness of the aorta. Aneurysms sometimes occur in more distal vessels, but those cases are generally much less serious because the blood pressure pushing on the vessels is much lower as it gets further away from the heart.

An occasional complication of a major heart attack is an aneurysm in the left ventricle of the heart itself. The damage to myocardium reduces elasticity to the point that chronic pressure will cause the wall of the ventricle to bulge. The force of the contractions becomes weaker, and the risk of developing heart failure is very high. (See *heart attack* and *heart failure*, this chapter.)

Causes

Several different factors can contribute to the chances of developing an aneurysm.

• *Compromised smooth muscle.* Atherosclerotic plaques invade and weaken aortal muscle (see *atherosclerosis*, this chapter). Aortic aneurysms are a serious complication of atherosclerosis and *high blood pressure* (this chapter).

- *Smoking.* The damage incurred to endothelium by carbon monoxide from cigarette smoke and a rise in blood pressure from nicotine makes smoking a leading risk factor for aortic aneurysm.

- *Congenitally weak arterial wall muscle.* Sometimes the tissue simply is not strong enough to put up with normal blood pressure, and with no warning, an aneurysm can rupture. This happens most often in the arteries at the base of the brain. When a high school basketball player drops dead on the court, this is usually the kind of situation that causes it. (See *stroke*, Chapter 3.)

- *Inflammation.* A few diseases, such as **polyarteritis nodosa** or **bacterial endocarditis**, can cause inflammation and weakening of the aortal tissue. Fortunately, these conditions are relatively rare; it is unlikely that someone with them will come looking for massage.

- *Untreated syphilis* (see *sexually transmitted diseases* Chapter 10) can lead to damage in the aorta, sometimes decades after the initial infection.

- *Trauma.* Mechanical trauma, such as a car accident in which a person is injured by a steering wheel, may sometimes damage the outer layers of the aorta while leaving the inner one intact. This results in the characteristic bulging and stretching of the most delicate arterial tissue.

Types of Aneurysms

Aneurysms come in a variety of shapes and sizes, some of which are particular to where the lesion occurs (Figure 4.7).

- *Saccular.* These are usually the case with thoracic or abdominal aortic aneurysms. The aortal wall bulges like a small (or large) rounded sack, which throbs and pushes against neighboring organs and other structures.

- *Fusiform.* This is also common for aortic aneurysms; in this case, the bulge is less round and more tubular, as if the aorta were widened like a sausage for a few inches.

- *Berry.* This is a term for small aneurysms in the brain (Figure 4.8).

- *Dissecting.* Also called "false aneurysm," this is the least common and most painful type of aortic damage. In this situation, the blood pressure actually *splits* the layers of the aorta between the tunica intima (innermost layer) and the tunica media (muscular layer). In some cases, this type of bulge can seal itself off when the blood trapped inside the split coagulates and solidifies.

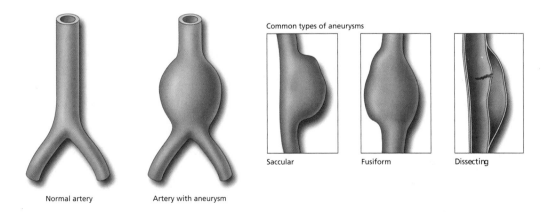

Figure 4.7. Several types of aneurysms.

Figure 4.8. A berry aneurysm in a cerebral artery.

Signs and Symptoms

Aneurysms can be difficult to identify by symptoms because they often are not painful until they are a medical emergency. This is certainly true of cerebral aneurysms. With aortic aneurysms, the swelling might create some warning signals; this usually happens when the bulge is pressing on something else or interfering with another organ's function. Thoracic aneurysms sometimes create difficulty with swallowing (*dysphagia*), chest pain, hoarseness, and coughing that is not relieved with medication, because the protrusion presses on and irritates the larynx. Abdominal aneurysms sometimes show as a throbbing lump near the umbilicus, loss of appetite, weight loss, reduced urine output and, if it pushes against the spine, severe backache.

    This should be extremely alarming to massage therapists! How is a person supposed to tell whether a client's backache is from a muscle spasm or an abdominal aneurysm? This is why it is vital to take a complete history before a first massage session. People with aneurysms will generally have a history of heart disease, atherosclerosis, or high blood pressure. If a client fits the profile for an aneurysm, it is necessary to explain to him that for his own benefit he needs to get medical clearance before receiving rigorous circulatory massage.

Diagnosis

Physical examinations often show signs of aneurysm; the turbulent movement of blood through the wide area of the aorta makes a specific sound in stethoscopes. Large aneurysms in thin people can be palpated as a pulsating mass. Otherwise, aneurysms are diagnosed by ultrasound, computed tomography (CT) scans, and magnetic resonance imaging (MRIs); approximately three fourths of the time, this happens when a patient undergoes tests for some other disorder, and the aneurysm is found by accident.

Complications

For those rare aneurysms that are *not* in the aorta or the brain, no serious complications may develop unless they get large enough to impede blood flow, which can lead to necrosis and gangrene. However, the more typical aneurysm at the very least presses against its neighbors, which can be uncomfortable or can even interfere with function. If blood pools in an aneurysm for any length of time, clots may form and then enter the bloodstream again (see *embolism*, *thrombus*, this chapter). And of course, a rupture leads to hemorrhaging in the best case, and shock followed by collapse of the circulatory system in the worst case. Most (75% to 80%) of the people whose aneurysms rupture die.

Treatment

Aneurysms *do not* spontaneously retreat because the pressure that causes them never lets up. They need to be repaired, either with open surgery or with *endovascular* surgery. Open surgery involves clamping off the artery above and below the lesion and attaching either a replacement graft or a Dacron substitute to the two ends. This is usually successful, but it has to be done *before* a rupture.

Endovascular surgery involves using a catheter through the femoral artery up to the aorta to insert a patch or stent at the aneurysm site. This is a much less invasive procedure with a lower risk of surgical complications, but it is new enough that long-term comparisons with open surgery cannot yet be made.

Some aneurysms do not require immediate intervention. Normal aortic size is approximately 2 cm; a dangerously distended aneurysm is approximately 5 to 6 cm. Many doctors recommend checking the growth of small aneurysms by ultrasound every 6 months until the benefits of intervention outweigh the risks.

Massage?

If a massage therapist works with a client who subsequently experiences a ruptured aneurysm and dies, it is conceivable that the therapist could be held responsible. Even if the aneurysm might have eventually ruptured regardless of massage, it is important to avoid raising even the *possibility* that massage might be responsible for a client's death.

Any condition involving damaged blood vessels requires extreme caution for circulatory massage. *Massage changes the internal environment.* It dilates some blood vessels and constricts others. It reroutes circulation, mechanically through compression and friction on the skin, via the parasympathetic nervous system, and by changing hormonal balance (reducing adrenaline), which shifts blood from the skeletal muscles (a sympathetic state) to the internal organs (a parasympathetic state). If a client cannot keep up with having his internal environment shifted in terms of blood vessel dilation, chemical distribution, and autonomic state, he is not a good candidate for circulatory massage.

If a client has been diagnosed with a stable aortic aneurysm and he wants to receive massage, the therapist should choose modalities that aim to lower blood pressure and support that parasympathetic state without putting undue mechanical force on this person's circulatory system.

Atherosclerosis

Definition: What Is It?

Arteriosclerosis refers to a "hardening of the arteries" from any cause. *Atherosclerosis* is a subtype of arteriosclerosis. It is a condition in which deposits of cholesterol and other substances infiltrate and weaken layers of large blood vessels, particularly the aorta and coronary arteries. It is compounded by the fact that damage to these blood vessels can cause them to spasm, while blood clots form at the site of these deposits. These features contribute to the occlusion of the diameter or *lumen* of the arteries (Figure 4.9), as well as to the risk of creating and loosening blood clots on the arterial side of the systemic circuit.

Atherosclerosis in Brief

Pronunciation
ath′er-ō-skler-ō′sis

What is it?
Atherosclerosis is a condition in which the arteries become inelastic and brittle because of atherosclerotic plaques.

How is it recognized?
Atherosclerosis has no symptoms until it is very advanced. However, it is connected to several other types of circulatory problems, including hypertension, arrhythmia, coronary artery disease, cerebrovascular disease, and peripheral vascular disease.

Is massage indicated or contraindicated?
Advanced atherosclerosis systemically contraindicates rigorous circulatory massage, but other modalities may offer many benefits with a minimum of risks.

Figure 4.9. Atherosclerosis.

Coronary artery disease (CAD) is atherosclerosis specifically located in the coronary arteries that supply the heart muscle (Figure 4.10).

Demographics: Who Gets It?

Random samplings of arteries taken from autopsies of people who died of something other than heart disease indicate that the incidence of atherosclerosis is very high in the United States, although it does not always become symptomatic. Cultures exist in which this disease is completely unknown, but they are generally in countries where dietary diseases are related to famine rather than to excess.

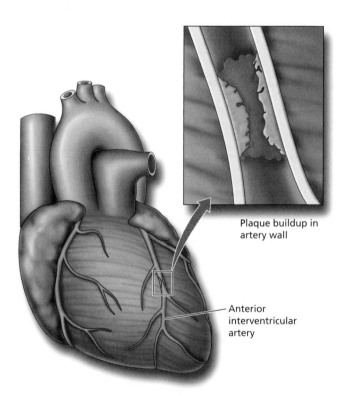

Figure 4.10. Coronary artery disease.

Certain populations carry a higher possibility of developing atherosclerosis. This is discussed in detail in the *Risk Factors* section of this article.

Etiology: What Happens?

The process of developing atherosclerosis is a complex one that is not yet completely understood. Several theories have been formed; however, as research reveals more secrets about this condition, the reality may turn out to be quite different from what people have always believed.

Theory 1   One theory for the development of atherosclerosis maps out various steps beginning with damage to the endothelial layer of the aorta. Deviations in the order of events in the disease process may occur for different people, but these are the basics:

- *Endothelial damage.* The inside layer of arteries is sometimes called the *tunica intima*. It is made of delicate epithelial tissue and subject to a lot of abuse. A variety of occurrences may hurl the first insult at the tunica intima: constant *hypertension* (this chapter) in the aorta and arteries surrounding the heart; carbon monoxide from cigarette smoke; high levels of circulation low-density lipoproteins (LDLs) and triglycerides; even a high level of iron in the blood may produce oxygen free radicals that begin the process of endothelial erosion.

- *Monocytes arrive.* These are small white blood cells that are attracted to any site of damage in the body. The monocytes infiltrate the epithelial layer and turn into *macrophages*: "big eaters."

- *Macrophages take up LDL.* The reasons for this are unclear. For a quick overview, LDLs are the low-density lipoproteins that are the "bad guys" of the cholesterol world. Actually, they have an important job, which is to escort usable cholesterol to all of the cells in the body. When those cells do not need any more cholesterol, however, they stop accepting it. This leaves those LDLs with nowhere to go. They are consumed by the white blood cells in the tunica intima, which are then called "foam cells." This is the beginning of the development of fatty streaks that characterize atherosclerosis.

- *Foam cells infiltrate and damage smooth muscle tissue.* Foam cells secrete growth factors; this causes the smooth muscle cells in the arterial wall to proliferate all around them. The grayish-white lumps of plaque that are inside dissected arteries are made of these extra muscle cells and cholesterol-filled macrophages. Furthermore, these foam cells can release enzymes that damage arterial walls and cause bleeding and clot formation.

- *Platelets arrive.* Attracted by the changing texture of the arterial wall, platelets come and release their chemicals, which do three unpleasant things:

  - *growth factors* are secreted, which reinforce the proliferation of new smooth muscle cells

  - *clots form*

Heart Disease in the United States: Sobering Statistics

The statistics for all varieties of cardiovascular disease are not generally separated from each other because most of these conditions exist in a circular relationship. A person is unlikely to have atherosclerosis without high blood pressure, for instance, and a person is unlikely to have a heart attack without the predisposing factor of atherosclerosis.

Statistics for cardiovascular disease as a whole in the United States are sobering. Approximately 2,600 people die of heart disease every day. That amounts to one death every 34 seconds. This group of diseases is the leading cause of death in the United States today, accounting for 38.5% of all deaths, or a ratio of one death out of every two and a half, although it is listed as a primary or contributing factor in close to 60% of all deaths. Heart disease and stroke account for 6 million hospitalizations per year, at a cost of $351 billion in direct and indirect health care costs.

Here is a breakdown of reported heart disease statistics[2,3]:

Condition	Prevalence
High blood pressure	50,000,000
Coronary artery disease	13,200,000
Myocardial infarct	7,800,000
Angina pectoris	6,800,000
Stroke	4,800,000
Congestive heart failure	5,000,000

When these numbers are adjusted for overlap, the prevalence of cardiovascular disease in the United States is over 64 million, or approximately one fourth of the adult population. But that is not all: the Centers for Disease Control and Prevention estimate that up to 90% of middle-aged adults in the United States will experience high blood pressure, but fewer than 30% will treat it successfully. Although these conditions are often associated with age, approximately 150,000 Americans who die of heart disease each year are younger than 65 years old.

[2] Heart Disease and Stroke Statistics—2004 Update. Copyright © American Heart Association. Available at: http://www.americanheart.org/downloadable/heart/1072969766940HSStats2004Update.pdf. Accessed winter 2004.

[3] Heart Disease and Stroke: The Nation's Leading Killers—The Burden of Heart Disease and Stroke. Centers for Disease Control and Prevention, National Center for Chronic Disease Prevention and Health Promotion. Available at: http://www.cdc.gov/nccdphp/aag/aag_cvd.htm. Accessed winter 2003.

- *vascular spasm* occurs because the chemical that inhibits it cannot get through all the plaque. This leads to a temporary lack of oxygen in the myocardium, and the gripping chest pain called ***angina pectoris***.

When vascular spasm and clots combine, partial or total occlusion of the artery can occur. Symptoms of this depend on the location of the blockage and the amount of tissue that is affected.

Theory 2   Another explanation of the development of atherosclerosis begins with the deposition of LDL cholesterol in the subendothelial spaces of the arteries. There it undergoes some chemical changes (oxidation), which makes it impossible to leave the artery wall. Circulating monocytes are attracted to the LDL deposits. They infiltrate the arterial wall and literally gorge themselves on the embedded cholesterol, becoming foam cells.

The monocytes can eat so much they rupture, releasing their contents in the area. Among the chemicals released are growth factors that stimulate smooth muscle cell proliferation in the arterial wall. These sites become raised lesions or *plaques*. Calcium is eventually deposited there. The rough texture created by plaques attracts passing thrombocytes, which then contribute to clot formation and the subsequent dangers discussed above.

Risk Factors

Risk factors for atherosclerosis can be divided into situations that can be modified and others over which a person has little or no control.

Non-Modifiable Risk Factors

- *Heredity, genetics.* This is one factor no one can control. Higher than average incidence of heart disease within families is clearly demonstrable. But a family history is not a death sentence; controlling modifiable factors will significantly reduce the chance of developing problems.

- *Gender.* Simply being a male increases the risk of atherosclerosis. Female hormones also seem to have some influence, because postmenopausal women have higher rates than premenopausal women.

- *Age.* The incidence of heart disease rises with age, but it is important to remember that nearly half of all those released from the hospital for cardiovascular problems every year are younger than 65 years of age.

- *Kidney disorders.* Atherosclerosis can sometimes lead to kidney problems. However, if the kidney problems predate the circulatory ones, high blood pressure brought about by kidney failure can be a precipitating cause of atherosclerosis. (See *renal failure*, Chapter 9.)

- *Signs of inflammation.* A new risk factor for atherosclerosis and cardiovascular disease in general has recently been identified in high levels of ***C-reactive protein*** (CRP). This is a liver enzyme secreted in the presence of an inflammatory response. It has become a dependable predictor for heart attack, stroke, and other conditions related to atherosclerosis, although the mechanism that links general, nonspecific inflammation to these risks is not clearly understood.

A Brief Digression on Cholesterol

Cholesterol is a fatty substance that is produced in the liver and is also available in any animal product. Saturated fats are particularly rich in easily absorbable cholesterol.

Cholesterol by itself has no access to the body's cells. Just as glucose must be escorted into cells by insulin, cholesterol must be escorted by ***lipoproteins***, other chemicals also produced by the liver. When a cholesterol measurement is taken, it is actually the lipoproteins that are being counted.

Three varieties of lipoproteins are involved with the movement of cholesterol: low-density lipoproteins (LDLs), high-density lipoproteins (HDLs), and triglycerides. The LDLs ("bad cholesterol") deliver cholesterol to the body's cells. They are only "bad" when the body's cells have no more need for their cargo. At that point, the LDLs will deposit the cholesterol in artery walls. The HDLs ("good cholesterol") are involved in a process called "reverse cholesterol transport." In this process, cholesterol is moved out of the arteries and back to the liver for metabolic processing. The third variety, triglycerides, are chemicals that help to convert fats and carbohydrates into energy for muscles. Studies have shown that elevated triglyceride levels contribute to plaque formation, so it is desirable to keep their numbers down.

When a person gets a cholesterol reading, it is useful to know not just what his or her overall levels are, but in what ratios the fat types occur. An ideal reading would find total levels below 200 milligrams per deciliter (mg/dL), with a relatively high proportion of HDLs (over 35 mg/dL) and lower numbers of LDLs and triglycerides (less than 130 mg/dL combined).

Unfortunately, in the United States, less than half the adult population can make this claim. More than 100 million people have cholesterol readings over 200 mg/dL, and approximately 40% of those people read over 240 mg/dL. The overall average is 215 mg/dL for women, and 211 mg/dL for men. Women have a slightly higher reading because menstruation tends to temporarily raise HDL levels.

Studies show that lowering cholesterol levels not only reduces the risk of developing atherosclerosis but actually extends life expectancy. Men with cholesterol readings of 200 mg/dL or below live an average of 3.8 to 8.7 years longer than men with cholesterol readings above 240 mg/dL.

Modifiable Risk Factors

- *Smoking.* Carbon monoxide from cigarette smoke is extremely corrosive to endothelium. Furthermore, nicotine causes the release of epinephrine and norepinephrine, leading to vasoconstriction and high blood pressure. Studies show that cigarette smokers have a 2 to 4 times higher risk of dying by heart disease than the general public.

- *High cholesterol levels.* A predictable statistical link has been established between high cholesterol levels and the development of pathologic atherosclerosis. Over 52% of Americans have cholesterol readings above the recommended maximum of 200 mg/dL. Over 20% have readings over 240 mg/dL. For more details on cholesterol, see sidebar, "A Brief Digression on Cholesterol".

- *High blood pressure.* Chronic uncontrolled high blood pressure contributes to endothelial damage, which opens the door to the formation of plaques.

- *Sedentary lifestyle.* Regular, moderate cardiovascular exercise, perhaps more than any other factor, can reduce the risk of atherosclerosis. It keeps arteries elastic and pliable, reduces weight, raises high-density lipoprotein (HDL) levels for the reduction of plaques, reduces the risk of diabetes, and lowers blood pressure.

- *Diabetes.* People with uncontrolled diabetes are especially susceptible to atherosclerosis because of the way their bodies metabolize food. However, if the diabetes is controlled, the risk of atherosclerosis is much lower.

Other risk factors are somewhat harder to quantify. The way a person responds to stress, for instance, has a lot to do with his health profile. If stress makes him eat poorly, smoke more, and raises his blood pressure, then his risk for developing atherosclerosis will be higher than for someone who deals with stress in different ways. *Depression* (Chapter 3) is another reliable predictor of heart disease. Finally, *metabolic syndrome* (Chapter 8) is a collection of physical properties that, when seen together, drastically increase the risk for cardiovascular disease.

Signs and Symptoms

What are the symptoms of atherosclerosis? Until the damage has progressed to dangerous levels, *there are none!* An artery has to be *75% to 80% occluded* before the person has any awareness of a problem. This is largely because the body does not depend on any single artery to do a job. Most parts of the body have two or three alternate vessels that can be pressed into service if one of them becomes clogged.

Once signs begin to develop, they revolve around poor delivery of oxygen to the heart and consequently poor delivery of blood to the rest of the body. Low stamina, shortness of breath, and a host of predictable complications are all signs and symptoms of advanced atherosclerosis.

Complications

The complications of atherosclerosis are sometimes the first symptoms of the disease. They include but are not limited to

- *High blood pressure.* Hypertension is both a cause and a result of this disease; it contributes to the original damage to the tunica intima, and it is made worse when the arterial walls are too brittle to adjust to the constant changes in blood volume flowing through them.

- *Aneurysm* (this chapter). When the wall of an artery is rendered inelastic and defective, it can bulge, become thin and weak, and become susceptible to rupture (this chapter).

- *Arrhythmia.* Advanced arteriosclerosis can contribute to the development of irregular or uncoordinated beating of the cardiac muscle, as blood supply through the coronary arteries is periodically interrupted. Arrhythmia can cause clots to form in the atria when there is incomplete emptying of the chamber. These clots can travel anywhere the aorta takes them.

- *Thrombus or embolism, peripheral circulatory damage.* A thrombus is a stationery clot; an embolism is a traveling clot (see *embolism, thrombus,* this chapter). Thrombi are the link between atherosclerosis and *stroke* (Chapter 3) or TIA (transient ischemic attack) when they travel to the brain, and between atherosclerosis and heart attack when they lodge in the coronary arteries. If a clot lodges in the renal artery, kidney damage occurs. Clots on the arterial side of the system also may end up in peripheral blood vessels, where they can cause stasis dermatitis, gangrene, and skin ulcers (Figure 4.11).

- *Angina pectoris.* The process of developing atherosclerotic plaques also creates a higher risk of short-term vascular spasm, which leads to intermittent heart and chest pain.

- *Heart attack* (this chapter). When rough plaques form on smooth artery walls, they attract clotting factors. If a clot or fragment of a clot breaks free from a plaque in the coronary artery, it travels until its blood vessel becomes too small to let it pass. All the myocardium that should have been supplied by that artery will then die: a myocardial infarction, or heart attack.

Diagnosis

The traditional way to check for *stenosis*, or narrowing of arteries, is to inject them with dye and take a series of x-rays to watch the movement of fluid through the tubes in a procedure called an *angiogram*. A faster, less intrusive test, called an ultrafast CT scan, takes clear pictures of arteries with approximately 1 chest x-ray's worth of radiation. It is not as complete a test as an angiogram, but it can be used to screen out high-risk patients who have no symptoms but who want to find out at what stage their disease exists.

Treatment

Treatment for atherosclerosis starts simply. If the situation is caught before it gets out of hand, it can often be dealt with by changing eating and exercise habits.

Some drugs and other substances, notably niacin and chromium, have been found to increase HDL levels and reduce LDL levels in the blood. Lipid-lowering agents can be successful, but they often have side effects. Unfortunately, plaques that have been long in place are only approximately 15% soluble fats; the rest are composed of cellular debris, connective tissue, foam cells, and hypertrophic smooth muscle cells.

More advanced cases, and more standardized medical approaches, often involve drugs or surgery. The drugs are generally smooth muscle relaxants that cause the blood vessels to dilate. Aspirin has been found to be useful as an anticoagulant, but many people experience stomach irritation with it. Specially coated tablets have been designed for the control of CAD that do not irritate the digestive system.

Surgical intervention for atherosclerosis used to be automatic bypass surgery. That is, surgeons would remove the damaged piece of coronary artery and replace it with something else, often a graft from the internal mammary artery or a piece of femoral vein. A single, double, triple or however-many bypass refers to how many sections of artery are being replaced.

Angioplasty is a less intrusive option that is useful for some patients. In this procedure, the artery may first be treated with a laser, which vaporizes plaques (laser angioplasty), and then a small balloon is inflated to widen the artery (balloon angioplasty). Unfortunately, the scarring that occurs when the balloon is removed ("restenosis") can

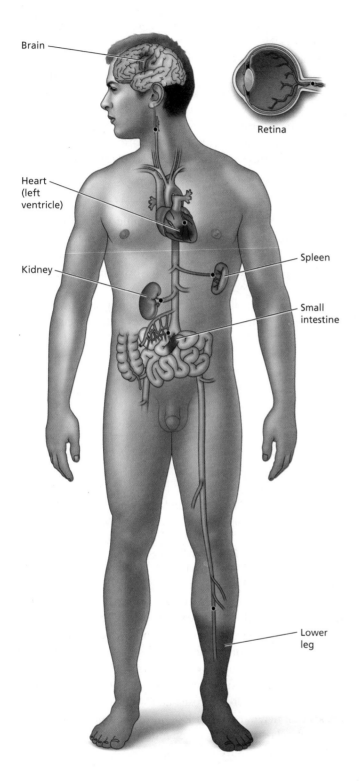

Figure 4.11. Arterial infarction sites.

be a difficult, even dangerous complication of this procedure; new cells rapidly proliferate where the endothelium was scraped. Low doses of radiation inside the artery may be used to limit restenosis. A small rigid coil, called a ***stent***, is inserted to keep the artery widened, and in some procedures a laser heats up and "welds" the inside of the artery into a permanently smooth shape.

In yet another type of procedure, *catheter atherectomy*, a tiny rotating drill is inserted into clogged arteries to shave off plaque. The shavings are then trapped and removed. This is sometimes used for carotid arteries when the risk of stroke is high.

With the exception of bypass surgery, all of these procedures can be done by inserting special tubes into arteries in the arms or legs and guiding the equipment to where it needs to go. Obviously the amount of shock to the system is less, and the recovery process is much easier than it used to be. However, new emphasis is being put on *maintaining* the structural changes brought about by intervention; if the patient reverts to former eating and exercise habits, his or her arteries can reach the same sorry state in just a few years.

Massage?

It is impossible to tell whether a client has a subclinical build-up of plaque. The deciding factor is whether the client can adjust to the changes in internal environment that massage will bring about. In other words, if his ability to maintain homeostasis is going to be overly challenged by rigorous movement of fluid through his system, he is not a good candidate for circulatory massage.

If a client is taking *any* kind of medication for circulatory problems, it is important to clearly understand why and to adjust massage modalities to fit the circulatory limitations of the client.

Hypertension

Definition: What Is It?

Hypertension in Brief

What is it?
Hypertension is the technical term for high blood pressure.

How is it recognized?
High blood pressure has no dependable symptoms. The only way to identify it is by taking several blood pressure measurements over time.

Is massage indicated or contraindicated?
For borderline or mild high blood pressure, massage may be useful as a tool to control stress and increase general health, but other pathologic conditions having to do with kidney or cardiovascular disease must be ruled out. High blood pressure that accompanies other cardiovascular disease may be inappropriate for circulatory massage, but may respond well to other modalities.

Hypertension is a technical term for *high blood pressure*. It is defined as blood pressure persistently elevated above 140 mg Hg systolic, or 90 mg Hg diastolic.

The animation "Hypertension" can be found on the Student Resource CD-ROM that accompanies this book.

Demographics: Who Gets It?

Approximately 50 million people in the United States have high blood pressure: that is 1 in every 4 adults. It strikes men more often than women, until women reach the age of 65. Then it evens out and affects both genders equally. African Americans have higher hypertension rates than other races. Age is a predisposing factor; approximately half of all people over 60 years old have high blood pressure.

Other predisposing factors include obesity, smoking, high cholesterol levels, atherosclerosis, and water retention. A genetic predisposition may raise the risk of high blood pressure, but sometimes it is hard to know what has been inherited: high blood pressure genes or high blood pressure habits.

Etiology: What Happens?

In hypertension, internal or external forces put pressure on the blood vessels. To understand how these forces can cause damage, it is necessary to take a brief look at exactly what blood pressure is.

Anatomy Review   A *sphygmomanometer* is an instrument that measures the pressure blood exerts against arterial walls at two different moments: ventricular contraction (*systole*) and ventricular relaxation (***diastole***). The blood pressure cuff converts the pressure in the arteries to millimeters of mercury (mm Hg).

The variables involved in measuring blood pressure are fourfold: total blood volume; pressure from *inside* the vessel (which would be increased if there were any buildup of material inside); pressure from the *outside* of the vessel (which would be increased by having excess fluid pressing all around); and blood vessel diameter. If any of these factors is out of balance, it will influence total body blood pressure, which will in turn influence the health and longevity of blood vessels.

Types of High Blood Pressure

Two types of high blood pressure have been identified: *essential*, which means "not due to some other pathology" and *secondary*, which is a temporary complication of some other condition such as pregnancy, kidney problems, adrenal tumors, or hormonal disorders. Secondary high blood pressure clears up when the precipitating cause is dealt with. Approximately 95% of all hypertension is essential. For both essential and secondary high blood pressure, another variable is possible: *malignant hypertension*. In this condition, the diastolic pressure rises very quickly, over a matter of weeks or months. It is extremely damaging to the circulatory system, a high risk for ischemic or hemorrhagic *stroke* (Chapter 3), and left untreated is often fatal. Malignant high blood pressure is a medical emergency.

Blood Pressure Readings   Here are some basic guidelines for rating the severity of hypertension in adults, based on the averages of more than two readings taken at each of more than two visits after an initial screening.[4]

Category	Systolic BP (mm Hg)	Diastolic BP (mg Hg)
Optimal	<120	<80
Prehypertension	120–139	80–89
Hypertension		
Stage 1 (mild)	140–159	90–99
Stage 2 (moderate)	160+	100+

Massage therapists are not generally required to take blood pressure measurements; these numbers are just an indicator of possible trouble. Be aware also that blood pressure can change significantly from hour to hour. It is not uncommon to see it shoot up from anxiety while a person is in a doctor's office; this is known as "white coat hypertension."

Signs and Symptoms

This disease, which is often called "the silent killer," has few recognizable symptoms. A few subtle signs are occasionally observed, however, so they are included here: shortness of breath after mild exercise; headaches or dizziness; swelling of the ankles, especially during the daytime; excessive sweating or anxiety. Any combination of these symptoms is an indicator that a visit to the doctor would be a good idea.

Complications

This is a very important list. Having high blood pressure can shorten a person's life span. Here is how:

- *Edema*. High blood pressure forces extra fluid out of the capillaries at the nutrient/waste exchange sites. This adds to overall levels of interstitial fluid, causing

---

[4] What Is High Blood Pressure? Available at: http://www.nhlbi.nih.gov/health/dci/Diseases/Hbp/HBP_WhatIs.html. Accessed winter 2003.

edema. In a typically vicious circle, edema further raises blood pressure by exerting external force on blood vessels. See more in *edema*, Chapter 5.

- *Atherosclerosis.* Having blood pushing against arteries in an unceasing torrent simply wears out the walls, especially when the arteries have naturally lost some of their resiliency from age. The moment there is the slightest damage for a platelet to cling to, the atherosclerotic process will begin. This reinforces high blood pressure by narrowing arterial diameters. See more in *atherosclerosis*, this chapter.

- *Stroke.* Someone with hypertension is 4 times more likely to have stroke than someone who does not have hypertension. The stroke may be from an embolism, or it may be from ruptured arteries in the brain. See more in *stroke*, Chapter 3.

- *Enlarged heart, heart failure.* Making the heart push against narrowed arteries causes the left ventricle to grow considerably, but the coronary arteries do not grow with it to handle the extra load. The muscle fibers also lose elasticity. Therefore, the contractions are actually weaker because the muscle is not well supplied with blood, and it cannot contract fully. This can also cause angina, or heart pain. When the ventricles of the heart are so overtaxed that they simply cannot keep up with the workload, the patient risks heart failure. This condition is 6 times more likely to happen to someone who is hypertensive than someone who is not. See more in *heart attack* and *heart failure*, this chapter.

- *Aneurysms.* This is the result of high blood pressure causing a bulge in the arteries. See more in *aneurysm*, this chapter.

- *Kidney disease.* In a way this is the most interesting complication of high blood pressure, because of the circular relationship between hypertension and kidney dysfunction. Problems can start in either place: the kidneys or the circulatory system. If it starts with the circulatory system, here is the process: hypertension causes atherosclerotic plaques to form in the renal arteries, which are subject to *huge* blood pressure. This causes reduced blood flow into the kidney, which impairs kidney function, leading to kidney damage, systemic edema, and yet more pressure exerted against vessel walls from that edema.

    If the problem starts in the kidneys, decreased kidney function will be an issue (see more under *renal failure*, Chapter 9). This is often accompanied by extra release of **renin**, the kidney-based hormone that regulates some electrolyte balance. Excess renin results in vasoconstriction, water and salt retention, increased edema, increased blood volume, and high blood pressure.

- *Vision problems.* Chronic high blood pressure can damage the blood vessels that supply the eyes, causing them to become thickened and less elastic. Reduction of blood flow to eyes results in permanent visual distortion.

Treatment

Hypertension is a highly treatable disease, but because it has virtually no symptoms until it has progressed to very dangerous levels, it is frequently untreated or incompletely treated (i.e., someone not taking his medication because he feels fine).

Diet is the first way to manage this condition. The National Heart Lung and Blood Institute (NHLBI) conducted research about dietary factors and blood pressure. Their findings have led to the DASH (Dietary Approaches to Stop Hypertension) diet: a combination of high-fiber, low-fat foods that provides higher than normal levels of calcium, magnesium, and potassium, while cutting sodium by approximately 20%. Following the DASH diet (which is useful for anyone, not just hypertension patients) has been found to be just as effective as many varieties of blood pressure medication, without side effects or long-term health risks. The DASH diet reduces systolic readings by anywhere from 6 to 11 points, and diastolic readings from 3 to 6 points within 2 weeks of initiating the change in eating habits.

Exercise is also crucial for the development of healthy new blood vessels, as well as for weight control. Losing even a small percentage of body weight for obese or overweight patients can have a profound affect on blood pressure and cardiovascular health.

Medication, if called for, includes diuretics, vasodilators, and beta-blockers, which decrease the force of ventricular contraction. Medicating high blood pressure is a bit problematic. Because the disease itself has no strong symptoms, and because the medicines often have unpleasant side effects (including dizziness, insomnia, impotence, and others), it has been difficult to get hypertension patients to be consistent with their medications. Recent statistics indicate that in the United States only one third of the people who have hypertension are aware of it, and less than a third of people diagnosed with hypertension treat it successfully.

Massage?

If a client knows that he has high blood pressure but he is *not* required to take medication for it, circulatory massage is probably fine, especially if the client is physically active, or encouraged to become physically active. Massage can help to lower general blood pressure and the stress that contributes to it. It is important, however, to rule out kidney and other advanced cardiovascular problems before beginning. Watch especially for signs that massage is over-challenging the body: clamminess, bogginess, and possible edema in the days after the treatment.

If a client *does* take medication for high blood pressure, circulatory modalities are strongly cautioned. Techniques that do not strongly influence fluid flow may be appropriate, but rigorous, fast-paced work may be too much of a challenge for an impaired ability to maintain homeostasis. As always, judgments about massage must be made by comparing the challenges of bodywork to activities of daily living.

Regardless of whether the client is on blood pressure medication, *deep abdominal work is contraindicated for high blood pressure.* This is because it is possible to accidentally trip the vasovagal reaction. Unintentionally overstimulating the vagus nerve can result in amplified parasympathetic reactions. This leads to systemic vasodilation and faintness from lack of blood to the brain. Another possibility is that the body could experience a sympathetic rebound effect. Ordinarily a vasovagal reaction is unpleasant but not dangerous—*unless* the blood vessels are not equipped to handle a rapid demand to dilate and constrict. Once again, a client's health is determined by his ability to maintain a stable internal environment during massage.

Raynaud's Syndrome
Definition: What Is It?

Raynaud's syndrome is a condition involving the status of the arterioles in the hands and feet, although it also can affect the nose, ears, and lips. Primary Raynaud's disease is a simple vasoconstriction disorder, whereas secondary Raynaud's phenomenon is a complication of an underlying problem.

Demographics: Who Gets It?

Raynaud's disease that is unrelated to underlying conditions usually affects women between 14 and 40 years of age; this population group

Raynaud's Syndrome in Brief

Pronunciation
rā-nō′

What is it?
Raynaud's syndrome is defined by episodes of vasospasm of the arterioles, usually in fingers and toes, and occasionally in the nose, ears, and lips.

How is it recognized?
Affected areas will often go through marked color changes of white or ashy gray for dark-skinned people, to blue to red. Attacks can last for less than a minute or several hours. Numbness or tingling may follow during recovery.

Is massage indicated or contraindicated?
Massage is indicated for Raynaud's syndrome that is *not* associated with an underlying pathologic condition. Otherwise, follow the guidelines for the precipitating condition.

makes up 75% of all primary Raynaud's patients. Secondary Raynaud's is often linked to autoimmune disorders, which women also experience in greater numbers than men, so women are more likely to be affected by either type of problem. Estimates vary, but it is projected that some variety of Raynaud's syndrome affects up to 5% to 10% of the general population.

Etiology: What Happens?

In both primary and secondary Raynaud's syndrome, the arterioles in the extremities experience vasospasm: contraction of smooth muscle tissue. It occurs in temporary episodes at first, but the vasoconstriction can become a permanent situation.

Causes (Primary)

Raynaud's disease is a primary problem, that is, unconnected to underlying pathologic conditions. It is may be attributable to emotional stress (the autonomic nervous system routes blood away from the skin during emergencies), cold, or because of a mechanical irritation, such as operating machinery that influences blood vessel dilation. Pianists and typists are particularly vulnerable. Raynaud's disease generally has a slow onset, and the attacks are less severe than when the symptoms occur as a secondary problem. If a person is prone to Raynaud's disease, both her feet and hands tend to be affected.

Causes (Secondary)

Occasionally extreme vasoconstriction is a complication of some other disorder. In this case the condition is called *Raynaud's phenomenon*. It generally has a much faster onset than Raynaud's disease, and the risk of serious complications is much higher. Some conditions associated with Raynaud's phenomenon are:

- Arterial diseases that involve occlusions, such as *diabetes* (Chapter 8), *atherosclerosis* (this chapter) and **Buerger's disease** (another rare situation involving inflammation and blood clots in the arteries);
- Connective tissue diseases such as *scleroderma* (Chapter 1), *lupus* (Chapter 5), and *rheumatoid arthritis* (Chapter 2).
- Sensitivity to some drugs including beta-blockers and ergot compounds;
- Neurovascular compression, as seen with *carpal tunnel syndrome* (Chapter 2).

Signs and Symptoms

Raynaud's syndrome is usually bilateral. During an attack, the skin goes through a characteristic cycle of colors: white, as the blood is shunted away from the area (on dark-skinned people the skin looks ashy gray); blue, as the cells are starved for oxygen; and red as the attack subsides, the arterioles re-open, and the blood returns to the affected area (Figure 4.12).

Attacks of Raynaud's phenomenon can last anywhere from less than a minute to several hours. Secondary Raynaud's can be so extreme and long-lasting that a wasting of flesh and ulcerations on the starved skin may develop. The fingers may taper, and the skin can become thin, smooth, and shiny. Gangrene is a rare but possible complication for these extreme cases.

Treatment

Treatment depends on whether the patient has a primary or secondary case of Raynaud's. Generally a noninvasive approach is taken first, at least to primary Raynaud's disease.

Figure 4.12. Raynaud's syndrome.

Quitting smoking, soaking in warm water, dressing appropriately for the weather, protecting the hands when working with cold or frozen foods, making sure that shoes are not too tight, even moving to a warmer climate are all suggested before more intervention is suggested.

Because primary Raynaud's disease can be exacerbated by emotional upset, patients are often encouraged to find productive ways to manage stress. This can range from learning biofeedback techniques to exercising regularly, to receiving massage.

If results are unsatisfactory, or if tissue damage from chronically impaired blood flow is a risk, the next step is medication to dilate the blood vessels. Other drugs work to counteract norepinephrine, the stress-related hormone that initiates vasoconstriction. Unfortunately, medical intervention is often unsuccessful for secondary Raynaud's phenomenon.

Massage?

The good news about Raynaud's is that though the primary version of the syndrome is fairly common, the secondary version is rather rare. If the Raynaud's is a part of lupus, scleroderma, or another vascular problem, the guidelines for massage must follow the cautions for the precipitating causes.

If any dangerous underlying causes for the vasoconstriction have been ruled out, primary Raynaud's syndrome indicates massage. Massage can work mechanically with local blood vessels and reflexively with the parasympathetic nervous system to stimulate vasodilation.

Varicose Veins

Definition: What Are They?

Varicose veins are distended, often twisted or "ropey," superficial veins. They are caused by damage to the internal valves whose job is to make sure that blood only goes one way: toward the heart. When blood backs up along the system, the affected vein is stretched,

Varicose Veins in Brief

What are they?
Varicose veins are distended veins, usually in the legs, caused by vascular incompetence and the poor return of blood to the heart.

How are they recognized?
Varicose veins are ropey, slightly bluish, elevated veins that twist and turn out of their usual course. They happen most frequently in branches of the saphenous veins on the medial side of the calf, although they are also found on the anterior and posterior aspects of the calf and thigh.

Is massage indicated or contraindicated?
Massage is locally contraindicated for extreme varicose veins, and anywhere distal to them. Mild varicose veins contraindicate deep, specific work but are otherwise safe for massage.

distorted, and generally weakened (Figure 4.13). Varicose veins can happen at the anus (*hemorrhoids*), at the esophagus (*esophageal varices*), or at the scrotum (*varicoles*). But most often they are in the legs (Figure 4.14), which is the focus of the rest of this discussion.

Demographics: Who Gets Them?

Women get varicose veins more often than men; this is largely due to estrogen, which can weaken venous walls, and to a history of pregnancy: a fetus can obstruct fluid return through the femoral vein, which can set the stage for later problems (see *pregnancy*, Chapter 10). It is estimated that approximately 1 in 10 people will have varicosities at some point, mostly after 50 years of age. Approximately 80 million people in the United States have some variety of venous disorder.

Figure 4.13. Varicose veins.

Figure 4.14. Varicose veins may change the contours of the skin.

Etiology: What Happens?

Anatomy Review The veins in the legs have a fascinating construction that assists the heart in getting the blood from the toes all the way back to the chest. Small veins pick up the blood from the internal muscle capillaries. These veins tend to run on the superficial aspect of muscles. They feed into larger veins that perforate the muscle bellies, and then into the really big deep veins that run under the muscles, close to the bones. When the leg muscles contract, the perforating veins are squeezed, sending their contents to the deep veins. When the leg muscles relax, the perforating veins draw in new blood from the smaller veins. The contraction and relaxation of the leg muscles (especially the soleus— "sump pump of the leg") is crucial to blood return. The valves inside the perforating veins and the deep veins ensure that blood will not collect in the smaller, weaker superficial veins.

Causes

What can damage the valves in the veins? It could be simple wear and tear: being on one's feet for many hours a day, especially if the legs muscles are not allowed to fully contract and relax during that time, weakens the veins. It also could be a mechanical obstruction to returning blood: knee socks that are too tight, a knee brace, or a fetus that presses on the femoral vein. Systemic congestion from kidney problems or liver backups has been seen to cause problems too. Finally, it could be simply congenitally weak veins. Once a valve sustains damage, blood puts pressure on the next valve down. Vascular incompetence will ultimately cause the weakest superficial veins to become distorted, dilated, and twisted off their regular pathway. This weakening process seldom affects the biggest, deepest veins, because their walls are thicker and the leg muscles act as built-in support hose.

Signs and Symptoms

Varicose veins look like lumpy bluish wandering lines on the surface of the skin. They are often visible on the back of the calf, but more often they affect the great saphenous vein, where they show up anywhere from the ankle to the groin on the medial side. They may be visible only when the patient is standing.

Varicose veins may itch or cause throbbing pain, especially at the end of the day when legs feel tired and heavy. They can contribute to edema around the ankles as fluid backs up in the lower leg.

Complications

Although varicosities are seldom anything more than annoying, occasionally they can create some unpleasant side effects. Chronically impaired circulation may result in varicose ulcers, which do not heal until circulation is restored. Skin irritation from poor circulation occasionally leads to a type of *eczema* (Chapter 1) that does not resolve until the varicosity is relieved. Interruptions in blood flow increase the likelihood of annoying night cramps (see *spasms, cramps,* Chapter 2). Stagnant blood in a distended vein may coagulate, raising the possibility of clotting. Most clots that form in varicose veins are superficial and melt easily, however, so they are usually a lesser threat than clots that form in deeper leg veins (see *thrombophlebitis,* this chapter). Be aware, however, that the presence of grossly distended varicose veins may indicate an increased risk of deep vein thrombosis.

Treatment

Mild varicose veins are usually treated with good sense. Using support hose or elastic bandages can give extra help to damaged veins and avoiding long periods of standing up without full contraction and relaxation of the muscles is often recommended. Reclining with the feet slightly elevated also reduces symptoms. Whether the veins can actually *heal* is somewhat controversial. If the damage has not progressed too far, relieving the mechanical stresses while strengthening the smooth muscle tissue (with hydrotherapy, for instance) can yield good results.

Surgery for mild varicose veins is not generally recommended as a purely cosmetic intervention. However, varicose veins are a progressive condition; they do not usually spontaneously reverse, and left untreated their complications can be serious. Therefore, a certain number of patients will eventually seek treatment for health, rather than cosmetic concerns.

Several strategies for reducing varicose veins have been developed. The traditional approach is surgery to remove the affected vein ("stripping"). ***Ambulatory phlebectomy*** ("mini-stripping") is a similar treatment that removes only small sections of the affected veins. ***Sclerosing*** involves injections of chemicals (salt or sugar solutions) into the vein that cause it to completely close down. Treatments to heat up and collapse vein walls are also gaining popularity. In all of these treatments, the body's remarkable ability to generate new blood vessels quickly accommodates the closure or removal of the affected vein.

Massage?

Massage is a local contraindication for varicose veins, particularly for veins that are elevated from the skin and that have visibly been distorted from their original pathway. Not only is the tissue injured and delicate, but it is inappropriate to push a lot of blood through vessels that may not be able to accommodate it. Heavy massage distal to these veins is cautioned as well.

Clients with very extreme varicosities that have a high risk of complications should be under a doctor's care and should be regularly checked for signs of deep vein thrombosis.

If the vein is only slightly darkened and not elevated or causing any pain, it is still wise to avoid local heavy pressure, but otherwise massage is safe. Tiny reddened spider veins (***telangiectasias***) are slightly dilated venules and are safe for massage.

HEART CONDITIONS

Heart Attack

Definition: What Is It?

A heart attack is damage to some portion of the cardiac muscle as a result of ischemia, which starves and kills some of the muscle cells. The ischemia is usually caused by coronary artery disease (CAD), or *atherosclerosis* (this chapter), of the coronary arteries, which supply the cardiac muscle with oxygen and nutrition. If these arteries are completely occluded by plaque, thrombi, or any combination of the two, some piece of the muscle dies (Figure 4.15). The muscle tissue does not grow back; it is replaced by inelastic, noncontractile scar tissue. The damaged area is referred to as an *infarct*. Another term for heart attack is *myocardial infarction* (MI).

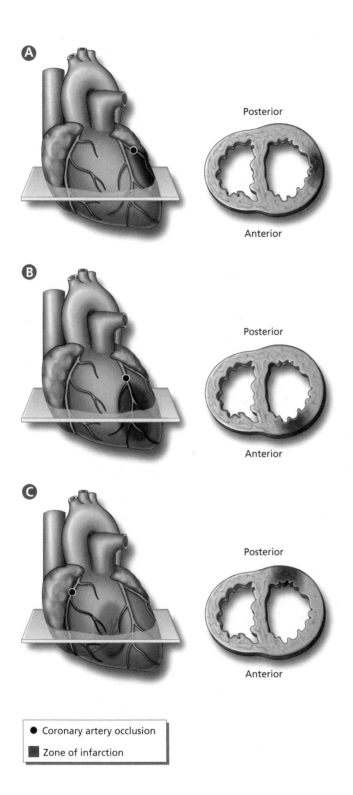

Figure 4.15. A–C. Heart attacks affecting the left ventricle.

Heart Attack in Brief

What is it?
A heart attack, or myocardial infarction, is damage to the myocardium caused by a sudden obstruction in blood flow through the coronary arteries, which results in permanent myocardial damage.

How is it recognized?
Symptoms of most heart attacks include a sensation of great pressure on the chest, spreading pain, and lightheadedness, dizziness, and nausea. Sometimes symptoms vary, and occasionally a minor heart attack may occur with no symptoms at all.

Is massage indicated or contraindicated?
Patients recovering from recent heart attacks are not candidates for circulatory massage. After they have completely recovered, they *may* be able to receive massage, depending on the rest of their cardiovascular health.

Demographics: Who Gets Them?

Coronary artery disease and heart attack is the leading cause of death in the United States, claiming over half a million lives every year, or one in every five deaths. Over a million heart attacks occur every year, and approximately half of them result in death. Close to 13 million heart attack or angina survivors are alive in the United States today.

Most people are familiar with the high-risk profile for heart attack victims: being sedentary, having *hypertension* (this chapter), having high cholesterol levels, smoking, being overweight. Being male, having a family history of cardiovascular disease, or being a woman over 35 who takes birth control pills all increase the chances of a heart attack.

That said, note that approximately one fourth of all heart attack patients have no previous symptoms or warning signs on record.

Etiology: What Happens?

A heart attack occurs when a portion of the cardiac muscle is killed off from lack of oxygen: an ischemic attack. Usually it comes from a blockage in the coronary artery that may be from a loosened blood clot or a broken or torn piece of atherosclerotic plaque. Rarely, a heart attack may occur when a coronary artery goes into prolonged spasm; this is seen most often in cocaine or other drug overdoses.

Examinations of exactly which plaques pose the greatest risk of heart attack have indicated that the size of the plaque evidently has little to do with its chances of breaking off or causing a heart attack. The more pertinent factor is how stable the plaque is. Older, harder plaques are relatively stable, but newer, softer plaques have a higher risk of breaking open and letting go of clots or atherosclerotic fragments that then block the coronary artery.

When a portion of the cardiac muscle is killed off by ischemic attack, the ability to contract with coordination and efficiency is badly damaged. If a heart attack is severe enough to trigger ventricular fibrillations, the risk of immediate death is very high.

The seriousness of a heart attack is determined by the size and location of the blockage. If it is relatively small and blood flow is impaired to an area that does not have to work especially hard, the heart attack is not a serious one. However, if the infarct, or area of damaged tissue, is large enough to weaken the heart's ability to contract, or if the damaged tissue contains the electrical conduction system for the heart, major intervention is necessary to aid in recovery.

Signs and Symptoms

Heart attacks can have a variety of signs and symptoms, some of which are extremely subtle, and some of which feel very severe. Three of the most common and dependable signs are:

- *Pressure, pain in the chest*
- *Spreading pain.* This may spread to the shoulder, arm, neck, and jaw of the left side of the body: the referred pain pattern for the dermatome shared by the heart.
- *Lightheadedness, nausea, sweating.* These usually occur along with chest pain. When they occur *without* chest pain they may still indicate a heart attack, but it is a less common presentation.

Other symptoms can include shortness of breath with or without chest pain, unexplained nausea, anxiety or weakness, fainting, palpitations, and cold sweat. Even stomach and abdominal pain may sometimes be signs of a heart attack.

Angina pectoris (literally, "chest pain") is one of the few early warning signs for the risk of heart attack. Three types of angina have been identified; each one, although not specifically leading directly to a heart attack, does indicate a significantly increased risk.

- *Angina pectoris.* This is the simplest and most common form of angina. It affects approximately 6.6 million people a year. In this form of angina, the heart can get enough oxygen to perform regular tasks, but any extra effort, such as carrying something heavy or running up a flight of stairs, demands too much of the clogged coronary arteries. The result is moderate to severe chest pain that is relieved with rest or angina medication: drugs that help blood vessels to expand.

- *Angina variant.* This is type of angina can occur *without* unusual physical activity. It often appears in the night, with very extreme but short-lived chest pain. It is caused by vascular spasm at or near the site of atherosclerotic plaques. This variety of angina is a reliable predictor of incipient heart attack.

- *Microvascular angina.* This type of chest pain is caused by dysfunction of the smallest blood vessels that come off the coronary arteries. It can be present even without signs of major atherosclerotic blockage, which distinguishes it from the other types of angina.

Compare and Contrast
CHEST PAIN, CHEST PAIN, CHEST PAIN

Not all chest pain means heart attack, although in a culture in which almost 40% of all deaths are related to cardiovascular disease, it seems logical to jump to that conclusion. What follows is a comparison of types of chest pain with some indications for what might be heart attack and what probably is not. It is important to point out, however, that heart attack symptoms are notoriously variable and it is *always* a good idea to consult a health care professional when the source of chest pain is not clear.

ANGINA

Duration
Chest pain lasts several minutes, and then subsides.

Trigger
Chest pain is usually triggered by activity.

Activity
Chest pain stops when activity stops.

Causes
Chest pain is caused by transient ischemia—the heart muscle doesn't get enough oxygen to function, temporarily.

HEART ATTACK

Duration
Chest pain does not subside within several minutes; in fact, it gets progressively worse.

Trigger
Chest pain may or may not be immediately triggered by activity.

Activity
Chest pain does not stop when activity stops, but continues to get worse.

Causes
Chest pain is caused by permanent ischemia—a blockage deprives cells of oxygen, and the heart is irrevocably damaged.

CHEST PAIN, CHEST PAIN, CHEST PAIN, *continued*

PULMONARY EMBOLISM	OTHER
Duration Chest pain does not subside within several minutes; in fact, it gets progressively worse.	**Duration** Chest pain subsides in less than a minute.
Trigger Chest pain may or may not be immediately triggered by activity.	**Trigger** Chest pain may or may not be immediately triggered by activity.
Activity Chest pain does not stop when activity stops, but continues to get worse.	**Activity** Chest pain stops when the person drinks water, changes position, or takes a deep breath.
Causes Chest pain is caused by a blood clot in the lungs. A small clot may have little impact. A large clot may lead to pulmonary and circulatory collapse.	**Causes** Chest pain is caused by any number of factors, including musculoskeletal injury, or gastroesophageal reflux.

Complications

Several of these conditions are expounded on elsewhere in this chapter; diseases of the cardiovascular system are highly interrelated. Furthermore, with heart disease it is hard to say what comes first: the infarct or the thrombus. In other words, the chronology of how these problems develop is often circular, rather than linear.

- *Embolism.* A heart attack can cause blood clots to form in the heart itself, which then exit through the aorta and travel to wherever the bloodstream takes them; these are arterial emboli, and they can land in the brain, causing a *stroke* (Chapter 3), or the renal arteries, where they can contribute to *renal failure* (Chapter 9). Prolonged bed rest can also promote *deep vein thrombosis* (this chapter), which then carries a risk for pulmonary embolism (see *embolism, thrombus*, this chapter). Pulmonary embolism also may occur if clots form on the right side of the heart and are carried out by the pulmonary artery.

- *Atrial and ventricular fibrillations:* These are rapid, incomplete, and weak attempts at contraction of the chambers. They occur most often if any part of the sinoatrial node, the heart's electrical "pacemaker," has been damaged. These inefficient contractions allow blood to pool and thicken in the chambers of the heart and may contribute to the risk of stroke from the left side, or pulmonary embolism from the right side. Ventricular fibrillations, because they interfere with blood flow to the entire body, may result in death if they are not treated quickly.

- *Aneurysm.* Weakened cardiac tissue can create a bulge in the heart muscle itself similar to aortic *aneurysms* (this chapter).

- *Heart failure.* Heart failure means that the muscle is no longer strong enough to do its work, and the body pays the price. See *heart failure*, this chapter.

- *Shock.* In shock, the circulatory system swings reactively from a sympathetic to a parasympathetic state, opening all of the arteries to a maximum diameter in the process. The main danger with shock is loss of blood to the brain from radically decreased blood pressure.

Diagnosis

With all the new technologies that have been developed to deal with cardiovascular disease, the ability to identify and treat heart attacks *before* damage occurs is extraordinarily limited. Most of the time, the best that can be done is to wait until the heart attack is over, and then take stock of the damage.

Screening for high-risk patients is usually conducted by angiogram: a flexible catheter is inserted into the femoral artery and snaked up to the coronary arteries. A contrast dye is injected into the artery and pictures are taken to see how blood flows through occluded sections. Unfortunately, this is an invasive procedure whose accuracy is somewhat limited. Although it can give useful information about arterial diameter, it does not measure risk for heart attack.

Much emphasis is currently being put on imaging techniques that will help to identify who is at most risk for having a heart attack, and where that risk will come from, *before* the heart is irrevocably damaged. Among the options that are becoming available are high-speed CT scans of the coronary arteries, contrast echocardiograms, blood tests for C-reactive protein (an enzyme associated with inflammation), and MRIs that can examine not only where plaques have developed, but how dense they are, and how deeply they penetrate into arterial walls.

Treatment

The first priority with heart attack patients is to identify where the blockage is, and to get rid of it as quickly as possible. This is done with clot-dissolving drugs, which can take effect in 90 minutes or less, and with immediate balloon angioplasty, which can open up most clogged arteries in approximately an hour. The technical term for this procedure is **percutaneous transluminal coronary angioplasty**, or PTCA. Other immediate care options include the administration of oxygen and pain management with nitroglycerin or morphine.

Later care usually includes more clot-dissolvers, and nitroglycerin, which works to relax the smooth muscle tissue in the arteries. After the emergency has passed, the main treatment for heart attacks is observation. A barrage of tests is conducted to determine the location and extent of damage to the cardiac muscle. These tests will then indicate one of three future courses of action: that the infarct was minor and requires no further medical intervention; that prescriptive anticoagulants are indicated; or that a serious and permanent narrowing of a coronary artery requires surgery to open and repair it. This surgery may be a more complete version of the angioplasty, or it may be coronary bypass surgery in which damaged sections of the coronary artery are replaced with grafts of healthy vessels from elsewhere in the body.

Treatment in heart attack and heart surgery recovery also must embrace the lifestyle changes that will support a healthier future: eating sensibly, exercising regularly, controlling high blood pressure, and quitting smoking are the most important factors.

Some studies have indicated that taking aspirin regularly can decrease the chance of a repeat heart attack for people with a history of heart disease. Specially coated tablets have been designed to minimize gastrointestinal problems, but this intervention carries a slight possibility of an increased chance of subdural hemorrhage, so patients must consider carefully all the implications of taking aspirin on a daily basis.

Massage?

The appropriateness of massage for heart attack survivors absolutely depends on the individual, the extent of the damage they survived, and how long ago it occurred. Some survivors of mild heart attacks may make themselves healthier than they ever were before, whereas others will accumulate high levels of plaque on their arteries within just a few years of surgery. The safety of circulatory massage depends on how easily the client can withstand those changes in internal environment that this work will bring about.

Case History 4.2

Heart Attack

Bob, Age 49: "The Wake-Up Call"

About 15 years ago my mom, who was 60 years old, had bypass surgery. I knew that having a female relative diagnosed with cardiovascular disease at 60 years old put me in a high-risk category for heart problems, especially since I've had type 2 diabetes for about 10 years. I know I didn't eat the healthiest diet in the world. At that time, my regular lunch was a quarter-pounder and a bag of fries.

Last summer my mother went through a series of angina attacks followed by an angioplasty and having a stent inserted. After watching her, I began to seriously think of my own condition. I talked to my doctor, and he set me up with a low-cost on-site stress test that just used an exercise bike. He said if I could pass that I'd be okay. I took it, and in the words of the technician, "my heart was not happy with what I was doing to it." So my doctor scheduled me with a cardiologist for a full treadmill test.

After that first test, I went out for what I knew would be my last double quarter-pounder with cheese.

I didn't last long on the treadmill. When it was over, my blood pressure dropped and I had some really unpleasant symptoms, like dizziness, nausea, and a general feeling of crappiness. My doctor called my wife in from the waiting room and with both of us together he said, "My recommendation is to put you in the hospital now. We'll do an angiogram along with anything else that needs to be done."

"Well," I said, "I have a couple of things I need to finish up. Can I take care of them and come right back?"

"I'd rather you didn't."

I checked right in.

I went into the hospital the Tuesday after Labor Day. On Wednesday, I had the angiogram followed by an angioplasty. They found that the main section of the left coronary artery was 100% blocked. They had trouble pushing a wire through it, but when they got that done, they put in the balloon, and then a titanium stent. (They said it wouldn't set anything off, but I can't get into Target anymore without having all the alarms go off.)

They told me that they found evidence of a recent heart attack—one that was a fraction of an inch away from what they call a "widow-maker." This was amazing to me, because I have no memory of any chest pains. The only thing I can remember was when I went on a trip with my family at the beginning of the summer. I'd hiked around a little that day. That night in the motel I had a migraine headache. I felt sick, and threw up. I took some ibuprofen and went to bed. That's the only time I can think of that I had any symptoms at all.

Three days after the angioplasty, I went home. They started my cardiac rehab right away. I go to the hospital to exercise under supervision. I am next door to an emergency room, and medical staff is in the room with me, so if anything happens, the response time will be really quick. When I first started, I was hooked up to a heart monitor with four patches to measure my blood pressure before, during, and after my exercise. The first time I tried to exercise, they made me quit because I was about to go into ventricular fibrillation. Now I go exercise three times a week. I use the treadmill, the bike, weight machines, and free weights. I walk a lot at work, but I can't walk at home; it's too steep around my house. My doctors tell me I can't ever let my heart rate get over 120 beats per minute. If it gets any higher than that, I run the risk of forming clots around the stent.

Heart Attack, *continued*

I'm on several medications now. Some control my diabetes (I don't take insulin), and I'm also taking anticoagulants for 3 months, along with beta blockers, and calcium channel blockers. And of course I've changed my diet. I eat so much chicken I feel like I'm growing feathers. It's all baked or grilled, and I take off the skin. We have little or no fried food, so no more french fries. Since I've made these changes my blood glucose has been much more under control—I average about 115 now, and normal is anywhere from 80 to 120.

This episode was a real wake-up call for me. I'm the youngest man at my job, and the last one they expected to have heart trouble. My identical twin went in for his own stress test and came back fine, but he was a couple of years later than me in developing his diabetes too, so he'll still have to keep an eye on it. I did some research about my situation and I found that what I had—silent ischemia—is especially common in diabetic men over 40. I hope any man with type 2 diabetes over 40 or 45 will be sure to get his heart checked. You never know what you might find.

Other Heart Conditions

Heart murmurs
The heart can make several types of noises during its contractions. These are referred to as murmurs. They often, but not always, point to some type of valvular dysfunction within the heart. A client with a persistent heart murmur may have an inefficient pump and may not be able to keep up with rigorous circulatory massage.

Angina pectoris
Literally "chest pain," this is a description of the symptoms that can occur when the heart muscle does not receive adequate oxygen. Angina pectoris is frequently a consequence of coronary arteries that are severely occluded, but other possible causes of chest pain include severe anemia or hyperthyroidism. This condition may involve severe pain or a feeling of heavy pressure around the chest, left shoulder, and arm and into the jaw and back.

Angina is typically brought on by periods of extreme stress or exertion and is relieved by rest and drugs that dilate coronary vessels (nitroglycerin) and that reduce heart rate (beta-blockers), among others.

Angina itself does not imply that a heart attack is happening; however, it does suggest cardiovascular problems that may put a person at risk for myocardial infarction.

Hypertrophy of the heart
This condition, which is seen most dramatically in the left ventricle, is brought about by chronically high systemic pressure in the blood vessels. If the heart has to fight against constricted arteries to push blood through the body, it will hypertrophy, or grow larger. It may increase in strength as well, for a while, but as the need for oxygen outgrows the supply from the coronary arteries, the tissue will eventually experience ischemia, possible myocardial infarction, and eventually congestive heart failure.

Congenital heart problems
Thirty-five different structural problems may affect the heart at birth, most of them focusing around valve function. Approximately 32,000 people a year are born with these problems, although new surgical techniques with infants (and even babies still in utero) are making it rarer and rarer to see adults with debilitating congenital heart defects.

Rheumatic fever
Rheumatic fever is an autoimmune complication of exposure to streptococcus in which antibodies attack the heart valves, especially the mitral valve. It affects approximately 1.3 million Americans, and is responsible for close to 6,000 deaths per year. Mitral valve damage will affect the way the heart can pump blood through the body. It can lead to arterial emboli or congestive heart failure.

Infectious diseases of the heart
Different varieties of streptococcus may prey on endocardium. If they find a way in (which can happen from something as innocuous as an abscessed tooth but is more often a complication of open heart surgery), they will *also* cause clots that are then released into the arterial system.

Massage?
Most of these conditions systemically contraindicate circulatory massage. Work that mechanically pushes fluid through the system will hinder, rather than help, these damaged structures.

Heart Failure in Brief

What is it?
Heart failure is a condition in which the heart no longer can function well enough to keep up with the needs of the body. It is usually slowly progressive, developing over a number of years before any changes in function may be noticeable.

How is it recognized?
Different symptoms are present, depending on which side of the heart is working inefficiently. Left-sided heart failure results in fluid congestion in the lungs with general weakness and shortness of breath. Right-sided heart failure results in fluid backups throughout the system, which shows as edema especially in the ankles and legs. Both varieties of heart failure will lead to chest pain, cold, sweaty skin, a fast, irregular pulse, coughing, especially when the person is lying down, and very low stamina.

Is massage indicated or contraindicated?
Circulatory massage is inappropriate for clients with heart failure, as it has the goal of pushing fluid through a system that is incapable of adjusting to those changes. Energetic work may be more appropriate to help clients lower stress and cope with the challenges of severely restricted circulation.

Heart Failure

Definition: What Is It?

Heart failure is a term for the progressive loss of cardiac function that accompanies age and a history or cardiovascular disease. It does *not* mean that the heart has stopped working altogether (that would be "cardiac arrest"); it simply means that the heart cannot keep up with the needs of the body.

💿 *The animation "Congestive Heart Failure" can be found on the Student Resource CD-ROM that accompanies this book.*

Demographics: Who Gets It?

The statistics on the incidence of heart failure in the United States are alarming but understandable, considering the changes in the health profile of the current population. Heart failure is on a dramatic rise in this country; it currently affects approximately 5 million people, and is expected to rise to 15 to 20 million people within the next 5 years. Approximately 400,000 new cases are diagnosed every year. Most of those cases are among people who have survived other cardiovascular crises: heart attacks, coronary artery disease, aneurysm, and others. Whereas many years ago these problems would have killed these patients, they now survive and their hearts simply wear out from progressive damage to the cardiovascular system.

More men have heart failure than women, and it affects black men approximately twice as often as whites. The incidence for heart failure rises dramatically with age: it affects approximately 1% of the population at age 50, and up to 5% of the population aged 75 years and older. Acute decompensated heart failure accounts for roughly 1 million hospitalizations per year.

Etiology: What Happens?

When the heart is asked to pump 2,000 gallons of blood each day through vessels that are progressively narrowed and resistant, it goes through a series of changes that ultimately limit its ability to function. Unfortunately, the heart will enter early stages of heart failure with no signs or symptoms.

As resistance in the cardiovascular system increases, the heart seems to grow; the muscle becomes bigger and the myocardial fibers thicken to overcome vascular narrowing. When this compensation is no longer adequate (this is "decompensated heart failure"), the heart begins to beat faster, pushing less blood with each contraction. Finally, the muscle simply wears out and functions so inefficiently that blood flow to the rest of the body is insufficient for the most basic kinds of activities: climbing a set of stairs, walking across a room, even getting out of bed.

Most cases of heart failure are related to underlying cardiovascular disease. A history of atherosclerosis or heart attack with resulting scar tissue in the heart muscle increases the risk of developing heart failure. High blood pressure, untreated *diabetes* (see Chapter 8), smoking, alcohol, and drug abuse can all be contributing factors as well. An especially potent setup for heart failure is any combination of these risk factors: uncontrolled high blood pressure along with smoking, for instance.

A smaller number of heart failure patients do not have a history of cardiovascular disease but have sustained damage to the heart muscle for other reasons. Cardiomyopathy, valve diseases, infections of the valves or heart muscle, or congenital problems may all be factors in these cases.

Types of Heart Failure

Heart failure is classified according to which side of the heart is affected. Signs, symptoms, and possible complications vary according to which side of the heart is worn out the most.

- *Left-sided heart failure.* In this situation, resistance in the systemic circuit leads to a backup in the pulmonary circuit, and the seepage of fluid back into the alveoli. This condition, if it becomes severe and is not corrected, results in pulmonary edema (Figure 4.16). Symptoms of left-sided heart failure include severe shortness of breath and stubborn coughing, perhaps with bloody sputum. One serious complication of this condition is the risk of *pneumonia* (Chapter 6) in the functionally impaired lungs.

- *Right-sided heart failure.* In the absence of left heart failure, this is called ***cor pulmonale.*** It commonly results from pulmonary disease and high vascular resistance

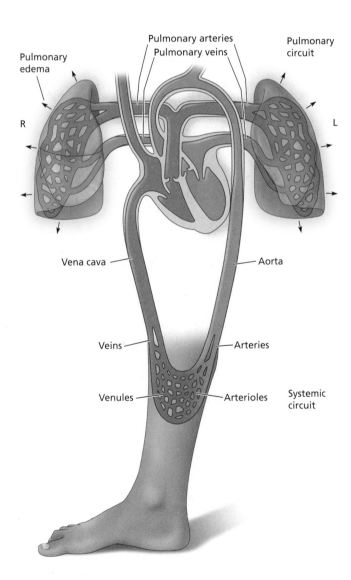

Figure 4.16. Left-sided heart failure leads to pulmonary edema.

in the lungs (see *chronic bronchitis* and *emphysema*, Chapter 6). In other words, it becomes difficult to pump blood through the pulmonary circuit. Here the backup is felt through the rest of the body. Symptoms include severe *edema* (Chapter 5), especially in the legs (Figure 4.17). Someone with this type of heart failure has ankles that look like they are spilling over the sides of her shoes. If the patient is bedridden, the edema may occur in the abdomen or low back: wherever gravity is pulling most. Right-sided heart failure is also closely linked to enlarged liver (**hepatomegaly**) and *renal failure* (see Chapter 9); as blood flow to the kidneys is reduced, the kidneys begin to retain water, which systemically increases blood pressure and makes the heart work even harder to push blood through narrow tubes.

- *Biventricular heart failure*. This is both left- and ride-sided failure simultaneously. It is the end stage of the disease, and if the patient does not respond to medications, he or she may be a candidate for a heart transplant or other surgery.

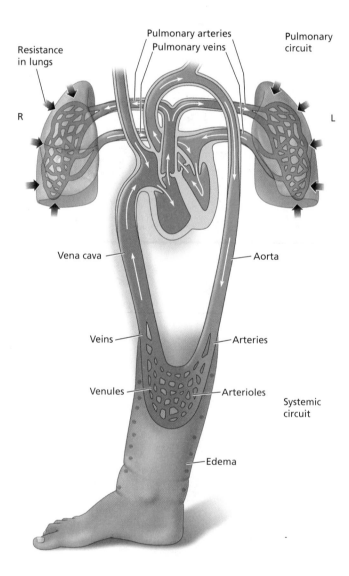

Figure 4.17. Right-sided heart failure leads to systemic edema.

Signs and Symptoms

Signs of heart failure depend on which side of the heart is dysfunctional, as described above. Along with shortness of breath (this is often exacerbated by lying down), low stamina, and distal edema, heart failure patients may also experience chronic chest pain, indigestion, arrhythmia, visibly distended veins in the neck, cold, sweaty skin, and restlessness.

Diagnosis

Heart failure is not difficult to diagnose. It is often done through observation of systemic edema and *auscultation*: listening to heart sounds, and to the lungs for indications of fluid retention. An x-ray may be required to look for cardiac enlargement, and an electrocardiogram may be conducted to analyze the efficiency of the heartbeat. An *echocardiogram* can show valve function if damage to these structures is suspected.

Treatment

The treatment options for heart failure depend on how severe it is, and which side of the heart has been affected. Early interventions include rest, changes in diet, and modifications in physical activity so that the heart can be exercised without becoming overly stressed. Drugs for heart failure may include beta-blockers, digitalis, diuretics, and vasodilators.

If a patient does not respond well to these noninvasive treatment options, surgery may be considered. Surgery can range anywhere from repair to damaged valves to wrapping a strong mesh bag around the heart, to a complete heart or heart-and-lung transplantation.

Massage?

Heart failure means that the heart cannot function in a way that provides for essential needs. Most heart failure patients have other cardiovascular problems that contribute to their disease. Circulatory massage, which works with the intention of mechanically increasing blood flow through a basically healthy system, is inappropriate for clients whose blood vessels and heart cannot accommodate these changes in internal environment.

Energetic work that invites (rather than forces) the body to positive change may help to reduce blood pressure and perceived stress, and so may be useful for heart failure patients, although it is not realistic to claim that massage can undo the extensive damage seen with these clients.

CHAPTER REVIEW QUESTIONS

1. Describe the process of the development of atherosclerosis.

2. Why are fatigue and low stamina signs of anemia?

3. Where do all emboli from the venous side of the systemic circuit go? Why?

4. Name three places arterial emboli can go to cause significant damage.

5. Heart attacks involve blockages where: in the heart itself, or in the coronary arteries?

6. What is a term for uncoordinated contractions of heart chambers?

7. Why is hypertension called "The Silent Killer"?

8. Describe the relationship between high blood pressure and kidney dysfunction.

9. Describe how a person may experience any three of the following conditions at the same time: high blood pressure, chronic renal failure, edema, atherosclerosis, diabetes, aortic aneurysm, stroke.

10. A client has ropy, distended varicose veins on the medial aspect of the right knee. Distal to the knee the tissue is clammy and slightly edematous. Pressing at the ankle leaves a dimple, which takes several minutes to disappear. What cautions must be exercised with this client? Why?

 Answers to these questions can be found on the Student Recource CD-ROM that accompanies this book.

Bibliography

General Resources, Circulatory System Conditions

1. de Dominico G, Wood E. Beard's Massage. Philadelphia: WB Saunders, 1997.
2. Damjanou I. Pathology for the Health-Related Professions. Philadelphia: WB Saunders, 1996.
3. Travell J, Simons DG. Myofascial Pain and Dysfunction: The Trigger Point Manual. Baltimore: Williams & Wilkins, 1983.
4. Clemente CD. Anatomy: A Regional Atlas of the Human Body. 3rd Ed. Baltimore: Urban & Schwarzenburg, 1987.
5. Tortora GJ, Anagnostakos NP. Principles of Anatomy and Physiology. 6th Ed. New York: Harper & Row, 1990.
6. Taber's Cyclopedic Dictionary. 14th Ed. Philadelphia: FA Davis, 1981.
7. Stedman's Medical Dictionary. 26th Ed. Baltimore: Williams & Wilkins, 1995.
8. Memmler RL, Wood DL. The Human Body in Health and Disease. 5th Ed. Philadelphia: JB Lippincott, 1983.
9. Juhan D. Job's Body: A Handbook for Bodywork. Barrytown, NY: Station Hill Press, 1987.
10. Kunz JRM, Finkel AJ, eds. The American Medical Association Family Medical Guide. New York, NY: Random House, 1987.
11. Marieb EM. Human Anatomy and Physiology. Redwood City, CA: Benjamin/Cummings, 1989.
12. Field T. Touch Therapy. London: Churchill Livingstone, 2000.

Anemia

1. Aplastic Anemia. Harvard Medical School. Available at: http://www.intelihealth.com/IH/ihtPrint/WSIHW000/9339/408/228842.html?d=dmtHealthAZ&hide=t&k=basePrint. Accessed winter 2003.
2. Sickle-Cell Anemia. Harvard Medical School. Available at: http://www.intelihealth.com/IH/ihtPrint/WSIHW000/9339/408/195959.html?d=dmtHealthAZ&hide=t&k=basePrint. Accessed winter 2003.
3. JAMA Patient Page: Facts About Sickle Cell Anemia. Copyright Copyright © 1999 American Medical Association. Available at: http://www.medem.com/search/article_display_for_printer.cfm?path=\\TANQUERAY\M_ContentItem&mstr=/M_ContentItem/ZZZWUBQQJAC.html&soc=JAMA/Archives&srch_typ=NAV_SERCH. Accessed winter 2003.
4. Anemia Overview. Copyright © 1998–2003 Mayo Foundation for Medical Education and Research (MFMER). Available at: http://www.mayoclinic.com/invoke.cfm?id=DS00321. Accessed winter 2003.
5. Aplastic Anemia Overview. Copyright © 1998–2003 Mayo Foundation for Medical Education and Research (MFMER). Available at: http://www.mayoclinic.com/invoke.cfm?id=DS00322. Accessed winter 2003.
6. Myelofibrosis. Copyright © 1998–2003 Mayo Foundation for Medical Education and Research (MFMER). Available at: http://www.mayoclinic.com/invoke.cfm?id=AN00474. Accessed winter 2003.
7. Polycythemia. Copyright © 1998–2003 Mayo Foundation for Medical Education and Research (MFMER). Available at: http://www.mayoclinic.com/invoke.cfm?id=HQ01231. Accessed winter 2003.
8. Anemia. Copyright © 1996–2004 MedicineNet, Inc. Available at: http://www.medicinenet.com/Anemia/article.htm. Accessed winter 2003.
9. Pernicious Anemia. Copyright © 1996–2004 MedicineNet, Inc. Available at: http://www.medicinenet.com/Pernicious_Anemia/article.htm. Accessed winter 2003.
10. Anemia. Merck Manual. Available at: http://www.merck.com/pubs/mmanual_home2/sec14/ch172/ch172a.htm. Accessed winter 2003.

Embolism Thrombus

1. Ask The Expert. James Louis Januzzi, Jr., M.D. Available at: http://www.intelihealth.com/IH/ihtPrint/WSIHW000/9339/8481/313327.html?d=dmtATD&hide=t&k=basePrint. Accessed winter 2003.
2. Atrial Fibrillation. Harvard Medical School. Available at: http://www.intelihealth.com/IH/ihtPrint/WSIHW000/9339/408/213152.html?d=dmtHealthAZ&hide=t&k=basePrint. Accessed winter 2003.
3. JAMA Patient Page Pulmonary Embolism. Copyright © 2001 American Medical Association. Available at: http://www.medem.com/medlb/article_detaillb_for_printe

r.cfm?article_ID=ZZZDQHMZUIC&sub_cat=575. Accessed winter 2003.

4. Heart Arrhythmias Overview. Copyright © 1998–2003 Mayo Foundation for Medical Education and Research (MFMER). Available at: http://www.mayoclinic.com/invoke.cfm?id=DS00290. Accessed winter 2003.

5. Pulmonary Embolism Overview. Copyright © 1998–2003 Mayo Foundation for Medical Education and Research (MFMER). Available at: http://www.mayoclinic.com/invoke.cfm?id=DS00429. Accessed winter 2003.

6. Pulmonary Hypertension Overview. Copyright © 1998–2003 Mayo Foundation for Medical Education and Research (MFMER). Available at: http://www.mayoclinic.com/invoke.cfm?id=DS00430. Accessed winter 2003.

7. What is a deep vein thrombosis and a pulmonary embolism? Copyright © 1996–2003 MedicineNet, Inc. Available at: www.medicinenet.com/Deep_Vein_Thrombosis. Accessed winter 2003.

8. The Merck Manual of Diagnosis and Therapy. Section 6. Pulmonary Disorders. Chapter 72. Pulmonary Embolism. Available at: http://www.merck.com/mrkshared/mmanual/section6/chapter72/72a.jsp. Accessed winter 2003.

Hemophilia

1. Factor XI Deficiency (Hemophilia C, plasma thromboplastic antecedent or Rosenthal Syndrome). National Hemophilia Foundation. Available at: http://www.hemophilia.org/bdi/bdi_types9.htm. Accessed winter 2003.

2. Hemophilia. NHLBI (National Heart, Lung, and Blood Institute, NIH (National Institutes of Health. Available at: http://www.nhlbi.nih.gov/health/public/blood/other/hemophel.htm. Accessed winter 2003.

3. Hemophilia A (Factor VIII Deficiency). National Hemophilia Foundation. Available at: http://www.hemophilia.org/bdi/bdi_types1.htm. Accessed winter 2003.

4. Hemophilia B (Factor IX Deficiency). National Hemophilia Foundation. Available at: http://www.hemophilia.org/bdi/bdi_types2.htm. Accessed winter 2003.

5. Hemophilia, Overview. Dimitrios P Agaliotis, MD. Copyright © 2003, eMedicine.com, Inc. Available at: http://www.emedicine.com/med/topic3528.htm. Accessed winter 2003.

6. Hemophilia Overview. Copyright © 1998–2003 Mayo Foundation for Medical Education and Research (MFMER). Available at: http://www.mayoclinic.com/invoke.cfm?id=DS00218. Accessed winter 2003.

7. Factor XIII deficiency. Copyright © 1998–2003 Mayo Foundation for Medical Education and Research (MFMER).

Available at: http://www.mayoclinic.com/invoke.cfm?id=AN00508. Accessed winter 2003.

8. Bernard-Soulier Syndrome. Available at: http://www.medicinenet.com/Bernard-Soulier_Disease/article.htm. Accessed winter 2003.

Leukemia

1. What You Need To Know About™ Leukemia. Available at: http://www.nci.nih.gov/templates/page_print.aspx?viewid=57b3abc6-4b52-41b0-8762-9372062313de. Accessed winter 2003.

2. Leukemia Facts 2003. Copyright © 2003–2004 The Leukemia & Lymphoma Society. Available at: http://www.leukemia-lymphoma.org/all_mat_detail.adp?item_id=87311&sort_order=3&cat_id=1204. Accessed winter 2003.

3. Leukemia. Harvard Medical School. Available at: http://www.intelihealth.com/IH/ihtPrint/WSIHW000/9339/408/216748.html?d=dmtHealthAZ&hide=t&k=basePrint. Accessed winter 2003.

4. Leukemia Facts & Statistics. Copyright © 2003–2004 The Leukemia & Lymphoma Society. Available at: http://www.leukemia.org/all_page?item_id=12486. Accessed winter 2003.

5. Leukemia Classifications—What is Leukemia? Available at: http://www.cancer.org/docroot/CRI/content/CRI_2_6X_Leukemia_Classifications_24.asp. Accessed winter 2003.

6. Chronic lymphocytic leukemia. Copyright © 1998–2003 Mayo Foundation for Medical Education and Research (MFMER). Available at: http://www.mayoclinic.com/invoke.cfm?id=AN00191. Accessed winter 2003.

7. Leukemia Overview. Copyright © 1998–2003 Mayo Foundation for Medical Education and Research (MFMER). Available at: http://www.mayoclinic.com/invoke.cfm?id=DS00351. Accessed winter 2003.

8. The Different Types of Leukemia. Copyright © 2003 American Cancer Society, Inc. Available at: http://www.cancer.org/docroot/CRI/content/CRI_2_2_1X_The_different_types_of_leukemia_62.asp?sitearea=. Accessed winter 2003.

Deep Vein Thrombosis

1. Cardiology Patient Page—Pulmonary Embolism and Deep Vein Thrombosis. Samuel Z. Goldhaber, MD; Ruth B. Morrison, RN, BSN, CVN. Available at: http://circ.ahajournals.org/cgi/reprint/106/12/1436.pdf. Accessed winter 2003.

2. Thrombophlebitis. Harvard Medical School. Available at: http://www.intelihealth.com/IH/ihtPrint/WSIHW000/9339/408/201930.html?d=dmtHealthAZ&hide=t&k=basePrint. Accessed winter 2003.

3. Treatment of Thrombosis—Deep venous thrombosis. Copyright © 1996–1999 by the American College of Surgeons, Chicago, IL. Available at: http://www.facs.org/jacs/articles/sumpioend.html. Accessed winter 2003.

4. Thrombophlebitis Overview. Copyright © 1998–2003 Mayo Foundation for Medical Education and Research (MFMER). Available at: http://www.mayoclinic.com/invoke.cfm?id=DS00223. Accessed winter 2003.

5. Deep Vein Thrombosis and Pulmonary Embolism. Copyright © 1996–2004 MedicineNet, Inc. Available at: http:// www.medicinenet.com/Deep_Vein_Thrombosis/article.htm. Accessed winter 2003.

Aneurysm

1. Aneurysm, Brain. William R Fraser, DO. Copyright © 2003, eMedicine.com, Inc. Available at: http://www.emedicine.com/aaem/topic17.htm. Accessed winter 2003.

2. Aneurysm, Abdominal. Robert O'Connor, MD, MPH. Copyright © 2003, eMedicine.com, Inc. Available at: http://www.emedicine.com/emerg/topic27.htm. Accessed winter 2003.

3. Aneurysm, Great Vessels. Bryan Hoynak, MD. Copyright © 2003, eMedicine.com, Inc. Available at: http://www.emedicine.com/aaem/topic18.htm. Accessed winter 2003.

4. Aneurysms. Copyright © 1996-2003 Texas Heart Institute. Available at: http://www.tmc.edu/thi/aneurysm.html. Accessed winter 2003.

5. Aortic Aneurysm. Harvard Medical School. Available at: http://www.intelihealth.com/IH/ihtPrint/WSIHW000/9339/31040.html?hide=t&k=basePrint. Accessed winter 2003.

6. Aortic Aneurysm Overview. Copyright © 1998–2003 Mayo Foundation for Medical Education and Research (MFMER). Available at: http://www.mayoclinic.com/invoke.cfm?id=DS00017. Accessed winter 2003.

7. Thoracic aortic aneurysm. Allan S. Stewart, M.D., Department of Surgery, University of Pennsylvania Medical Center, Philadelphia, PA. NLM (National Library of Medicine), NIH (National Institutes of Health). Copyright © 2002 A.D.A.M., Inc. Available at: http://www.nlm.nih.gov/medlineplus/ency/article/001119.htm. Accessed winter 2003.

Atherosclerosis

1. Plasma fatty acid composition and depression are associated in the elderly: the Rotterdam Study. Tiemeier H, van Tuijl HR, Hofman A, et al. Available at: http://www.ncbi.nlm.nih.gov/entrez/query.fcgi?cmd=Retrieve&db=PubMed&list_uids=12816769&dopt=Abstract. Accessed winter 2003.

2. Atherosclerosis. James L Orford, MBChB; Andrew P Selwyn, MD. Copyright © 2003, eMedicine.com, Inc. Available at: http://www.emedicine.com/med/topic182.htm. Accessed winter 2003.

3. Cholesterol. Copyright © 1996–2003 Texas Heart Institute. Available at: http://www.tmc.edu/thi/choleste.html. Accessed winter 2003.

4. Heart Disease and Stroke: The Nation's Leading Killers—The Burden of Heart Disease and Stroke. Centers for Disease Control and Prevention, National Center for Chronic Disease Prevention and Health Promotion. Available at: http://www.cdc.gov/nccdphp/aag/aag_cvd.htm. Accessed winter 2003.

5. Atherosclerosis. Harvard Medical School. Available at: http://www.intelihealth.com/IH/ihtPrint/WSIHW000/9339/408/221482.html?d=dmtHealthAZ&hide=t&k=basePrint. Accessed winter 2003.

6. Coronary Artery Disease. Harvard Medical School. Available at: http://www.intelihealth.com/IH/ihtPrint/WSIHW000/9339/408/216672.html?d=dmtHealthAZ&hide=t&k=basePrint. Accessed winter 2003.

7. JAMA Patient Page: Cholesterol and Atherosclerosis. Copyright © 2001 American Medical Association. Available at: http://www.medem.com/search/article_display_for_printer.cfm?path=\\TANQUERAY\M_ContentItem&mstr=/M_ContentItem/ZZZ2ONRXHMC.html&soc=JAMA/Archives&srch_typ=NAV_SERCH. Accessed winter 2003.

8. Blood tests: Seeking clues about your heart's health. Copyright © 1998–2003 Mayo Foundation for Medical Education and Research (MFMER). Available at: http://www.mayoclinic.com/invoke.cfm?id=HB00016. Accessed winter 2003.

9. Cardiovascular disease: A blueprint for understanding the leading killer. Copyright © 1998-2003 Mayo Foundation for Medical Education and Research (MFMER). Available at: http://www.mayoclinic.com/invoke.cfm?id=HB00032. Accessed winter 2003.

10. Chest Pain Overview. Copyright © 1998–2003 Mayo Foundation for Medical Education and Research (MFMER). Available at: http://www.mayoclinic.com/invoke.cfm?id=DS00016. Accessed winter 2003.

Hypertension

1. What Is High Blood Pressure? Available at: http://dci.nhlbi.nih.gov/Diseases/Hbp/HBP_WhatIs.html. Accessed winter 2003.

2. About High Blood Pressure. Copyright ©2002 American Heart Association, Inc. Available at: http://www.americanheart.org/presenter.jhtml?identifier=2152. Accessed winter 2003.

3. Essential Guide to Hypertension: Hypertension in Special Groups. Copyright © 1998 American Medical Association. Available at: http://www.medem.com/search/article_display_for_printer.cfm?path=\\TANQUERAY\M_ContentItem&mstr=/M_ContentItem/ZZZT9VFDJMC.html&soc=AMA&srch_typ=NAV_SERCH. Accessed winter 2003.

4. High Blood Pressure Statistics. Copyright © 2002 American Heart Association, Inc. Available at: http://www.americanheart.org/presenter.jhtml?identifier=4621. Accessed winter 2003.

5. High Blood Pressure (Hypertension). Harvard Medical School. Available at: http://www.intelihealth.com/IH/ihtPrint/WSIHW000/8059/11159/195803.html?d=dmtHealthAZ&hide=t&k=basePrint. Accessed winter 2003.

6. Secondary Hypertension. Harvard Medical School. Available at: http://www.intelihealth.com/IH/ihtPrint/WSIHW000/8059/11159/197427.html?d=dmtHealthAZ&hide=t&k=basePrint. Accessed winter 2003.

7. High Blood Pressure Overview. Copyright © 1998–2003 Mayo Foundation for Medical Education and Research (MFMER). Available at: http://www.mayoclinic.com/invoke.cfm?id=DS00100. Accessed winter 2003.

8. High blood pressure definitions. Copyright © 1998–2003 Mayo Foundation for Medical Education and Research (MFMER). Available at: http://www.mayoclinic.com/invoke.cfm?id=HI00031. Accessed winter 2003.

9. Medical conditions that cause secondary hypertension. Copyright © 1998–2003 Mayo Foundation for Medical Education and Research (MFMER). Available at: http://www.mayoclinic.com/invoke.cfm?id=HQ01345. Accessed winter 2003.

10. The "Dash" Eating Plan (Dietary Approaches to Stop Hypertension). NIH (National Institutes of Health), NHLBI (National Heart, Lung, and Blood Institute. Available at: http://www.nhlbi.nih.gov/health/public/heart/hbp/dash/new_dash.pdf. Accessed winter 2003.

Raynaud's Syndrome

1. Raynaud Phenomenon. Jeffrey R. Lisse, MD, FACP. Copyright © 2003, eMedicine.com, Inc. Available at: http://www.emedicine.com/med/topic1993.htm. Accessed winter 2003.

2. Raynaud's Phenomenon. Harvard Medical School. Available at: http://www.intelihealth.com/IH/ihtPrint/WSIHW000/9339/10964.html?hide=t&k=basePrint. Accessed winter 2003.

3. Raynaud's Disease Overview. Copyright © 1998–2003 Mayo Foundation for Medical Education and Research (MFMER). Available at:

http://www.mayoclinic.com/invoke.cfm?id=DS00433. Accessed winter 2003.

Varicose Veins

1. Varicose Veins. Harvard Medical School. Available at: http://www.intelihealth.com/IH/ihtPrint/WSIHW000/9339/10960.html?hide=t&k=basePrint. Accessed winter 2003.

2. Varicose Veins Overview. Copyright © 1998–2003 Mayo Foundation for Medical Education and Research (MFMER). Available at: http://www.mayoclinic.com/invoke.cfm?id=DS00256. Accessed winter 2003.

3. Varicose Veins and Spider Veins. Available at: http://www.4woman.gov/faq/varicose.htm. Accessed winter 2003.

4. Varicose Veins and Spider Veins. Craig Feied, MD, FACEP, FAAEM; Robert Weiss, MD; Robert B Hashemiyoon, MD. Copyright © 2003, eMedicine.com, Inc. Available at: http://www.emedicine.com/derm/topic475.htm. Accessed winter 2003.

Heart Attack

1. Causes of Heart Attack. Harvard Medical School. Available at: http://www.intelihealth.com/IH/ihtPrint/WSIHW000/9339/408/152220.html?d=dmtContent&hide=t&k=basePrint. Accessed winter 2003.

2. Heart Attack (Myocardial Infarction). Harvard Medical School. Available at: http://www.intelihealth.com/IH/ihtPrint/WSIHW000/9339/408/213077.html?d=dmtHealthAZ&hide=t&k=basePrint. Accessed winter 2003.

3. Blood tests: Seeking clues about your heart's health. Copyright © 1998–2003 Mayo Foundation for Medical Education and Research (MFMER). Available at: http://www.mayoclinic.com/invoke.cfm?id5HB00016. Accessed winter 2003.

4. Chest Pain Overview. Copyright © 1998–2003 Mayo Foundation for Medical Education and Research (MFMER). Available at: http://www.mayoclinic.com/invoke.cfm?id=DS00016. Accessed winter 2003.

5. Heart Attack Overview. Copyright © 1998–2003 Mayo Foundation for Medical Education and Research (MFMER). Available at: http://www.mayoclinic.com/invoke.cfm?id5DS00094. Accessed winter 2003.

Heart Failure

1. Heart Failure. Michael E Zevitz, MD. Copyright © 2003, eMedicine.com, Inc. Available at: http://www.emedicine.com/med/topic3552.htm. Accessed winter 2003.

2. Cardiomyopathy. Harvard Medical School. Available at: http://www.intelihealth.com/IH/ihtPrint/WSIHW000/9339/408/213081.html?d5dmtHe

althAZ&hide5t&k5basePrint. Accessed winter 2003.

3. Congestive Heart Failure. Harvard Medical School. Available at: http://www.intelihealth.com/IH/ihtPrint/WSIHW000/9339/9755.html?hide5t&k5basePrint. Accessed winter 2003.

4. Myocarditis. Harvard Medical School.

Available at: http://www.intelihealth.com/IH/ihtPrint/WSIHW000/9339/408/266766.html?d=dmtHealthAZ&hide=t&k=basePrint. Accessed winter 2003.

5. Congestive Heart Failure Overview. Copyright © 1998–2003 Mayo Foundation for Medical Education and Research (MFMER). Available at: http://www.mayoclinic.com/invoke.cfm?id=DS00061. Accessed winter 2003.

6. Heart Disease and Stroke Statistics—2004 Update. Copyright © American Heart Association. Available at: http://www.americanheart.org/downloadable/heart/1072969766940HSStats2004Update.pdf. Accessed winter 2004.

LYMPH AND IMMUNE SYSTEM CONDITIONS

5

Chapter Objectives

After reading this chapter, you should be able to . . .

- Identify the one type of edema that indicates massage.
- Identify three types of edema that contraindicate massage.
- List two types of lymphoma.
- Explain why lymphoma causes anemia.
- Describe one risk of working with clients who have mononucleosis.
- Describe two central nervous system components seen with most chronic fatigue syndrome patients.
- Explain three benefits of not interfering with fever.
- Describe the three stages of HIV infection
- State the most common symptom or complication associated with lupus.
- Describe the four cardinal signs of inflammation.

INTRODUCTION: LYMPH SYSTEM

The lymphatic system is a critically important system for massage practitioners to understand. It is a bit peculiar: its components are not even vaguely symmetric, and it functions as a sort of subsystem to both the circulatory and immune systems. The conditions listed under this heading may be influenced by either of the other two systems. Here is a brief overview of how the lymphatic system works.

Lymph System Structure

As blood travels away from the heart, it goes through progressively smaller tubes—the aorta branches into the arteries, which branch into arterioles, which finally divide into the very tiny and delicate capillaries.

343

The pressure and speed with which blood travels decreases as it gets further away from the heart. Still, everything keeps moving at a good pace; a blood cell can complete its journey through the systemic circuit approximately every 60 seconds.

The walls of the capillaries are made of one-cell-thick squamous epithelium, designed for maximum efficiency of diffusion. The diameter, or lumina, of capillaries is so tiny that the red blood cells must line up one by one to pass through. This is the moment for the transfer of nutrients and wastes in the tissue cells. This is also where, having dropped off oxygen and picked up carbon dioxide, the vessels turn from arterial capillaries into venous capillaries. And finally, this is the moment when fluid from the arterial blood is squeezed out of the capillaries. In other words, *this* is the origin of interstitial fluid.

Interstitial fluid is absolutely vital! It is the medium by which all of the body's nutrients and wastes travel. It needs to keep moving, however; if it stagnates, toxins can accumulate there and cause problems. Interstitial fluid keeps moving through the system by flowing into a different type of capillary: a lymphatic capillary. Lymphatic capillaries are similar to circulatory capillaries in construction, with one major difference: they are part of an *open* system. That is, interstitial fluid and even small particles can flow into lymphatic capillaries at almost any point along the length of that capillary (Figure 5.1). (Circulatory capillaries are *closed* to the extent that red blood cells are *not* able to come and go unless the vessel has been damaged.)

When interstitial fluid is drawn into a lymphatic capillary, it is officially called *lymph*. Lymph is composed mainly of plasma that has been pressed out of the bloodstream, loads of metabolic wastes that have been exuded by hardworking cells, and some chunks of particulate waste as well.

The new lymph is routed to a series of cleaning stations called *nodes*, where the wastes are neutralized and any small particles are filtered out. The nodes are also home to most of the body's specific immune response cells, so if any pathogens have been picked up and marked by macrophages in the lymph, this is where the specific immune response begins. Eventually the cleaned-up fluid is deposited back into the circulatory system; this happens just above the right atrium of the heart where the right and left thoracic ducts empty into the right and left thoracic veins respectively.

Lymph System Function

Lymph flows through the lymphatic capillaries into bigger and bigger vessels, usually against the pull of gravity, and without the aid of the heart's direct pumping action. What moves it along? Several factors contribute:

- *gravity*: gravity helps to move lymph if the limb is elevated;
- *muscle contraction*: when muscle fibers squeeze down around lymphatic vessels, they push fluid through just like a hand squeezes around a tube of toothpaste;
- *alternating hot and cold*: hydrotherapy applications can cause contractions in the smooth muscle tissue of lymphatic vessels to move fluid along;

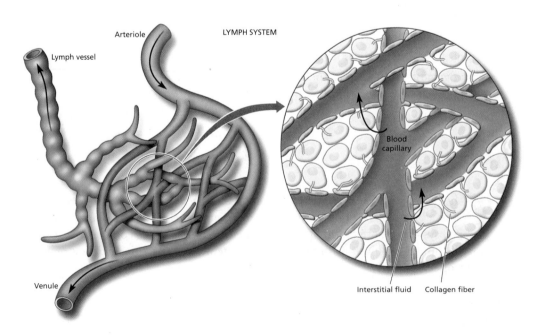

Figure 5.1. The origin of lymph.

- *breathing*: deep breathing draws lymph up the thoracic duct like an expanding bellows during inhalation and squeezes it muscularly during exhalation;

- *massage*: big mechanical manipulative strokes such as pétrissage and deep effleurage can increase lymph flow, but small, extremely superficial reflexive strokes also can cause fluid to be drawn into lymphatic capillaries.

If everything works well, fluid levels in the tissues should be constant, but not stagnant. When plasma leaves the circulatory capillaries to become interstitial fluid, a nearly equivalent amount of fluid is drawn back in. The leftover, approximately 10%, stays between the cells and is eventually drawn into the lymph system; this is called Starling's equilibrium. A back-up anywhere in the system could result in major changes in fluid balance. If lymph vessels or nodes are blocked, for instance, fluid accumulates between tissue cells. The stagnant fluid quickly becomes a hindrance to diffusion and other chemical reactions, rather than the transfer medium it is designed to be. This is the problem with many of the diseases of the lymph system, and this is a serious situation for massage practitioners, who generally should *not* be trying to push fluid through a system that is already overtaxed.

Immune System Function

The immune system is unique in that it is not composed of a collection of organs each performing a task for a coordinated total effort, like the cardiovascular, muscular, nervous, or other systems in the body. Instead, it is a nebulous, incredibly complex collection of cells and chemicals distributed all over the body whose coordinated function is not to turn food into energy or to distribute oxygen, but to do something even more fundamental: to keep the whole organism safe.

⊙ *The animation "Immune System" can be found on the Student Resource CD-ROM that accompanies this book.*

The primary function of the immune system is to distinguish what is "self" from what is "non-self" and to eradicate anything that is "non-self" as quickly as possible. Immune system devices range from being very general to highly specific in identifying exactly which pathogens they will attack. Some white cells will attack anything; others will simply ignore a pathogen if it is not their particular target. Most of the nonspecific immune devices such as intact skin and the acidity of the gastric juices are not discussed here, but it is worthwhile to look at some of the specific immune machinery because when it is working well it is positively miraculous, and when it is not working well, or when it makes mistakes, things can go terribly wrong.

T-Cells and B-Cells

The two interlocking branches of the specific immune responses are cellular immunity (T-cells) and humoral immunity (B-cells). Neither of these extremely complicated systems can work at all unless their target pathogen is displayed by a macrophage. So *that* is the first step in fighting off an infection: a macrophage must find, eat, and display a piece of the microorganism in question. Fortunately, macrophages are distributed generously all through the blood and interstitial fluid, and they are concentrated in places such as the superficial fascia, lymph nodes, lungs, and liver, where the chance of meeting pathogens is especially high.

Consider what happens when someone touches a contaminated doorknob and then picks his teeth: rhinovirus 14 has just been introduced into the body. A passing macrophage eats the pathogen, and it is drawn through lymphatic capillaries into a nearby lymph node, for instance in the submandibular group. A T-cell is waiting there. It just happens to be especially designed to recognize the flag of rhinovirus 14. The T-cell gets very busy, replicating itself into several different forms, which go out into the bloodstream in search of more viruses to attack. In the process, the original T-cell stimulates its B-cell partner. This B-cell clones, and the new cells start producing rhinovirus 14–specific antibodies at a mind-boggling pace: 2,000 antibodies per second! Antibodies are *not* alive. They are Y-shaped chemicals that are forged especially to lock onto their target pathogen and "retire" it. This can happen in several different ways, depending on the pathogen and the antibodies involved.

Back when the T-cells and B-cells were first becoming active, they each made a few copies of themselves that would outlive the infection and circulate through the body on the lookout for future attempts by the same pathogen to invade. These are *memory cells*, and thanks to them people very seldom get sick with the same pathogen twice. If rhinovirus 14 gains access to the body again, an immune attack will mobilize against it so quickly that a person might never know he had been invaded.

The immune system is miraculous in how the T- and B-cells can somehow recognize their own special pathogen and launch just the right attack against it. B-cells have been shown to produce antibodies that can disable *manmade* pathogens that do not occur in nature. *That* is being prepared! The immune system occasionally makes mistakes, however. Sometimes it launches a full-scale attack, with an inflammatory response, antibody production, and the all of the rest, against an antigen that is not really dangerous: cat dander or pollen, for instance; this is called an allergic reaction. The other slip the immune system can make is to mistake a part of the body for a dangerous pathogen, that is, it fails to distinguish self from nonself. Conditions involving this type of mistake are called autoimmune disorders.

That is a very brief summary of specific immunity, and it is a lot more than was known just 25 years ago. One of the most exciting discoveries about immune system function is

Different White Blood Cells for Different Functions

White blood cells come in different sizes, classes, and strengths. Each type of leukocyte has a specific role in the immune system and inflammatory response. As researchers learn more about how these cells work and communicate with each other, we gain the ability to influence their activities.

Neutrophils are the smallest, fastest, and most common of the white blood cells. They are produced in bone marrow, and chemicals that leak from damaged cells stimulate their production in even greater numbers. Neutrophils have a short life span; they sacrifice themselves to disable potential invaders.

Monocytes begin as small white blood cells, but they have the power to change. When they are released into the blood stream from the bone marrow, they circulate until they reach a target tissue. Then they leave the circulatory system to infiltrate that tissue and grow into *macrophages*: big eaters that can devour pathogens and display bits of cell membrane that begin the specific immune response.

Monocytes and macrophages move slowly; they are usually involved in the subacute or chronic phases of inflammatory response.

Eosinophils and *basophils* are not well-understood inflammatory agents. They have been observed most often in the context of allergic reactions and responses against invading parasites.

Lymphocytes include B-cells, T-cells, and natural killer cells. These are manufactured in both bone marrow and lymphoid tissue and are most often engaged in specific immune system responses to pathogens. These are the agents that allow us to develop immunity to infections.

---

that immune system cells actually *talk* to each other, discussing in a language made of chemicals called *cytokines* what their strategies are in fighting off infection. These chemical messages are beginning to be deciphered, and some of them have been found to say things like "act like me," "come over here," and "eat this." This opens whole new treatment options, as we decipher these chemical codes and begin to manufacture medicines that can influence immune system behavior by mimicking specific cytokines.

Furthermore, it turns out that immune system cells do not just talk to each other. Some of the chemical messages they send out are picked up and acted on by other systems in the body, especially the nervous and endocrine systems. White blood cells have receptors for central nervous system chemicals, for instance. In other words, the nervous system can "talk" directly to the immune system. Some of the *lymphokines* secreted by white blood cells are similar, even identical, to the neurotransmitters previously assumed to exist only in the central nervous system. Other lymphokines, specifically *interleukin-1*, are secreted by macrophages, but relay information to the hypothalamus. This creates some major implications about how health and resistance to disease are related to mental and emotional state. Intuitively this makes a lot of sense, and for the first time there is a way to back up these theories with empiric evidence. A branch of science called *psychoneuroimmunology* has developed specifically to explore these relationships. Bit by bit, that imaginary division between "mind" and "body" is disappearing.

 # LYMPH AND IMMUNE SYSTEM CONDITIONS

Lymph System Conditions

Edema
Lymphangitis
Lymphoma
Mononucleosis

Immune System Conditions

Allergic Reactions
Chronic Fatigue Syndrome
Fever
HIV/AIDS

Inflammation
Lupus

LYMPH SYSTEM CONDITIONS

Edema

Definition: What Is It?

Edema is the accumulation of fluid between cells. It may be associated with inflammation or poor circulation. In either case, the stagnant fluid needs to be pulled into lymphatic capillaries and processed by the lymph system.

Etiology: What Happens?

The Starling equilibrium states that the forces that cause fluid to leave blood capillaries should *almost* equal the forces that cause fluid to be reabsorbed by blood capillaries, and that anything left over (which should be about 10%) should be taken in and processed by the lymph system. Lymph capillaries are perfectly designed to pick up excess interstitial fluid: each squamous cell is anchored to surrounding tissue by a collagen filament. When excess fluid accumulates in any area, these anchoring filaments pull back on the squamous cells, thus increasing the lymph capillary's ability to take in fluid. Sometimes, though, more fluid builds up in the tissues than the circulatory and lymph systems combined can take in, and this is called edema. This occurs in conditions in which blood or lymph return is somehow impaired, so fluid accumulates between the cells. Edema is not generally noticeable until interstitial fluid volume is approximately 30% above normal.

Causes

Edema can have several causes; most of them are a combination of chemical and mechanical factors. Mechanical factors may involve a weakened heart or an obstruction of some kind; chemical causes of edema usually have to do with the accumulation of proteins in the interstitial fluid, which causes the area to retain water.

Massage?

Most types of systemic edema, and *every* instance of pitting edema, contraindicate circulatory massage because of the impact this kind of bodywork has on fluid flow. Pitting edema is identified when pressure on a body part leaves an indentation because fluid refill is slow (Figures 5.2a, 5.2b).

Contraindicated Edemas

- If the heart is overtaxed (i.e., *heart failure*, Chapter 4) and is not pumping the volumes it should be, fluid accumulates in the tissues. Massage will not improve this situation and could quite possibly make it worse by putting an even greater load on the system.
- If the kidneys are not filtering blood fast enough or completely enough because of chemical imbalance or mechanical obstruction, edema develops, and massage could make the situation much worse. (See *renal failure*, Chapter 9.)

Edema in Brief

Pronunciation
ĕ-dē′mă

What is it?
Edema is the retention of interstitial fluid because of electrolyte or protein imbalances or because of mechanical obstruction in the circulatory or lymphatic systems.

How is it recognized?
Edematous tissue is puffy or boggy. It may be hot, if associated with local infection, or quite cool, if it is cut off from local circulation.

Is massage indicated or contraindicated?
Most edemas contraindicate circulatory massage. This is especially true of pitting edema, where the tissue does not immediately spring back from a touch. Edemas that indicate massage include those due to subacute soft tissue injury or temporary immobilization caused by some factor that does *not* contraindicate massage.

Figure 5.2a. Pitting edema, before thumb pressure. **Figure 5.2b.** Pitting edema, after thumb pressure.

- If the liver is congested, the puffiness and bogginess of typical edema may be less visibly apparent, but the same rules apply: pushing blood through a system that is chemically or mechanically impaired will only do damage. (See *cirrhosis*, Chapter 7.)

- If edema accumulates because of local infection, massage is contraindicated because of the risk of pushing pathogens into the lymphatic and circulatory systems before the body has had a chance to marshal appropriate defenses. (See *inflammation*, this chapter.)

- If a mechanical blockage develops anywhere in the circulatory system, massage is contraindicated because it can damage delicate structures, or worse, it could break loose a blood clot. Some examples of mechanical blockages include edema associated with *pregnancy* (Chapter 10), *thrombus, embolism*, or *deep vein thrombosis* (see Chapter 4).

- One specific type of water retention, called *lymphedema*, is a complication of losing lymph nodes for cancer staging. It is discussed in the *cancer* section of Chapter 10.

Indicated Edemas

All this is not to say that every kind of edema absolutely contraindicates every kind of massage under every circumstance. Edema is a red flag for massage therapists, and it calls for caution before proceeding. However, if a client has fluid retention related to a subacute musculoskeletal injury, skilled massage is *very* appropriate and in fact could be vital to the healing process (see *sprains*, Chapter 2). Likewise, if a client is confined to bed or is even partially immobilized for some reason that does *not* contraindicate massage, bodywork can be valuable to the health of his or her injured tissues as long as the risk of blood clotting has been ruled out.

Bodywork modalities with minimal impact of fluid flow are more appropriate for edema than Swedish or other types of massage, but even practitioners of energy work need to know *why* their clients are retaining water to make the best possible choices for their care. Similarly, practitioners of any type of lymphatic work need to be fully informed about the causative factors for edema before they influence this system.

Lymphangitis

Definition: What Is It?

Lymphangitis is an infection with inflammation in the **lymphangions**: lymphatic capillaries.

Demographics: Who Gets It?

People with depressed immunity or poor circulation are especially susceptible to lymphangitis and **lymphadenitis** (inflammation of the lymph nodes) because their white blood cell activity is likely to be sluggish, making any available bacteria able to set up shop.

Massage practitioners have a much greater chance of developing lymphangitis than most clients do. This condition is an occupational hazard for bodywork professions because repeated immersions of the hands in soapy water may lead to hangnail formation, and drying and cracking of nail beds, in combination with exposure to the pathogens that inhabit even healthy clients' skin.

Etiology: What Happens?

In lymphangitis, the lymph capillaries become infected, usually with some of the colonies of streptococcus bacteria that congregate on the skin. This condition can be a complication of *cellulitis*, or from a viral or fungal infection such as *herpes simplex* or *ringworm* (see Chapter 1). If the pathogens are successful, they can set up an infection in the lymph vessel before macrophages or other white blood cells can stop them. Infections that invade the lymph nodes are called *lymphadenitis*.

Signs and Symptoms

Symptoms of lymphangitis start with signs of local infection: pain, heat, redness, and swelling. The infected lymph vessel often shows a visible scarlet track running proximally from the portal of entry, which is usually some lesion in the skin such as a hangnail, a knife cut, or an insect bite (Figure 5.3). If the infection is unchecked by white blood cells, it quickly moves further into the lymph system, leading to swollen nodes, fever, and a general feeling of misery. This can happen surprisingly quickly; lymphangitis can become a systemic infection in a matter of hours.

Complications

Lymphangitis is an infection of the *lymph* system, not the circulatory system. However, if even a few bacteria get past the filtering action of the lymph nodes, the infection *will* enter the bloodstream at the right or left subclavian veins. Then the situation changes to a much more serious one: *septicemia*, or blood poisoning, which is life threatening. This is why, if lymphangitis is a possibility, medical intervention is advisable at the earliest possible opportunity.

Lymphangitis in Brief

What is it?
Lymphangitis is an infection of lymph capillaries. If it gets into the nodes, it is called *lymphadenitis*. If it gets past the lymphatic system, it is called blood poisoning (*septicemia*), and it can be life threatening.

How is it recognized?
Lymphangitis has all the signs of local infection: pain, heat, redness, swelling. It also may show red streaks from the site of infection running toward the nearest lymph nodes.

Is massage indicated or contraindicated?
Lymphangitis contraindicates circulatory massage until the infection has been completely eradicated.

Figure 5.3. Lymphangitis: an infection of lymph capillaries.

Treatment

Lymphangitis is usually treated successfully with antibiotic therapy. Treatment must begin soon after the infection has been identified, however, or the infection may complicate into blood poisoning.

Massage?

Lymphangitis patients feel so sick so fast that it is highly unlikely that an infected client would try to keep an appointment. Although a client who has lymphangitis is contraindicated to *receive* massage, a practitioner who has it is likewise contraindicated to *give* massage. Therefore, massage therapists must keep their hands clean and own a good pair of cuticle scissors. They must *not* allow hangnails and other lesions to go uncovered or untrimmed, and perhaps most importantly, they must *not* allow their health to degenerate to the point that they are vulnerable to this kind of infection.

If a massage therapist has an open hangnail or other wound on a finger, the threat of lymphangitis is an excellent reason to cover it with a "finger cot" or other device during appointments.

Case History 5.1

Lymphangitis

Ruth, Age 24: "It Was the Most Miserable Night of My Life."

There was a winter when I was working four jobs at once. I was a tutoring for a massage school, I was setting up a small practice of my own, I was a nanny during the afternoons, and I was also working in a theater company, doing anything that needed doing, which was usually a lot.

I remember it was the week before Christmas, which was a really busy time for the theatre company—we went on tour doing shows for young children. I had also done several massage treatments that week, which was unusual for me. I was working in the light booth at the theater one morning when I noticed that a hangnail on my right index finger suddenly seemed swollen, hot, and tender. There was not anything I could do about it. I remember sitting there for about an hour watching it get bigger, redder, and more painful.

Lymphangitis, *continued*

That afternoon I had to leave town to be with my family over the holidays. The airport had been socked in with fog for 3 days, which delayed all the flights, so I missed my connection and had to spend the night on the floor of O'Hare Airport in Chicago. It was one of the most miserable times I can remember. I was feverish and shaking, and my hand hurt like hell.

By the time I finally reached D.C., all I wanted to do was go to bed. I spent practically the entire holiday flat on my back. The swelling at my finger finally subsided, but not before I broke out in intensely painful blisters all over my mouth. My doctor back home told me they were probably just an opportunistic outbreak while my defenses were low. All I know is they made it impossible to eat and I missed all my favorite foods.

I found out much later that I had probably had lymphangitis, and that I was very lucky it didn't develop into blood poisoning, especially since I didn't see a doctor until the whole thing was over. If I had it to do over again, I'd make sure I *never* let myself get so run-down, and I'd be sure to cover any noticeable hangnails before doing massage. I wouldn't wish an experience like that on my worst enemy.

Lymphoma

Definition: What Is It?

Lymphoma is any type of cancer of the lymph nodes. Like *leukemia* (see Chapter 4), lymphoma involves a mutation of the DNA in specific white blood cells. However, these cells are all based in lymph nodes rather than bone marrow, which makes the appearance and the progression of the disease very different from those of leukemia.

Lymphoma is usually categorized as Hodgkin's lymphoma (HL), and non-Hodgkin's lymphoma (NHL). Under the heading of NHL, many different subtypes of lymphoma have been identified.

Demographics: Who Gets It?

Approximately 61,000 people in the United States are diagnosed with lymphoma every year: 7,600 with HL, and 53,400 with NHL. Between 1975 and 2000, lymphoma increased approximately 2.5% per year, rising a total of 71% over that time.[1] The reasons for this are not clearly understood, although one subtype of NHL has a close association with infection with human immunodeficiency virus (HIV) and Epstein-Barr virus, both of which have become much more common in the past three decades.

Although lymphoma does occur in children, most patients are adults. Hodgkin's lymphoma most commonly affects adults in their

Hodgkin's Disease:

Thomas Hodgkin (1798–1866) was a British physician who documented this disorder.

Lymphoma in Brief

What is it?
Lymphoma is any variety of cancer that grows in lymph nodes. Several types have been identified, some of which are aggressive and very threatening, others of which may progress more slowly.

How is it recognized?
Painless swelling of lymph nodes is the cardinal sign of lymphoma, along with the possibility of anemia, fatigue, low-grade fever, night sweats, itchiness, abdominal pain, and loss of appetite, all of which last for 2 weeks or more.

Is massage indicated or contraindicated?
Rigorous circulatory massage is generally not recommended for a person who is fighting lymphoma, although this may be a case-by-case decision. Persons who have been free from lymphoma for 5 years or more are considered "cured." Noncirculatory types of massage may be appropriate for lymphoma patients, although it is recommended that the therapist participate as part of an integrated health care team.

---

1 The Leukemia & Lymphoma Society's Facts & Statistics 2003. The Leukemia & Lymphoma Society. Available at: http://www.leukemia-lymphoma.org/all_page?cat_id5&item_id512486&image_number50 &image_dir5&viewmode5print. Accessed winter 2004.

20s or those over 50. Non-Hodgkin's lymphoma is most common among people 60 to 70 years of age.

Lymphoma causes almost 25,000 deaths per year: 23,400 from NHL and 1,300 from HL.

Etiology

Lymphoma is cancer that originates in lymph nodes. Like leukemia, this disease begins with a mutation of the DNA of the affected cells, which in this case is some type of T-cell, B-cell, or natural killer cell. The mutated cell begins to replicate, producing massive numbers of nonfunctioning lymphocytes. This causes the lymph nodes to enlarge, and it initiates the other symptoms associated with lymphoma, namely, anemia, night sweats, itchy skin, and fatigue, among others.

The seriousness of the lymphoma depends on what type of cell has mutated, and how quickly it replicates. More than 30 different types of lymphoma have been identified, and they are categorized mainly by the appearance of the mutated cells.

Types of Lymphoma

- *Hodgkin's lymphoma.* This disease involves the mutation of B-cells into large, malignant, multinucleate cells called **Reed Sternberg cells.** It is seen most often in the submandibular nodes but also can occur at the axillary and inguinal nodes. Eventually the growths metastasize to organ tissues, particularly the liver or bone marrow. HL accounts for approximately 10% of all lymphoma cases.
- *Non-Hodgkin's lymphoma.* These cancers, which account for 90% of all lymphomas, involve the mutation of lymphocytes into many different forms. They are classified as low-grade, intermediate, and high-grade lymphomas according to their aggressiveness. Some sources call low-grade lymphomas "indolent lymphomas," whereas intermediate and high-grade lymphomas are called "aggressive lymphomas." A short list of the 30 or so NHL includes the following:
  - *Low-grade lymphomas:*
    - Lymphocytic lymphoma
    - Follicular cleaved-cell lymphoma
    - Follicular mixed-cell lymphoma
  - *Intermediate lymphomas:*
    - Follicular large-cell lymphoma
    - Diffuse mixed-cell lymphoma
    - Diffuse large-cell lymphoma
  - *High-grade lymphomas:*
    - Immunoblastic lymphoma
    - Lymphoblastic lymphoma
    - Burkitt's lymphoma
    - Non-Burkitt's lymphoma

Risk Factors

The increasing incidence of lymphoma in the last 30 years has raised the distinct possibility that this cancer can be linked to environmental exposures. Some research finds statistical relationships between lymphoma and exposure to insecticides, herbicides, fertilizers, and even hair dye, but the direct cause-and-effect relationships have not yet been established.

Other environmental factors that increase the risk of developing certain types of lymphoma involve infection with specific pathogens. The incidence of lymphoma is 50 to 100 times higher among HIV-positive patients than it is among the general population. Epstein-Barr Virus, which is associated with *mononucleosis* (this chapter), has been linked to Burkitt's lymphoma. ***Human T-cell lymphotropic virus*** (HTLV) is associated with T-cell lymphoma. Having the *Helicobacter pylori* bacterium (see *ulcers*, Chapter 7) raises the risk of developing lymphoma that originates in the stomach wall. One study shows that people with *psoriasis* (Chapter 1) have 3 times the risk of developing lymphoma as the general population. Whether this is an issue with the disease itself or with complications of disease treatments has not yet been explored.

Signs and Symptoms

The primary symptom of any kind of lymphoma is painless, nontender swelling of lymph nodes, especially in the neck, axilla, and inguinal area (Figure 5.4). Other symptoms include *anemia* (see Chapter 4), fatigue, weight loss, night sweats, itchy skin, and loss of appetite. If symptoms persist for 2 weeks or more, testing for lymphoma will probably be conducted.

Late-stage lymphoma involves decreased immunity and susceptibility to secondary infection such as shingles (see *herpes zoster*, Chapter 1), *flu*, or *pneumonia* (Chapter 6).

Diagnosis

The diagnosis of lymphoma begins with manual palpation of enlarged lymph nodes. If symptoms persist for 2 weeks or more, tests may be run to evaluate the node or nodes, and computed tomography (CT) scans or magnetic resonance imaging (MRIs) may be used to look for signs of growth in the chest or abdomen, so the cancer can be accurately staged.

Treatment

Treatment choices for lymphoma depend on several factors, including exactly which type of cells are affected, the progression of the disease, and whether it is a "type A" or "type B" presentation (see sidebar, "Lymphoma Staging").

Lymphoma Staging

Lymphoma is staged by its degree of progression. In addition to a numerical stage, lymphoma is also classified by whether symptoms other than enlarged glands accompany it. In other words, Stage I-A means that the cancer is localized and not accompanied by fever, night sweats, or weight loss. Stage II-B means that the cancer has spread to nearby lymph nodes, and the patient also has fever, night sweats, and loss of appetite.

I. The cancer is found in only one area—and that area is *not* the abdomen or the thoracic cavity.
II. The cancer is found in only one area plus the nearest lymph nodes, *or* it is found in two sets of lymph nodes, but they are on the same side of the diaphragm, *or* the cancer is found in the digestive tract with or without lymph node involvement.
III. Tumors and affected lymph nodes are found on both sides of the diaphragm, *or* the cancer begins in the lymph nodes in the chest, *or* the cancer is in multiple places in the diaphragm, *or* the cancer is found in the central nervous system.
IV. The cancer is found in the bone marrow or in the central nervous system.

Recurrent lymphoma is cancer that reappears after a full course of treatment.

Figure 5.4. Hodgkin's lymphoma: cervical and submandibular lymph nodes are visibly enlarged.

A Massage Therapist's Guide to Pathology

Chemotherapy and radiation are the usual choices, but some other options are finding success in dealing with lymphoma, including allogenic and autologous bone marrow transplants and *radioimmunotherapy*: a process in which special antibodies that have been treated with radioactive iodine are injected into the body, where they attack and destroy cancer cells.

Prognosis

The prognosis for lymphoma depends on the type of cancer, the stage at which it is diagnosed, the age of the patient, and several other factors. Interestingly, the slower-growing types of lymphoma do not tend to respond as well to chemotherapy as the more aggressive varieties, which are considered more treatable.

The overall 5-year survival rate for lymphoma is over 56%, but the survival rate among children is as high as 78%. Hodgkin's lymphoma is considered the most survivable of all blood cancers; up to 80% of HL patients who are diagnosed early make it to the 5-year goal, and 70% make it to 15 years or longer.

Presently approximately 445,000 lymphoma survivors live in the United States.

Massage?

Rigorous circulatory massage is inappropriate for clients whose lymph nodes may be malfunctioning, regardless of whether it is possible for massage to speed up metastasis. Noncirculatory work may be more appropriate because the client may reap many supportive benefits without the risks of pushing a lot of fluid through a system that does not work smoothly. Massage is used increasingly to help ameliorate the side effects of chemotherapy and radiation. Nonetheless, it is always a good idea to work as part of a fully informed health care team when a client is going through long-term, complicated, and life-threatening challenges to health.

Mononucleosis

Definition: What Is It?

Mononucleosis is a viral infection of the salivary glands and throat, which then moves into the lymphatic system by way of B-cells. The causative agent in 85% to 90% of all cases is the Epstein-Barr Virus (EBV), a member of the herpes family. Other pathogens that can cause mononucleosis are also members of *herpesviridiae*: specifically, *cytomegalovirus* (CMV) and *human herpesvirus 6* (HHV6).

Demographics: Who Gets It?

EBV is everywhere. Random blood studies show that the rate of infection with EBV in the United States and elsewhere is 90% to 95% by the time people reach 40 years of age. Not everyone who has been exposed to EBV develops the symptoms associated with mononucleosis, or "mono," however.

Mono is diagnosed in the United States at a rate of approximately 50 out of every 100,000 people. It is especially prevalent among adolescents and young adults; most cases are found in people between 15 and 25 years old. Mono is diagnosed in as many as 5% of college-aged people every year.

Mononucleosis in Brief

Pronunciation
mon'ö-noo-klē-ö'sis

What is it?
Mononucleosis is an infection, usually with the Epstein-Barr Virus (EBV) but occasionally with cytomegalovirus (CMV) or other agents. The virus attacks B-cells in the epithelial tissue in the salivary glands and throat first, and then invades the liver, spleen, and lymph nodes.

How is it recognized?
The three leading symptoms for mononucleosis are fever, swollen lymph nodes, and sore throat. Other symptoms may include profound fatigue, low stamina, enlarged spleen, and enlarged liver.

Is massage indicated or contraindicated?
Mononucleosis contraindicates circulatory massage in the acute stage when the body is fighting hard to beat back this viral attack. In later stages, as long as circulation is healthy and the spleen and liver are not congested, circulatory massage may improve recovery time. Noncirculatory types of bodywork may be appropriate, as long as the possibility of lymphatic congestion is considered.

Etiology: What Happens?

Mononucleosis from EBV spreads most efficiently through direct contact. This virus is fragile outside of a human host, and although it may remain viable for a short time on a dish or suspended in a droplet of mucus in the air, the most dependable way to catch it is through intimate saliva-to-saliva contact; it is not called the "kissing disease" for nothing.

Like many viral infections, mononucleosis moves through the body in two stages. In the first stage, the virus attacks B-cells in the epithelial tissue of the throat and salivary glands. It can take a long time for the infection to get established; incubation can last up to 60 days, during which time the patient is contagious but not strongly symptomatic. Once established well in the epithelial tissue of the throat, however, the virus moves on to infect B-lymphocytes in the lymph nodes, liver, and spleen.

The effect of the virus on its target B-cells is to make them immortal: that is, instead of dying at the end of a normal life span, the infected cells live on to replicate and produce a variety of antibodies, including antibodies to the virus itself, but also nonfunctioning antibodies called *heterophils*. Changes to the infected B-cells cause them to resemble monocytes: an entirely different type of white blood cell. It is their resemblance to monocytes that led to the name *mononucleosis*.

As infected B-cells proliferate, the body responds by producing high numbers of cytotoxic T-cells. These T-cells eventually establish control over the rogue B-cells, and ultimately the virus becomes dormant in epithelial tissue of the throat. This process can take a long time, however; active virus has been found in the saliva of some patients many months after the acute stage of the infection had passed. The efficiency of the T-cell response is now being investigated as a predictor in whether EBV exposure carries a risk of developing into any type of *lymphoma* (this chapter).

Once a person is infected with EBV, the virus is present forever, although usually dormant. It may intermittently reactivate, however. During these episodes, it is likely to be contagious but asymptomatic.

Signs and Symptoms

Mononucleosis is notorious for presenting different symptoms in different patients. The younger a person is when he is exposed to EBV, the subtler his symptoms tend to be. Young children often go through exposure, infection, and recovery with no discernible symptoms at all.

In older patients, particularly adolescents and young adults, the symptoms are more dependable. The prodromic stage, as the infection is becoming established but creates no strong symptoms, may be marked by general fatigue and *malaise*; the patient often does not feel well, but he may not feel sick, either. This may last anywhere from a few days to several weeks. As the infection becomes more aggressive, the leading triad of symptoms appears: fever of 102°F to 104°F, an extremely sore throat from the initial viral infection, and lymph nodes that are swollen from the production of massive numbers of B-cells and T-cells. The cervical lymph nodes are usually affected worst; however, submandibular, axillary, and inguinal lymph nodes also may be palpably swollen and tender.

Puffy, swollen eyelids are a common complaint among mono patients. *Splenomegaly* (enlargement of the spleen) occurs in approximately half of all patients. Approximately 20% also experience inflammation of the liver (see *hepatitis*, Chapter 7). A small percentage of mono patients develop a splotchy, measle-like rash—especially if they are concurrently taking *amoxicillin* or *ampicillin*: two penicillin-family antibiotics that could be prescribed for strep throat. Most mono patients on these medications develop painful, alarming rashes.

Signs and symptoms of acute mononucleosis tend to last approximately 2 weeks before subsiding, but the whole infection is so wearing on the body that it can take several weeks or even months before a patient feels fully functional again.

Diagnosis

Diagnosing EBV is not difficult; the problem is in establishing the stage the infection is in. Several features of this virus make it problematic to label: mono presents differently in different patients, the incidence of EBV is nearly universal, and the virus can be present and active for many weeks or months after an infection. Furthermore, a person can have lifelong reactivations of the virus without symptoms. All of these issues can make it difficult to definitively state that a person's symptoms are due only or even primarily to this particular pathogen.

The starting place for a diagnosis of mono is a "monospot test": this looks for signs of heterophile antibodies. Complete blood counts also show abnormally high lymphocytes: both atypical B-cells and extra T-cells to fight them.

Ultimately, because no medical intervention alters the course of mononucleosis, knowing the exact phase of the infection is not important. It is important, however, to rule out some conditions that mimic this infection but that are either more serious or more treatable. Some of these possibilities include *rubella*, *HIV/AIDS* (this chapter), *diphtheria*, measles, and strep throat—which is also a possible complication of the disease.

Complications

For most people, mono is an unpleasant but basically benign, self-limiting infection. It can cause a significant disruption in a person's life because it has such a powerful effect on stamina, resiliency, and general strength, but it is seldom a life-threatening situation. A very small number of patients, however, do develop serious complications. These can involve infections in the central nervous system (see *encephalitis* and *meningitis*, Chapter 3), infection of the heart, and breathing problems when lymph nodes get so inflamed that they block air passageways.

One fairly common complication of mono is a streptococcal infection of the throat. It is important to be clear about what infection is causing which symptoms in this case because, although strep throat is easily treatable with antibiotics, mono is not.

Perhaps the greatest danger for most mononucleosis patients is the potential for damage to the spleen. This gland, which is sometimes described as "the body's largest lymph node," can become dangerously enlarged with lymphocytic activity. Because the spleen also breaks down and recycles dead red blood cells, it has a generous blood supply. If the enlarged organ is injured by a fall or other trauma, it could rupture, which leads to internal hemorrhage and rapid circulatory collapse. Persons recovering from mono are counseled to avoid contact sports for several weeks to reduce their risk of this kind of injury.

Treatment

Mononucleosis does not respond to antiviral medications. The typical approach is to treat the symptoms (*acetaminophen* to reduce fever and pain, good nutrition, and generous hydration), and wait for it to be over. At one time mono patients were confined to bed for several weeks. More recently it has been concluded that they simply need to curtail activities that exhaust them and to avoid situations that could put them at risk for damaging the spleen.

Massage?

A person in an acute stage of mononucleosis will have a fever, inflamed lymph nodes, and will feel generally sick and awful; all of these features contraindicate circulatory massage. When a person is in recovery from this infection, lymphatic congestion may linger; this is also a caution for circulatory massage and lymph drainage techniques. Energetic work that supports healing properties without taxing the lymph or immune systems may be a valuable addition to the lengthy healing process for mononucleosis.

A person with a history of mono but no current symptoms is a perfectly fine candidate for massage.

IMMUNE SYSTEM CONDITIONS

Allergic Reactions

Definition: What Are They?

Allergies are immune system reactions against stimuli that are not hazardous. In this situation, the immune system behaves as though an *antigen*, which could be oak pollen, cat dander, or another benign substance, were a potentially dangerous threat.

Demographics: Who Gets Them?

Allergies affect some 50 million Americans every year and are the 6th leading cause of chronic disease, costing approximately $18 billion per year to treat.

Different types of allergies affect different parts of the population. Research points to the "Hygiene Hypothesis" to explain why rates of allergic rhinitis ("hay fever"), asthma, eczema, and other allergies are on the rise in the United States. This theory suggests that overprotection from antigens in early childhood interferes with proper immune system development and makes people more susceptible to allergies later in life. Children raised in homes with pets, and who spend time in daycare with other children in their first year of life, have lower rates of allergies than others.

Repeated exposure to some substances, especially latex, can lead to allergic reactions later in life as well.

Multiple chemical sensitivity syndrome (Chapter 11) develops most often in people who undergo prolonged exposure to toxic substances, and who consequently develop progressively more extreme reactions to other substances as well.

Etiology: What Happens?

Antibodies are the Y-shaped proteins manufactured by activated B-cells against specific pathogens. Some classes of antibodies and some types of T-cells are particularly reactive to noninfectious antigens, causing acute or chronic allergic symptoms. These hypersensitivity reactions have been classified as four distinct types. For details on types of hypersensitivity reactions, see sidebar "Hypersensitivity Reactions."

Several conditions involving allergic reactions are discussed elsewhere in this book, depending on which system is most significantly affected. *Eczema/dermatitis* and *hives*

Allergic Reactions in Brief

What are they?
Allergic reactions are immune system mistakes in which an inflammatory immune system response becomes potentially dangerous as it overreacts or reacts inappropriately to a variety of triggers.

How are they recognized?
The most dangerous acute sign of an allergic reaction is swelling around the face and throat that may obstruct airflow. This may be accompanied by decreased blood pressure and bronchospasm. Other signs can include hives and other rashes, gastrointestinal discomfort with food allergies, and, in the case of multiple chemical sensitivity, headache, disorientation, cognitive difficulties, joint pain, and other symptoms.

Is massage indicated or contraindicated?
Most hypersensitivity reactions contraindicate massage in the acute stage, because increasing blood flow to areas that are already congested is counterproductive. Between episodes, persons with allergies need to be careful about massage lubricants, essential oils, perfumes, candles, and other equipment that therapists often use but that may trigger a reaction.

Hypersensitivity Reactions

Four types of hypersensitivity reactions have been classified. Because two of them can involve the skin and the other two can involve systemic disorders, it is useful for massage therapists to be familiar with them.

- *Type I*

  A Type I hypersensitivity reaction is an immediate reaction to an antigen, or particle of "non-self." In this situation, IgE, a specific class of antibody, quickly sensitizes nearby mast cells to the presence of an "enemy"—which could be a fragment of pollen, the proteins from peanuts or shellfish, or a droplet of bee venom. The alerted mast cells then release histamine and other chemicals that create dramatic changes in vascular permeability and that attract other white blood cells to the area. This inflammatory response creates the symptoms that are associated with typical allergic reactions: redness, swelling, itching, weepy eyes, and runny nose with hay fever; or nausea, vomiting, and diarrhea with certain food allergies.

- *Type II*

  Type II hypersensitivity reactions are far less common than type I. They involve inflammatory cytotoxic ("cell killing") reactions against a specific substance that may or may not belong to the body.

  Examples of type II reactions include *myasthenia gravis* (Chapter 2), hemolytic *anemia* (Chapter 4), and reactions to the transfusion of mismatched blood.

- *Type III*

  In type III reactions, antibodies bind with antigens, but the particles they form are too small to be phagocytized. These tiny conglomerates are eventually caught in the body's most delicate fluid filters: in the kidneys, the eyes, the brain, and the serous membranes surrounding the heart, lungs, and abdominal cavity. There they stimulate immune system activity, which results in inflammation and damage to these very delicate structures.

  Examples of type III reactions include *systemic lupus erythematosus* (this chapter), a specific type of *glomerulonephritis* (Chapter 9), and possibly *rheumatoid arthritis* (Chapter 2).

- *Type IV*

  Type IV, or "delayed," reactions are cell-mediated; they rely on T-cells to stimulate an immune response to an irritant. In some cases, large clumps of immune system cells called granulomas are formed. In other cases, an immune system overreaction occurs without the formation of granulomas.

  Contact *dermatitis* (Chapter 1) is an example of a type IV hypersensitivity reaction. In this case, an inflammatory reaction appears on the skin after exposure to an irritating substance such as plant toxins (e.g., poison ivy), certain dyes, soaps, metals, or latex. This is usually a delayed reaction, and may occur 24 to 48 hours after exposure.

(Chapter 1) affect the skin; *asthma* and allergic *sinusitis* (Chapter 6) affect the respiratory system; and allergic *gastroenteritis* (Chapter 7) affects the digestive system. This article addresses two examples of multisystem hypersensitivity reactions: anaphylaxis and angioedema.

- *Anaphylaxis:* **Anaphylaxis** is an acute, severe, systemic allergic reaction leading to the release of massive amounts of histamine from previously sensitized mast cells. The result is a sudden decrease in blood pressure (hypotension) and accumulation of fluid in the tissues (edema). If the reaction centers in the respiratory tract, it can dangerously interfere with breathing.

  Some of the most common triggers include antibiotics, blood products, the contrast medium used in diagnostic imaging, latex, stings of wasps, ants, and honeybees, and some foods such as peanuts and other nuts, soybeans, cow's milk, eggs, fish, and shellfish.

  The first exposure to a trigger may not cause a significant allergic reaction; however, repeated exposures lead to increased antibody activity, complement activation, and mast cell activity, which causes and reinforces inflammation. Anaphylaxis is distinguished from angioedema because it occurs both at the site of exposure and systemically through the body.

- *Angioedema:* **Angioedema** is the rapid onset of localized swelling. The swelling can occur in the skin, genitals, extremities, or in the gastrointestinal tract. If it occurs in the tongue, larynx, or pharynx, angioedema can interrupt airflow, which is a life-threatening condition.

  Allergens commonly associated with angioedema include peanuts or tree nuts, chocolate, fish, tomatoes, eggs, fresh berries, milk, and food preservatives. Medicines associated with this condition include aspirin, angiotensin-converting enzyme (ACE) inhibitors, and some other hypertension medications.

Signs and Symptoms

Anaphylaxis in the skin creates hives, itchiness, and flushing. Excessive edema can cause respiratory symptoms, including shortness of breath, coughing, and wheezing. A person may have so much swelling around the throat that swallowing becomes difficult; this is dysphagia. Gastrointestinal symptoms include nausea, vomiting, cramps, bloating, and diarrhea. In extreme circumstances, a person may experience slowed heart rate, hypotension, fainting, and shock.

Signs of angioedema depend on where the inflammation takes place. The skin may be puffy and hot, although if it appears without hives it may not be itchy. It is often asymmetric and will affect only one part of the lip, for instance, or one side of the face. It has a rapid onset, but usually resolves within 72 hours (Figure 5.5).

Diagnosis

Diagnosis of angioedema and anaphylaxis is straightforward: visible swelling of various tissues (most often around the face and throat), along with shortness of breath or gastrointestinal symptoms, indicates exposure to a triggering allergen.

Treatment

Angioedema and anaphylaxis are typically treated with diphenhydramine (Benadryl) or epinephrine in the short term, and steroidal anti-inflammatories after the crisis has passed. People at risk for anaphylactic reactions are trained to keep medication, usually injectable epinephrine, close at hand in case of emergency. When these allergic reactions are caused by insect stings, a long-term course of desensitization may be recommended.

Massage?

Obviously, a person in the midst of an angioedema or anaphylaxis episode is not a good candidate for Swedish massage; this person needs to seek medical intervention if

Hypersensitivity Reactions and Massage Oil

Type I hypersensitivity reactions typically occur within several seconds to a few minutes of exposure to an irritating substance. However, a late-phase type I reaction can sustain allergic symptoms long after the irritation has been removed. *Arachidonic acid* is a substance associated with late-phase type I reactions, especially in the form of bronchial asthma. The significance of this for massage therapists is that some types of massage oils can break down into arachidonic acid on the skin. A client who is sensitive to this type of reaction may have no immediate skin symptoms but may wonder several hours later why he is coughing, wheezing, and feeling short of breath.

Oils that are particularly prone to breaking down into arachidonic acid are composed mostly of omega-6–sized molecules. These include safflower, soy, almond, sunflower, and corn oils. Although they can be pleasant and convenient to use for massage, they are the most likely to cause skin irritation and allergic reactions. Therefore, when it is important to avoid potentially irritating oils for certain conditions, these are the ones to eliminate first.

Figure 5.5. Angioedema.

breathing becomes impaired and may consider massage only after the crisis has passed. At that point, the massage therapist should be aware of this person's history and choose a hypoallergenic lubricant without the use of essential oils or perfumes to reduce the risk of triggering another attack.

Chronic Fatigue Syndrome

Definition: What Is It?

Chronic fatigue syndrome (CFS) is a recently recognized distinct collection of signs and symptoms that affect multiple systems in the body. It varies in severity from being mildly limiting to being completely debilitating.

This condition was officially named in 1988 by scientists at the Centers for Disease Control. They purposely kept the name vague because this disease affects different people in very different ways, and by getting any more specific about causes or symptoms they feared they would exclude some people who are badly affected by this condition. Nonetheless, some people feel this title trivializes their condition, and CFS is therefore also called CFIDS (*chronic fatigue immune dysfunction syndrome*). In Europe, a condition called **myalgic encephalomyelitis**, or ME, is sometimes referred to as a synonym for CFS, but whether it is actually the same disease is not certain.

CFS has probably been documented since at least the 19th century. Florence Nightingale suffered from debilitating fatigue for decades; it is suspected that she had CFS. This also may be the condition behind other vague diagnostic labels such as "neurasthenia" and, more recently, "yuppie flu."

Chronic Fatigue Syndrome in Brief

What is it?
Chronic fatigue syndrome (CFS) is a collection of signs and symptoms that affect many systems in the body and result in debilitating fatigue.

How is it recognized?
The central symptom to CFS is fatigue that is not restored by rest. It may be accompanied by swollen nodes, slight fever, muscular and joint aches, headaches, excessive pain after mild exercise, and nonrestorative sleep.

Is massage indicated or contraindicated?
Massage is indicated for CFS and can be a very helpful part of a treatment plan.

Demographics: Who Gets It?

Statistics on the incidence of CFS are difficult to gather, for several reasons. First, it is probably drastically underreported, because not all people who are affected will attempt to be treated. CFS looks like several other disorders, any of which may be happening simultaneously, so a definitive diagnosis is sometimes difficult to get. Finally, statistics gathered from different cities show some vast differences in racial, gender, and age distribution of the disorder, which means that although diagnostic criteria have recently been redefined for clarity, some disparity still exists in when and where it is identified.

When all this disparate information is processed, estimates suggest that this disorder (or other CFS-like disorders) probably affects 500,000 to 800,000 Americans. It is diagnosed most often in white women, but some areas report a higher incidence in other groups. CFS-like symptoms are sometimes observed in children, but it is assumed that these symptoms probably arise for other reasons in people younger than 12 years old, and so it is not officially diagnosed among that population.

Etiology: What Happens?

Chronic fatigue syndrome is not well understood. It seems clear that it arises from a combination of factors that may or may not involve infectious agents. In most cases, it does *not* appear to be a contagious condition, but isolated incidents of whole communities coming down with CFS-like symptoms may point to exceptions to that rule.

Causes

Possible causes of CFS are a subject of intense scrutiny. Rather than focusing on any single causative factor, researchers have come to the conclusion that CFS is usually the result of a combination of factors that may vary significantly from one patient to another. The factors may include viral exposure, stress, central nervous system problems, or any combination of issues.

For several years the leading theory was that a person was infected with a common virus (probably Epstein-Barr, the herpes family virus that causes most cases of *mononucleosis*, this chapter) and then her body simply continued to behave as though the infection were acute long after the danger had passed. Although blood studies of persons with CFS often show some immune system abnormalities (levels of an inflammatory cytokine called interleukin-1 are very high, whereas natural killer cell levels are unusually low), it now seems clear that not all CFS cases begin with a viral infection.

Other pathogenic exposures have been implicated in CFS, specifically *candidiasis* (see Chapter 7), **mycoplasmas** (a particular kind of bacteria-like pathogen), some enteroviruses, and other infectious agents. No single agent has been found to be present in most CFS patients, however, and most people who have been exposed to these agents do *not* develop CFS symptoms.

Two central nervous system components seem to be consistent problems for most CFS patients:

- *A hypothalamus-pituitary-adrenal axis (HPA) dysfunction:* This can lead to a sluggish but tenacious stress response (see sidebar "The Stress Response System," Chapter 3), and eventually to adrenal depletion.

- *Neurally mediated hypotension:* This is a situation in which impulses from the brain to the circulatory system do not keep the blood vessels contracted enough to maintain a normal blood pressure. This condition is connected to an inappropriate response to adrenaline.

A dysfunctional connection between the central nervous system and the endocrine system seems to be at the center of most CFS difficulties. People with CFS typically have lower than normal levels of cortisol in the blood, which indicates adrenal exhaustion as a part of the picture. Furthermore, many people with CFS report moderate to severe allergies: a further example of inappropriate immune response and adrenal depletion.

Signs and Symptoms

Fatigue is the central symptom of CFS: fatigue that is unending and not restored by sleep or rest. Other symptoms vary but may include general muscular or joint pain, low-grade fever, swollen lymph nodes, short-term memory loss, problems with concentration, sore throat, and nonrestorative sleep.

Other symptoms may include abdominal bloating, nausea, diarrhea, and cramping, chest pain, irregular heartbeat, coughing, dizziness, dry eyes and mouth, weight loss, jaw pain, morning stiffness, night sweats, and psychological problems related to living with chronic illness (see *depression* and *anxiety disorders*, Chapter 3).

This list of symptoms points to an important feature of CFS: this condition closely resembles two other chronic stress-related conditions: *fibromyalgia syndrome (FMS)* (Chapter 2) and *irritable bowel syndrome (IBS)* (Chapter 7), and it frequently occurs along with them. In fact, so much crossover exists between these conditions that many people who experience aspects of all three disorders are simply diagnosed with whatever syndrome's primary features appear first: IBS for gastrointestinal discomfort; FMS for leading muscle and joint pain; or CFS if the leading symptom is unrelenting fatigue.

Diagnosis

No particular marker in the blood identifies CFS. This condition is diagnosed first by ruling out other diseases with a similar profile. Once that has been accomplished, CFS is diagnosed based on the following criteria:

- The patient has unexplained persistent fatigue that is out of proportion to physical exertion. Fatigue is not alleviated by rest, it leads to a curtailment of normal activities, and its pattern is different from previous experience.

- At least four of the following additional symptoms must be present. They must not predate the onset of fatigue, and they must be a consistent problem for 6 months or more:

Short term memory loss	Confusion, difficulty with concentration	Sore throat
Tender lymph nodes	Muscle pain	Joint pain without inflammation
Pain that exceeds 24 hours after mild exercise	Nonrestorative sleep	Headaches of a new type or pattern since the onset of symptoms

Differential Diagnoses

One thing that makes getting a clear diagnosis of CFS so difficult is that many other disorders can cause long-term unexplained fatigue. It is important to rule some of these out, because they may be more serious than CFS, and sometimes they can be successfully treated and resolved.

Some of the disorders that are ruled out when looking for a solid diagnosis include

Hypothyroidism (See Chapter 8)	*Hepatitis B or C* (See Chapter 7)	*Lupus* (this chapter)
Postpolio syndrome (See Chapter 3)	*Lyme disease* (See Chapter 2)	*Sleep apnea or narcolepsy* (See *sleep disorders*, Chapter 3)
Cancer (See Chapter 11)	*Diabetes* (See Chapter 8)	*Eating disorders* (See Chapter 3)
Bipolar disease (See *depression*, Chapter 3)	Alcohol or substance abuse (See *chemical dependency*, Chapter 3)	Severe obesity
Reactions to medications	General autoimmune dysfunction	Dementia (See *Alzheimer's disease*, Chapter 3)
Chronic, subacute infection	Schizophrenia	

Treatment

The primary treatment for CFS is making lifestyle choices that support the body as fully as possible. This means avoiding stress as much as possible (here "stress" means any stimulus—emotional or physical—that requires that the body adapt to a change); moderating dietary choices to minimize stimulants (caffeine, sugar) and depressants (alcohol) as much as possible; and exercising *very* gently, within tolerance, so as not to exacerbate symptoms. Some people with CFS have some success with addressing nutritional deficiencies. Magnesium, copper, and zinc are minerals that are frequently reported to improve CFS symptoms.

An important part of treatment for CFS patients is education; the more patients learn about their condition, the better equipped they are to handle its challenges.

Medical intervention can be helpful, but it can be difficult to find exactly the right combination of drugs. Many CFS patients are extremely hypersensitive to chemicals, and they often find that one-quarter of regular dosage is adequate. A powerful combination for many people is immune-suppressant drugs combined with low-dose tricyclic anti-depressants.

Massage?

Massage stimulates a parasympathetic response, cleanses tissues, and stimulates circulation when exercise may be too much to handle; it can relieve muscle and joint pain, and it can improve sleep. Studies show that people diagnosed with CFS report lower levels of anxiety and better quality sleep after receiving massage.[2] Because CFS does not appear to be contagious or a condition that spreads through the circulatory system, gentle massage is a safe and appropriate choice for these people.

Fever

Definition: What Is It?

Here is a condition that can be recognized at a glance (or touch). Massage therapists are not, by the way, usually required to keep thermometers in their offices.

Fever is an abnormally high body temperature, usually brought about by bacterial or viral infection, but sometimes stimulated by

---

Fever in Brief

What is it?
Fever is a controlled increase in core temperature, usually brought about by immune system reactions, often in response to pathogenic invasion.

How is it recognized?
Fever is identifiable by readings on a thermometer.

Is massage indicated or contraindicated?
Most fever contraindicates massage because it is an indication that the body is fighting an infection and should be allowed to do its work undisturbed.

Types of Hyperthermia

Fever is a systemic rise in body temperature that is carefully controlled by the hypothalamus. It has the advantages of speeding up immune system activity, while slowing and starving infectious agents. Fever is an extraordinarily efficient system to fight infection.

Sometimes, however, a person's core temperature can rise without hypothalamic control. This generally occurs when a person generates more heat than he or she can release. In this case, the body temperature continues to rise until external factors work to cool off the person. If environmental factors do not allow this to happen, the person could be at risk for brain damage or death.

The three levels of hyperthermia are heat cramps, heat exhaustion, and heat stroke. They are most commonly seen in people who are physically very active in warm, humid environments. Massage therapists who work at sporting events can expect to see any of these manifestations of hyperthermia.

- *Heat cramps:* Muscle cramping is a frequent result of the dehydration that accompanies excessive heat production. The body sweats in an attempt to lower its temperature, and the result is a deficit in interstitial fluid. This makes it more difficult for the calcium ions that stimulate muscle contractions to be reabsorbed into their storage containers. Consequently, muscle contractions are sustained and uncontrolled. Fortunately, massage along with rehydration is an excellent way to mechanically move fluid back into the muscle bellies and stimulate the chemical and neurologic reactions that reduce the spasm.

- *Heat Exhaustion:* This situation occurs when muscular activity generates more heat than a person can release. It is marked by excessive sweating, headache, vasodilation, and dehydration. Excessive sweating may lead to low blood pressure, light-headedness, and fainting.

- *Heat Stroke:* Heat stroke is the final stage of hyperthermia. In this condition, body temperature rises to dangerous levels (around 104°F for adults). Prolonged dehydration may lead to the *lack* of sweating and circulatory shock from loss of water and electrolytes. The person may become confused or delirious. Heat stroke can be fatal if the core temperature is not quickly but carefully reduced to safe levels.

- *Malignant Hyperthermia:* This is not a sports-related problem, but rather a genetic anomaly that allows the body temperature to rise to dangerous, even fatal levels, with a minimum of muscular work. It is sometimes seen as part of an allergic reaction to anesthesia. Many people do not know they are at risk for this disorder until they have a dangerous episode.

[2] Field T. Touch Therapy. London: Churchill Livingstone, 2000:165.

other types of tissue damage. It is a controlled change in temperature, which distinguishes it from other types of hyperthermia (see sidebar "Types of Hyperthermia").

Etiology: What Happens?

Several steps are involved in the development of a fever:

- A person is infected with some microorganism: bacteria, for instance.

- White blood cells find and eat those invaders.

- Some pieces of the bacterial cell membranes are displayed by the macrophages. They stimulate other white blood cells to secrete a lymphokine called *interleukin-1*. Other lymphokines and substances that are secreted include interleukin-6 and *tumor necrosis factor* (TNF).

- Interleukin-1 circulates through the system, ending up in the brain. It causes a series of chemical reactions involving prostaglandins that tell the hypothalamus to reset the body's thermostat to a higher level. In this situation, interleukin-1 is acting as a *pyrogen*: a *fever-starter*.

- Orders from the hypothalamus ripple downward through the body, setting up the muscular and glandular reflexes to raise the core temperature. These reflexes include shivering, constriction of superficial capillaries, and increased metabolism.

The characteristic shivering and "chills" that go along with a rising fever are part of the mechanism to increase the core temperature. Once that goal has been met, the shivering stops, but the body processes keep working to maintain the increased temperature until the stimulating chemicals have been removed. Reaching this peak is called the *crisis* of the fever. When the crisis has passed, the body's cooling mechanisms take over: sweating and capillary dilation. That is the sign that the worst is over and the fever is broken.

This culture has a strange and troubling discomfort with discomfort. In general, people would rather *hide* a symptom than *feel* it and figure out what it is trying to tell them. This is particularly true with fever, which can be disagreeable and inconvenient. In rare cases, it can get high enough to do some serious damage. However, most of the time fever is a sign that the body is working in the most efficient possible way to get rid of invading pathogens. Some of those mechanisms include:

- The presence of interleukin-1 and other cytokines will not only help to reset the body's thermostat; it will stimulate T-cell production. Increased T-cell production then stimulates B-cells and the production of antibodies.

- In the presence of fever, *interferon*, a powerful antiviral agent, is much more active.

- Increased temperature limits iron secretion from the liver and spleen, starving off and slowing bacterial and viral activity.

- Increased temperature raises the heart rate (10 beats per minute per degree), which in turn increases the distribution of white blood cells throughout the body.

- Increased temperature increases cell wall permeability and speeds chemical reactions. This promotes faster recovery for damaged tissues.

Sometimes people will even use a sauna to induce an "artificial fever" in an attempt to stimulate immune system activity.

Aspirin, ibuprofen, and acetaminophen all work to inhibit fever by interrupting the action of prostaglandins on the hypothalamus to reset the thermostat.

Complications

Fever occasionally can complicate into a dangerous situation, particularly when the temperature rises over 104°F. The most common complications are *dehydration* (from prolonged sweating), *acidosis* (the blood gets too acidic), and possibly brain damage. Death from fever occurs somewhere around 112°F to 114°F for adults. If a fever comes down too fast, it can quickly dilate blood vessels. This situation can turn into *shock*, which can be dangerous, especially to older patients.

Massage?

Fever systemically contraindicates massage. Energetic techniques that do not impact blood flow may be helpful for someone having a hard time getting past her crisis point, as long as the therapist is safe from the threat of a contagious condition.

HIV/AIDS

Definition: What Is It?

AIDS, or acquired immune deficiency syndrome, was first recognized as a specific disease in the United States in 1983, but research since then indicates that it has been present here since 1979, and in Africa and the Caribbean since long before that. This virus, which is called HIV-1 (human immunodeficiency virus), attacks various agents of the immune system, with disastrous results.

Demographics: Who Gets It?

Worldwide: As of 2003, the World Health Organization estimates that 40 million people are HIV positive; most are adults, but approximately 2.5 million HIV patients are children younger than 15 years old. Women, formerly thought to be less at risk for the disease, now constitute 50% of the people infected.

Approximately 5 million new HIV infections occur every year: 14,000 per day. Sub-Saharan Africa has the fastest growing AIDS population in the world; 70% of new infections occur there, whereas South and Southeast Asia is the site of 17% of new HIV infections. More than 80% of new AIDS infections worldwide are the result of heterosexual intercourse.

United States In the United States, 886,000 people have been identified as HIV positive. Many thousands more are probably HIV positive but do not know it yet. Approximately 40,000 new infections begin every year in this country: 70% are among men, and 30% are among women. Approximately half of all new infections are among people younger than 25 years of age. Close to 10,000 children younger than age 13 are infected with HIV.

Among men, 60% of new infections are the result of homosexual intercourse, 25% are the result of sharing contaminated drug needles, and 15% of new infections are from heterosexual intercourse. Among women, 75% of new infections are from heterosexual intercourse, and 25% are from drug use.

Rates of HIV infection decreased steeply in the late nineties, but more recently they have leveled off and even slightly increased. AIDS is currently the fifth leading cause of death among people 25 to 44 years old and the leading cause of death among black men in that age group.

HIV/AIDS in Brief

What is it?
Acquired immune deficiency syndrome (AIDS) is a disease caused by the human immunodeficiency virus (HIV), which attacks and disables the immune system. This leaves a person vulnerable to a host of diseases that are usually not a threat to uninfected people.

How is it recognized?
Most people with HIV experience a week or two of flu-like symptoms within several weeks of being infected, followed by an interval with no symptoms. When the virus has successfully inactivated the immune system, infection by opportunistic pathogens such as herpes simplex and zoster, cytomegalovirus, or *Pneumocystis carinii* occurs.

Is massage indicated or contraindicated?
All stages of HIV infection indicate massage as long as the practitioner is healthy and does not pose any risk to the client, and the client is able to keep up with the changes that massage brings about in the body.

A Virus Primer

Viruses consist of a protein coat of variable complexity wrapped around a core of DNA or RNA. Outside of a host cell, viruses have no metabolic functions and cannot replicate. Inside a host cell, the virus shoots its core into the nucleus and reprograms the functions of that cell to replicate more viruses. In other words, the host cell becomes a virus factory. When the factory is full of inventory, it literally bursts at the seams, releasing hordes of new viruses in search of other hosts. Enormous amounts of damage occur with any viral infection, not only to the cells attacked by the virus, but also to the cells the body sacrifices to fight back.

Most viruses cause short-term acute infections that spread easily. The coughing and sneezing seen with respiratory tract infections such as cold and flu are remarkably efficient distributors of virus. Likewise, the diarrhea that occurs with intestinal infections is an effective way to spread virus through fecal contamination. The immune system response to these viruses is severe and usually successful; most infections are curtailed and the viruses are expelled in short order.

A few viruses, however, cause long-term chronic infections, instead of short-term acute illness. Hepatitis B and C, herpes, and HIV are notorious among these. For a virus to live in a body for a prolonged period, it must be able to hide from immune system cells to escape attack and destruction. It is precisely the ability of HIV to hide from typical immune system activity that makes it so difficult to fight. In addition to being good hiders, chronic infectious viruses have been seen to produce "decoy" particles that draw antibody attack away from themselves, and to secrete "fake cytokines": chemical messengers that confuse and slow down immune system response.

As we learn more about how chronic infectious viruses pool in hidden reservoirs in the body, our ability to fight back will improve. We may someday be able to eradicate these hidden invaders permanently.

Etiology: What Happens?

HIV enters the body by way of body fluids: blood (including contaminated transfusions and shared needles) semen, vaginal secretions, and breast milk.

HIV invades a target cell through a molecular portal of entry on the membrane called CD4, along with co-receptor sites, which vary. Monocytes and macrophages have this molecular doorway, and so are called CD4+ cells. HIV pools in nonspecific monocytes and macrophages, using them as a transport to the secondary sites of infection: the helper T-cells that are also CD4+. These cells are stationed throughout the body in the lymph nodes, spleen, tonsils, and adenoids.

These targets are significant for a couple of reasons. First, when the virus pools in macrophages before moving up in the immune system hierarchy, its presence does not immediately trigger the production of antibodies, which makes it difficult to identify in a blood test. Second, consider the consequences of a virus that targets, as its ultimate goal, the helper T-cells. Helper T-cells are the vital link between humoral and cell-mediated immunity. They tell the B-cells when to produce plasma cells and antibodies; they govern the activities of macrophages and monocytes through the secretion of lymphokines; they also stimulate killer T-cells and natural killer cells. Without helper T-cells, the entire immune system collapses and leaves the body vulnerable to a wide array of opportunistic diseases.

Most viruses invade active cells and enlist all of that activity to produce new viruses. One of the more mysterious aspects of AIDS is that HIV works at a different pace. In addition to invading active cells, it also invades *inactive* T-cells and lies in wait, its protein strands floating in the cytoplasm, until the day when the T-cell is activated by the presence of its target pathogen. Then the virus wakes up as well, invades the nucleus, and effectively disables the T-cell.

Blood-borne HIV can move from the bloodstream into a target cell through CD4 receptors and co-receptors on the membranes of helper T-cells, but it also can move directly from one infected cell to another. In addition, it has been found that HIV can pool in specialized cells in the core of lymph nodes, where it eventually causes the cells to break down and the lymph node to lose function. HIV has also been found in astrocytes and microglial cells in the central nervous system. This breaks down the blood-brain barrier, so toxic accumulations can lead to neurologic symptoms.

The HIV is composed of RNA rather than DNA, which holds the blueprints for our own cells. This retrovirus uses an enzyme called *transcriptase* to convert is RNA to DNA during replication. In the process, the virus is often minutely altered—just enough to make it resistant to identification or treatment. Some drug treatments for AIDS focus on interrupting the complex processes of viral transcription and replication inside the host cells.

Progression

Each stage of this disease is associated with decreasing numbers of active helper T-cells and increased viral *titers* (counts of virus). The typical pattern looks like this:

- *Phase 1:* A person is infected with HIV. The virus is present in the body but may be pooling in white blood cells rather than eliciting an immune response. Consequently, tests are negative, no symptoms are present, but the person can transmit the disease because her "viral load," that is, levels of virus in the blood, is very high. This incubation phase can last a year or more, although the average is 3 weeks to 6 months in sexually transmitted cases.

- *Phase 2:* In the acute primary HIV infection, antibodies become detectable in blood tests. Approximately 70% of people experience fatigue, swollen glands, fever, weight loss, headaches, drowsiness, and confusion within several weeks of exposure. These symptoms usually last approximately 2 weeks and are often mistaken for the *flu* (Chapter 6) or *mononucleosis* (this chapter).

- *Phase 3:* This is the asymptomatic period of infection. No symptoms or opportunistic diseases are obvious. Although the virus is busy replicating while decimating immune system cells, the body is able to keep up with the process. It is during this phase that medical intervention limits viral growth and prolongs life expectancy. The length of the asymptomatic phase varies widely, depending on the initial health of the person, what kind of treatment is given, and several other factors. It can last anywhere from 1 to 15 years, with a median average of 10 years.

- *Phases 4 and 5:* During this time, symptoms of opportunistic diseases or AIDS-related cancers become apparent and eventually debilitating. A normal helper T-cell count is 800 to 1,000 cells/mL blood. AIDS is diagnosed when these levels drop to 200 cells/mL or below, and indicator diseases begin to develop.

HIV Resistance

Recent research has focused on the variables that determine how long a person who is HIV positive can keep the virus under control. Some people who are infected with HIV never develop symptoms, or develop them much more slowly than most people. These "long-term nonprogressors" can provide important clues for how the virus may be fought once infection has been established. Three main factors have been identified.

- *Host resistance:* Some HIV patients have a genetic mutation in their immune systems that creates fewer receptor sites on their macrophages and T-cells for the virus to latch on to. It takes more exposure over a longer period to establish an infection in these people because the chance for a successful invasion is so much lower.

- *Immune system response:* When most cells are invaded by a virus, they display a fragment of that virus on their membrane. This serves as a signal to immune system agents that the cell is compromised and should be destroyed. The human immunodeficiency virus is capable of slowing down this "display" reaction, or of hiding from it altogether by mimicking normal cell membranes. If the efficiency of the display mechanism is improved, immune system response is more aggressive.

- *Virulence of the virus:* Sometimes HIV is partially weakened by medication or an immune system response but remains transmittable to another person. Infection with a weakened virus generally means the new host is better able to control it. Relative virulence of individual viruses is difficult to measure, however.

Most long-term nonprogressors or very slow progressors probably have a combination of these factors working in their favor.

Signs and Symptoms

Signs and symptoms of HIV depend on the stage of infection. Specific guidelines have been given in the discussion of phases of the disease.

Communicability

HIV is spread from one person to another through the exchange of intimate fluids. These include blood (as from contaminated blood products, shared needles, or maternal–fetal circulation), semen, vaginal secretions, and breast milk. HIV does not accumulate in concentrations high enough to cause infection in other body fluids such as sweat, saliva, or tears. The virus is unstable outside a human host, so it is not transmissible through contaminated surfaces, or through insect vectors such as mosquitoes, ticks, or bedbugs.

Certain situations increase the communicability of HIV. Infection with syphilis, chlamydia, or gonorrhea (see *sexually transmitted diseases*, Chapter 10) greatly increases the chance of infection. Acute mononucleosis has recently been seen to increase infection risk as well.

Complications

When HIV has virtually disabled normal immune function, the body is incapable of fending off attacks from pathogens that healthy people have no problems with. A whole list of formerly obscure diseases are now so closely associated with AIDS they are called "indicator diseases." Here are some of the most common and serious ones:

- *Pneumocystis carinii pneumonia* (PCP): This is a protozoal infection of the lungs.
- *Cytomegalovirus* (CMV): This member of the herpes family can cause retinitis and blindness, colitis, pneumonia, and infection of the adrenal glands.
- *Kaposi's sarcoma* (KS): This is a type of skin cancer (Figure 5.6).
- *Non-Hodgkin's lymphomas*: HIV has been found to specifically initiate the cancer cell replication with a variety of lymphomas, as well as KS (this chapter).

Other opportunistic diseases associated with AIDS include toxoplasmosis, which can cause encephalitis or pneumonia; *candida*, a yeast infection that can cause thrush or esophagitis (see Chapter 5); and *cryptococcus neoformans*, a fungal infection that can cause meningitis and pneumonia. In addition to these "indicator diseases," people with AIDS are highly susceptible to gastrointestinal disturbances, *herpes simplex* (Chapter 1), *meningitis* and *shingles* (Chapter 3), *cervical cancer* (Chapter 10), *hepatitis C*, (Chapter 7) and many other conditions. Of special note is that when *tuberculosis* (Chapter 7) occurs simultaneously with HIV, the risk of having tuberculosis become an active, potentially contagious condition rises exponentially with each year of co-infection.

Figure 5.6. Kaposi's sarcoma.

Although it is difficult to catch HIV from an infected person without some kind of intimate contact, it is *not* difficult to catch some of the contagious complications of AIDS. Tuberculosis, herpes, and other infections do not always discriminate between HIV-positive and -negative persons.

Diagnosis

Infection with HIV is determined by the presence of antibodies in the blood. This is a bit problematic because the peculiar nature of this pathogen prevents the body from tagging it and initiating antibody production until the virus is widespread. To get a truly dependable diagnosis, HIV tests must be conducted up to 6 months after the last incidence of high-risk behavior: sharing IV drug needles, unprotected sex with a potentially infected partner, or the use of blood or blood products.

Typically, the first blood test given is an *ELISA* (enzyme-linked immunosorbent assay) test. Because this extremely sensitive test sometimes yields false positives, a positive reading is followed by a second ELISA test and/or a Western Blot test. If both tests are negative and the person is clearly in a high-risk population and showing signs of being sick, tests may be conducted to look for signs of the virus itself in the blood, rather than antibodies to the virus.

Treatment

One of the factors that makes finding a cure for AIDS so difficult is that in the process of converting its core from RNA to DNA, the virus can minutely change, just enough to make it resistant to drugs as well as to immune system activation. The answer to that problem has been to combine various drugs to anticipate the mutations of the virus. This has been highly successful in laboratory settings; however, these drug combinations are often prohibitively toxic to the actual patients.

The most successful AIDS treatments so far have involved interrupting viral replication. The use of *highly active antiretroviral therapy* (HAART) has been seen to slow progression in many patients; however, it cannot access the virus when it hides in long-lived cells such as memory T-cells, which have a life expectancy of 60 years or more. Although the goal of fully eradicating the virus from an infected person is still a long way off, studies of patients who manage to control their infections efficiently continue to point the way to better treatment options.

The picture for people with AIDS in this country is rosier than it has been since the disease was identified in 1983. Although treatment can cost $15,000 to $20,000 per year, many people with AIDS in the United States at least have access to care. This is not the case in developing countries, where AIDS statistics are growing the fastest. Some 90% of the world's AIDS patients have little or no access to treatment.

Massage?

HIV is spread through the exchange of bodily fluids: semen, breast milk, blood, and vaginal secretions. No research has ever shown that it can be transmitted through sweat or casual contact. Obviously, the person most at risk for getting sick when an AIDS patient receives massage is not the therapist; it is the client. Therefore, care must be taken that the practitioner does not carry active pathogens that may put a client with AIDS at risk.

Massage for HIV-positive clients who are asymptomatic is absolutely indicated. Although in advanced stages of AIDS, opportunistic diseases can make circulatory massage problematic, other types of work may reduce stress, which in turn strengthens the immune system. It can be a very appropriate treatment option and an important source of support and comfort for people who are often rejected, ignored, or actively persecuted by society.

The Language of Inflammation

Massage therapists are well trained in recognizing the basic signs of inflammation: pain, heat, redness, swelling, and sometimes loss of function. This litany has a long and venerable history beginning with the earliest practitioners of the healing arts. The traditional names for signs of inflammation come from Latin:
Dolor (pain)
Calor (heat)
Rubor (redness)
Tumor (swelling)
Functio Laesa (loss of function)

Inflammation in Brief

What is it?
Inflammation is a protective device in response to injury or infection. It involves localized vascular, cellular, and chemical reactions to isolate the area and to resolve the damage through immune system response.

How is it recognized?
The signs of inflammation are redness, pain, swelling, heat, and loss of function. These can be localized or systemic.

Is massage indicated or contraindicated?
Acute inflammation contraindicates circulatory massage; however, bodywork may be appropriate for subacute situations, depending on the causative factors. Inflammation due to infection obviously carries a higher risk to the client and the practitioner than inflammation in response to musculoskeletal injury.

Inflammation

Definition: What Is It?

Inflammation is a tissue response to the threat of bodily injury or invasion by antigens: bits of "nonself." The inflammatory response is controlled by chemical, cellular, and vascular functions that have the remarkable ability to adjust that response to the severity of the threat.

Etiology: What Happens?

When a person sustains tissue damage, cells are injured, ripped open, destroyed. The damage may occur from mechanical or thermal stress (a sprain, a laceration or a burn, for instance), or it may be caused by pathogenic invasion, or tissue may be injured by toxic chemicals. When cells are injured, a chain of events begins to minimize damage and threat of invasion. This chain of events is called inflammation: a reaction of injured tissue to defend and protect the body from invasion. The different aspects of this reaction are specifically designed to achieve three basic goals: to dispose of pathogens and cellular debris; to prevent the spread of pathogens in the body; and to prepare the injured area for healing.

Three components contribute to all stages of inflammation. The *chemical* components include inflammation mediators released from nearby cells such as histamine and cytokines: chemicals that participate in cell-to-cell communication. The *vascular* components of inflammation involve vasodilation, vasoconstriction, and changes in the permeability of vessel walls to allow the migration of certain blood cells. The *cellular* component of inflammation includes platelet and white blood cell movement to the area of infection or injury, clotting, and phagocytosis as those white blood cells consume pathogens and debris.

Progression

Step 1: The Injury—Acute Vascular Response   For the sake of simplicity, consider a basic laceration or puncture wound as a model, although the same principles hold true for any kind of local injury. (See Figures 5.7a and 5.7b.) In the *very first moments*, especially if it was a very serious injury, vasoconstriction occurs. This is a protective mechanism against excessive bleeding. The vasoconstrictive stage is over within a few seconds for a minor injury, and several minutes for a more serious one.

A period of capillary vasodilation follows vasoconstriction. This is the most important step in the whole inflammatory process. Stimulated cells, especially mast cells, which are stationed in superficial fascia and epithelial membranes, release a host of chemicals that increase the permeability of blood vessel walls and promote capillary dilation.

Step 2: Immediate Cellular Response   When vasodilating chemicals have acted on local capillaries, substances can quickly get *out* of the bloodstream and *into* the damaged area. Specifically, neutrophils are usually the first white blood cells to arrive on the scene, but they are accompanied by antibodies, platelets, and clotting factors that are equally crucial in the inflammatory process. In addition to bringing new material in, this increased fluid flow also flushes wastes out, including dead cells and pathogenic toxins.

Figure 5.7a. Many cellular changes happen with the inflammatory response to protect the body from infection and to prepare the area for healing.

Figure 5.7b. *continued*

A complicated chain of events causes certain plasma proteins in the nearby capillaries to form fibrous nets. These nets serve a double purpose of making a clot to close off any broken blood vessels and to catch loose pathogens before they enter the bloodstream. Blood clots help to isolate infection from the rest of the body.

Step 3: Long-Term Cellular Response   Slower-moving white blood cells arrive later in the inflammatory process. They include monocytes, macrophages, and lymphocytes. These immune system agents are bigger than the neutrophils; they have bigger appetites and can disable multiple pathogens, whereas the neutrophils can only serve once. Macrophages eat pathogens as well as cleaning up the body's own dead and damaged cells.

The result of all this cellular mopping up is the formation of *tissue exudates*. Exudates are any fluids that can be expressed from tissues that are in the process of healing. Pus is one example; it is composed of dead and living white blood cells, along with whatever pathogens they have managed to kill. Pus is usually walled in by the thickened connective tissues surrounding the infection site. It can be expressed through the surface of the skin, aspirated, or, if left alone long enough, it will usually be reabsorbed by the body (macrophages eventually clean it up).

Another type of cell that is drawn to areas of inflammation in this phase is fibroblasts: collagen-producing cells. These lay down a weak, delicate version of collagen to begin knitting together damaged tissues. This collagen is reinforced and realigned later in the healing process.

Step 4: Resolution and Maturation   In this stage, any residual blood clots are dissolved. New scar tissue becomes tougher and stronger and, depending on the type of tissue that was injured, it may align itself with the direction of forces put on it (see *sprains*, Chapter 2). The tissue is restored to as close to a normal state as possible.

Steps 1 and 2 happen in what would be considered the acute phase of infection: they begin within moments of the injury and remain the primary activity for up to 3 days, depending on the severity of the damage.

Steps 3 and 4 involve the rebuilding of damaged tissue. This usually begins 3 to 4 days after the injury, and continues for 2 weeks or more. The maturation phase, when the scar tissue molds and changes according to the stresses put on it, can last up to 2 years, depending on the severity of the injury, the general health of the person, and other variables.

Signs and Symptoms

Every massage therapist should know this litany: the symptoms of inflammation are pain, heat, redness, swelling, and sometimes loss of function. In some cases, itching, clotting, and pus formation could be added to the list.

It is easy to see how each of these symptoms comes about. Vasodilation brings about the redness, heat, and swelling by drawing extra blood to a small area. Pain and itching can be the result of several factors: edematous pressure, damaged nerve endings, irritating pathogenic toxins, and irritating chemicals released by other cells. If the inflammation limits movement, the patient experiences loss of function. Clotting and pus formation have already been discussed. Not all of these symptoms are present in all cases of inflammation.

With long-lasting infectious inflammations, the types of white blood cells present will vary, and it may take days or weeks to completely eradicate all traces of the pathogens. Some pathogens are never completely eradicated but simply become dormant: see *herpes zoster*, Chapter 3. Also, some types of pathogens cause a systemwide inflammatory reaction with *fever* (this chapter).

Treatment

The typical treatment for inflammation is no surprise: anti-inflammatories. These can be steroidal, for example, cortisone, or nonsteroidal, such as aspirin. Regardless of their chemical impact on the body, anti-inflammatories may have significant impact on massage: they may hide the results of over-treatment, thus raising the risk that massage could cause injury. If a client is taking anti-inflammatories for a condition that does *not* contraindicate massage, suggest that she make her appointment just as her dose is wearing off. That way, it will be possible to get much more accurate information about what massage is actually doing to her body.

Massage?

Acute localized infections at very least locally contraindicate circulatory massage. Thickened fascial walls will isolate the infection to a certain extent, but working anywhere around a badly infected knee may be asking for trouble. For a view of a worst-case scenario, see *lymphangitis*, this chapter. If the infection is systemic, as in *influenza* (Chapter 6), it is also a systemic contraindication, at least in the acute stage.

Inflammation does not always imply the presence of infection. *Sprains* (Chapter 2) and *dermatitis* (Chapter 1) are two examples among many conditions in which an inflammatory process occurs without invading pathogens. When inflammation is present without infection, the general rule for circulatory massage is to wait for the subacute stage, when bringing more fluid to the area is not likely to make matters worse. Lymph draining techniques may be safe and appropriate in earlier stages of noninfectious inflammation.

Bodywork may be helpful in flushing out debris and improving sluggish and congested circulation in the post-acute stages of infection and inflammation.

Lupus

Definition: What Is It?

Lupus is an autoimmune disease in which the various types of tissues are attacked by the body's own antibodies. Lupus has the potential to be life threatening. In extreme cases this disorder can attack the heart, the lungs, the kidneys, and the brain, with devastating results.

Demographics: Who Gets It?

Statistics on this disease vary greatly. Population surveys estimate that the incidence of lupus in the United States is between 1.4 and 2 million people. African Americans, Native Americans, and Asians have higher rates than whites, and Caribbean Blacks have the highest rates of all. The incidence of this disease is between 40 and 50 out of every 100,000 people.

Lupus affects people at any age, but it is most common in women of childbearing age. It affects women far more than men; depending on the age group studied, women with lupus outnumber men by as much as 9 to 1.

Etiology: What Happens?

Three varieties of lupus have been identified: drug-induced lupus erythematosus, discoid lupus erythematosus, and systemic lupus erythematosus.

- *Drug-induced lupus* is a situation in which some rarely prescribed medications for high blood pressure, heart arrhythmia, and epilepsy can create lupus symptoms. These symptoms disappear when the medications are discontinued.

- *Discoid lupus erythematosus* (DLE) is a chronic skin disease. It can involve small scaly red patches with sharp margins that do not itch, or it can create the characteristic "butterfly rash" of redness over the nose and cheeks (Figures 5.8 and 5.9). The skin can become very thin and delicate, or lesions may become permanently discolored and thickened. If the lesions affect deep layers of the skin, scar tissue may lead to permanent hair loss. More commonly, acute flares lead to temporary hair loss. Approximately 10% of people with DLE go on to develop systemic lupus erythematosus.

- *Systemic lupus erythematosus* (SLE) is a condition in which antibody attacks are launched against a variety of tissues throughout the body. This can result in *arthritis* (Chapter 2), *renal failure* (Chapter 9), *thrombosis* (Chapter 4), psychosis, *seizures* (Chapter 3), inflammation of the heart, and *pleurisy*. SLE can be a very serious disorder that usually can be controlled, but at this time it cannot be cured. SLE sometimes begins as DLE, but not always. The rest of this discussion focuses on SLE, which creates the most far-reaching and long-lasting symptoms of the three varieties of lupus.

Causes

The precise cause or causes of lupus are unknown. A genetic link is sometimes a factor; however, a child of a parent with lupus has only a 5% chance of developing the disease.

 Lupus:

From the Latin word for "wolf," this name could have come about for a couple of reasons. It could refer to the characteristic "butterfly mask" on the face that looks like the facial markings of a wolf, or it could refer to the circular lesions that may appear on the face or elsewhere on the body that were thought to resemble wolf bites.

Lupus in Brief

What is it?
Lupus is an autoimmune disease in which antibodies attack various types of tissue throughout the body. Three distinct types of lupus exist; however, systemic lupus erythematosus (SLE) is both the most common and the most serious.

How is it recognized?
Eleven specific criteria have been determined for a diagnosis of lupus. They include, among other things, arthritis in two or more joints, pleurisy, pericarditis, kidney, and nervous system dysfunction.

Is massage indicated or contraindicated?
When lupus is in a state of acute flare, circulatory massage could exacerbate symptoms. When the condition is in remission, bodywork of any kind could be very helpful to reduce pain and anxiety, and to help maintain flexibility.

Figure 5.8. Discoid lupus.   **Figure 5.9.** Malar rash.

When one identical twin develops SLE, the other twin may not. This indicates that although a genetic susceptibility may be inherited, environmental factors also probably contribute to the development of the disease. Environmental factors may include exposure to certain viruses, ultraviolet light, certain medications, and high levels of estrogen. Women with lupus often report a change in symptoms with their menstrual cycle, and recent research shows that estrogen replacement therapy that is employed to reduce the risk of *osteoporosis* (Chapter 2) can increase the risk of lupus for some women.

One branch of research is examining the role of a specific enzyme whose job is to help clean up dead and dying cells. When this enzyme is weak or in low supply, the dead cells can trigger an autoimmune reaction against even healthy cells, which then becomes generalized throughout the body. Another area of inquiry is in the individual's response to the immune system substance interferon; persons with lupus tend to have bigger, more tenacious inflammatory responses when this chemical is present.

Signs and Symptoms

Lupus can affect virtually every system in the body (Figure 5.10). Sometimes the problems associated with lupus are not serious, or even detectable. At other times, they can be life threatening. Because some of the features of this disease make profound changes in health, it is worth looking at how SLE affects several systems.

- Integumentary System: The characteristic butterfly or discoid rash that is seen with lupus has already been mentioned. These rashes, which can appear anywhere on the body, may be exacerbated by sunlight in a condition called photosensitivity. Lupus also can cause ulcers in the mucous membranes, particularly in the nose, throat, and mouth. Lupus-related rashes may be acute or subacute; subacute rashes tend to be photosensitive but do not leave permanent scars. Photosensitive rashes can be prevented or reduced with the use of sunscreen and avoiding sun exposure during peak hours.

  When SLE causes superficial blood vessels to become inflamed, symptoms may appear on the skin in the shape of welts, red lines, and painful bumps.

- *Musculoskeletal System*: Eighty percent to ninety percent of all people with lupus eventually develop arthritis. Joint pain usually occurs at the hands and feet, and seldom in the spine. Interestingly, even someone with longstanding lupus will *not* usually show signs of internal joint damage.

  Nonspecific muscle pain is another common symptom, and many lupus patients also may meet the criteria for *fibromyalgia* (Chapter 2).

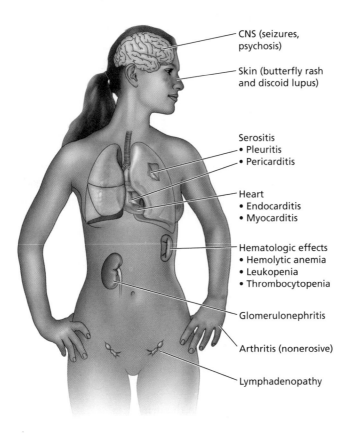

Figure 5.10. Sites affected by systemic lupus erythematosus.

- *Nervous System*: Twenty-five percent of people with lupus will have some nervous system dysfunction. This can range from extreme headaches to psychosis to high fever or seizures (see *seizure disorders* , Chapter 3), depending on which part of the brain is being adversely affected by blood vessel inflammation. When the clotting disorders that may accompany this disorder occurs in the brain, the result is cerebrovascular accident, or *stroke* (Chapter 3).

- *Cardiovascular System*: Lupus can lead to inflammation and damage of major blood vessels, opening the door to *atherosclerosis* (Chapter 4), even in young people. It is also associated with a specific clotting disorder that involves slow clot formation and slow clot dissolving. This problem can lead to *thrombophlebitis* or *pulmonary embolism* (Chapter 4).

  In addition to blood vessel damage, lupus also may affect the serous membranes of the heart. This results in inflammation, arrhythmia, and severe chest pain.

  Anemia (Chapter 4) is a frequent complication of long-term inflammation and bone marrow suppression. Thrombocytopenia, or a shortage of platelets, may occur when lupus antibodies have attacked thrombocytes. *Raynaud's phenomenon* (Chapter 4) is a sign of vasculitis: inflammation of the blood vessels.

- *Respiratory System*: A common complication of lupus is pleurisy: inflammation and fluid accumulation in the serous membranes that line the lungs. This causes pain on inhalation and restricted movement of the lungs.

- *Excretory System*: Tissue damage in the kidneys leads to *glomerulonephritis* (Chapter 9): a condition seen in 50% of people with lupus. Kidney damage can accumulate without symptoms until the kidneys are on the brink of renal failure.

• *Reproductive System*: The clotting disorder associated with lupus can make it difficult to carry a child to term. Repeated spontaneous miscarriages are sometimes the first sign of the disease that will lead to a diagnosis. Pregnant women with lupus face special challenges, because the medications that control symptoms are sometimes not safe for the baby.

Diagnosis

It is clear from this long and varied list of symptoms that lupus can look like a lot of different diseases. Fortunately, it leaves some specific clues in the blood that can help to identify the disease. Unfortunately, those clues are sometimes present in people *without* lupus, so they cannot be used as a definitive diagnosis.

A collection of 11 signs and symptoms has been developed as a diagnostic criterion.[3] If any four of these criteria are present at any time, a positive diagnosis of lupus can be made. The four signs do *not* need to be present simultaneously.

• Malar (butterfly) rash
• Discoid skin rash (can cause permanent scarring)
• Photosensitivity
• Mucous membrane ulcers, particularly in the mouth, nose, or throat
• Arthritis in more than two joints, specifically in the hands or feet (*not* in the spine)
• Pleurisy or pericarditis
• Kidney problems: blood or protein in the urine
• Brain irritation: seizures or psychosis
• Blood count abnormalities: low red blood cells, white blood cells, or platelets
• Immunologic disorders: special antibodies or lupus anticoagulants are present in the blood
• *Antinuclear antibodies* (ANA) present in the blood

This condition, like other autoimmune conditions, is exacerbated by certain kinds of stimuli. Exposure to certain drugs, including penicillin, sulfa, and tetracycline, may initiate an attack. So might excess exposure to ultraviolet light, emotional stress, injury, infection, or trauma. Someone who has lupus must identify those stimuli that are particularly potent for her and avoid them carefully.

Treatment

The treatment strategy for lupus is to minimize the negative impact of inflammation during flares. Lupus patients have essentially four levels of medical recourse in the effort to manage this condition. Each intervention has inherent risks, however, which must be weighed against the benefits.

If the case is not very severe, it may be managed with NSAIDs. These drugs are inexpensive and easily accessible, and they are often effective against inflammation. Unfortunately, they are also associated with chronic stomach irritation (see *ulcers*, Chapter 7), and long-term use can also irritate and damage the kidneys, which is of greater concern for lupus patients, many of whom end up sustaining kidney damage from the disease process, and who do not want to speed that progression with medication.

Steroidal anti-inflammatories are sometimes prescribed for short-term use, especially during flares. These are very powerful anti-inflammatories, but they are also

[3] Systemic Lupus Erythematosus. Systemic Lupus Erythematosus. Copyright © 2003 American College of Rheumatology. Available at: http://www.rheumatology.org/public/factsheets/sle.asp. Accessed winter 2004.

associated with many dangerous side effects, including mood changes, weight gain, liver damage, bone thinning, and *osteonecrosis*: death of bone and joint tissue, especially in the hips and shoulders (see *avascular necrosis*, Chapter 2).

Anti-malarial drugs have found success in treating some of the symptoms of lupus, especially skin rashes and ulcers of mucous membranes. Some anti-malarial drugs cause changes in eye function; therefore, an ophthalmologist must closely monitor their use.

In very severe cases of lupus, *cytotoxic* drugs that entirely disable the immune system may be recommended. This of course leaves the patient vulnerable to secondary infections because her immune system has been suppressed to keep it from attacking her own tissues.

Other treatment options for lupus depend on the presenting symptoms. Acute rashes may be treated with topical steroid creams or ointments. If a patient experiences blood clotting problems, anticoagulants may be administered. It is a high priority to treat lupus symptoms quickly as they arise; early intervention can reduce the amount of damage that accrues during flares, and keep the body functioning at normal levels during periods of remission.

The treatment options for lupus sound alarming, but in truth this disease is usually manageable. When this disease was first recognized, most patients died within 5 years of diagnosis. Now, thanks to these medical interventions, 80% to 90% of all lupus patients can expect a normal life span.

Massage?

Active flares of lupus mark periods of inflammation that can damage the heart, the lungs, the kidneys, and the joints. Circulatory massage during these acute episodes may exacerbate symptoms and put unhealthy stress on an inflamed cardiovascular system. Energy work during these episodes, however, may be supportive and helpful.

Circulatory massage is more appropriate during remission, especially as a treatment strategy against the stress that can trigger attacks, but care must be taken to ensure that the circulatory system is capable of handling the changes in internal environment that massage brings about.

CHAPTER REVIEW QUESTIONS

1. What is an allergy?
2. What is an autoimmune disease? Give two examples
3. What are cytokines, and what do they do?
4. What type of cell is the initial target for HIV?
5. Who is most at risk for getting sick when a massage therapist works with an AIDS patient? Why?
6. What is the link between chronic fatigue syndrome and the central nervous system?
7. Describe how the inflammatory process causes pain, heat, redness, and swelling.
8. What are the dangers of working with a client who is taking anti-inflammatories?
9. How is lupus generally treated medically? Why?
10. Why are massage therapists particularly at risk for lymphangitis?

 Answers to these questions can be found on the Student Resource CD-ROM that accompanies this book.

Bibliography

General Resources, Lymph and Immune System

1. de Dominico G, Wood E. Beard's Massage. Philadelphia: WB Saunders, 1997.
2. Damjanou I. Pathology for the Health-Related Professions. Philadelphia: WB Saunders, 1996.
3. Travell J, Simons DG. Myofascial Pain and Dysfunction: The Trigger Point Manual. Baltimore: Williams & Wilkins, 1983.
4. Clemente CD. Anatomy: A Regional Atlas of the Human Body. 3rd Ed. Baltimore: Urban & Schwarzenburg, 1987.
5. Tortora GJ, Anagnostakos NP. Principles of Anatomy and Physiology. 6th Ed. New York: Harper & Row, 1990.
6. Taber's Cyclopedic Dictionary. 14th Ed. Philadelphia: FA Davis, 1981.
7. Stedman's Medical Dictionary. 26th Ed. Baltimore: Williams & Wilkins, 1995.
8. Memmler RL, Wood DL. The Human Body in Health and Disease. 5th Ed. Philadelphia: JB Lippincott, 1983.
9. Juhan D. Job's Body: A Handbook for Bodywork. Barrytown, NY: Station Hill Press, 1987.
10. Kunz JRM, Finkel AJ, eds. The American Medical Association Family Medical Guide. New York, NY: Random House, 1987.
11. Marieb EM. Human Anatomy and Physiology. Redwood City, CA: Benjamin/Cummings, 1989.
12. Field T. Touch Therapy. London: Churchill Livingstone, 2000.

Edema

1. Edema and Water Retention. Copyright © 1998 The Country Doctor™. Available at: http://www.thecountrydoctor.com/prescriptions/edema.htm. Accessed winter 2004.
2. Revis DR, Jr. Lymphedema. Copyright © 2003, eMedicine.com, Inc. Available at: http://www.emedicine.com/med/topic2722.htm. Accessed winter 2004.
3. Lymphedema: A Brief Overview. Copyright © 2002 National Lymphedema Network. Available at: http://www.lymphnet.org/whatis.html. Accessed winter 2004.
4. Rockson SG. When It's Not Lymphedema. Copyright © 2003 National Lymphedema Network. Available at: http://www.lymphnet.org/lymphlink1099.html. Accessed winter 2004.

Lymphangitis

1. Pitetti RD. Lymphangitis. Copyright © 2003, eMedicine.com, Inc. Available at: http://www.emedicine.com/ped/topic1336.htm. Accessed winter 2004.
2. Lymphadenitis and lymphangitis. Copyright © 2002 A.D.A.M., Inc. Available at: http://www.nlm.nih.gov/medlineplus/ency/article/001301.htm. Accessed winter 2004.

Lymphoma

1. Detailed Guide: Childhood Non-Hodgkin's Lymphoma. What Are the Key Statistics for Childhood Non-Hodgkin's Lymphoma? American Cancer Society. Available at: http://www.cancer.org/docroot/CRI/content/CRI_2_4_1x_What_are_the_key_statistics_for_childhood_non_Hodgkins_lymphoma_9.asp?sitearea=CRI&viewmode=print&. Accessed winter 2004.
2. Detailed Guide: Lymphoma, Non-Hodgkin's type. What Are The Key Statistics About Non-Hodgkin's Lymphoma? American Cancer Society. Available at: http://www.cancer.org/docroot/CRI/content/CRI_2_4_1X_What_are_the_key_statistics_for_non-Hodgkins_lymphoma_32.asp?sitearea=CRI&viewmode=print&. Accessed winter 2004.
3. Detailed Guide: Childhood Non-Hodgkin's Lymphoma. What's New in Childhood Non-Hodgkin's Lymphoma Research and Treatment? American Cancer Society. Available at: http://www.cancer.org/docroot/CRI/content/CRI_2_4_6x_Whats_new_in_childhood_non_hodgkins_lymphoma_research_and_treatment_9.asp?sitearea=CRI&viewmode=print&. Accessed winter 2004.
4. Complementary & Alternative Therapies For Leukemia, Lymphoma, Hodgkin's Disease, & Myeloma. Available at: http://www.leukemia-lymphoma.org/all_mat_toc.adp?cat_id=&item_id=9882&viewmode=print. Accessed winter 2004.
5. The Leukemia & Lymphoma Society's Facts & Statistics 2003. Available at: http://www.leukemia-lymphoma.org/all_page?cat_id=&item_id=12486&image_number=0&image_dir=&viewmode=print. Accessed winter 2004.
6. Lymphoma (Hodgkin Disease And Non-Hodgkin Lymphoma). Harvard Medical School. Available at: http://www.intelihealth.com/IH/ihtPrint/WSIHW000/8096/24763.html?k=basePrint. Accessed winter 2004.
7. Non-Hodgkin Lymphoma. The Leukemia & Lymphoma Society. Available at: http://www.leukemia.org/all_page?item_id=8965. Accessed winter 2004.
8. Hodgkin's Disease Overview. Copyright © 1998–2003 Mayo Foundation for Medical Education and Research (MFMER). Available at: http://www.mayoclinic.com/invoke.cfm?id=DS00186. Accessed winter 2004.
9. Study Links Psoriasis to Lymphoma Cancers. Copyright © 2003 Reuters Health Information. Available at: http://www.nlm.nih.gov/medlineplus/news/fullstory_14715.html. Accessed winter 2004.
10. AIDS-Related Lymphoma. National Cancer Institute. Available at: http://www.cancer.gov/templates/page_print.aspx?viewid=85D2A0CC-431A-4B84-88F9-B8CC124184F1&version=patient. Accessed winter 2004.
11. What You Need To Know About™ Non-Hodgkin's Lymphoma. Available at: http://www.cancer.gov/cancerinfo/wyntk/non-hodgkins-lymphoma. Accessed winter 2004.

Mononucleosis

1. Cunha BA. Infectious Mononucleosis. Copyright © 2003, eMedicine.com, Inc. Available at: http://www.emedicine.com/med/topic1499.htm. Accessed winter 2004.
2. Infectious Mononucleosis. Harvard Medical School. Available at: http://www.intelihealth.com/IH/ihtPrint/WSIHW000/24479/10351.html?k=basePrint. Accessed winter 2004.
3. Gardner A. HealthDay Reporter. Mono Virus Tied to Hodgkin's Disease. Copyright © 1994–2000 HealthCentral.com. Available at: http://www.healthcentral.com/PrintFormat/PrintFullText2.cfm?id=515343. Accessed winter 2004.
4. Mononucleosis and Epstein-Barr: Are they related? Copyright © 1998–2003 Mayo Foundation for Medical Education and Research (MFMER). Available at: http://www.mayoclinic.com/invoke.cfm?id=AN00661. Accessed winter 2004.
5. Mononucleosis UPS Risk for HIV Infection. Copyright © 2003 Reuters Health Information. Available at: http://www.nlm.nih.gov/medlineplus/news/fullstory_14831.html. Accessed winter 2004.
6. Weston RL. MONO = Infectious Mononucleosis. Available at:* Accessed winter 2004.
7. Epstein-Barr Virus and Infectious Mononucleosis. National Center for Infectious Diseases. Centers for Disease Control and Prevention. Available at: http://www.cdc.gov/ncidod/diseases/ebv.htm. Accessed winter 2004.

Allergic Reactions

1. Hawkins HM. Acupuncture and allergies. AcupunctureToday. Available at: http://www.acupuncturetoday.com/archives2001/feb/02hawkins.html. Accessed winter 2004.
2. The Immune System in Health and Disease. Allergy and Hypersensitivity. Copyright © 2001 by Garland Publishing. Available at: http://www.ncbi.nlm.nih.gov/books/bv.fcgi?tool=bookshelf&call=bv.View..ShowSection&searchterm=hypersensitivity&rid=imm.section.1756. Accessed winter 2004.
3. Allergy Statistics. National Institute of Allergy and Infectious DiseasesNational Institutes of Health. Available at: http://www.niaid.nih.gov/factsheets/allergystat.htm. Accessed winter 2004.
4. Krause RS. Anaphylaxis. Copyright © 2003, eMedicine.com, Inc. Available at: http://www.emedicine.com/EMERG/topic25.htm. Accessed winter 2004.

5. Reid M, Euerle B. Angioedema. Copyright © 2003, eMedicine.com, Inc. Available at: http://www.emedicine.com/med/topic135.htm. Accessed winter 2004.

6. Abnormal Medical Tests and Physical Signs Associated with Multiple Chemical Sensitivity. Copyright © 2000, MCS Referral & Resources. Copyright © 2000, MCS Referral & Resources.

7. Commonly Asked Questions about Anaphylaxis. Copyright © 2004, the Food Allergy & Anaphylaxis Network. Available at: http://www.foodallergy.org/anaphylaxis.html. Accessed winter 2004.

8. Begany T. Hygiene Hypothesis Gains Support in the United States and Europe. Available at: http://www.respiratoryreviews.com/jan03/rr_jan03_hygiene.html. Accessed winter 2004.

9. Magill MK, Suruda A. Multiple Chemical Sensitivity Syndrome. Copyright © 1998 by the American Academy of Family Physicians. Available at: http://aafp.org/afp/980901ap/magill.html. Accessed winter 2004.

10. Multiple Chemical Sensitivity: A 1999 Consensus. Heldref Publications, Helen Dwight Reid Educational Foundation. Available at: http://heldref.org/html/Consensus.html. Accessed winter 2004.

11. Angioedema. Copyright © 2002 A.D.A.M., Inc. Available at: http://www.nlm.nih.gov/medlineplus/ency/article/000846.htm. Accessed winter 2004.

12. Ross GH. Treatment Options in Multiple Chemical Sensitivity. Toxicology and Industrial Health, 8(4), 87–94. Available at: http://www.aehf.com/articles/treatment_options_mcs.html. Accessed winter 2004.

Chronic Fatigue Syndrome

1. Cunha BA. Chronic Fatigue Syndrome. Copyright © 2003, eMedicine.com, Inc. Available at: http://www.emedicine.com/med/topic3392.htm. Accessed winter 2004.

2. Chronic Fatigue Syndrome, CFS Information. Centers for Disease Control and Prevention, National Center for Infectious Diseases. Available at: http://www.cdc.gov/ncidod/diseases/cfs/info.htm#Demo. Accessed winter 2004.

3. Chronic Fatigue Syndrome, CFS Definition. Centers for Disease Control and Prevention. National Center for Infectious Diseases. Available at: http://www.cdc.gov/ncidod/diseases/cfs/defined/defined2.htm. Accessed winter 2004.

4. Byron Marshall Hyde M.D. Are Myalgic Encephalomyelitis and Chronic Fatigue Syndrome Synonymous Terms? Copyright Nightingale Research Foundation. Available at: http://www.nightingale.ca/ICaustralia2.html. Accessed winter 2004.

5. Treatment of Patients with Chronic Fatigue Syndrome. Centers for Disease Control and Prevention, National Center for Infectious Diseases. Available at:

http://www.cdc.gov/ncidod/diseases/cfs/treat.htm. Accessed winter 2004.

Fever

1. Fever Overview. Copyright © 1998–2003 Mayo Foundation for Medical Education and Research (MFMER). Available at: http://www.mayoclinic.com/invoke.cfm?id=DS00077. Accessed winter 2004.

HIV/AIDS

1. Basic Statistics. National Center for HIV, STD and TB Prevention. Divisions of HIV/AIDS Prevention. Centers for Disease Control & Prevention. Available at: http://www.cdc.gov/hiv/stats.htm. Accessed winter 2004.

2. HIV/AIDS Statistics. National Institute of Allergy and Infectious DiseasesNational Institutes of Health. Available at: http://www.niaid.nih.gov/factsheets/aidsstat.htm. Accessed winter 2004.

3. Frye RE, Rivera DM. Human Immunodeficiency Virus Infection. Copyright © 2003, eMedicine.com, Inc. Available at: http://www.emedicine.com/ped/topic1027.htm. Accessed winter 2004.

4. Frequently Asked Questions and Answers about Coinfection with HIV and Hepatitis C Virus. Centers for Disease Control & Prevention. National Center for HIV, STD, and TB Prevention. Available at: http://www.cdc.gov/hiv/pubs/facts/HIV-HCV_Coinfection.htm. Accessed winter 2004.

5. Hart L. Fighting AIDS today. Produced by the BMJ Publishing Group Ltd of the BMA. Copyright © 2003 BMJ. Available at: http://www.studentbmj.com/back_issues/1202/education/449.html. Accessed winter 2004.

6. HIV and Its Transmission. Centers for Disease Control & Prevention. National Center for HIV, STD, and TB Prevention. Available at: http://www.cdc.gov/hiv/pubs/facts/transmission.htm. Accessed winter 2004.

7. A Glance at the HIV Epidemic. Centers for Disease Control & Prevention. Available at: http://www.cdc.gov/nchstp/od/news/At-a-Glance.pdf. Accessed winter 2004.

8. Human Immunodeficiency Virus Type 2. Centers for Disease Control & Prevention. National Center for HIV, STD, and TB Prevention. Available at: http://www.cdc.gov/hiv/pubs/facts/hiv2.htm. Accessed winter 2004.

9. HIV/AIDS Overview. © 1998–2003 Mayo Foundation for Medical Education and Research (MFMER). Available at: http://www.mayoclinic.com/invoke.cfm?id=DS00005. Accessed winter 2004.

10. How HIV Causes AIDS. National Institute of Allergy and Infectious DiseasesNational Institutes of Health. Available at: http://www.niaid.nih.gov/factsheets/howhiv.htm. Accessed winter 2004.

11. The Deadly Intersection Between TB and HIV. Centers for Disease Control &

Prevention. National Center for HIV, STD, and TB Prevention. Available at: http://www.cdc.gov/hiv/pubs/facts/hivtb.htm. Accessed winter 2004.

Inflammation

1. Friedlander E. Pathologist. Inflammation and Repair. Available at: http://www.pathguy.com/lectures/inflamma.htm#intro. Accessed winter 2004.

2. Hypertension May Be Inflammatory Disease-study. Copyright © 2003 Reuters. Available at: http://www.nlm.nih.gov/medlineplus/news/fullstory_15071.html. Accessed winter 2004.

Lupus

1. Greenspun B. Systemic Lupus Erythematosus. Copyright © 2003, eMedicine.com, Inc. Available at: http://www.emedicine.com/pmr/topic135.htm. Accessed winter 2004.

2. Handout on Health: Systemic Lupus Erythematosus. National Institutes of Health (NIH). National Institute of Arthritis and Musculoskeletal and Skin Diseases (NIAMS). Available at: http://www.niams.nih.gov/hi/topics/lupus/slehandout/index.htm. Accessed winter 2004.

3. Lupus Erythematosus. Copyright © 2004 University of Washington. Available at: http://www.orthop.washington.edu/arthritis/types/lupus/01. Accessed winter 2004.

4. The enemy within: Women and autoimmune diseases. © 1998–2003 Mayo Foundation for Medical Education and Research (MFMER). Available at: http://www.mayoclinic.com/printinvoker.cfm?objectid=228367C1-61A8-45EF-A649741F1DFC372E. Accessed winter 2004.

5. Arthritis News. Prolonged Remission In Lupus Is Rare, Continued Observation Necessary. Copyright © 2003 American College of Rheumatology. Available at: http://www.nlm.nih.gov/medlineplus/lupus.html. Accessed winter 2004.

6. Autoantibodies Precede Disease in Lupus Patients. National Institutes of Health (NIH). National Institute of Arthritis and Musculoskeletal and Skin Diseases (NIAMS). Available at: http://www.niams.nih.gov/ne/press/2003/11_05.htm. Accessed winter 2004.

7. Genetic "Signature" Linked to Severe Lupus Symptoms. National Institutes of Health (NIH). National Institute of Arthritis and Musculoskeletal and Skin Diseases (NIAMS). Available at: http://www.niams.nih.gov/ne/press/2003/02_11.htm. Accessed winter 2004.

8. Statistics about Lupus. Copyright © 2001 Lupus Foundation of America, Inc. Available at: http://www.lupus.org/education/stats.html. Accessed winter 2004.

9. Systemic Lupus Erythematosus. Copyright © 2003 American College of Rheumatology. Available at: http://www.rheumatology.org/public/factsheets/sle.asp. Accessed winter 2004.

RESPIRATORY SYSTEM CONDITIONS

Chapter Objectives

After reading this chapter, you should be able to. . .

- Cite what percentage of calories a healthy person invests in the act of respiration while at rest.
- Describe three muscles involved in respiration.
- Identify the difference in causative factors between acute and chronic bronchitis.
- Identify two differences between influenza and common cold.
- Explain why the flu vaccine does not impart lifelong immunity.
- Name three causative agents for pneumonia.
- Cite what percentage of tuberculosis exposures turn from primary to secondary disease.
- Identify three risk factors for developing emphysema.
- Explain why persons with asthma, chronic bronchitis, and emphysema are often encouraged to be vaccinated against the flu.
- Cite the average 5-year survival rate for lung cancer.

INTRODUCTION

Structure

The easiest way to discuss the structure of the respiratory system is to follow a particle of air through it (Figure 6.1). Take a deep breath: air drawn in through the nose encounters mucous membranes. Mucous membranes line any cavity in the body that communicates with the outside world: the respiratory system, the digestive system, and the reproductive and urinary systems. In the respiratory system, the mucous membranes start inside the nose and mouth, and they line the sinuses and throat, all the way down into the smaller tubes in the lungs. The wet, sticky mucous membranes in the respiratory system are responsible for warming, moistening, and filtering all the air that passes by.

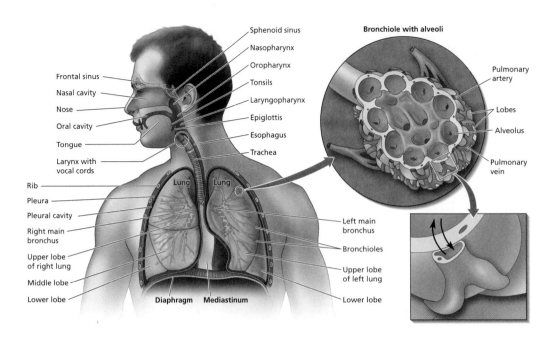

Figure 6.1. Overview of the respiratory system.

Once past the nose and mouth, air enters first the pharynx, then the larynx, the trachea, then the bronchi. The bronchi are asymmetric: the right bronchus is bigger, wider, and straighter, leading into the three right lobes of the lungs. The left bronchus, however, is smaller in diameter, and it curves off to the side to reach the two lobes of the left lung. This is significant because if anything should ever get inhaled into the lungs, it almost always follows the path of least resistance to the right side. The next section of tubing is the bronchioles, which subdivide 23 times until finally ending in microscopic *alveoli*. These little grape-shaped clusters of epithelium are like tiny balloons surrounded by blood capillaries. Gaseous exchange occurs through the alveoli. If for any reason they are impaired or not functioning correctly, the body cannot make an efficient trade of carbon dioxide for oxygen.

The structure of the lungs themselves is well suited for fighting off infection. Each lung has two or three separate lobes, and each of those lobes has smaller separate segments. This isolation of different areas makes it difficult for pathogens to infect the whole structure. The whole tract is lined with mucous membrane, which traps pathogens and other particles. Then the "mucous blanket" slowly creeps toward the mouth and nose for expulsion. Smooth muscle tissue lines all of the tubes down to the smallest bronchi; once an irritant has gotten into these tubes, a healthy cough reflex quickly moves it out of the body.

Function

Air cycles through the lungs anywhere from 12 to 20 times per minute. The lungs themselves do not have any muscle tissue to make them fill up or empty; they are simply two limp-walled sacs that inflate or deflate according to the air pressure inside and outside of them. A change in air pressure is brought about by a change in the shape of the thoracic cavity. If the cavity is made larger, the air pressure inside is low until air rushes in to equalize it. In other words, the act of inhaling is simply filling a vacuum. When the pressure inside and outside of the lungs has been equalized, air eases out again: exhalation. Exhalation is usually a passive process; it does not involve muscular activity unless a person specifically tries to remove air from his lungs.

The kinds of conditions examined in this chapter mostly have to do with how vulnerable the respiratory system can be to infection. Fortunately, thanks to the sticky mucous membranes and lungs that have carefully isolated segments, those infections seldom get a strong enough grip on to do lasting damage.

RESPIRATORY SYSTEM CONDITIONS

Infectious Respiratory Disorders

Acute Bronchitis
Common Cold
Influenza
Pneumonia
Sinusitis
Tuberculosis

Chronic Obstructive Pulmonary Diseases

Asthma
Bronchiectasis
Chronic Bronchitis
Emphysema

Other Respiratory Disorders

Cystic Fibrosis
Lung Cancer

INFECTIOUS RESPIRATORY DISORDERS

Acute Bronchitis

Definition: What Is It?

Acute bronchitis is a self-limiting infection and inflammation of the respiratory tract, specifically of the bronchial tree. It is usually a complication of the common *cold* or *flu* (this chapter), but the causative factors are often difficult to identify. Acute bronchitis is a self-limiting disorder; it is usually resolved within 10 days to several weeks of onset. This helps to distinguish it from chronic bronchitis (this chapter), which is an irreversible condition.

Demographics: Who Gets It?

An estimated 12 million cases of acute bronchitis are diagnosed every year in the United States. Most cases are identified among young children, but adults are certainly susceptible. Adults who smoke or work in environments with dust, fumes, or other pollutants are at higher risk for developing acute bronchitis than others.

Etiology: What Happens?

When the bronchi are irritated or infected by any kind of pathogen, an inflammatory response ensues. The tubes swell, the cilia are damaged, excessive mucus is produced, and the result is coughing and wheezing as air moves through obstructed passageways. The big mystery with infectious acute bronchitis is the source of the infection. Most cases are complications of a cold or flu, in which the viruses simply move from the upper respiratory system to the bronchial tubes. Other causative agents may include a variety of bacteria, fungi, or noninfectious irritants such as fumes, air pollutants, and other contaminants. Chronic reflux from the esophagus can also irritate the bronchi (see gastroesophageal reflux disorder, Chapter 7).

Acute Bronchitis in Brief

What is it?
Acute bronchitis is an infection and inflammation of the bronchial tree anywhere between the trachea and the bronchioles. If inflammation extends into the bronchioles and alveoli, it is called bronchopneumonia.

How is it recognized?
The hallmark of acute bronchitis is a persistent productive cough along with sore throat, nasal congestion, fatigue, and fever. Whereas other symptoms generally subside within 10 days, the cough may last for several weeks while the bronchi heal.

Is massage indicated or contraindicated?
Acute bronchitis, like all acute infections, contraindicates circulatory massage. If the infection has passed and the cough is the only lingering symptom, massage may be appropriate as long as the client is comfortable on the table.

Signs and Symptoms

The primary sign of acute bronchitis is a persistent productive cough. Sputum may be clear or opaque. Wheezing, nasal congestion, headache, low fever, muscle aches, chest pain, and fatigue also may be present. Most of the symptoms of acute bronchitis subside within approximately 10 days of onset, but the cough may persist for several weeks while the delicate lining of the bronchial tubes heals.

Diagnosis

Acute bronchitis is usually diagnosed by the presence of its distinctive symptoms. However, several other respiratory disorders can create similar symptoms. Bacterial sinusitis, mild pneumonia, and asthma (this chapter) can all involve wheezing and productive coughs. These disorders should be ruled out to be sure that treatment options are as effective as possible.

Treatment

The best treatment options for most cases of acute bronchitis are the same as those for cold or flu: plenty of rest, lots of fluids, and warm, humid air to liquefy mucus and aid in its expulsion. Antibiotics are not effective in most cases of acute bronchitis, but they are appropriate when the causative agent has been identified as bacterial.

Bronchodilators and cough suppressants can help to ameliorate some of the symptoms of acute bronchitis, but they do not eradicate the infection or speed recovery.

Massage?

Circulatory massage is inappropriate for someone in the acute stage of a bronchial infection. When the infection has passed, however, and the person is left with a persistent cough while the bronchial tubes heal, massage may be appropriate as long as the client is comfortable on the table.

Common Cold

Common Cold in Brief

What is it?
The common cold (or upper respiratory tract infection, URTI) is a viral infection from any of approximately 200 different types of viruses.

How is it recognized?
The symptoms of colds are nasal discharge, sore throat, mild fever, dry coughing, and headache. Symptoms last anywhere from 2 days to 2 weeks.

Is massage indicated or contraindicated?
Colds indicate circulatory massage only when the acute stage has passed, and even then massage may exacerbate symptoms as the healing process may be accelerated. Energetic types of bodywork may be supportive and helpful if a person has a hard time getting past the peak of a cold.

Definition: What Is It?

This condition is brought about by any of approximately 200 different viruses. Over the course of a lifetime, people are exposed to multitudes of cold viruses. They get sick, they establish immunity to that particular pathogen, and they move on to the next infection. Much of this happens in childhood; by adulthood people have encountered most of what they are likely to see, and the frequency of infections generally subsides. However, no single infectious agent causes the so-called "common cold," and the viruses themselves keep mutating and changing. This is why there may never be an effective cure for this condition.

Demographics: Who Gets It?

It is difficult to project just how common the common cold really is. One estimate suggests that approximately 1 billion infections with common cold virus occur in the United States in an average year. Children are most at risk for these infections, until their immune systems have built up a collection of resistant antibodies. Children have an average of 6 to 10 colds a year, and adults generally have 2 to 4 per year. People older than 60 years old may have fewer than 2 colds per year.

Colds are a major cause of school and work absenteeism, and cost untold millions of dollars in health care and lost productivity.

Etiology: What Happens?

The viruses that cause the common cold have a specific target cell: mucus-producing cells that line the throat and respiratory tract. When a virus gains access to its target, it infiltrates that cell and takes over its processes until the cell literally bursts with new viruses.

Although the damage that cold viruses cause is substantial, it pales in comparison with the damage caused by the immune system when it is fighting off a cold virus. Special signals released by infected cells attract immune system agents, which cause the area to be flooded with inflammatory chemicals and aggressive immune systems cells. It is the immune system response to a viral threat that causes most of the discomfort that is associated with common cold symptoms.

Contrary to popular belief, being cold has nothing to do with catching cold. Extensive research has shown that a person's susceptibility to a cold virus has little to do with temperature, diet, exercise, or even whether her tonsils are enlarged. Instead, the leading risk factors for catching cold are being under psychological stress, having respiratory allergies that make mucous membranes vulnerable to infection, and the stage of menstrual cycle.

Signs and Symptoms

The symptoms of a cold are probably familiar to everyone: runny nose, sneezing, sore throat, dry coughing, headache, and perhaps a mild fever. Colds are typically limited to the upper respiratory tract, which is why they are sometimes called URTIs, for *upper respiratory tract infections*. Symptoms generally last less than 2 weeks, although the virus may be present in the body for up to 3 days before symptoms begin. This incubation period is also a contagious period, which can make the spread of infection hard to control.

Complications

Colds are seldom dangerous except when they complicate into another disorder. The compromised integrity of the membranes and the accumulations of mucus, a perfect growth medium, leave the body vulnerable to a bacterial onslaught that can include ear infections, laryngitis, *acute bronchitis*, *sinusitis*, and *pneumonia* (this chapter).

Prevention

Cold viruses can live for up to 3 hours outside the body. The viruses are airborne after an infected person coughs or sneezes, but they are much more readily spread when someone gets a virus on her hand or face, and it finds access into the body through a portal of entry: the mouth or the nose. Picking up a virus on the hands or from a light switch, a doorknob, or a piece of money, and then rubbing the nose is a very efficient way to spread the disease.

The best way to prevent the spread of colds and other infectious diseases is by frequently washing the hands, focusing on the cuticles and nails, using soap or detergent and scrubbing for 10 seconds or more before rinsing.

Treatment

Because these are viral infections, antibiotics are useless for treating colds. Getting extra rest, drinking lots of fluids, and isolating oneself from family, classmates, and co-workers who could get infected are all high priorities. Using a humidifier may relieve some of the irritation to mucous membranes, although it is important to be aware that some types of humidifiers can be breeding grounds for bacteria, and it is important to keep them scrupulously clean. Over-the-counter drugs can relieve the symptoms of a cold, but they do *not* reduce recovery time. In fact, by inhibiting the ways a body fights off infection (reducing fever, drying up the sinuses), over-the-counter drugs have been shown to actually increase the amount of time the infection is present in the body. Some research shows that aspirin also can increase the concentration of virus shed in nasal secretions, thus increasing the possibility of spreading the disease.[1]

Concerns have arisen over the prescription of "just in case" antibiotics. Only a small percentage of colds complicate into bacterial infections, and the frequent administration of needless antibiotics does not improve recovery time but can contribute to the creation of new and more drug-resistant strains of bacteria.

Alternative health care strategies for dealing with colds include plenty of vitamin C, echinacea, lysine (an amino acid with antiviral properties), zinc lozenges (also antiviral), and perhaps licorice root as an expectorant. Some of these interventions have been shown to reduce recovery time, but their efficacy as cold preventatives has yet to be proved. Hydrotherapy options include artificial fevers to boost immune function (see *fever*, Chapter 5) and cold double-compresses or packs.

Massage?

A synonym for flu is grippe, from the French *gripper*, to seize.

Circulatory bodywork is appropriate for colds only after the fever has peaked. If someone receives massage in the acute stage of a cold, it can spread it through the body *much* more effectively than would happen naturally, and that is *not* a benefit. Conversely, if someone is on the post-acute side of an infection, massage may help to speed recovery time. It is important to ask permission, however, because this sometimes makes the person feel as though she is having a relapse. It is, after all, squeezing 3 days of recovery into 1 day of feeling crummy again.

Influenza

Definition: What Is It?

Influenza or "flu" is a viral infection of the respiratory tract. Most of the time it is a relatively benign, self-limiting infection, but it can become life threatening if an aggressive virus is paired up with a vulnerable patient.

Demographics: Who Gets It?

Everyone can get the flu and probably does at least a few times over a lifetime. It is estimated that anywhere from 10% to 20% of the population has at least one bout of flu each year. Children are 2 to 3 times more likely to contract flu than adults.

Influenza in Brief

What is it?
Influenza ("flu") is a viral infection of the respiratory tract.

How is it recognized?
The symptoms of flu include high fever and muscle and joint achiness that may last for up to 3 days, followed by a runny nose, coughing, sneezing, and general malaise.

Is massage indicated or contraindicated?
Massage is indicated for the flu in the subacute stage only.

[1] The Common Cold Fact Sheet. National Institute of Allergy and Infectious Diseases, National Institutes of Health.

For most people, flu is a significant inconvenience but not a serious problem. For the very young, the very old, people with chronic heart or lung disease, people who are immune suppressed, or people who spend a lot of time in hospitals or long-term care facilities, an outbreak of flu can be deadly. Flu and its complications hospitalize 114,000 people and kill 36,000 Americans each year.

Etiology: What Happens?

Flu viruses work in the usual way of infectious agents: they gain access to the body (flu virus is usually inhaled as airborne particles) and then they invade and attack their target cells, in this case, mucus-producing cells that line the respiratory tract. Once the infection becomes established, the immune system response causes most of the extreme symptoms. White blood cells attack infected mucous cells, causing sore throat and coughing. They also release the chemicals that stimulate *fever* (see Chapter 5). It can take 2 or 3 days for symptoms to appear, but the person is shedding virus in oral and mucous secretions all the time. The peak of communicability is usually around day 4 of the infection. The person will continue to shed virus throughout the acute and subacute stages, up to 7 days after symptoms have subsided.

Three different classes of flu virus have been identified. The type A viruses are the most virulent and are responsible for the major epidemics that claimed millions of lives in the early part of this century. Type A viruses mutate quickly, and so can cause repeated infections in the same person. Type B flu viruses can also spread, but they are not as aggressive or widely spread as type A viruses. Type C flu viruses are not associated with epidemics, and they are relatively stable. They create much less severe symptoms than the other types.

Type A flu viruses are remarkably adaptable. They can infect several species besides humans, including birds, pigs, seals, whales, and horses. The flu appears to pass from one species to another and undergoes some minor changes to its enzymes that allow it to invade its new host. In some cases, the transmission may occur directly from animals to humans without mutation. So far, only type A viruses have been seen to be capable of this process.

Flu viruses also have the ability to mutate as they develop resistance to attack. This makes it impossible for the body to establish permanent immunity; each time it is exposed, the pathogen is different.

We Are All Under the Influence: The History of Flu

Symptoms of the infectious disease now called flu have been documented since the 5th century BC. In those early days of medicine, this disorder was seen to spread throughout a population, but symptoms sometimes would not appear for a few days after exposure, and it continued to spread for several days after all symptoms were gone among the original patients. Because its course seemed so mysterious, it was assumed that this disease was controlled by the influence of the planets and stars. In the early 1500s, the Italian term for influence ("*influenza*") became the common name for this disorder.

The first recorded pandemic of flu virus is known from records from Europe from 1580. The 20th century saw three pandemics of flu infections and a strong threat of a fourth.

1918: The "Spanish Lady" was a flu virus that swept across the globe. In the course of 3 years it killed half a million people in the United States, and 20 million people worldwide.

1957: The Asian Flu

1968: The Hong Kong Flu

1977: The Russian Flu: these flu viruses killed a total of 1.5 million people worldwide.

1997: In Hong Kong, another new flu virus was identified. This one had a previously unknown feature: it seemed to be directly communicable from birds to people. It infected 18 people and killed six, but if it had escaped Hong Kong it could have killed millions more. It was controlled largely by an aggressive public health effort that ended in the slaughter of all of Hong Kong's domestic poultry to limit the potential spread of the virus.

Today flu is not considered much of a menace by most of the population, but for those people who live in confined situations such as nursing homes or other long-term care facilities, those who live with chronic lung or heart disease, or those who are immune suppressed, flu can be a life-threatening infection.

Signs and Symptoms

Flu symptoms can range from being subtle to causing death within hours or days. For most common infections, the symptoms look like a really bad cold: respiratory irritation with runny nose and dry cough, sore throat, headache, chills, and a long-lasting high fever (it is not unusual for flu-related fevers to go over 102°F in adults, and they may last for 3 days or more). Most flu infections cause symptoms that affect more than the upper respiratory tract, however. Many patients experience aching muscles and joints, as well as debilitating fatigue. (One area that flu viruses generally *will not* attack, however, is the gastrointestinal tract. What is commonly referred to as "stomach flu" is far more likely to be infection with rotavirus or a case of food poisoning.) For more information on how the flu differs from the common cold, see sidebar "Compare and Contrast: Is It a Cold? Is It the Flu? Does It Matter?"

Flu symptoms usually appear approximately 3 days after exposure to the virus, and they may persist for up to 2 weeks. If they persist longer than that, or if the coughing begins to produce a lot of phlegm, it may be that the original viral infection has complicated to a secondary bacterial infection of the lungs.

Complications

The greatest danger with flu is the possibility of an opportunistic bacterial infection in the shape of pneumonia or acute bronchitis. This is a particular danger for high-risk populations: the very young, the very old, heavy smokers, diabetics, people who are immune-suppressed, people living in long-term care facilities, or people with chronic lung or heart problems.

Compare and Contrast
IS IT A COLD? IS IT THE FLU? DOES IT MATTER?

Colds and flu are both caused by viral attacks on mucus cells in the respiratory tract. They have similar symptoms, and they carry similar cautions about working with clients who have these infections. Still, flu infections can be much worse than colds, they are more contagious, and they can linger in the body much longer. Therefore it is useful to have a clear idea of which pathogen a client is battling.

PRESENTATION	COMMON COLD	INFLUENZA
Duration	Usually less than a week.	Could be 10 days or more.
Fever	Usually low (under 102°F) and short-term (resolves within 48 hours).	Usually high (over 102°F) and long-term (may persist for 3 days or more).
Location	Symptoms are strictly in the upper respiratory tract.	Symptoms may be felt systemically as muscle and joint pain, inflamed lymph nodes, and debilitating fatigue.
Complications	If complications occur, they will usually be in the shape of sinus or ear infections.	If complications occur, they will usually affect the lower respiratory tract as bronchitis or pneumonia.
Communicability	Cold virus is usually spread by hands contacting contaminated surfaces. Colds are contagious but do not usually create widespread epidemics.	Flu virus is usually spread by inhalation of airborne virus. Flu viruses are often highly virulent and may infect high proportions of the population.
Resolution of the infection	Cold viruses are quickly eliminated from the body; when symptoms are over, it is no longer contagious.	Flu virus may linger in the body several days after symptoms have abated; it continues to be communicable at this time.

Treatment

As a viral infection, flu is unaffected by antibiotics. Good sense measures include rest, liquids, alternative regimens, and lots of chicken soup. Over-the-counter drugs may abate the symptoms but will not speed healing. They can be useful, however, if the symptoms are preventing a person from getting the sleep she needs to heal.

Some antiviral medications are finding use among flu patients. *Amantadine* can reduce the duration of symptoms of flu if they are caused by a type A virus, but it is associated with central nervous system side effects, including sleeplessness, restlessness, and confusion: especially among elderly patients. A closely related medication, *rimantadine*, usually has fewer side effects. Neither amantadine nor rimantadine is effective against types B or C viruses, and both medications have been seen to allow the mutation of flu virus into more dangerous drug-resistant strains.

Every year the Food and Drug Administration distributes a vaccine to fight a combination of type A and type B viruses. These vaccines are composed approximately a year ahead of when "flu season" (November through March) hits. Consequently, the vaccine may or may not be fully effective against the viruses that are circulating when it is administered. Furthermore, because viruses mutate so quickly, flu vaccines need to be updated every year. Nonetheless, flu vaccines are highly recommended for high-risk populations.

Massage?

A person with flu who receives circulatory bodywork in the early stages of infection may find himself with a much more serious infection than he would otherwise have. A person who receives massage after the infection has peaked and he is on the mend may find that he recovers more quickly. Two cautions must be kept in mind, however. One is, squeezing several days of recovery into 1 or 2 days may make the client feel sick again; he should know that this is a possibility. The other is that a person who is recovering from the flu may still be shedding virus up to 7 days after symptoms have disappeared. This puts the massage therapist at risk for getting sick.

Pneumonia

Definition: What Is It?

Pneumonia is a general term for inflammation of the lungs, usually caused by an infectious agent.

Demographics: Who Gets It?

Pneumonia can affect the entire age range of the population, from infants to senior adults. Because it is an opportunistic infection that takes advantage of weak immune systems, it combines with flu to be the seventh leading cause of death in the United States. Every year, between 3 and 5 million people in the United States get pneumonia; half a million of them receive hospital care, and approximately 60,000 people die. Severity of the infection ranges from being not much worse than a bad cold to being a cause of death within 24 hours.

Etiology: What Happens?

The alveoli are the most vulnerable structures in the lungs. They are the tiny air balloons with walls made of squamous epithelium. They are surrounded by the capillaries of the

Pneumonia:

The Greek root of this word is *pneumon*, which means lung. The suffix *-ia* indicates "condition."

Pneumonia in Brief

What is it?
Pneumonia is an infection in the lungs brought about by bacteria, viruses, or other pathogens.

How is it recognized?
The symptoms of pneumonia include coughing that may be dry or productive, high fever, pain on breathing, and shortness of breath. Extreme cases may show cyanosis or a bluish caste to the skin and nails.

Is massage indicated or contraindicated?
Depending on the causative factor and the general resiliency of the person, pneumonia may indicate massage in the subacute stage.

pulmonary circuit for the exchange of O_2 and CO_2 in the bloodstream. When an infectious agent is aspirated into the lungs, these tiny air balloons fill up with dead white blood cells, mucus, and fluid seeping back from the capillaries. Eventually, diffusion of gases is impossible. Abscesses may form, and capillary damage may occur, allowing bleeding into the alveoli, and eventually into the sputum.

In some forms of pneumonia, fibrin, a blood protein responsible for clotting, thickens the fluid in the alveoli until it becomes a gelid mass. This is known as *consolidation*. In most cases, the alveolar exudate remains liquid; however, it is still a hindrance to diffusion. Edema is not always limited to the alveoli. In extreme cases, fluid may be found between the visceral and parietal layers of the pleurae. This can lead to *pleurisy*: scarring and limitation of movement between the pleurae during breathing.

Causes of Pneumonia

Several infectious agents can cause pneumonia. Each one of them has a different symptomatic profile, including what kind of sputum they create and how they may appear on chest x-rays. It is also possible for more than one type of pathogen to be present at a time, a fact that sometimes makes diagnosis and treatment of this condition a challenge.

- *Viruses:* Viral infections account for approximately half of all pneumonia cases. Influenza *A* and *B* (this chapter) and *syncytial* virus are the most common culprits. Other viruses include cytomegalovirus, *herpes simplex* (Chapter 1), and adenovirus. The incubation period of viral pneumonia is 1 to 3 days. Viral pneumonia tends to be short-lived and not serious. It appears most frequently in children.

- *Staph and Strep:* Varieties of these bacteria often live harmlessly in the throat, but when resistance is low they may invade the lower respiratory tract to set up an infection in the lungs. The toxins released by the bacteria initiate an inflammatory response, leading to edema in the alveoli and a reduced ability to draw oxygen into the system. This kind of infection usually responds well to antibiotics.

- *Mycoplasma:* **Mycoplasma** are the smallest free-living agents ever found. They are neither bacteria nor viruses, although they share characteristics of each. The incubation period for mycoplasma pneumonia is quite lengthy: 1 to 4 weeks, and because it tends not to be as severe as bacterial or viral types of infection, it is sometimes called "walking pneumonia." Fortunately, like bacterial pneumonia, mycoplasma pneumonia responds well to antibiotics.

- *Pneumocystis carinii:* **Pneumocystis carinii** is an infection almost exclusively associated with immunosuppressed patients such as those with HIV/AIDS (Chapter 5) and those receiving cancer chemotherapy or immunosuppressive drugs to prevent the rejection of organ transplants.

- *Others:* Other pathogens that can cause pneumonia include chlamydia, rickettsia, and tuberculosis bacilli.

Forms of Pneumonia

Pneumonia appears in several forms. Each one may have different presentations or cautions attached to it, so it is worthwhile to be familiar with the most common types.

- *Primary pneumonia* is relatively rare. In this case, no predisposing factor has weakened the patient; it is simply an attack directly on the lungs.

- *Secondary pneumonia* is by the far the most common situation. In this, a pathogenic assault on lung tissue is successful because the body's immune system is weakened by another disease. Even if the primary disease is viral, the accumulation of mucus is a perfect growth medium for bacteria, leaving the patient vulnerable to this kind of infection.

Within the headings of primary or secondary, pneumonia also may be classified by the location of the infection.

- *Bronchopneumonia.* This type starts as a bronchial inflammation and spreads into the lungs. It appears in a patchy pattern all over the lungs, not segregated to a specific area.
- *Lobar pneumonia.* This type is restricted to one lobe of the lungs. Consolidation occurs there, and gradually the whole lobe may be affected.
- *Double pneumonia* affects both lungs. It can be bacterial or viral.

A final classification for pneumonia determines the source of the infectious agent.

- *Community-acquired pneumonia* is the most common form, and is usually a bacterial infection of *Streptococcus pneumoniae* (also called **pneumococcus**), **Haemophilus influenzae**, or from influenza type A or B.
- *Nosocomial* or *hospital-acquired pneumonia* is an infection in a person who has been a hospital inpatient for at least 72 hours within the previous 1 to 3 weeks.

Signs and Symptoms

Symptoms of pneumonia can vary widely, depending on the causative factor and how much of the lung is affected. Some of the possible symptoms of pneumonia include coughing, very high fever, chills, sweating, delirium, chest pains, cyanosis, thick and colored sputum, shortness of breath, muscle aches and pains, and pleurisy.

Pneumonia can have a sudden or gradual onset. Very often it follows the same course as flu, but instead of getting better, the respiratory symptoms get rapidly worse, along with fever up to 104°F.

Diagnosis

Pneumonia is usually diagnosed by clinical examination and a description of symptoms. Both viral and bacterial pneumonia have sudden onset with a rapid development of symptoms, whereas mycoplasma pneumonia may take weeks for symptoms to reach their peak. Different types of bacterial pneumonia produce different colors of sputum, from opaque green to rust-colored to "currant jelly" sputum, so these are often helpful diagnostic clues. Cultures of bacterial are rarely taken because they take a long time to grow and they are often incorrect.

A diagnosis is sometimes confirmed with an x-ray, which shows where areas of the lungs have become pathologically dense. Again, different types of lung infections have particular patterns in x-rays, so this is another helpful diagnostic clue.

Treatment

Treatment depends entirely on what type of pneumonia is present. Bacterial and mycoplasma pneumonias generally respond well to antibiotics, but viral infections do not respond to these medications.

Symptomatic relief and supportive therapy include breathing humidified air, drinking ample fluids, and supplementing oxygen if necessary.

Prevention

Two main methods exist to prevent some of the most common types of pneumonia infections. Flu vaccines, if they are effective against the circulating flu viruses of the year, prevent flu infections from complicating into viral or bacterial pneumonia. A vaccine has been developed against the most common type of bacterial pneumonia, *Streptococcus pneumoniae*. This vaccine is recommended mainly for high-risk patients and for people who live or work in long-term care facilities or hospitals.

Prognosis

Considering the delicacy of the epithelium in the lungs, it is amazing that if a pneumonia infection is short-lived, it is completely reversible. The body can reliquefy and absorb the consolidated matter in affected alveoli, as it can reabsorb the fluid from any inflamed part of the lung. If a patient is basically healthy, he or she can expect to recover fully within 2 weeks.

In long-standing cases in which fibrosis and scar tissue accumulate, permanent damage to the elasticity of the epithelial tissue may occur, or the freedom with which the lungs move in the pleural cavity may be compromised. This can raise the risk for future infections.

When people develop this condition as a complication of a more serious underlying disorder, pneumonia can be life threatening. Secondary pneumonia is an opportunistic disease. It kills more people every year than any other kind of infection because it takes advantage of low defenses. It is often the final complication of other serious diseases, even noninfectious ones. People who have had a stroke, heart failure, alcoholism, or cancer die of pneumonia more often than of any other disease. People who are bedridden or paralyzed are susceptible too, because their cough reflex is often impaired; they cannot expel mucus easily. Having a preexisting chest problem such as flu, bronchitis, emphysema, or asthma is an open invitation. And finally, being immune-suppressed because of tissue transplants, acquired immune deficiency virus (AIDS), steroids, leukemia, or cytotoxic drugs makes a person particularly vulnerable to pneumonia.

Massage?

This is a serious and complicated condition that frequently accompanies other serious conditions. Under the right circumstances, post-acute pneumonia can respond very well to the mechanical impact of percussive massage. Tapotement on the chest and back can help to move mucus from the alveoli into the bronchial tubes, where muscle action and the cough reflex can take over to expel it from the body. Massage therapists working with pneumonia patients would do well to be part of a well-informed health care team, rather than working alone.

Sinusitis

Definition: What Is It?

Sinusitis, as the name implies, is a condition in which the mucous membranes that line the sinuses become inflamed and swollen.

Demographics: Who Gets It?

Sinusitis statistics are rising quickly. It is estimated that over 30 million sinus infections occur in the United States each year and that 15% or more of the population experiences chronic sinusitis at one time or another.

Etiology: What Happens?

Sinuses are hollow areas located lateral to, above, and behind the nose (Figure 6-2). Sinuses are meant to be hollow. They provide resonance for the voice, and they lighten

Sinus:

From the Latin for channel, hollow place, or tunnel.

Sinuses

| ■ Frontal sinus | ■ Ethmoidal air cells | ■ Sphenoidal sinus | ■ Maxillary sinus |

Figure 6.2. Sinusitis.

the weight of the head considerably. The mucous membranes lining sinuses are provided with cilia: tiny hairs that move the mucus along at a rate of about 16 beats per second, so that trapped pathogens and particulate matter can be swallowed instead of reaching the lower respiratory system.

When the cilia break down, often as a result of viral infection or environmental irritants, pathogen-laden mucus lingers over delicate epithelial cells, stimulating an inflammatory response. Soon the hollow areas fill with sticky, pus-filled mucus that cannot drain. Inflamed, infected sinuses can be a source of tremendous pain and discomfort.

Alternatively, the cilia may remain intact and highly functional, but the mucous membranes are stimulated to respond to oak pollen or cat dander as if they were life-threatening organisms. Inflammation ensues, with itchiness, production of huge amounts of thin, runny mucus, puffy, itchy eyes, and all of the symptoms now associated with *allergic rhinitis*, or "hay fever."

Sinusitis in Brief

What is it?
Sinusitis is inflammation of the paranasal sinuses from allergies, infection, or physical obstruction.

How is it recognized?
Symptoms include headaches, localized tenderness over the affected area, runny or congested nose, facial or tooth pain, headache, fatigue, and if it is related to an infection, thick opaque mucus, fever, and chills.

Is massage indicated or contraindicated
Acute infections contraindicate massage, but in chronic or noninfectious situations, it can be appropriate for bodywork as long as the client is comfortable on the table.

Causes

Sinusitis comes in two varieties: noninfectious and infectious. Noninfectious sinusitis may also be called allergic rhinitis. Infectious sinusitis involves a pathogenic invasion followed by an inflammatory response that creates a vicious circle: the body creates excessive mucus to help remove infectious agents, but the inflamed tissues make drainage of that mucus (which is an ideal growth medium for many types of bacteria and other pathogens) impossible.

- *Noninfectious sinusitis: allergic rhinitis*: Hay fever causes inflammation of the sinus membranes, but it happens without underlying infection. Hay fever is often distinguished from infectious sinusitis by the lack of congestion and by the quality of the nasal discharge: it tends to be thin and runny rather and thick and sticky. Hay fever is the only variety of sinusitis that may be safely treated with antihistamines.

  It is always a possibility that the irritation to sinuses caused by hay fever can open the door to a secondary bacterial infection, which makes the sinusitis infectious as well as allergic.

- *Infectious sinusitis*: Infectious sinusitis can be acute, in which symptoms develop just as a respiratory infection subsides, and continue to get worse for 6 to 8 weeks, or it can be a chronic situation in which symptoms may be less severe but more prolonged: episodes of chronic sinusitis can last 8 weeks or more and can happen several times a year.

  Many pathogens may contribute to infectious in acute sinusitis, often in combinations. Some of the most common presentations include. . .

  - *Viruses and bacteria:* The most common types of sinusitis begin as viral infections (see *common cold,* this chapter). When defenses are low, the bacteria that normally colonize the skin and mucous membranes take advantage of the situation and begin to multiply. The bacteria most commonly associated with these infections are *Streptococcus pneumoniae* and *Haemophilus influenzae*. Dental work may very occasionally cause sinusitis if the contents of an abscessed tooth are somehow released into the nasal cavity.

  - *Fungi and bacteria:* Recent research has shown that some people with chronic sinusitis have significant amounts of fungal growth in their sinuses. One theory is that sensitivity to fungi stimulates an inflammatory response that then allows naturally occurring bacteria to grow and cause a chronic infection. This is a problem particularly for persons with *diabetes* (Chapter 8), HIV/AIDS (Chapter 5), or other types of immunosuppression.

  - *Structural problems:* A deviated septum or the growth of nasal polyps can obstruct the flow of mucus out of the sinuses. This is not an infectious situation to begin with, but mucus held back from normal flow is a perfect growth medium for bacteria, so what begins as a simple structural anomaly can become a true infection.

  - *Environmental irritants:* Exposure to cigarette smoke (first- or second-hand), indoor and outdoor pollutants, cocaine, or other irritants can destroy cilia and create a high risk for infection.

  - *Other conditions:* Acute and chronic sinusitis is frequently seen with other conditions. Severe dental caries (cavities) raises the risk of sinusitis, probably from the availability of local bacteria. *Asthma* (this chapter) is associated with sinusitis, because both conditions have to do with excessive mucus production and a hyperreactive inflammatory response. *GERD* (Chapter 7) is also associated with sinusitis, which is less well understood. Still, treating GERD successfully often reduces sinusitis symptoms, so these conditions are often dealt with simultaneously.

Signs and Symptoms

Symptoms of sinusitis vary according to the cause of the inflammation and which sinuses are involved. Severe headache is a key feature, especially on waking. Bending over makes it much worse because that position increases pressure on already stressed membranes. The affected area may be extremely painful to the touch, and swelling or puffiness around the eyes or cheeks may be visible. Fever and chills may accompany an acute bacterial infection. Sore throat, coughing (caused by post-nasal drip), and congestion or runny nose may appear with any type of sinus irritation, and regardless of whether it is an infectious or allergic situation, people with sinusitis are likely to experience fatigue and general malaise because the body is fighting hard to cast off an invader.

The mucus expressed with a sinus infection is likely to be streaked or completely opaque in shades that range from pale green to yellow to brown. It tends to be thick and sticky. The mucus expressed with hay fever, conversely, tends to be thin, runny, and clear.

Complications

It is rare but not unheard of for sinus infections to spread and become very serious situations. The infection can infiltrate facial bones, causing *osteomyelitis* and permanent bone damage, or it can gain access to the central nervous system and cause *meningitis* (Chapter 3).

Treatment

Treatment for sinusitis begins with self-help measures: staying in humid air or breathing steam to help moisturize and liquefy the clogged mucus is an important step. Increasing daily water intake and reducing the use of alcohol, caffeine, and other diuretics also may help to soften and loosen thick, sticky mucus. Using air filters to remove irritating particles from the air also can help.

Drugs prescribed for this disorder begin with antibiotics if the infection is bacterial. Sinuses are difficult to access, and the bacteria associated with most cases of sinusitis tend to be drug resistant, so this condition often requires long-term courses of specialized antibiotics.

Decongestants are sometimes recommended to shrink the mucous membranes, but these are only appropriate for short-term use because they can create a terrible "rebound effect" when usage is stopped. Corticosteroids in nasal spray form can reduce swelling, but they are also best used in short-term doses. In very extreme cases, surgery is recommended. This involves inserting a tube through the nose and enlarging sinus passages, removing polyps, repairing a deviated septum, and doing anything else that may assist the mucus to drain freely.

Antihistamines are specifically avoided with sinus infections. These substances simply dry up the mucus and allow it to cling to the membrane walls, thus improving bacterial access. Allergies *without* signs of infection may be treated with antihistamines to limit the inappropriate immune response that causes inflammation.

Massage?

Massage is fine for allergic sinusitis because the client has no bacterial or viral infection to spread, catch, or complicate into a more serious condition. (It can be uncomfortable to be completely horizontal for extended periods, however.)

When a client has an acute sinus infection, however, and especially if he is feverish and achy, circulatory bodywork is contraindicated.

Chronic sinus infections are probably safe for most types of bodywork, as long as the client is comfortable. Face holes or cradles may put pressure on sensitive parts of the face and exacerbate symptoms.

Tuberculosis:

From the Latin *tuber*, a swelling or bump (or potato), plus *-osis*, condition. The word *tubercle*, an anatomic term denoting a bump or protrusion, has the same root.

Tuberculosis

Definition: What Is It?

"Tubercle" means *bump*, as in the greater tubercle of the humerus. Tuberculosis (TB) is a disease involving pus and bacteria-filled *bumps*, usually in the lungs, but sometimes in other places too.

Demographics: Who Gets It?

The World Health Organization reports that TB affects one third of the world's population. Eight million people are infected with it every year, and two to three million people die; that is more than the deaths from AIDS, malaria, and all tropical diseases combined.

In the United States, it was considered virtually conquered because in the 1950s a series of antibiotics was developed that finally managed to kill it. It steadily declined until 1986 when suddenly it began to rise again. Between 1986 and 1993, TB statistics in the United States rose alarmingly. When public health efforts became more focused, rates of new TB infection began to decline. However, approximately 15 million Americans are infected with the disease, and approximately 16 thousand have it in the active phase, during which it is highly infectious.

The distribution of TB in the United States is not demographically even. It occurs in highest numbers among the poor, people of color, people with limited access to health care, people in prisons or homeless shelters, and recent immigrants. For more information on TB statistics, see sidebar, "Tuberculosis: Worldwide Statistics, U.S. Statistics."

Etiology: What Happens?

Tuberculosis is an airborne disease. It is caused by *Mycobacterium tuberculosis*. This is a microorganism with a peculiar waxy coat that gives it many advantages over regular bacteria. This pathogen exists quite happily outside of the body. When a person with an active infection coughs or sneezes, bacteria are expelled into the air. The tiny bacteria, protected from drying out by their waxy covering, simply drift until another host comes along. Ordinary antiseptics and disinfectants are ineffective because it rarely clings to surfaces. Even boiling it is not dependable. The only thing that will always kill *mycobacterium tuberculosis* is prolonged, direct sunlight.

Progression

Tuberculosis moves in the body in two phases.

- *Primary phase:* A person inhales some bacteria. (It usually takes prolonged exposure to begin a new infection because these bacteria grow slowly.) The bacteria travel all the way to the alveoli, where they are engulfed by macrophages. The waxy coating on the pathogens makes them resistant to the macrophage's digestive enzymes. Instead, they take up residence inside the macrophages and slowly build up whole colonies of bacteria. Unable to expel these invaders, the body instead builds a protective fibrous wall around the site of infection: a tubercle. Tubercles are usually found in the lungs, but if some of the bacteria seep out into the bloodstream or lymph, they set up the

---

Tuberculosis in Brief

What is it?
Tuberculosis (TB) is a bacterial infection that usually begins in the lungs but may spread to bones, kidney, lymph nodes, or elsewhere in the body. It is a highly contagious airborne disease.

How is it recognized?
Infection with the TB bacterium may produce no initial symptoms. If the infection turns into the active disease, symptoms may include coughing, bloody sputum, fatigue, weight loss, and night sweats.

Is massage indicated or contraindicated?
Active TB disease contraindicates massage, unless the client has been on consistent medication for several weeks and has medical clearance. Massage for clients with TB infection but no disease is fine, but these people should be under medical supervision as well.

Tuberculosis: Worldwide Statistics, U.S. Statistics

Tuberculosis (TB) has a long history in medical and cultural tradition. It was called "consumption" and "the white plague" for many years because it literally consumed its victims with fever and bacterial invasion, causing them to become ghostly pale in the process. In the 19th century, it was the leading cause of death by infectious disease in the United States. It was such an integral part of the cultural scene that it appeared in opera, literature, theatre, and music, from *La Bohème* to *A Long Day's Journey into Night*.

For years the only dependable treatment for TB was to retire to a sanatorium, often a luxurious retreat where patients who could afford it would be given excellent food, good rest, and lots of sunshine for several months. If they outlived their disease, they were able to return home. Many sanatoria that began as TB treatment centers are now health and spa resorts.

The causative agent for TB, *Mycobacterium tuberculosis*, was first isolated and identified in 1882. In the 1950s, the development of a series of antibiotics that could successfully eradicate the disease completely changed its place in the medical community. From being a life-threatening scourge, it became all but unknown in the United States.

The confluence of several events has led to a resurgence of TB both in the United States and especially in developing nations, where antibiotic therapy is harder to access. The national and worldwide statistics on TB are cause for concern, but also point out that with the right kinds of intervention, the "white plague" can indeed become a thing of the past.

Worldwide Statistics[2]:

Approximately 2 billion people have been infected with TB. That is a worldwide incidence of approximately one in three.

Of those infections, 4.4 million are among HIV-positive patients, in whom the risk of active infection and contagion is very high.

More than 8 million new infections occur every year. Tuberculosis has become the leading cause of death from AIDS around the world, but especially in sub-Saharan Africa and Southeast Asia.

The institution of DOTS treatment protocols limits the spread of both regular and multi–drug-resistant TB. Because this has been implemented in several key countries, some have moved off the World Health Organization's high-risk list; others are very close.

U.S. Statistics[3]:

Approximately 15 million Americans are infected with TB. Recent immigrants constitute 40% of all TB infections in the United States.

Approximately 16,000 Americans have active TB infections.

Approximately 100,000 Americans have coexisting HIV and TB infections.

Multi–drug-resistant TB has been reported in 43 states and the District of Columbia.

Between 1984 and 1993, the rates of TB in the United States rose by 16%. Now they are consistently going down.

[2] Tuberculosis Summary. Copyright © 2001 World Health Organization / Organisation mondiale de la Santé. Available at: http://www.who.int/gtb/publications/globrep01/summary.html. Accessed winter 2004.
[3] Questions and Answers About TB. Available at: http://www.cdc.gov/nchstp/tb/faqs/pdfs/qa.pdf. Accessed winter 2004.

same process elsewhere in the body. Kidneys, the spine, and the central nervous system are the most common other choices.

A single undetectable capsule in the lung is where it all stops for most people. This is tuberculosis infection, but *not* the active disease. Within 10 to 12 weeks, T-cells are activated, and a specific immune response will ensue. Antibodies are produced that will react to another contact with the bacillus, as in the "scratch test" that looks for past exposure. The inhaled bacteria remain stuck inside their tidy fibrous package until something happens to set them free, usually a future depression in immune system function.

- *Secondary phase:* Approximately 10% of the people exposed to TB will develop the active disease later in life. The bacteria escape and spread into other areas in the lungs, or wherever else in the body they may be stationed. The body attempts to surround the new sites with bigger and bigger fibrous capsules, which can cause permanent scarring. Pleurisy, the scarring and sticking of the pleurae, is nearly always a complication of tuberculosis. Inside the capsules, the bacteria are destroying cells, and the tissue is necrotic, or dead (Figure 6.3).

New tubercles eventually take up enough room in the lungs to impede function. A cough begins and gradually produces bloody sputum; this phlegm actually contains detached pieces of the bacteria-infested tubercles, which is why tuberculosis is so very contagious. If several of the tubercles join together, their necrotic centers can cause a cavity in the lung. Surrounding blood vessels may hemorrhage into the cavity, leading to coughing up blood or *hemoptysis*. Similar cavities can develop in the kidneys if the tubercles form there. Infections in the bones tend to destroy articular cartilage.

Figure 6.3. Tuberculosis: fibrous capsules
surround necrotic tissue.

Risk Factors

The major risk factor for TB infection without active disease is any kind of long-term exposure to someone with active disease. Travelers to parts of the world where TB is most common are at risk, as are people who spend time with immigrants from those same areas, or other groups where the disease may be rampant, such as prisons, nursing homes, and homeless shelters.

Once a person has been exposed to TB, the next question is what will increase his or her risk of developing the active infection. Several risk factors for this process have been identified.

HIV puts people very much at risk for active TB. In an otherwise healthy person, the bacterium would enter the body and be largely controlled by the immune system. TB infection turns into TB disease in 1 of every 2 or 3 people who are HIV positive, and these people can then, in turn, infect others. In fact, TB is the only airborne sickness that AIDS patients can transmit to healthy people.

Other risk factors for progressing to active TB infection include other conditions in which the immune system is compromised: poor nutrition, substance abuse, alcoholism, advanced age, and limited access to health care.

Factors that contribute to the prevalence of TB in the United States include the vulnerability of HIV-positive patients, high numbers of immigrants from countries with high rates of TB (40% of the U.S. population with TB are immigrants), increasing levels of poverty, injection drug use, and homelessness, poor compliance with treatment plans, and growing numbers of elderly people living in long-term care facilities.

Signs and Symptoms

The primary phase of TB is so benign a person may never know she has been exposed; the symptoms, if there are any, are the same as for a mild flu. However, the active disease shows much more severe symptoms. They include fever, sweating, weight loss, and exhaustion. Chest pain and shortness of breath are common. A stubborn cough that starts dry and becomes productive of bloody or pus-filled phlegm is a cardinal sign. Other symptoms arise if other organs have been infected as well.

Diagnosis

Identifying people who have been exposed to the TB bacterium is not difficult. Within several weeks of infection, enough antibodies to the pathogen will have been produced that a "scratch test" will create a characteristic welt.

When the disease becomes active, however, it becomes surprisingly difficult to catch early, because its symptoms mimic pneumonia, lung abscesses, and fungal infections. X-rays can show the tubercles in the lungs, but it is not until bacteria are expelled in bloody sputum that the disease can be reliably identified and the pathogens analyzed for which medications will be most effective.

Treatment

In the old days, wealthy TB patients were sent to sanitoria where it was hoped that sunlight, rest, and good food would enable them to outlive their infection. That is still a good approach, but it is even better when it is combined with the right antibiotics. More than 90% of TB patients have full recovery if their treatment is completed.

Anyone who has been exposed to TB, regardless of whether the infection is dormant or active, can receive successful antibiotic treatment. The problem is that these antibiotics need to be taken with unfailing consistency. In addition, several different types of antibiotics may be prescribed to circumvent the bacteria's resistance to any single variety. This can mean up to 13 pills a day for 6 to 9 months. Not surprisingly, studies indicate that approximately one third of all patients do not take their medication as directed.

Multi–Drug-Resistant TB

When patients do not take all of their TB medication properly, the bacterium may mutate into a form that most drugs cannot affect. Whoever is infected with this new strain will be likewise difficult to treat. This mutation is called multi–drug-resistant TB, or MDR-TB.

It costs approximately 10 times more to treat MDR-TB than to treat regular TB. It requires 18 to 24 months of intensive drug therapy that is highly toxic and has many unpleasant side effects. The death rate of MDR-TB that is treated in this way is approximately the same as the death rate for completely untreated regular TB: 40% to 60%.

MDR-TB has been reported in 43 states and the District of Columbia.

DOTS

In a study done of "directly observed therapy, short-course" (DOTS), that is, when social workers directly observed their clients taking their medication for each and every dose, the rate of acquired drug resistance sank to 2.1%, down from 14%. DOTS is now considered the gold standard for TB treatment. Fortunately, although progress is slow, DOTS is being used more and more frequently. Thanks to DOTS, some of the countries on the World Health Organization's list of at-risk locations have been able to move off the list; several more are on the brink.

A successful DOTS program depends on several factors, including governmental commitment, reliable detection of infection, a dependable and affordable source of medication, and a good reporting system. Populations that are mobile, such as war refugees and homeless people, are difficult to track and treat successfully.

Massage?

TB is an infection that can travel in the blood and lymph. If a client has the active disease, massage can spread it through the body and help to set up tubercles where they would not otherwise have occurred. TB is also contagious; therapists will not do their clients much good if their own careers are cut short by this condition. However, if a client has been exposed to the bacterium and is under medication or if a client has had the active disease but has been under medication for several weeks, massage may be appropriate, with medical clearance to assure that the risk of contagion has been eliminated.

CHRONIC OBSTRUCTIVE PULMONARY DISEASES

Asthma

> ### Asthma in Brief
>
> **What is it?**
> Asthma is the result of spasmodic constriction of bronchial smooth muscle tubes in combination with chronic local inflammation and excessive mucus production.
>
> **How is it recognized?**
> Asthma attacks are sporadic episodes involving coughing, wheezing, and difficulty with breathing, especially exhaling.
>
> **Is massage indicated or contraindicated?**
> Massage is indicated for anyone with asthma who is not in the throes of an attack. Between episodes, massage can be useful to reduce stress and deal with some of the muscular problems that accompany difficulty with breathing.

Definition: What Is It?

Asthma is a chronic disorder that may be triggered by external factors such as allergens or pollutants but is also directly linked to internal factors such as emotional stress. In asthma, someone is exposed to a stimulus that causes a sympathetic reaction, which is followed by a parasympathetic overreaction.

Asthma is considered by some in the medical field to be part of a collection of lung problems called *chronic obstructive pulmonary disease* (COPD) because in some extreme cases it can cause structural changes in the lungs that open the door to two other COPD problems: *chronic bronchitis* and *emphysema* (this chapter). In most cases, however, asthma does not cause irreversible damage to the lungs. Therefore, some professionals do not put it in the COPD category.

Demographics: Who Gets It?

Asthma affects some 20 million people in the United States, from young infants to elderly people. Approximately 12 million asthma attacks are reported each year, with approximately half a million hospitalizations. Asthma is responsible for an estimated 5,000 deaths per year: a statistic that has more than doubled since 1979, in spite of new and improved treatment options.

Children are more often affected by asthma than adults. Persons who have asthma as a child are very likely to continue to have symptoms well into adulthood.

Etiology: What Happens?

Rising asthma statistics over the past two decades have drawn a lot of attention to the quality of indoor air. As buildings become "tighter" to conserve energy, the amount of airborne irritants in them can accumulate to levels that are dangerous to some people. Specific substances such as pet-related allergens, cockroach wastes, cigarette smoke, and dust mites have been found to be especially potent asthma triggers.

Some researchers have questioned how exposure to common asthma triggers during infancy and early childhood may impact the incidence of this disease, but statistics show both increases and decreases linked to early exposure, leading to the conclusion that the hyperreactivity of asthmatics' bronchioles develops because of many unpredictable factors.

All bronchioles are sensitive to foreign debris, but asthmatics' bronchioles are extremely irritable. Furthermore, the bronchial tubes of a person with asthma appear to be in a state of chronic inflammation, always ready to begin an attack when appropriately stimulated. When the right trigger comes along, an asthmatic person's bronchioles first dilate (a sympathetic reaction), and then the body overcompensates by sending the bronchioles into spasm. The irritated membranes lining these tubes swell up and secrete extra mucus (Figure 6.4). People with asthma find it very difficult to breathe, especially to exhale, during an attack.

Three common types of asthma have been identified, along with a few others that occur more rarely.

- *Extrinsic asthma*: This is a typical example of a type 1 hypersensitivity reaction. In this situation, the mast cells that are thickly distributed in the mucous membrane secrete excessive histamine. Histamine causes vasodilation, increases cell permeability, and, in the respiratory system, initiates excess mucus production.

- *Intrinsic asthma*: This situation is more common in adults than in children. It involves attacks that may have no known origin or that may be related to exercise, upper respiratory tract infection (see common cold, this chapter) or emotional stress.

- *Mixed asthma*: This combination or extrinsic and intrinsic factors is probably the most common situation.

- *Others*: A few other types of asthma exist but are less common They include *occupational asthma*, which is a reaction to work-related substances such as detergents, plastics, resins, and fumes, and *cardiac asthma*, which is related to congestive heart failure (see Chapter 4), and the resulting excess fluid in the lungs. Other forms of asthma may be related to irritation from *GERD* (Chapter 7) or *sinusitis* (this chapter).

Signs and Symptoms

Symptoms of asthma include dyspnea (shortness of breath), wheezing (the sound of air moving through tightened and clogged up bronchioles), and coughing that may or may not be productive. It feels especially difficult to *expel* air; the bronchioles are constricted, so the alveoli do not empty easily.

Figure 6.4. Asthma: Normal bronchiole (A) and bronchiole under attack (B)

Asthma can show symptoms in several different ways. *Bronchial asthma* is a typical episode with tight bronchioles with excess mucus production and wheezing; *exercise-induced* asthma occurs with physical exertion, sometimes hours later; *silent asthma* shows no symptoms leading up to an episode, and then the patient suddenly finds himself dangerously short of breath; *cough variant asthma* shows coughing alone as its primary symptom.

If the symptoms are extreme and prolonged, the asthmatic person may start to feel panicky, adding sweating, increased heart rate, and anxiety to the list of symptoms. In emergency situations, the lips and face may take on a bluish cast (cyanosis) when access to oxygen is severely restricted.

Asthma attacks are sporadic, lasting anywhere from a few minutes to a few days. Between attacks, the lungs are generally normal. Someone who has had asthma for a long time may develop structural changes in the lungs that raise the risk of other respiratory disorders, particularly chronic bronchitis and emphysema.

Diagnosis

Asthma is typically diagnosed by ruling out other lung infections or disorders and by measuring lung capacity and airflow through a series of spirometry tests. One other disorder, called *vocal cord dysfunction*, shares many symptoms with asthma but does not respond to the same treatments, so it is important to consider that in a diagnosis.

Treatment

Treatment for asthma begins with managing the stimuli that are known to trigger attacks. Patients are also taught to recognize the warning sign of an attack so it can be treated as quickly as possible.

Medical intervention is available in several forms. Steroidal anti-inflammatories can quell the inflammatory nature of the bronchioles. Oral or intravenous steroids are associated with several serious side effects, but inhaled steroids are reported to be much safer. Bronchodilators relax the smooth muscles of the bronchiole tubes; these come in several forms. It has been found that the most effective treatment for most people is to combine steroids with bronchodilators and to administer treatment at the first signs of an episode. This approach can limit the severity of the episode and decrease the risks associated with very severe asthma attacks.

Other medications alter the way immune system chemicals work in the respiratory tract, but these are generally reserved for patients for whom the standard approaches are unsuccessful.

Massage?

A person who has asthma can derive great benefit from massage, as long as he is not in the midst of an attack. No one who is fighting for breath will be comfortable on a massage table. Someone who struggles with this problem will probably have a number of different muscular reflections of it that massage can help with. Watch for hypertonic intercostals, scalenes, serratus posterior inferior, and diaphragm with asthmatic clients. These muscles of inspiration will be chronically tight for someone who does not breathe easily, and that tightness will further interfere with his breathing.

Be aware, however, that many asthma patients have other allergies, including allergies to certain types of oils or perfumes. Clients with asthma typically derive the best benefit from the use of hypoallergenic lubricants.

Case History 6.1

Asthma

Richard L., Age 52: "A Smog Problem"

I didn't contract asthma until I was 22, after I got back from Viet Nam. I was living in Los Angeles, and I got real bad bronchitis. I was diagnosed then with just a common smog problem.

Then I moved to Corvallis, Oregon, and ran into the Willamette Valley Crud: they have pollination 10 months out of the year there. I saw an allergist who gave me skin tests, and I came up positive to 95% of the things he tested me for. Then I realized it wasn't just the smog; I had a lung problem.

At that time, I started taking desensitization shots. I did that for about 5 years, but it didn't really help. I ended up quitting, and just medicating myself with aspirin, Sudafed, and over-the-counter inhalants. I didn't have any really bad episodes that I couldn't handle, but I was working in construction, and I knew that I couldn't be sawing or working in a closed room because I would stop breathing; my lungs would just shut down.

Then I moved to Bellingham, Washington, and went into a roofing business. I was working with hot tar, and this stuff called "torch down" that's pretty fumey. A couple of times I ended up in the emergency room with breathing problems. They gave me a prescription inhalant and prednisone.

When I moved to Seattle, I wound up with an asthma specialist who's been really good for me. I've had a few bouts down here; one time a cold put me in the hospital for about a week. I work in a shipyard now. I can stay away from the worst of the fumes, but about once a year I get a bad attack and go on prednisone until it clears up.

I've been doing massage since the 60s but just recently went to school and got licensed. I'm really sensitive to perfumes, and massage schools are 90% female, so I'd always choose where to sit, to be away from anyone wearing perfume. But I never thought about massage oils until we got into it. I knew to stay away from oils and lotions that are scented at all. When I got a massage with almond oil, I noticed my skin would turn really red, but it wasn't until someone worked on my chest and back that I noticed about an hour later my breathing was affected.

Asthma affects my life in all kinds of ways. My lung capacity is only about 65% of normal. I like to go listen to music, but the venues where the good bands play are always too smoky. I have to stay away from stale flower shops. It was almost impossible to go into a mall because you have to walk past the perfume counter to get through the big department stores, but that seems to be less of a problem now. Asthma really limits my social life too. When someone asks us over to dinner, our first question has to be, "Do you have any pets?"

As my massage clientele builds, I'm able to cut back at the shipyard. Eventually I'll be able to do massage full time. My focus now is on controlling my environment—keeping out the things I know will trigger an attack and trying to stay as healthy as possible.

Bronchiectasis

Definition: What Is It?

Bronchiectasis is a chronic obstructive pulmonary disease in which the bronchi of the lungs are damaged and lose the ability to constrict and to clear mucus from their surface.

Bronchiectasis in Brief

Pronunciation
brong-kē-ek'tă-sis

What is it?
Bronchiectasis is a condition in which the bronchial tubes become structurally damaged, leading to permanent dilation and excessive production of mucus.

How is it recognized?
This condition usually follows congenital diseases or repeated severe lung infections. Its symptoms include chest pain, shortness of breath, productive coughing, and possible clubbing of the fingers.

Is massage indicated or contraindicated?
Bronchiectasis contraindicates massage if acute infection is present, but otherwise massage (with percussion on the chest) may be appropriate if the client is comfortable and if the therapist works as part of a well-informed health care team.

Demographics: Who Gets It?

Bronchiectasis, which is often related to a history of extreme and repeated respiratory tract infections, is on the decline in this country. In young people, it is usually connected to a congenital lung disorder such as *cystic fibrosis* (this chapter), whereas in older people it is more likely to be the result of recurring injury and insult to the lungs.

Etiology: What Happens?

Bronchiectasis is a classic example of a vicious circle. Typically it begins when bronchial tissue has been repeatedly damaged through infection, aspiration of food, exposure to toxic pollutants, or other triggers. The smooth muscle tissue and elastin fibers in the bronchioles eventually break down, and the tubes become permanently dilated, although the passage is usually obstructed with abnormally large deposits of mucus. Because the smooth muscle tissue is no longer functional, the mucus cannot be dislodged. It becomes an inviting growth medium for secondary bacterial infection, which further damages the bronchial tubes and adds to the progress of bronchiectasis.

This condition is usually discussed as a congenital problem or an acquired disease. Sometimes the respiratory system does not fully develop in a growing fetus, and bronchiectasis may be a result of this weakness. Cystic fibrosis also opens the door to this disorder. Alpha-1 antitrypsin deficiency is a situation in which the alveoli of the lung lack an important lubricant. This makes a person more susceptible to *emphysema* (this chapter) and bronchiectasis.

Acquired bronchiectasis is usually attributable to a severe infection such as viral or bacterial *pneumonia* or *tuberculosis* (this chapter). An allergic reaction to *inhaled aspergillosis* can irritate the bronchial tubes enough to initiate the disease process, as can inhaled irritants such as cigarette smoke, sulfur dioxide, and ammonia. Repeated gastric aspiration related to *GERD* (Chapter 7) is another predisposing factor.

Signs and Symptoms

Symptoms of bronchiectasis can include fever, shortness of breath, chest pain, and a chronic productive cough, sometimes with foul-smelling sputum. *Auscultation* of the chest reveals several different lung sounds, including wheezing, *rales*, and crackles. If the condition has been present for a long time, "clubbing" of the fingers may develop; this is a change in the structure of the furthest extremities that occurs when oxygen is in short supply.

Untreated bronchiectasis raises the risk of dangerous lung infections and right-sided heart failure as the pulmonary circuit develops resistance to blood flow from the heart.

Diagnosis

Bronchiectasis is diagnosed with a clinical history to screen for past infections or congenital diseases, along with various imaging techniques that may range from x-rays to computed tomography (CT) scans to magnetic resonance imaging (MRI) of the lungs. Because it is on the decline in the United States, and because it can be difficult to differentiate from asthma or pneumonia, a correct diagnosis may sometimes be missed. This becomes a problem when a person is treated incorrectly while his disease progresses to affect more tissue.

Treatment

Bronchiectasis is difficult to treat because the damage to the bronchial tubes may be permanent or difficult to reverse. Limiting the risk of further infection is a high priority, as is helping to clear the tubes of excessive mucus. Consequently, bronchodilators, postural drainage, appropriate antibiotics, and possibly surgery to remove damaged tissue may be recommended.

Massage?

A person with bronchiectasis may not be comfortable lying flat on a table because that position often aggravates coughing. If this issue can be addressed and if no infection is current at the time of an appointment, massage is appropriate for a person with this disorder. Postural drainage along with cupping may be appropriate to try to dislodge deposits of mucus; this is best done as part of a well-informed health care team.

Chronic Bronchitis

Definition: What Is It?

Chronic bronchitis is part of a group of closely connected lung problems called chronic obstructive pulmonary disease (COPD). Chronic bronchitis, as its name implies, involves long-term irritation of the bronchi and bronchioles, which may occur with or without infection. It is a progressive disorder that may be halted or slowed but not reversed. It often occurs simultaneously or as a predecessor to emphysema (this chapter).

Demographics: Who Gets It?

Approximately 9.2 million people in the United States have chronic bronchitis. Men have it more often than women, and it appears more frequently in whites than any other racial group.

Smokers are more vulnerable to any type of COPD than nonsmokers; approximately 15% of all smokers develop chronic bronchitis.

COPD, which includes chronic bronchitis, emphysema, and sometimes asthma, is the fourth leading cause of death in the United States, killing approximately 120,000 people every year.

Etiology: What Happens?

This disorder is the result of long-term irritation to bronchial tubes. When the delicate lining of the respiratory tract is chronically insulted with cigarettes (first-hand, second-hand, or side-stream smoke), air pollutants, industrial chemicals, or other contaminants, an inflammatory response ensues. Attacks against the bronchial lining destroy elastin fibers, cause the overgrowth of mucus-producing cells and the excessive production of mucus, and increase resistance to the movement of air in and out of the system. Eventually the damage to the bronchioles is permanent; chronic bronchitis is an irreversible progressive disorder.

As resistance to air flow in the bronchioles increases, less oxygen enters the body with each breath. The heart has to work harder to push enough blood into the lungs to

---

Chronic Bronchitis in Brief

What is it?
Chronic bronchitis is one of the lung disorders classified as chronic obstructive pulmonary disease (COPD). It involves long-term inflammation of the bronchi with or without infection, leading to permanent changes in the bronchial lining. Chronic bronchitis frequently occurs as a prelude to or simultaneously with emphysema.

How is it recognized?
Chronic bronchitis is diagnosed when a person experiences a productive cough that occurs most days for 3 months or more, for at least 2 consecutive years. Other common signs are a susceptibility to respiratory tract infections, cyanosis, and pulmonary edema.

Is massage indicated or contraindicated?
Massage can be appropriate for chronic bronchitis patients, as long as they are not fighting acute respiratory infection at the time, and as long as heart function is not compromised.

The lungs are particularly vulnerable to infection, stationed as they are at the receiving end of everything that enters the body through the nose. They have some structural features that make it easy to isolate sites of infection, and they are well stocked with stationary immune system cells to fight off incoming invaders, but they are susceptible to a variety of infectious disorders that can cause both short-term and long-term damage.

Acute bronchitis often accompanies upper respiratory infections or flu. This is a viral attack directly on the bronchi, although it can also complicate into a bacterial infection. Chronic bronchitis involves long-term irritation to the bronchial lining, all the way down to the terminal bronchioles. This irritation can cause the lining to become permanently thick with excessive mucus production that can make it difficult to breathe. Finally, bronchiectasis is a disorder brought about by repeated lung infections that cause structural changes to the bronchial tubes: they become permanently widened. When the bronchi become unable to move mucus out of the body, it pools in the lungs, creating a risk for further infection and more structural damage.

If a lung disorder is present, it is useful for the massage therapist to have a clear idea of the situation, so that the client may be made as comfortable as possible on the table, and the risk of spreading infection is minimized.

	ACUTE BRONCHITIS	CHRONIC BRONCHITIS	BRONCHIECTASIS
Cause	Viral attack on lungs; often accompanies cold or flu	Long-term lung irritation, e.g., cigarette smoke, pollution, particles in the air	A history of multiple lung infections, including acute bronchitis and pneumonia
Symptoms	A productive cough with clear sputum (if the sputum is colored, suspect a secondary bacterial infection), along with fever, aches and pains	A productive cough with clear sputum (if the sputum is colored, suspect a secondary bacterial infection). Excessive mucus production, requiring lots of throat clearing. Susceptibility to lung infections. Wheezing, shortness of breath, cyanosis.	A frequent cough with a large amount of green or yellow sputum, especially when lying down.
Prognosis	If the patient is basically healthy, full recovery with no long-term problems.	If the irritation to the lungs is halted, the problem may not progress, but it is not reversible. If it does progress, it may develop into right-sided heart failure, respiratory failure, or emphysema.	Patient must avoid lung irritants and the possibility of further lung infections, which may cause further damage to the bronchi.
Implications for massage	This client should not receive massage until the infection has been resolved.	This client may receive massage, as long as he can be positioned on the table in a way that does not exacerbate his symptoms. Care must be taken to rule out the possibility of circulatory stress.	This client may receive massage, as long as he can be positioned on the table in a way that does not exacerbate his symptoms.

supply the body with fuel. At the same time, red blood cell production may increase, in an effort to provide more access to any oxygen that can seep into the capillaries. The blood may become thicker with excess erythrocytes (this is called *polycythemia*), and so the heart has to work even *harder* to push it through the pulmonary circuit. Eventually right-sided *heart failure* (see Chapter 4) may develop, leading to *edema*, especially in the legs and ankles.

Signs and Symptoms

Signs and symptoms of chronic bronchitis develop slowly, often taking months or years before they are severe enough to attract attention. The process usually begins with a mild cough, perhaps following a typical flu or cold infection. The cough lingers long after the infection has cleared. It is present most days for 3 months or more and produces thick, clear sputum. This pattern occurs for at least 2 years in a row.

The person may be aware that he must clear his throat very often, especially in the morning; this reflects the excessive production of mucus in his lungs. Shortness of breath gets progressively worse, and the chronic bronchitis patient becomes highly vulnerable to any respiratory infections to which he may be exposed.

Later in the process, the chronic bronchitis patient may develop signs of oxygen deprivation: cyanosis and eventually edema from right-sided heart failure.

Complications

Complications of this situation are obvious. Bronchi that are chronically inflamed and producing loads of mucus are highly vulnerable to viral or bacterial infection. A person with chronic bronchitis can develop pneumonia from cold or flu viruses much more easily than the general population.

The long-term risk of right-sided heart failure has already been discussed. This serious prognosis is the reason it is important to try to stop the progression of chronic bronchitis as soon as it can be recognized.

Diagnosis

Chronic bronchitis is diagnosed through a variety of methods, including patient history, physical examination, and a test of pulmonary function called *spirometry*. In this test, the patient exhales into a container that measures lung volume. Additional tests may be conducted to measure levels of oxygen and carbon dioxide in the blood.

Treatment

People with chronic bronchitis are especially susceptible to viral and bacterial infections of the respiratory tract. If a bacterial infection arises, aggressive treatment with antibiotics may be recommended to prevent the situation from developing into life-threatening pneumonia. Chronic bronchitis patients are encouraged to be vaccinated against pneumococcus pneumonia and to get yearly flu shots for the same reason.

Other than preventing worse infections from happening, treatment for chronic bronchitis focuses on halting the progression of the damage and keeping the patient as comfortable as possible. Quitting smoking, if that is an issue, is the single most important step a chronic bronchitis patient can take. Patients should avoid polluted air and known triggers of bronchial spasm. Bronchodilators in spray or pill form may be prescribed to keep the smooth muscle tissue of the respiratory tract relaxed and open. Oxygen may be supplemented in a medical emergency; however, most chronic bronchitis patients do not need to supplement oxygen on a regular basis.

Massage?

If a chronic bronchitis patient has a healthy circulatory system and no current infections, massage, including circulatory massage, should probably be fine. Someone in an advanced stage of the disease may not be able to keep up with the internal changes to blood flow that circulatory modalities bring about; the clients would require bodywork that does not intend to move a lot of fluid, and may have some special requirements for positioning to keep comfortable.

Emphysema in Brief

What is it?
Emphysema is a condition in which the alveoli of the lungs become stretched out and inelastic. They merge with each other, decreasing surface area, destroying surrounding capillaries, and limiting oxygen–carbon dioxide exchange.

How is it recognized?
Symptoms of emphysema include shortness of breath with mild or no exertion, a chronic dry cough, rales, cyanosis, and susceptibility to secondary respiratory infection.

Is massage indicated or contraindicated?
Emphysema indicates massage with caution for circulatory complications, secondary infection, and positioning the client for maximum comfort.

Emphysema

Definition: What Is It?

Emphysema, along with bronchial asthma and chronic bronchitis, is the third of a group of the classic chronic obstructive pulmonary disease, or COPD, triad. The name *emphysema* means "blown up" (as in inflated, not exploded), and this is a very apt description of the disease process.

Demographics: Who Gets It?

An estimated 32 million Americans have some form of COPD. Approximately 2 million people have emphysema. Most emphysema patients are between 65 and 75 years old. More than 80% of emphysema cases can be traced to cigarette smoking, but other cases may develop from occupational hazards: working with grain dust, in coal mines, or in quarries can increase risk. A small percentage of emphysema patients have a genetic lack of the alpha-1 antitrypsin protein that protects alveolar walls. These people generally develop the disease before they are 50 years old.

Etiology: What Happens?

When the delicate epithelium that lines the respiratory tract is constantly irritated (cigarette smoke and air pollution are the two biggest culprits), the cilia, which are supposed to trap pathogens and particles, eventually disintegrate. Then the bronchioles produce excess mucus in an effort to fight off environmental irritations: this is *chronic bronchitis* (this chapter), and it involves damage proximal to the terminal bronchioles. When the damage spreads further, or when it originates distally to the terminal bronchioles, the delicate alveoli are vulnerable.

Three hundred million alveoli in the lungs provide sites for oxygen–carbon dioxide exchange. Each one has a circulatory capillary to allow the exchange of oxygen and carbon dioxide. All alveoli are meant to be supplied with a specific substance called alpha-1 antitrypsin (AAT): this is a protein that protects the delicate tissue from damage by environmental forces. Long-term exposure to cigarette smoke or other pollutants overcomes the protective abilities of AAT, resulting in the destruction of the alveolar elastin fibers. The alveoli become less elastic, and they fill up with mucus, which interferes with their ability to exchange oxygen and carbon dioxide. Instead of emptying and filling with every breath, they only partially empty, or stay altogether full. This usually begins in a small area, but if the irritation continues, it spreads throughout the lung. The alveolar walls eventually break down and merge with each other, forming larger sacs, called *bullae* (Figure 6.5). These sacs have less volume and less surface area for gaseous exchange than the uninjured alveoli did. Although most bullae stay under

Normal alveoli   Overinflated
                      alveoli (bulla)

Figure 6.5. COPD/emphysema.

4 cm, some can become "giant bullae" and inflate enough to obstruct 30% of lung volume.

As the alveoli fuse and surface area for gaseous exchange is lost, the emphysema patient has to work much harder to move air in and out of the lungs. A person with healthy lungs expends approximately 5% of his energy in the effort of breathing. A person with advanced emphysema puts closer to 50% of his energy into this job, and he must do this every minute, 24 hours a day.

Less gaseous exchange means reduced oxygen levels in the blood, or *hypoxia*. This situation is toxic to brain cells. It also causes the epithelial walls of the alveoli to thicken into tough fibrous connective tissue, which allows even less diffusion. As breathing becomes more difficult (the emphysema patient must *consciously* exhale—it no longer happens spontaneously), the respiration rate slows. This leads to even higher concentrations of carbon dioxide in the blood. The blood vessels supplying the damaged alveoli also sustain damage; it becomes harder to pump blood through the pulmonary artery. Hypoxia also leads to spasm of pulmonary blood vessels. All of these factors may contribute to pulmonary hypertension and right-sided *heart failure*, or *cor pulmonale* (see Chapter 4). Eventually the untreated emphysema patient experiences respiratory and circulatory collapse.

Signs and Symptoms

It can take many years for emphysema to advance to a stage in which a person seeks medical help. Because it usually affects people older than 65 years of age, early symptoms are often assumed to be normal signs of aging. Symptoms of emphysema include pain with breathing, shortness of breath, a dry cough, and wheezing. Weight loss often occurs, because a person who must exert so much energy in breathing has little interest in eating. "Rales," a characteristic bubbling, rasping sound of air moving through a narrowed passage, may occur with some cases. Difficulty in exhaling also may be reflected in a spirometry test. Exhalation takes longer, and the patient may develop a habit of pushing air out through pursed lips. This is an attempt to push against increasing back-pressure in the lungs. Because the lungs no longer deflate normally with each breath, the diaphragm becomes permanently flattened. The emphysema patient often develops "barrel chest"; that is, the intercostals lock into a position that holds the rib cage out as wide as possible.

Complications

Emphysema patients are extremely vulnerable to influenza and pneumonia (this chapter) because they have lost much of the ability to resist secondary infection. Another complication occurs if the bullae should rupture. This allows air into the pleural space (which is supposed to be a vacuum) and ends in total lung collapse. Finally, the stress to the circulatory system if the lungs sustain this kind of damage is very great. The right ventricle, trying to pump blood through the partially collapsed pulmonary circuit, enlarges and eventually leads to heart failure. The risk of blood clots forming somewhere in the circuit is also high, which results in pulmonary *embolism* (see Chapter 4).

Treatment

Emphysema is basically an irreversible disease. If it is found and treated early, further damage can be avoided. Once the alveoli have begun to break down, however, they cannot be rebuilt. The first course of action, of course, is to remove the irritating stimulus; usually this is cigarette smoke. Drugs may be administered to dilate the bronchi and take pressure off the alveoli, to remove mucus and edema from the lungs, and to ward off potential lung infections. Oxygen supplementation may be recommended during sleep or after exercise. Surgery called bullectomy, lung volume reduction surgery, or lung shaving removes only damaged portions of the lung. This increases thoracic capacity for the diaphragm to work and improves circulation. Statistics on how it affects longevity, however, are not yet available. In rare cases, a heart and lung transplant may be necessary.

Emphysema and other COPD patients are often strongly urged to be vaccinated against pneumococcus pneumonia and to get a yearly flu shot because they are at higher risk for serious lung infections than the general population.

Massage?

If a client is in the early stages of this disease and his tissues are healthy and responsive (that is, his skin shows signs of normal blood flow by appropriate temperature and color changes with massage) and if he has no heart problems or secondary infection, massage may be very beneficial. Back, neck, and chest massage may be especially helpful to help reduce any muscular resistance to the movement of air in and out of the body.

Advanced cases, in which a client is experiencing difficulty with breathing and shortness of breath, may not be appropriate for rapid, vigorous Swedish strokes; however, calming reflexive work may be excellent for dealing with anxiety and the stress of quitting smoking, as well as the inevitable fatigue these people experience. Massage also can address the muscular contribution to "barrel chest." Emphysema and other COPD patients often cannot tolerate lying completely prone or supine; they may be more comfortable receiving work in a reclining chair or on a massage chair.

Case History 6.2

Emphysema

Roberta F., Age 68

Roberta is 5'2" and weighs 100 pounds. She started smoking in 1947, and quit in 1984. She first experienced pulmonary symptoms in the mid 1980s. She noticed that she was frequently short of breath, she had low energy, and she had consistent headaches on rising each morning. She was unable to walk far, or fast. In an effort to catch her breath, she hyperventilated easily, which only made matters worse. She experienced a lot of stress and frustration that breathing was so difficult, and that she could no longer accomplish the things she wanted to do.

Roberta's original doctor diagnosed her with chronic obstructive pulmonary disease (COPD) and chronic bronchitis. She then saw a pulmonary specialist, who diagnosed her with emphysema. This finding was based on a number of tests, including a chest x-ray, spirometry, an analysis of arterial blood gases, and a measurement of the air volume she was able to expel.

Emphysema makes it hard for Roberta to do anything. The activities of daily living are difficult, and all daily routines have to be altered to accommodate the disease. Stairs and hills are especially challenging. Emphysema dulls the thinking by depriving the brain of oxygen. It reduces the appetite, and the lack of oxygen reduces the benefit from what food is eaten. It also strains the heart, because it has to work harder to push more blood, which contains less oxygen, through the body.

When Roberta was x-rayed for emphysema, it was found that she also has some degree of osteoporosis. This condition, in combination with her breathing difficulties, has significantly altered her posture. Her shoulders rise to her ears in an attempt to get more air. Also the shoulders tend to roll forward. Because of the increased tension Roberta experienced while trying to breathe, some muscle stiffness and pain was occasionally a problem.

Another aspect of Roberta's experience with emphysema is how it has seriously affected her resistance to disease. Some medicines Roberta takes to help her breathe weaken her immune system, so it is harder for her to ward off respiratory ailments. In March of 1997, she had a crisis that hospitalized her for 10 days. At that time, she began supplementing oxygen by nose. She was in a rehabilitation facility for 2 weeks, working with physical and occupational therapists, who taught her ways to accomplish more with less energy.

In June 1997, she had a bad cold, which put her in the hospital for 4 days.

In January 1998, Roberta contracted pneumonia, which was confirmed by chest x-ray. She was in the hospital for 5 days. The pneumonia cleared up with antibiotics, and she returned home.

Roberta is now feeling improved. She still supplements oxygen, and her daily activities have become a little easier. She tries to keep up with her exercises, eat properly, and reduce stress. She also attends Better Breathing Club meetings sponsored by the American Lung Association to keep up with new information about techniques to deal with her disease, and she sees her pulmonary specialist regularly.

*Author's note: Roberta passed away from pneumonia in 2002. Many thanks to her and her family for generously sharing her story.

OTHER RESPIRATORY DISORDERS

Cystic Fibrosis

Definition: What Is It?

Cystic fibrosis (CF) is an autosomal recessive genetic disorder of exocrine glands, causing the production of thick, viscous secretions. It affects the digestive, integumentary, and reproductive system glands but has its greatest impact on the respiratory system.

Demographics: Who Gets It?

CF is the most common lethal inherited disease of whites; it is rarer among other races. It occurs approximately once out of every 4,000 births, or roughly 2,500 times per year in the United States. Carriers of the CF genes are more common; however, an estimated that 10 to 12 million people have the CF gene and could potentially pass it to a child.

Approximately 30 thousand people in the United States currently have CF. The average age at diagnosis is 3 years; the average lifespan is just over 30 years, although that number is rising. Approximately 40% of all CF patients today are older than 18 years. Men tend with CF tend to live longer than women.

Etiology: What Happens?

The genetic mutations that cause CF were isolated in 1989. Several hundred slightly different changes can happen, but the net result is that the transmembrane conductance regulator gene (CFTR) is altered so that cell membranes in secreting tissues cannot conduct chloride. This leads to abnormally thick, sticky secretions in many exocrine glands, but most particularly in the respiratory tract, digestive tract, skin, and reproductive tract (see Figure 6.6).

- CF usually has its most profound effects on the respiratory system. The changes in mucous membrane function cause mucus in the respiratory tract to become thick, gluey, and difficult to dislodge. This provides a rich growth medium for bacterial infection, and because of the genetic dysfunction, *neutrophilic* action against pathogens reinforces the inflammatory response, which causes more damage and supports rather than suppresses the infection. A variety of bacterial agents may create chronic infection; the one that is the most difficult to eradicate is an infection with *Pseudomonas aeruginosa*.

  Other respiratory system changes include the growth of nasal polyps and the development of chronic rhinitis.

- Digestive system dysfunction can affect both the gastrointestinal (GI) tract and the accessory organs. A warning sign for CF is a baby born with an intestinal obstruction; this happens because the mucus in the small and large intestines does not move well. Poor absorption in the small intestine also leads to a failure to thrive. Poor access to vitamins creates symptoms as well.

  CF can interfere with the normal production of bile, and the drainage of bile into the small intestine, leading to enlarged spleen, *gallstones*, portal hypertension, liver con-

Cystic Fibrosis in Brief

What is it?
Cystic fibrosis is a congenital disease of exocrine glands that causes their secretions (mainly mucus, digestive enzymes, bile, and sweat) to become abnormally thick and viscous.

How is it recognized?
Cystic fibrosis is a multisystem disease, but its effects on the respiratory system are typically the most common and most acute. Symptoms include chronic lung infections, shortness of breath, productive cough, along with digestive difficulties and failure to thrive in very young children.

Is massage indicated or contraindicated?
Persons with cystic fibrosis receive intensive physiotherapy to dislodge mucus from the lungs, and they are recommended to exercise within tolerance to build lung capacity and immune system resilience. Massage certainly does not tax the body any more than these measures, but day-by-day judgments must be made based on the client's health and the presence of acute or chronic infection.

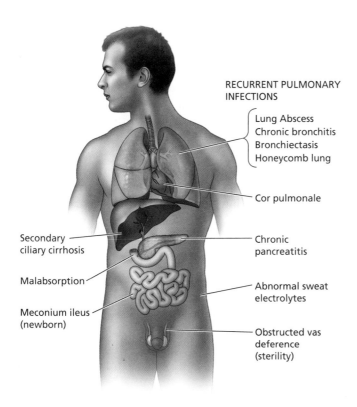

RECURRENT PULMONARY
INFECTIONS

Lung Abscess
Chronic bronchitis
Bronchiectasis
Honeycomb lung

Cor pulmonale

Secondary
ciliary cirrhosis

Chronic
pancreatitis

Malabsorption

Meconium ileus
(newborn)

Abnormal sweat
electrolytes

Obstructed vas
deference
(sterility)

Figure 6.6. Complications of cystic fibrosis.

gestion, or *cirrhosis*. Poor secretion of bicarbonate from the pancreas can lead to *pancreatitis* and *peptic ulcers* in the duodenum (see all of these conditions in Chapter 7).

- CF affects sweat glands in the skin, leading to abnormally thick, salty perspiration and the risk of heat stroke and salt depletion, especially in infants.

- Men with CF are almost always sterile. This occurs because the epididymis cannot secrete normally, or because the vas deferens does not form completely. Women with CF often have a normal reproductive system and can have successful pregnancies.

- The leading cause of death for people with CF is respiratory infection or collapse. Liver disease is the second cause of death, followed by transplant complications and suicide.

Signs and Symptoms

Signs and symptoms of CF vary by which system is affected most severely. Respiratory symptoms are most common. They include a dry or productive cough, shortness of breath, wheezing, chest pain, cyanosis, hemoptysis (coughing up blood), and clubbing of fingers, which occurs with oxygen deprivation in the extremities.

Symptoms affecting other systems are discussed in the etiology section above.

Diagnosis

CF is usually diagnosed with a skin test to analyze the secretions of the sudoriferous glands. Other tests may be conducted to look for the specific defect in the CFTR gene or to look for characteristic changes in the epithelial lining of the upper respiratory tract. The average age at diagnosis is 3 years.

Complications

Complications of CF are related to the exocrine gland dysfunction of the affected system. Respiratory complications include chronic, intractable bacterial infection; *bronchiectasis* (this chapter); the development of resistance in the pulmonary circuit; pneumothorax; and a risk of right-sided *heart failure* (Chapter 4).

Digestive system dysfunction tends to be less severe than respiratory problems, but the complications are wide reaching. They include cirrhosis, gallstones, duodenal ulcers, intestinal obstruction with or without rectal prolapse, a risk of pancreatitis or *diabetes* (Chapter 8) from a damaged pancreas, and vitamin and mineral deficiencies from poor absorption; this can lead to *osteoporosis* (Chapter 2) in adults with CF.

Complications of CF for the integumentary system are discussed above: they include a risk of salt depletion or heat stroke. The group most at risk for these problems is infants.

The male reproductive system is more vulnerable to CF than the female. As stated above, men with CF are almost always sterile.

Treatment

Cystic fibrosis is not a curable disease; at this point, treatment options focus on dealing with symptoms and complications. Taking food in easily digestible forms and exercising to increase or maintain lung function are recommended for people who are not able to fight acute infection or intestinal blockages. Supplementing pancreatic enzymes and vitamins is usually recommended as well.

Bronchodilators, mucus-dissolving drugs (*mucolytics*), antibiotics to fight infection, and anti-inflammatories are typical interventions for CF patients. Advanced cases may be good candidates for lung transplantation, although this procedure has a high rejection rate.

Genetic therapists continue to explore ways to introduce healthy CFTR genes into the tissues of patients with CF. This field is in its infancy, but the future of CF treatment may lie in this direction.

Massage?

The role of massage for a client who has CF must be guided by the health and resilience of the client, which may vary greatly from one day to the next. Many children and adults with CF undergo intense physiotherapy to dislodge deposits of mucus in the lungs, and when no acute infection is present, they are recommended to exercise within tolerance to build stamina and strength. Massage is probably safe and appropriate under these circumstances as long as the therapist works with the rest of the health care team, is healthy, and does not share any virulent pathogens with his or her client.

Lung Cancer

Definition: What Is It?

Lung cancer is the growth of malignant cells in the lungs. These cells eventually form tumors, but because they have extremely easy access to both the circulatory and lymph systems, they are capable of spreading before tumors are detectable.

Lung cancer is an example of epithelial cancer that tends to grow where tissue is vulnerable to repeated irritation and damage.

Lung Cancer in Brief

What is it?
Lung cancer is the development of malignant cells in the lungs. These cells have easy access to blood and lymph vessels and quickly spread to other organs in the body.

How is it recognized?
The early symptoms of lung cancer are virtually indistinguishable from normal irritation from cigarette smoke: a chronic cough, blood-stained sputum, and recurrent bronchitis or pneumonia.

Is massage indicated or contraindicated?
Sadly, most people diagnosed with lung cancer will not survive. Massage has a place in cancer recovery care, as well as in terminal care, but these situations call for specific precautions to achieve maximum benefit with minimal risk.

Demographics: Who Gets It?

Statistics in the United States vary, but an estimated 160,000 to 175,000 new cases of lung cancer are diagnosed, and approximately 160,000 people die of this disease, each year. Although it was once considered a "men's disease," the social acceptability of women smoking has led to rising numbers of women being diagnosed with lung cancer, whereas statistics for men are beginning to fall off. The average lung cancer patient, therefore, is a man or a woman in the sixth to seventh decade of life, who has smoked for 20 years or more.

Cancer in general is the second leading cause of death in the United States, and lung cancer accounts for nearly 30% of all cancer deaths. Some statistics show that it is the cause of more deaths than breast, colon, and prostate cancers (the next three runners-up) combined.

Etiology: What Happens?

Lung cancer occurs in epithelial cells that are chronically irritated by environmental contaminants. Although cigarette, pipe, and cigar smoke are responsible for 85% to 90% of all cases of lung cancer, other causes have also been identified. Exposure to radon, a naturally occurring inert gas that is released when rocks and soil are moved for construction, is the second leading cause of lung cancer, followed by exposure to asbestos, uranium, arsenic, and other carcinogens.

When the epithelial cells that line the respiratory tract have a long history of exposure to these highly toxic substances, their orderly pattern of replication and repair is finally disrupted. Abnormal cells accumulate in uncontrolled and disorganized patches. A rich supply of blood and lymph vessels allows mutated cells to travel out of their immediate area before a detectable tumor appears; this is why lung cancer is seldom caught before metastasis.

The lymph nodes in the mediastinum are often the first site of metastasis for lung cancer. From there the cells have access to distant places in the body. The liver, bone tissue, the skin, the adrenal glands, and the brain are frequently invaded.

Two genetic patterns have been identified as especially important in the development of lung cancer. One involves the presence of specific oncogenes, or cancer-causing genes; the other involves the inactivation of tumor-suppressor genes. The ability to investigate the genetic patterns in cancer patients may eventually lead to earlier diagnoses among high-risk individuals and a better overall long-term prognosis for this disease.

Types of Lung Cancer

Different types of lung cancer tend to grow at different rates, and in different parts of the lung. Several types of lung cancer have been identified; they break down into two basic groups: small cell carcinoma and non–small cell carcinoma.

- *Small cell carcinoma:* This is also called "oat cell" carcinoma. It is responsible for about 25% of all lung cancers. Small cell lung cancer grows fast, spreads quickly, and is rarely operable. The 5-year survival rate for small cell carcinoma patients is less than 1%.

- *Non–small cell carcinoma:* This includes several different types of cancers, depending on which cells they affect first. Non–small cell carcinomas account for 75% of all lung cancers. They include squamous cell carcinoma, adenocarcinoma, large cell carcinoma, and several others (Figure 6.7). Most of these grow more slowly than small cell carcinoma, but the symptoms they create are so subtle that diagnosis does not usually

Bronchiolar carcinoma
infiltrating growth

Figure 6.7. Lung cancer.

happen until long after the cancer has spread beyond its original area. The 5-year survival rate for all non–small cell carcinoma patients is less than 30%.

Risk Factors

The most obvious risk factor for lung cancer is smoking. Cigarette smoke contains more than 40 known carcinogens, and the tar in cigarettes holds the damaging chemicals close to the delicate linings of the lungs. Light smokers are approximately 10 times more likely to get this disease than nonsmokers; heavy smokers are 25 times more susceptible. Almost 90% of all lung cancer patients are smokers or people exposed to second-hand or side-stream smoke. (Side-stream smoke is the smoke coming directly from lit cigarettes; not from the smokers.) Every year, an estimated 3,000 Americans die of lung cancer connected to side-stream or second-hand smoke; that is more deaths than those from all other air pollutants combined.

Lung cancer is also an occupational risk for people working with asbestos insulation, coal miners, and people who work with other toxic chemicals. Exposure to radon, excessive radiation, or a history of TB, COPD, or other lung infections also can increase risk.

Signs and Symptoms

One of the biggest problems with lung cancer is that it is extremely difficult to identify early. The growth of abnormal cells in alveoli, bronchial linings, or mucous membranes stimulates virtually no changes in function or sensation. A persistent "smoker's cough" is one early sign, along with bloodstained phlegm, chest pain, and possibly shortness of breath. None of these symptoms is particular cause for alarm, because a smoker or someone who works with irritating chemicals will probably have them regardless of the health of their respiratory cells.

Later signs of lung cancer may be more revealing. If a tumor is growing near the apex of the lung, it may put mechanical pressure on the brachial plexus, leading to symptoms that mimic *thoracic outlet syndrome* (Chapter 2). A tumor that presses on the superior vena cava may cause facial swelling and dilated blood vessels in the neck and face; this is called *superior vena cava syndrome*. If a tumor protrudes on the esophagus or larynx, a person may experience chronic hoarseness. Tumors that press on the phrenic nerve can cause the paralysis of the diaphragm.

Diagnosis

Once a tumor has formed in the lung, it is not hard to find; any imaging technique, from x-rays to CT scans to MRIs can locate growths. An analysis of sputum might reveal abnormal cells, but then again it might not. Radiographic studies of bronchiole tubes can show where obstructions are growing, and needle biopsies of suspicious areas can help to pinpoint a diagnosis. The problem is that this type of cancer often metastasizes *before* detectable tumors have grown. This makes it difficult to identify early enough to catch. In fact, only 20% of all detected lung cancers are caught before they have spread to elsewhere in the body. Approximately 25% of all diagnoses catch the cancer while it is still in the thorax but may be in both lungs. More than 55% of all patients have tumors growing in distant areas at the time of diagnosis.

Treatment

Treatment for lung cancer depends on what kind of cancer is growing and how far it has progressed. For the lucky few that find their cancer while it is still localized, surgery followed by radiation may be adequate. The surgery could involve the removal of a small section of lung tissue (a wedge resection), the removal of an entire lobe (a lobectomy), or even the removal of an entire lung (a pneumonectomy). These are options for non–small cell carcinoma.

Small cell carcinoma grows so fast and spreads so quickly that it is generally treated with radiation and chemotherapy alone; surgery usually has no chance of containing the extent of the growth.

New therapies for lung cancer are always in development. One of them is ***photodynamic therapy***: a process in which a laser-sensitive chemical is injected into the cancerous area, absorbed into abnormal cells, and then activated by a laser, which causes the chemicals to destroy the cancerous cells. Even when all of the identified abnormal cells of a lung cancer patient are caught and removed or destroyed, the chance of having the cancer recur is high. Despite many advances in cancer identification and treatment, the prognosis for most lung cancer patients remains very poor.

Massage?

Massage can be a useful stress reliever for a person undergoing cancer treatment; it stimulates immune system activity, reduces pain and fatigue, and generally adds to the quality of life. Fears about the possibility of spreading cancer cells through the circulatory or lymph systems can be allayed by using noncirculatory techniques. Of course, certain cautions must be observed when working with people who are receiving radiation or chemotherapy, or who have had recent surgery. For more details, see *cancer*, Chapter 11.

If a client's condition is terminal, massage still has a useful place in comfort care protocols. Even when a person is too fragile to receive most types of bodywork, energy work, gentle stroking of hands and feet, or simple laying on of hands can all contribute to feelings of peace and well-being. In these situations, the massage therapist may want to teach family members and loved ones of the patient some simple techniques that may enrich their time together.

CHAPTER REVIEW QUESTIONS

1. What is the purpose of mucous membranes? Where are they found?
2. How does the structure of the lungs work to limit the spread of infection?
3. Explain the sympathetic/parasympathetic swing that occurs with asthma.
4. What is the best defense against catching or spreading the cold virus?
5. What is the danger associated with taking broad-spectrum antibiotics "just in case"?
6. What are the repercussions of having alveoli fuse together, as happens with emphysema?
7. Why is the prognosis for lung cancer generally so poor?
8. What feature of the TB bacterium distinguishes it from most other pathogens?
9. What happens when prescriptions of antibiotics for tuberculosis (or other bacterial infections) are not completed as directed? Why is this a particular danger for TB?
10. Why is CF associated with a high risk of lung infection?
11. What is the relationship between chronic bronchitis and acute bronchitis?
12. A client has sinusitis. Her mucus is thick, opaque, and sticky. She has had a headache and a mild fever for several days. Is she a good candidate for massage? Why or why not?

 Answers to these questions can be found on the Student Resource CD-ROM that accompanies this book.

Bibliography

General Resources, Respiratory System

1. de Dominico G, Wood E. Beard's Massage. Philadelphia: WB Saunders, 1997.
2. Damjanou I. Pathology for the Health-Related Professions. Philadelphia: WB Saunders, 1996.
3. Travell J, Simons DG. Myofascial Pain and Dysfunction: The Trigger Point Manual. Baltimore: Williams & Wilkins, 1983.
4. Clemente CD. Anatomy: A Regional Atlas of the Human Body. 3rd Ed. Baltimore: Urban & Schwarzenburg, 1987.
5. Tortora GJ, Anagnostakos NP. Principles of Anatomy and Physiology. 6th Ed. New York: Harper & Row, 1990.
6. Taber's Cyclopedic Dictionary. 14th Ed. Philadelphia: FA Davis, 1981.
7. Stedman's Medical Dictionary. 26th Ed. Baltimore: Williams & Wilkins, 1995.
8. Memmler RL, Wood DL. The Human Body in Health and Disease. 5th Ed. Philadelphia: JB Lippincott, 1983.

9. Juhan D. Job's Body: A Handbook for Bodywork. Barrytown, NY: Station Hill Press, 1987.
10. Kunz JRM, Finkel AJ, eds. The American Medical Association Family Medical Guide. New York, NY: Random House, 1987.
11. Marieb EM. Human Anatomy and Physiology. Redwood City, CA: Benjamin/Cummings, 1989.
12. Field T. Touch Therapy. London: Churchill Livingstone, 2000.
13. Foundation for Medical Education and Research (MFMER). Available at: Pleurisy Overview. Copyright © 1998-2003 Mayo Foundation for Medical Education and Research (MFMER). Available at: http://www.mayoclinic.com/invoke.cfm?id=DS00244. Accessed winter 2004.
14. Respiratory syncytial virus Overview. Copyright © 1998-2003 Mayo Foundation for Medical Education and Research (MFMER). Available at: http://www.

mayoclinic.com/invoke.cfm?id=DS00414. Accessed winter 2004.
15. Using antibiotics sensibly. Copyright © 1998–2003 Mayo Foundation for Medical Education and Research (MFMER). Available at: http://www.mayoclinic.com/invoke.cfm?id=FL00075. Accessed winter 2004.
16. Viral vs. bacterial infection: What's the difference? Copyright © 1998–2003 Mayo Foundation for Medical Education and Research (MFMER). Available at: http://www.mayoclinic.com/invoke.cfm?id=AN00652. Accessed winter 2004.
17. Severe acute respiratory syndrome Overview. Copyright © 1998–2003 Mayo http://www.mayoclinic.com/invoke.cfm?id=DS00501. Accessed winter 2004.
18. Severe Acute Respiratory Syndrome (SARS). Available at: http://www.theberries.ns.ca/SPRING2003/SARS.html. Accessed winter 2004.

Acute Bronchitis

1. Acute Bronchitis. Copyright © 2001 American Academy of Family Physicians. Available at: http://familydoctor.org/677.xml. Accessed winter 2004.
2. Qarah S, Hmidi A. Bronchitis. Copyright © 2003, eMedicine.com, Inc. Available at: http://www.emedicine.com/med/topic247.htm. Accessed winter 2004.
3. Bronchiolitis Overview. Copyright © 1998–2003 Mayo Foundation for Medical Education and Research (MFMER). Available at: http://www.mayoclinic.com/invoke.cfm?id=DS00481. Accessed winter 2004.
4. Bronchitis Overview. Copyright © 1998–2003 Mayo Foundation for Medical Education and Research (MFMER). Available at: http://www.mayoclinic.com/invoke.cfm?id=DS00031. Accessed winter 2004.

Common Cold

1. The Common Cold. National Institute of Allergy and Infectious Diseases. National Institutes of Health. Available at: http://www.niaid.nih.gov/factsheets/cold.htm. Accessed winter 2004.
2. Greene A. Cold and Flu Differences. Copyright © 2003 Greene Ink, Inc. Available at: http://websites2.medseek.com/websitefiles/drgreene/body.cfm?id=21&action=detail&ref=577. Accessed winter 2004.
3. Flu and Cold: Statistics. Copyright © 2003 American Lung Association®. Available at: http://lungusa.org/press/lung_dis/asn_c&f_1802b.html. Accessed winter 2004.
4. Cold Overview. Copyright © 1998–2003 Mayo Foundation for Medical Education and Research (MFMER). Available at: http://www.mayoclinic.com/invoke.cfm?id=DS00056. Accessed winter 2004.
5. Colds, coughs and runny noses: Children's resistance comes with time. Copyright © 1998–2003 Mayo Foundation for Medical Education and Research (MFMER). Available at: http://www.mayoclinic.com/invoke.cfm?id=CC00005. Accessed winter 2004.

Influenza

1. Flu. National Institute of Allergy and Infectious Diseases. National Institutes of Health. Available at: http://www.niaid.nih.gov/factsheets/flu.htm. Accessed winter 2004.
2. Derlet R, Lawrence R. Influenza. Copyright © 2003, eMedicine.com, Inc. Available at: http://www.emedicine.com/med/topic1170.htm. Accessed winter 2004.
3. Key Facts About the Flu. Available at: http://www.cdc.gov/flu/keyfacts.htm. Accessed winter 2004.
4. Influenza Overview. Copyright © 1998–2003 Mayo Foundation for Medical Education and Research (MFMER). Available at: http://www.mayoclinic.com/invoke.cfm?id=DS00081. Accessed winter 2004.

5. Flu Spreads Across U.S. But No Epidemic Yet: CDC. Copyright © 2003 Reuters. Available at: http://www.nlm.nih.gov/medlineplus/news/fullstory_15203.html. Accessed winter 2004.

Pneumonia

1. Smith IM. Diagnosing Pneumonia a Tough Call. Copyright © 1992–2003 the Author(s) and The University of Iowa. Available at: http://www.vh.org/adult/patient/internalmedicine/aba30/1992/pneumonia-diagnosis.html. Accessed winter 2004.
2. Cunha BA. Pneumonia, Community-Acquired. Copyright © 2003, eMedicine.com, Inc. Available at: http://www.emedicine.com/med/topic3162.htm. Accessed winter 2004.
3. Sharma S. Pneumonia, viral. Copyright © 2003, eMedicine.com, Inc. Available at: http://www.emedicine.com/med/topic1854.htm. Accessed winter 2004.
4. Pneumonia Overview. Copyright © 1998–2004 Mayo Foundation for Medical Education and Research (MFMER). Available at: http://www.mayoclinic.com/invoke.cfm?id=DS00135. Accessed winter 2004.
5. Pneumocystis infection. Parasites and Health. Available at: http://www.dpd.cdc.gov/dpdx/HTML/Pneumocystis.htm. Accessed winter 2004.
6. Pneumonia. Copyright © 2003 American Lung Association®. Available at: http://www.lungusa.org/diseases/lungpneumoni.html. Accessed winter 2004.

Sinusitis

1. Davidoff TQ, Cunningham M. Sinusitis, Acute. Copyright © 2003, eMedicine.com, Inc. Available at: http://www.emedicine.com/med/topic2555.htm. Accessed winter 2004.
2. Grossan M. Asthma and Sinusitis. Copyright © 2003, eMedicine.com, Inc. Available at: http://www.emedicine.com/ent/topic516.htm. Accessed winter 2004.
3. Bajracharya H, Hinthorn D. Sinusitis, Chronic. Copyright © 2003, eMedicine.com, Inc. Available at: http://www.emedicine.com/med/topic2556.htm. Accessed winter 2004.
4. Acute sinusitis Overview. Copyright © 1998–2003 Mayo Foundation for Medical Education and Research (MFMER). Available at: http://www.mayoclinic.com/invoke.cfm?id=DS00170. Accessed winter 2004.

Tuberculosis

1. Questions and Answers About TB. Available at: http://www.cdc.gov/nchstp/tb/faqs/pdfs/qa.pdf. Accessed winter 2004.
2. Anand MKN, Reddy JJM. Tuberculosis, Gastrointestinal. Copyright © 2003, eMedicine.com, Inc. Available at: http://www.emedicine.com/radio/topic885.htm. Accessed winter 2004.
3. Agrawal A, Agrawal A. Lung, Postprimary Tuberculosis. Copyright © 2003,

eMedicine.com, Inc. Available at: http://www.emedicine.com/radio/topic412.htm. Accessed winter 2004.
4. Herchline T, Amorosa J. Tuberculosis. Copyright © 2003, eMedicine.com, Inc. Available at: http://www.emedicine.com/med/topic2324.htm. Accessed winter 2004.
5. Tuberculosis Overview. Copyright © 1998-2003 Mayo Foundation for Medical Education and Research (MFMER). Available at: http://www.mayoclinic.com/invoke.cfm?id=DS00372. Accessed winter 2004.
6. Resistant tuberculosis (MDR-TB). Copyright © 2003 World Health Organization (WHO). Available at: http://www.who.int/gtb/policyrd/DOTSplus.htm. Accessed winter 2004.
7. TB Summary. Copyright © 2003 World Health Organization (WHO). Available at: http://www.who.int/gtb/publications/globrep01/summary.html. Accessed winter 2004.
8. Tuberculosis. Copyright © 2003 World Health Organization (WHO). Available at: http://www.who.int/mediacentre/factsheets/who104/en/. Accessed winter 2004.
9. What is DOTS? WHO publications on DOTS. (World Health Organization publications on Directly Observed Therapy). Available at: http://www.who.int/gtb/dots/whatisdots.htm. Accessed winter 2004.

Asthma

1. Basic Facts about Asthma. CDC/National Center for Environmental Health. Available at: http://www.cdc.gov/nceh/airpollution/asthma/faqs.htm. Accessed winter 2004.
2. Canaday P, Collins J. Asthma. Copyright © 2003, eMedicine.com, Inc. Available at: http://www.emedicine.com/radio/topic59.htm. Accessed winter 2004.
3. Saglimbeni AJ. Exercise-Induced Asthma. Copyright © 2003, eMedicine.com, Inc. Available at: http://www.emedicine.com/sports/topic155.htm. Accessed winter 2004.
4. Inhaled and Oral Corticosteroids. Copyright © 2003 National Jewish Medical and Research Center. Available at: http://asthma.nationaljewish.org/treatments/longterm/inhaled_oral.php. Accessed winter 2004.
5. Patel A. Adult-onset asthma: An interview with a Mayo Clinic specialist. Copyright © 1998-2003 Mayo Foundation for Medical Education and Research (MFMER). Available at: http://www.mayoclinic.com/invoke.cfm?id=HQ00190. Accessed winter 2004.
6. Asthma and the cockroach connection. Copyright © 1998–2003 Mayo Foundation for Medical Education and Research (MFMER). Available at: http://www.mayoclinic.com/invoke.cfm?id=HQ01512. Accessed winter 2004.
7. Asthma Overview. Copyright © 1998–2003 Mayo Foundation for Medical Education and Research (MFMER). Available at: http://www.mayoclinic.com/invoke.cfm?id=DS00021. Accessed winter 2004.

8. Cold and flu: What to do if you have asthma. Copyright © 1998–2003 Mayo Foundation for Medical Education and Research (MFMER). Available at: http://www.mayoclinic.com/invoke.cfm?id =AA00011. Accessed winter 2004.
9. Enzyme May Play Unexpected Role in Asthma. National Institute of Allergy and Infectious Diseases. National Institutes of Health. Available at: http://www.niaid.nih.gov/newsroom/releases/asthma-june03.htm. Accessed winter 2004.

Bronchiectasis

1. Chow JS, Snyder B, Hunsaker A. Bronchiectasis in Cystic Fibrosis. Copyright © 1994–2003 BWH Radiology. Available at: http://brighamrad.harvard.edu/education/online/tcd/tcd.html. Accessed winter 2004.
2. Mysliwiec V, Pina JS. Bronchiectasis: the 'other' obstructive lung disease. Copyright © 1994–2003 BWH Radiology. Available at:* Accessed winter 2004.
3. Emmons EE, Ouellette DR. Bronchiectasis. Copyright © 2003, eMedicine.com, Inc. Available at: http://www.emedicine.com/med/topic246.htm. Accessed winter 2004.
4. Bronchiectasis. Copyright © National Jewish Medical and Research Center. Available at: http://nationaljewish.org/. Accessed winter 2004.

Chronic Bronchitis

1. Chronic Bronchitis. Copyright © 2003 American Lung Association®. Available at: http://www.lungusa.org/diseases/lungchronic.html. Accessed winter 2004.
2. Chronic Obstructive Pulmonary Disease. What Are Chronic Bronchitis and Emphysema? Available at: http://www.nhlbi.nih.gov/health/public/lung/other/copd/bronemph.htm. Accessed winter 2004.
3. Chronic Obstructive Pulmonary Disease. National Institutes of Health. National Heart, Lung, and Blood Institute. Available at: http://www.nhlbi.nih.gov/health/public/lung/other/copd_fact.pdf. Accessed winter 2004.
4. Mink BD. Exercise and Chronic Obstructive Pulmonary Disease: Modest Fitness Gains Pay Big Dividends. Copyright © 1997. The McGraw-Hill Companies. Available at: http://www.physsportsmed.com/issues/1997/11nov/mink.htm. Accessed winter 2004.

5. Bronchitis Overview. Copyright © 1998–2004 Mayo Foundation for Medical Education and Research (MFMER). Available at: http://www.mayoclinic.com/invoke.cfm?id=DS00031. Accessed winter 2004.

Emphysema

1. Kleinschmidt P. Chronic Obstructive Pulmonary Disease and Emphysema. Copyright © 2003, eMedicine.com, Inc. Available at: http://www.emedicine.com/emerg/topic99.htm. Accessed winter 2004.
2. Sharma S. Chronic Obstructive Pulmonary Disease. Copyright © 2003, eMedicine.com, Inc. Available at: http://www.emedicine.com/med/topic373.htm. Accessed winter 2004.
3. Facts About Chronic Obstructive Pulmonary Disease (COPD). Available at: http://www.cdc.gov/nceh/airpollution/copd/copdfaq.htm. Accessed winter 2004.
4. Emphysema: Does it increase the risk of lung cancer? Copyright © 1998–2003 Mayo Foundation for Medical Education and Research (MFMER). Available at: http://www.mayoclinic.com/invoke.cfm?id=HQ00617. Accessed winter 2004.
5. Emphysema Overview. Copyright © 1998–2003 Mayo Foundation for Medical Education and Research (MFMER). Available at: http://www.mayoclinic.com/invoke.cfm?id=DS00296. Accessed winter 2004.

Cystic Fibrosis

1. Sharma G. Cystic Fibrosis. Copyright © 2003, eMedicine.com, Inc. Available at: http://www.emedicine.com/ped/topic535.htm. Accessed winter 2004.
2. New Theory Proposed for Cystic Fibrosis Infections. National Institutes of Health. National Institute of Allergy and Infectious Diseases. Available at: http://www.nih.gov/news/pr/nov2001/niaid-19.htm. Accessed winter 2004.
3. Machalek AZ. Bacterial Slime Clogs Cystic Fibrosis Lungs. The National Institute of General Medical Sciences. Available at: http://www.nigms.nih.gov/news/releases/brief_greenberg.html. Accessed winter 2004.
4. Facts About Cystic Fibrosis. National Heart, Lung, and Blood Institute. Available at: http://www.nhlbi.nih.gov/health/public/lung/other/cf.htm. Accessed winter 2004.
5. do Pico GA. Cystic Fibrosis. Copyright © 1998 American College of Chest Physicians.

Available at: http://www.chestnet.org/education/online/pccu/vol12/lessons19_20/lesson20.php. Accessed winter 2004.
6. About Cystic Fibrosis. What is CF. Cystic Fibrosis Foundation. Available at: http://www.cff.org/about_cf/what_is_cf.cfm?CFID=1340246&CFTOKEN=5072069. Accessed winter 2004.

Lung Cancer

1. Cigarette Smoking-Related Mortality. Available at: http://www.cdc.gov/tobacco/research_data/health_consequences/mortali.htm. Accessed winter 2004.
2. Maghfoor I, Perry M. Lung Cancer, Non-Small Cell. Copyright © 2003, eMedicine.com, Inc. Available at: http://www.emedicine.com/med/topic1333.htm. Accessed winter 2004.
3. Irshad A, Ravenel J. Lung Cancer, Small Cell. Copyright © 2003, eMedicine.com, Inc. Available at: http://www.emedicine.com/radio/topic405.htm. Accessed winter 2004.
4. Sharma S. Cancer, Lung. Copyright © 2003, eMedicine.com, Inc. Available at: http://www.emedicine.com/aaem/topic84.htm. Accessed winter 2004.
5. Hassan I. Lung, Metastases. Copyright © 2003, eMedicine.com, Inc. Available at: http://www.emedicine.com/radio/topic404.htm. Accessed winter 2004.
6. Murphy TD. Passive Smoking and Lung Disease. Copyright © 2003, eMedicine.com, Inc. Available at: http://www.emedicine.com/ped/topic2625.htm. Accessed winter 2004.
7. Lung cancer Overview. Copyright © 1998–2003 Mayo Foundation for Medical Education and Research (MFMER). Available at: http://www.mayoclinic.com/invoke.cfm?id=DS00038. Accessed winter 2004.
8. Non-Small Cell Lung Cancer. National Cancer Institute. Available at: http://www.cancer.gov/templates/page_print.aspx?viewid=1b299ff5-e610-4d11-a121-b32aefc7ec2c&version=patient. Accessed winter 2004.
9. Questions and Answers About Beta Carotene Chemoprevention Trials. Available at: http://cis.nci.nih.gov/fact/4_13.htm. Accessed winter 2004.
10. Small Cell Lung Cancer. National Cancer Institute. Available at: http://www.cancer.gov/templates/page_print.aspx?viewid=0c22f1bd-4315-4727-8330-79549c8237f3&version=patient. Accessed winter 2004.

DIGESTIVE SYSTEM CONDITIONS

7

Chapter Objectives:

After reading this chapter, you should be able to . . .

- Name the most dangerous complication of gastroenteritis.
- Describe a comfort measure for working with clients who have GERD.
- Identify the parts of the alimentary canal that can be affected by Crohn disease.
- Explain the relationship between stress and peptic ulcers.
- Name a risk factor for colorectal cancer.
- Describe the difference(s) between diverticulosis and diverticulitis.
- Explain why anemia can be a complication of ulcerative colitis.
- List three complications of cirrhosis.
- Describe the primary methods of communicability for hepatitis A, B, and C.
- Explain why statistics for hepatitis C have recently surged upward.

INTRODUCTION

The Digestive Tract: Structure and Function

The best way to discuss how the digestive tract works is to follow a piece of food through the system (Figure 7.1).

When the teeth grind a bite of food, it is broken into small pieces so that the digestive enzymes in the saliva and the rest of the gastrointestinal tract have more access to the nutrients. The food moves from the mouth, down the esophagus, and into a wide place in the tube: the stomach. Here it is further pulverized by powerful muscular contractions, while being exposed to more chemicals. Accessory organs make their chemical contributions as the former food, now referred to as *chyme*, moves into the small intestine. By now the barrage of digestive enzymes has reduced the meal into its most primitive building blocks: sugars, fats, and proteins. The secretion of digestive enzymes anywhere in the upper gastrointestinal tract is largely a function of the vagus nerve, the biggest contributor to the parasympathetic

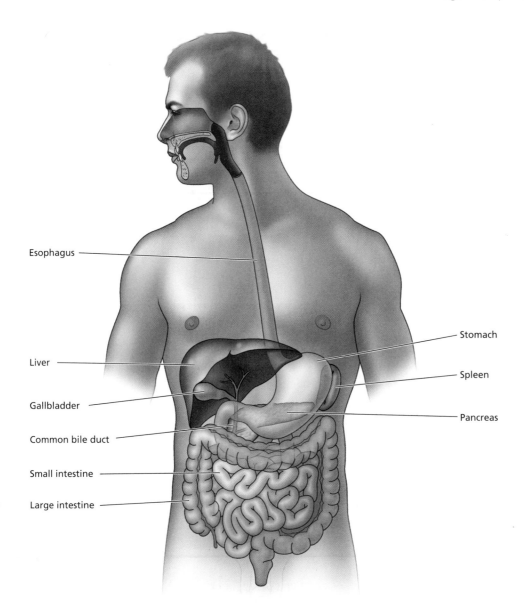

Figure 7.1. Overview of the digestive system.

nervous system. In this way, the efficiency of digestion depends on whether a person is in a sympathetic or parasympathetic state.

The small intestine loops and twirls around the abdomen, secured by sheets of connective tissue membrane called the *mesentery*, a part of the peritoneum. It is lubricated on the outside by other layers of the peritoneum, which allow it to move freely as a person twists, squirms, and changes positions. The inside of a healthy small intestine looks like velvet or velour, with millions of tiny villi, each one supplied with blood and lymph capillaries for the absorption of nutrients; amino acids and glucose go into the bloodstream, while

fats are drawn into the lymph system. Rhythmic waves of smooth muscle contraction gently ease the chyme along the tube until, at the distal end of the small intestine, it passes through the ileocecal valve: the entryway to the colon.

The colon is a much shorter and wider section of tubing than the small intestine, and it differs also in the absence of villi and the presence of anchoring pieces of connective tissue that bind the colon down at the four flexures, or corners of the abdomen. A healthy colon has segments called *haustra*. In this part of the tube, water is squeezed out of the chyme, which is now called a *bolus*. Water is reabsorbed back into the body; this is also the site of vitamin K synthesis. The colon functions like a trash compactor; everything left of a meal that makes it this far is condensed and excreted.

The Accessory Organs: Structure and Function

The continuous tube that winds from mouth to anus is only one part of the digestive system; the *accessory organs* contribute to the process of turning food into energy or building blocks as well. These organs include the liver, gallbladder, and pancreas, each of which produces or releases chemicals into the digestive tract. Here is a brief review of each of these organs.

The Liver

This is an organ of immense complexity, with literally hundreds of functions. One of the things that make the liver unique is its powers of regeneration; hepatocytes, or liver cells, are remarkably adaptable. Livers that have been partially removed can recover full functional size within weeks of surgery, and small pieces of liver that have been transplanted into other hosts can often grow to full function within a similar short period. The liver is also special in that it has twice the blood supply of most other organs; between the hepatic artery delivering oxygen and the portal vein delivering fresh products of digestion from the small intestine, it is no wonder that this organ is hot and dark red. Although the internal blood pressure is relatively low, cellular activity in the liver is very high.

The liver is the largest gland in the body. It is the destination of the portal system detour, receiving all the vitamins, amino acids, and glucose that are extracted from the small intestine and not immediately needed in the body. By storing glucose as *glycogen* until it is called for, the liver also acts as a sugar buffer, preventing some of the radical swings in blood glucose levels that would happen if there were no intermediate stop for sugar. The liver is also the site for much of the most vital protein synthesis in the body. Many of the enzymes that sponsor cellular activity are born here; this is also the origin of blood proteins that regulate intracellular fluid and blood clotting.

Detoxification functions of the liver are well known. The liver alters many drugs into a form that is less toxic or that can be excreted. A functioning liver prevents many substances, including alcohol, from reaching toxic levels. It also processes the poisonous wastes generated by protein digestion, changing them to uric acid to be excreted by the kidneys. In addition to these functions, the specialized leukocytes in the liver called *Kupffer cells* are constantly watching for any pathogens that they can eradicate. Finally, the liver helps to recycle the *heme* from dead red blood cells into *bilirubin*, a major component of bile, a substance that is vital for the digestion of fats. The liver produces up to 3 cups of bile each day. Bile leaves the liver via the cystic duct and enters the gallbladder.

The Gallbladder

This is a small bright green sack that hangs off the liver about halfway along the costal angle on the right side of the body. Its function is fairly simple: it receives bile from the liver, stores it, and concentrates it. The gallbladder can hold up to 1 cup of bile at a time. On hormonal command, it releases the bile into the duodenum via the common bile duct. There the bile helps to emulsify fats: the fats are held in tiny globules to make them easier to digest. The gallbladder and its ducts are susceptible to dysfunction, which can have serious repercussions.

The Pancreas

This is a fascinating gland that holds the distinction of being both an exocrine gland, releasing digestive juices into the intestine via the pancreatic duct, and an endocrine gland, releasing hormones directly into the bloodstream. Its exocrine secretions are so alkaline they can be corrosive. Any blockage in the pancreatic duct can lead to very serious tissue damage because the pancreas is quite capable of digesting itself.

Gastrointestinal Problems and Massage

Most of the gastrointestinal (GI) tract problems that respond well to massage are related to autonomic imbalance; when a person is under stress, digestion becomes a low priority. If this state of affairs goes on for a long time, problems will develop. The most common disorders of this type are spastic or flaccid constipation, indigestion, and gas.

The first concern, however, is to eliminate the possibility of more serious conditions that contraindicate circulatory massage. Massage practitioners are sometimes put in the position of deciding whether their work is going to help people get over the stress-related stomachache or put them in the hospital. Symptoms that are a red light for something very serious include severe localized pain, bloody stools, anemia, bloating, and fever. A general rule is that if symptoms have persisted for 3 weeks or more, it is time to visit the doctor.

Problems in the GI tract are impossible to pin down without diagnostic tests, and, fortunately, this is not within the scope of practice of massage therapy. Massage should not be performed when the client has any unexplained or undiagnosed pain. Any relief that a massage provides may delay the client from getting medical assistance for a serious and acute illness. Symptoms of simple, short-term problems are often indistinguishable from very serious illness in the GI tract. Although spastic constipation is not inherently dangerous, colon cancer is—and massage therapists are not equipped to tell the difference.

DIGESTIVE SYSTEM CONDITIONS

Disorders of the Upper Gastrointestinal Tract

Celiac Disease
Crohn Disease
Esophageal Cancer
Gastroenteritis
Gastroesophageal Reflux Disorder
Stomach Cancer
Ulcers

Disorders of the Large Intestine

Appendicitis
Colorectal Cancer
Diverticular Disease
Irritable Bowel Syndrome
Ulcerative Colitis

Disorders of the Accessory Organs

Cirrhosis
Gallstones
Hepatitis
Jaundice
Liver Cancer
Pancreatic Cancer
Pancreatitis

Other Digestive System Conditions

Candidiasis
Peritonitis

DISORDERS OF THE UPPER GASTROINTESTINAL TRACT

Celiac Disease

Definition: What Is It?

Celiac disease is a condition in which the intestinal villi are flattened or destroyed altogether as part of an immune system reaction in the presence of *gluten*, a protein present in many types of grains. It is also known as celiac sprue, nontropical sprue, or gluten-sensitive enteropathy.

Demographics: Who Gets It?

The incidence of celiac disease in the United States is a topic of some controversy. Although it is diagnosed in 1 of approximately every 4,700 people, recent studies indicate that it may affect about 1 of every 133 people. It is most common among people of European descent and occurs in much lower rates among African, Chinese, and Japanese populations.

A genetic link for celiac disease is clearly demonstrable; it occurs in approximately 10% of all first-degree relatives of diagnosed people. The fraternal twin of an affected person has a 30% chance

Celiac Disease in Brief

Pronunciation
sē'lē-ak

What is it?
Celiac disease is a condition in which a damaging inflammatory response follows the consumption of any food containing gluten. This leads to the destruction of intestinal villi and poor access to ingested nutrients.

How is it recognized?
Celiac disease can develop in childhood or adulthood, and its symptoms vary greatly from one person to another. Most symptoms are related to malabsorption (many nutrients are not absorbed and so pass through to the stools) or malnutrition (complications related to vitamin and nutrient deficiencies).

Is massage indicated or contraindicated?
Celiac disease is not directly affected by bodywork, although as with all situations involving intestinal discomfort, clients should be encouraged to seek a diagnosis if symptoms are persistent—even if massage provides temporary relief.

of developing the disease, whereas an identical twin of an affected person has a 70% chance. The exact location of the genetic mutation that leads to this condition is still under investigation.

Etiology: What Happens?

Some sources list celiac disease as an autoimmune disease, whereas others suggest it is an allergic reaction to the components of gluten. The truth is probably somewhere in the middle, and ongoing research continues to reveal more about how this condition causes the problems associated with it.

Gluten is a protein found in many grains, including wheat, rye, barley, spelt, and others. When gluten is consumed by a person without celiac disease, it is broken down by digestive enzymes into small chains of amino acids that are absorbed into the intestinal villi and then used by the body. When celiac disease is present, gluten is broken into its component pieces, including a long chain of amino acids called *gliadin*, but this substance resists any further enzyme action to break it into smaller pieces. For reasons that are not completely clear, gliadin is absorbed into the villi of people with celiac disease, where intracellular enzymes interact with it and trigger a mild or severe inflammatory response.

Eventually repeated inflammatory attacks on intestinal villi cause them to degenerate, lay flat, or disappear altogether. The person then loses access to absorbable nutrition not only from sources of gluten, but from other sources as well. Glucose from dairy products is often particularly difficult to digest, leading to symptoms of lactose intolerance, although the problem is not with the lactose itself but with the villi that are meant to absorb it. Fats become similarly unavailable, and they pass through the digestive system to be expelled in the stools. Poor uptake leads to signs of malabsorption and malnutrition, although the diet of a person with celiac disease may be identical to that of an average person.

Celiac disease frequently occurs concurrently with some other autoimmune disorders, including type 1 *diabetes, hypothyroidism, hyperthyroidism* (all in Chapter 8); *lupus* (Chapter 5); *rheumatoid arthritis* (Chapter 2); and others. In addition to these conditions, many people with celiac disease develop a painful rash on their extremities, buttocks, neck, truck, and scalp called *dermatitis herpetiformis*.

A genetic link in celiac disease is easy to trace, because the incidence within families is significantly higher than that in the general population. Age at onset varies significantly, however, with some people developing symptoms in early childhood, whereas others develop symptoms after a significant stressful trigger in adulthood, such as surgery, childbirth, or trauma. Still others may go throughout life with symptoms so mild they are ignored or misdiagnosed as other gastrointestinal disorders. Statistics show, however, that people who do not manage their celiac disease have a shorter lifespan than the general population, and they are more susceptible to a variety of problems ranging from non-Hodgkin's *lymphoma* (see Chapter 5), to surgeries for *appendicitis* (this chapter), *hernia* (Chapter 2), and tonsillitis.

Signs and Symptoms

Signs and symptoms of celiac disease typically center on malabsorption of nutrients and malnutrition. Whereas many patients experience pain or discomfort in the gastrointestinal tract, many others only experience the results of poor vitamin and nutrient uptake.

Gastrointestinal symptoms include gas, bloating, and diarrhea. Stools are often high-volume, pale, and foul-smelling because they contain much of the fat and other material that would normally have been absorbed in the small intestines.

Related symptoms include weight loss (or failure to gain weight in children), anemia, irritability, depression, behavior changes, muscle cramps and weakness, poor stamina, tooth discoloration, and the dermatitis described above.

Although some people with celiac disease experience very severe symptoms whenever they are exposed to gluten, others have such mild symptoms they may never be recognized. This does not rule out damage to the intestines, however, and these people are just as susceptible to the complications of celiac disease as persons with discernible symptoms.

Complications

The complications of celiac disease also have to do with malabsorption and malnutrition. Poor uptake of iron and vitamins leads to anemia, folic acid deficiency, and a high risk of neural tube defects in a growing fetus (see *spina bifida*, Chapter 3). Poor uptake of calcium leads to osteomalacia (weak bones) in children, or *osteoporosis* (Chapter 3) in adults, as well as a particular kind of *kidney stones* (Chapter 9), muscle weakness, and chronic spasm. Behavioral changes, irritability, and a risk of seizures can be linked to a vitamin B_{12} deficiency.

Young children with celiac disease experience delayed growth and development, and frequently never reach their projected height.

Constant irritation and inflammation of the gastrointestinal tract raises a significant risk of *adenocarcinoma* or *lymphadenoma* in the small intestine. Non-Hodgkin's lymphoma is a significant cause of death for persons who never identify their celiac disease.

Diagnosis

The diagnosis of celiac disease recently became much easier, as the presence of certain antibodies in the blood can be traced with a blood test. A positive blood test is not definitive, however; a scope and a biopsy of the lining of the jejunum are typically conducted to confirm a diagnosis.

According to studies of the general population, celiac disease probably occurs more than 30 times more frequently in the United States than it is diagnosed. This discrepancy seems unreasonable: how could it go undiagnosed so often? The answer may lie in the fact that mild cases of celiac disease, while causing damage to the intestinal wall and raising the risk of serious complications, may never cause severe enough independent symptoms to warrant a directed search. Myriad other gastrointestinal disorders may create the same symptoms, including *irritable bowel syndrome* (this chapter) and simple stress-related indigestion. To make matters more complicated, irritable bowel syndrome may exist concurrently with celiac disease, making the process of distinguishing between symptoms problematic.

Other disorders frequently confused with celiac disease include *Crohn disease, ulcerative colitis, gastroenteritis* (all this chapter), *chronic fatigue syndrome* (Chapter 5), and depression (Chapter 3).

Treatment

No treatment for celiac disease exists, except to avoid gluten in any form. Gluten is present in many grains, including wheat, rye, barley, spelt, triticale, and kamut. Many (but not all) people with celiac disease are also sensitive to oats, although whether this grain actually contains gluten or is frequently contaminated with it is somewhat questionable. Gluten is also used in many other products, including vitamins or other pills, cosmetics (especially lipstick), and as a thickener in many processed foods.

Gluten is not present in corn, potatoes, beans, or soy; flour made from these foods can frequently be substituted to help constitute a gluten-free diet. Other gluten-free foods include fruits, vegetables, and meats. It is possible to have a varied and well-balanced gluten-free diet, but eating processed foods or at restaurants may be problematic.

Most celiac disease patients who avoid all sources of gluten for months or years can heal completely and achieve the complete rebuilding of their intestinal villi. However, this reconstruction can easily be undone if gluten-rich foods are consumed; a person with celiac disease must commit to a lifelong dietary adjustment.

Massage?

Massage has no impact on the health of intestinal villi. It can, however, temporarily relieve gastrointestinal discomfort. Although this is usually a benefit, it may lead to a delay in seeking a diagnosis. Celiac disease, like many other intestinal diseases, has the best prognosis when it is identified early. Consequently, if a client reports recurring symptoms that persist for more than a few days or weeks, that person should be referred to another medical professional as soon as possible.

If a client has been diagnosed with celiac disease and manages it successfully through dietary changes, he or she is a fine candidate for massage. Abdominal work should be conducted strictly within the comfort level of the client, of course.

Crohn Disease

Definition: What Is It?

Crohn disease is a progressive inflammatory disorder that can affect any part of the gastrointestinal tract, from the mouth to the anus. Advanced cases also may involve tissues outside the digestive system.

Crohn disease and *ulcerative colitis* (this chapter) are often described together under the umbrella term "inflammatory bowel disease" because of the way they affect tissues, but they are etiologically quite different. Although Crohn disease can and often does affect the large intestine as well as the upper GI tract, it is discussed in this section to help distinguish it from ulcerative colitis. For more information on how these two conditions are alike and dissimilar, see "Compare and Contrast, Crohn Disease and Ulcerative Colitis."

Demographics: Who Gets It?

Crohn disease affects about 500,000 Americans; men and women are affected more or less equally. It can develop in young children, but most patients are diagnosed in their 20s or 30s; the average age of onset is 27.

The geographic distribution of this condition is interesting. It is especially common in the United States, Canada, and Scandinavia. It is somewhat less common in the United Kingdom and Western Europe, followed by Australia and South Africa. It is rare in all other countries.

A genetic susceptibility is evidently part of the Crohn disease profile; approximately 20% of all patients have a first-degree relative (parent, child, or sibling) who also has an inflammatory bowel disease. Statistically it occurs in higher numbers among Ashkenazi Jews than in other populations. Whites are most at risk for this disorder; it happens among this population four times more often than among nonwhites.

Crohn Disease in Brief

What is it?
Crohn disease is a progressive inflammatory condition that may affect any part of the GI tract. It involves the development of deep ulcers, blockages, and the formation of abnormal passageways (fistulae) in the small and large intestine.

How is it recognized?
The primary symptom of Crohn disease is abdominal pain, especially in the lower right quadrant (the distal end of the ileum). Cramping, diarrhea, and pain at the anus also may accompany active flares of this disease.

Is massage indicated or contraindicated?
Massage is appropriate for Crohn disease patients when their condition is in remission. During flares they also may benefit from noncirculatory work, but abdominal work will be uncomfortable.

Compare and Contrast
CROHN DISEASE AND ULCERATIVE COLITIS

Crohn disease and ulcerative colitis are two conditions linked under the description, "inflammatory bowel disease," or IBD. This may create the impression that these two disorders are slightly different manifestations of the same problem, but current research indicates that they are significantly different in etiology, progression, and long-term prognosis. Although differentiating between these conditions has little impact on a massage therapist's decision, it may have big impact on the life of the client.

CROHN DISEASE

Area affected
Often begins in the ileum but can spread distally into the colon, or proximally into the rest of the small intestine. Seldom affects the rectum.

Pattern of progression
Progresses in unpredictable, disconnected patches that may appear anywhere along the GI tract.

Depth of lesions
Ulcers may burrow through the mucosa, into the muscular or serous wall of the GI tract. Perforation is not uncommon.

Complications
Can lead to liver problems, skin and mouth ulcers, eye inflammation, peritonitis, bladder infections, and colon cancer.

Surgery
Surgery can remove affected areas, but it often continues to attack healthy tissue; surgery often needs to be repeated.

ULCERATIVE COLITIS

Area affected
Always begins in the rectum. May spread proximally up the colon, but never all the way to the small intestine.

Pattern of progression
Progresses in a continuous connected series of lesions.

Depth of lesions
Ulcers penetrate only the mucosa or submucosa of the colon; they seldom cause perforation.

Complications
Significantly raises the risk of colon cancer; other complications include liver inflammation, arthritis, skin rashes, and anemia.

Surgery
Surgery to remove the affected area is curative.

Etiology: What Happens?

Crohn disease involves the development of inflamed areas in the large and small intestine. Many cases begin in the distal portion of the small intestine, the ileum, but this progressive disease can affect upper regions of the GI tract, as well as the colon and anus.

One of the distinguishing features of Crohn disease is that the areas it affects are not continuous; the inflamed regions appear in an unpredictable patchwork anywhere in the GI tract (Figure 7.2). These lesions may then develop ulcers that affect deep layers of the intestinal wall, even to the point of perforation. Eventually these ulcers can cause accumulations of scar tissue that partially block the intestine, or they can stimulate the development of abnormal connecting tubes from the colon to other organs, such as the

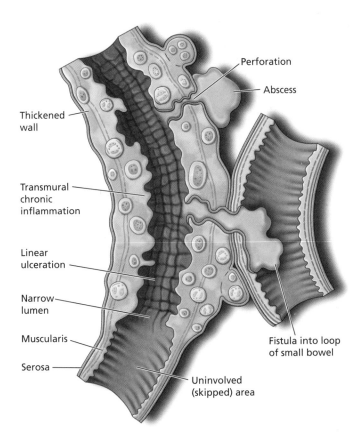

Figure 7.2. Crohn disease.

bladder or even to the surface of the skin. These tubes are called *fistulae*, and they allow intestinal contents to exit the GI tract.

In some cases of Crohn disease, massive accumulations of scar tissue cause the GI tract to become dangerously narrow; this is called *stenosis*. Stenosing Crohn disease can also lead to the formation of fistulae, as the body tries to reroute digestive system contents that have become blocked.

Causes

Crohn disease is, so far, an idiopathic disease. Several theories about its causes are being pursued. An inappropriate inflammatory response is part of the picture, but it is unclear whether that response is the cause or the result of the disease. Some speculation about an initial exposure to a common mycobacterium, *paratuberculosis*, is gaining momentum (see the sidebar "Crohn Disease History"); the fact that some patients have success with early aggressive doses of antibiotics lends some credence to this approach. Although this condition may be linked to bacterial exposure, it does *not* appear to be contagious. Regardless of the initial trigger, the development of Crohn disease depends on a genetic susceptibility to this kind of inflammatory response.

Food sensitivities and stress have been seen to exacerbate Crohn disease symptoms, but they have not been identified as direct causes.

Another new branch of research focuses on the immune system chemicals that are predominant in the patches of inflamed tissue during Crohn disease flares. Several

Crohn Disease History

Throughout the 20th century, Crohn disease has gone through several incarnations. It has been called *granulomatosis enteritis* for the presence of white blood cell conglomerates called granulomas. It has been called *regional enteritis* for its patchy appearance throughout the small and large intestines. It has also been labeled *terminal ileitis* because it often begins at the distal end of the ileum.

One of the first researchers to document this disorder was a Scottish doctor named Thomas Kennedy Dalziel. In 1913, he noted its similarity to certain inflammatory conditions found among livestock, and he proposed that it might be caused by the same pathogen—*Mycobacterium paratuberculosis*.

In 1932, a team of researchers, including Dr. Burrill Crohn (1884–1983), were unable to find significant signs of bacteria in the lesions, and so the theory of bacterial infection was dropped. Instead, the disease was studied as some kind of immune system dysfunction involving inappropriate inflammatory attacks against digestive system tissue. Not until 1959 was the disease clearly distinguishable from the closely related ulcerative colitis.

In 1985, new tests showed that particles of *M. paratuberculosis* can indeed be found in Crohn disease ulcers. Early treatment with the correct antibiotics shows promising results with many Crohn disease patients, although some of them require these antibiotics for a prolonged period.

M. paratuberculosis is a common pathogen that most people encounter early in life, when it usually causes a short-term bout of diarrhea. Crohn disease patients simply seem to have a genetic susceptibility to creating a lifelong inflammatory response to this pathogen that causes significant and extensive damage to the digestive tract.

cytokines that exacerbate the inflammatory response have been identified, including tumor necrosis factor, interleukin 10, and interleukin 12. The good news about these discoveries is that mechanisms to inactivate these chemicals are available and are currently under investigation as future Crohn disease treatment options.

Signs and Symptoms

Crohn disease occurs in periods of flare and remission, which implies an autoimmune component. During periods of remission, a patient may have no symptoms at all, but during a flare the most common symptoms include abdominal pain, especially at the distal end of the ileum in the lower right quadrant, along with cramping, diarrhea (often with blood), and bloating. Weight loss, fever, joint pain, small ulcers in the mouth and throat, and characteristic lesions on the skin also may accompany acute flares. Many Crohn disease patients also experience severe pain around the anus, along with anal fissures and localized infections.

Complications

Crohn disease disrupts normal digestion in several ways. Inflammation in the intestines means a patient has less access to ingested nutrition. When Crohn disease occurs in young children, this can lead to stunted growth and delayed development; in children and adults, it can lead to serious malabsorption and malnutrition. This disease can cause bowel obstruction or perforations, leading to *peritonitis* (this chapter); adhesions between layers of the peritoneum can form; it can cause abscesses in the GI tract or around the anus; it can cause intestinal hemorrhage if the ulcers erode into blood vessels. If fistulae form into the bladder, leaking fecal material can cause bladder infections. Chronic irritation to epithelial cells in the GI tract also increases the risk of developing colon cancer.

Crohn disease has been linked to problems outside the GI tract as well. It can cause inflammation at the bile duct, leading to *cirrhosis* and *jaundice* (this chapter). It has been linked with acute inflammation affecting the liver, eyes, and joints. It can cause the outbreak of ulcers called *aphthae* in the mouth, and characteristic lesions on the skin as well; these open sores most often appear around the ankles and lower legs.

Treatment

The damage to the whole length of the digestive system that Crohn disease can cause is significant, and so it is usually treated aggressively. Treatment during flares usually begins with steroidal anti-inflammatories and immunosuppressant drugs to quell the inflammatory reaction. Other drugs that inhibit the activity of inflammatory cytokines are under investigation. Many Crohn disease patients end up having surgery to remove affected sections of intestine, but this surgery is not curative; new patches of inflamed tissue may arise in other places, which then requires further surgery.

Crohn disease patients have to be extraordinarily careful about their diet, especially during flares. High-fiber, bulky foods can exacerbate symptoms and create obstructions if scar tissue has narrowed the passageway. Sometimes high-calorie liquid diets are recommended during these episodes. In extreme cases, the patient may take in all nutrients by IV to give the whole system a break from the stress of digesting food.

Massage?

When this condition is in remission and the digestive tract is not under inflammatory attack, massage is a supportive and appropriate choice for clients with Crohn disease. Deep abdominal work should probably be avoided, but anything that creates a parasympathetic response for increased efficiency of digestion and nutrient absorption would probably be useful.

During flares, a client with Crohn disease will probably be uncomfortable on the table, and circulatory work may exacerbate symptoms. Other types of bodywork, however, may be welcome and helpful in the effort to reduce pain and distress.

Esophageal Cancer

Definition: What Is It?

Esophageal cancer is the development of malignant cells in the esophagus. These cells have a slightly different pattern depending on whether they grow at the proximal end (squamous cell carcinoma of the esophagus) or at the distal end (adenocarcinoma of the esophagus). Esophageal cancer is a relatively rare but serious disease that is difficult to detect early.

Demographics: Who Gets It?

The occurrence of esophageal cancer has some specific demographic patterns. Although it is relatively rare in the United States, it is common in developing countries. In the United States, African American men are more at risk than any other population group for squamous cell carcinoma, whereas white men lead the statistics for adenocarcinoma. Men of all races outnumber women with esophageal cancer by about 8 to 1.

Approximately 13,500 cases of esophageal cancer are diagnosed in this country, and an estimated 12,500 people die of the disease annually. The prognosis for esophageal cancer is usually poor; the overall 5-year survival rate is less than 10%.

Etiology: What Happens?

The esophagus is a tube approximately 10 inches long. It runs from the throat to the lower esophageal valve, which opens into the stomach. It is composed of four layers of tissue: the mucous membrane that lines the tube, the submucosa that provides blood and lymph support for the active mucus-producing cells, the muscularis that provides strong wave-like contractions to move a food bolus from the throat into the stomach, and the adventitia: a connective tissue outer layer. The esophagus lacks a serous membrane covering.

When malignant cells grow in the upper or middle parts of the esophagus, they tend to appear in squamous epithelial cells; this is called squamous cell carcinoma of the esophagus. This condition is closely related to smoking or alcohol use; smoking in combination with alcohol use increases the risk of malignancies by a large margin. Until

---

Esophageal Cancer in Brief

What is it?
Esophageal cancer is the growth of malignant cells in the esophagus. It is classified as squamous cell carcinoma, which usually occurs at the proximal end of the esophagus, and adenocarcinoma, which occurs at the distal end, near the lower esophageal valve.

How is it recognized?
Esophageal cancer is rarely recognized in early stages. In later stages a growth may obstruct the esophagus, leading to a feeling of food or liquid "getting stuck" on the way to the stomach. Pain and difficulty with swallowing along with unintended weight loss are the symptoms that usually prompt people to seek a diagnosis.

Is massage indicated or contraindicated?
As with other cancers, the guidelines for massage and esophageal cancer are determined largely by what stresses or complications cancer treatments may cause. Surgery, radiation, chemotherapy, and other options all carry specific cautions and concerns for massage therapists.

recently, squamous cell carcinoma of the esophagus was by far the most common type of esophageal cancer, accounting for 85% or more of all cases.

When malignant cells grow in glandular tissue, the growth is called adenocarcinoma. This is the case when esophageal cancer originates at the distal end of the tube, close to the lower esophageal valve. A condition called Barrett's esophagus is usually a predisposing factor for adenocarcinoma of the esophagus. Barrett's esophagus is a complication of *gastroesophageal reflux disease* (GERD) (this chapter), and is considered a precancerous state for esophageal cancer. Although once rare, adenocarcinoma of the esophagus is now diagnosed more often than squamous cell carcinoma.

Malignant cells from esophageal cancer can invade other tissues through a number of different venues. Because the esophagus has no serous membrane cover, any tumor that penetrates through all four layers of the esophagus may then be able to spread easily to nearby structures. The trachea, diaphragm, aorta, and vena cava are most susceptible. A generous supply of lymphatic capillaries in the esophageal submucosa means that lymphatic spread of the disease is also a risk. The lymph system can then carry malignant cells to nearby nodes and other tissues, including the lungs, liver, and bones. Esophageal cancer also can spread through the bloodstream, although this appears to happen less often than other routes for metastasis.

Risk Factors

The primary risk factors for esophageal cancer are age, gender, and race: issues that are not controllable. However, several other risk factors can be controlled: use of tobacco products and use of alcohol have been seen to increase the risk for squamous cell carcinoma of the esophagus; this risk is compiled when alcohol and tobacco use occur simultaneously.

The main risk factor for adenocarcinoma is damage to the esophageal lining when it is exposed to a chronic, repeating barrage of gastric juices. The cells of the esophageal mucosa change to resemble cells that line the stomach. This raises the risk for malignancy so significantly that many physicians recommend surgery or other interventions even before cancer is confirmed.

Other risk factors for esophageal cancer include a history of any other head or neck cancer, exposure to toxic substances (i.e., ingesting lye or other poisons), exposure to asbestos, and a lifetime habit of drinking extremely hot beverages. Worldwide studies also show that a shortage of vitamins A, B, and C, and the minerals magnesium and zinc are common among esophageal cancer patients.

Signs and Symptoms

Early signs and symptoms of esophageal cancer are practically nonexistent, which is why this disease has such a high mortality rate; it is often undetected until a tumor is large enough to create a mechanical obstruction, and metastasis to other nearby organs or lymph nodes has already occurred.

The symptoms that most often cause people to go to the doctor include a feeling of food or liquid "getting stuck" on its way to the stomach, pain with swallowing, hoarseness, and unplanned weight loss. A chronic cough, with or without blood, also may occur.

Diagnosis

The diagnostic procedure for esophageal cancer typically begins with a barium swallow. This test shows exactly where a lesion or tumor might have developed. Various depths and techniques of scopes may follow, along with a positron-emission tomography (PET) scan, a computed tomography (CT) scan, or ultrasound to check for signs of lymphatic involvement. For more information on staging esophageal cancer, see sidebar, "Staging Esophageal Cancer."

Treatment

Treatment for esophageal cancer ranges from surgery to chemotherapy, radiation, or other options. Photodynamic therapy is sometimes employed in this situation: special drugs are absorbed into cancerous cells and then activated by a laser to destroy the target cells.

Recovery from treatment for esophageal cancer is often problematic because it requires good nutrition to heal from such invasive procedures, and eating is often very difficult.

Massage?

The guidelines for massage and esophageal cancer are the same as for massage and any other type of cancer. Benefits and risks must be weighed in the context of the stresses brought about by cancer treatment as much as by the cancer itself. Although massage can improve sleep and appetite, care must be taken not to overwhelm the system of a person undergoing an extraordinarily stressful process. For more information about massage in the context of cancer, see Chapter 11.

Gastroenteritis

Definition: What Is It?

Gastroenteritis is inflammation of the GI tract, specifically the stomach or small intestine.

Demographics: Who Gets It?

Anyone of any age can get gastroenteritis, although it is most dangerous for the very young, the very old, and people whose immune systems are compromised. Although only approximately 10% of all affected people seek medical consultation, some estimates suggest that each year some 100 million cases of gastroenteritis occur in the United States. It is responsible for over 200,000 hospitalizations of children and about 10,000 deaths each year.

Etiology: What Happens?

Gastroenteritis can have several causes. Although each factor may create slightly different symptoms, the basics (nausea, vomiting, diarrhea) are consistent.

- *Viruses:* The most common cause of GI inflammation is an infection with *rotavirus* or *Norovirus* (a group that includes Norwalk virus). Any of the hepatitis viruses also can cause it, as

---

Staging Esophageal Cancer

Testing for esophageal cancer usually begins with a barium swallow or endoscopy to look for the reasons behind the earliest symptom: a feeling of something being "stuck in the throat." If suspicious tissue is found, a CT scan or ultrasound test follows, to look for signs of metastasis in the nearby lymph nodes, as well as the trachea, lungs, and liver.

Esophageal cancer is staged using the TNM classification. These findings are then applied to stages 0 through 4 as follows:

Tumor	Node	Metastasis
Tx: unassessable	Nx: unassessable	Mx: unassessable
T0: no evidence of a primary tumor	N0: no nodal involvement	M0: no distant metastasis
T-IS: in situ tumor (affects the innermost lining of the esophagus only)	N1: nearby nodes are involved	M1: distant metastasis
T1: tumor invades the mucosa or submucosa		
T2: tumor invades the muscularis		
T3: tumor invades the adventitia		
T4: tumor invades nearby structures, notably the trachea		

Stage	T	N	M	5-year survival rate
O	T-IS	N0	M0	75%
I	T1	N0	M0	60%
IIA	T2-T3	N0	M0	40%
IIB	T1-T2	N1	M0	20%
III	T3-T4	N1	M0	15%
IV	Any	Any	M1	<5%

Gastroenteritis in Brief

What is it?
Gastroenteritis is any form of gastrointestinal inflammation. This may be attributable to a viral or bacterial infection, a parasite, fungus, food intolerance, or other cause.

How is it recognized?
The symptoms of gastroenteritis are nausea, vomiting, and diarrhea. Fever, blood in the stools, and other signs may be present, depending on the cause.

Is massage indicated or contraindicated?
Acute gastroenteritis contraindicates massage, especially when it is caused by an infectious agent. Chronic situations may be appropriate for bodywork, as long as the cause of the problem is clearly understood.

can any member of the enterovirus family. Viral gastroenteritis is highly contagious and can reach epidemic levels in environments such as daycare centers, where most infants have not yet developed antibodies against infection and the chance of fecal–oral contamination is very high. It is estimated that viruses cause anywhere from 50% to 70% of all cases of gastroenteritis in the United States.

- *Bacteria:* Common bacterial pathogens include *Salmonella, Shigella, Campylobacter,* and several varieties of *Escherichia coli.* Bacterial gastroenteritis is usually spread through improperly stored or prepared food, or contaminated water or ice. "Travelers' diarrhea" is almost always from the *E. coli* bacterium. One form of bacterial irritation is caused by *Helicobacter pylori,* the pathogen associated with gastric *ulcers* (this chapter). Bacterial gastroenteritis accounts for 15% to 20% of all cases.

- *Others:* Other causes of gastroenteritis include parasites (i.e., *Giardia* and *Cryptosporidium*), fungal infections (i.e., candidiasis, this chapter), toxins (i.e., poisonous mushrooms or poison shellfish), dietary problems (i.e., food allergies), medications (i.e., antibiotics or magnesium-containing laxatives or antacids), or other conditions such as *celiac disease, appendicitis, Crohn disease, ulcerative colitis, irritable bowel syndrome,* or *diverticulitis* (this chapter). Weakness at the pyloric valve may allow contents of the duodenum to back up into the stomach, causing local irritation. This is called "bile reflux."

Once a pathogen, allergen, or toxic substance has gained access to the digestive tract, it can affect the function of the stomach and intestines in several ways. Some pathogens, such as Shigella and Campylobacter, directly invade the mucosal lining. Others, such as some varieties of *E. coli,* produce wastes that are highly toxic and destroy digestive system cells indirectly. Certain animal and plant poisons are cytotoxic: they kill any intestinal cells to which they are exposed. When the GI tract is damaged or inflamed, absorption of nutrients and water is severely limited. This causes the loss of both water and valuable electrolytes through diarrhea and vomiting.

Signs and Symptoms

Different causative factors of gastroenteritis can lead to various symptoms, but the basic trio of intestinal inflammation includes abdominal pain, nausea and vomiting, and diarrhea. These are appropriate responses to infection because they are efficient methods of clearing out the GI tract, but several of these diseases are spread through oral–fecal contamination, so hygiene becomes critical when dealing with these symptoms.

Other signs that may develop with gastroenteritis include bloating, cramps, gas, and mucus or blood in the stools.

Complications

The most serious complication of gastroenteritis is dehydration from the massive fluid and mineral loss that goes along with diarrhea and vomiting. The loss of critical fluid and electrolytes can be fatal; gastroenteritis is a leading cause of death in many developing nations. In the United States, the people most at risk for this extreme reaction are infants, immune-compromised persons, and the elderly, whose systems are less able to cope with this extreme change in internal environment. Signs of dangerously progressed dehydration include sunken eyes, lack of urination, and skin tenting: when the skin is pinched, it does not immediately contract back to its original position.

Some gastroenteritis factors can cause other complications as well. Campylobacter bacteria have been linked with *Guillain-Barré* syndrome (Chapter 3), and Salmonella can complicate into *meningitis* (Chapter 3), or blood poisoning. Some forms of *E. coli* are highly toxic and can lead to renal failure (Chapter 9).

Diagnosis

Diagnosis of gastroenteritis is often a problem. Taking stool samples is the most efficient way to identify infectious agents, but this is a time-consuming and expensive process. Conversely, treating bacterial infections with the wrong antibiotics can lead to more extreme symptoms and more resistant pathogens. To complicate matters further, it is possible to continue carrying the infectious agents long after symptoms have subsided. This has serious repercussions for food handlers and childcare and health care workers, who are in positions to spread their infection to many other people.

Treatment

Gastroenteritis is usually an acute, self-limiting condition and is not generally treated with anything more sophisticated than rest and fluid and electrolyte replacement. Viruses do not respond to antibiotics, and antibiotics for bacterial infections may make intestinal inflammation worse. The use of anti-diarrhea medications is often discouraged because the body is shedding pathogens: interfering with that process may prolong the infection.

If supplementing fluids by mouth aggravates vomiting, it may be necessary to use intravenous fluid replacement in a hospital setting.

Gastroenteritis is much easier to prevent than to treat. When gastroenteritis occurs in outbreaks, it is often due to some specific source of contamination: a shipment of infected meat, a contaminated well, or some shellfish harvested from contaminated water. Because foodstuffs are now shipped quickly all over large areas, it is a constant public health challenge to track down the source of infection and to limit its spread among the rest of the population.

Prognosis

Most cases of gastroenteritis resolve within 2 to 3 days without medical intervention. If symptoms persist longer than 2 to 3 weeks, it is no longer considered an acute infection, but a chronic condition. This would lead medical professionals to look for an underlying condition such as food allergies, irritable bowel syndrome, diverticulitis, Crohn disease, ulcerative colitis, or human immunodeficiency virus/acquired immune deficiency syndrome (HIV/AIDS).

Massage?

Acute gastroenteritis contraindicates circulatory massage for several reasons: an infection may be present and could be exacerbated; the infection may be communicable; and the client is unlikely to be comfortable because he will probably be feeling nauseous at the time.

If a client has chronic digestive system irritation that is unrelated to infection, cancer, or other dangerous causes, bodywork could be helpful in creating a parasympathetic state that would improve efficiency and comfort.

Gastroesophageal Reflux Disease (GERD)

Definition: What Is It?

Gastroesophageal reflux disease (GERD) is a condition involving damage to the squamous epithelial lining of the esophagus when it is chronically exposed to digestive juices released from the stomach. It is usually associated with weak muscular action at the lower esophageal sphincter, but several factors may contribute.

Demographics: Who Gets It?

Heartburn, the predecessor to GERD, is astonishingly common in this country. It is estimated that 7% to 10% of all Americans experience heartburn every day, and up to 40% of all Americans have it at least once a month. GERD is diagnosed when heartburn becomes a chronic, ongoing situation, especially in the presence of structural changes to the esophageal lining or to the lower esophageal sphincter. GERD can happen to any person at any age. It has been documented among infants, the elderly, and every age in between, but it is most common among mature people.

Etiology: What Happens?

Most cases of GERD are connected to some combination of three problems: the lower esophageal sphincter (LES) is too relaxed; the LES does not allow appropriate clearing of acids in the esophagus; or the stomach is slow to empty, adding to back-pressure at the LES.

Any one of these problems allows stomach contents, including highly corrosive hydrochloric acid (and occasionally bile and pancreatic enzymes that have backed up through a weak pyloric valve) to enter the esophagus, which lacks the thick layers of mucus that protect the stomach from acid exposure.

Chronic irritation of the esophageal lining can cause several reactions.

- *Respiratory injury* may occur if gastric secretions reach up to the larynx. It is not uncommon for these substances to be aspirated into the lungs, especially by infants and young children.

- *Ulcers* may form in the esophagus. These lesions may become infected, or they may bleed into the GI tract.

- *A stricture* may form. This is a thickening of the esophageal wall with scar tissue in response to irritation (Figure 7.3). Strictures may make it difficult to swallow normally.

- *Barrett's esophagus* may develop. This is a pathologic change in the normal esophageal squamous cells; they mutate into cells that resemble the stomach lining. Barrett's esophagus has been identified as a possible precancerous condition, opening the door to adenocarcinoma, one increasingly common type of *esophageal cancer* (this chapter).

Risk Factors

A number of risk factors for developing GERD have been identified. Some of these are modifiable, which gives most GERD patients some influence over their disease process. Risk factors for GERD include:

- *Pregnancy*. Most pregnant women experience some heartburn, especially when the baby is big enough to put mechanical pressure on the stomach. Some pregnant women go on to develop significant structural changes in the esophagus.

- *Obesity*. Being clinically overweight can cause the abdominal contents to put ongoing mechanical pressure on the diaphragm and esophageal sphincter.

- *Smoking*. Smoking has been seen to weaken and loosen the esophageal sphincter.

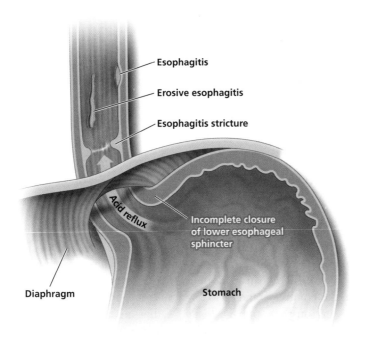

Figure 7.3. Gastroesophageal reflux disease.

- *Diet.* A diet high in fatty or spicy foods, as well as the ingestion of caffeine, alcohol, chocolate, and highly acidic foods, can exacerbate GERD.

- *Connective tissue diseases.* Diseases such as *lupus* (Chapter 5) or *scleroderma* (Chapter 2) may result in inflammation and weakening of the LES.

- *Hiatal hernia.* A hiatal hernia (an enlargement of the opening in the diaphragm where the esophagus passes through to the stomach) may catch and irritate the superior part of the stomach. Most people with hiatal hernias experience GERD, although not all GERD patients have hiatal hernias.

- *Delayed stomach emptying.* Some diseases, including *diabetes* (Chapter 9), *ulcers* (this chapter), and *spinal cord injuries* (Chapter 3), cause reduced peristalsis and sluggish movement of substances through the GI tract. When stomach contents linger too long, the accumulation of pressure and gastric juices can cause them to put back-pressure on the esophagus.

- *Other risk factors.* These include exposure to radiation for chest tumors, infection of the esophagus, and certain medications.

Signs and Symptoms

Signs and symptoms of GERD are largely created by the action of gastric juice on the delicate esophageal lining. A bitter taste, a feeling like some food has been regurgitated, gas, indigestion, bloating, and pain in the chest behind the sternum are common symptoms. It is not unusual for the pain of GERD to be mistaken for *heart attack* (see Chapter 4) or angina. Symptoms are reliably aggravated by lying down.

Other GERD symptoms that occur less frequently include trouble swallowing, coughing, wheezing, and coughing up blood if ulcers in the esophagus have eroded into a blood vessel.

Diagnosis

Diagnostic tests for GERD reveal very precise information about the nature and location of structural changes to the stomach and esophagus. They include barium x-rays, endoscopy, a test for pH balance in the esophagus, and possibly a biopsy to examine suspicious-looking cells. Approximately 10,000 GERD patients per year develop Barrett's esophagus, which may be precancerous.

Treatment

Treatment for GERD falls into two categories: management of the problem and repairing the problem. Managing GERD so that it does not get worse includes strategies such as losing weight if the patient is overweight, eating smaller portions so the stomach does not get as full, not lying down within 2 hours after a meal, avoiding caffeine, alcohol, and nicotine, raising the bed approximately 6 inches at the head, loosening clothing that puts pressure around the waist, and putting a heating pad on the stomach when it is painful.

Medication for GERD can work in a variety of ways. Antacids neutralize stomach acid, but over-the-counter brands also may cause the stomach to expand with gas, putting more pressure on the esophageal valve. Other medications can block receptors in the stomach that stimulate acid production, increase stomach motility to assist in sluggish movement, and block the release of hydrogen ions that contribute to the stomach's acidic environment.

Surgery for GERD usually focuses on strengthening the esophageal sphincter and taking pressure off the stomach. If the esophagus is limited by the development of a scar tissue stricture, this may be stretched and dilated. A portion of the stomach may be wrapped around the sphincter to give it external support in a procedure called a *fundoplication*. Of course, if a hiatal hernia puts pressure on the stomach, surgery may be performed to correct it.

Newer options to treat Barrett's esophagus include the use of photodynamic therapy, electrocautery, and laser surgery.

Massage?

Massage usually improves digestive function and efficiency through the parasympathetic response. With GERD patients, however, this may not be a benefit when gastric acid can splash back up into the esophagus. Therefore, it is important to work with clients who have GERD in a way that does not exacerbate symptoms. This may mean not working within 2 hours of the client having eaten, it may mean working with a massage chair or in a semi-reclined position, or it may mean putting 6-inch blocks under the head-end of the massage table. Although clients with GERD can benefit from bodywork, their special needs may require imaginative accommodations on the part of their massage therapists.

Clients who successfully control their GERD with medication are perfectly fine for massage, although abdominal work around the area of the stomach should be conservative.

Stomach Cancer

Definition: What Is It?

Stomach cancer is the development of malignant tumors in the stomach that can block the passage of food through the digestive system, and can spread, either through cells directly moving into the peritoneal space, or through blood and lymph flow, to other organs.

Demographics: Who Gets It?

Stomach cancer is on a dramatic decline in the United States. However, in much of the rest of the world, especially in countries in Asia and South America, stomach cancer is the second leading cause of death by cancer (lung cancer is first).

In the United States, approximately 24,000 people are diagnosed with stomach cancer every year, and approximately 14,000 people die. Most stomach cancer patients are in their 60s or 70s, and men with the disease outnumber women by almost 2:1.

Etiology: What Happens?

Although several different types of cancer have been observed to grow from stomach cells, most stomach cancer tumors are adenocarcinomas; in other words, they arise from epithelial tissue. It is not always clear what triggers the growth of these tumors, but the clear difference in U.S. statistics compared with those of Asia and Latin America have yielded some useful clues about the development of this disease.

Stomach cancer rates in the United States began to decline in the 1930s, about the time that refrigeration became accessible for the majority of Americans. The average diet shifted away from smoked, pickled, and salted foods, and toward more fresh meats and fresh, canned, or frozen vegetables. In countries in which stomach cancer is very prominent, the consumption of salted, smoked, or pickled foods is significantly higher than it is in the United States.

Studies of the *Helicobacter pylori* bacteria associated with ulcers (this chapter) show that these bacteria can convert some of the chemicals in high-risk foods into carcinogens. Most stomach cancer patients test positive for *H. pylori*. In fact, the World Health Organization suggests that up to 50% of all cases of stomach cancer are related to *H. pylori* infection. Infection rates of this not-well-understood bacterium are relatively low in the United States.

Any situation that impedes the production of gastric digestive secretions increases the risk of stomach cancer. This can include a history of *H. pylori* infection, stomach surgery, pernicious anemia, and other factors. When the environment in the stomach is insufficiently acidic, ingested materials do not break down properly, and many become carcinogenic.

As the stomach wall is assaulted with chronic exposure to carcinogenic substances, minute changes in the tissues may develop. These precancerous changes are virtually silent and are almost never detected. Malignant cells can grow into tumors large enough to obstruct the passage of food through the digestive tract or they can invade and completely perforate the stomach wall, allowing them to spread to nearby abdominal organs.

By the time stomach cancer is detected, it has usually spread through the portal vein to the liver, or into the lymph system. Almost half of all stomach cancer patients experience metastasis in the peritoneum, and approximately one third discover cancerous cells in the liver.

Risk Factors

The major risk factors for developing stomach cancer include the following:

- *H. pylori infection:* Most stomach cancer patients have *H. pylori* in their digestive tract. These bacteria have been seen to convert certain food products into carcinogens.

Stomach Cancer in Brief

What is it?
Stomach cancer is the development of malignant tumors in the stomach, which may then metastasize directly to other abdominal organs, or through blood and lymph flow to distant places in the body.

How is it recognized?
Symptoms of stomach cancer include a feeling of fullness after only a little food, heartburn, unintentional weight loss, blood in the stools, vague abdominal pain above the navel, and occasionally vomiting, constipation, or diarrhea.

Is massage indicated or contraindicated?
The prognosis for stomach cancer, which is rarely found before metastasis, is generally not promising. Most clients who know that they have stomach cancer will probably be undergoing a series of treatments including surgeries, chemotherapy, and radiation. Bodywork to alleviate the discomforts of cancer treatment may be appropriate, as long as the risks involved with each type of intervention are respected.

- *Diet:* Diets that are high in smoked food, salted fish and meats, and pickled vegetables increase the risk of developing stomach cancer. Nitrates used as food preservatives also contribute to this risk. Diets heavy in red meats (more than 13 portions per week) are seen to double stomach cancer risk.
- *Tobacco and alcohol use:* These products have been associated with the development of stomach cancer, especially in the proximal portion of the stomach.
- *Other factors:* A wide variety of other factors increase stomach cancer risk, including having had previous stomach surgery, having type A blood, being male, being between 60 and 79 years old, and having the genes that have been associated with *colorectal cancer* (this chapter).

Signs and Symptoms

Signs and symptoms of stomach cancer are mostly related to having a physical obstruction in the digestive tract. They include a feeling of fullness after only a little food; vague abdominal pain above the navel; unintentional weight loss; heartburn and other ulcer symptoms; nausea and vomiting; and the development of ascites: the accumulation of excessive fluid in the peritoneal space. Tumors may bleed slightly, leading to small amounts of blood in the stool. This is detected with a fecal occult blood study.

Diagnosis

Because the early changes that occur with stomach cancer are so subtle, it is very seldom identified before metastasis in the United States. In Japan, where it occurs approximately 5 times more frequently, mass screenings are conducted to try to find the cancer in earlier stages.

Diagnostic techniques for stomach cancer include endoscopy and biopsy; a barium wash of the upper GI tract followed by radiographs; and an endoscopic ultrasound, CT scan, or magnetic resonance imaging (MRI) of the stomach wall to assist in the staging process. For information on staging stomach cancer, see sidebar, "Staging Stomach Cancer."

Staging Stomach Cancer

Like other digestive cancers, stomach cancer is diagnosed with endoscopy followed by more detailed imaging methods to find the extent of metastasis. The TNM classification system is used to describe the cancer's progress. These findings are then applied to stages 0 through 4 as follows:

Tumor	Node	Metastasis
T-IS: In situ cancer, affecting the mucosa only	N0: No nodal involvement	M0: no distant metastasis
T1: Tumor affects the submucosal layer	N1: 1–6 nearby nodes have been invaded	M1: Distant metastasis
T2a: Tumor affects the muscularis	N2: 7–15 nearby nodes have been invaded	
T2b: Affects the subserosa	N3: More than 15 nearby nodes have been invaded	
T3: The stomach is perforated		
T4: Adjacent organs or blood vessels have been infiltrated		

Stage	T	N	M	5-year survival rate
O	T-IS	N0	M0	89%
IA	T1	N0	M0	78%
IB	T1	N1	M0	58%
II	T1	N2	M0	34%
II (alternate)	T2 a or b	N0	M0	34%
IIIA	T1-T3	N1–N2	M0	20%
IIIB	T3	N2	M0	8%
IV	Any	Any	M1	7%

Stomach cancer is rarely found in early stages, however, so the overall 5-year survival rate is approximately 20%.

Treatment

Stomach cancer is treated with the same arsenal of tools used against most cancers: chemotherapy, radiation, and surgery. Because it is not usually found in early stages, many stomach cancer patients will undergo combinations of therapies in an attempt to limit the spread of the cancer through the rest of the body.

Massage?

If a client knows that he has stomach cancer, he will probably be engaged in a combination of treatments to try to limit the spread of the disease. Cancer treatments can be extraordinarily harsh and taxing for the body to accommodate; massage has a place in reducing pain, improving sleep, and generally supporting the process for cancer patients, as long as the cautions that accompany various cancer treatment options are respected. For more information about this topic, see *cancer*, Chapter 11.

Ulcers

Definition: What Is It?

Peptic ulcers of the esophagus, stomach, and duodenum are discussed in this section, but an ulcer is an ulcer, whether it is in the GI tract or on the skin. An ulcer is the result of tissue damage that, because it is subject to constant irritation and the healing process may be somehow impeded, never gets better. Cells die, are sloughed off, and a crater develops but does not crust over. An ulcer is a perpetually open sore, and an invitation to infection. For more information on skin ulcers, see *decubitus ulcers* (Chapter 1).

Demographics: Who Gets Them?

Ulcers are a common malady in the United States, although their occurrence has recently begun to decline. It is estimated that approximately 10% of all Americans will have at least one ulcer in their lifetime. Approximately 25 million Americans have diagnosed ulcers today. Between 500,000 and 850,000 new cases are diagnosed each year, leading to over 1 million hospitalizations. Men with ulcers outnumber women about 2:1.

Etiology: What Happens?

Ulcers in the esophagus, stomach, or small intestine are called peptic ulcers, named for the protein-digesting enzyme pepsin that contributes to their development (Figure 7.4). Esophageal ulcers typically develop as a complication of *gastroesophageal reflux disease* (this chapter). The general understanding of how stomach and duodenal ulcers come about has undergone some radical changes in the last several years.

For as long as ulcers have been understood as sores on the stomach or intestinal wall, they have been treated with the assumption that they arise from too much stress or spicy food. Ulcer patients have been counseled to eat bland food and avoid getting upset or overly excited. Many found that their ulcers eventually healed but would recur later; ulcers were essentially a lifelong affliction.

Contributing Factors: Stress　The link between stress and ulcers turns out to be a significant factor, but probably not in the way that had always been assumed. Furthermore, the incidence of ulcers across the population does not follow demographics that are associated with high-stress situations; therefore, some variables in stress coping mechanisms have evidently never been addressed.

The normal environment inside a stomach has features that can be classified as "aggressive" and others that are "defensive." Aggressive features include the production of hydrochloric acid and pepsin, which help to digest proteins. Defensive features include a generous blood supply to the stomach wall, which serves to help damaged cells regenerate quickly, as well as stimulating mucus production; a lining that protects the stomach wall from acid and pepsin; and the production of bicarbonate to neutralize acid. These aggressive and defensive mechanisms work best when they keep each other in balance.

Ulcers in Brief

What are they?
Ulcers are sores that for various reasons do not go through a normal healing process; they remain open and vulnerable to infection. Peptic ulcers occur in the esophagus, stomach, or duodenum: the proximal portion of the small intestine.

How are they recognized?
The symptoms of peptic ulcers include general burning or gnawing abdominal pain between meals that is relieved by taking antacids or eating. Other symptoms can include bloating, burping, gas, and consistent vomiting after meals.

Is massage indicated or contraindicated?
Specific work on the abdomen may exacerbate symptoms of peptic ulcers, so they are at least a local contraindication for mechanical types of bodywork. Other modalities, and massage away from the upper abdomen, are certainly indicated for ulcer patients.

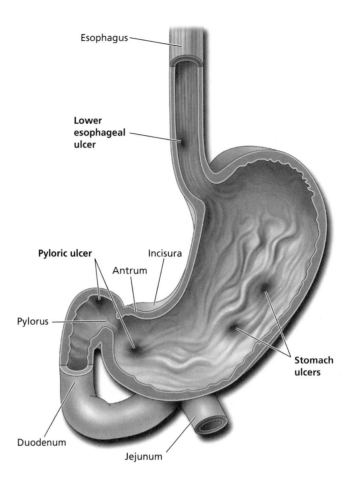

Figure 7.4. Sites of ulcers.

Recall that when a person is in a sympathetic state, blood supply to the whole digestive tract is suppressed while blood is rerouted toward skeletal muscle to support the "flight or fight" reaction. Stomach activity is suspended during a sympathetic reaction. Lack of blood flow means that mucus production is slowed, but so is acid and pepsin production; the two mechanisms stay in balance. When stress is lifted, however, and a person shifts back into a relaxed, parasympathetic state, stomach activity is stimulated again. The problem is that the stomach produces acid and pepsin much faster than it rebuilds a thinned, delicate mucous lining. This imbalance between aggressive and defensive features leaves the stomach wall vulnerable to damage. In other words, ulcers seem to be more related to the *relief* of stress than to the presence of stress![1]

Contributing Factors: *Helicobacter pylori* Stress is only part of the ulcer picture, however. In 1982, a remarkable discovery revealed an unexpected phenomenon: a bacterium that can survive and thrive in the highly acidic environment of the stomach. This bacterium, called *Helicobacter pylori*, is found in many biopsies of ulcers. It is an organism with spiral-shaped flagella that invades the mucous membrane of the stomach when structural weak spots appear. The identification of *H. pylori* led to the conclusion that

[1] This realization often prompts the question, "Shouldn't we just stay in stress all the time then, to avoid ever getting an ulcer?" The answer is that living in chronic low-grade stress opens the door to hosts of other diseases that are far more life-threatening than peptic ulcers.

imbalances in stomach chemistry can initiate tissue damage to the stomach wall, but bacterial infection makes the ulcer a long-term chronic problem. For more information on *H. pylori*, see sidebar, "What is *Helicobacter pylori*?"

The presence of *H. pylori* bacteria in most ulcer biopsy specimens led to a whole new understanding of how peptic ulcers develop and how to treat them. The addition of antibiotics to ulcer treatments leads to a successful, permanent solution for many ulcer patients. This finding was so conclusive that in 1994 the National Institutes of Health issued a statement asserting that up to 90% of all peptic ulcers were related to *H. pylori* infection. A certain population, however, have ulcers that are unrelated to bacteria.

Contributing Factors: NSAIDs   The use of nonsteroidal anti-inflammatory drugs (NSAIDs) for everything from headaches to back pain to heart disease and stroke prevention has led to some significant disruption of stomach function for many patients. Aspirin, ibuprofen, and naproxen sodium all interrupt the "defensive" aspects of stomach activity. They interfere with blood flow to the mucous membrane, they slow mucus production, and they inhibit the production of bicarbonate. An estimated 10% of all diagnosed peptic ulcers arise from long-term NSAID use instead of from bacterial infection, although it is also possible that NSAID damage and *H. pylori* could be present simultaneously.

Signs and Symptoms

The primary symptom of peptic ulcers is a gnawing, burning pain in the chest or abdomen. It can last anywhere from 30 minutes to 3 hours. The pain that occurs in relation to eating varies greatly from one person to the next (it can depend on the location of the ulcer), but it is generally relieved by antacids or eating more food.

Other signs of ulcers can include nausea, vomiting, loss of appetite, and bleeding into the GI tract.

Complications

Complications of ulcers can be serious. When ulcers erode into capillaries, bleeding occurs, leading to *anemia* (see Chapter 4). If the eroded blood vessel is a larger arteriole or artery, hemorrhaging can lead quickly to shock and death if left untreated. Ulcers also can perforate, or eat all the way through, the organ wall, releasing bacteria and partially digested food into the peritoneal space (see *peritonitis*, this chapter). Perforation happens more often with duodenal than stomach ulcers. Ulcers can create a combination of scar tissue and inflammation that causes the pyloric valve to spasm, thus completely obstructing the digestive tract. If this situation is not quickly resolved, surgery may be required to reopen the digestive tract.

What Is *Helicobacter pylori*?

Helicobacter pylori is a bacterium that is admirably designed to withstand and even thrive in the corrosively acidic environment of the stomach. The bacterium has several anatomic features that allow it to infect the mucous membranes of the stomach wall.

Until 1984, it was never even considered that a bacterium could survive in the stomach. When pioneer researchers Barry Marshall and Robin Warren proposed the possibility, they were all but laughed offstage. But when biopsies of ulcerative tissue consistently showed the presence of *H. pylori* bacteria, the laughter quieted. And when ulcer patients found that combining appropriate antibiotics with other acid-limiting medications led to a permanent cure for their ulcers—something that was unheard of at the time—the approach to treating this common condition completely changed. In 1994, the National Institutes of Health issued a statement that it was clear that *H. pylori* does indeed cause most peptic ulcers and is also a contributing factor to stomach cancer and lymphoma.

So what is *H. pylori*, and where does it come from? Little is well understood about this pathogen. It is a short, microaerophilic gram-negative bacillus, with spiraling flagella. Its presence can be easily determined by a blood test for antibodies, although this test does not indicate whether the infection is acute or long-standing. It is sensitive to common antibiotics such as tetracycline and amoxicillin. Worldwide, it is estimated that up to two-thirds of all adults have been infected with *H. pylori*. In the United States, most infections have been documented among older adults, African Americans, Hispanics, and people in lower socioeconomic classes.

The discovery of *H. pylori* and its role in peptic ulcers has raised as many questions as it has answered:

- How is the bacterium communicated? No one knows, but it could be through oral–fecal contamination or through oral–oral contact.

- How can it be prevented? It is impossible to prevent the spread of *H. pylori* without knowing how it gets from one person to another.

- If it is sensitive to common antibiotics, why is it not eradicated when a person takes amoxicillin or tetracycline for something else? Antibiotics for *H. pylori* seem to work only when an ulcer has been formed, or when the infected person has acute gastritis from bacterial irritation.

- Does the presence of *H. pylori* contribute to general indigestion? It is unclear, but taking antibiotics for indigestion definitely does not clear up an *H. pylori* infection, or relieve symptoms of dyspepsia.

- What diseases are associated with *H. pylori*? This one we know. This bacterium has been definitively associated with an assortment of serious conditions, including chronic active gastritis, stomach cancer, peptic ulcers, and lymphoma that begins in the stomach.

Finally, having a peptic ulcer raises the risk of developing *stomach cancer* (this chapter) by 2 to 6 times. Although stomach cancer is on the decline in the United States, it is still the second leading type of cancer worldwide. Another type of cancer, ***mucosal-associated lymphoid type lymphoma*** is also associated with *H. pylori* and a history of peptic ulcers.

Diagnosis

Blood tests for *Helicobacter* are a useful tool, but they do not indicate a stage of infection. For that reason, ulcers are often diagnosed by having a patient drink a barium preparation and then taking a series of x-rays of the gastrointestinal tract. This reveals not only the presence but also the precise location of the ulcers. Once the presence of an ulcer has been determined, a biopsy of the affected tissue shows whether a bacterial infection is part of the picture.

Treatment

Treatment for most ulcers includes antibiotics for the *H. pylori*, bismuth, which protects the delicate stomach lining, and several medications that limit acid production. Patients who complete this treatment have up to a 90% chance of permanent recovery.

Ulcers caused by the use of NSAIDs do not respond to antibiotic therapy. The only way to limit them is to suspend the use of the medications that are damaging the stomach lining.

Massage?

Massage is unlikely to make an ulcer any worse, unless the therapist mechanically manipulates the stomach or intestines. Consider the abdomen a local contraindication for deep specific work. Otherwise, both circulatory and noncirculatory massage can be helpful in reestablishing the autonomic balance that promotes permanent healing.

DISORDERS OF THE LARGE INTESTINE

Appendicitis

Appendix:

The Latin root of appendix is appendo, which means, "hang something on." This refers to the appendix's location, hanging off the cecum of the large intestine.

Definition: What Is It?

Appendicitis describes the inflammation, usually with infection, of the vermiform appendix: a structure approximately the size of a little finger that dangles off the cecum.

Demographics: Who Gets It?

Appendicitis can affect anyone of any age, but it is most common in people between 11 and 20 years old. The incidence of appendicitis in the United States is approximately 1 out of every 1,000 people per year. Ultimately, approximately 7% of the U.S. population will eventually have appendicitis.

Etiology: What Happens?

In some animals, the appendix performs a vital role in digestion and immunity. In humans, however, its function is not completely understood. In fact, it used to be standard procedure to remove the appendix during any abdominal surgery, just in case it should someday cause a problem. More recently, it has been recognized that the lymphatic follicles lining the appendix may help to produce some types of immunoglobulins, so the appendix is only taken out when leaving it in poses significant danger.

Inflammation of the appendix is generally precipitated by an obstruction of the opening into the cecum. Many cases are related to the development of *fecaliths*: small petrified stools that block the connection between the appendix and the large intestine. When the appendix cannot drain appropriately, the risk of bacterial infection is very high. Once an infection begins, the appendix becomes inflamed and may develop internal or external abscesses. Left untreated, the infected appendix may reach the point of perforation or rupture, releasing bacteria and pus into the peritoneum.

Appendicitis in Brief

What is it?
Appendicitis is inflammation of the vermiform appendix. It is usually a result of infection after a blockage at the opening of the appendix. The blockage may be caused by a hardened piece of fecal matter or by lymphatic inflammation.

How is it recognized?
The symptoms of appendicitis are widely variable but include general abdominal pain that gradually settles in the lower right quadrant. Rebound pain is usually severe. Fever, nausea, vomiting, food aversion, constipation, and diarrhea may be present.

Is massage indicated or contraindicated?
Acute appendicitis contraindicates massage. This condition may complicate into peritonitis if it is neglected.

Signs and Symptoms

Symptoms of appendicitis are notoriously variable. They cover a wide range of possibilities, and not all patients experience all symptoms. The classic symptoms of appendicitis are a combination of food aversion and general central abdominal pain, which eventually settles into severe pain in the right lower quadrant of the abdomen. This pain is especially severe during palpation and release: "rebound pain." However, only approximately 50% of all appendicitis patients report these symptoms.

Nausea, vomiting, diarrhea, and constipation may be present when the appendix is inflamed. Pain is often aggravated by coughing, sneezing, or abdominal movement. Patients may develop a low fever. If the appendix ruptures, the pain may temporarily subside, because the pressure has been relieved, and the infection can take a few hours to completely take over the system.

Complications

In a worst-case scenario, the appendix may completely rupture, leaking its colonies of bacteria into the peritoneal cavity, where peritonitis is a near certainty. Occasionally the greater omentum may be positioned to smother a perforated appendix, which can temporarily localize the infection. However, this generally leads to internal adhesions and abscesses, which, without medical intervention, would probably rupture as well.

In some situations, the appendix may develop abscesses: small, painful, localized infections. In this case, the risk of infection being released by surgery is high, so the abscesses must be drained or resolved by antibiotic therapy before the appendix is removed.

Diagnosis

Although the ability to identify intestinal disorders has taken quantum leaps forward with CT scans, ultrasounds and laparoscopes, appendicitis remains extremely difficult to identify. Young children, elderly people, and pregnant women are especially difficult to diagnose correctly for appendicitis.

Appendicitis resembles several other serious conditions, including *kidney stones* or *urinary tract infection* (Chapter 8), *Crohn disease*, *gastroenteritis*, *diverticular disease* or *gallstones* (this chapter), *pelvic inflammatory disease, fibroid tumors*, ectopic *pregnancy*, and *ovarian cysts* (Chapter 10). Several of the tests used to identify appendicitis (white blood cell counts, urinalysis, x-rays, barium enemas, and CT scans) are designed to find the cause of the blockage and to rule out these common misdiagnoses.

Treatment

Once infection in the appendix has been identified, surgery is performed to remove it. This has traditionally been done through an incision close to the site of the appendix, but recent advances have made laparoscopies a viable option. The advantage to this technique is that the wound is much smaller and recovery time is much shorter than those for traditional abdominal surgery.

It is best to perform this simple surgery in the early stages of inflammation before gangrene, rupture, or abscesses can create further complications.

In situations in which doing surgery is impractical, it is occasionally possible to treat appendicitis with antibiotics. However, a large percentage of patients treated this way experience a resurgence of their infections within a year.

Massage?

Someone with acute appendicitis needs immediate care, not massage. Even a chronic low-grade infection can flare up quickly, and the risk of rupture and peritonitis is very high. For guidelines about working with someone recovering from an appendectomy, see *postoperative conditions*, Chapter 11.

Colorectal Cancer

Definition: What Is It?

Colorectal cancer is the development of tumors anywhere in the large intestine from the ascending right side to the rectum. Although the two conditions are linked, malignant colon or rectal cancer is not the same thing as the presence of *adenomas* or colon polyps.

Demographics: Who Gets It?

Statistics on colon and rectal cancers vary, but most suggest that approximately 135,000 cases of these diseases are diagnosed each year, and they cause roughly 56,000 deaths each year. This makes colorectal cancer the second leading cause of death by cancer in the United States (only lung cancer is higher).

Although it has traditionally be perceived as a "men's disease," colorectal cancer affects men and women almost evenly. The leading demographic for developing these diseases is age: 90% of all colorectal patients are older than 50 years old.

Racial statistics for these diseases show some predictable patterns. Native Alaskans have the highest incidence of colon and rectal cancer among both men and women. African Americans are diagnosed slightly more often than whites. Native Americans, Vietnamese, and Filipinos show the lowest average rates of developing both colon and rectal cancers. Within these ethnic groups, however, within two generations of following a Western diet, rates of colon cancer climb to approach the national average, which means that ultimately close to 6% of all Americans will have colon or rectal cancer.

Colorectal Cancer in Brief

What is it?
Colorectal cancer is the development of malignant tumors in the colon or rectum. Growths can block the bowel or metastasize to other organs, particularly the liver.

How is it recognized?
Colorectal cancer creates different symptoms depending on what part of the bowel is affected. The most dangerous symptoms are extreme changes in bowel habits, including diarrhea or constipation lasting more than 10 days. Other symptoms include blood in the stool, iron-deficiency anemia, and unintentional weight loss.

Is massage indicated or contraindicated?
If a client is diagnosed with colon or rectal cancer in the early stages, some types of massage may be a useful supportive therapy to help deal with the side effects of cancer treatment. Colorectal cancer survivors are good candidates for massage, although the presence of a colostomy bag requires some adjustments.

Etiology: What Happens?

The colon, or bowel, is the last and widest section of the digestive tract. In this 6-foot long piece of tubing, the remnants of food are compacted, needed water is reabsorbed into the body, and feces are stored in the rectum until they are expelled. The inner lining of the colon is composed of epithelium, which, as has been seen in other discussions of cancer, is particularly susceptible to uncontrolled cell growth.

Most colon cancers begin with the development of adenomas: small polyps in the bowel. Minor chromosome damage is believed to cause the formation of these polyps: the cells in the mucosa of the colon simply multiply without any reason and create these small pile-ups of excess tissue (Figure 7.5). But if the polyps are present for a long period of time, two things happen: *oncogenes* are activated, and tumor suppressor genes are inactivated. The net result is that cells on the surface of the colon mucosa continue to replicate and refuse to die off. They can invade the deeper layers of the bowel and even erode all the way through it, they can obstruct the movement of fecal matter through the GI tract (Figure 7.6), and they can metastasize through the lymph system to other places in the body: notably, the brain, liver, and lungs. This is the transition from polyps to colon cancer, and it generally happens without warning.

Causes

No one knows what prompts common colon polyps, which occur in 30% to 40% of older Americans, to become malignant. Large polyps and ones that have been present for long periods are the most likely to become cancerous (10% of polyps bigger than 1 cm

Figure 7.5. Colon polyps.

Figure 7.6. Colorectal cancer.

are positive for cancer cells), but what actually causes the shift is still a mystery. One theory is that high-fat foods linger in the colon longer than others, and some of their by-products are carcinogenic. This theory also suggests that diets that are high in fiber cause matter to move through the colon faster and more completely, "scrubbing" the bowel walls of damaging or irritating materials.

Recent research indicates that insoluble fiber itself may not be the major cancer-fighting aspect of eating grains, fruits, and vegetables; it may be the presence of phytochemicals that suppresses the malignant changes in colon polyps.

Regardless of the specific cancer-fighting mechanism, the relationship between diet and colon cancer is demonstrable in population studies that show colon cancer rates are much higher in cultures that follow a western diet (North America, Australia, and Europe) than in cultures that do not (South America, Africa, and Asia). Furthermore, colon cancer rates are increasing in countries that are currently moving toward a westernized diet standard. However, when it gets down to individual cases, no specific study proves that any particular diet will prevent or even decrease the chances of developing this disease. This is not to say that no connection exists between diet and colon cancer; it merely points out that no one has yet defined exactly what the connection is.

Risk Factors

As with many diseases, the risk factors for developing colorectal cancer include issues that can be controlled and other issues that cannot.

- *Obesity:* People who are obese have a statistically higher chance of developing colon cancer. The leading theories behind this suggest that excessive fat in the omentum (an "apple" shape, as opposed to fat in the superficial fascia of the buttocks and thighs in a "pear" shape) changes metabolism and stimulates the growth of new cells in the colon. This issue is also addressed in *metabolic syndrome* (Chapter 8).

- *Family history:* **Familial adenomatous polyposis** (FAP) and **hereditary nonpolyposis colorectal cancer syndrome** (HNPCC) are two genetic conditions that predispose some people toward the development of colon cancer. Although these people have a much greater than average chance of developing the disease, they constitute only 5% of all colorectal cancer patients. Most colon cancer cases are found in people who are not part of these high-risk groups.

- *Inflammatory bowel disease: Ulcerative colitis* and *Crohn disease* (this chapter) are very highly connected with colon cancer. The younger a person is when diagnosed with either of these problems, the greater her chances will be of eventually developing colon cancer. The risk is so high that for some people preventive surgery to remove the whole colon is suggested before the cancer has a chance to develop.

- *Age:* The chances of having colon cancer rise with age. Ninety percent of all colon cancer patients are older than 50 years.

Signs and Symptoms

Like so many other types of cancer, colon cancer does not often show distinctive symptoms until it has progressed to dangerous levels. Symptoms also vary according to where tumors are growing. Cancer in the spacious ascending colon is often first manifested as unexplained anemia: tumors can bleed continuously into the colon, making less iron, and therefore less oxygen, available to body cells. Iron-deficiency anemia, especially among men and postmenopausal women, is a warning sign for colon cancer.

Growths in the more constricted descending colon, however, are experienced as extreme constipation or narrowed stools. Other signs of colon cancer that a person may or may not be aware of are blood in the stools (sometimes it is obvious and bright red; sometimes it occurs in invisible, microscopic amounts), lower abdominal pain, a feeling that bowel movements are incomplete, and unintentional weight loss.

Diagnosis

Colon cancer is not difficult to diagnose, but it requires some simple tests that many people choose to avoid, even though they are not dangerous or painful. Because of this, only 37% of all colon cancers are found before the growths have invaded dangerously deeply into the colon wall. Nonetheless, aggressive public information campaigns, more consistent early testing, and better treatment options have resulted in a steady decline of colon cancer deaths in the last several years.

Basic screening for colon cancer begins with a digital rectal examination. This procedure, which is the same as that for prostate cancer, reveals masses in the rectum. Fecal occult blood studies, examinations of stool samples that will indicate the presence of microscopic amounts of blood in the stool, are another early screening technique. Although several conditions can involve blood in the stool, this is a serious sign that must be investigated.

If a digital examination indicates an abnormality or stool samples are positive for abnormal levels of blood, the next step is usually a barium enema, which shows through x-rays any particular masses in the colon. A sigmoidoscopy also may be used: this is an exploration of the colon via a small tube with a camera attached. This scope looks for polyps that may have become malignant. The sigmoidoscopy is limited to the sigmoid colon; a full colonoscopy can be performed if tumors are suspected higher up in the structure.

If any test reveals the presence of suspicious polyps, tissue samples must be obtained to examine them for cancerous cells. The advantage of sigmoidoscopies and colonoscopies is that tissue biopsies can be performed at the same time as the initial examination. Although barium enemas are cheaper and easier to perform, a positive test always requires surgery to extract a tissue sample.

A new option, an ultra-fast CT scanner, has been applied to colon screenings. This test is much shorter and more comfortable than other screening techniques, but so far it has been imprecise in providing exact information about the location, size, and depth of possible colon cancer growths.

All of these screening techniques sound to many people almost worse than having the disease itself. However, the statistics that compare survival rates for people who are diagnosed early compared with those who found their cancer later are a convincing

Staging Colorectal Cancer

The TNM classification system identifies the progress of tumors, lymph node involvement, and the extent of metastasis. The numeric classification is based on combinations of TNM staging, as follows:

Tumor	Node	Metastasis
Tx: unassessable	Nx: unassessable	Mx: unassessable
T0: no evidence of a tumor	N0: no nodal involvement	M0: no distant metastasis
T-IS: in situ tumor (affects the mucosa only)	N1: 1–3 nodes are involved	M1: distant metastasis
T1: tumor invades the submucosa	N2: 4 or more nearby nodes are involved	
T2: tumor invades the muscularis	N3: nodes may be involved nearby or distantly	
T3: tumor invades the subserosa		
T4: tumor invades the serosa and may extend into other organs		

Stage	T	N	M	5-year survival rate
I	T-IS–T2	N0	M0	72%
II	T3-T4	N0	M0	54%
III	Any	N2–N3	M0	39%
IV	Any	Any	M1	7%

The overall 5-year survival rate for colorectal cancer is 50%.

reason to follow the basic guidelines for colon cancer screening. The National Cancer Institute[2] recommends that people older than 50 years who are not at high risk for colorectal cancer should have annual digital rectal examinations and fecal occult blood tests. They should have a sigmoidoscopy or a barium enema every 5 years. Regular colonoscopies are recommended for 10-year intervals.

If a polyp is found to be cancerous, the next step is to determine how far the cancer has progressed. Several staging methods have been developed to identify the progression of colon cancer. For the colorectal cancer staging protocol, see sidebar, "Staging Colorectal Cancer."

Treatment

Treatment for colon cancer depends on the stage at which it is identified. Stage I or II cancer is generally treated with surgery to remove the affected section of bowel. The remaining bowel may be sewn together if possible, or the healthy section may be connected to a colostomy bag for exterior storage and disposal of wastes.

Stage III colorectal cancer requires surgery to remove the affected length of bowel, as well as chemotherapy to reduce the chance of metastasis through the lymph system.

Stage IV colorectal cancer is treated in much the same way as stage III, but with more aggressive chemotherapy and radiation to limit growths at distant sites.

Massage?

Clients who are fighting colorectal cancer need all the support they can get. Massage can be an important and useful addition to their therapy, to help balance out the challenges of surgery, chemotherapy, and radiation, as long as the cautions that accompany those treatments are respected. (See *cancer*, Chapter 11).

Colon cancer survivors are good candidates for massage. If they use a colostomy bag, special compensations may be needed for comfort and practicality, but massage may still be appropriate. The best person to consult in this situation is the client.

 Diverticulum:

This is a Latin word from *deverto*, meaning "to turn aside." Diverticula are byroads or detours in the large intestine.

Diverticular Disease

Definition: What Is It?

Diverticular disease is a condition of the small intestine or colon in which the mucosa and submucosa layers of the gastrointestinal tract bulge through the outer muscular layer to form a small sac or diverticulum. It happens most often in the descending section or sigmoid bend of the colon. These bulges may become infected, leading to diverticulitis.

[2] National Cancer Institute Trial Yields New Data on Colon Cancer Screening. Available at: http://www.cancer.gov/newscenter/pressreleases/PLCO. Accessed winter 2004.

Demographics: Who Gets It?

Diverticular disease is a common condition, affecting up to half of the U.S. population aged 60 to 80 years, and two thirds or more of all people older than 85 years. Men and women are equally affected.

It is most common in countries where diets are based on animal fats and processed grains. Interestingly, it was first documented in the early 1900s, just when new technology had been developed to remove the bran from wheat, and the American diet shifted to rely heavily on low-fiber white flour.

Diverticular disease is rare in countries where the diet is built around whole grains, fruits, and vegetables.

Etiology: What Happens?

Diverticula in the colon form during a special type of smooth muscle contraction in the large intestine called *segmentation*. These contractions are very strong, but without adequate bulk (supplied by soluble and insoluble fiber) to press against, the pressure causes colon walls to bulge. The mucosa and submucosa of the colon may herniate through the outer muscular layer to form small sacs, or diverticula. These sacs can be filled with fecal matter and bacteria, and the potential for infection is high (Figure 7.7). Approximately 20% of the people diagnosed with diverticulosis eventually develop diverticulitis, or inflammation of the diverticula.

Most diverticula form in the sigmoid flexure or descending colon, but they have been recorded throughout the alimentary canal, all the way up to the esophagus. They can range from approximately the size of a kernel of corn to the size of a walnut or even larger.

Signs and Symptoms

Symptoms of diverticulosis may be nonexistent. When infection is present, however, symptoms include nausea, fever, cramping, and severe pain on the lower left side of the

---

Diverticular Disease in Brief

What is it?
Diverticul*osis* is the development of small pouches that protrude from the colon or small intestine. Diverticul*itis* is the inflammation that happens when these pouches become infected. Collectively these disorders are known as diverticular disease.

How is it recognized?
Diverticulosis is generally silent. It occurs much more often in the colon than the small intestine. When inflammation (diverticulitis) is present, lower left side abdominal pain, cramping, bloating, constipation, or diarrhea may occur.

Is massage indicated or contraindicated?
Deep abdominal massage is locally contraindicated if the client knows diverticula have developed. Acute infection of diverticula systemically contraindicates circulatory massage.

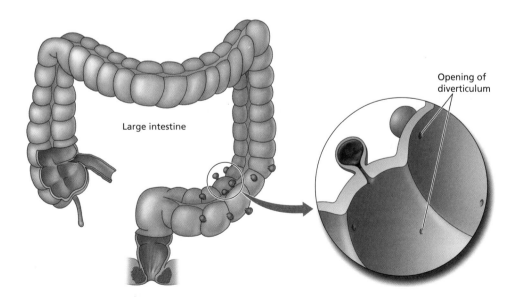

Figure 7.7. Diverticular disease.

abdomen. Diarrhea or constipation also may occur. Symptoms of diverticulitis often have a sudden onset and become rapidly worse, but some people experience several days of mild discomfort before severe infection sets in.

Complications

Complications of diverticulitis are rare, but they can be serious enough to become life threatening in a short amount of time. They can include. . .

- *Bleeding.* Sometimes capillaries get stretched over the dome of the protrusion, and they may tear open and bleed into the colon.

- *Abscesses.* Infected diverticula may develop localized collections of pus and dead white blood cells. If any of these abscesses rupture, their contents may be released into the peritoneum, causing *peritonitis* (this chapter).

- *Perforation.* Diverticula may tear open and release their contents into the peritoneum. This is a medical emergency and requires immediate care.

- *Blockage.* The accumulation of scar tissue where diverticula have formed and become infected may block the colon. A partial blockage requires medical attention but is not an emergency, but a total blockage requires immediate intervention.

- *Fistulae.* Areas in the digestive tract that are damaged by inflammation have the potential to become abnormally joined to other abdominal or pelvic organs. Small passageways or *fistulae* may develop between the two organs, allowing the passage of fecal matter into spaces where it does not belong. Diverticula may do this with the urinary bladder, small intestine, or uterus.

Diverticular disease has not been associated with an increased risk of developing *colorectal cancer* (this chapter); however, this condition can make colon cancer more difficult to identify early. Therefore, diverticular disease patients need to take extra care to get regular screenings for colorectal cancer.

Treatment

Treatment for diverticulosis alone is not usually necessary because the symptoms are so mild, or do not exist at all. Although the diverticula are not reversible, further growths can be prevented with changes toward a higher-fiber diet and exercise.

Treatment for diverticulitis starts with antibiotics and a strictly controlled diet. If substantial tissue damage has occurred, including a bowel obstruction, uncontrolled bleeding, perforation, large abscesses, or fistulae, surgery may be performed to resolve the situation. Depending on the seriousness of the condition, surgery may involve a simple resection of the colon, removing the infected or damaged area, or it may require a temporary or permanent colostomy.

Massage?

A client probably will not know whether she has diverticulosis unless her colon has been scanned for some other reason. If the condition has already been diagnosed, conduct deep abdominal work with caution; the muscular wall of the colon is already structurally impaired, and the colon is pinned down at the flexures, and therefore vulnerable to entrapment. Acute infection of diverticula, identified by local pain with fever, chills, nausea, and diarrhea or constipation, systemically contraindicates circulatory bodywork.

Case History 7.1
Diverticulitis

Cathy S., Age 50: "Try Warm Prune Juice"

Cathy is a 50-year-old speech and language pathologist with a number of problems involving a hyperreactive immune system. She was recently diagnosed with multiple sclerosis. In addition to systemic arthritis, Cathy has spondylosis: a degeneration of the articular facets between L5 and S1 resulting in hypermobility of the low back, chronic pain, and a fragile state of balance that is easily disrupted by a minor force such as a cough or sneeze.

My husband's mother had colon cancer. We knew what it was like to have to deal with this disease, so last August we all got checked. I had a colorectal scope that showed a very large diverticulum—the doctor said it was big enough that he could double up the scope hose into it. I had no pain, and there was no infection. I did not think much more about it.

For the last 10 years, I've had problems with bowel movements, just being regular. I didn't think much of it. I had a hysterectomy 5 years ago and at that time I asked what would be the best way to become regular. I was told to take warm prune juice. I did it, and that took care of the problem for quite a while.

I didn't really know there was anything wrong until last April—Good Friday, as a matter of fact. It was a day worse than most days at work. I didn't have time to eat properly, so I snacked on graham crackers all day. By 2:00 I was just about bent over double—still charting patients, mind you, but bent over double. I just couldn't get any relief.

I continued to work until 6:00, at which point I was just about screaming. (But, of course, not telling anybody.) I went to the after-hours clinic, and they gave me prescription-strength Zantac and an antibiotic. Within half an hour the pain went away—or at least resolved to the point where I could stand myself.

Having had that experience, I decided I better see a gastroenterologist. I had the upper and lower scope: a colonoscopy and endoscopy, and that's when they found the diverticulum again, although there was no longer any infection.

I was diagnosed with diverticulosis along with "chronic inflammatory disease," which may go along with my generally hyperactive immune system.

These days I stick with a low-fat diet, and I drink *lots* of water—64 ounces a day, minimum. I eat small meals. I take Zantac every night, along with Relafen for arthritis pain, and I've never had another episode. I receive massage regularly. Deep psoas work can often help to relieve my lower back pain, but I can't do it every time—some days I'm just too tender.

Irritable Bowel Syndrome

Definition: What Is It?

Irritable bowel syndrome (IBS) is a recently acknowledged and little understood condition involving digestive system dysfunction without structural changes. It has also been known as *spastic colon*, *irritable colon*, *mucus colitis*, and *functional bowel syndrome*.

Demographics: Who Gets It?

IBS statistics vary, but most agree that this is a relatively common condition. Twenty percent to 30% of the U.S. population may have IBS symptoms at some point in their

Irritable Bowel Syndrome in Brief

What is it?

Irritable bowel syndrome (IBS) is a collection of signs and symptoms that indicate a functional problem with the digestive system, specifically with the colon. It is aggravated by stress and diet.

How is it recognized?

The symptoms of IBS include alternating bouts of constipation and diarrhea, bloating or abdominal distension, and moderate to severe cramping abdominal pain that is relieved with defecation.

Is massage indicated or contraindicated?

IBS indicates massage, as long as bodywork does not exacerbate symptoms.

lives. Women are affected approximately 3 times more often than men. IBS accounts for some 5 million doctor visits each year.

Etiology: What Happens?

In a normal colon, fecal matter is squeezed and compacted while needed water and salts are reabsorbed back into the bloodstream. Material moves back and forth through the colon, but eventually strong contractions move the formed stools into the rectum, where they are stored until another bout of strong colon contractions moves them out of the body altogether.

The development of IBS symptoms probably varies by individual, but some general observations have determined that the digestive tract as a whole and the colon in particular are hyperreactive in IBS patients. That is, small stimuli create major contractions for no discernible reason. In IBS, peristalsis, which should be smooth and rhythmic, becomes uncoordinated and irregular.

Studies of the central nervous systems of IBS patients compared with those of healthy patients show that at least part of this syndrome may be connected to a dysfunction of the "brain–gut axis": the link of continuous feedback between GI tract sensation and motor response. Neurotransmitters and their receptors function differently in people with IBS than in those without. Interestingly, many people with IBS also have other smooth muscle tissue dysfunction, including a tendency toward orthostatic hypotension a condition noted in the majority of *chronic fatigue syndrome* (Chapter 5) patients. IBS frequently appears simultaneously with chronic fatigue syndrome and another chronic pain syndrome, *fibromyalgia* (Chapter 2).

IBS very often goes hand-in-hand with anxiety and stress. Most people with this condition report flare-ups in conjunction with threatening situations: job interviews, examinations, major life changes, and so on. The development of IBS probably has little to do with the presence of stress per se and more to do with how the individual handles it. Whereas some people lose sleep under stress, IBS patients lose coordinated bowel function.

Signs and Symptoms

IBS can manifest in a variety of ways: cramps, abdominal pain, gas, bloating, constipation and diarrhea (usually in cycles), and a frequent need to defecate, although a feeling of incomplete evacuation is often present. Abdominal pain is usually relieved after bowel movements.

The changes brought about by IBS are purely functional; no structural anomalies develop because of this disorder. For this reason, if a person with IBS develops a fever or has blood in her stool, IBS is *not* the cause, and this is reason for concern.

Diagnosis

IBS can range from being occasionally inconvenient to being severely debilitating, but it is not a life-threatening disease. Its symptoms can mimic several serious digestive system conditions, however. In particular, *colon cancer*, *ulcerative colitis*, and *Crohn disease* (all in this chapter) must be eliminated as possibilities. Other GI tract problems that can look like IBS include parasitical infestations (i.e., *Giardia*), food allergies, and chronic infections.

Case History 7.2

Irritable Bowel Syndrome

Debbie T., Age 29: "It's Just Something You Ate."

I had my first attack of IBS in January 1991. I woke up out of a dead sleep. I thought I had appendicitis or something. I had diarrhea, I was throwing up, I had never hurt that bad. There was no warning, no build-up, it was just there. I hurt so bad I passed out. My husband called the ambulance and I went to the hospital. In the ambulance they asked about my sunburn—I was completely covered with a red rash. The rash only happened the first time.

At the hospital, they gave me something through an IV that was supposed to coat my stomach. They said I probably had food poisoning.

Four months later, it happened again. I woke up out of a dead sleep, and ended up in the hospital. Four months later, there I was again. It was so painful, I was really noisy, but I didn't care. They took a bunch of blood samples, but they didn't show anything. "It's just something you ate," they kept saying. It got to where they would recognize me coming in, and knew exactly what to do.

When the attacks started happening more and more frequently, I finally went to see a gastroenterologist. He said, "Write down everything you eat, and call me from the hospital next time it happens." I knew it wasn't anything I was eating—I'd get attacks after a bowl of cereal! And I didn't want another attack to happen. People said it was lactose intolerance, but I have milk all the time—my attacks didn't happen all the time.

The next time was 2 months later. I was in the hospital, and they decided to do a blood gas test—they have to stick the needle into an artery to do that. It is no fun. I couldn't have any medication; I was supposed to lie completely still. Well, they couldn't get the needle in. My gastroenterologist said, "If you can't get the blood gas, I won't see you again." That's when I switched to a different doctor.

I told my new doctor what was happening, and he scheduled me for a colonoscopy right away. He looked at that; he was looking for ulcers or tumors or something, but there was nothing, and he diagnosed me with irritable bowel syndrome. He put me on 25 mg amitriptyline, a mild anti-depressant, and it cleared right up.

The only problem with the medicine was that I wanted to get pregnant again. I tried to go off it, but found I couldn't go more than 1 day without another attack.

It was only after all this that I was finally told that IBS is a stress-related disease. I had sort of noticed a pattern: every time I had company, I would have an attack. Whenever my sister came to visit, she would stay with my son while my husband would take me to the hospital. Every time I went on vacation, I'd get so stressed because I didn't know where the hospital was, and sure enough, I'd need to go to one. My doctor said, "Get biofeedback." Well, I'd never even heard of biofeedback, and my insurance company wouldn't cover it. I didn't know what to do.

When I went through a divorce, I stopped taking the amitriptyline, and I didn't have any more major attacks. I went to counseling for a long time to help with other things, and now I'm taking a different antidepressant. I haven't seen my gastroenterologist in over a year.

These days I will occasionally have a mild episode. Really greasy food tends to aggravate my stomach. I have found that if I can wake up before my stomachaches get really bad, and if I can make myself breathe slow and deep, I can make them go away—it takes about 20 minutes. But if I get all worked up and I lose control, they just get worse and worse, and I have to go to the hospital. I haven't had to do that for a long time.

No definitive test identifies IBS; it is diagnosed in the absence of other conditions that may cause similar symptoms. Fortunately, with the advent of colonoscopes, this is not difficult to do. A colonoscopy can confirm that no structural change or damage to the colon has occurred, and it also may show the characteristic uncoordinated contraction of the colon to aid in diagnosis.

Treatment

Treatment for IBS depends on the individual. The first recourse is to consider dietary and stress factors. Nicotine, caffeine, alcohol, and dairy products have been found to be particularly irritating, but no particular food or drink is a definitive trigger for IBS attacks for all patients. Some doctors recommend fiber supplementation; the addition of bulk to the diet can fill the colon more completely and help to limit spasm.

Drug intervention usually involves anti-spasmodics, anti-diarrheals, antacids, and antidepressants. Although these medicines may offer some relief, IBS is generally considered to be a lifelong condition, and so patients are encouraged to find their own best ways to cope through dietary changes, therapy, and relaxation techniques.

Massage?

Massage is useful for many IBS patients, if the individual welcomes this kind of stimulus. It is important to treat these clients very conservatively, especially with any mechanical work around the abdomen, but many of them respond well to the autonomic balancing that bodywork provides.

Ulcerative Colitis in Brief

What is it?
Ulcerative colitis is a condition in which the mucosal layer of the colon becomes inflamed and develops shallow ulcers.

How is it recognized?
Symptoms of acute ulcerative colitis include abdominal cramping pain, chronic diarrhea, blood and pus in stools, weight loss, and mild fever.

Is massage indicated or contraindicated?
Acute ulcerative colitis contraindicates circulatory massage at least locally; massage is systemically contraindicated in the presence of fever. In subacute situations, *gentle* abdominal massage may be helpful, but only within the tolerance of the client.

Ulcerative Colitis

Definition: What Is It?

Ulcerative colitis (UC) is a disease of the colon involving progressive inflammation and ulceration. The inflammation is limited to the large intestine, however, which distinguishes it from *Crohn disease* (this chapter), which is a different condition listed as a type of "inflammatory bowel disease." (See Compare and Contrast, "Crohn Disease and Ulcerative Colitis.")

Demographics: Who Gets It?

Ulcerative colitis affects men and women about equally. Most patients are diagnosed between the ages of 15 and 25, or between the ages of 55 and 65. An estimated 1 million Americans have some type of inflammatory bowel disease, and they are more or less evenly split between ulcerative colitis and Crohn disease.

Etiology: What Happens?

The initial cause of ulcerative colitis is a subject of some debate. Although no definitive trigger has been identified, most researchers now agree that it is an autoimmune condition. It occurs in unpredictable flares followed by periods of remission: a pattern similar to that of other autoimmune conditions such as *lupus* (Chapter 5) or *rheumatoid arthritis* Chapter 2).

Ulcerative colitis begins in the rectum when immune system cells attack the most superficial layer of the colon. The resulting inflammation kills tissue and results in the formation of shallow ulcers: open sores that may never fully heal. Colon function is extremely limited, and the patient experiences chronic bloody diarrhea. The sores may become infected, leading to the release of blood and pus in the stools.

Ulcerative colitis is a progressive disease. Although it begins in the rectum, it may spread to affect the whole colon. Lesions are continuous, however, and do not appear in the unpredictable patchy patterns seen with Crohn disease.

Signs and Symptoms

Symptoms of ulcerative colitis depend largely on how much of the bowel is affected: the greater the extent of inflammation, the worse the symptoms will be. During flare-ups, the primary symptom is painful, chronic diarrhea, with blood and pus in the stools. Abdominal cramping, loss of appetite, and mild fever also may occur during acute episodes.

The inflammatory nature of this disease often affects other systems in the body. A person with ulcerative colitis may also experience liver inflammation (see *hepatitis*, this chapter) symptoms of *osteoarthritis*, *osteoporosis* (see Chapter 2), *anemia* from blood loss (see Chapter 4), and *kidney stones* (see Chapter 9) from the disruption in electrolyte balance and chronic dehydration that accompany long-term diarrhea. *Uveitis*, or inflammation of structures in the eye, may result in permanent vision loss if it is not treated. Some skin disruptions are also associated with ulcerative colitis; these may occur in connection with flares or may outlive a flare to be a chronic infection.

Between acute episodes, the ulcerative colitis patient may experience only minimal abdominal pain but must be careful to avoid any triggers of abdominal cramping or discomfort.

Diagnosis

Ulcerative colitis is diagnosed through a variety of tests. Blood tests show signs of anemia and possible infection during flares; stool samples show whether rectal bleeding is taking place. A colonoscopy shows specific sites of ulcers, which may then be examined by biopsy to examine them for signs of infection or cancer.

It is important to reach a clear diagnosis for ulcerative colitis because the other two conditions that its symptoms sometimes mimic require different courses of treatment. The two conditions occasionally confused with ulcerative colitis are *irritable bowel syndrome* (this chapter) and *Crohn disease*.

Complications

In addition to the disorders listed among symptoms, patients with ulcerative colitis that involves the whole colon are at significantly more risk of developing *colorectal cancer* (this chapter) than the general population. This risk goes up significantly 8 to 10 years after diagnosis with ulcerative colitis. In very rare situations, the colon may swell up to the point that it is in danger of rupture. This is called **toxic megacolon** and is a medical emergency.

Treatment

Treatment options for ulcerative colitis begin with a class of medications that lessen the severity of flare-ups and prolong periods of remission. If these do not control the inflammation satisfactorily, steroidal anti-inflammatories may be prescribed for short periods. Immune suppressive drugs and, surprisingly, nicotine patches also have been found to improve symptoms.

If a patient does not get relief with these options, or if inflammation of the colon has progressed to a dangerous degree, surgery is the only permanent solution for ulcerative colitis. Anywhere between 20% and 40% of all ulcerative colitis patients eventually require surgery. Several surgical options have been developed, but all of them involve the removal of the entire bowel. External colostomy bags, internal colostomy bags, or the joining of the small intestine to the muscles of the rectum are options for ways to replace the main functions of the colon.

Massage?

Ulcerative colitis contraindicates local mechanical, circulatory massage. Deep abdominal work is inappropriate for a client with ulcerative colitis in any stage; so is any kind of work that would reflexively increase blood flow to the pelvic cavity. Massage is systemically contraindicated in the presence of fever. In periods of remission, *gentle* massage to the abdomen may be useful, within the client's tolerance, and any other work to balance the autonomic nervous system is highly called for.

DISORDERS OF THE ACCESSORY ORGANS

Cirrhosis:

This is a Greek word from the roots kirrhos (yellow) and osis, (condition). Thus, it is easy to see the association between cirrhosis and a related condition, jaundice, which comes from the French word for yellow.

Cirrhosis

Definition: What Is It?

Cirrhosis is a result of a disease process, rather than a disease itself; it involves the death and replacement of healthy liver cells with nonfunctioning scar tissue. Cirrhosis can interfere with virtually every function of the liver, with potentially fatal repercussions.

Demographics: Who Gets It?

Cirrhosis and other connected liver diseases affect some 25 million Americans, and it kills between 25,000 and 35,000 of them. It is the eighth leading cause of death in the United States.

Etiology: What Happens?

The liver is composed of highly organized layers of epithelial hepatocytes: cells that produce a myriad of vital chemicals for metabolism and survival. Bile is produced here, which helps to metabolize fats; other enzymes that metabolize proteins and carbohydrates are manufactured here as well. Clotting factors, proteins that maintain the proper balance of tissue fluid, and cells that help filter and neutralize toxins and hormones are all produced in the liver.

Under normal circumstances, the liver is a remarkably forgiving organ with great powers of regeneration. However, some situations involving chronic, long-term irritation or infection suppress the regeneration of healthy, organized cells and stimulate the proliferation of extracellular matrix: that is, collagen and other substances that are meant to provide structural support for the active hepatocytes. When this happens, the tiny channels that are meant to direct fluid flow to the appropriate vessels become blocked, and the liver, the largest gland in the body, becomes congested with blood, lymph, bile, and other fluids.

Cirrhosis in Brief

Pronunciation
sir-rō'-sis

What is it?
Cirrhosis is a condition in which normal liver cells become disorganized and dysfunctional; many of them are replaced or crowded out by scar tissue. Cirrhosis is often the final stage of chronic or acute liver diseases.

How is it recognized?
Early symptoms of cirrhosis include loss of appetite, nausea, vomiting, and weight loss. Later complications may include muscle wasting, jaundice, *ascites*, vomiting blood, and mental and personality changes.

Is massage indicated or contraindicated?
Advanced cirrhosis involves difficulties with fluid flow in the body. Bodywork that challenges this ability may not be appropriate. Some cirrhosis patients experience muscle wasting as their ability to metabolize proteins diminishes. Exercise and physical therapy are recommended for these patients for maintenance of strength and function, and massage as part of a health care team may have a role in this process as well.

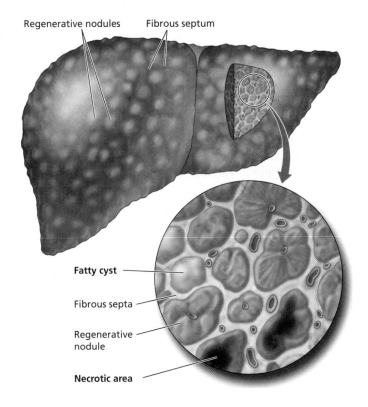

Figure 7.8. Cirrhosis: scarring of the liver.

Cirrhotic deposits of scar tissue are interspersed with small nodules of functioning cells, giving the liver a characteristically knobby, bumpy appearance, hence the nickname "hobnailed liver" (Figure 7.8). In the early stages, cirrhosis causes the liver to enlarge. As the connective tissue contracts, however, the liver sometimes returns to a normal size, though not to normal function.

Causes

Until recently, alcoholism (see *chemical dependency*, Chapter 3) was the leading cause of cirrhosis in the United States. Now alcoholism is rivaled by *hepatitis C* (this chapter) as the leading cause. Cirrhosis can also arise from types B, D, drug-related, and autoimmune hepatitis. Any obstruction of the bile duct can cause cirrhosis, including *gallstones* (this chapter) or pancreatic tumors. Some inherited liver diseases can also cause it. Long-term exposure to environmental toxins can contribute to cirrhosis, as can congestive *heart failure* (see Chapter 4).

Signs and Symptoms

Cirrhosis is often a silent disease until it is quite advanced. Early symptoms are vague and can be attributed to any number of other common disorders. They include nausea, vomiting, weight loss, and the development of red patches on the skin of the upper body. At this time blood tests may be normal; no clear signs may point directly to cirrhosis. Later symptoms are usually identified by the complications discussed below.

Complications

As the liver loses more and more function, complications arise according to the parts of the liver affected and the speed of progression. The complications may vary from one patient to another; it all depends on which part or parts of the liver are under attack. At the center of several complications is a condition called *portal hypertension*. This happens when the liver becomes so congested that it cannot freely accept blood delivered from the digestive and accessory organs via the portal system, and pressure accumulates in the portal system veins. Other complications arise as the liver simply no longer produces enough vital blood components, or does not adequately filter and neutralize toxic materials.

- *Splenomegaly (enlarged spleen):* The spleen enlarges because it cannot drain through the portal vein. The danger with splenomegaly is that when fluid backs up in this organ the risk of rupture and internal hemorrhage is high.

- *Ascites:* When pressure in the portal system increases, plasma seeps out of the veins and lymphatic vessels into the peritoneal space, causing the abdominal distension known as ascites (Figure 7.9). The bacteria that normally inhabit the abdomen may set up an infection in this fluid, causing spontaneous bacterial *peritonitis* (this chapter), a life-threatening infection.

- Internal varices: Pressure in abdominal veins grows as fluid backs up through the system. This can lead to internal venous distensions and varicosities, especially in the esophagus and stomach. Varicose veins can hemorrhage during vomiting, leading to bloody vomit, shock, or death. Ruptured *varices* are the second leading cause of death by cirrhosis.

- *Bleeding, bruising:* When the liver no longer produces adequate clotting factors, the ability to heal from minor injury is severely impaired. Cirrhosis patients may bruise extensively and bleed for abnormally long periods.

- *Muscle wasting:* When the enzymes that aid in protein metabolism are in short supply, a cirrhosis patient may experience progressive atrophy or wasting of his or her skeletal muscles. Physical therapy and exercise are often recommended to patients with this problem, to minimize permanent loss of bulk and function.

- *Jaundice:* Bilirubin (a by-product of dead red blood cells) is produced in the spleen, and it is meant to be recycled in the liver to be a component of bile. When cirrhosis

Figure 7.9. Cirrhosis can lead to abdominal distention called ascites.

interferes with this process, water-soluble components of bilirubin accumulate in the bloodstream. Bilirubin is strongly pigmented, and it can turn the sclera of the eyes and the skin a yellowish color. It also can cause rashes and itching, as some people have an extreme reaction to this unfamiliar chemical in their skin.

- *Systemic edema:* One of the critical proteins for maintaining fluid balance in the body, albumin, is significantly lowered in advanced cirrhosis. Without albumin, the body cannot maintain proper fluid levels, and edema accumulates systemically in all interstitial spaces. (See *edema*, Chapter 5.)

- *Hormone disruption:* Men with cirrhosis have livers that no longer inactivate their normal low levels of estrogen; feminizing characteristics such as breast development, loss of chest hair, impotence, and atrophy of the testicles soon follow. For women, hormonal changes include the cessation of periods, infertility, and the growth of body hair. Both men and women with cirrhosis can expect decreased sex drives.

- *Encephalopathy:* When cirrhosis is very advanced, the detoxifying agents in the liver are out of commission. No more protection from the chemicals (ammonia, for instance) that are produced whenever protein is metabolized is provided. Furthermore, the blood-brain barrier that usually keeps the central nervous system safe becomes much less effective with cirrhosis. Metabolic toxins accumulate in the blood and eventually cause brain damage. Symptoms here include somnolence, confusion, tremors, hallucinations, even coma and death. Up to 70% of all cirrhosis patients experience some level of encephalopathy.

- *Kidney failure:* Advanced cirrhosis can reduce blood flow to the kidneys, resulting in kidney failure. *Hepatorenal syndrome* is an emergency situation that requires a liver transplant for a person to survive. (See *Kidney Failure*, Chapter 9.)

Treatment

The prognosis for someone in the early stages of cirrhosis caused by alcoholism is excellent, *if* the damage can be stopped. That is the main treatment objective: *stop the damage.* Medication is sometimes administered to counteract the complications of the disease: diuretics for edema, antacids for intestinal discomfort, *levulose*, an undigestible sugar, to bind with ammonia so that it can be excreted. Vitamins are recommended to guard against malnutrition. Cirrhosis due to hepatitis is treated with interferon as an antiviral measure. Steroids for inflammation due to autoimmune hepatitis are occasionally prescribed.

New advances with transplant surgery are making it possible to restore normal health to people in end-stage cirrhosis; approximately 5,300 liver transplants are performed yearly in the United States. Transplants are recommended for alcoholic patients only when they have not suffered extensive damage to other organs, and when they are in long-term recovery (6 months or more). The rising numbers of hepatitis C patients in end-stage liver failure has resulted in longer waiting lists for liver transplants; approximately 12,000 people are on the waiting list at any given time.

Massage?

Advanced cirrhosis contraindicates rigorous circulatory massage, because the circulatory system is simply not equipped to handle the changes this work brings about. Noncirculatory work may be helpful and supportive, and massage with the goal of helping to maintain muscle health also may be appropriate. Bodywork for cirrhosis patients should be administered as part of an integrated health care effort.

Gallstones

Gallstones in Brief

What are they?
Gallstones are crystallized formations of cholesterol or bile pigments in the gallbladder. They can be as small as grains of sand or as large as a golf ball.

How are they recognized?
Most gallstones do not cause symptoms. When they do, pain that may last several hours develops in the upper right side of the abdomen. Pain may refer to the back between scapula and the right shoulder. Gallstones stuck in the ducts of the biliary system may cause jaundice or pancreatitis.

Is massage indicated or contraindicated?
Silent stones have little impact on overall health and function, so massage for these clients is certainly appropriate, although draining strokes over the liver are contraindicated. Clients recovering from gallbladder surgery may need some special considerations (see *postoperative conditions,* Chapter 11). A client with a history of gallstones but no current symptoms is fine for massage.

Definition: What Are They?

The technical term for gallbladder is *cholecyst* because it is a cyst (holding tank) that collects, among other things, cholesterol.

The formation of tiny crystals or stones in the gallbladder itself is called *cholelithiasis.*

Inflammation of the gallbladder from having a stone get stuck or other causes is called *cholecystitis.*

When stones become lodged in the common bile duct, the condition is called *choledocholithiasis.*

Inflammation of any of the ducts in the biliary system (the exocrine ducts of the liver, gallbladder and pancreas) is called *cholangitis.*

Although these terms are fun to understand and decipher, they actually have little to do with making a decision about massage for a client who has gallstones.

Demographics: Who Gets Them?

Gallstones are a fairly common condition, affecting some 20 million people in the United States; 1% to 3% of all affected people have symptoms within a given year.

Women are far more prone to developing gallstones than men; they outnumber men by about 2:1. Some races show a predilection for gallstones; Northern Europeans, Native Americans, and Latin Americans all have higher incidences of gallstones than other population groups. Other contributing factors for developing gallstones are discussed shortly.

Etiology: What Happens?

Bile is produced in the liver and delivered to the gallbladder through the hepatic duct and the cystic duct (Figure 7.10). When a person eats a high-fat meal, hormonal commands cause the gallbladder to release its contents into the cystic duct. The bile then flows into the common bile duct, into the small intestine. Pancreatic secretions also use the common bile duct for access to the small intestine.

The purpose of bile is to hold particles of fat in tiny, discreet pieces so that they can be absorbed into the lacteals: lymphatic projections in the intestinal villi. Without bile, fat particles tend to stick together in indigestible clumps. This reduces access to important fat-soluble vitamins and nutrients.

Bile is primarily made up of water, bile salts (which help in fat digestion), bilirubin from recycled red blood cells, and cholesterol, which is filtered out of the bloodstream by the liver. When either cholesterol or bilirubin occurs in higher than normal concentrations in bile, they can precipitate out of the liquid to become tiny granules called "bile sludge" or larger stones (Figure 7.11).

Most gallstones (80%–90%) are composed of cholesterol. The others are made of bilirubin, the coloring agent for feces. Bilirubin stones are also called "pigment stones." They are usually a sign of some type of blood dysfunction that causes premature destruction of red blood cells, resulting in abnormally high levels of bilirubin in the blood and in the liver.

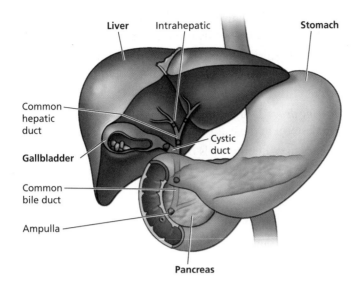

Figure 7.10. Gallstones may become lodged anywhere in the duct system.

Contributing Factors

Cholesterol stones are the most common type of gallstones. Several factors can increase the risk of developing cholesterol stones, including the following:

- *Obesity*. Obesity reduces the amount of bile salts in bile, resulting in high levels of cholesterol.

- *Estrogen*. Estrogen tends to increase the amount of cholesterol in bile while decreasing gallbladder activity, which allows the cholesterol to crystallize. Estrogen levels may be related to pregnancy, birth control pills, or hormone replacement therapy.

Figure 7.11. Gallstones.

- *Race*. Northern Europeans, Native Americans, and Latin Americans have the highest incidence of gallstones of any specific racial groups.
- *Gender*. Women with gallstones outnumber men by approximately 2:1.
- *Age*. The incidence of gallstones rises with age; most gallstone patients are older than 60 years.
- *Cholesterol-lowering drugs*. Drugs that are designed to lower blood cholesterol help to concentrate cholesterol in the gallbladder, increasing the risk of forming stones.
- *Diabetes*. Diabetics have higher levels of triglycerides, which raises the risk for gallstones.
- *Rapid weight loss*. Rapid weight loss causes the liver to metabolize fat for fuel, resulting in higher levels of cholesterol in the bile.
- *Fasting*. Fasting reduces gallbladder emptying, so bile becomes concentrated and cholesterol precipitates out into stones.

Signs and Symptoms

An estimated 80% of all people who have gallstones experience no symptoms. The only reason a person *would* have symptoms would be if a stone got lodged in the hepatic duct, the cystic duct, or lower down in the common bile duct. In this situation the pain is excruciating and is referred to as "biliary colic." ("Colic" is the spasmodic contraction of involuntary muscle, in this case in the common bile duct.) This extreme local pain will often last for hours, building to a peak and then gradually subsiding when the stone moves either back into the gallbladder sack or into the duodenum. The pain may be intense enough to induce nausea and vomiting. If the stone gets immovably stuck, the patient may require hospitalization to have it surgically removed.

The gallbladder refers pain between the shoulder blades and over the right shoulder. Although most patients experience pain in the upper right-hand quadrant of the abdomen, some may feel it primarily in the back or shoulder where, mysteriously, the most gifted massage in the world will not relieve it.

Complications

Gallstones in themselves are not usually a serious threat, but they can create some unpleasant or even life-threatening complications. The most obvious is an obstruction of the cystic or hepatic duct, which can lead to *jaundice* (this chapter). If the clog is distal to where the pancreas adds its secretions to the common bile duct, the pancreas can also sustain damage from a back-up of its highly corrosive digestive juices; this is acute *pancreatitis* (this chapter), and gallstones are the leading cause of this disorder. The pooling of stagnant bile also can lead to infection of the gallbladder, or cholecystitis. It is possible for an infected gallbladder to rupture, releasing its contents and causing *peritonitis* (this chapter).

Treatment

Surgery is the most common intervention to deal with gallstones. The whole gallbladder is removed, thereby preventing the formation of future gallstones. Recent advances in laparoscopic surgery have made it possible to remove the gallbladder using a series of very small incisions, instead of through open surgery. This minimizes general trauma to the body, and radically reduces recovery time. Approximately half a million gallbladder surgeries are performed every year; 80% are by laparoscopy.

Another new surgical intervention is the *endoscopic retrograde cholangiopancreatography* (ERCP). This is a scope on a thin tube that is inserted through the mouth, down the esophagus, through the stomach, and into the small intestine and biliary duct system. It is often used as a diagnostic measure, but in some cases a special tool can be attached to the scope to remove or dislodge gallstones without removing the gallbladder.

If a person loses her gallbladder, she can still produce bile, but it is dripped into the duodenum in a steady stream rather than being saved for high-fat meals. The only real concern is that she may lose some access to important fat-soluble vitamins. Fortunately, digestive supplements can aid in the digestion of fats (See Sidebar, "Lose the Gallbladder, Keep the Fat").

Massage?

Acute biliary colic; e.g., a gallbladder attack, contraindicates massage, especially if signs of an infection (fever, chills, sweating) are present. If a client *knows* she has gallstones but they are silent, consider the costal angle on the right side a local caution. Otherwise, people with gallstones, or people with a history of gallstones or gallbladder surgery, are fine for massage.

Lose the Gallbladder, Keep the Fat

Bile, manufactured in the liver and stored in the gallbladder, has the function of suspending consumed fats in tiny pieces so the body can absorb and digest them in the small intestine. If a person loses her gallbladder then she has less access to incoming fat, and so she absorbs less fat from her diet.

Why, then, do gallbladder surgery patients *not* lose a lot of weight after surgery? (We know they *do not* because if they did, having one's gallbladder taken out would probably beat liposuction as the most popular form of elective surgery!)

It turns out that to *burn* fat that is stored in the body's lipid cells, we need to *consume* certain kinds of fats that will help to soften those lipid cells' membranes. When a person loses her gallbladder and she loses access to incoming nutrition in the form of fats, it actually becomes *harder* to lose weight because her body retains whatever fat is in her lipid cells much more tenaciously. Because obesity is a leading contributor to the formation of gallstones, losing one's gallbladder makes it doubly hard to resolve problems with being overweight.

Hepatitis

Definition: What Is It?

Hepat-itis means *inflamed liver*. It can be caused by drug reactions or exposure to certain toxins, but it is most often one of a variety of viral infections that can mildly or severely impair liver function. Seven types of viral hepatitis have been so far identified: hepatitis A through hepatitis G. Hepatitis A, B, and C cause approximately 90% of all cases in the United States; they are the focus of this discussion.

Etiology: What Happens?

Hepatitis in Brief

What is it?
Hepatitis is inflammation of the liver, usually caused by viral infection.

How is it recognized?
All types of hepatitis produce the same symptoms, with variable severity. Symptoms, when any occur at all, include fatigue, abdominal pain, nausea, diarrhea, and jaundice.

Is massage indicated or contraindicated?
Acute hepatitis contraindicates circulatory massage. For clients with chronic hepatitis, the appropriateness of massage depends on their general health.

Hepatitis A, B, and C all involve viral attacks against liver cells. Each type of virus is unique, however. Exposure to one type of hepatitis does *not* impart immunity to any other type of hepatitis.

Methods of transmission and communicability of each type of virus are discussed in the individual headings. Once the virus has gained access to the body, however, it attacks liver cells and stimulates an immune system response. Hepatitis can be identified and diagnosed by the presence of antibodies in the blood and also by the presence of specific enzymes that indicate liver damage.

The viral attack on liver cells leads to the characteristic signs and symptoms of liver dysfunction: malaise, fatigue, nausea, and for many patients, *jaundice* (this chapter): the result of a back-up of bilirubin because the liver cannot send it to the gallbladder as usual. Hepatitis infections may be acute or chronic. The severity of symptoms varies widely from one person to another, depending on the phase of the infection, the general health of the patient, and the type of virus involved.

Hepatitis A

What Is It?

This used to be called infectious hepatitis. It is a short, acute infection, it usually causes no lasting damage, and it creates lifelong immunity.

Demographics: Who Gets Hepatitis A?

Hepatitis A occurs among all age groups. Estimates suggest that approximately 180,000 people in the United States are infected every year. Up to 30% of Americans have antibodies to hepatitis A, showing that they have been exposed to this virus.

Risk groups for hepatitis A include travelers to places where water contamination is likely, daycare workers, intravenous drug users, and people who have unprotected sex with hepatitis A patients.

Communicability of Hepatitis A

Hepatitis A virus concentrates in the feces of an infected person; therefore it is most easily transmitted through oral–fecal contact, often through contaminated food or water. Hepatitis A is the reason for those huge signs about hand washing in restaurant bathrooms. Raw or undercooked shellfish grown in contaminated water can spread the disease to humans.

Oral–fecal contact is the most common transmission route for hepatitis A, but it also can be carried in the blood and body fluids, so shared drug needles or unprotected sex with hepatitis A patients also can spread the infection.

Signs and Symptoms of Hepatitis A

Symptoms of hepatitis A are similar to those of the rest of the hepatitis family, but they tend to be the most severe and the shortest in duration. They include weakness, nausea, fever, anorexia, and possible jaundice that is accompanied by dark urine and pale stools. This virus incubates for 2 to 6 weeks before symptoms appear, but it is contagious during this period. Once symptoms appear, the virus is present in the system for another 2 to 3 weeks, although a person may not feel fully restored to health for up to 6 months.

Treatment for Hepatitis A

Treatment for hepatitis A is a combination of rest, fluids, and good sense. Ninety-nine percent of hepatitis A patients recover without medical intervention. In some cases, gamma globulin shots are recommended to provide short-term protection when a specific source of infection has been identified, such as a contaminated restaurant. A vaccine against this infection is available for people traveling, working, or living in places where the virus is prevalent.

Massage for Hepatitis A?

Acute hepatitis contraindicates circulatory massage. The liver is a keystone for fluid management in the body; to push more fluid through a system that is not functioning well could lead to some serious repercussions. Noncirculatory techniques, however, may be welcome and very supportive during a long recuperation.

Hepatitis B

What Is It?

Hepatitis B virus (HBV) works very differently from hepatitis A. It causes long-term chronic infections with much subtler symptoms. Hepatitis B carries risks and possible complications that are much more serious than those associated with hepatitis A.

Most people who are exposed to hepatitis B recover fully with immunity and no serious problems. However, approximately 5% of those exposed develop chronic infections and may be long-term carriers of the virus. Within that group of patients, the risk of developing other liver diseases later in life is higher than that of the general population.

Demographics: Who Gets Hepatitis B?

High-risk groups for hepatitis B include any person who comes in contact with someone else's body fluids. This includes people who live or work with hepatitis B patients, anyone who has unprotected sex with a hepatitis B patient, infants born to hepatitis B–positive mothers, immigrants from countries where hepatitis B is prevalent, and IV drug users.

Approximately 200,000 new cases of HBV are diagnosed each year in the United States. Most new cases are among people between 15 and 39 years old, and most of those are among newly sexually active teenagers. Between 1 and 1.25 million Americans currently carry the hepatitis B virus in a chronic infection; all of these people are capable of spreading the virus to others.

Communicability of Hepatitis B

Hepatitis B is communicable primarily through body fluids. It does *not* appear to spread through the digestive system, like hepatitis A. Hepatitis B virus is found most densely in blood, semen, and vaginal fluid, but viral particles also may be found in saliva.

Unlike many pathogens, this virus is quite sturdy. It remains viable for a week at temperatures above 100°F, and up to 6 months at room temperature. Furthermore, it occurs in high concentrations, so limited exposure can cause an infection. For this reason, it is especially important to sterilize any instruments that come in contact with human blood: tattoo needles, body piercing equipment, acupuncture needles, and professional medical and dental tools all fall into this category.

Infants born to mothers with hepatitis B are at particularly high risk for infection; 90% of all such infants become infected. If they are not treated immediately, most infants with hepatitis B will develop chronic liver disease early in life.

Signs and Symptoms of Hepatitis B

Symptoms of hepatitis B are basically the same as those of hepatitis A, but the onset is slower, and they last for a much longer time. The incubation period is 2 to 6 months in this case (it is contagious during all that time), and it can stay in the system for months or years. The severity and duration of the viral attack is largely determined by the general health of the infected person. Long-term carriers of hepatitis B may have no symptoms at all.

Complications of Hepatitis B

Approximately 5% of the people who get hepatitis B develop chronic infections. Chronic liver inflammation can lead to the development of varicose veins on the stomach and esophagus, which may rupture and bleed. Liver failure, *cirrhosis*, and *liver cancer* (this chapter) are other possibilities.

Treatment of Hepatitis B

Hepatitis B treatments are only sporadically successful. Interferon is effective slightly more than half the time, but it carries a lot of unpleasant and even dangerous side effects. Another antiviral agent, *lamivudine*, is better tolerated by most patients, but tends to be less effective against viral activity.

Prevention of Hepatitis B

A vaccine series against hepatitis B has been developed. People who work in hospitals, prisons, and long-term care facilities are often required to get it. People traveling to high-risk areas or people living with an infected person are also targeted. Some areas recommend the series for children to guard against the spread of the disease when they become sexually active.

Massage for Hepatitis B?

Hepatitis B contraindicates circulatory massage in the acute stage, when the liver is already overtaxed with cellular damage. If a client has a chronic version of the disease, the decision about circulatory massage must be determined based on that person's overall health and resiliency. The benefits include improved immune system activity as well as the restoration of autonomic balance, and so on, but the risks could involve stressing a weak system that is incapable of adapting to the changes circulatory massage brings about and exposure to a pathogen that occurs in high concentrations in the blood and is sturdy outside of a host. Noncirculatory massage may provide many of the benefits, while minimizing the possible risks.

   Clients who have recovered from hepatitis B infections with no other problems are fine for massage.

Hepatitis C

What Is It?

Before the viruses D, E, F, and G were discovered, this disorder was called hepatitis non-A non-B. Although it has been investigated since the late 1970s, the causative virus was not identified until 1989.

   Like hepatitis B, hepatitis C causes long-term chronic infections. Unlike hepatitis B, however, the percentage of hepatitis C patients who develop long-term problems is very high. Only 5% to 25% recover spontaneously; the other 75% to 95% percent of hepatitis C patients will experience a chronic infection. Of those with chronic hepatitis C, approximately 15% will develop cirrhosis within 10 to 20 years, and the risk of liver cancer is much higher than that for the general population. The presence of other illnesses, specifically HIV, hepatitis B, or alcoholism, raises the risk of complications from long-term hepatitis C infections.

   Hepatitis C is estimated to cause approximately 8,000 to 10,000 deaths per year.

Demographics: Who Gets Hepatitis C?

Hepatitis C is something of a silent epidemic; although many people have never heard of it, this virus is the most common blood-borne infection in the United States. It is carried by close to 4 million Americans today, and almost 3 million people have the disease as a chronic infection.

The primary risk group for new hepatitis C infections is intravenous drug users. An estimated 38,000 new infections occur among this group every year. Happily, that number is on the decline; statistics in the early 1990s were much more severe.

Another risk group for hepatitis C infections is people who received transfusions of blood or blood clotting factors before 1987. Since then, improved screening techniques has made the public blood supply much safer.

Communicability of Hepatitis C

Blood-to-blood contact is the most reliable way to transmit hepatitis C, although in approximately 10% of all cases the mode of transmission is unclear. Blood-to-blood contact can come about in the form of shared drug needles, accidental needle sticks in medical settings, or contaminated medical, tattoo, or body-piercing instruments.

Signs and Symptoms of Hepatitis C

Symptoms of hepatitis C are weakness, fever, nausea, and possible jaundice, but they are generally milder than those seen with hepatitis A or B, and they often do not appear until many years after infection. Many people may never know that they have been infected with the hepatitis C virus until 20 or 30 years later, when the liver can no longer compensate for the damage that has accumulated.

Treatment for Hepatitis C

Treatment of hepatitis C is good sense (rest, fluids, and good nutrition) and close monitoring to watch for signs of complications. No vaccine has been developed against this virus. Interferon and ribavirin may be prescribed separately or together to try to control the severity of the viral attack. Almost half of all the liver transplantations conducted in the United States every year are to correct the damage brought about by hepatitis C infections.

Massage for Hepatitis C?

As with other hepatitis infections, circulatory massage is contraindicated in the presence of acute disease. When the infection is chronic, judgments must be made based on the overall health and circulatory resiliency of the client.

Other Types of Hepatitis

Hepatitis may be caused by factors other than viruses A, B, and C. Hepatitis D is an incomplete virus that can only work in the presence of hepatitis B. Hepatitis E, F, and G are rare viruses that are uncommon in the United States.

It is also possible for other viruses to cause liver inflammation, often as a complication of a different primary infection. Epstein-Barr virus (see *mononucleosis*, Chapter 5) and cytomegalovirus are two examples.

Nonviral hepatitis has been seen as a reaction to certain medications, or as an autoimmune disease launched against hepatocytes.

Massage and Other Types of Hepatitis?

The same rules apply here as for other types of hepatitis: acute infection contraindicates circulatory massage, although energetic work may be supportive and helpful. Chronic situations may be determined by the overall health and ability to adapt to changes of the client.

Jaundice

Definition: What Is It?

Jaundice, from the French *jaune* (yellow), is not a disease in itself, but a symptom of some underlying liver or gallbladder pathologic condition leading to the accumulation of bilirubin in the blood.

Etiology: What Happens?

One of the functions of the liver is to accept the by-products of dead red blood cells, including bilirubin, delivered from the spleen through the portal system. It synthesizes the bilirubin into bile. Bile drips from the liver into a storage tank: the gallbladder. Bile is used for the digestion and absorption of fats and fat-soluble vitamins. Eventually all of the bilirubin gets into the digestive tract and is a coloring agent for feces, which makes it a useful diagnostic tool.

When bilirubin cannot leave the liver for a variety of reasons, it backs up into the bloodstream. Eventually bilirubin can visibly stain the skin, mucous membranes, and the sclera of the eyes.

Several types of jaundice have been identified, each one categorized by the pathologic condition that created the problem. Jaundice is treated according to the underlying causes.

- *Neonatal jaundice:* This is a fairly common condition for newborns. Their livers are not yet mature and cannot keep up with the turnover of fetal red blood cells. It takes a few days to process this extra load to catch up. Treatment is usually exposure to "bili-lights:" full-spectrum lights that stimulate liver activity.

- *Hemolytic jaundice:* This is a rare condition that is specifically related to hemolytic anemia. In this situation, red blood cells die off too fast, and although the liver may be functioning at normal levels, it cannot keep up with the volume. (See *anemia*, Chapter 4.) Hemolytic anemia and jaundice may be caused by infection or incompatible blood transfusions. One hallmark of this situation is that the liver has not processed the bilirubin into a water-soluble form, so it is not excreted by the kidneys. Consequently, although the skin may be discolored with this type of jaundice, the urine is not.

- *Hepatic jaundice:* This covers any jaundice caused by other liver dysfunction: *cirrhosis*, *hepatitis* (this chapter), malaria, or, more rarely, a congenital malfunction of liver enzyme systems. In any case, the liver is compromised by scar tissue or inflammation, and it is incapable of processing the bilirubin delivered from the portal system.

- *Extrahepatic jaundice:* This is jaundice caused by a mechanical obstruction somewhere *outside* the liver; gallstones, pancreatic tumors, or gastrointestinal tract tumors may be responsible. Advanced pregnancy also can constrict the gallbladder in a way that prevents the drainage of bile. The pooling of fluid because of blockage can lead to infection and permanent liver damage. Extrahepatic jaundice not caused by pregnancy may require surgery to excise the obstruction.

Signs and Symptoms

Jaundice indicates that bilirubin, instead of passing from the liver into the duodenum, accumulates in the bloodstream and is distributed throughout the body. Skin, mucous membranes, and eyeballs take on a characteristic yellow color (Figure 7.12), and urine gets unusually dark as the kidneys excrete excessive bilirubin. However, fecal matter, no longer colored by bilirubin, gets lighter instead of darker. One of the symptoms of jaundice is light or "clay colored" stools.

Figure 7.12. Yellowing sclera of the eye with jaundice.

Complications

Although jaundice is simply a signal of some other problem, it can itself create some difficulties. Without adequate secretion of bile, little or no absorption of fats is possible, so access for important fat-soluble vitamins is limited. One of the most serious short- term consequences of this problem is bleeding disorders caused by a shortage of vitamin K.

Massage?

Jaundice does not occur in a vacuum; it always accompanies some other kind of liver dysfunction, which may range from being very mild to being life threatening. An episode of jaundice would indicate, however, that even chronic situations are in a severe state, so circulatory massage may not be an appropriate choice.

When massage therapists understand the underlying factors contributing to a client's jaundice, they will be in a better position to make an informed choice about which modalities offer maximum benefits with minimum risk.

Liver Cancer

Definition: What Is It?

Primary liver cancer, also called **hepatocellular carcinoma,** is cancer that originates in the liver. This is distinguished from secondary liver cancer, or metastatic liver disease, which is a result of cancer that originates elsewhere and leads to tumors in the liver.

Demographics: Who Gets It?

Worldwide, liver cancer is one of the most common and most deadly forms of cancer. In the United States, it is relatively rare, affecting approximately 15,000 people per year, and causing roughly the same number of deaths. This number is expected to rise as more people are diagnosed with hepatitis C. Asian populations, especially recent immigrants from Viet Nam, have the highest rates of liver cancer in the United States. Hispanics and African Americans have higher rates than whites.

Liver Cancer in Brief

What is it?
Primary liver cancer is the growth of malignant cells within hepatocytes. Liver cancer is aggressive and usually silent in early stages, leading to late diagnoses and a generally poor prognosis.

How is it recognized?
Liver cancer is silent in early stages, but as tumors grow and interfere with function symptoms may include vague to intense abdominal pain, ascites, muscle wasting, fever, unintended weight loss, and jaundice.

Is massage indicated or contraindicated?
A person with liver cancer may undergo extensive and intrusive treatment options; any bodywork must be adjusted to respect the challenges of these treatments. Other liver cancer patients may be in the process of dying, and massage may be an important and welcome comfort measure in this situation.

Men have liver cancer more frequently than women. Depending on the population group, up to 80% of all liver cancer patients may be men. In the United States, most diagnoses occur among people older than 60 years.

Etiology: What Happens?

Liver cancer develops when hepatocytes replicate out of control. A history of viral irritation, especially over several decades (see *hepatitis*, this chapter), alcoholism, and *cirrhosis* (this chapter) are all contributing factors to uncontrolled cellular activity. This is especially true when any combination of these factors coexist within a single person.

Liver cancer tumors may develop singly, or they may occur in several disconnected areas throughout the left and right lobes of the liver. They tend to be highly invested with blood vessels, which raises the risk for distant metastasis (usually to the lungs) before signs and symptoms lead to a diagnosis.

Risk Factors

Several risk factors for liver cancer have been identified. They are especially potent when they appear in combinations.

- *Hepatitis B (HBV) infection:* This is an example of a virus that has specifically been seen to *cause*, not just appear frequently with, a specific type of cancer. Genetic material from HBV can be found in the malignant cells of liver cancer. HBV is an especially high risk for liver cancer when the infection is chronic and was contracted in childhood. Persons infected with HBV as adults have a lower risk of developing liver cancer, although cirrhosis is still a strong possibility.

- *Hepatitis C (HCV) infection:* The relationship between HCV and liver cancer is not completely understood; some research indicates that the virus may actually cause the cancer, and other studies suggest that liver cancer develops indirectly through the cirrhosis associated with hepatitis C. Nonetheless, approximately 5% to 10% of all people diagnosed with hepatitis C eventually develop liver cancer. Because HCV currently infects approximately 4 million people in the United States, it is expected that rates of liver cancer will consequently rise within the next several years.

- *Alcoholism:* Alcohol abuse, especially in combination with hepatitis B or C, greatly raises the risk of liver cancer. Interestingly, it appears that it is the cessation of alcohol use that triggers the cellular mutation: when a person stops drinking and the liver begins to regenerate, cells are more likely to become malignant. (Studies show, however, that alcoholics who stop drinking and later develop liver cancer live an average of 10 years longer than those who do not stop drinking and die of causes other than cancer.) See more in *chemical dependency*, Chapter 3.

- *Hemochromatosis:* This is a genetic blood disorder involving the production of too many red blood cells. Persons with untreated **hemochromatosis** are at high risk to develop cirrhosis and then may go on to liver cancer.

- *Cirrhosis:* This condition is the result of long-term liver damage and develops in the presence of chronic viral infection, alcoholism, and toxic exposure. It is possible for liver cancer to develop without cirrhosis, but it is not the usual presentation.

- *Aflatoxin B$_1$:* This is a chemical from a mold called *Aspergillus flavus*. This mold grows on peanuts and grains stored in hot, humid conditions. **Aflatoxin B$_1$** is an extremely potent carcinogen and is probably responsible for most liver cancer cases in Asia and sub-Saharan Africa.

Signs and Symptoms

When tumors grow in the liver, they interfere with normal function. Because hepatitis or cirrhosis probably are also present, these signs may be missed or ignored. The most commonly reported signs and symptoms of liver cancer include vague abdominal pain that becomes progressively more intense; unintended weight loss and food aversion; muscle wasting; ascites (which may obscure signs of weight loss); fever; an abdominal mass, and, if the bile duct is blocked, *jaundice* (this chapter). Blood tests may indicate signs of liver dysfunction. One specific substance, alpha fetoprotein, is present in the blood approximately 60% of the time when liver cancer is present. Other blood tests may show unusual hormonal activity as cancerous cells secrete chemicals usually restricted to other cells.

Diagnosis

Liver cancer is generally diagnosed through a combination of imaging techniques that include CT scans with or without contrast medium, ultrasound, and MRIs, along with a biopsy of suspicious cells. One of the challenges of liver cancer diagnosis is that primary liver cancer cells appear similar to secondary liver cells that have metastasized from another location. These two problems require a different treatment approach, so it is important to distinguish between them.

Staging

Liver cancer staging is typically not discussed in stages 0 through IV as other cancers are; instead it is often discussed in terms of best treatment options.

- *Localized resectable cancer* indicates that a single tumor under 2 cm without signs of spreading to blood or lymph vessels has been found.
- *Localized unresectable cancer* means that although metastasis is not obvious, the liver is too damaged by cirrhosis or other factors to make surgery a safe choice. These patients are often treated with surgical alternatives discussed below.
- *Advanced cancer* indicates that distant metastasis has occurred, and although chemotherapy and radiation may slow the progress, the cancer is probably not curable.
- *Recurrent cancer* is cancer that returns after previous treatments.

Treatment

Even when liver cancer is caught in its earliest recognizable stages, survival for more than 5 years is rare. Most survivors of liver cancer surgery have a recurrence within several months. This cancer is aggressive and difficult to control, and liver cancer patients tend to have serious underlying liver disease that makes them poor candidates for many types of surgery. Furthermore, liver cancer tends not to respond well to chemotherapy or radiation. Consequently, a number of treatment options have been developed that try to control the growth of the cancer without invasive surgery. These include techniques to burn or freeze tumors through laparoscopic or percutaneous instruments; injections of ethanol to destroy tumor cells; and the use of drugs or implements to block the blood vessels that supply tumors. No single treatment option shows outstanding promise for a long-term cure for liver cancer, however, and the 5-year survival rate for this disease is under 10%.

Surgery typically involves a resection of the liver (removing the portion or portions in which tumors are present), or liver transplantation. The fact that many liver cancer patients have a long history of cirrhosis or hepatitis makes both resections and transplant surgeries difficult.

Massage?

A person who has been diagnosed with liver cancer is unlikely to survive the disease. If that person is undergoing therapy, side effects may make some types of bodywork uncomfortable or even dangerous; therapists should consult with the client's health care team to get information about any risks. If a person seeks massage as a comfort measure as they face the end of life, bodywork can be a wonderful, nurturing, and supportive experience. Massage therapists may wish to teach family members and friends some simple techniques to improve the quality of time spent between the dying person and his or her loved ones.

Pancreatic Cancer in Brief

What is it?
Pancreatic cancer is the growth of malignant cells in the pancreas. It is usually a cancer of the exocrine cells, which normally produce digestive enzymes, but it occasionally grows in the islets cells where hormones are produced.

How is it recognized?
Early signs of pancreatic cancer are subtle and not usually alarming: abdominal discomfort, unintended weight loss, and loss of appetite are frequently reported. Later signs may include jaundice, hepatomegaly or splenomegaly, ascites, and signs of distant metastasis, which vary according to location.

Is massage indicated or contraindicated?
Pancreatic cancer is almost always fatal within a few months of diagnosis. Massage is appropriate as a comfort measure, particularly as part of a health care team working for pain relief and palliative effects.

Pancreatic Cancer

Definition: What Is It?

Pancreatic cancer begins as the mutation of certain genes that sponsor uncontrolled growth of cells in the pancreas. It usually grows in the exocrine ducts of this gland, but occasionally grows in the endocrine-producing cells. Pancreatic cancer is aggressive, metastasizes easily, and is difficult to detect in early stages; consequently it is the fifth leading cause of death by cancer in this country.

Demographics: Who Gets It?

Pancreatic cancer is diagnosed approximately 30,000 times per year in the United States. The average life expectancy after diagnosis is 4 to 6 months. Consequently, it is the cause of roughly the same number of deaths every year.

Men get pancreatic cancer slightly more often than women, but in recent years that statistic has been shifting; this may reflect an increasing number of women smokers who are now within the most common age range for a diagnosis of pancreatic cancer. African American men and women get pancreatic cancer slightly more often than whites. Other ethnic groups have a generally lower risk.

Etiology: What Happens?

The pancreas is a small, spongy gland located behind the stomach. It produces digestive enzymes that collect in an extensive duct system and eventually enter the duodenum. It also manufactures hormones related to the maintenance of blood sugar levels.

Pancreatic cancer has been studied extensively. Several exact mutations of specific genes in the endocrine ducts of the organ have been identified, all of which lead to the growth of invasive, aggressive, life-threatening tumors.

When these tumors arise in the exocrine ducts, they are referred to as adenocarcinomas. When they grow in the islet cells, they are called *neuroendocrine* tumors. In either case, the tumors tend to grow quickly and easily invade nearby tissues simply by spreading out. The duodenum, stomach, and peritoneal wall are often affected by these local extensions. When cells invade the abdominal lymph system, the liver is often the first site of metastasis.

Risk Factors

Exact causes or triggers of pancreatic cancer have not been identified, but a number of risk factors have been seen to increase the chance that pancreatic genes might mutate. The primary risk factors for pancreatic cancer are age (most diagnoses are among people 60–80 years old); gender (men are diagnosed more often than women); race (it occurs slightly more frequently among African Americans); a history of smoking (this may be responsible for up to 30% of genetic mutations); a history of type 2 *diabetes* (see Chapter 8) or chronic *pancreatitis* (this chapter); diet (high in fats and low in fresh fruits and vegetables); and inherited characteristics: people with a family history of familial adenomatous polyposis (see *colorectal cancer*, this chapter), melanoma (see *skin cancer*, Chapter 1), or the BRCA-2 gene (see *breast cancer*, Chapter 10) have a higher risk for pancreatic cancer than others.

Signs and Symptoms

Early pancreatic cancer creates such subtle symptoms that people rarely consult their doctors about them: abdominal discomfort, loss of appetite, and unintended weight loss typically occur for 2 months or more before most people seek a diagnosis.

If a tumor obstructs the common bile duct, *jaundice* (this chapter) may occur as the bilirubin that would normally enter the digestive tract accumulates in the bloodstream. Jaundice may be accompanied by systemic *pruritus* (itching). Other late-stage signs of adenocarcinoma of the pancreas include difficulty with digestion, ascites, and enlargement of the liver and spleen. If the cancer affects the endocrine cells, difficulty with the regulation of blood glucose may arise.

Diagnosis

Pancreatic cancer can be difficult to accurately diagnose and stage. A number of different techniques have been developed, each with advantages and disadvantages. Various types of ultrasound and CT scans with or without a contrast medium are usually used. These often can predict whether a person is *not* a good candidate for surgery, but not whether he or she *is*. Laparoscopies and needle biopsies, while yielding very precise information, carry the risk of shedding cancer cells further throughout the abdominal cavity.

Staging

The staging protocol for most cancers does not apply as well to pancreatic cancer. Rather than labeling a person's cancer from stage 0 to stage IV, pancreatic cancer is more often discussed in three states:

- *Potentially respectable:* In this situation, a growth is isolated to a particular area that is accessible through surgery for removal. A small percentage of patients are diagnosed at this stage (15%–20%), but life expectancy is much better if it is caught while operable.
- *Locally advanced:* Pancreatic tumors reach out and invade local tissues such as the stomach, liver, and peritoneum. This often happens before distant metastasis.
- *Metastatic:* In this stage, the cancer has invaded the lymph system, and tumors may be growing far from their site of origin.

Treatment

A small percentage of people diagnosed with pancreatic cancer are good candidates for resection, but those who are have a better prognosis than others. That said, surgery for this condition is invasive, often requires taking not only parts of the pancreas, but also a piece of the small intestine, and the chance of recurrence is very high. The average lifespan of a person who has this surgery is 12 to 19 months, rather than the 4 to 6 months for untreated pancreatic cancer.

If it is determined that a person has inoperable cancer, various combinations of chemotherapy and radiation may be used to slow the tumor's growth and prolong life. In some rare cases, the combination of chemotherapy and radiation has successfully reduced a growth to the point that it could be surgically excised.

Surgery to relieve some of the symptoms of pancreatic cancer may be performed. This may include procedures to bypass the exocrine ducts, to insert a stent to keep ducts open, or to sever the local nerves and thereby reduce pain.

Ultimately the treatment options for pancreatic cancer will probably include hospice care for a dying person. At this point, any comfort measures are appropriate and welcomed.

Massage?

If a person is diagnosed with pancreatic cancer, he or she is probably dying. This person may seek out massage as a way to cope with the fear, pain, and anxiety that this process brings about, or as a way to help better tolerate the challenges of chemotherapy and radiation. Many types of bodywork are appropriate and supportive during this process, as long as the fragility of this person's body is respected. For more information on massage and cancer in general, see *cancer*, Chapter 11.

Pancreatitis in Brief

What is it?
Pancreatitis is the inflammation of the pancreas. It has an acute and chronic form.

How is it recognized?
Constant or episodic pain high in the abdomen is the leading sign of pancreatitis. This pain often refers into the back. Other signs have to do with pancreatic dysfunction: poor absorption of food leading to weight loss, secondary diabetes mellitus, and jaundice are all possible signs of pancreatitis.

Is massage indicated or contraindicated?
Undiagnosed abdominal pain that persists for more than a few days requires medical attention. Massage is unlikely to make pancreatitis worse unless a therapist works deeply high in the abdomen, but this is a potentially dangerous disease; it is important that a temporary relief in symptoms that massage might bring about not delay a person's getting an accurate diagnosis. After an episode of pancreatitis has passed and the client, doctor, and therapist have a clearer idea of the cause of symptoms, massage may be more appropriate as long as it does not cause pain.

Pancreatitis

Definition: What Is It?

Pancreatitis is the inflammation of the pancreas. Acute pancreatitis could be triggered by gallstones, toxic exposures, blunt trauma, or other factors; chronic pancreatitis is usually related to long-term abuse of alcohol.

Demographics: Who Gets It?

Fifty thousand to 80,000 people a year are diagnosed with acute pancreatitis in this country. People with AIDS are more prone to acute pancreatitis because of susceptibility to infection and the toxicity of the medications they may take. Numbers on chronic pancreatitis are more difficult to gather. It is most common among long-term alcoholics.

Etiology: What Happens?

The pancreas manufactures both endocrine and exocrine secretions. Its exocrine products are composed of bicarbonate to neutralize material exiting the highly acidic stomach and digestive enzymes that break down carbohydrates, proteins, and fats into absorbable particles. If the ducts in the pancreas are blocked, or if the gland develops cysts or abscesses, these functions are lost—or may even turn back to destroy the pancreas tissue itself; this is called **autodigestion**.

- *Acute pancreatitis*. In acute pancreatitis, a sudden onset of symptoms indicates that part of the extensive ductwork of the gland has been blocked. This can be brought about by alcohol use, a blunt trauma, a congenital malformation of the pancreas, an infection (usually with mumps or cytomegalovirus), having *gallstones* (this chapter) become lodged in the common bile duct, exposure to ethanol or other toxins, or from *cystic fibrosis* (Chapter 6). The net result is that the pancreatic secretions cannot be released into the duodenum.

Acute pancreatitis is usually mild, short-lived, and has an uneventful recovery. But when it is a severe situation, a number of complications may develop, including cyst-like pockets on the gland, abscesses, necrosis of pancreatic tissue, and the release of dangerous toxins into the bloodstream that could lead to circulatory shock, renal failure, or adult respiratory distress syndrome.

- *Chronic pancreatitis.* In chronic pancreatitis, long-term wear and tear lead to permanent damage to the delicate epithelial tissue of the gland. Calcifications of the ducts may become dense enough to be easily observed on a standard x-ray. Chronic pancreatitis is almost always related to alcohol abuse (see *chemical dependency,* Chapter 3), although other factors, including heredity, autoimmune dysfunction, and gallstones, also can be triggers. The main complications of chronic pancreatitis include constant pain that begins in the abdomen but then penetrates through to the back, malabsorption of nutrients, and the onset of secondary *diabetes* mellitus (see Chapter 8). The pain associated with chronic pancreatitis can be so persistent and extreme that addiction to narcotic painkillers is a significant risk for these patients.

Signs and Symptoms

Upper abdominal pain is the leading symptom of acute and chronic pancreatitis. With acute pancreatitis, the pain is extreme and has a sudden onset. With chronic pancreatitis, the pain may be episodic, lasting for hours, days, or more, and then subsiding until the next attack. Episodes get progressively closer together until the pain is unremitting. Pancreatic pain often refers into the back, which is an issue of concern for massage therapists, of course.

Other symptoms indicate the loss of pancreatic enzymes and hormones: unintended weight loss, difficulties with the regulation of blood glucose, and the possibility of jaundice if the obstruction of the pancreatic duct also affects the common bile duct.

Diagnosis

Several varieties of imaging techniques can yield important information about pancreatitis, depending on whether the problem is in the head, neck, or tail of the organ. CT scans, MRIs, x-rays, and needle biopsies all may be used to identify the source of pancreatic pain. Blood tests may be conducted to look for heightened levels of amylase or other pancreatic enzymes in the blood.

Treatment

Pancreatitis is treated according to the cause. If it is related to gallstones, these are removed so the ducts can flow freely. If abscesses form, these are drained or removed. If tissue has died because of autodigestion, that is also removed. The pancreatic duct may be surgically re-opened or a stent may be inserted. Digestive enzymes may be taken orally to relieve the pancreas of the work of producing them. Finally, if the pain from chronic pancreatitis is unresponsive to any other interventions, surgery may be performed to sever the sensory nerves from the gland.

Massage?

Pancreatitis is a relatively rare condition that usually self-resolves without major complications. Sometimes, however, it can be life-threatening, and because it refers pain into the back, clients may not realize the source of the problem. This is an example of a situation in which undiagnosed abdominal discomfort or pain that persists for more than a few days should be referred to another medical professional.

A person undergoing treatment for pancreatitis may receive massage if he or she is comfortable on a table, but obviously abdominal work must be conducted with caution. A client with a history of pancreatitis but no current symptoms or complications is a fine candidate for massage.

OTHER DIGESTIVE SYSTEM CONDITIONS

Candidiasis

Candidiasis in Brief

What is it?
Candidiasis is a condition in which the normally occurring *Candida albicans* fungi that colonize the GI tract become invasive and disrupt normal function of the digestive system and other systems in the body.

How is it recognized?
Signs and symptoms of candidiasis can be severe and acute, involving mouth and skin lesions as well as systemic blood infections, or subtle and chronic, involving fatigue, impaired mental ability, food and chemical sensitivities, and several other symptoms in varying degrees of severity.

Is massage indicated or contraindicated?
Chronic candidiasis indicates massage, but therapists should understand that many acute candidiasis patients experience compromised immune system function, and so should take care to protect clients from the threat of infection.

Definition: What Is It?

Candida albicans is one type of many yeast-like fungi that inhabit the digestive tract, often from the mouth to the anus (Figure 7.13). They are usually beneficial organisms that live in balance with other flora and fauna of the GI tract. Under certain circumstances, that balance can be upset and *Candida* can replicate too easily, leading to a variety of problems. This condition of having normal levels of *Candida* grow out of control is called candidiasis.

Demographics: Who Gets It?

Candidiasis affects different people in different ways, and its incidence as a health problem is largely a matter of opinion. Some experts only recognize an imbalance in people who are very extremely affected. These would include groups whose immune systems are generally weaker than normal, such as infants, AIDS patients, diabetics, organ transplant recipients, and the elderly.

Other experts suggest that candidiasis affects a much broader population in a much more subtle way, and that the symptoms of an imbalance are either too subtle to identify or attributed to other problems such as allergies, chronic fatigue syndrome, chronic yeast infections, hypothyroidism, and other disorders.

Figure 7.13. *Candida albicans*, the yeast that causes candidiasis.

Etiology: What Happens?

Under normal circumstances, a balanced environment of flora (plant-like organisms) and fauna (animal-like organisms) peacefully coexist in the GI tract. The flora keep the fauna from replicating too much, and the fauna do likewise for the flora. These organisms live in symbiosis: a mutually beneficial relationship with their human hosts.

When a disruption in the balance of the GI tract occurs, either plants or animals can dominate. When bacteria are suppressed, candida in the GI tract change their form from being benign, helpful yeast-like organisms, to more aggressive fungi. In the absence of balancing bacteria, the fungi have more opportunity to reproduce and spread. Because candida live in virtually every human digestive tract, the exact delineation between colonization and infestation is not always clear. Opinions vary about how extensive a candida colonization has to be before it causes symptoms (see Sidebar, "Is It Candidiasis?").

Candidiasis Triggers

Often the trigger for intestinal imbalance is the prescription of antibiotics: medications designed to kill harmful bacteria but that also kill beneficial bacteria as well. (This is why many health care providers recommend supplementing lactobacilli along with antibiotic prescriptions.) Other well-accepted causes of candidiasis include disorders involving genetic immune system dysfunctions, thymus tumors, and hormonal imbalances. Studies of patients with chronic candidiasis show that their immune systems are often severely disabled and incapable of targeting this pathogen.

Some experts propose that candida overgrowth can also be a result of taking birth control pills or steroidal anti-inflammatories and having a diet that is high in simple sugars, wheat, and alcohol: all favorite foods for the growing fungi.

Is It Candidiasis?

Two schools of thought dominate the discussion of candidiasis. The more conservative allopathic approach generally assumes that the overgrowth of candida is not a problem until very severe symptoms occur, which may involve the skin, mucous membranes, or invasive candidiasis, a systemic infection of the blood.

Many naturopathic and holistic practitioners propose that milder overgrowths of candida also can cause many chronic, low-grade symptoms. The fungi may grow and spread throughout the intestines, sinking root-like structures into the walls. They produce waste products that can be highly irritating to the host. Invasion of the intestinal wall may also allow substances to enter into the bloodstream, where immune system responses launched against incompletely digested material may be extreme. Between losing access to nutrition because the fungi get it first, dealing with their metabolic wastes, and immune system responses against digestive contents, a person with chronic, low-grade candidiasis could develop a number of subtle or severe symptoms.

The practitioners who deal with candidiasis as a contributor to many other chronic conditions often report success when helping their patients change their diets and lifestyles in ways that restore balance to intestinal flora and fauna. This clinical evidence has yet to be reproduced in a formal research setting, however, which leads to resistance to the acceptance of candidiasis as a common, chronic disorder responsible for symptoms that range from fatigue to menstrual pain to food allergies.

Signs and Symptoms

- *Mouth lesions:* Severe candida infections can take several forms. Thrush, an outbreak of whitish, usually painless lesions in the mouth, is one form that is commonly seen in infants and immune-suppressed people. Candidiasis may also create red, sore areas in the mouth and on the tongue.

- *Anal lesions:* Babies with candida can develop painful and persistent "diaper rash"—in this case it is not irritation caused by exposure to the ammonia in urine, but a skin reaction to the fungi colonizing the rectum and anus. In adults this may take the form of "jock itch" or tinea cruris (see *fungal infections*, Chapter 1).

- *Other skin lesions:* Systemic candidiasis may affect finger and toenails, causing them to become thickened and discolored, often with edema around the cuticles. Lesions sometimes occur on the scalp, leading to baldness.

- *Systemic symptoms (acute infection):* Fever and chills that do not respond to antibiotics may indicate invasive candidiasis, in which the organisms have directly entered the bloodstream through compromised capillaries in the intestines. Invasive candidiasis can be a very serious problem, as the organisms can affect and impair function in virtually any organ. The rise of invasive candidiasis has been cause for concern because the introduction of powerful antibiotics and other immunosuppressants have made many people, especially those with compromised immune systems, susceptible to candida overgrowth.

- *Systemic symptoms (chronic infection):* If a person has an imbalance of fungi in the GI tract, he or she may experience any combination of the following: food and chemical sensitivities: headaches (including migraines), chronic yeast and urinary tract infections, fatigue, reduced resistance to infection, acne, and many others.

Diagnosis

The sheer number and variety of symptoms that a candida imbalance can induce makes this condition a challenge to identify and treat. Many clinicians do not recognize that many common and persistent signs and symptoms may be fungi-related, and many patients may read about candida symptoms and assume (rightly or wrongly) that this is the source of all their problems. For all but the most extreme versions of the condition, it may be difficult to get an accurate diagnosis or successful treatment.

Diagnosis for extreme versions of candidiasis involves skin biopsies to examine obvious lesions for signs of fungal infection. For chronic cases of this condition, a stool sample is often examined to look for signs of intestinal imbalance. Not many facilities test for this kind of subtle problem, however, and the process can be time-consuming and expensive. Furthermore, no diagnostic criteria have been developed to distinguish the difference between asymptomatic amounts of yeast that may normally appear in the stool and a symptomatic case of candidiasis.

Treatment

Various topical antifungal medications may be recommended for severe versions of candidiasis, along with treatment for whatever underlying conditions may be contributing to the disorder.

For subtler versions of the disorder, internal antifungals are sometimes recommended, although these can take a long time to work, and some people have very severe reactions to them. Reestablishing internal flora bacteria to balance out the fungi is a high priority. Research is being conducted into how to inhibit the transformation of the relatively passive yeast form of the organism into the more aggressive fungal form.

Massage?

A person with a severe candidiasis infection is likely to be under medical care for any of a variety of immune-compromising conditions. Massage in this situation depends on the health of the skin, and whatever underlying disorders might be present.

Massage for someone who may be trying to overcome a less severe, chronic infestation of candida is appropriate, and may aid in the attempt to rid the body of yeast-related toxins.

 Peritoneum:

This is a Latin word derived from a Greek root. *Periteino* means "to stretch over," which is an apt description of the peritoneum, which stretches over all of the abdominal contents.

Peritonitis

Definition: What Is It?

Peritonitis is an infection that has become established in the peritoneal space (Figure 7.14), where it is dark, moist, and just about 100°F: a perfect growth medium. Bacteria also may thrive in the peritoneal space because some key immune devices are absent: white blood cells have no direct access. Other irritants also may cause inflammation of the peritoneum, including gastric juice from a perforated peptic ulcer, or bile from the gallbladder or injured liver.

Etiology: What Happens?

The bacteria that cause peritonitis can gain access to the peritoneal space through a variety of sources:

* *Rupture* of an organ is one possibility. This is a complication of *appendicitis*, perforated *ulcers*, and *diverticulitis* (all in this chapter).

* *Pelvic or abdominal abscesses* such as those seen with *ulcerative colitis* (this chapter) or *pelvic inflammatory disease* (Chapter 10) can release bacteria into the peritoneal space, leading to systemic infection.

* *Mechanical perforation* of the abdomen can introduce bacteria from the outside, with a knife wound, for instance. This is an occasional complication of intestinal or colon surgery, and the possibility of peritonitis is the reason behind the heavy doses of antibiotics that are prescribed before such surgeries take place.

* *Spontaneous peritonitis* is an occasional complication of advanced *cirrhosis* (this chapter) and other liver diseases, in which ascites, the seepage of plasma into the abdomen, may carry intestinal bacteria along with it.

Peritonitis in Brief

What is it?
Peritonitis is inflammation, usually caused by bacterial infection, of the peritoneal lining of the abdomen.

How is it recognized?
Acute peritonitis usually shows the signs of systemic infection: fever and chills, along with abdominal pain, rigidity of abdominal muscles, distension, nausea, and vomiting.

Is massage indicated or contraindicated?
Acute peritonitis is a medical emergency and contraindicates massage.

Figure 7.14. Peritonitis is an infection in the peritoneal space.

- *Peritoneal dialysis* is a method of kidney dialysis for people with advanced kidney failure. It uses the peritoneal membrane as a filter to clean the blood. One of the risks of peritoneal dialysis is the contamination of the tubing that connects to the peritoneum: this can cause peritonitis.

Signs and Symptoms

The symptoms of peritonitis vary, depending on the original cause. Abdominal pain is usually part of the picture. It tends to begin as diffuse pain, but it localizes at the original site of infection. Nausea and vomiting are usually present, and if the infection is untreated, severe dehydration may result. Many patients experience reduced urine output, and difficulty passing gas or bowel movements. After 2 or 3 hours, the abdomen will swell and pain may subside, but this is not a sign of improvement; rather, it is an indication that the intestines have gone into paralysis. At this point, death is not far away unless the patient gets immediate hospital care.

Treatment

Treatment for peritonitis varies according to cause and severity. At the very least, antibiotics are needed. Emergency situations will require abdominal surgery to remove or repair the ruptured organ, and to wash out the peritoneal cavity as fully as possible. When peritonitis is caught early, it usually responds well to treatment, but if it is left too long, it can be deadly.

Massage?

Any form of acute peritonitis systemically contraindicates massage until all signs of infection have passed.

 # CHAPTER REVIEW QUESTIONS

1. Describe how ongoing stress can contribute to digestive system problems.
2. Why is the appendix no longer routinely removed in the course of other abdominal surgery?
3. What is ascites? How can liver dysfunction cause it?
4. Why might someone with ulcerative colitis be at a higher risk of developing colon cancer than the general population?
5. Describe the leading theory behind the development of colon cancer.
6. What is the difference between diverticula and colon polyps?
7. Most people with gallstones never have symptoms. What finally causes symptoms to occur?
8. Why are oral antibiotics often ineffective for dealing with a bacterial infection of the gastrointestinal tract?
9. What is a possible cause of ulcers that does not involve the *Helicobacter pylori* bacterium?
10. A client is recovering from a bout with hepatitis A. His skin has a yellowish tone and the sclera of his eyes is yellow too. What condition is probably present? Is this client a good candidate for circulatory massage? Why?

 Answers to these questions can be found on the Student Recource CD-ROM that accompanies this book.

Bibliography

General Resources, Digestive System

1. de Dominico G, Wood E. Beard's Massage. Philadelphia: WB Saunders, 1997.
2. Damjanou I. Pathology for the Health-Related Professions. Philadelphia: WB Saunders, 1996.
3. Travell J, Simons DG. Myofascial Pain and Dysfunction: The Trigger Point Manual. Baltimore: Williams & Wilkins, 1983.
4. Clemente CD. Anatomy: A Regional Atlas of the Human Body. 3rd Ed. Baltimore: Urban & Schwarzenburg, 1987.
5. Tortora GJ, Anagnostakos NP. Principles of Anatomy and Physiology. 6th Ed. New York: Harper & Row, 1990.
6. Taber's Cyclopedic Dictionary. 14th Ed. Philadelphia: FA Davis, 1981.
7. Stedman's Medical Dictionary. 26th Ed. Baltimore: Williams & Wilkins, 1995.
8. Memmler RL, Wood DL. The Human Body in Health and Disease. 5th Ed. Philadelphia: JB Lippincott, 1983.
9. Juhan D. Job's Body: A Handbook for Bodywork. Barrytown, NY: Station Hill Press, 1987.
10. Kunz JRM, Finkel AJ, eds. The American Medical Association Family Medical Guide. New York, NY: Random House, 1987.
11. Marieb EM. Human Anatomy and Physiology. Redwood City, CA: Benjamin/Cummings, 1989.
12. Field T. Touch Therapy. London: Churchill Livingstone; 2000.

Celiac Disease

1. Celiac Disease May Be Underrecognized in America, Clinician Reviews®. Copyright © 2003 Clinicians Group, LLC. Available at: http://www.medscape.com/viewarticle/452468. Accessed fall 2003.
2. Celiac Disease. Available at: http://digestive.niddk.nih.gov/ddiseases/pubs/celiac/index.htm. Accessed fall 2003.
3. Celiac Sprue Association, Celiac Disease defined. Available at: http://www.csaceliacs.org/celiacdisease.html. Accessed fall 2003.
4. Celiac Sprue Association, Celiac Disease The Diagnoses. Available at: http://www.csaceliacs.org/diagnosis.html. Accessed fall 2003.
5. Celiac disease. Copyright © 1998–2003 Mayo Foundation for Medical Education and Research (MFMER). Available at: http://www.mayoclinic.com/invoke.cfm?id=DS00319. Accessed fall 2003.
6. Lee D. Celiac Sprue (Gluten Enteropathy). Copyright © 1996–2003 MedicineNet, Inc. Available at: http://www.medicinenet.com/Celiac_Sprue/article.htm. Accessed fall 2003.
7. Jennings JSR, Howdle PD. New Developments in Celiac Disease. Copyright © 2003 Lippincott Williams & Wilkins. Available at: http://www.medscape.com/viewarticle/450313. Accessed fall 2003.

Crohn Disease

1. Introduction to Crohn Disease. Copyright © 2004 Crohn's & Colitis Foundation of America (CCFA). Available at: http://www.ccfa.org/research/info/aboutcd. Accessed winter 2004.
2. Crohn's Disease. National Institute of Diabetes and Digestive and Kidney Diseases, National Institutes of Health. Available at: http://digestive.niddk.nih.gov/ddiseases/pubs/crohns/index.htm. Accessed winter 2004.
3. Minerd J. Crohn's Disease-New Experimental Treatment. The National Institutes of Health Word on Health. Available at: http://www.nih.gov/news/WordonHealth/dec2001/story02.htm. Accessed winter 2004.
4. Does Mycobacterium paratuberculosis cause Crohn's Disease? Paratuberculosis Awareness & Research Association. Available at: http://alan.kennedy.name/crohns/welcome.htm. Accessed winter 2004.
5. Nachimuthu S, Piccione P. Crohn Disease. Copyright © 2003, eMedicine.com, Inc. Available at: http://www.emedicine.com/med/topic477.htm. Accessed winter 2004.
6. Chen Y, Zhou D. Crohn Disease. Copyright © 2003, eMedicine.com, Inc. Available at: http://www.emedicine.com/radio/topic197.htm. Accessed winter 2004.
7. Coping with Crohn's disease: One man's story. Copyright © 1998–2003 Mayo Foundation for Medical Education and Research (MFMER). Available at: http://www.mayoclinic.com/invoke.cfm?id=DG00001. Accessed winter 2004.

Esophageal Cancer

1. How is esophagus cancer diagnosed? Copyright © 2003 American Cancer Society, Inc. Available at: http://www.cancer.org/docroot/cri/content/cri_2_4_3x_how_is_esophagus_cancer_diagnosed_12.asp?sitearea=cri&viewmode=print&. Accessed fall 2003.
2. Smith RP. Esophageal Cancer. The Abramson Cancer Center of the University of Pennsylvania. Copyright © 1994–2003 University of Pennsylvania Cancer Center. Available at: http://www.oncolink.com/custom_tags/print_article.cfm?Page=2&id=9465&Section=Cancer_Types. Accessed fall 2003.
3. Esophagus: U.S. Racial/Ethnic Cancer Patterns. National Cancer Institute. Available at: http://www.nci.nih.gov/statistics/cancertype/esophagus-racial-ethnic. Accessed fall 2003.
4. How is esophagus cancer staged? Copyright © 2003 American Cancer Society, Inc. Available at: http://www.cancer.org/docroot/CRI/content/CRI_2_4_3X_How_is_esophagus_cancer_staged_11.asp?sitearea=. Accessed fall 2003.

5. Harris BL, Kernstine KH. All contents copyright © 1992–2003 the Author(s) and The University of Iowa. Available at: http://www.vh.org/adult/provider/surgery/EsophagealCarcinoma/EsophagealCarcinoma.html. Accessed fall 2003.
6. What You Need To Know About™ Cancer of the Esophagus. National Institutes of Health. Available at: http://www.nci.nih.gov/cancerinfo/wyntk/esophagus. Accessed fall 2003.

Gastroenteritis

1. Sepulveda AR, Dore MP. Gastritis, Chronic. Copyright © 2003, eMedicine.com, Inc. Available at: http://www.emedicine.com/med/topic852.htm. Accessed winter 2004.
2. Diskin A. Gastroenteritis. Copyright © 2003, eMedicine.com, Inc. Available at: http://www.emedicine.com/emerg/topic213.htm. Accessed winter 2004.
3. Gastroenteritis Overview. Copyright © 1998–2003 Mayo Foundation for Medical Education and Research (MFMER). Available at: http://www.mayoclinic.com/invoke.cfm?id=DS00085. Accessed winter 2004.
4. Gastritis Overview. Copyright © 1998–2003 Mayo Foundation for Medical Education and Research (MFMER). Available at: http://www.mayoclinic.com/invoke.cfm?id=DS00488. Accessed winter 2004.

Gastroesophageal Reflux Disorder

1. Patti M, Diener U. Gastroesophageal Reflux Disease. Copyright © 2003, eMedicine.com, Inc. Available at: http://www.emedicine.com/med/topic857.htm. Accessed winter 2004.
2. Khan AN, Chandramohan M. Hiatal Hernia. Copyright © 2003, eMedicine.com, Inc. Available at: http://www.emedicine.com/radio/topic337.htm. Accessed winter 2004.
3. Sawyer MAJ, Patel TH. Gastroesophageal Reflux. Copyright © 2003, eMedicine.com, Inc. Available at: http://www.emedicine.com/radio/topic300.htm. Accessed winter 2004.
4. Qureshi WA. Hiatal Hernia. Copyright © 2003, eMedicine.com, Inc. Available at: http://www.emedicine.com/med/topic1012.htm. Accessed winter 2004.
5. Jailwala J, Shaker R. Reflux Laryngitis. Copyright © 2003, eMedicine.com, Inc. Available at: http://www.emedicine.com/ent/topic355.htm. Accessed winter 2004.
6. Barrett's esophagus Overview. Copyright © 1998–2003 Mayo Foundation for Medical Education and Research (MFMER). Available at: http://www.mayoclinic.com/invoke.cfm?id=HQ00312. Accessed winter 2004.

7. Heartburn/GERD Overview. Copyright © 1998–2003 Mayo Foundation for Medical Education and Research (MFMER). Available at: http://www.mayoclinic.com/invoke.cfm?id=DS00095. Accessed winter 2004.
8. Hiatal hernia Overview. Copyright © 1998–2003 Mayo Foundation for Medical Education and Research (MFMER). Available at: http://www.mayoclinic.com/invoke.cfm?id=DS00099. Accessed winter 2004.

Stomach Cancer

1. What's New in Stomach Cancer Research and Treatment? Copyright © 2003 American Cancer Society, Inc. Available at: http://www.cancer.org/docroot/cri/content/cri_2_4_6x_whats_new_in_stomach_cancer_research_and_treatment_40.asp?sitearea=cri. Accessed winter 2004.
2. How Is Stomach Cancer Staged? Copyright 2003 © American Cancer Society, Inc. Available at: http://www.cancer.org/docroot/cri/content/cri_2_4_3x_how_is_stomach_cancer_staged_40.asp?sitearea=cri. Accessed winter 2004.
3. Isaac Hassan, MBChB, DMRD, FRCR. Gastric Carcinoma. Copyright © 2003 eMedicine.com, Inc. Available at: http://www.emedicine.com/radio/topic787.htm. Accessed winter 2004.
4. Stomach cancer Overview. Copyright © 1998–2003 Mayo Foundation for Medical Education and Research (MFMER). Available at: http://www.mayoclinic.com/invoke.cfm?id=DS00301. Accessed winter 2004.
5. Too Much Salt May Hike Stomach Cancer Risk. Copyright © 2004 by United Press International. Available at: http://www.nlm.nih.gov/medlineplus/news/fullstory_15459.html. Accessed winter 2004.
6. What You Need To Know About™ Stomach Cancer. National Cancer Institute. Available at: http://www.cancer.gov/cancerinfo/wyntk/stomach. Accessed winter 2004.

Ulcers

1. Shayne P. Gastritis and Peptic Ulcer Disease. Copyright © 2003, eMedicine.com, Inc. Available at: http://www.emedicine.com/emerg/topic820.htm. Accessed winter 2004.
2. Shrestha S, Lau D. Gastric Ulcers. Copyright © 2003, eMedicine.com, Inc. Available at: http://www.emedicine.com/med/topic849.htm. Accessed winter 2004.
3. Jatinder PS, Ahluwalia MD, Graber MA, et al. Gastroenterology and hepatology: peptic ulcer disease. Copyright © 1992–2004 the Author(s) and The University of Iowa. Available at: http://www.vh.org/adult/provider/familymedicine/FPHandbook/Chapter05/02-5.html. Accessed winter 2004.
4. Helicobacter pylori and Peptic Ulcer Disease. Centers for Disease Control and Prevention, National Center for Infectious Diseases, Division of Bacterial and Mycotic Diseases. Available at: http://www.cdc.gov/ulcer/md.htm. Accessed winter 2004.
5. Helicobacter pylori Diseases, Asymptomatic Patients. Helicobacter Foundation. Available at: http://www.helico.com/. Accessed winter 2004.
6. Peptic Ulcer Overview. Copyright © 1998–2003 Mayo Foundation for Medical Education and Research (MFMER). Available at: http://www.mayoclinic.com/invoke.cfm?id=DS00242. Accessed winter 2004.
7. Dubois A. Spiral Bacteria in the Human Stomach: The Gastric Helicobacters. Digestive Diseases Division, Department of Medicine, Uniformed Services University of the Health Sciences Bethesda, Maryland, USA. Available at: http://www.cdc.gov/ncidod/EID/vol1no3/dubois.htm. Accessed winter 2004.

Appendicitis

1. Craig S. Appendicitis, Acute. Copyright © 2003, eMedicine.com, Inc. Available at: http://www.emedicine.com/emerg/topic41.htm. Accessed winter 2004.
2. Appendicitis Overview. Copyright © 1998–2003 Mayo Foundation for Medical Education and Research (MFMER). Available at: http://www.mayoclinic.com/invoke.cfm?id=DS00274. Accessed winter 2004.

Colorectal Cancer

1. Colon and Rectum: U.S. Racial/Ethnic Cancer Patterns. Available at: http://www.cancer.gov/statistics/cancertype/colon-and-rectum-racial-ethnic. Accessed winter 2004.
2. Cirincione E, Cagir B. Rectal Cancer. Copyright © 2003, eMedicine.com, Inc. Available at: http://www.emedicine.com/med/topic1994.htm. Accessed winter 2004.
3. Hassan I. Colon, adenocarcinoma. Copyright © 2003, eMedicine.com, Inc. Available at: http://www.emedicine.com/radio/topic182.htm. Accessed winter 2004.
4. Colorectal Cancer Overview. Copyright © 1998–2003 Mayo Foundation for Medical Education and Research (MFMER). Available able at: http://www.mayoclinic.com/invoke.cfm?id=DS00035. Accessed winter 2004.
5. National Cancer Institute Trial Yields New Data on Colon Cancer Screening Test. National Cancer Institute. Available at: http://www.cancer.gov/newscenter/pressreleases/PLCO. Accessed winter 2004.

Diverticular Disease

1. Joffe S, Kachulis A. Colon, Diverticulitis. Copyright © 2003, eMedicine.com, Inc. Available at: http://www.emedicine.com/radio/topic183.htm. Accessed winter 2004.
2. Sherif A, Perez N. Diverticulitis. Copyright © 2003, eMedicine.com, Inc. Available at: http://www.emedicine.com/med/topic578.htm. Accessed winter 2004.
3. Adediji OA, Ozick L. Diverticulosis, Small Intestinal. Copyright © 2003, eMedicine.com, Inc. Available at: http://www.emedicine.com/med/topic3102.htm. Accessed winter 2004.
4. Diverticulitis Overview. Copyright © 1998–2003 Mayo Foundation for Medical Education and Research (MFMER). Available at: http://www.mayoclinic.com/invoke.cfm?id=DS00070. Accessed winter 2004.

Irritable Bowel Syndrome

1. Ulcerative Colitis. National Institute of Diabetes and Digestive and Kidney Diseases, National Institutes of Health. Available at: http://digestive.niddk.nih.gov/ddiseases/pubs/colitis/. Accessed winter 2004.
2. El-Baba MF. Irritable Bowel Syndrome. Copyright © 2003, eMedicine.com, Inc. Available at: http://www.emedicine.com/ped/topic1210.htm. Accessed winter 2004.
3. Rowe WA. Inflammatory Bowel Disease. Copyright © 2003, eMedicine.com, Inc. Available at: http://www.emedicine.com/med/topic1169.htm. Accessed winter 2004.
4. Irritable bowel syndrome. Copyright © 1998–2004 Mayo Foundation for Medical Education and Research (MFMER). Available at: http://www.cnn.com/HEALTH/library/DS/00106.html. Accessed winter 2004.
5. Irritable bowel syndrome Overview. Copyright © 1998–2003 Mayo Foundation for Medical Education and Research (MFMER). Available at: http://www.mayoclinic.com/invoke.cfm?id=DS00106. Accessed winter 2004.
6. Whitehead WE, Palsson O, Jones KR. Systematic Review of the Comorbidity of Irritable Bowel Syndrome with Other Disorders: What Are the Causes and Implications? Copyright © 2004 Pro Health, Inc. Available at: http://www.immunesupport.com/library/showarticle.cfm/id/3468/T/Both/. Accessed winter 2004.

Ulcerative Colitis

1. Mallory MA, Raugi GJ. Dermatologic Manifestations of Gastrointestinal Disease. Copyright © 2003, eMedicine.com, Inc. Available at http://www.emedicine.com/derm/topic545.htm. Accessed winter 2004.
2. Shapiro W. Inflammatory Bowel Disease. Copyright © 2003, eMedicine.com, Inc. Available at: http://www.emedicine.com/emerg/topic106.htm. Accessed winter 2004.
3. Khan AN, Macdonald S. Toxic Megacolon. Copyright © 2003, eMedicine.com, Inc. Available at: http://www.emedicine.com/radio/topic702.htm. Accessed winter 2004.
4. Al-Ataie MB, Shenoy VN. Ulcerative Colitis. Copyright © 2003, eMedicine.com, Inc. Available at: http://www.emedicine.com/med/topic2336.htm. Accessed winter 2004.
5. Rowe WA. Inflammatory Bowel Disease. Copyright © 2003, eMedicine.com, Inc. Available at: http://www.emedicine.com/med/topic1169.htm. Accessed winter 2004.

6. Inflammatory bowel disease Overview. Copyright © 1998–2003 Mayo Foundation for Medical Education and Research (MFMER). Available at: http://www.mayoclinic.com/invoke.cfm?id=DS00104. Accessed winter 2004.

7. Ulcerative colitis: Any link to arthritis? Copyright © 1998–2003 Mayo Foundation for Medical Education and Research (MFMER). Available at: http://www.mayoclinic.com/invoke.cfm?id=AN00301. Accessed winter 2004.

Cirrhosis

1. Cirrhosis and Portal Hypertension. Copyright © 1997–2003 American Academy of Family Physicians. Available at: http://familydoctor.org/x1808.xml?print-xml. Accessed winter 2004.

2. Cirrhosis of the Liver. National Institute of Diabetes and Digestive and Kidney Diseases, National Institutes of Health. Available at: http://digestive.niddk.nih.gov/ddiseases/pubs/cirrhosis/index.htm. Accessed winter 2004.

3. Shah R, Spears JM. Ascites. Copyright © 2003, eMedicine.com, Inc. Available at: http://www.emedicine.com/med/topic173.htm. Accessed winter 2004.

4. Guillen S, Black M. Transplant, Liver. Copyright © 2003, eMedicine.com, Inc. Available at: http://www.emedicine.com/aaem/topic458.htm. Accessed winter 2004.

5. Taylor CR. Cirrhosis. Copyright © 2003, eMedicine.com, Inc. Available at: http://www.emedicine.com/radio/topic175.htm. Accessed winter 2004.

6. Cirrhosis Overview. Copyright © 1998–2003 Mayo Foundation for Medical Education and Research (MFMER). Available at: http://www.mayoclinic.com/invoke.cfm?id=DS00373. Accessed winter 2004.

7. Nonalcoholic fatty liver disease: A common but preventable condition. Copyright © 1998–2003 Mayo Foundation for Medical Education and Research (MFMER). Available at: http://www.mayoclinic.com/invoke.cfm?id=MC00012. Accessed winter 2004.

Gallstones

1. Khan AN, Macdonald S. Cholecystitis, Acute. Copyright © 2003, eMedicine.com, Inc. Available at: http://www.emedicine.com/radio/topic158.htm. Accessed winter 2004.

2. Gilroy R, Mukherjee S. Biliary Colic. Copyright © 2003, eMedicine.com, Inc. Available at: http://www.emedicine.com/med/topic224.htm. Accessed winter 2004.

3. Yakshe P. Biliary Disease. Copyright © 2003, eMedicine.com, Inc. Available at: http://www.emedicine.com/med/topic225.htm. Accessed winter 2004.

4. Bonheur JL, Ells P. Biliary Obstruction. Copyright © 2003, eMedicine.com, Inc.

Available at: http://www.emedicine.com/med/topic3426.htm. Accessed winter 2004.

5. Santen S. Cholecystitis and Biliary Colic. Copyright © 2003, eMedicine.com, Inc. Available at: http://www.emedicine.com/emerg/topic98.htm. Accessed winter 2004.

6. Gladden D, Migala AF. Cholecystitis. Copyright © 2003, eMedicine.com, Inc. Available at: http://www.emedicine.com/med/topic346.htm. Accessed winter 2004.

7. Santen S. Cholelithiasis. Copyright © 2003, eMedicine.com, Inc. Available at: http://www.emedicine.com/emerg/topic97.htm. Accessed winter 2004.

8. Snyder GB. Mirizzi Syndrome. Copyright © 2003, eMedicine.com, Inc. Available at: http://www.emedicine.com/radio/topic451.htm. Accessed winter 2004.

9. Vijayaraghavan R. Gallbladder Mucocele. Copyright © 2003, eMedicine.com, Inc. Available at: http://www.emedicine.com/med/topic2817.htm. Accessed winter 2004.

10. Jensen SW. Postcholecystectomy Syndrome. Copyright © 2003, eMedicine.com, Inc. Available at: http://www.emedicine.com/med/topic2740.htm. Accessed winter 2004.

11. Brunetti JC. Cholelithiasis. Copyright © 2003, eMedicine.com, Inc. Available at: http://www.emedicine.com/radio/topic163.htm. Accessed winter 2004.

12. Gallstones Overview. Copyright © 1998–2003 Mayo Foundation for Medical Education and Research (MFMER). Available at: http://www.mayoclinic.com/invoke.cfm?id=DS00165. Accessed winter 2004.

13. Gallbladder cancer Overview. Copyright © 1998–2003 Mayo Foundation for Medical Education and Research (MFMER). Available at: http://www.mayoclinic.com/invoke.cfm?id=DS00425. Accessed winter 2004.

Hepatitis

1. Turner LC. Hepatitis A. Copyright © 2003, eMedicine.com, Inc. Available at: http://www.emedicine.com/ped/topic977.htm. Accessed winter 2004.

2. Pyrsopoulos NT, Reddy KR. Hepatitis B. Copyright © 2003, eMedicine.com, Inc. Available at: http://www.emedicine.com/med/topic992.htm. Accessed winter 2004.

3. Dhawan VK. Hepatitis C. Copyright © 2003, eMedicine.com, Inc. Available at: http://www.emedicine.com/med/topic993.htm. Accessed winter 2004.

4. Autoimmune hepatitis. Copyright © 1998–2003 Mayo Foundation for Medical Education and Research (MFMER). Available at: http://www.mayoclinic.com/invoke.cfm?id=AN00024. Accessed winter 2004.

5. Hepatitis A Overview. Copyright © 1998–2003 Mayo Foundation for Medical Education and Research (MFMER). Available at: http://www.mayoclinic.com/invoke.cfm?id=DS00397. Accessed winter 2004.

6. Hepatitis B Overview. Copyright © 1998–2003 Mayo Foundation for Medical Education and Research (MFMER). Available at: http://www.mayoclinic.com/invoke.cfm?id=DS00398. Accessed winter 2004.

7. Hepatitis C Overview. Copyright © 1998–2003 Mayo Foundation for Medical Education and Research (MFMER). Available at: http://www.mayoclinic.com/invoke.cfm?id=DS00097. Accessed winter 2004.

8. Liver cancer Overview. Copyright © 1998–2003 Mayo Foundation for Medical Education and Research (MFMER). Available at: http://www.mayoclinic.com/invoke.cfm?id=DS00399. Accessed winter 2004.

9. Toxic hepatitis. Copyright © 1998–2003 Mayo Foundation for Medical Education and Research (MFMER). Available at: http://www.mayoclinic.com/invoke.cfm?id=AN00374. Accessed winter 2004.

10. Body piercing and tattoos: More than skin deep. Copyright © 1998–2003 Mayo Foundation for Medical Education and Research (MFMER). Available at: http://www.mayoclinic.com/invoke.cfm?id=MC00020. Accessed winter 2004.

Jaundice

1. Christensen J. Jaundice. Copyright © 1992–2004 the Author(s) and The University of Iowa. Available at: http://www.vh.org/adult/provider/internalmedicine/BedsideLogic/ch6.html. Accessed winter 2004.

2. Weisiger RA. Hyperbilirubinemia, Conjugated. Copyright © 2003, eMedicine.com, Inc. Available at: http://www.emedicine.com/med/topic1065.htm. Accessed winter 2004.

Liver Cancer

1. Adult Primary Liver Cancer. National Cancer Institute. Available at: http://www.cancer.gov/cancerinfo/pdq/treatment/adult-primary-liver/healthprofessional/. Accessed fall 2003.

2. Introduction to Liver Cancer. Copyright © 1994–2003 Trustees of the University of Pennsylvania. Available at: http://www.oncolink.com/types/article.cfm?c=5&s=15&ss=113&id=1738. Accessed fall 2003.

3. Liver and Intrahepatic Bile Duct: U.S. Racial/Ethnic Cancer Patterns. National Cancer Institute. Available at: http://www.nci.nih.gov/statistics/cancertype/liver-racial-ethnic. Accessed fall 2003.

4. Irwin K. Unraveling the mysteries of liver cancer.

5. Fong T-L. Hepatocellular Carcinoma (Liver Cancer). Copyright © 1996–2003 MedicineNet, Inc. Available at: http://www.medicinenet.com/Liver_Cancer/article.htm. Accessed fall 2003.

6. Primary Liver Cancer. Copyright © 2001 RITA Medical Systems, Inc. Available at: http://www.livertumor.org/about.asp. Accessed fall 2003.

7. What You Need To Know About™ Liver Cancer. National Cancer Institute. Available at: http://www.cancer.gov/cancerinfo/wyntk/liver. Accessed fall 2003.

8. Zeroing in on Liver Cancer Treatment. Copyright © 2001 RITA Medical Systems, Inc. Available at: http://www.livertumor.org/more.asp. Accessed fall 2003.

Pancreatic Cancer

1. Confronting Pancreatic Cancer. Copyright © 2000–2003 Pancreatica.org—www.pancreatica.org. Available at: http://www.pancreatica.org/faq.html. Accessed fall 2003.

2. Pancreatic Cancer (Cancer of the Pancreas). Copyright © 1996–2003 MedicineNet, Inc. Available at: http://www.medicinenet.com/Pancreatic_Cancer/article.htm. Accessed fall 2003.

3. Yeo TP. Overview of Pancreas Cancer. July/August 2002;26(4). Copyright © 2003 The Johns Hopkins University, Baltimore, Maryland. Available at: http://pathology.jhu.edu/n.web?EP=N&FL=PANCREAS_INTRO. Accessed fall 2003.

4. Pancreatic cancer. Copyright © 1998–2003 Mayo Foundation for Medical Education and Research (MFMER). Available at: http://www.mayoclinic.com/printinvoker.cfm?objectid=606A404B-8078-4164-A5C4C829B75A978B. Accessed fall 2003.

5. Osterweil N. Pancreatic Cancer Vaccine Shows Promise in Early Trials. Medscape Medical News 2003. Copyright © 2003 Medscape. Available at: http://www.medscape.com/viewarticle/461922_print. Accessed fall 2003.

6. Erickson RA. Pancreatic Cancer. Copyright © 2003, eMedicine.com, Inc. Available at: http://www.emedicine.com/med/topic1712.htm. Accessed fall 2003.

7. What You Need To Know About™ Cancer of the Pancreas. National Institutes of Health. Available at: http://www.nci.nih.gov/cancerinfo/wyntk/pancreas. Accessed fall 2003.

Pancreatitis

1. Romero-Urguhart G, Phillips J. Pancreatitis, Acute. Copyright © 2003, eMedicine.com, Inc. Available at: http://www.emedicine.com/radio/topic521.htm. Accessed fall 2003.

2. Pancreatitis. Copyright © 1998–2003 Mayo Foundation for Medical Education and Research (MFMER). Available at: http://www.mayoclinic.com/invoke.cfm?id=DS00371. Accessed fall 2003.

3. Pancreatitis. Copyright © 1996–2003 MedicineNet, Inc. Available at: http://www.medicinenet.com/Pancreatitis/article.htm. Accessed fall 2003.

4. Khan AN, Macdonald S. Pancreatitis, Chronic. Copyright © 2003, eMedicine.com, Inc. Available at: http://www.emedicine.com/radio/topic522.htm. Accessed fall 2003.

Candidiasis

1. Chronic Candidiasis. Copyright © 2004 doctorfungus.org. Available at: http://www.doctorfungus.org/mycoses/human/candida/Chronic_Candidiasis.htm. Accessed winter 2004.

2. Hidalgo JA, Vazquez JA. Candidiasis. Copyright © 2003, eMedicine.com, Inc. Available at: http://www.emedicine.com/med/topic264.htm. Accessed winter 2004.

3. Bryan MG, Libow L. Candidiasis, Chronic Mucocutaneous. Copyright © 2003, eMedicine.com, Inc. Available at: http://www.emedicine.com/derm/topic569.htm. Accessed winter 2004.

4. Lambiase MC, Vaughan TK. Candidiasis, Cutaneous. Copyright © 2003, eMedicine.com, Inc. Available at: http://www.emedicine.com/derm/topic67.htm. Accessed winter 2004.

5. Scully C. Candidiasis, Mucosal. Copyright © 2003, eMedicine.com, Inc. Available at: http://www.emedicine.com/derm/topic68.htm. Accessed winter 2004.

6. Oral thrush overview. Copyright © 1998–2003 Mayo Foundation for Medical Education and Research (MFMER). Available at: http://www.mayoclinic.com/invoke.cfm?id=DS00408. Accessed winter 2004.

Peritonitis

1. Genuit T, Napolitano L. Peritonitis and Abdominal Sepsis. Copyright © 2003, eMedicine.com, Inc. Available at: http://www.emedicine.com/med/topic2737.htm. Accessed winter 2004.

2. Bandy SM, Tuttle A. Spontaneous Bacterial Peritonitis. Copyright © 2003, eMedicine.com, Inc. Available at: http://www.emedicine.com/emerg/topic882.htm. Accessed winter 2004.

ENDOCRINE SYSTEM CONDITIONS

Chapter Objectives

After reading this chapter, you should be able to

- List three hormones secreted by the pituitary gland and the tissues they affect.
- Name two hormones associated with changing levels of bone density.
- Identify two risks for working with clients who have acromegaly.
- Describe the difference(s) between type 1 and type 2 diabetes.
- Name three possible complications of inadequately treated type 2 diabetes.
- Describe three signs or symptoms of hyperthyroidism.
- Identify the major risk for hyperthyroidism treatment.
- Describe the hormone shifts that lead to hypoglycemia.
- Describe three signs or symptoms of hypothyroidism.
- List the five factors that contribute to metabolic syndrome.

INTRODUCTION

The endocrine system is a collection of glands that secrete hormones: chemical messages that instruct or stimulate other glands and tissues in the body to function in a variety of ways. Whereas the nervous system exerts electrical control over body functions, the endocrine system exerts chemical control. Interestingly, the control center for both systems is the same structure: the hypothalamus.

The hypothalamus is a nondescript mass of tissue deep in the middle of the brain. It has a generous blood supply, which allows it to monitor functions of the body. The hypothalamus is primarily responsible for maintaining homeostasis: that stable internal environment. It does so through electrical transmission to the brainstem to manage heart rate, blood pressure, temperature, and other functions, and also through chemical transmission to the pituitary gland, the so-called "Master Gland" of the endocrine system. The hypothalamus is located directly above and behind the pituitary, and it actually tells the pituitary what to secrete and when to secrete it, sometimes sending out some of its own hormones via a stalk called the *infundibulum* to be released into the blood by the pituitary gland.

Chemicals released by the hypothalamus and pituitary glands travel to their target glands through the blood. They stimulate those glands to release *their* hormones. When those secretions reach appropriate levels in the blood, the hypothalamus and pituitary stop sending out their signals; most of endocrine regulation is operated through a negative-feedback loop.

The cycle of hormone stimulation and suppression usually works best when it occurs in gentle, rhythmic fluctuation. For example, when a person's blood sugar gets low, two things happen: he perceives that he is hungry, and his pancreas secretes glucagon, a hormone that stimulates the liver to release stored glucose. He eats, his digestive tract absorbs sugar from his meal, his blood sugar rises. This stimulates the pancreas to release insulin to carry the sugar out of the blood and into cells, lowering blood sugar. When levels are low enough, the person feels hungry, eats, and the cycle begins again. The blood sugar/insulin cycle takes place several times a day; it only takes a few hours to move from one state to another. Other endocrine cycles move on a roughly 24-hour rotation (these are called circadian rhythms). The menstrual cycle also depends on rhythmic fluctuations, but this one takes approximately 4 weeks to complete. Other cycles, specifically those related to stress and perceived threat, depend on external circumstances to determine their frequency and duration.

Endocrine system glands secrete more than 50 different chemicals, each of which has specific target tissues and functions. Endocrine effects also may be determined by the frequency with which they are released into the bloodstream, and by the balance between each hormone and its antagonists.

Hormones fall into three chemical classes:

- *Peptides*. These are the most common types of hormones. They are made of chains of amino acids and are stored in various cellular holding tanks. Growth hormone, erythropoietin, and parathyroid hormone are types of peptide hormones.
- *Amines*. These are hormones derived from a specific amino acid, *tyrosine*. They are also stored in cellular deposits. Adrenaline and thyroxine are examples of amine hormones.
- *Steroids*: these are lipids, and are not stored; steroid levels are maintained by constant production levels. Cortisol and testosterone are steroid hormones.

It is useful for massage therapists to be able to recognize the names of most hormones and their actions, because this is a key feature of physiology. However, a few hormones are so strongly implicated in basic health issues that massage therapists may benefit from more than just passing familiarity.

- *Growth hormone*. Growth hormone is released from the pituitary gland and stimulates the conversion of fuel into new cells. Infants, children, and teenagers secrete massive amounts of growth hormone; adults secrete less. When a person has finished growing, the primary purpose of growth hormone is to stimulate the regeneration and repair of damaged tissue: in other words, healing. Growth hormone is secreted primarily in stage IV sleep. *Sleep disorders* can lead to a shortage of this important chemical (see Chapter 3).

- *Adrenaline*. Also called epinephrine, this steroid hormone comes from the adrenal gland medulla, along with a very similar hormone, noradrenaline. It is associated with short-term high-grade stress and acts to reinforce all of the reactions initiated by the sympathetic nervous system. A slow connection between the pituitary gland and the adrenal glands can cause a sluggish stress response system; this is discussed in the sidebar "The Stress Response System," Chapter 3.

- *Cortisol*. This steroid hormone is one of a group of *glucocorticoids* secreted by the adrenal cortex, and influences the metabolism of proteins. It is the hormone secreted under long-term, low-grade stress, and it is measurable in the saliva. Cortisol is important for several reasons: it is a very powerful anti-inflammatory, and it is sometimes used systemically or locally for that purpose; it dissolves connective tissues—people with systemically high levels of cortisol are more prone to musculoskeletal injury and osteoporosis; and it suppresses immune system response to disease and infection.

- *Mineralocorticoids*. These adrenal cortex secretions help to regulate electrolyte balance, and control fluid retention. *Aldosterone* is a major mineralocorticoid.

- *Insulin/glucagon*. These hormones work together to regulate blood glucose; insulin decreases it, and glucagon increases it. Both of these hormones are manufactured and released by the pancreas. Their relationship to endocrine pathologic conditions is discussed in the articles on diabetes mellitus and hypoglycemia.

- *Thyroxine*. This hormone is secreted by the thyroid gland in two different molecular forms: T3 and T4. It stimulates the metabolism of fuel into energy. Thyroid pathologic conditions have to do with overproduction or underproduction of thyroxine.

- *Calcitonin*. This thyroid secretion stimulates osteoblasts to extract calcium from the blood and add to bone density. In other words, it decreases blood calcium.

- *Parathyroid hormone.* This hormone comes from the tiny parathyroid glands located deep to the thyroid gland. It is the antagonist of calcitonin, stimulating osteoclast activity and pulling calcium off the bones to raise blood calcium.

- *Testosterone, estrogens, progesterone.* These hormones are released mainly by the gonads (testicles for men, ovaries for women) and have to do with secondary sexual characteristics, menstrual cycle, maintaining pregnancy, and a host of other issues. Anabolic steroid supplements are meant to increase muscle mass; this is why they are sometimes employed by athletes, often with unforeseen and dangerous results.

    The negative feedback loops in these hormone relationships seem to be especially precarious, possibly because environmental exposures to various types of hormones (in medications, dairy products, meat, plastics, pesticides, and other environmental toxins) overbalance the scales. A phenomenon called "estrogen dominance" is now being considered in the identification and treatment of symptoms relating to premenstrual syndrome, menopause, and other women's health issues. These are discussed further in Chapter 10.

- *Other hormones.* Other hormones have less implication for massage but big impact on how well the body works. One is **erythropoietin** or EPO, secreted by the kidneys. EPO stimulates the production of red blood cells. It can be artificially supplemented to increase the oxygen-carrying capacity of the blood but also may increase the risk of blood clots. **Thymosin** is a hormone from the thymus; it is involved with the maturation of T-cells. **Melatonin** comes from the pineal gland, and helps to create wake/sleep cycles. **Prostaglandins** are hormones produced by almost any kind of cell for local action. Prostaglandins create a myriad of effects in the body, including smooth muscle contraction and increased pain sensitivity.

Endocrine glands release their secretions (often under direction of the pituitary/hypothalamus unit) directly into the blood. This distinguishes them from exocrine glands, which send their secretions into ducts for release in very specific localized areas. Some glands, such as the liver, the pancreas, and the stomach, produce both endocrine and exocrine secretions. The hormones circulate systemically through the body but attach to specific receptor sites on their target tissues. Then they stimulate the target tissue to perform some function, such as to make red blood cells (erythropoietin from the kidneys acting on red bone marrow), or to pull calcium off the bones (parathyroid hormone acting on osteoclasts).

Endocrine system disorders usually have to do with imbalances in the hormones being produced. Autoimmune attacks or tumors often stimulate or suppress certain glands, leading to problems with creating an efficient negative feedback loop. When too much or too little of any hormone is present in the blood, symptoms can be felt throughout the body. Other endocrine disruptions occur when circulating hormone levels are normal but target tissues have developed resistance to their action.

Existing methods to measure and evaluate hormone balance are as accurate as scientists can make them, but it is likely that subtle dysfunctions are often missed in diagnosis, leading to chronic low-grade symptoms that may never successfully be resolved. Fortunately, most extreme endocrine problems are fairly rare and not seriously impacted by massage. Most clients with endocrine disorders can receive great benefits from bodywork.

ENDOCRINE SYSTEM CONDITIONS

Acromegaly	Hyperthyroidism	Hypothyroidism
Diabetes Mellitus	Hypoglycemia	Metabolic Syndrome

ENDOCRINE SYSTEM DISORDERS

Acromegaly

Definition: What Is It?

Acromegaly is a disorder involving too much growth hormone. It is usually related to the development of a slow-growing benign tumor on the pituitary gland, although occasionally it can be connected to tumors elsewhere. It involves abnormal growth (*mego* is from the Greek for *large*) of many different body parts, especially the hands and feet (*acro* refers to extremities). When a tumor on the pituitary occurs in an adult, the resulting disorder is called acromegaly. When it occurs in a child, the condition is called *gigantism*.

Etiology: What Happens?

Among the many jobs of the pituitary gland is the secretion of growth hormone, under the command of the hypothalamus. The secretion of growth hormone stimulates in turn the release of another hormone, from the liver: *somatomedin C*, also known as insulin-like growth factor I (IGF-I). Growth hormone and IGF-I stimulate the metabolism of fuel into new cells for growth (in young people) and for repair (in older people).

When a tumor grows on the pituitary gland, excessive amounts of growth hormone are released, leading to an excessive secretion of IGF-I. This stimulates the production of masses of new tissues, resulting in bone enlargement, which often leads to joint distortion and pain, and enlargement and weakening of the heart. In addition, the tumor itself can exert mechanical pressure in the central nervous system, causing a variety of problems unrelated to hormonal disruption. The type of tumor associated with acromegaly is benign, but dangerous for the symptoms it causes.

Signs and Symptoms

Often the earliest noticed symptoms of acromegaly are headaches and vision problems brought about by mechanical pressure inside the cranium. Excessive growth hormone secretion in adulthood leads to enlargement of the hands and feet, facial changes including enlarged mandibles and spaces between teeth. Joint pain, fatigue, excessive sweatiness, and sleep apnea (see *sleep disorders*, Chapter 3) are frequent problems. If a tumor grows to a significant size, other central nervous system symptoms may occur, including cranial nerve damage.

The onset of acromegaly is typically so slow that an average time of 12 years elapses between the beginning of symptoms and a conclusive diagnosis.

Complications

Because the sudden growth of new tissues late in life puts a significant stress on the heart, many of the most serious complications of acromegaly have to do with cardiovascular stress. *High blood pressure* is a common complication, along with a pathologic enlargement of the heart. Eventually, many acromegaly patients experience *heart failure* (see Chapter 4).

Some acromegaly patients develop diabetes mellitus and insulin resistance, and some research indicates a higher incidence of certain types of cancer, especially *colon cancer* (see Chapter 7) among acromegaly patients.

Diagnosis

Acromegaly is diagnosed when abnormal growth is detected and when both growth hormone and IGF-I levels are elevated.

Pituitary tumors often grow slowly, so the symptoms of acromegaly develop over a prolonged period. More than 90% of all diagnoses are made when the tumor is larger than 1 cm, which makes surgical removal more difficult.

Treatment

Surgery for acromegaly is most successful when the pituitary tumor is smaller than 1 cm, but only a minority of cases are diagnosed at this stage. Other therapies focus on attempts to balance the growth hormone/IGF-I balance that is lost when the pituitary gland becomes hyperactive. Various medications inhibit growth hormone secretion or uptake in target tissues. If an acromegaly patient can begin treatment with these medications before developing circulatory problems, the disease can be manageable and not necessarily a life-shortening condition.

Massage?

High blood pressure, enlargement of the heart, and congestive heart failure are key complications of acromegaly. Swedish massage, sports massage, or other modalities that focus on moving a lot of fluid through the system may not be appropriate for these clients.

Joint pain and arthritis are other common complications of acromegaly. Although bodywork cannot reverse these changes, it may be able to alleviate some of the musculoskeletal pain that they cause.

A massage therapist working with an acromegaly patient should be part of a well-informed health care team.

Diabetes Mellitus

Definition: What Is It?

Diabetes is not a single disease, but rather a group of related disorders that all result in hyperglycemia, or elevated levels of sugar in the bloodstream, which are then shed in the urine. Two main varieties of the disease are examined in this article: type 1 and type 2. These account for approximately 98% of all diabetes diagnoses.

Demographics: Who Gets It?

Diabetes is the sixth leading cause of death in the United States, contributing to approximately 213,000 deaths per year. An estimated 18 million Americans (over 6% of the U.S. population) have diabetes, but 5 million do not know it yet. Rates of diabetes have risen by 600% in the past four decades, and it is estimated that by 2050, 29 million people will have this disease. Researchers credit higher numbers of obese people coupled with sedentary lifestyles for this alarming increase.

 Diabetes Mellitus:

Diabetes comes from the Greek for "a siphon" or "to pass through," referring to the tendency for diabetics to urinate very frequently. *Mellitus* is from Latin for "sweetened with honey." Diabetes mellitus essentially means, "sweet pee."

Diabetes Mellitus in Brief

What is it?
Diabetes is a group of metabolic disorders characterized by glucose intolerance and disturbances in carbohydrate, fat, and protein metabolism.

How is it recognized?
Early symptoms of diabetes include frequent urination, thirstiness, and increased appetite, along with weight loss, nausea, and vomiting. These symptoms are often subtle enough that the first signs of disease are the complications it can cause: neuropathy, impaired vision, kidney dysfunction, or other problems.

Is massage indicated or contraindicated?
Diabetes indicates massage as long as tissues are healthy and circulation is unimpaired. Many people with advanced or poorly treated diabetes experience numbness, cardiovascular problems, or kidney failure. Circulatory massage in these situations would not be appropriate.

Diabetes, a largely treatable and even preventable disease, costs approximately $132 billion a year in direct medical costs and indirect costs of disability, lost wages, and premature mortality. It accounts for approximately 11% of all health care costs.

Type 2 diabetes occurs among all races but is most common among Native Americans and Alaskans, African Americans, Pacific Islanders, and Hispanic populations. Until recently, type 2 diabetes was a mature adult's disease; now many new diagnoses are among children between 9 and 19 years old. Diabetes is diagnosed in approximately 1.3 million people per year.

Etiology: What Happens?

Insulin is required to escort glucose into cells where it can be consumed to produce energy; insulin also aids in the removal of fat from the blood into storage lipid cells. In diabetes, glucose and fats build up in the blood either because insulin is in short supply, or because insulin receptor cells have developed resistance (or both). In the absence of insulin, the body cannot burn glucose; a remarkably clean fuel source, and must resort first to stored fat reserves, and then finally to proteins. Eventually, in the absence of any other fuel source, the body burns its own muscle tissue. These fuel sources do not burn cleanly. They leave behind a lot of toxic debris, which is largely responsible for the complications associated with diabetes.

Several types of diabetes mellitus have been identified; the two most common varieties are considered here:

Type 1 Type 1 diabetes, formerly known as "insulin-dependent diabetes mellitus" (IDDM), is an autoimmune disorder. It can be brought about by a number of different factors, including exposure to certain drugs and chemicals, or as a complication of some kinds of infections. Killer T cells of people with type I diabetes attack parts of the beta cells in the pancreas where insulin is produced. The destruction of these cells leads to a lifelong deficiency in insulin.

Type 1 diabetes usually shows symptoms before age 30, but one variety, called "latent autoimmune diabetes in adults" (LADA), may not be identified until later. Type 1 diabetes is the rarer, and more serious, of the two basic types of diabetes. Approximately 300,000 people in the United States have it, and approximately 30,000 new cases are diagnosed each year. It accounts for about 5% of all diabetes in this country. Because type 1 diabetes requires self-administered doses of insulin to take the place of the constant steady production provided by a healthy pancreas, type 1 diabetics can go through very extreme cycles of blood sugar levels—from very, very high, which can cause ketoacidosis and diabetic coma, to dangerously low, which can lead to insulin shock.

Type 2 This variety used to be called "non–insulin-dependent diabetes mellitus" (NIDDM), but that name is no longer accurate. It is more common for women than men. Approximately 80% of people with type 2 diabetes are overweight. It is especially prevalent in African Americans, Hispanics, Pacific Islanders, and Native American populations. Type 2 diabetes is usually controllable with diet, exercise, and possibly some anti-diabetes drugs, depending on how advanced it is when treatment begins, but many patients eventually have to supplement insulin.

The exact cause of adult-onset diabetes is uncertain and is probably different for different people. For some, it seems clear that a lifelong habit of a high-carbohydrate diet simply wears out the pancreas, and makes the insulin-producing cells less efficient. In others, the insulin production may be at normal levels, but the incoming flood of glucose is too much to deal with. And for still others, insulin production may be normal or even above normal, but for some reason, the target cells have fewer receptor sites to receive the insulin (see *metabolic syndrome*, this chapter). In any case, the results are the same: frequent urination, excessive thirst, and excessive hunger, along with the possibility of dangerous accumulations of atherosclerotic plaques and other serious complications.

Other types of diabetes include *gestational diabetes* (see *pregnancy*, Chapter 10), in which a woman develops a transient case while being pregnant. Somewhere between 2% and 5% of all pregnancies involve gestational diabetes. This condition can cause birth defects in the child, as well as routing massive amounts of blood sugar to the developing baby, resulting in very high birth weights and a high incidence of cesarean section surgeries. Women who have gestational diabetes and their babies also have an increased risk of developing type 2 diabetes later in life. *Secondary diabetes* may develop with damage or trauma to the pancreas, or as a symptom of some other endocrine disorder such as *acromegaly* (see this chapter) or Cushing syndrome (hyperactive adrenal glands). *Diabetes insipidus* is a dysfunction of the pituitary gland and insufficient production of *antidiuretic hormone* (ADH).

Signs and Symptoms

Three defining "polys" are common to all types of diabetes. *Polyuria*, or frequent urination, results from elevated blood sugar, which acts as a diuretic; it pulls water from the cells in the body, then excess water is expelled in the urine. *Polydipsia* means excessive thirst, which accompanies the loss of water with polyuria. *Polyphagia* refers to increased appetite because diabetics must get most of their energy from fats and proteins instead of carbohydrates, which are the most efficient kind of fuel. Other symptoms of diabetes include fatigue, weight loss, nausea, and vomiting.

Very often, signs of diabetes are missed until the disease has caused permanent damage to other organs in the body. These problems are discussed in the *Complications* section of this article.

Diabetic Emergencies

People with diabetes are vulnerable to specific medical emergencies, any of which can be fatal if not treated promptly.

- *Ketoacidosis* involves a critical *shortage* of insulin and lack of glucose in the cells. In this situation, the body partially metabolizes fats for fuel, and the acidic by-product of that metabolism (ketones) dangerously changes the pH balance of the blood. *Ketoacidosis* is identifiable by a characteristic sweet or fruity odor to the breath. Diabetics can test themselves for ketoacidosis with test strips that look for signs of ketones in the urine. Ketoacidosis can be brought on by stress, infection, or trauma and can lead to shock, coma, and death. It occurs only in people with type 1 diabetes.

Insulin Resistance: Silent and Dangerous

Insulin resistance (IR) is a condition in which a given concentration of insulin does not have the expected effect on cellular uptake of blood glucose. It is typically related to decreased numbers of insulin receptors on cell membranes, often in conjunction with postreceptor problems inside the cell. Meanwhile, blood sugar levels climb, stimulating the production of more insulin. In this way, hyperglycemia and hyperinsulinemia (the presence of excessive insulin in the blood) occur simultaneously. This situation, along with the excessive release of glucose from the liver, opens the door to type 2 diabetes mellitus.

Insulin resistance is also considered a causative factor for another situation, called *metabolic syndrome* (this chapter). Metabolic syndrome is associated with a dangerously increased risk of many forms of *heart disease* (Chapter 4).

Insulin resistance itself is often a silent disorder. Some patients with IR develop a skin discoloration called **acanthosis nigricans**: velvety brown patches appear around skin folds, especially at the axilla. It is thought that excessive insulin interacts with skin cells to produce this sign. Episodes of *hypoglycemia* (this chapter) occasionally affect people with IR; this indicates that antibodies have destroyed damaged insulin receptor sites, thus temporarily causing a sudden uptake of blood glucose.

Insulin resistance may be identified by testing blood glucose or insulin after fasting, when levels should be low. Other experts suggest that a glucose tolerance test, which measures glucose in the blood 2 hours after a patient ingests 75 mg sugar, is more indicative of the early stages of this disorder.

Statistics vary, but most suggest that anywhere from 3% to 33% of the U.S. population may have some level of insulin resistance.

- *Hyperosmolality* is a situation in type 2 diabetics also related to high blood sugar. The imbalance in the pH of the blood associated with ***hyperosmolality*** can lead to shock, coma, and death.

- *Insulin shock* is an emergency at the other end of the scale. In this case, *too much* insulin is circulating, either because too much has been administered or because a skipped meal, sudden exertion, stress, infection, or trauma has resulted in the consumption of all available blood sugar. The consequence of having too much available insulin is a dangerously low blood sugar level, or hypoglycemia. Symptoms of diabetic shock include dizziness, confusion, weakness, and tremors. It too can lead to coma and death if not treated (with juice, milk, candy, or non-diet soda to replace blood sugar) quickly.

Complications

Complications of diabetes are many and serious.

- *Cardiovascular disease.* Diabetics are especially prone to these problems because residue left from the metabolism of fats and proteins contributes to high rates of *atherosclerosis* (see Chapter 4). Unlike many atherosclerosis patients, diabetics do not simply accumulate plaque on coronary arterial walls but systemically throughout the body. Diabetes increases the risk of *stroke* (Chapter 3), *hypertension*, and *aneurysm*. (Chapter 4). Some degree of cardiovascular disease is present in 75% of all diabetes-related deaths. Approximately 65% of people with diabetes have high blood pressure.

- *Edema.* This condition develops in the extremities because of sluggish blood return. This can also give rise to stasis dermatitis. (See *dermatitis*, Chapter 1.)

- *Ulcers, gangrene, amputations.* Imagine what happens if *all* of the body's blood vessels were caked with plaque. Absence of blood flow carrying nutrients and white blood cells makes it difficult or impossible to heal from even minor skin lesions. Ingrown toenails can become life-threatening for diabetics; instead of healing, they become gangrenous. The tissue either dies of starvation or is infected with pathogens that are impossible to fight off, forming characteristic diabetic ulcers, usually on the feet (Figure 8.1). Diabetes leads to approximately 60% of the thousand lower extremity amputations every year.

- *Kidney disease.* Renal vessels get clogged with plaques very readily, because they are one of the first diversions from the descending aorta. Excess blood sugar, which acts as a powerful diuretic, is also hard on the kidneys, eventually causing reduced

Figure 8.1. Diabetic ulcers.

formation of glomerular filtrate and a thickening of the basement membrane in the Bowman's capsule. Not surprisingly, then, diabetes is the leading cause of renal failure and of the need for kidney transplants (see *renal failure*, Chapter 9).

Renal failure is the leading cause of death for people with diabetes. Research indicates that *very* frequent monitoring and adjustments of blood sugar can significantly reduce the amount of glomerular build-up in diabetic kidneys, thus reducing the risk of secondary hypertension by approximately 50%.

- *Impaired vision.* The capillaries of the eyes of diabetic persons can become abnormally thickened, depriving eye cells of nutrition. Diseased capillaries leak blood and proteins into the retina. Microaneurysms can form that also cut off circulation. All of these contribute to diabetic **retinopathy**. Excess glucose also binds with special proteins in the lens, causing first cataracts, then blindness. This disease is the leading cause for new blindness in the United States.

  Approximately half of all diabetes patients will experience some level of visual impairment within 10 years of being diagnosed. Close to 80% have some vision loss within 15 years.

- *Neuropathy.* Lack of capillary circulation and excess sugar in the blood both contribute to nerve damage. Symptoms of peripheral neuropathy include tingling or pain and eventual numbness. Neuropathy of the autonomic motor system can lead to an inability to maintain postural blood pressure, poor emptying of the stomach, diarrhea, constipation, or sexual impotency. Neuropathy generally appears approximately 10 to 20 years after diabetes is diagnosed. It is estimated that up to 25% of all diabetes patients will experience some degree of neuropathy.

- *Others.* Diabetes affects just about every body system in some way. It is linked to *urinary tract infections* (Chapter 9), *candidiasis* (Chapter 7), birth defects, and higher than normal rates of gum disease and tooth loss.

Diagnosis

Normal fasting blood sugar (a measurement that is taken before eating in the morning) is 110 mg/dL of blood. Diabetes is diagnosed when fasting levels rise over 125 mg/dL for 2 or more consecutive days.

Another test, called the hemoglobin A1c test, measures how much sugar sticks to the hemoglobin in circulating erythrocytes. This is often considered a better long-term test, because it reflects general blood sugar levels for periods of 3 months or more, instead of in increments of several hours. A normal reading is 4% to 5.9%; diabetes is diagnosed when A1c tests show 8% or greater amounts of glucose.

Treatment

Before the development of insulin in 1921, the diagnosis of diabetes was a death knell. Most people lived only a few years after the disease was identified. Now diabetes is a highly treatable disease, although it is estimated that only approximately 12% of all diagnosed people treat it aggressively enough to prevent the development of complications. Furthermore, successful treatment rates have remained static in spite of the availability of more products and an aggressive public relations campaign to focus attention on diabetes diagnosis and treatment.

The goals for diabetes treatment are fourfold: to improve insulin production in the pancreas when possible, to inhibit the release of glucose from the liver, to increase the sensitivity of target cells to insulin, and to decrease the absorption of carbohydrates in the small intestines. In addition to these measures, special care of eyes and feet can reduce the risk of blindness and amputations associated with the disease.

Type 1 diabetes is treated primarily with insulin. New techniques of administering insulin more frequently have been developed to minimize the dangerous roller coaster ride of too much to too little blood sugar that these people experience. These include insulin pens, which deliver a measured dose under the skin without a hypodermic needle, and insulin pumps, which feed a steady drip into the body through a plastic tube.

Type 2 diabetes is first addressed with changes in diet and exercise. In fact, it has been estimated that in overweight people with prediabetic blood sugar levels, a 5% to 7% loss of weight loss could completely prevent the disease. Approximately 35% of type 2 diabetes patients are treated with insulin supplementation. Hypoglycemic agents also may be prescribed.

Many diabetes patients eventually develop renal insufficiency: their kidneys simply cannot keep up with their needs. *Hemodialysis* is a treatment that involves rerouting the blood through a "kidney machine" that removes excess water and waste products before returning the blood to the body. Dialysis of any kind is usually a stop-gap measure while a person is waiting for a kidney to become available for transplant.

A kidney transplant may be recommended for people with advanced renal disease. Occasionally a kidney and pancreas are transplanted together for type 1 diabetics. Pancreas transplants have a high rejection rate, however. A new option of transplanting beta cells from a donor into the liver of the diabetic person is being explored with some success, but it is not widely available at this time.

Massage?

Massage may be appropriate for people with diabetes, under the right circumstances. The main condition is that the client must have healthy, responsive tissue with good blood supply. For clients with advanced diabetes, kidney failure, and atherosclerosis,

Case History 8.1

Type 2 Diabetes

Maureen, Age 43: "A Do-It-Yourself Project"

Maureen, age 43, had experienced gestational diabetes while pregnant with two of her three children. One year ago she had been experiencing chronic yeast infections, unintentional weight loss, blurred vision, and unusual thirstiness when she went for her annual checkup. She was not happy, but also not surprised, to be diagnosed with type 2 diabetes.

At first Maureen was intimidated by the glucose testing equipment she had to use, and she was terrified by the long-term complications that often develop with diabetes. But as she did more research, she came to the conclusion that diabetes is very much a "do it yourself" project. She found that proper control can be achieved through education, hard work, and stress reduction.

She tests her blood frequently and sees immediate relationships between her glucose levels and how much stress she's going through and how much exercise she gets. Since her diagnosis, Maureen's diabetes medication has been cut in half, and she is able to maintain reasonable glucose levels by being proactive about her health. Although she is still upset about her disease, she is thankful that she was diagnosed early enough to take control of her situation and change it for the better.

circulatory massage is probably out of the question, but energetic techniques are certainly appropriate.

Some researchers suggest that the best time to schedule a massage with a person who supplements insulin is *not* at the peak of insulin activity. Massage lowers blood sugar as well, so the risk of a hypoglycemic episode is significant. Diabetic clients who get regular massage would be well advised to measure their blood glucose before and after their sessions, to determine whether they would benefit from eating a small meal before receiving massage. Massage therapists who have diabetic clients may want to keep high-sugar snacks (juice, milk, candy, non-diet soda) available in case a client shows signs of hypoglycemia.

Massage therapists should be aware that diabetic neuropathy can involve lack of sensation. Someone with type 2 diabetes may be completely unaware of her condition until someone points out her ulcers, which often occur on the feet.

Graves disease is named after an Irish physician, Robert J. Graves (1796-1853), who first documented the relationship between an enlarged thyroid gland (goiter) and the symptoms it produces (excessive production of energy from fuel and bulging eyes).

Hyperthyroidism

Definition: What Is It?

Hyperthyroidism is a condition in which the thyroid gland produces excessive amounts of two forms of thyroxine, a hormone that stimulates metabolism of fuel into energy. Most cases of hyperthyroidism are related to autoimmune attacks against the whole thyroid gland. In these cases it also may be called *Graves disease* or *diffuse toxic thyroid*. More rarely, thyroid hyperactivity may be confined to one or more localized nodes, or it may be caused by thyroid infection.

Demographics: Who Gets It?

Hyperthyroidism is a common disorder, affecting between 1% and 2% of all people in the United States at some time in their lives. Approximately 500,000 new cases are diagnosed every year. Women are affected more often than men, by a margin of approximately 3–4 to 1. Most cases are diagnosed between the ages of 20 and 40 years.

A strong genetic link has been established in Graves disease; if one person has this disorder, it is likely that some kind of thyroid dysfunction will be present in some other first- or second-degree relative. Studies of identical twins show that if one twin develops Graves disease, the other twin probably will as well, although the leading signs and symptoms could be significantly different.

Etiology: What Happens?

Hyperthyroidism in Brief

What is it?
Hyperthyroidism is a condition in which the thyroid gland produces too much of its hormones that stimulate metabolism of fuel into energy. It is usually related to an autoimmune attack against the whole thyroid gland, but it can be caused by small, localized hyperactive nodules, or infection.

What does it look like?
Signs and symptoms of hyperthyroidism involve too much production of energy from available fuel: restlessness, sleeplessness, irritability, dry skin and hair, rapid heartbeat, tremor, unintended weight loss, and for women, irregularity of menstrual periods.

Some hyperthyroid patients experience complications involving eye problems or skin rashes. A severe and acute episode of hyperthyroidism is called a thyroid storm.

Is massage indicated or contraindicated?
Most people with hyperactive thyroid glands respond well to massage, which may help, at least temporarily, to ameliorate some of the stress-related symptoms that they experience.

Hyperthyroidism is usually caused by one of three things: a thyroid infection, a nodule or group of nodules that become hyperactive for unknown reasons (this is called *toxic nodular* or *multinodular goiter*), or an autoimmune attack against the thyroid gland that causes it to secrete excessive amounts of metabolic hormones.

Autoimmune hyperthyroidism, or Graves disease, is by far the most common variety of this disorder, accounting for some 70% to 80% of all cases. In this situation, antibodies called thyroid-stimulating immunoglobins (TSI) mistakenly attack the thyroid gland, causing it to grow to huge dimensions (this is called goiter) and to secrete excessive levels of both forms of thyroxine.

Under normal circumstances, pituitary secretions of thyroid-stimulating hormone (TSH) tell the thyroid when and how much to metabolize fuel into energy. When Graves disease is well established, the TSIs can chemically mimic TSH, so circulating levels of this hormone drop significantly. The result is that the conversion of fuel into energy increases by 60% to 100%.

Whereas genetics clearly plays a major part of developing Grave's disease, its onset often seems to be connected to a stressful situation such as a death in the family or a job change. Other risk factors for developing this disorder include exposure of the thyroid to x-rays, or having taken antiviral medications such as interferon or interleukin.

Signs and Symptoms

The primary symptom of Graves disease is the development of goiter: the gland becomes enlarged enough to create a visible, painless swelling in the neck. Other signs and symptoms are mostly related to the secretion of thyroid hormones (Figure 8.2). They include anxiety, irritability, insomnia, rapid heartbeat, tremor, increased perspiration, sensitivity to heat, and unintentional weight loss. Skeletal muscles, especially in the arms and pelvis, often become weak. Other symptoms may include a lighter flow during menstrual periods, dry skin and brittle nails, and problems specifically with the skin and eyes, discussed later in this section.

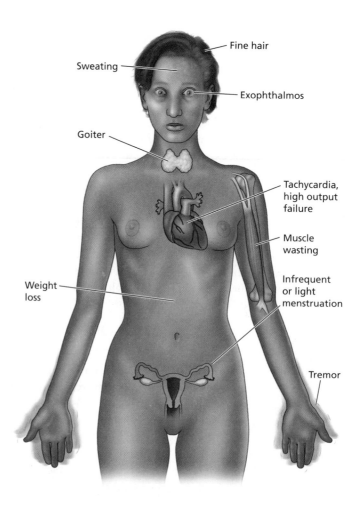

Figure 8.2. Systemic effects of hyperthyroidism.

Figure 8.3. Hyperthyroidism: exophthalmos.

Complications

The thyroid is not the only tissue that may be attacked in Graves disease. Some other sites of tissue damage include the eyes and the skin on the feet and lower legs. Hyperthyroidism can affect the eyes in a couple of different ways. One fairly common situation involves the elevation of eyelids in a way that makes the eyes seem to bulge. Protrusion of the eyes is known as *exophthalmos* or *proptosis* (Figure 8.3).

Another eye problem related to Graves disease is a rare disorder called *Graves ophthalmopathy*. This causes the eyeball to protrude beyond its protective orbit because tissues and muscles behind it swell. The front surface of the eye can dry out, causing light sensitivity, double vision, decreased freedom of movement within the orbit, pain, and excessive tearing.

Some Graves disease patients develop red raised patches of skin on their shins, feet, or elsewhere. These rashes, caused by the deposition of *mucopolysaccharides* in the dermis, are called *pretibial myxedema*, and they are generally not painful or dangerous.

In addition to eye and skin problems, some Graves disease patients experience occasional episodes of especially high metabolism called thyroid storms. In these episodes, symptoms become suddenly acute and may include rapid heartbeat, fever without infection, intolerance to heat, confusion, agitation, and finally shock. Thyroid storms can be medical emergencies and require immediate intervention to slow the heart and bring down the fever.

Diagnosis

Graves disease is usually diagnosed through a physical examination, a blood test, and an examination of the way the thyroid takes up radioactive iodine.

The physical examination concentrates on issues such as goiter, temperature, heart rate, muscle weakness, and tremor.

Blood tests look for low levels of TSH combined with high levels of TSI, along with abnormally high levels of thyroxine.

The ingestion of radioactive iodine shows how quickly the thyroid absorbs iodine (a primary component of thyroxine), as well as which parts of the thyroid appear to be hyperactive. This test helps to delineate between Graves disease and nodular hyperthyroidism.

Treatment

Hyperthyroidism can be treated in a number of ways, depending on the underlying causes and the severity of the symptoms.

- *Radioactive iodine:* Although this is also a diagnostic tool, radioactive iodine also can be used to kill off a portion of the hyperactive thyroid, to bring levels of thyroxine to within safe and normal standards. Many Graves disease patients find that their symptoms are abated with only one or two doses of radioactive iodine, although most develop signs of *hypothyroidism* (this chapter) in later months or years. Hypothyroidism is easier to manage than hyperthyroidism and so is considered the lesser of the two evils.

- *Antithyroid medications:* Several classes of medications have been developed that prevent the thyroid from producing too much thyroxine or that prevent the thyroxine from having major impact on the body. Sometimes these medications are used to prepare a patient for surgery or radioactive iodine treatment, but occasionally they are successful by themselves.

- *Surgery:* Patients who cannot take antithyroid drugs or radioactive iodine may consider a thyroidectomy: a surgery in which most of the thyroid is removed. This is a risky procedure, however, because the parathyroids, which control calcium metabolism, are often damaged in the process, along with the vocal cords and laryngeal nerves. Surgery for hyperthyroidism is generally avoided if at all possible.

Massage?

As long as the person's skin is healthy and intact, massage of all kinds may be beneficial to clients with hyperactive thyroid glands. The calm, relaxed response that massage creates may provide a welcome change to the sympathetic-like symptoms of hyperthyroidism.

Hypoglycemia

Hypoglycemia in Brief

Pronunciation
hī′pö-glī-sē′mē-ă

What is it?
Hypoglycemia is the condition of having abnormally low levels of blood glucose, so cells have no access to important fuel.

What does it look like?
Signs and symptoms of a hypoglycemic episode include dizziness, confusion, chills and sweating, hunger, headache, and pallor. Symptoms pass when a person eats or drinks something with available glucose.

Is massage indicated or contraindicated?
A person in a hypoglycemic episode needs to replace glucose first, get a massage second. Once the symptoms have passed, bodywork is a fine choice. If a person experiences ongoing hypoglycemic symptoms, or frequent acute episodes, he or she should find out why.

Definition: What Is It?

Hypoglycemia is the condition of having an inadequate amount of glucose circulating in the blood to fuel all the body's needs. It is usually a complication of other problems, especially *diabetes* mellitus (this chapter), but it occasionally stands alone as a primary disorder.

Demographics: Who Gets It?

Many people experience occasional hypoglycemic episodes, when they have been stressed, have not eaten enough, or are otherwise unbalanced. However, outside of the context of diabetes, this is a relatively unusual problem for someone to have to deal with in an ongoing, chronic context. It can happen with fasting and some rare genetic diseases that interfere with glucose digestion.

Etiology: What Happens?

The cyclic nature of blood glucose levels is an excellent example of an efficient negative-feedback loop. The pancreas secretes two hormones: insulin and glucagon. Insulin *lowers* blood sugar by escorting glucose into hungry cells. Glucagon *raises* blood sugar by stimulating the liver to release stored glucose into the blood. When blood sugar levels are slightly higher than usual, for instance, after a meal, the pancreas releases insulin to lower them. When they get too low, the pancreas releases glucagon to raise them.

Hypoglycemia occurs when blood glucose levels get abnormally low. The "normal" range is 60 to 120 mg/dL of blood; hypoglycemia is suspected when blood glucose drops below 50 mg/dL. Although the pancreas may release glucagon in an attempt to raise blood glucose, the liver may simply not be able to comply, or it complies too slowly. The body, in need of fuel, cannot function normally and begins to become distressed. Very extreme episodes of hypoglycemia can lead to loss of consciousness or even coma.

Hypoglycemia is an occasional reaction to fasting, infection, or stressful situations. When it occurs in diabetes patients, it is in reaction to a dose of insulin that has not been matched by adequate nutrition.

Signs and Symptoms

Signs and symptoms of hypoglycemia are created by cells, especially in the brain, that are starving for glucose. They include dizziness, hunger, headache, confusion, blurred vision, and a decreased ability to concentrate. Sweating and chills, pallor, shakiness, increased heart rate, and nausea also may occur. If a person in a hypoglycemic episode does not eat something in short order, she may lapse into unconsciousness or coma.

Massage?

As stated previously, many people experience occasional episodes of hypoglycemia caused by stress, infection, or temporary under-eating. Clients in a bout of a hypo-glycemic attack are better off drinking some juice or eating something high in carbohy-drates than they are receiving a massage. When the symptoms have subsided, massage is a perfectly appropriate choice.

If a client reports repeated hypoglycemic episodes, that person would be well advised to pursue the reasons with a nutritional expert. It may be that her ability to regulate blood glucose is failing and that she is in the early stages of diabetes; it may be that she is showing signs of a hereditary disorder; or it may be that she simply needs to change her eating habits so that her body experiences less stress in the ongoing job of supplying her cells with fuel.

Hypothyroidism

Definition: What Is It?

Hypothyroidism is a condition in which circulating levels of thyroid hormones are abnormally low. This interferes with the body's ability to generate energy from fuel.

Demographics: Who Gets It?

Statistics on hypothyroidism vary widely. Although some sources suggest that it affects approximately 2% of all women and 1% of all men, others indicate that the incidence is much higher. Regardless, hypothyroidism is seen most often in mature people; an estimated 6

Hypothyroidism in Brief

What is it?
Hypothyroidism is a condition in which the thyroid gland produces an inadequate supply of the hormones that regulates metabolism of fuel into energy. Some cases of hypothyroidism are the result of an autoimmune attack on the thyroid gland, but others are related to the long-term complications of treatment for hyperthyroidism or other factors.

What does it look like?
Symptoms of hypothyroidism are subtle and often missed. They include fatigue, weight gain, depression, intolerance of cold, and for women, heavy menstrual periods.

Is massage indicated or contraindicated?
One of the complications of hypothyroidism, especially in elderly patients, is the accelerated development of athero-sclerosis. As long as this condition is recognized and respected, massage can be a supportive and positive experience for hypothyroidism patients.

to 7 million Americans, mainly women over 40 years old, have been diagnosed with this condition.

Etiology: What Happens?

The thyroid gland produces thyroid hormone in two different forms: T3 (*triiodothyronine*) and T4 (*thyroxine*). It does this under the direction of the pituitary gland, which releases TSH. When adequate amounts of T3 and T4 are circulating in the blood, secretion of TSH is suppressed. Thus, thyroid and pituitary secretions keep each other in balance.

The purpose of thyroid hormones is to stimulate the conversion of fuel (oxygen and calories) into energy. In hypothyroidism, inadequate amounts of thyroid hormones are produced, so incoming fuel is simply stored and never used. In a typical early case of hypothyroidism, the pituitary gland releases excessive thyroid-stimulating hormone, but circulating levels of T4 are converted to T3 very quickly. Consequently, TSH levels are high, T4 levels are significantly low, but T3 levels are close to normal.

Several different contributing factors of hypothyroidism have been identified:

- *Hashimoto's thyroiditis.* **Hashimoto's thyroiditis** is an autoimmune attack against the thyroid gland that results in the suppression of thyroid secretions (as opposed to the autoimmune attack that stimulates excessive thyroid secretions seen with Graves disease).

- *Complication of treatment for hyperthyroidism.* Most hyperthyroidism patients who use radioactive iodine to suppress thyroid activity eventually develop hypothyroidism.

- *Congenital birth defect.* Some babies are born with abnormally small thyroid glands, or no thyroid gland at all. If these children are not treated, they will experience stunted growth and mental retardation.

- *Medications.* Some medications, specifically lithium (used to treat bipolar depression) or iodides (used as a form of iodine), can suppress thyroid function.

- *Exposure to radiation.* Persons who have been exposed to radiation in the neck for cancer treatment, or in more general ways, have a high risk of developing hypothyroidism. This has been an issue for survivors of the Chernobyl nuclear plant accident.

- *Idiopathic.* Some cases of hypothyroidism do not seem to be related to any specific underlying disorder but simply arise without known cause. This situation seems to be especially prevalent among middle-aged women. This type of hypothyroidism is often linked with other chronic conditions, including *chronic fatigue syndrome* (see Chapter 5) and *fibromyalgia* (see Chapter 2).

Whatever the cause for hypothyroidism, the net result is that a person has difficulty turning fuel into energy. The body tends to absorb nutrition and store it indefinitely, either as fat in lipid cells or as cholesterol in atherosclerotic plaques (see *atherosclerosis*, Chapter 4).

Signs and Symptoms

Signs and symptoms of hypothyroidism are often subtle but steadily progressive (Figure 8.4). A person may not realize the extent of her problem until someone points it out to her. The result of not being able to convert fuel into energy means that a person is likely to gain weight, feel fatigued and depressed, and have a sluggish digestive system with chronic constipation. She may have poor tolerance of cold, and her skin will be puffy, but dry. She may have many symptoms of fibromyalgia, *depression* (see Chapter 3), or chronic fatigue syndrome. Her hair may be flat and brittle, and may even fall out.

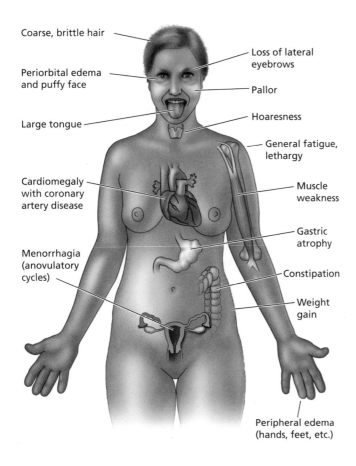

Coarse, brittle hair

Loss of lateral eyebrows

Periorbital edema and puffy face

Pallor

Large tongue

Hoaresness

General fatigue, lethargy

Cardiomegaly with coronary artery disease

Muscle weakness

Gastric atrophy

Menorrhagia (anovulatory cycles)

Constipation

Weight gain

Peripheral edema (hands, feet, etc.)

Figure 8.4. Systemic effects of hypothyroidism.

Menstrual periods tend to be heavy and long-lasting. Some hypothyroidism patients develop goiter: a painless enlargement of the thyroid.

It is common for hypothyroid patients to develop atherosclerosis because liver function to produce the chemicals that expel cholesterol from the body is sluggish. The heart may become enlarged as well. Fluid retention in the arms and wrists raises the risk of *carpal tunnel syndrome* (see Chapter 3); fluid retention in the neck along with goiter may cause chronic hoarseness. Very severe cases may cause a patient to become so cold and drowsy that she becomes unconscious. This is called ***myxedema coma***, and it is a rare but dangerous complication of hypothyroidism among elderly patients.

Diagnosis

Blood tests can identify when TSH levels are abnormally high. Hypothyroidism is the only disease that causes this change in an ongoing way, so this test is very useful for beginning a diagnosis.

Physical examinations for hypothyroidism look for goiter, along with a significantly slowed heart rate. Reflexes are often slower in hypothyroid patients.

It is especially important for pregnant women to be tested for thyroid function. Pregnancy can hide some symptoms of hypothyroidism, which can create serious repercussions for the unborn child. Most newborns are tested for thyroid function as a matter of course; early intervention in the rare cases when thyroid function is subnormal can prevent stunted growth and mental retardation.

Controversy is developing over what is considered "normal" levels of circulating thyroid hormones. The standards now employed often do not seem to reflect the true needs of many people who live with hypothyroidism at levels that are too subtle to be detected by current tests. As research continues into this condition, scales of normality may be developed to meet the needs of individuals more accurately than current standards do.

Treatment

The treatment for hypothyroidism is to supplement thyroid hormones. Desiccated thyroid glands of a variety of animals have traditionally been prescribed to treat hypothyroidism, but the doses are difficult to regulate, because potency varies widely. Thyroid hormone is usually replaced with a synthetic version, but only in the form of T4. Although many people experience relief with this treatment, others must explore other options to find the right supplement of both T3 and T4.

Massage?

Outside the risk of atherosclerosis (which is a risk for many mature clients regardless of thyroid function), massage is a perfectly appropriate choice for hypothyroidism clients. Although it is unlikely to stimulate normal production of thyroxine, massage can certainly improve the quality of life of people who feel chronically drained and lethargic.

Metabolic Syndrome

Metabolic Syndrome in Brief

What is it?
Metabolic syndrome is a collection of problems that indicates a high risk of several serious diseases, including diabetes, heart attack, atherosclerosis, and stroke.

How is it recognized?
Metabolic syndrome is recognized though its combined associated conditions, including disruptions in cholesterol, hypertension, central obesity, and others.

Is massage indicated or contraindicated?
The appropriateness of massage for a person with metabolic syndrome depends on his or her cardiovascular health. If exercise is recommended for weight loss and improved insulin function, then massage is probably also safe. If, however, these conditions have led to severe cardiovascular problems, massage must be adjusted to accommodate circulatory weakness.

Definition: What Is It?

Metabolic syndrome, sometimes called "syndrome X" or "insulin resistance syndrome," is a condition involving several signs that seen alone are not especially alarming, but when they appear in conjunction with each other, the risk of cardiovascular disease is very high.

Demographics: Who Gets It?

Estimates of the incidence of metabolic syndrome vary widely. Some researchers suggest that it affects some 16 million Americans, although most are unaware of it. Others suggest that up to 44% of all people over 50 years old meet the diagnostic criteria for metabolic syndrome.[1] Regardless of the exact numbers, it is clear that metabolic syndrome is a common, silent, often-ignored condition.

Etiology: What Happens?

Metabolic syndrome is identified as a cluster of five main features, including high triglycerides, low high-density lipoproteins (the "good" cholesterol), hypertension, central obesity (fat retention in the omentum more than in superficial fascia), and high fasting blood glucose levels. Other possible features

[1]Alexander CM, Landsman PB, Teutsch SM, et al. NCEP-Defined Metabolic Syndrome, Diabetes, and Prevalence of Coronary Heart Disease Among NHANES III Participants Age 50 Years and Older. Copyright © 2003 American Diabetes Association, Inc. Available at: http://www.medscape.com/viewarticle/453709_print. Accessed winter 2004.

in metabolic syndrome include a high risk of blood clotting, and polycystic ovary disease in women (see *ovarian cysts*, Chapter 10). These factors are not particularly alarming when they appear alone, but in combinations they set the stage for an extremely elevated risk of *atherosclerosis, heart attack, heart failure, aneurysm* (all Chapter 4), *stroke* (Chapter 3), or other cardiovascular disease.

Many researchers suggest that insulin resistance causes metabolic syndrome, although it is not clear whether that happens through direct damage to arterial walls from circulating blood glucose or from secondary problems associated with *diabetes* (this chapter). Insulin resistance with hyperglycemia is such a prevalent contributor to metabolic syndrome that most researchers label this condition as an endocrine disorder, even though most of its worst repercussions affect the cardiovascular system.

Signs and Symptoms

Metabolic syndrome typically appears as central obesity (most of the body weight is carried around the abdomen in an "apple" rather than a "pear" shape), along with disruptions in cholesterol, hypertension, and blood glucose, as described above. Outside of excessive body weight, however, metabolic syndrome does not typically cause specific symptoms; its other components are silent.

Diagnosis

Metabolic syndrome is diagnosed when three of five risk factors are simultaneously present:

- High-fasting blood glucose (over 110 mg/dL after 9 hours of fasting)
- Abdominal obesity (a waist measurement of over 35" for women, or over 40" for men)
- Elevated triglyceride levels (over 150 mg/dL)
- Low levels of high-density lipoproteins (under 40 mg/dL for men; under 50 mg/dL for women)
- Hypertension (systolic over 130; diastolic over 85)

Treatment

Studies show that persons with neither diabetes nor metabolic syndrome have a low risk of heart disease; people with well-controlled diabetes (i.e., diabetes without metabolic syndrome) have a risk of heart disease similar to those without metabolic syndrome. However, people with metabolic syndrome, and especially people with metabolic syndrome along with diabetes, are at a significantly increased risk for heart disease. These findings are important, because they point to the importance of managing risk factors *before* they lead to significant disability.

The first, best option for a person with metabolic syndrome is to exercise and lose weight. Reducing body weight by 5% to 7% (this is only 10–14 pounds for a 200-pound person) significantly reduces the risk of complications caused by insulin resistance, and exercise improves insulin action and decreases blood glucose. Limiting alcohol use and quitting smoking are other important steps.

If these lifestyle changes are insufficient to control this disorder, medications that improve insulin uptake or stimulate more insulin production may be prescribed.

Massage?

The appropriateness of massage in the context of metabolic syndrome depends entirely on the health and resilience of the client. If this person works successfully to control his or her disease through diet and exercise adjustments, massage is probably safe and appropriate. If this person has developed any of the serious complications associated with these conditions, judgments must be made to accommodate possible weaknesses of the circulatory system.

CHAPTER REVIEW QUESTIONS

1. Describe the negative-feedback loop between insulin and glucagon.
2. Both the autonomic nervous system and the endocrine system are controlled by what structure?
3. How can diabetes contribute to heart disease? Kidney disease? Blindness?
4. What are three symptoms of abnormally low levels of thyroxine?
5. What are three symptoms of abnormally high levels of thyroxine?
6. How can hyperthyroidism lead eventually to hypothyroidism?
7. Describe the signs and symptoms of a person experiencing a hypoglycemic attack.
8. Name five features associated with metabolic syndrome.
9. Describe how successfully treating metabolic syndrome can prevent other serious health problems.

 Answers to these questions can be found on the Student Recource CD-ROM that accompanies this book.

Bibliography

General Resources, Endocrine System

1. de Dominico G, Wood E. Beard's Massage. Philadelphia: WB Saunders, 1997.
2. Damjanou I. Pathology for the Health-Related Professions. Philadelphia: WB Saunders, 1996.
3. Travell J, Simons DG. Myofascial Pain and Dysfunction: The Trigger Point Manual. Baltimore: Williams & Wilkins, 1983.
4. Clemente CD. Anatomy: A Regional Atlas of the Human Body. 3rd Ed. Baltimore: Urban & Schwarzenburg; 1987.
5. Tortora GJ, Anagnostakos NP. Principles of Anatomy and Physiology. 6th Ed. New York: Harper & Row; 1990.
6. Taber's Cyclopedic Dictionary. 14th Ed. Philadelphia: FA Davis; 1981.
7. Stedman's Medical Dictionary. 26th Ed. Baltimore: Williams & Wilkins; 1995.
8. Memmler RL, Wood DL. The Human Body in Health and Disease. 5th Ed. Philadelphia: JB Lippincott; 1983.
9. Juhan D. Job's Body: A Handbook for Bodywork. Barrytown, NY: Station Hill Press; 1987.
10. Kunz JRM, Finkel AJ, eds. The American Medical Association Family Medical Guide. New York, NY: Random House; 1987.
11. Marieb EM. Human Anatomy and Physiology. Redwood City, CA: Benjamin/Cummings, 1989.
12. Field T. Touch Therapy. London: Churchill Livingstone, 2000.

Acromegaly

1. Centurion SA, Schwartz RA. Acromegaly. Copyright © 2004, eMedicine.com, Inc. Available at: http://www.emedicine.com/derm/topic593.htm. Accessed winter 2004.
2. Khandwala HM, Friend K. Acromegaly. Copyright © 2004, eMedicine.com, Inc. Available at: http://www.emedicine.com/med/topic27.htm. Accessed winter 2004.
3. Acromegaly Overview. Copyright © 1998–2004 Mayo Foundation for Medical Education and Research (MFMER). Available at: http://www.mayoclinic.com/invoke.cfm?id=DS00478. Accessed winter 2004.
4. Growth hormone to prevent aging: Is it a good idea? Copyright © 1998–2004 Mayo Foundation for Medical Education and Research (MFMER). Available at: http://www.mayoclinic.com/invoke.cfm?id=HA00030. Accessed winter 2004.

Diabetes Mellitus

1. Mathur R. Diabetes Mellitus. Copyright © 1996–2004 MedicineNet, Inc. Available at: http://www.medicinenet.com/script/main/art.asp?articlekey=343&pf=3&track=qpa343. Accessed winter 2004.
2. Preventing Chronic Diseases: Investing Wisely in HealthPreventing Diabetes and Its Complications. Centers for Disease Control and Prevention. Available at:

http://www.cdc.gov/nccdphp/pe_factsheets/pe_ddt.htm. Accessed winter 2004.
3. Diabetes & Women's Health Across the Life Stages. Centers for Disease Control and Prevention. Available at: http://www.cdc.gov/diabetes/pubs/pdf/womenshort.pdf. Accessed winter 2004.
4. Diabetes statistics. Centers for Disease Control and Prevention. Available at: http://www.cdc.gov/nchs/fastats/diabetes.htm. Accessed winter 2004.
5. Ezzo J, Donner T, Nickols D, et al. Is Massage Useful in the Management of Diabetes? A Systematic Review. Copyright © 2001 by the American Diabetes Association. Available at: http://spectrum.diabetesjournals.org/cgi/content/full/14/4/218. Accessed winter 2004.
6. Soman SS, Soman AS. Diabetic Nephropathy. Copyright © 2004, eMedicine.com, Inc. Available at: http://www.emedicine.com/med/topic549.htm. Accessed winter 2004.
7. Diabetic Neuropathies: The Nerve Damage of Diabetes. National Institutes of Diabetes and Digestive and Kidney Diseaes (NIDDK), National Institutes of Health (NIH). Available at: http://diabetes.niddk.nih.gov/dm/pubs/neuropathies/index.htm. Accessed winter 2004.
8. Islet cell transplantation: The diabetes treatment frontier. Copyright © 1998–2004 Mayo Foundation for Medical Education

and Research (MFMER). Available at: http://www.mayoclinic.com/invoke.cfm?id=DA00046. Accessed winter 2004.

9. National Diabetes Fact Sheet. Centers for Disease Control and Prevention (CDC). Available at: http://www.cdc.gov/diabetes/pubs/estimates.htm. Accessed winter 2004.

10. Fradkin J, Cowie C, Saydah S. Most People with Diabetes Do Not Meet Treatment Goals. National Institute of Diabetes and Digestive and Kidney Diseases (NIDDK), National Institutes of Health (NIH). Available at: http://www.nih.gov/news/pr/jan2004/niddk-20.htm. Accessed winter 2004.

11. NIH Reports Progress in Diabetes Research. National Institute of Diabetes and Digestive and Kidney Diseases (NIDDK), National Institutes of Health (NIH). Available at: http://www.niddk.nih.gov/welcome/releases/10-23-02.htm. Accessed winter 2004.

Hyperthyroidism

1. Yeung SCJ, Chiu AC. Graves Disease. Copyright © 2003, eMedicine.com, Inc. Available at: http://www.emedicine.com/med/topic929.htm. Accessed winter 2004.

2. Graves' disease Overview. Copyright © 1998–2003 Mayo Foundation for Medical Education and Research (MFMER). Available at: http://www.mayoclinic.com/invoke.cfm?id=DS00181. Accessed winter 2004.

3. NINDS Thyrotoxic Myopathy Information Page. The National Institute of Neurological Disorders and Stroke (NINDS), National Institutes of Health (NIH). Available at: http://www.ninds.nih.gov/health_and_medical/disorders/thyrotoxic_myopathy.htm?format=printable. Accessed winter 2004.

4. Floyd JL. Thyrotoxicosis. Copyright © 2004, eMedicine.com, Inc. Available at: http://www.emedicine.com/radio/topic315.htm. Accessed winter 2004.

Hypoglycemia

1. Hoffman R. Hypoglycemia. Copyright © 2004, eMedicine.com, Inc. Available at: http://www.emedicine.com/ped/topic1117.htm. Accessed winter 2004.

2. Hypoglycemia. National Institute of Diabetes and Digestive and Kidney Diseases (NIDDK), National Institutes of Health (NIH). Available at: http://diabetes.niddk.nih.gov/dm/pubs/hypoglycemia/index.htm. Accessed winter 2004.

3. Hypoglycemia Overview. Copyright © 1998–2004 Mayo Foundation for Medical Education and Research (MFMER). Available at: http://www.mayoclinic.com/invoke.cfm?id=DS00198. Accessed winter 2004.

Hypothyroidism

1. Echeverry DM, Kedlaya D. Hypothyroid Myopathy. Copyright © 2004, eMedicine.com, Inc. Available at: http://www.emedicine.com/pmr/topic57.htm. Accessed winter 2004.

2. Orlander PR, Woodhouse WR. Hypothyroidism. Copyright © 2003 eMedicine.com, Inc. Available at: http://www.emedicine.com/med/topic1145.htm. Accessed winter 2004.

3. Hypothyroidism Overview. Copyright © 1998–2004 Mayo Foundation for Medical Education and Research (MFMER). Available at: http://www.mayoclinic.com/invoke.cfm?id=DS00353. Accessed winter 2004.

4. Citkowitz E. Myxedema Coma or Crisis. Copyright © 2003, eMedicine.com, Inc. Available at: http://www.emedicine.com/med/topic1581.htm. Accessed winter 2004.

Metabolic Syndrome

1. Findings and Recommendations from the American College of Endocrinology Conference on the Insulin Resistance Syndrome. Copyright © 2003 American Association of Clinical Endocrinologists (AACE). Available at: http://www.aace.com/pub/BMI/findings.php. Accessed winter 2004.

2. Deadly Quartet of Metabolic Risk FactorsIncreases Mortality from Coronary Artery Disease. Copyright © Cleveland Clinic Foundation 5/01. Available at: http://www.clevelandclinic.org/heartcenter/pub/professionals/cardiacconsult/2001/spring/syndromex.htm. Accessed winter 2004.

3. Hyperinsulinemia. Copyright © 1998–2003 Mayo Foundation for Medical Education and Research (MFMER). Available at: http://www.mayoclinic.com/invoke.cfm?id=HQ00896. Accessed winter 2004.

4. Incremental Lifestyle Changes Can Ward Off Syndrome X. Copyright © The Cleveland Clinic 2003. Available at: http://www.clevelandclinic.org/health/health-info/docs/3000/3053.asp?index=10807. Accessed winter 2004.

5. Insulin Resistance and Hyperinsulinemia. Copyright © 2004 The Health Alliance. Available at: http://www.health alliance.com/hospitals/Jewish/glueck/insulin_resistance.htm. Accessed winter 2004.

6. Olatunbosun S, Dagogo-Jack S. Insulin Resistance. Copyright © 2003, eMedicine.com, Inc. Available at: http://www.emedicine.com/med/topic1173.htm. Accessed winter 2004.

7. Mandava P, Palm ML. Metabolic Disease & Stroke: Hyperglycemia/Hypoglycemia. Copyright © 2004, eMedicine.com, Inc. Available at: http://www.emedicine.com/neuro/topic581.htm. Accessed winter 2004.

8. Kendall P. Syndrome X and Insulin Resistance. Copyright © Colorado State University Cooperative Extension 1995–2003. Available at: http://www.ext.colostate.edu/pubs/columnnn/nn971022.html. Accessed winter 2004.

9. Metabolic syndrome and type 2 diabetes mellitus: focus on peroxisome proliferator activated receptors (PPAR). Copyright © 2003, Tenenbaum et al; licensee BioMed Central Ltd. Available at: http://www.pubmedcentral.nih.gov/articlerender.fcgi?artid=153546. Accessed winter 2004.

10. Alexander CM, Landsman PB, Teutsch SM, et al. NCEP-Defined Metabolic Syndrome, Diabetes, and Prevalence of Coronary Heart Disease Among NHANES III Participants Age 50 Years and Older. Copyright © 2003 American Diabetes Association, Inc. Available at: http://www.medscape.com/viewarticle/453709_print. Accessed winter 2004.

11. Insulin Resistance and Pre-Diabetes. National Institute of Diabetes and Digestive and Kidney Diseases, National Institutes of Health. Available at: http://diabetes.niddk.nih.gov/dm/pubs/insulinresistance/index.htm. Accessed winter 2004.

12. Type 2 Diabetes and Syndrome X. Copyright © 1997–2003 Diabetic-Lifestyle. Available at: http://www.diabetic-lifestyle.com/articles/jun00_whats_1.htm. Accessed winter 2004.

13. Syndrome X. Copyright © 1998–2003 Mayo Foundation for Medical Education and Research (MFMER). Available at: http://www.mayoclinic.com/invoke.cfm?objectid=31F72990-F5EC-48A8-87DB7539FB6EA84E. Accessed winter 2004.

URINARY SYSTEM CONDITIONS

Chapter Objectives

After reading this chapter, you should be able to. . .

- Describe the four major structures that constitute the urinary system.
- Name a hormone produced by the kidneys and describe its function.
- Identify the primary causative factor for most kidney stones.
- Identify the causative agent in most cases of pyelonephritis.
- Describe two types of renal failure.
- Name two contributing factors for acute renal failure.
- Identify the most commonly recognized factor in the development of bladder cancer in industrialized countries.
- Explain why females get urinary tract infections more often than males.
- Explain why a urinary tract infection in a male can indicate a serious problem.
- Describe the difference(s) between interstitial cystitis and a bladder infection.

INTRODUCTION

Function and Structure

The urinary system is a relatively small system in the body, composed of the kidneys, the ureters, the bladder, and the urethra.

The huge renal artery comes directly off the aorta and enters the kidneys. It rapidly decreases in diameter to form thousands of capillaries. Each of these is entangled with another type of epithelial tube: the nephron, which surrounds the knot-like capillary glomerulus with the Bowman's capsule and winds a complicated pathway all around the capillary loop (Figure 9.1). The constant force of blood pressure from the renal artery forces movement of fluids from circulatory capillaries into the nephrons. Chemical exchanges are made back and forth at this point. Waste products and water are squeezed out of the capillaries and into the nephrons, and then later in the loop the capillaries reabsorb whatever water and salts are needed to keep the blood properly diluted. The nephron then takes its load of wastes and excess

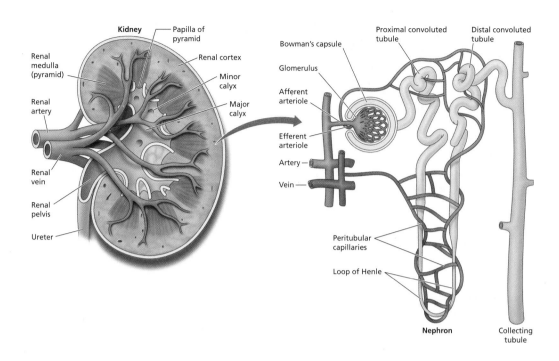

Figure 9.1. Overview of the urinary system.

water to the renal pelvis where it delivers everything that the body needs to expel. The renal pelvis empties into the ureters; they lead to the bladder, which acts as a holding tank. When enough urine has accumulated, it is expelled through the urethra. The cleansed blood, now relieved of excess water, nitrogenous wastes, uric acid, and other debris, exits the kidney through the renal vein.

The kidneys have another function that is not directly involved in the filtering of waste products from the blood. *Erythropoietin* (EPO), a hormone that stimulates red blood cell production, is produced in the kidneys. Damage to these delicate organs can therefore sometimes be identified by changes in red blood cell production.

Kidneys are constructed primarily of epithelial tissue, which makes them vulnerable to injury. This is why tapotement along the inferior edge of the rib cage is not recommended; it is unlikely, but possible, to injure the kidneys here. When the kidneys have been damaged, red blood cells leak from capillaries into the nephrons. This shows as blood in the urine (*hematuria*) and is evidence of trauma, infection, or other potentially dangerous situations in the kidneys.

Filtration, the movement of substances through a membrane by external mechanical pressure (in this case the blood pressure), is the mechanism by which most substances are exchanged between the circulatory system and the urinary system. It is clear how carefully intertwined blood pressure and kidney health must be. If blood pressure is consistently high (see *hypertension*, Chapter 4), then the kidneys will sustain damage and become less efficient. Conversely, if the kidneys are not functioning adequately, the body accumulates excess fluid, which forces blood pressure to rise. Some of the conditions discussed in this chapter have to do with the complicated relationship between the urinary and circulatory systems. Other conditions considered here will be related to the vulnerability of the urinary system organs to infection.

URINARY SYSTEM CONDITIONS

Kidney Disorders

Glomerulonephritis
Kidney Stones
Pyelonephritis
Renal Failure

Bladder and Urinary Tract Disorders

Bladder Cancer
Interstitial Cystitis
Urinary Tract Infection

KIDNEY DISORDERS

Glomerulonephritis

Definition: What Is It?

Glomerulonephritis is a relatively rare but serious situation involving inflammation and scarring of the glomeruli (microscopic knots of epithelial tissue that are surrounded by capsules). Several types of glomerulonephritis have been classified. Many of them have no known cause, some are related to other specific diseases, and some are complications of or autoimmune reactions to other infections in the body.

Demographics: Who Gets It?

Different age groups are at risk for different types of glomerulonephritis. Children may experience this disease as a complication of a streptococcal infection. Adults may experience glomerulonephritis as a spontaneous event or as a part of an autoimmune disorder, an allergy, or a reaction to toxic exposure.

Etiology: What Happens?

The semipermeable membranes that separate the circulatory capillaries from the nephrons act as filters to keep vital blood components in the bloodstream while allowing water and wastes to exit into the urinary system. An acute or chronic inflammatory reaction in these filters can compromise their effectiveness and allow important substances to leave the body through the urine, while allowing toxins to accumulate in the bloodstream. Glomerulonephritis is defined by an inflammatory reaction, usually in association with immune system dysfunction. The chronic inflammation leads to an accumulation of scar tissue where only soft, pliable epithelium should be; this means the kidneys become progressively less able to manage fluids in the body, and it may lead to chronic *renal failure* (this chapter).

Some experts discuss glomerulonephritis in two subgroups:

- *Acute postinfectious glomerulonephritis* is a situation that follows a few weeks after an infection (usually with some type of streptococcus, as seen with strep throat or *impetigo* [Chapter 1]).

- *Mesangial glomerulonephritis* involves immune system abnormalities and the loss of erythrocytes into the urine. *Mesangial glomerulonephritis* is associated with human immunodeficiency virus/acquired immune deficiency syndrome (*HIV/AIDS*), *mononucleosis* (Chapter 5), *celiac disease*, and *cirrhosis* (Chapter 7).

When the body launches a specific immune system attack against an invader, a variety of things can happen. One mechanism involves the formation of "immune complexes": sticky bits of antigens and antibodies, often accompanied by *complement* (a series of immune system chemicals that are meant to aid in the destruction of invading pathogens). Under normal circumstances, these clumps of material would be consumed by macrophages. Occasionally they can develop in or get caught by the glomeruli, leading to a localized inflammatory reaction. This seems to be the case in many types of glomerulonephritis.

It is not always clear what leads to the development of immune complexes in the kidneys. For some people, this is connected to autoimmune dysfunction; glomerulonephri-

 Glomerulus

This is the diminutive form of the Latin word *glomus*, for "ball of yarn," which is an excellent description of the tufts of capillary loops that allow for diffusion and filtration in the kidneys.

Glomerulonephritis in Brief

Pronunciation
glö-mär'ū-lö-nef-rī'tis

What is it?
Glomerulonephritis is a condition in which the glomeruli (small structures that are part of the nephron–capillary unit) become inflamed and cease to function efficiently.

How is it recognized?
Early signs and symptoms of glomerulonephritis include high blood pressure, dark or rust-colored urine, or foamy urine. Later symptoms indicate chronic renal failure and include systemic edema, fatigue, headaches, decreased urine output, rashes and discoloration of the skin, and general malaise.

Is massage indicated or contraindicated?
Symptomatic glomerulonephritis systemically contraindicates circulatory massage. This is an inflammatory condition that impairs the body's ability to manage fluid exchanges. Bodywork that does not significantly impact circulation may be appropriate.

tis is a possible complication of *lupus* (Chapter 5) or other autoimmune diseases. Many people who have glomerulonephritis have also been exposed to environmental toxins (notably hydrocarbons, silicon, mercury, and lithium), which opens the possibility that this disorder may arise as a kind of hypersensitivity reaction along with an inflammatory response to immune complexes.

Prognosis

Depending on the cause, glomerulonephritis can be a short-term acute infection with complete recovery (this is usually the case when it accompanies a streptococcal infection), or a long-term progressive condition in which the kidneys are slowly destroyed, leading to end-stage renal failure and dependence on dialysis. No preventive or curative measures have been developed. Some varieties of this disease have been known to recur even after the kidneys have been replaced.

Signs and Symptoms

When the kidneys function inefficiently, the repercussions are felt throughout the rest of the body. However, it may take a long time to see the results. Early symptoms of glomerulonephritis are abnormalities in the urine such as high protein levels or red blood cells. Hematuria, or blood in the urine, can be observed as dark or rust-colored urine. Protein in the urine makes it look foamy. Occasionally, no observable signs develop. Glomerulonephritis is sometimes found only when a routine analysis reveals higher-than-normal levels of protein or blood in the urine.

Another indicator of glomerulonephritis is *hypertension* (Chapter 4). This is both a symptom and a complication of most chronic kidney disorders because a disruption in urine output causes fluid retention and external pressure on all blood vessels. Hypertension that does not respond to normal interventions can sometimes lead to a diagnosis of glomerulonephritis.

Later symptoms of glomerulonephritis are indicators of renal failure, including general malaise, skin discoloration, itching, fatigue, anemia, low urine output, systemic edema, and, in very severe cases, lethargy, confusion, and coma.

Treatment

The treatment for this disease depends entirely on the cause and is generally geared toward symptom abatement. Controlling high blood pressure is the first priority; this may be done with diuretics or angiotensin-converting enzyme (ACE) inhibitors. If glomerulonephritis is a complication of a general infection, antibiotics may lead to a complete recovery. If it is an autoimmune or other inflammatory problem, steroids may be used to limit damage to the nephrons. Cytotoxic drugs also are used to inhibit the damaging effects of an immune system attack against the kidneys.

Massage?

This is a condition in which the kidneys are inflamed from a pathogen, an autoimmune reaction, or some unknown reason. The result is a person who may have an infection, who probably has high blood pressure, and who is incapable of processing fluids under normal conditions, much less under the increased volume that massage may produce. Glomerulonephritis systemically contraindicates circulatory massage, although many noncirculatory techniques can yield important benefits without challenging fluid flow.

Kidney Stones

Definition: What Are They?

Also called renal calculi or ***nephrolithiases***, kidney stones are crystals that sometimes develop in the renal pelvis. The size of kidney stones varies widely, depending on how long they have been developing and what they are made of. Most stones range between the size of grains of sand to approximately 1 inch in diameter. Some stones are much larger, growing into the cortex of the kidney, forming what is called a *staghorn calculus* (Figure 9.2).

Small stones may pass through the urinary tract with no symptoms, but larger ones may get stuck in the ureters. The technical name for them in this location is ***ureterolithiases***.

Demographics: Who Gets Them?

Kidney stones usually form in the absence of adequate fluids. Thus, they are very common in tropical environments where people tend to lose more liquid through sweat than they replace. Peak months for the diagnosis of kidney stones in the United States are June through August, for the same reason. The incidence of kidney stones in the United States is rising, particularly in the southeast. This has given rise to the term "stone belt" for this part of the country.

Men with kidney stones outnumber women by approximately three to one. Kidney stones happen more frequently among whites than among other races. Every year, approximately 1 million people in the United States pass a stone; this accounts for almost half a million emergency room visits per year. It is predicted that about 10% of all

Figure 9.2. Staghorn calculus.

Americans will pass a stone at some time. Most people who are susceptible to kidney stones get their first one between 20 and 30 years of age, and 75% of them will experience at least one repeat stone sometime in their lifetime.

Etiology: What Happens?

Kidney stones can be composed of several different substances, each one indicative of a different type of metabolic problem.

- **Calcium oxalate** *or* **calcium phosphate** *stones.* These account for the largest majority of kidney stones, from 75% to 85%. They are associated with parathyroid dysfunction (too much calcium is pulled off the bones into the bloodstream), too much Vitamin D, abnormally high rates of calcium absorption in the gastrointestinal tract, abnormal leakage of calcium or phosphate into the nephrons, or other problems.
- **Struvite** *stones.* These stones are associated with chronic *urinary tract infection* (this chapter). Approximately 5% to 15% of all kidney stones are struvite stones.
- *Uric acid stones.* These stones form in the kidneys of people whose blood is abnormally acidic. Accounting for about 5% to 15% of all kidney stones, uric acid stones are associated with a diet high in meat and purines. People who have uric acid kidney stones are also at high risk for *gout* (Chapter 2).
- *Cystine stones.* These stones are relatively rare, constituting only 2% of all kidney stones. They are directly related to a genetic dysfunction with the metabolism of cystine, an amino acid.
- *Other stones.* A tiny percentage of all kidney stones fall outside the four main categories. Genetic problems with metabolism or the use of protease inhibitors (see *HIV/AIDS*, Chapter 5) are usually the causes of these stones.

Signs and Symptoms

Most kidney stones are completely silent: 85% or more of them pass through the ureters without pain. When they get stuck or when they are large enough to scrape the delicate lining of the urinary tract, however, kidney stones cause a typical extreme "grabbing pain." The ureters contract in irritation, causing renal colic. The pain has a sudden onset, comes and goes in waves, and can be so severe that it causes nausea and vomiting as a sympathetic reaction. The pain often refers into the groin area. Occasionally the stone may be caused by or may lead to an infection in the kidneys; in these instances, fever and chills accompany the severe pain.

Complications

Most kidney stones that are big enough to cause problems are excruciatingly painful, but they do eventually pass into the bladder and out in the urine without causing long-lasting damage to the urinary system. Occasionally, however, a stone can grow to be of a size to seriously disrupt kidney function. This may lead to chronic or acute *renal failure* (this chapter).

Diagnosis

Many silent kidney stones are found during routine abdominal x-rays. People reporting kidney stone pain may undergo a computed tomography (CT) **urogram**. This is a highly sensitive test that can identify the size and location of any kidney stones, and can rule out

Case History 9.1

Kidney Stones

Walter B, Age 77: "Once You've Had a Kidney Stone, You Never Forget It."

I've had kidney stone attacks since 1939, then in 1944, and so on and so forth. The first time I was 19 years old. I'd been horseback riding the day before, so when the pain started we figured I had just thrown my back out somehow. The director of the hospital finally detected what it really was.

In 1944 I had an attack at night, in bed. Once you've had a kidney stone attack, you never forget what it feels like. I knew immediately what was happening, and they rushed me via command car to the military hospital, 20 miles away from the Battle of the Bulge. The renal surgeon authorized an attempt to remove the stone with an uteroscopic tube. Back in those days the tube was metal, not flexible—hence the discomfort, which I've never forgotten. The procedure was unsuccessful because somehow I had already passed the stone.

The doctor said that I had "anomalous kidneys."

"What the hell does that mean?" I asked.

"It just means they're unlike any kidneys I've ever seen," he said.

After these two incidents, I wasn't given any further treatment or medication. I was just told to drink plenty of liquids.

I had another attack in the 1960s. I was visiting a friend in Swampscott and had to try to drive 25 miles into Boston without killing myself or anyone else—quite an ordeal. But I never passed a whole stone; they all turned to gravel.

Then in the Blizzard of '78, I had my last attack. Boston was digging out from a huge snowstorm. No one was allowed to drive; the streets had to be clear for ambulances and fire trucks. The pain was God-awful, just unbearable. They always say it's like having a baby—you just wouldn't believe it. I couldn't get to the hospital right away, so the doctor told me to drink some whiskey to dull the pain. Finally, I was given special dispensation to take a taxicab to the hospital.

In the hospital, they put a tube up the urethra to try to "basket" the stone. That was the only one they ever got. I remember, I was laying on my side with the sheet like a big tent draped over me. I just had a local anesthetic, and when the doctor finally got the stone, he dropped it on my sheet—it sounded just like a pebble dropping.

When the stone was basketed at the hospital, it was sent to the kidney stone lab, where it was identified as a calcium stone. The medication consisted of Allopurinol tablets and hydrochlorothiazide pills taken daily. There's been no sign of an attack since then.

About 4 years ago, I had another uteroscopic procedure as part of a regular examination. The urologist used a new flexible tube (not like the metal one from 1944!). The whole thing took about 4 minutes and involved a minimum of discomfort. Several of my friends, though, have had attacks within the past year or two, and their treatment and recovery seemed to be much more painful and prolonged than mine, in spite of all the new techniques available.

any other disorders that may mimic kidney stones, including gallstones, abdominal aneurysm, diverticular disease, pancreatitis, and others.

Other tests to look for kidney stones include x-rays, ultrasound, and *intravenous pyelography*: a test in which dye is injected and observed for how it moves through the kidneys.

Treatment

The pain of kidney stones is so intense that long ago people operated on them without anesthesia; "cutting for stone" was considered worth living through, just to get rid of them. Nowadays several other options are available, and only a small percentage of kidney stone patients have to go through major surgery. Three main interventions for kidney stones have been developed. Which one is appropriate is determined by the stones' size, location, and the general health of the patient.

- *Percutaneous nephrolithotomy* is a surgery conducted through a tiny tunnel in the back leading to the stone, which is either extracted or subjected to sonic waves that reduce its size.
- *Uteroscopic stone removal* uses a flexible tube that is inserted into the urethra and snakes up to where the stone is lodged to remove it from the ureters.
- *Extracorporeal shockwave lithotripsy* is the use of sound waves to break up stones into a size that can be passed through the ureters with minimal risk for getting stuck. This procedure can leave the patient feeling bruised and battered from the extremity of the shock waves that are required to break up stones, but it can treat larger deposits than either of the other two options.

Preventive treatments for persons susceptible to kidney stones depend on what constitutes the stones. This is why it is necessary for patients to catch their stones as they pass with the urine. The stones are then analyzed, as is the urine passed, within a 24-hour period after the stone passes. A treatment program is developed based on these findings.

Some interventions include surgery to remove the parathyroid glands, medication to regulate metabolism, dietary adjustments, and most importantly adequate hydration. Kidney stone patients need to drink up to 1 gallon of water every day to keep stones moving through the system before they become big enough to cause problems. Patients are also frequently recommended to limit caffeine, alcohol, and oxalate-rich foods (dark leafy vegetables, nuts, and chocolate) to reduce the risk of future stones.

Massage?

Massage for people with a history of kidney stones but who no present symptoms is perfectly appropriate. However, a person with or without a history of kidney stones who is experiencing *any* symptoms of renal colic is not a good candidate for massage.

Pyelonephritis

Pyelonephritis in Brief

What is it?
Pyelonephritis is an infection of the kidney or renal pelvis.

How is it recognized?
Symptoms of acute pyelonephritis include burning pain with urination, back pain, fever, chills, nausea, and vomiting. Chronic infections may show no symptoms.

Is massage indicated or contraindicated?
Kidney infections systemically contraindicate circulatory massage until the infection has been completely eradicated.

Definition: What Is It?

As the name implies, *pyelonephritis* is an infection of the nephrons in the kidney, although the renal pelvis also may be involved. Acute infections present severe symptoms, but chronic infections may be silent while kidney function progressively diminishes.

Etiology: What Happens?

Most kidney infections are a complication of an *Escherichia coli* infection in the urinary tract that travels up the ureters to set up an infection in the kidneys (see *urinary tract infection*, this chapter). Other kidney infections can develop from more obscure pathogens. They also can be related to *diabetes* (Chapter 8) or pregnancy, they can arise from a neurogenic bladder (a bladder that has no motor control and so empties passively into a bag), or they can come from surgical or medical instrumentation such as catheters or cystoscopes. Some kidney infections can be a complication of a *kidney stone* (this chapter) or an enlarged prostate that blocks the ureters (see *benign prostatic hyperplasia* and *prostate cancer*, Chapter 10).

Signs and Symptoms

Acute pyelonephritis usually involves the rapid onset of symptoms that begin with a urinary tract infection and move deeper into the body. They include fever, burning and frequency of urination, cloudy urine, extreme back pain, fatigue, nausea, and vomiting. Symptoms typically develop over a 1- to 2-day period.

Chronic pyelonephritis in adults is often a situation in which an acute infection has been incompletely treated, and so bacterial invasion of the kidney continues but in a quieter fashion. Therefore, many chronic kidney infections are silent; they create no symptoms, but damage accumulates in the kidney. When chronic pyelonephritis occurs in children, it is typically related to a structural anomaly at the vesicoureteral valve. This condition, called *vesicoureteral reflux* (VUR), allows urine to back up into the kidney, which creates a high risk of long-term, silent, cumulative damage.

Complications

Regardless of whether the situation is chronic or acute, if pyelonephritis is recurrent, it can cause scarring and long-lasting kidney damage. Insufficient kidney activity leads to *hypertension* (Chapter 4) and *renal failure* (this chapter). Another possible complication of a very acute infection is sepsis (blood poisoning from the infection leaking into capillaries). This is a life-threatening situation that can lead rapidly to dangerously *low* blood pressure and death.

Diagnosis

Urinalysis to look for signs of infection, combined with symptoms that describe pain higher and more extreme than found with a typical urinary tract infection, is usually enough information for a diagnosis of kidney infection. If the infectious agent is something unusual, more tests may be needed. CT scans or intravenous pyelograms are sometimes used to look for kidney stones or tumors that might be causing problems or abscesses on the kidneys that can create similar symptoms.

Treatment

Most kidney infections clear up satisfactorily with antibiotic therapy. If the infection is very extreme, the patient may need to be hospitalized to monitor how well he or she is processing fluids. Some patients need to be monitored especially closely; these include people with *diabetes*, *spinal cord injury* survivors (Chapter 3), and kidney transplant recipients.

Prevention

Acute pyelonephritis is almost always related to bacteria that enter the body at the urethral opening. Let this be a lesson, ladies: always wipe front to back.

Massage?

Acute kidney infections contraindicate circulatory bodywork. The risk of making the situation worse is matched only by the patient's inability to lie still because the pain is so extreme. Chronic kidney infections are less dramatic, but the kidneys are still vulnerable to damage. The safest course is to avoid any circulatory work until all signs of infection have been eradicated.

Renal Failure

Renal Failure in Brief

What is it?
Renal failure is a situation in which the kidneys are incapable of functioning at normal levels. It may be an acute or a chronic problem, and it is potentially life-threatening.

How is it recognized?
Symptoms of acute and chronic renal failure differ in severity and type of onset, but some things they have in common are reduced urine output, systemic edema, and changes in mental state brought about by the accumulation of toxins in the blood.

Is massage indicated or contraindicated?
Acute and chronic renal failure systemically contraindicate circulatory massage.

Definition: What Is It?

Renal failure means that for various reasons the kidneys are not functioning adequately. If the kidneys slow down suddenly (e.g., in response to shock or systemic infection), this is referred to as *acute renal failure*. If they sustain cumulative damage over the course of many months or years, this is called *chronic renal failure*. In either case, although the name implies that they have ceased functioning altogether, the truth is that the kidneys are still working, but they are simply unable to keep up with the body's demands.

Demographics: Who Gets It?

Statistics for renal failure vary according to whether it is an acute or chronic problem. Risk factors for developing chronic renal failure are having chronic *hypertension* (Chapter 4), *diabetes* (Chapter 8), or *glomerulonephritis* (this chapter). Some incidence of renal failure is determined by geographic distribution, suggesting the influence of environmental toxins. Race is also a determining factor: African-Americans are far more likely to experience both chronic high blood pressure and chronic renal failure than whites.

Some researchers suggest that as many as 20 million Americans are in early stages of kidney disease, although at this stage this condition is silent, so it usually goes undiagnosed. Statistics for end-stage renal disease (ESRD) are also alarming. This serious condition is diagnosed approximately 89,000 times each year, and an estimated 366,000 people in the United States currently live with it. The incidence of ESRD has risen 7% per year since 1978.

Etiology: What Happens?

Although the kidneys are able to heal from most short-term abuse, any chronic or severe recurrent problems may eventually cause permanent damage to the delicate tissues, thereby interfering with kidney function. Fortunately, the human body is equipped with approximately twice as much kidney as it absolutely needs, so people can tolerate a large extent of damage before problems develop.

Kidneys have several important functions: they produce EPO, the hormone that stimulates blood cell production; they manage electrolyte levels in the blood; they concentrate urine; and they manage overall fluid levels. One of the important functions of the kidneys, controlling the levels of certain minerals, is extremely compromised during renal failure. Consequently, circulating levels of calcium, phosphorus, and potassium are dangerously changed. This has important impact on bone density, digestive capabilities, the inflammatory process, and heart rhythms.

Kidney failure is classified as acute or chronic.

Acute Renal Failure

Acute renal failure (ARF) is identified when kidney function suddenly drops to 50% or less of normal levels; this may take place over several hours or days. Causes of acute renal failure usually fall into one of three categories.

- *Prerenal problems.* This means something prevents blood flow into the kidneys, so the glomeruli and nephrons essentially collapse from lack of fluid volume. Prerenal problems can include reduced blood volume, low blood pressure from septicemia or traumatic shock, extreme dehydration, or an embolism that blocks the renal artery.

- *Intrarenal problems.* These are pathologic conditions that arise within the kidneys themselves, including glomerulonephritis, an embolism caught inside the kidney, an *E. coli* infection that produces tissue-damaging toxins (this is also called **hemolytic uremic syndrome**), drug reactions, and other problems.

- *Postrenal problems.* When fluid is prevented from leaving the kidneys, damage to the delicate nephrons can accumulate to dangerous levels. *Kidney stones* (this chapter), *enlarged prostate* (Chapter 10), or tumors can create this kind of problem.

Acute renal failure is generally a short-term problem that may become life-threatening. Its mortality rate is usually connected to the general health and resiliency of the patient. It may last for days or weeks, but if the contributing factors are controllable, kidney function may be restored. Some patients, however, eventually develop chronic renal failure.

Chronic Renal Failure

Chronic renal failure (CRF) is an impairment in kidney function that may persist for months or years before it causes any symptoms.

Kidney function is measured in terms of **glomerular filtration rate** (GFR), that is, how efficiently fluid moves from the glomeruli into the nephrons.

- Normal GFR is 120 mL/minute.

- Chronic renal insufficiency, a silent condition, is identified with GFR of 30 to 70 mL/minute.

- Chronic renal failure as diagnosed with GFR is under 30 mL/minute.

- End-stage renal disease occurs when GFR is under 10 mL/minute.

Diabetes mellitus is the most common cause of CRF, followed by chronic hypertension, glomerulonephritis, and other more obscure causes.

Signs and Symptoms

Because the kidneys have so many functions, symptoms of renal failure affect virtually every major organ system of the body. Symptoms include decreased urine output, systemic *edema* from salt and water retention (Chapter 5), arrhythmia from potassium retention, *anemia* from the lack of EPO (Chapter 4), and osteomalacia (bone thinning) from the lack of vitamin D (which is necessary for calcium metabolism). Rashes and skin discoloration arise from the retention of toxic pigments in the blood. Other symptoms include lethargy, fatigue, headaches, loss of sensation in the hands and feet, tremors, seizures, easy bruising and bleeding, muscle cramps, and changes in mental and emotional states as the accumulation of wastes in the blood affects the brain.

Treatment

Treatment for acute and chronic renal failure is determined by whatever underlying pathologic conditions caused the damage. Treatment goals are to control the symptoms, prevent further complications, and slow the progress of the disease. This often means aggressively controlling blood pressure and blood sugar levels (if diabetes is part of the picture). Medication to control potassium levels in the blood is important to avoid heart problems. Fluid and salt intake may be restricted until kidney function can keep up with the body's demands. Diuretics are sometimes prescribed to help the kidneys process fluids.

If a patient's kidneys are simply incompetent regardless of these interventions, dialysis may become necessary. This routes the blood through a machine or through the peritoneum to extract wastes from the blood. Approximately 200,000 people in the United States use kidney dialysis to stay alive.

Kidney transplants replace a damaged organ with a healthy kidney from an appropriate donor. They can be successful if the new tissue is not rejected. Unfortunately, the shortage of suitable donated organs means that among the 52,000 people waiting for kidney transplants this year, only 15,000 operations will be performed.

Massage?

Any stage of renal failure contraindicates circulatory massage, although energy work may be supportive and helpful. If a client has a history of renal failure, the massage therapist should inform the health care team that the client wishes to receive massage.

Massage for transplant recipients may be appropriate, if it fits within the stresses of normal activities of daily living. Therapists should be aware that organ transplant recipients commit to a lifetime of immunosuppressant medications, and so they are at risk for some infections that the rest of the population does not have to worry about.

BLADDER AND URINARY TRACT DISORDERS

Bladder Cancer

Definition: What Is It?

Bladder cancer is the development of malignant cells in the urinary bladder.

Demographics: Who Gets It?

Bladder cancer is a relatively common disease. It is the fourth leading cancer among men (following lung, prostate, and colorectal cancers), and the eighth leading cancer among women. Approximately 54,000 new cases are diagnosed each year, and it causes an estimated 12,000 deaths each year in the United States. Rates of diagnosis of this disease increased by 36% per year between 1984 and 1993. Currently approximately 300,000 people in the United States live with bladder cancer.

Bladder cancer occurs in men approximately 3 times more often than in women. It affects white men more than any other group, but women and African-American men usually have poorer survival rates than white men. It is usually a disease of older people; the average age at diagnosis is 68 years.

Bladder Cancer in Brief

What is it?
Bladder cancer is the growth of malignant cells in the urinary bladder. Most bladder cancer starts in the superficial layer of transitional epithelium.

How is it recognized?
The earliest sign of bladder cancer is the appearance of blood in the urine, which may be red or rust colored. Bladder cancer is painless at this point. In later stages the bladder may become irritable. Painful urination, reduced urination, or increased urinary frequency all may occur.

Is massage indicated or contraindicated?
As with most varieties of cancer, massage with its parasympathetic effects and immune system support has a place in the recovery process. Bladder cancer has a high recurrence rate and most patients undergo surgery at some point. As long as these issues are respected and the massage therapist works as part of a well-informed health care team, bodywork may be appropriate for these patients.

Etiology: What Happens?

Like most types of cancer, most cases of bladder cancer involve epithelial cells, in this case, the transitional epithelium that lines the urinary bladder. Constant, repetitive damage to this epithelium causes the mature cells to die. This stimulates rapid replication in the basal layer, and soon new colonies of immature cells migrate to the surface. These new cells are easily disrupted by genetic mutations and may become malignant growths that cause bleeding into the bladder.

Causes of bladder cancer vary according to medical history and geographic region. Persons who have undergone pelvic radiation for other problems are at an increased risk for developing bladder cancer, as are people who have had chronic infections, bladder stones, or catheter use. In Africa, Asia, and South America, bladder cancer is associated with a specific parasitic infestation, *Schistosoma haematobium*.

In the United States and European countries, most cases of bladder cancer are directly related to more controllable factors. The transitional epithelium of the bladder seems to be particularly susceptible to damage from environmental toxins. Several genetic mutations that limit the body's ability to inhibit tumor growth or invasion have been linked to bladder cancer. These mutations are frequently triggered by exposure to carcinogenic substances. Approximately half of all bladder cancer cases are believed to be related to cigarette smoking. Other contributing factors include exposure to aromatic amines (chemicals used in dry cleaning fluid, hairdressing chemicals, and textile and rubber industries). The relationship between bladder cancer and carcinogenic substances is one of the most clearly demonstrable links between environmental exposures and cancer. The good news is that bladder cancer is probably a completely preventable disease, if exposure to the carcinogenic substances is limited or eradicated.

Signs and Symptoms

The earliest and most dependable sign of bladder cancer is hematuria, or blood in the urine. The urine of a bladder cancer patient is often visibly reddened or rust colored, although the patient experiences no particular pain in the early stages of the disease. If the tumors continue to grow and invade deeper layers of the bladder, secondary symptoms may develop that are related to mechanical pressure, including bladder irritability (painful urination, increased urinary frequency, reduced urine output) and compression on the rectum, pelvic lymph nodes, and any other structures that happen to be in the way. For information about the staging protocol for bladder cancer, see sidebar, "Staging Protocols for Bladder Cancer."

Diagnosis

If a person in his 60s or 70s has no pain, but his urine is bright red or rusty, the immediate conclusion most doctors will come to is that he has bladder cancer. Urine samples may be tested to look for shedding cancer cells, and a digital rectal

---

Staging Protocols for Bladder Cancer

Bladder cancer is staged based on the depth of invasion of new growths. Many specialists now use the TNM staging system to help define stages 0 through IV. This protocol shows how bladder cancer without distant metastasis may be diagnosed as stage IV, indicating the high risk of recurrence and deep invasion.

Tumor	Node	Metastasis
Tx: unassessable	Nx: unassessable	Mx: unassessable
T0: no evidence of a tumor	N0: no nodal involvement	M0: no distant metastasis
Ta: noninvasive papillary carcinoma		
T-IS: in situ ("flat tumor")	N1: 1 node is involved; it is under 2 cm in diameter	M1: distant metastasis
T1: tumor invades the subepithelial connective tissue	N2: 1 node is involved; it is between 2 and 5 cm; *or* multiple nodes under 5 cm.	
T2: tumor invades the muscular layer of the bladder	N3: nodes over 5 cm may be involved	
T3: tumor invades the perivesical tissue (tissue around the bladder) bladder)		
T4: tumor invades the prostate, uterus, vagina, pelvic wall, or abdominal wall		

Stage	T	N	M
0a	Ta	N0	M0
0-IS	T-IS	N0	M0
I	T1	N0	M0
II	T2	N0	M0
III	T3–T4	N0	M0
IV	T3–T4	N1-N3	M0-M1

examination (or pelvic examination if the patient is a woman) provides information about tumors. Other diagnostic techniques include using dye to stain the urine and make the bladder easy to radiograph; using a cystoscope, with which a physician visually examines the bladder through a tube inserted through the urethra; and performing local biopsies to examine abnormal tissue for signs of metastasis.

Treatment

Bladder cancer treatment depends on what stage it is in when it is diagnosed. Surgeons can use a small wire loop on the end of a cystoscope to remove abnormal tissue, or another tool may be used to burn the tumor away with electricity. More invasive surgeries may remove part or all of the bladder, and if signs of pelvic metastasis are present, other tissues as well. Men may lose the prostate gland; women may lose the uterus, ovaries, and parts of the vaginal wall. Pelvic lymph nodes are also removed, leading to the risk of lymphedema in the legs. Urine flow may be routed out of the body through a stoma, or a variety of surgeries have been developed to form artificial bladders from parts of the large or small intestines.

In addition to surgery, radiation and chemotherapy may be used to battle bladder cancer. Chemotherapy may be administered intravenously, orally with pills, or through a site-specific bladder wash to distribute the medication directly to the target tissues.

Prognosis

Most bladder cancer cases are diagnosed before the cells have moved out of the bladder. This is excellent news, of course, because the survival rate for cancers caught early is much better than for cancers caught in stage 3 or later. Nevertheless, bladder cancer has an unusual habit of growing in several places at the same time, so although it may be possible to catch one or two tumors, the invisible third, fourth, and fifth tumors may not become symptomatic for another several months. This means that the recurrence rate for bladder cancer is surprisingly high: up to 80% of all patients have at least one recurrence of their cancer during their lifetime.

Overall, the 5-year survival rate for bladder cancer is 76% for whites and 55% for African-Americans. All bladder cancer patients must follow up their treatment with lifelong regular examinations to guard against recurrence.

Massage?

The main issues of concern in working with bladder cancer patients are the high rates of recurrence and the frequency with which surgery is an early treatment intervention. The rules for massage and bladder cancer are the same as the rules for massage and any kind of cancer. Although the benefits that bodywork has to offer in the way of immune system strengthening, pain reduction, anxiety reduction, and general support are powerful, massage therapists need to be working as part of a team, sharing information and concerns with the rest of the client's health care staff.

Interstitial Cystitis

Definition: What Is It?

Interstitial cystitis (IC) is a condition in which the urinary bladder becomes small and inelastic. It is not to be confused with ordinary cystitis, which is a complication of a *urinary tract infection* (this chapter).

Demographics: Who Gets It?

Statistics on IC have been difficult to gather, but it is estimated that somewhere between 700,000 and 1 million Americans have it. Of those, 90% are women, 10% are men. IC is rare in children. The population group most at risk is women between 20 and 50 years of age; the average age at onset is 43.

Etiology: What Happens?

The bladder, a hollow organ, is designed to shrink when it is empty and expand when it is full. A healthy bladder can hold about 1 to 1.5 cups of urine. The average adult passes approximately 1 to 1.5 quarts of urine every day, depending on how much liquid has been consumed and a number of other factors.

Normal urine is composed of water, excess salts extracted from the blood, nitrogenous wastes such as urea and uric acid, and other debris. It should not contain any living microorganisms. Fragments of white blood cells or pathogens indicate an infection somewhere in the urinary system. The bladder itself is shielded from the acidity of urine by a lining of protective mucus.

IC occurs when the inner lining of the bladder no longer protects the organ from urine. Most IC patients develop tiny bleeding areas called pinpoint hemorrhages in the bladder wall. Approximately 10% of patients develop a particular lesion called a Hunner's ulcer inside the bladder. As the problem progresses, the muscular walls of the bladder become fibrotic and inelastic. Patients find that they have little capacity for storing urine; it is not unusual for them to have to use the bathroom about every 20 minutes.

The cause of IC is a mystery. One theory is that this may be an autoimmune disease or allergy that weakens the protective mucous membrane in the bladder's epithelium. In this way, irritating chemicals from urine can infiltrate and damage the bladder wall. The presence of abnormal numbers of mast cells in some IC patients supports this theory. A pathologic thinning of the mucous membrane on the bladder wall is another factor to consider. Other researchers are considering the possibility that the causative agent for IC may be some pathologic agent that has yet to be identified. IC does not respond to antibiotic therapy, so it is clear that no known strain of bacteria causes this problem.

Signs and Symptoms

Symptoms of IC include chronic pelvic pain, pain and burning on urination, increased frequency, urgency, and painful intercourse. Symptoms tend to progressively worsen for about 5 years and then stabilize. Some patients find that symptoms occur in periods of flare and remission; others find that their daily experiences are all about the same.

Diagnosis

IC is diagnosed by a process of exclusion. Conditions that must be ruled out for a positive diagnosis include *urinary tract infections*, vaginitis, *bladder cancer*, *kidney stones* (this chapter), *endometriosis* for women, and *prostatitis* (both in Chapter 10) for men. Once other pathologic conditions have been ruled out, a cystoscopic examination may be conducted to look for ulcers or bleeding spots, which can only be seen when the bladder is fully distended.

Interstitial Cystitis in Brief

Pronunciation
in-ter-stish'ăl

What is it?
Interstitial cystitis (IC) is a chronic inflammation of the bladder involving scar tissue, stiffening, decreased capacity, pinpoint hemorrhages, and sometimes ulcers in the bladder walls.

How is it recognized?
Symptoms of IC are very much like those of urinary tract infections: burning, increased frequency and urgency of urination; decreased capacity of the bladder; and pain, pressure, and tenderness.

Is massage indicated or contraindicated?
IC is a poorly understood condition that seems to be exacerbated by stress. Bodywork may be a helpful and supportive choice for IC patients, although it probably does not work to reverse the situation.

Treatment

Because this is a disease without a known cause, it is also without a known cure. IC treatment is generally aimed at symptomatic relief and the development of coping skills. Often the diagnostic tool of bladder distension can give relief, as can a "distillation" or bladder wash. This is done with *dimethyl sulfoxide* (DMSO), which can pass into the bladder wall to act as an anti-inflammatory and block pain sensation. Other bladder washes using hyaluronic acid or heparin are being explored. An oral medication to help rebuild the mucous lining has recently been approved for use. Aspirin and other painkillers may be recommended, as are exercise, smoking cessation, and dietary changes. No single intervention is successful for all patients, however, and nothing has yet provided a permanent solution. IC may recur after months or even years of remission.

Some patients have such severe problems that surgery becomes an option. They may have a new bladder constructed from a segment of the colon, or they may have the bladder removed altogether and replaced with a stoma and external bag.

Massage?

Among the interventions IC patients may need to explore are options to reduce the stress and anxiety that accompany chronic, painful conditions. Acupuncture, hypnotherapy, biofeedback, and other therapies may be recommended. Massage can be a useful tool in this effort too, as long as the client's need for frequent urination can be met.

Urinary Tract Infection

Definition: What Is It?

Urinary tract infections (UTIs) are infections that may occur anywhere in the urinary system, from the kidneys to the bladder to the urethra. Because kidney infections are discussed elsewhere (see *pyelonephritis*, this chapter), this section focuses on infections of the lower urinary tract: the urethra (urethritis) and the bladder (cystitis).

Demographics: Who Gets It?

UTIs are the cause of approximately 7 million visits to the doctor every year. Estimates vary, but somewhere between 20% and 50% of all women will have a UTI at least once. It is almost always a women's disorder because the female urethra is so short and located close to the anus, where bacteria that are harmless in the digestive tract can create problems if they gain access to the urinary tract.

Although women, particularly sexually active young women, are most at risk for UTIs, other populations also may have this problem. It is certainly possible for men to have a UTI; this is sometimes the warning sign of something potentially serious, such as prostate problems (see *prostate cancer* and *benign prostatic hyperplasia*, Chapter 10). People who must drain their bladder with a catheter are virtually assured of eventually having a UTI; their chances rise an estimated 5% per day of catheter use.

Urinary Tract Infection in Brief

What is it?
A urinary tract infection (UTI) is an infection of the urinary tract, usually from bacteria that live harmlessly in the digestive tract.

How is it recognized?
Symptoms of UTI include pain and burning sensations during urination, increased urinary frequency, urgency, and cloudy or blood-tinged urine. Abdominal, pelvic, or low back pain may occur. In the acute stage, fever and general malaise may be present.

Is massage indicated or contraindicated?
Acute UTIs contraindicate circulatory massage, as do all acute infections. Massage may be appropriate in the subacute stage, although deep work on the abdomen is still locally cautioned until all signs of infection are gone.

Etiology: What Happens?

Under normal circumstances, the environment in the bladder is sterile. The urine contains waste products to be expelled from the body, but no living microorganisms should be present. Furthermore, the bladder is lined with a protective mucus-producing layer of cells that works to prevent infectious or noxious agents from harming the bladder walls.

Sometimes foreign microorganisms are introduced into the urethra. If the circumstances are right, they can cling to the mucous lining of the urethra or the bladder, and set up an infection that may stay localized or may travel further into the urinary system.

Causes

Escherichia coli is the causative agent behind close to 90% of all UTIs. These strains of bacteria live normally and harmlessly in the digestive tract. Certain varieties of staphylococcus cause a small percentage of UTIs, and other agents including Klebsiella, Chlamydia, and Mycoplasma are behind a minority of infections. It is important to identify the correct causative agent, because not all of them respond to the same antibiotics.

Chronic irritation also can contribute to the development of UTIs. "Honeymoon cystitis" refers to inflammation and subsequent infection brought about by repeated friction and irritation of the urethra from sexual activity.

The relationship between stress and UTIs has much anecdotal support. Living in a sympathetic state may reduce blood flow to the bladder, which in turn may make it more susceptible to infection. However, clinical evidence shows that although stress may aggravate symptoms of UTIs, it has not been proved to cause them.

Risk Factors

Some women have been found to be more susceptible to UTIs than others, although the reasons for this are not completely clear. Some factors, however, are reliable predictors of who will develop a UTI:

- *Spermicides.* Spermicide foams and jellies used with diaphragms or alone have been shown to raise the risk of UTIs in some women.

- *Diaphragm use.* Women who use diaphragms show statistically higher rates of UTIs than women who do not.

- *Pregnancy.* Pregnant women do not necessarily get more UTIs than women who are not pregnant, but the risk of having a simple infection complicate into a more dangerous one is higher for these patients.

- *Diabetes.* Elevated sugar levels in the urine make a hospitable environment for bacteria to grow in the bladder.

- *Neurogenic bladder.* If a bladder has lost motor function, it does not empty as completely as a normal one. *Neurogenic bladder* raises the potential for infection, as does the presence of catheter tubes, which are used for people with limited bladder function.

Signs and Symptoms

The symptoms of UTIs are painful, burning urination; a frequent need to urinate; reduced bladder capacity; urgency; and blood-tinged or cloudy urine. Pelvic, abdominal, or low back pain also may occur. Men with UTIs may experience pain in the penis or scrotum. If severe flank or back pain and fever develop, a kidney infection should be suspected.

Complications

Bacteria that live in the digestive tract cause almost all UTIs. If the bacteria are able to travel up the system, they may set up an infection in the bladder (cystitis). (This is not to be confused with *interstitial cystitis*, this chapter). If the infection remains unchecked, it may move all the way up the ureters and into the kidneys, causing a kidney infection (see *pyelonephritis*, this chapter) Chronic UTIs may contribute to chronic renal failure (this chapter). Untreated kidney infections can lead to the release of infectious bacteria in the blood (life-threatening septicemia).

Unfortunately, not all UTIs show symptoms, so they may be neglected. It is possible for some people to experience extreme complications of this type of infection that can easily lead to permanent kidney damage or even to death.

Treatment

The first step in self-treatment of a UTI is to drown it: radically increasing fluid intake gives the body the much needed opportunity to fully and frequently empty the bladder—not only of urine but of bacteria as well. Drinking highly acidic liquids such as blueberry or cranberry juice is helpful for many women, because an acidic environment inhibits bacterial growth. These berries also contain chemicals that limit the ability of bacteria to cling to bladder walls. It is important, however, to avoid *sweetened* juice; the amount of sugar it takes to make cranberry juice sweet may actually make the bladder a more hospitable environment for infection. In chronic, subacute situations, hydrotherapy in the form of hot and cold sitz baths may be recommended.

UTIs usually respond well to a short course of antibiotics. In this case, 3 to 5 days' worth of medication is more appropriate than 2 weeks' worth because the body concentrates antibiotics in the urine. With bladder infections, as with all types of bacterial infections, it is especially important to take the *full* prescription of antibiotics. Stopping too soon often results in recurrent infections with more highly resistant bacteria.

People who experience low-grade chronic UTIs that do not clear up with normal treatments are sometimes successfully treated with long-term low doses of antibiotics. Structural problems with the way urine drains from the bladder may contribute to chronic infections; surgery may be recommended to correct these problems.

Prevention

Some basic precautions can help prevent UTIs, especially for women who are especially vulnerable to them. These include drinking *lots* of water and acidic juices; urinating whenever necessary rather than holding it for a more convenient time; wiping from front to back after a bowel movement to prevent the introduction of digestive bacteria into the urethra; taking showers rather than baths; emptying the bladder after sex; and avoiding feminine hygiene sprays and douches that can aggravate the urethra.

Massage?

Acute UTIs are sometimes accompanied by *fever* (Chapter 5), a systemic contraindication. A small but significant risk of spreading the infection to the kidneys should also be considered. Even in the post-acute stage (after signs of acute infection have subsided), the lower abdomen is a local contraindication for massage until all signs of infection have been eradicated.

CHAPTER REVIEW QUESTIONS

1. Describe how high blood pressure can lead to kidney dysfunction.

2. Describe how kidney dysfunction can lead to high blood pressure.

3. Why do people get kidney stones more often in hot environments than in other places?

4. Why are women more likely to get urinary tract infections than men?

5. How can renal failure lead to disconnected symptoms such as itching or mental incapacitation?

6. Describe the relationship between long-term stress and urinary tract infections.

7. A client complains of transient extreme pain on one side of her mid-back. Her muscles are not particularly tender, and she shows no signs of infection. What condition is likely to be present?

8. A client who is an elderly man mentions that he has been passing blood in his urine. What condition is likely to be present?

 Answers to these questions can be found on the Student Recource CD-ROM that accompanies this book.

Bibliography

General Resources, Urinary System

1. de Dominico G, Wood E. Beard's Massage. Philadelphia: WB Saunders, 1997.
2. Damjanou I. Pathology for the Health-Related Professions. Philadelphia: WB Saunders, 1996.
3. Travell J, Simons DG. Myofascial Pain and Dysfunction: The Trigger Point Manual. Baltimore: Williams & Wilkins, 1983.
4. Clemente CD. Anatomy: A Regional Atlas of the Human Body. 3rd Ed. Baltimore: Urban & Schwarzenburg, 1987.
5. Tortora GJ, Anagnostakos NP. Principles of Anatomy and Physiology. 6th Ed. New York: Harper & Row, 1990.
6. Taber's Cyclopedic Dictionary. 14th Ed. Philadelphia: FA Davis, 1981.
7. Stedman's Medical Dictionary. 26th Ed. Baltimore: Williams & Wilkins, 1995.
8. Memmler RL, Wood DL. The Human Body in Health and Disease. 5th Ed. Philadelphia: JB Lippincott, 1983.
9. Juhan D. Job's Body: A Handbook for Bodywork. Barrytown, NY: Station Hill Press, 1987.
10. Kunz JRM, Finkel AJ, eds. The American Medical Association Family Medical Guide. New York, NY: Random House, 1987.
11. Marieb EM. Human Anatomy and Physiology. Redwood City, CA: Benjamin/Cummings, 1989.
12. Field T. Touch Therapy. London: Churchill Livingstone; 2000.

Glomerulonephritis

1. Glomerulonephritis Overview. Copyright © 1998–2004 Mayo Foundation for Medical Education and Research (MFMER). Available at: http://www.mayoclinic.com/invoke.cfm?id=DS00503. Accessed winter 2004.
2. Kazzi AA, Tehranzadeh AD. Glomerulonephritis, Acute. Copyright © 2004, eMedicine.com, Inc. Available at: http://www.emedicine.com/emerg/topic219.htm. Accessed winter 2004.
3. Glomerulonephritis. Copyright © 1996–2003 Aetna InteliHealth Inc. Available at: http://www.intelihealth.com/IH/ihtIH/WSIHW000/9339/31198.html. Accessed winter 2004.
4. Uffe Ravnskov, MD, PhD. Glomerulonephritis and Chronic Renal Failure: The Crucial Role of Chemical Exposure. Copyright © Uffe Ravnskov. Available at: http://www.ravnskov.nu/index.htm. Accessed winter 2004.

Kidney Stones

1. Kidney Stone Analysis. Copyright © 1996–2004 WebMD Inc. Available at: http://my.webmd.com/content/healthwise/107/26535.htm?lastselectedguid={5FE84E90-BC77-4056-A91C-9531713CA348}. Accessed winter 2004.
2. Kidney Stones in Adults. National Institute of Diabetes and Digestive and Kidney Diseases, National Institutes of Health. Available at: http://kidney.niddk.nih.gov/kudiseases/pubs/stonesadults/index.htm. Accessed winter 2004.
3. Kidney stones Overview. Copyright © 1998–2004 Mayo Foundation for Medical Education and Research (MFMER). Available at: http://www.mayoclinic.com/invoke.cfm?id=DS00282. Accessed winter 2004.
4. Rineer S. Kidney Stones. Copyright © 2004, eMedicine.com, Inc. Available at: http://www.emedicine.com/aaem/topic280.htm. Accessed winter 2004.

Pyelonephritis

1. Asinger A. Acute Pyelonephritis. Copyright © 1992–2004 the Author(s) and The University of Iowa. Available at: http://www.vh.org/adult/provider/radiology/RCW/031397/031397.html. Accessed winter 2004.
2. Kidney infection (pyelonephritis). Copyright © 2002 A.D.A.M., Inc. Available at: http://www.nlm.nih.gov/medlineplus/ency/article/000522.htm. Accessed winter 2004.
3. Gowda A, Nzerue CM. Pyelonephritis, Chronic. Copyright © 2004, eMedicine.com, Inc. Available at: http://www.emedicine.com/med/topic2841.htm. Accessed winter 2004.
4. Pyelonephritis (Kidney Infection) in Adults.

National Institute of Diabetes and Digestive and Kidney Diseases (NIDDK), National Institutes of Health (NIH). Available at: http://kidney.niddk.nih.gov/kudiseases/pubs/pyelonephritis/. Accessed winter 2004.

Renal Failure

1. About Transplants: Fast Facts. Scientific Registry of Transplant Recipients (SRTR). Available at: http://www.ustransplant.org/facts.html. Accessed winter 2004.
2. Agraharkar M, Gupta R. Acute Renal Failure. Copyright © 2003 eMedicine.com, Inc. Available at: http://www.emedicine.com/med/topic1595.htm. Accessed winter 2004.
3. Analgesic Nephropathy (Painkillers and the Kidneys). National Institute of Diabetes and Digestive and Kidney Diseases, National Institutes of Health. Available at: http://kidney.niddk.nih.gov/kudiseases/pubs/analgesicnephropathy/index.htm. Accessed winter 2004.
4. Verrelli M. Chronic Renal Failure. Copyright © 2004, eMedicine.com, Inc. Available at: http://www.emedicine.com/med/topic374.htm. Accessed winter 2004.
5. Kidney Disease Facts & Statistics. American Society of Nephrology. Available at: http://130.94.125.192/data/modules/pbm/rendered/prevalence.asp. Accessed winter 2004.
6. Kidney Failure: Choosing a Treatment That's Right for You. National Institute of Diabetes and Digestive and Kidney Diseases, National Institutes of Health. Available at: http://kidney.niddk.nih.gov/kudiseases/pubs/choosingtreatment/index.htm. Accessed winter 2004.
7. Krause RS. Renal Failure, Chronic and Dialysis Complications. Copyright © 2004, eMedicine.com, Inc. Available at: http://www.emedicine.com/emerg/topic501.htm. Accessed winter 2004.
8. Kidney Failure Overview. Copyright © 1998–2004 Mayo Foundation for Medical Education and Research (MFMER). Available at: http://www.mayoclinic.com/invoke.cfm?id=DS00280. Accessed winter 2004.
9. Transplant Statistics: Annual Report : Kidney and Pancreas Transplantation. Scientific Registry of Transplant Recipients (SRTR). Available at: http://www.ustransplant. org/annual_reports/ar02/highlights/ar02_chapter_six.htm. Accessed winter 2004.

Bladder Cancer

1. Bladder Cancer. National Cancer Institute (NCI), National Institutes of Health (NIH). Available at: http://www.nci.nih.gov/cancerinfo/pdq/treatment/bladder/healthprofessional/. Accessed winter 2004.
2. Steinberg GD, Kim HL. Bladder Cancer. Copyright © 2003, eMedicine.com, Inc. Available at: http://www.emedicine.com/med/topic2344.htm. Accessed winter 2004.
3. What You Need To Know About™ Bladder Cancer. National Cancer Institute (NCI), National Institutes of Health (NIH). Available at: http://www.cancer.gov/templates/page_print.aspx?viewid=cddc0d3e-4fdc-4332-8f6b-1d6136ffdd5f. Accessed winter 2004.

Interstitial Cystitis

1. Metts JF. Interstitial Cystitis: Urgency and Frequency Syndrome. Copyright © 2001 by the American Academy of Family Physicians. Available at: http://www.aafp.org/afp/20011001/1199.html. Accessed winter 2004.
2. Rovner E, Sanchez-Ortiz R. Interstitial Cystitis. Copyright © 2004, eMedicine.com, Inc. Available at: http://www.emedicine.com/med/topic2866.htm. Accessed winter 2004.
3. Interstitial Cystitis. Copyright © 2001 National Kidney Foundation, Inc. Available at: http://www.kidney.org/general/atoz/. Accessed winter 2004.

Urinary Tract Infection

1. Important Facts About Urinary Tract Infections. Copyright © 2004 National Kidney Foundation, Inc. Available at: http://www.kidney.org/general/news/factsheet.cfm?id=10. Accessed winter 2004.
2. Rajavel S, Yuk-Kuen Kao R. Nephrology and Urology: Urinary Tract Infections: Females. Copyright © 1992–2004 the Author(s) and The University of Iowa. Available at: http://www.vh.org/adult/provider/familymedicine/FPHandbook/Chapter08/01-8.html. Accessed winter 2004.
3. Emmons WW, Tamminga CL. Urinary Tract Infection, Males. Copyright © 2003, eMedicine.com, Inc. Available at: http://www.emedicine.com/med/topic2346.htm. Accessed winter 2004.
4. Emmons WW, Tessier JM. Urinary Tract Infection, Females. Copyright © 2004, eMedicine.com, Inc. Available at: http://www.emedicine.com/med/topic2835.htm. Accessed winter 2004.
5. Orenstein R, Wong ES. Urinary Tract Infections in Adults. Copyright © 1999 by the American Academy of Family Physicians. Available at: http://www.aafp.org/afp/990301ap/1225.html. Accessed winter 2004.
6. Urinary Tract Infections in Adults. National Institute of Diabetes and Digestive and Kidney Diseases, National Institutes of Health. Available at: http://kidney.niddk.nih.gov/kudiseases/pubs/utiadult/index.htm. Accessed winter 2004.

REPRODUCTIVE SYSTEM CONDITIONS

10

Chapter Objectives

After reading this chapter, you should be able to . . .

- Describe where in the reproductive system fertilization usually occurs.
- Name the two most common types of breast cancer.
- List four treatment options for breast cancer.
- Explain the connection between endometriosis and anemia.
- Identify four risk factors for the development of ovarian cancer.
- Explain why ovarian cancer is extremely dangerous.
- Identify the most dangerous complication of pelvic inflammatory disease.
- Name two serious conditions associated with pregnancy.
- Describe the leading signs of benign prostate hyperplasia.
- Explain why difficulty with urination is one of the major signs for prostate cancer.

INTRODUCTION

Terminology for structures in the reproductive system can sometimes be confusing. Many researchers have recently moved toward labeling structures by their location or function rather than by their traditional names, which often refer to the physicians or anatomists who first recorded them. Thus, fallopian tubes, named for 16th century anatomist Gabriele Fallopio, may now be called oviducts or uterine tubes, which is more descriptive. Traditional names are still in common use, however. In this chapter, structures are referred to by both traditional and functional/locational names, so that practitioners trained in either terminology will feel at home.

What Is This Thing Called Estrogen?

Estrogen is not a single hormone, but a group of closely related chemicals that includes *estradiol*, *estriol*, and *estrone*. These chemicals are synthesized from cholesterol primarily in the ovaries during a woman's fertile years. After menopause, they continue to be manufactured in peripheral tissues in much smaller amounts, using root chemicals secreted by the adrenal cortex.

Estrogens are received by target tissues all over the body. They are not only associated with sex organ function; they influence the growth, health, and activity of many organs, including bones and the heart. They influence cell production and differentiation. Estrogens are also associated with mood swings and emotional responsiveness.

The liver makes estrogens chemically able to stimulate biologic activity in their target cells. This metabolism can occur in a variety of ways, which have great implications for long-term health. Some "bad" estrogen metabolites are associated with tissue proliferation (i.e., cancer) of the breast, uterus, cervix, ovaries, and thyroid. "Good" estrogen metabolites are associated with healthy bone maintenance and cardiovascular protection.

What determines which estrogen metabolites will be present in a woman's body? Two main factors are at work here: diet and estrogen exposure.

Diet: High-fat, low-fiber diets do several things to estrogen production. By providing excessive cholesterol, they allow the body to manufacture more estrogens to begin with. By providing a minimum of fiber, they prevent the binding of excessive estrogens to the molecules that would inactivate them. And by disrupting healthy balance of bacteria in the intestines, poor diets allow some estrogens to reenter the circulation.

Estrogen exposure: People are exposed to estrogen from internal production (endogenous estrogens) and external sources (exogenous estrogens). Endogenous estrogens have already been discussed as a function of diet and estrogen metabolism. Endogenous estrogen exposure is also increased by obesity; all body fat cells can contribute to estrogen production. Exogenous estrogen exposure is an issue that has only recently begun to be discussed. Oral birth control pills, hormone replacement therapy, and supplements found in meat and dairy products, as well as environmental chemicals such as pesticides, herbicides, plastics, and industrial solvents, all contribute to cumulative endogenous estrogen exposure.

Excessive estrogen exposure and the metabolism of "bad" estrogens have been identified as contributing factors in several cancers of hormone-dependent tissues.[1] In addition, estrogen dominance is being investigated as an issue in other reproductive system disorders, including premenstrual syndrome, endometriosis, uterine fibroids, and menopause. The good news is that estrogen exposure and metabolism can be influenced by diet and nutrition. Estrogen receptor sites in target tissues can bind with several different estrogen-like substances (*phytoestrogens*, including soy, legumes, and other sources), and some nutritional supplements can help disable free estrogen metabolites before they influence cell proliferation or differentiation.

Ultimately these reproductive system disorders may be treated or even prevented by having patients take greater control over how much estrogen they are exposed to, and how their bodies put that estrogen to use.

[1] Hall DC. Nutritional Influences on Estrogen Metabolism. Applied Nutritional Science Reports. Copyright © 2001 by Advanced Nutrition Publications, Inc.

Function and Structure: The Female Reproductive System:

Low in the female pelvis are two small structures called the ovaries. They are attached via the ovarian ligament to the uterus. The ovaries produce hormones, which are released into the bloodstream, and they produce eggs, usually one each month during ovulation, which are released into the peritoneal space. The fimbriae of the fallopian (uterine) tubes gently caress the ovaries, coaxing the egg toward them. Once inside tubes, the eggs make the 5-day journey to the uterus itself. If an egg is going to be fertilized, it will generally happen inside the uterine tube.

When the egg reaches the uterus, it finds itself inside a hollow organ that is built of criss-crossed layers of muscle. The inside surface of the uterus, the *endometrium*, is made of delicate epithelial tissue that holds vast billowy supplies of blood to provide a nest for that fertilized egg (Figure 10.1). If the egg is not fertilized, the uterus sheds the blood and egg with it in the menses. Then it will begin the process of building a new nest for next month's candidate.

The timing of the ripening and release of eggs from the ovaries and the building and shedding of the endometrial nest is under the control of the endocrine system. Hormones secreted from the ovaries themselves as well as the pituitary gland determine when and how these various events will happen. Birth control pills work by introducing artificial hormones into the blood. These trick the pituitary into believing that the woman is always pregnant, and so she never ovulates.

The relationship between the reproductive system and the endocrine system is extremely tight; the female reproductive cycle is under the control of hormone secretions. Several of the conditions discussed in this chapter could be considered endocrine system disorders, but the tissue changes occur in reproductive system organs, so they are discussed here. (See sidebar, "What Is This Thing Called Estrogen?")

Female reproductive conditions that have significance for massage therapists generally have to do with growths or local tenderness deep in the abdomen. Although working deeply in the vicinity of the uterus or ovaries is not generally practiced, sometimes these conditions can displace internal organs, making them vulnerable in places they would not ordinarily be found.

Function and Structure: The Male Reproductive System

The male reproductive system comprises the testes, the spermatic cord, other glands that contribute to the produc-

Figure 10.1. Overview of the female reproductive system.

tion of semen, and the urethra, which expels semen through the penis (Figure 10-2).

Sperm cells are among the smallest of human cells and the only ones equipped with flagella for locomotion. They are manufactured in specialized tubes in the testes, the *sem-*

iniferous tubules. Sperm cells grow and mature in the testes; they are suspended from the body in the scrotal sac because they flourish best when the temperature is slightly lower than internal body temperature. Mature sperm cells are stored in the *epididymis*: a long tube that is coiled up behind the testes

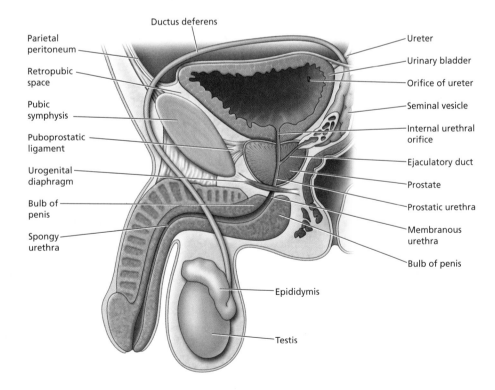

Figure 10.2. Overview of the male reproductive system.

in the scrotum. Sperm cells leave the epididymis through the left and *right vas deferens*, which carries them through the inguinal ring into the abdomen. Along the way other glands, including the seminal vesicles and prostate, contribute to the fluid that suspends and nourishes the sperm on their long journey toward the ovum. The left and right vas deferens join together at the urethra, and sperm leaves the penis during ejaculation.

The most common disorders of the male reproductive system have to do with the prostate gland, which is in a

position to obstruct the urethra during ejaculation or urination. Although "prostate massage" is typically conducted by a urologist through the wall of the rectum during an examination (and is therefore outside the scope of practice of massage therapists), prostate problems can seriously diminish a person's quality of life. Consequently, some clients may seek bodywork as a coping mechanism while he manages his disorder. Massage conducted to maximize the benefits of parasympathetic effect and improved immune system function can be a safe and appropriate choice.

REPRODUCTIVE SYSTEM CONDITIONS

Disorders of the Uterus

Abortion, Spontaneous and Elective
Cervical Cancer
Dysmenorrhea
Endometriosis
Fibroid Tumors

Disorders of Other Female Reproductive Structures

Breast Cancer
Ovarian Cancer
Ovarian Cysts

Disorders of the Male Reproductive System

Benign Prostatic Hypertrophy
Prostate Cancer

Prostatitis
Testicular Cancer

Other Reproductive System Conditions

Menopause
Pelvic Inflammatory Disease
Pregnancy
Premenstrual Syndrome
Sexually Transmitted Diseases

DISORDERS OF THE UTERUS

Abortion, Spontaneous and Elective

Definition: *What Are They?*

An elective abortion is the intentional termination of a pregnancy; a spontaneous abortion is an unintentional termination. In either case, the fetus and placenta are detached from the uterine wall and cannot continue to develop.

Etiology of Elective Abortion: *What Happens?*

A pregnancy can be terminated in different ways, depending on the stage. If it happens within the first 12 weeks, an elective abortion is usually conducted by vacuum suction. The walls of the cervix are dilated to allow a flexible tube into the uterus, which removes the fetal tissue. In the 13th to 15th weeks, a D&C, or *dilation and curettage*, may be performed; this is a more complicated procedure and requires more anesthetic and sometimes a hospital stay. Later termi-

Abortion, Spontaneous and Elective In Brief

What are they?
Spontaneous and elective abortions are pregnancies that are ended, unintentionally or intentionally, before the fetus is born naturally.

How are they recognized?
Generalized or pelvic pain may be present, along with vaginal bleeding. Often, however, no outward signs may show that a woman is recovering from a spontaneous or elective abortion.

Is massage indicated or contraindicated?
Massage is locally contraindicated (no deep abdominal work) for women recovering from a recent spontaneous or elective abortion until her bleeding has stopped and she is free of any signs of infection. Bodywork elsewhere can be supportive and helpful.

nations are brought about by inducing premature labor. They can be very difficult and always require hospitalization.

Nonsurgical interventions in early pregnancy have recently been approved for use in the United States. These include drugs that, when combined with carefully timed doses of prostaglandins, block cell division or counteract the activity of *progestin*: a hormone that supports the implantation of a fertilized egg.

Etiology of Spontaneous Abortion: What Happens?

Several unintentional factors may contribute to the disruption of a pregnancy. In many cases, it can be hard to discover exactly what causes a fetus to die, but many issues have been identified, some of which are controllable, but many of which are not.

Controllable factors that may raise the risk of spontaneous abortion or miscarriage include smoking, untreated infections of the reproductive tract (see *pelvic inflammatory disease*, this chapter), untreated *diabetes* or *thyroid disorders* (see Chapter 8), exposure to toxic chemicals, especially solvents, and progesterone deficiency in the early weeks of pregnancy before the placenta has begun to secrete its own supply of this hormone that allows fetal implantation. An immune system response that causes blood in fetal vessels to clot can be controlled with low doses of aspirin or other blood thinners.

Factors that a woman has no control over include structural problems in the uterus such as *fibroid tumors* (this chapter) or a weak cervix, the fertilization of multiple eggs, age, autoimmune disease (especially *scleroderma*, Chapter 2), an immune system rejection of fetal tissue, failure of the fetus to implant into the endometrium, or what is perhaps the most common cause of miscarriage: the fetus is simply missing key genetic information that would allow it to continue to develop. When the moment comes that the needed genes are missing, the fetus dies.

Miscarriages usually happen in the first 14 weeks of pregnancy, although the risk of miscarriage goes way down after the 8th week. If the fetus dies after the 20th week, it is no longer called a miscarriage or spontaneous abortion; it is called a stillbirth, but the principles are the same.

The frequency of spontaneous abortions is a subject of debate. It is estimated that up to 50% of all fertilized eggs are expelled from the body for one reason or another before a woman may know that she is pregnant at all. Of recognized pregnancies, anywhere from 25% to 30% of all fetuses are spontaneously aborted.

Signs and Symptoms

When the endometrial lining of the uterus is disrupted in any way but a normal menses, what is left is a large surface area of raw, bleeding epithelium. This is true for elective and spontaneous abortions, and also for childbirth. Symptoms of this trauma can include pain (local and referred), bleeding, and cramping. These are generally self-limiting; that is, the symptoms resolve themselves with time, unless complications develop.

Complications

Complications of abortions or miscarriages can include infection from incomplete shedding of the uterine lining; damage to the uterus, bladder, or colon from surgical instruments; and possible hemorrhaging. *Depression* (see Chapter 3) is also a frequent complication of these events. The later the gestational age of the fetus, the higher the risk of complications from elective or spontaneous abortion.

Treatment

The best treatment for a woman recovering from an elective abortion, a miscarriage, or successful childbirth is tender loving care. If any infection develops, or if uterine lining has not been shed completely, a D&C and antibiotics may be necessary.

Massage?

Deep abdominal massage is locally contraindicated for women recovering from spontaneous and elective abortions and postpartum situations, at least until the bleeding has stopped. Massage elsewhere is very much indicated, although the risk of blood clotting for pregnant women is quite high, so it is wisest to stick with noncirculatory modalities (see *pregnancy*, this chapter).

Cervical Cancer

Definition: What Is It?

Cervical cancer is the growth of malignant cells in the lining of the cervix. Although some types of abnormal cells grow slowly and do not present a serious threat, other types are aggressive and invasive.

Demographics: Who Gets It?

Approximately 13,000 women in the United States are diagnosed with invasive cervical cancer per year; estimates suggest that four times that many are diagnosed with noninvasive abnormal cervical cells. Cervical cancer kills approximately 4,000 American women each year.

The average age at which a woman may be diagnosed with precancerous changes in her cervix is 28 years, but cervical cancer can develop at any age, from the beginning of sexual activity to long after menopause.

Cervical Cancer in Brief

What is it?
Cervical cancer is the development of cancerous cells in the lining of the cervix. These may spread to affect the whole cervix, the rest of the uterus, and other pelvic organs.

How is it recognized?
Early stages of cervical cancer are virtually silent; this disease is detected by Pap tests before symptoms develop. Later signs and symptoms include bleeding or spotting outside a normal menstrual period, vaginal discharge, and pelvic pain.

Is massage indicated or contraindicated?
Most cases of cervical cancer are caught and eradicated before the woman is in serious danger of metastasis. These patients are good candidates for any kind of bodywork. For a woman dealing with advanced stages of cervical cancer, the massage therapist must make adjustments for the radiation, chemotherapy, or surgical procedures that may be part of her experience.

Cervical Cancer: History of a Disease

In the early part of the 20th century, cervical cancer was one of the leading causes of death by cancer for women in this country. This disease is virtually silent, creating no symptoms until it has spread throughout the pelvic cavity and into the lymph system—by which time it is practically impossible to survive.

Then from 1955 to 1992 a remarkable phenomenon occurred: rates of death by cervical cancer took a huge downswing, dropping by some 74%.

What made the difference? A simple examination: the *Papanicolaou test* (Pap smear), which makes it possible to detect precancerous cells in the cervix before they spread. Because of the Pap smear, women could have abnormal cells detected and removed before they had a chance to become malignant, and they could find and remove malignancies before they had a chance to

spread throughout the pelvic cavity. Consequently, the 5-year survival rate for cervical cancer is now close to 100% for preinvasive cells, 91% for early invasive cells, and 70% overall.

Today the recommended protocol for cervical cancer detection is to receive a Pap smear once a year. If a woman has 3 consecutive years without any sign of dysplasia, her doctor may recommend that she can have Pap smears less frequently. Higher mortality rates among nonwhite women and women of low socioeconomic status point out the fact that up to 30% of at-risk women still do not have access to this inexpensive and highly useful test.

Cervical cancer has been largely controlled in the United States, but worldwide it is still a leading cause of death by cancer in countries where women do not have access to Pap tests. Although no vaccine against dangerous types of HPV has been approved for humans, several are in development, and the future promises that one day cervical cancer may become a completely preventable disease.

Etiology: What Happens?

Cervical cancer is an example of a malignancy brought about directly by a viral infection, in this case with some of the 80 known varieties of human papilloma virus (HPV) family. Approximately 25 of these viruses are associated with genital warts, although not all types of HPV cause visible growths.

HPV is a sexually transmitted disease, transferred by direct skin-to-skin touching. It is *not* preventable by the use of condoms because other parts of the genitals still come in contact during sex. Statistics on the incidence of HPV infection in this country vary; some say approximately 6 million women are currently infected; others suggest that up to 40 million Americans are HPV carriers. Being infected with HPV is not a dependable indicator of cervical cancer, however; many of the viruses in this family are *not* associated with aggressive or invasive cancers.

When a woman is infected with HPV, the virus may trigger cellular changes in the lining of her cervix. Precancerous changes are called *dysplasia*, and they can be stimulated by both low-risk and high-risk types of HPV. A new test has recently been developed to help identify what type of HPV might be present.

If a woman happens to be infected with a low-risk type of virus, her abnormal cells may spontaneously resolve, and she may never know that anything had happened. However, if she is infected with an aggressive form of HPV, cancerous cells will grow in the lining of the cervix and then may spread throughout the uterus, the vagina, and into the pelvic cavity, affecting the bladder, colon, and inguinal lymph nodes. Ultimately the cancer may travel to distant parts of the body.

Exposure to HPV is the central risk factor for developing cervical cancer. However, other factors may contribute to the likelihood of having abnormal cells become malignant. Sexual activity at an early age may increase the transmission rate of HPV. Smoking raises cervical cancer risk by close to 300%. Being the daughter of a woman who took *diethylstilbestrol* (DES) to prevent miscarriage also increases risk, as does immune system suppression through human immunodeficiency virus (HIV) infection or immune-suppressant drugs. Co-infection with *herpes simplex* (Chapter 1) or other sexually transmitted infections (see *STDs*, this chapter) also raise the risk. Finally, socioeconomic standing is a major factor, as this often determines whether a woman has adequate access to early detection and care.

Signs and Symptoms

Early stages of cervical cancer have no symptoms to speak of. The cancer must be significantly advanced before any signs appear. These usually include bleeding or spotting between menstrual periods or after menopause, vaginal discharge, and pelvic or abdominal pain.

Diagnosis

The Pap smear is the current standard for early cervical cancer detection. In this test, a small scraping of cells and mucus from the cervix is extracted and analyzed. If abnormal cells are found, a follow-up test that visually examines the cervix for suspicious changes (a *colposcopy*) may be conducted. A biopsy removes the affected part of the cervix; if more suspicious cells are found, further tests may be conducted to stage the cancer and determine the best possible treatment options.

Pap tests are fast, cost-effective, and only mildly painful, but if the tissue sample happens to miss some abnormal cells, "false-negative" results may be returned. Fortunately, most types of cervical cancer grow slowly, and yearly examinations are usually adequate to insure protection from having dysplasia become cervical cancer. For specific information about cervical cancer staging, see sidebar, "Cervical Cancer Staging."

Cervical Cancer Staging

The staging protocols for cervical cancer can be confusing, and as they are constantly under review, they change frequently. The most current recommendations for cervical cancer divide this disease into precancerous and cancerous stages.

Precancerous staging:

Precancerous cellular changes of the cervix have two possible designations: *squamous intraepithelial lesions* (SIL), or *cervical intraepithelial neoplasia* (CIN). In either case, the term *intraepithelial* means that atypical cells are limited to the epithelial lining of the cervix and have not invaded deeper tissues.

The term *SIL* is qualified as being low-grade or high-grade. The term *CIN* is qualified as stages I, II, and III. The following table demonstrates how they interrelate:

SIL grade	CIN grade	Cellular changes
Low-grade	CIN-I	Mild dysplasia
High-grade	CIN-II	Moderate dysplasia
	CIN-III	Severe dysplasia, cancer in situ

Cancer staging:

The staging protocol for invasive cervical cancer follows a TNM pattern similar to that used for many cancers, but because this procedure was developed by the Federation Internationale du Gynecologie et d'Obstetrique, it is sometimes called the FIGO system. The staging system for cervical cancer has been developed in great detail; a simplified version is included here:

Tumor	Node	Metastasis
Tx: unassessable	Nx: unassessable	Mx: unassessable
T0: no evidence of a tumor	N0: no nodal involvement	M0: no distant metastasis
T-IS: in situ tumor (affects the mucosa only)	N1: nodes near the cervical area have been invaded	M1: distant metastasis
T1a (FIGO Ia): growth is under 5 mm in depth and 7 mm in width		

Tumor	Node	Metastasis
T1b (FIGO Ib): the growth is in the cervix only, and has penetrated to 4 mm or more.		
T2 (FIGO II): the growth is limited to the cervix or tissues close to the cervix		
T3 (FIGO III): the pelvic wall or lower 1/3 of the vagina have been invaded; obstruction of the ureters and subsequent enlargement of the kidneys may develop		
T4 (FIGO IV): the mucosa of the bladder or rectum have been invaded		

These TNM classifications translate into cervical cancer stages as seen below:

Stage	T	N	M
0	T-IS	N0	M0
I	T1	N0	M0
II	T2	N0	M0
III	T3	Any	M0
IV	Any	Any	M1

Treatment

Treatment for cervical cancer depends entirely on the stage in which it is diagnosed. Most cases are found in stage 0 or stage I, which means treatment can be limited to removing the abnormal cells and watching carefully for further changes. Surgical interventions to remove cervical dysplasia include cryotherapy, in which cells are frozen off; loop electrosurgical excision procedure (LEEP), in which electricity is passed through a loop of thin wire to slice off the suspicious tissue; laser surgery, and a cone biopsy.

Surgical procedures for cancer caught in later stages may range from full or partial hysterectomies to full pelvic *exenteration*, in which virtually all the pelvic organs are removed.

Radiation and chemotherapy also may be employed with advanced cases of cervical cancer.

Massage

Massage for a client who has cervical dysplasia is certainly fine, especially if she is receiving appropriate care. Clients who are dealing with advanced cases of cancer must cope not only with the disease process, but with the many complex and extremely unpleasant complications those treatments may involve. Carefully conducted bodywork that respects the many challenges of surgery, radiation, and chemotherapy can offer all of the benefits of massage, while minimizing any possible risks. See more on this topic in *cancer*, Chapter 11.

Dysmenorrhea

Definition: What Is It?

Dysmenorrhea is a technical term for painful menstrual periods. Generally a woman is said to have dysmenorrhea if she has to limit her regular activities or requires medication to function for 1 day or more every month.

Demographics: Who Gets It?

Most women have severe menstrual pain at least once in their life. An estimated 40% of all women in the United States experience regular painful periods, and approximately 10% of all women are incapacitated for 1 to 3 days each month. Dysmenorrhea is the leading cause of lost time from school or work for women of child-bearing age. Primary dysmenorrhea usually begins within a few years of menarche. It is generally not changed by childbearing.

Etiology: What Happens?

Dysmenorrhea in Brief
What is it? Dysmenorrhea is the technical term for menstrual pain that is severe enough to interfere with and limit the activities of women of childbearing age. It may be a primary problem, or secondary to some other pelvic pathologic condition.
How is it recognized? The symptoms of dysmenorrhea are dull aching or sharp severe lower abdominal pain preceding or during menstruation. Nausea and vomiting may accompany very severe symptoms. Secondary dysmenorrhea may create pelvic pain outside normal periods as well.
Is massage indicated or contraindicated? Massage is appropriate for primary dysmenorrhea, although the abdomen locally contraindicates deep work during days of heavy menstrual flow. The appropriateness of bodywork for secondary dysmenorrhea depends of the type of pathology involved, along with stage, severity, treatment, and other variables.

Dysmenorrhea can be primary; that is, it starts within the first 3 years of menstruation in an otherwise healthy woman, or secondary to some underlying pathologic condition.

Causes of Primary Dysmenorrhea

Several different factors can contribute to primary dysmenorrhea.

- *Prostaglandins*: These are chemicals produced all over the body, and especially in the uterus. They cause smooth muscle contractions, but they also sensitize the body to pain. Prostaglandins are found in higher concentrations in women who have menstrual pain than in women who do not.
- *Pain–spasm cycle*: When the uterus is in sustained contraction, oxygen cannot easily supply the muscle. Ischemia causes pain, which reinforces the spasm, and so on. This is often exacerbated by a shortage of calcium, which tends to make muscle spasms more tenacious.
- *Ligament irritation*: The uterine ligament, which anchors the uterus to the pelvic wall, can be pulled and irritated when the uterus is in spasm.

It is easy to see how physical or emotional stress fits into the picture of menstrual pain. Sympathetic reactions in the body exacerbate uterine ischemia, leading to pain, which reinforces the spasm. The emotional state of dreading the pain and discomfort of menstrual periods can then become a self-fulfilling prophecy: the stress of anticipating an unpleasant event works to make that event even more unpleasant.

Causes of Secondary Dysmenorrhea

Secondary dysmenorrhea is a complication of some other pelvic disorder. Some of the most common problems that cause menstrual pain include *pelvic inflammatory disease* (PID), *fibroid tumors*, *sexually transmitted diseases*, and *endometriosis* (all in this chapter). Pelvic adhesions, deposits of scar tissue from previous surgeries or trauma, also may contribute to menstrual pain.

Signs and Symptoms

Symptoms of dysmenorrhea vary. They can include dull aches in the abdomen and low back or sharp pains and cramping in the pelvis and abdomen. These usually happen early in menstruation, but some women have symptoms during their whole period. Headaches, nausea, vomiting, diarrhea, and constipation are all possibilities, along with a frequent need to urinate. If the dysmenorrhea is related to an underlying pathologic condition, pelvic pain may not be limited to the menstrual cycle; it can happen at any time.

Diagnosis

Ongoing debilitating menstrual pain is important to investigate because it could be indicative of serious underlying problems. Diagnosis often involves a laparoscopy to check for endometriosis, which is a leading cause of secondary dysmenorrhea. Ultrasounds to look for fibroid tumors may be performed. Cultures of vaginal secretions also may be examined to look for signs of PID, chlamydia, syphilis, or gonorrhea. In the absence of these conditions, painful periods can be treated without fear of ignoring some important underlying causes.

Treatment

For most cases of dysmenorrhea, painkillers such as ibuprofen, naproxen, or Cox-2 inhibitors work by inhibiting the secretion of prostaglandins. A thorough nutritional analysis also may reveal strategies for dealing with menstrual pain; this is a useful course for many women, but no specific nutritional supplements have been found to alleviate all cases of dysmenorrhea. Dietary changes to radically reduce fats and animal proteins while increasing fiber and calcium are often recommended. Exercise and stretches also can relieve the pain from the irritated uterine ligament, which is tugged on by a uterus in spasm.

For more serious situations in which where painkillers, heat, and stretching do not affect the pain, more aggressive interventions may be considered. Low-dose birth control pills prohibit ovulation, which in turn prohibits the secretion of prostaglandins in the uterus. If a structural issue such as fibroid tumors is at the root of the problem, surgery may be an option. Medications or laparoscopic surgery for endometriosis may alleviate symptoms.

Massage?

A woman who is in the middle of a painful period will probably not respond well to deep abdominal massage, but nurturing touch elsewhere is highly called for and beneficial. A woman who regularly has painful periods but who has no known pelvic pathologic conditions is a good candidate for abdominal massage when she is *not* menstruating; this may help to relieve tension, take stress off the uterine ligament, and even minimize abdominal adhesions that may contribute to pain.

Endometriosis

Definition: What Is It?

Endometriosis is a condition in which cells from the endometrium, the inner lining of the uterus, become implanted elsewhere in the body. They usually begin in the pelvic cavity but may spread further into the abdomen, and even above the diaphragm.

Demographics: Who Gets it?

Endometriosis is probably fairly common. An estimated 5 million or more American women deal with this problem, but statistics are difficult to gather because it cannot be diagnosed without surgery. It affects females as young as 9 years old, and postmenopausal women, but most patients are diagnosed between ages 20 and 45. Most endometriosis patients are women who have heavy, long-lasting menstrual periods, whose cycles occur in less than 28 days, and who have never had children.

Etiology: What Happens?

Endometriosis in Brief
What is it?
Endometriosis is the implantation and growth of endometrial cells in the peritoneal cavity (and possibly elsewhere) that grow and then decay with the menstrual cycle.
How is it recognized?
Endometriosis may have no symptoms. When it does, they generally include heavy, painful menstruation, pelvic and abdominal pain, difficulties with urination or defecation, painful intercourse, and other problems, depending on which tissues have been affected. Symptoms are worst during menstruation. Infertility is a frequent complication of endometriosis.
Is massage indicated or contraindicated?
If a client has endometriosis, deep abdominal or pelvic work may be painful, especially when it is close to her menstrual cycle. The supportive effects of massage, however, can be an important part of the coping mechanisms women with this disorder must develop.

Endometriosis involves the implantation and growth of endometrial cells anywhere outside the uterus. It was first described in 1921 by Dr. James Sampson, who noticed these growths in the peritoneal cavities of women undergoing abdominal surgery. He hypothesized that the endometrial cells got out of the uterus through retrograde backflow through the uterine tubes, or through circulatory or lymphatic dissemination. Eighty years later, these theories are still the basis for understanding the causes of this disorder.

Having endometrial cells find their way out of the uterus is not uncommon. In fact, up to 90% of all women have some endometrial cells in the pelvic cavity during menstruation. But not all of those women have those cells successfully colonize a pelvic organ. The differences in cellular activity between women who have endometriosis and women who do not yield some clues about how this disease develops.

Women who have endometriosis have some immune system anomalies that are not seen with other women. These include low levels of the killer T-cells and natural killer (NK) cells that would normally eradicate stray endothelial cells in the pelvic cavity. They have higher than normal levels of suppressor T-cells, which serve to quell an appropriate immune system response. Women with endometriosis have a high number of macrophages around their growths, but instead of phagocytizing the new material, these macrophages secrete chemicals that inhibit T-cell and NK cell activity, while stimulating the growth of new blood vessels, and the production of scar tissue. The activated B-cells of women with endometriosis do produce antibodies to attack the new tissue, but they do not seem to work very well outside the uterus. Unfortunately, these antibodies *do* work *inside* the uterus, which can increase symptoms and make the implantation of a fertilized egg difficult. Finally, women with endometriosis secrete unusually high levels of prostaglandins, which contribute to severe cramping and pain sensitization.

Endometrial growths usually become established on the outside of the uterus, on the uterine tubes, the broad ligaments, the ovaries, the bladder, or the colon (Fig. 10.3).

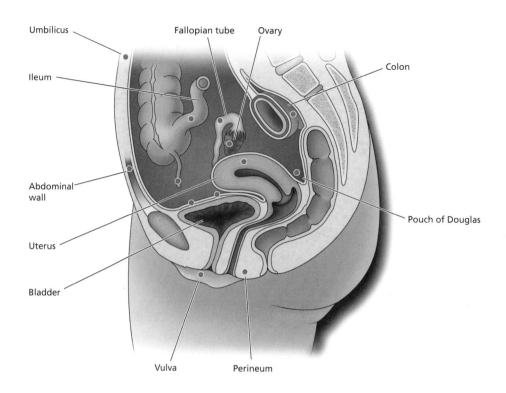

Figure 10.3. Sites of endometriosis.

Growths have been found as far away from the uterus as the lungs, and even the brain. Wherever they land, they stimulate the growth of supplying blood vessels, and they proliferate in accordance with the hormonal commands in the body. However, these growths cannot be shed with normal menstruation. Instead, they decay and accumulate in local areas, stimulating an inflammatory response. The body attempts to isolate them by surrounding the deposits with fibrous connective tissue. Eventually multitudes of fibrous "blood blisters" accumulate on whatever surfaces the endometrium can find.

Endometrial growths that are found early look like clear vesicles on whatever structures they have colonized. Later these vesicles become bright red. Over a course of 10 or more years they become thick, black, and scarred. Growths that have darkened over time are sometimes called "chocolate cysts."

Causes

Backflow through the uterine tubes or capillary and lymphatic dissemination of endometrial cells are still considered the leading initiators of endometriosis, but it is unclear why some women develop permanent growths and others do not. A genetic potential clearly exists, because women with mothers or sisters who have been diagnosed with endometriosis have a much higher chance of being diagnosed themselves. However, these statistics do not reflect variables such as the likelihood that these women will seek medical care, or whether their disease is brought about by genetic problems or by shared environmental factors, including environmental estrogens. One such environmental factor is exposure to dioxins: chemicals produced by the manufacture and use of pesticides, paper pulp, and the burning of hazardous waste.[2]

---

[2] What Is Endometriosis? Copyright © 2003 by IVF.com, Atlanta, GA, USA. Available at: http://www.ivf.com/endoassn.html. Accessed winter 2004.

Signs and Symptoms

Very often infertility is the symptom that brings a woman with endometriosis to a doctor for a first diagnosis. Other symptoms of endometriosis are often nonexistent, at least in the early stages, but premenstrual spotting, a sensation of urinary urgency with painful urination, and diarrhea and rectal bleeding during menstruation may occur. Some cases may show severe *dysmenorrhea* (this chapter) before, during, and *after* periods. Interestingly, the amount of pain a woman experiences has little to do with the size of her endometrial growths; many women with microscopic growths report more pain that other women with advanced deposits.

Symptoms of endometriosis are cyclical and reach a peak during menstruation. This feature has probably prevented a lot of women from seeking medical help because traditionally it has been assumed that painful menstruation is a normal and expected part of the having "the curse." As women have become more proactive about healthcare, they have discovered that painful menstruation is *not* a given and have become more willing to explore the causes and possible solutions to their pain.

Complications

Accumulations of bloody deposits and fibrous connective tissue can cause a lot of damage in the pelvic cavity. Scar tissue deposits can create adhesions in or on the uterine tubes and ovaries, which cause infertility or ectopic *pregnancy* (this chapter). The collecting of blood in these extra, unintentional deposits routes blood away from where it can be useful, resulting in *anemia* (see Chapter 4). Uterine hyperplasia is a condition that occasionally accompanies endometriosis; the normal endometrial lining becomes pathologically thickened, leading to excessive bleeding and further difficulties with fertility.

Diagnosis

Only one diagnostic test for endometriosis is definitive: laparoscopic surgery. Although patients may describe characteristic symptoms that become progressively worse and peak during menstruation, only a *laparoscopy* will specifically identify the lesions.

Treatment

Treatment for endometriosis depends on what outcome the woman desires. No permanent solution for this disorder has yet been developed; even a complete hysterectomy will not protect a patient from endometriosis if any microscopic deposits remain that may be stimulated with hormone replacement therapy.

Because many women wish to treat endometriosis to become pregnant, treatment options are often geared toward limiting symptoms and progression long enough to allow fertilization to take place. Symptoms disappear during pregnancy because no estrogen is secreted to stimulate the menstrual cycle, but they usually recur after a baby is born.

Four main goals are at the center of medical intervention for endometriosis. These are to relieve pain, to stop the progression of established growths, to prevent the establishment of any new growths, and to maintain or restore fertility, if that is the patient's wish. NSAIDs or other analgesics may be adequate for pain relief. Hormone therapy that disrupts the secretion of estrogen may be employed to limit growths. These may be used alone, or as a preparation for surgery. Surgical interventions may include the use of lasers or *electrocauterization* to *ablate* (remove the top layer of tissue) or cut out visible growths, and to reduce adhesions between pelvic organs.

Hysterectomy:

This comes from the Greek root *hystera*, which means womb or uterus. The word *hysteria* comes from the same root. In the early days of medicine, hysteria was assumed to be a woman's complaint, associated with womb-related disturbances.

Massage?

Endometriosis is one of those reproductive system disorders that can cause the pelvic organs to become displaced, as they are distorted with abnormal deposits and scar tissue. Consequently, deep abdominal massage is not appropriate for clients who know they have endometriosis, especially for those who are menstruating; the presence of inflammation and the threat that cells may break free and settle elsewhere in the pelvic cavity both make doing deep abdominal work problematic.

However, many women with endometriosis also live in a state of anxiety, stress, and frustration with their own bodies that may exacerbate their most painful symptoms. Massage therapy along with other relaxation techniques is frequently recommended for women who must learn to cope with the long-term consequences of a disorder that has no permanent solution.

Fibroid Tumors

Fibroid Tumors in Brief

What are they?
Fibroid tumors are benign growths in the muscle or connective tissue of the uterus.

How are they recognized?
Fibroid tumors are often asymptomatic. Some, however, cause heavy menstrual bleeding or may put mechanical pressure on other structures in the pelvis.

Is massage indicated or contraindicated?
Large, diagnosed fibroid tumors contraindicate deep abdominal massage. However, most fibroids are quite small and virtually symptomless, and massage will not have any impact on them at all. In these cases, massage is indicated for the benefit of the client, if not for the possibility of changing the state of her fibroid tumors.

Definition: What Are They?

Fibroid tumors, or *leiomyomas*, are benign tumors that grow in or around the uterus. They can grow within the smooth muscle walls or, more rarely, they can be suspended from a stalk into the pelvic cavity, or into the uterus. Some can even hang down into the vagina (Figure 10-4). Fibroids can grow singly or in clusters, and they vary in size from being microscopic to weighing several pounds and completely filling the uterus.

Demographics: Who Gets Them?

The number of women with fibroids is difficult to project, because they are usually silent. Some estimates suggest that although they are found in up to 20% of all fertile women, they may be present in up to 80%. Growth of fibroids seems to be stimulated by estrogen; after menopause many tend to shrink and ultimately disappear. Fibroids are far more common in African American women than they are in other populations.

Etiology: What Happens?

The pathophysiology of uterine fibroids is not well understood. Although they sometimes run in families, they are not strictly genetically linked. Many experts believe that they arise as a combination of genetic, environmental, and hormonal factors.

Fibroids are typically classified by their location. Submucosal fibroids grow under the mucous lining of the uterus; they are the deepest type. Intramural fibroids grow within layers of the muscular wall of the uterus. Subserosal fibroids grow on the superficial aspect of the uterus, but deep to the peritoneum.

Signs and Symptoms

Usually fibroids create no symptoms at all. In very extreme cases, the fibroid may grow large enough to put pressure on the sensory nerves inside the uterus or press on nearby structures such as the bladder, which can cause urinary frequency, or the rectum, which can cause difficulties with defecation. If they press on the fallopian (uterine) tubes they

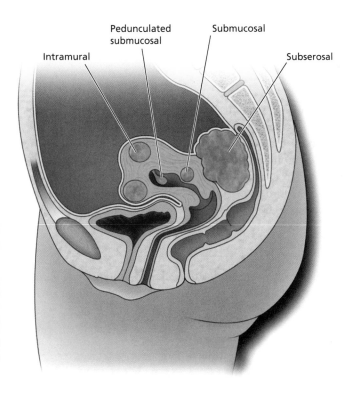

Figure 10.4. Leiomyomas (fibroid tumors).

may interfere with pregnancies. They can also cause heavy menstrual bleeding, and occasionally bleeding between menstrual periods.

Complications

Fibroids are very seldom a serious condition, but they can lead to some troubling consequences. The heavy periods they cause sometimes lead to *anemia* (see Chapter 4) from excessive blood loss. They can cause infertility by obstructing fallopian tubes or interfering with the implantation of a fertilized ovum. They also can interfere in pregnancies brought to term: if a fibroid is large enough, it will crowd the growing fetus or may block the exit through the cervix. These problems can lead to premature births and cesarean sections.

Pedunculate fibroids, the type that dangle into the uterus or vagina, have been known to twist on their stalks, which causes extreme pain and requires surgery to remove. It is also possible for very large fibroids to outgrow their blood supply. This will lead to a process called degeneration, in which tissue that is deprived of oxygen dies. The body slowly reabsorbs the necrotic mass, but it can be a long and painful process; more often, surgery is performed to remove the fibroid.

Diagnosis

Fibroids are generally found during pelvic examinations, when it is noted that the uterus is enlarged or irregularly shaped. The diagnosis usually can be confirmed by ultrasound or magnetic resonance imaging (MRI), but occasionally it can be difficult to tell whether it is the uterus that is distended, or if a cyst or tumor is growing on the ovaries: a potentially much more dangerous situation. If it is not clear what kind of growth is present, a CT scan or laparoscopy may be called for to rule out *ovarian cancer* (this chapter).

Fibroids typically grow slowly, but occasionally they can grow fast, doubling their size within a few months. In this situation, a biopsy is recommended to rule out the possibility of a uterine malignancy.

Treatment

Fibroids seldom require treatment unless they cause pain and excessive bleeding, or if they interfere with pregnancy.

Hormone therapy can shrink them, but they will grow back when medication is stopped. Surgical options range from minimally invasive procedures to shrink the growths with liquid nitrogen (*cryomyolysis*), to blocking off the supplying arteries (*uterine artery embolization*), to laser surgery, to partial or full hysterectomies. Fibroid tumors lead to between 170,000 and 300,000 hysterectomies in this country every year.

Massage?

Diagnosed fibroids locally contraindicate deep abdominal work. Undiagnosed fibroids are not impacted by massage to speak of, and so massage is indicated for the benefit of the client, if not for the improvement of her condition.

Disorders of Other Female Reproductive Structures

Breast Cancer

Breast Cancer in Brief

What is it?
Breast cancer is the growth of malignant tumor cells in breast tissue; these cells can invade skin and nearby muscles and bones. If they invade lymph nodes, they can metastasize to the rest of the body.

How is it recognized?
The first sign of breast cancer is a small painless lump or thickening in the breast tissue or near the axilla. The lump may be too small to palpate but may show on a mammogram. Later the skin may change texture, the nipple may change shape, and discharge from the nipple may be present.

Is massage indicated or contraindicated?
Breast cancer patients undergo treatment options that are extremely taxing on general health and physical and emotional well-being. As long as bodywork choices are made that respect these challenges, massage can be a wonderful, supportive, important coping mechanism for many breast cancer patients.

Definition: What Is It?

Breast cancer is the development of tumors in the epithelial or connective tissue of the breast. These growths may start out as nonmalignant but may become invasive if neglected for a prolonged period.

Demographics: Who Gets It?

The American Cancer Society estimates that about 216,000 new cases of invasive breast cancer are diagnosed in women and approximately 1,450 cases in men each year in the United States. In addition, approximately 60,000 cases of noninvasive ("in situ") breast cancer will be identified. Most women with breast cancer are mature; 77% of them are older than 50 years when diagnosed.[3]

Before 1980, the lifetime risk of contracting breast cancer was 1 in 11. Now it is 1 in 8, but some factors that may be falsely driving that number up, including women's increasing longevity (the chance of getting breast cancer increases significantly just with age) and the fact that breast cancer is being found and diagnosed earlier than ever before.

[3] Breast Cancer. Copyright © 2003 American Cancer Society, Inc. Available at: http://documents.cancer.org/104.00/104.00.pdf. Accessed winter 2004.

Breast cancer is the leading cause of death by cancer in women younger than 54 years and the second most common cause of death by cancer for women older than 54 (lung cancer is the first). It is responsible for the deaths of some 40,000 women each year, and approximately 500 men. An estimated 2 million women with breast cancer are alive today.

Etiology: What Happens?

Breasts are constructed of lobes, where milk is produced in lactating women; ducts, where milk is delivered to the nipple; and *stroma*: collagen, elastin, and fat cells that provide support and the bulk of breast tissue. The lobes and ducts are made of epithelial cells; the stroma is connective tissue and lipid cells. Although cancer grows in any of these tissues, the lobes and ducts are by far the most likely to develop malignant cells.

- *Ductal carcinoma.* This is the most common type of breast cancer, accounting for between 70% and 80% of all diagnoses. It can occur *in situ*, in which cells only affect the epithelial lining of the ducts, or it can become invasive. Ductal carcinoma in situ (DCIS) is associated with the development of small calcified deposits in the breasts.

- *Lobular carcinoma.* This is less common than ductal carcinoma, accounting for 5% to 10% of all tumors. It can be limited to the epithelial lining of the lobes (lobular carcinoma in situ, or LCIS), but this condition carries a high risk of becoming invasive. Lobular carcinoma also has a higher incidence of appearing in both breasts than ductal carcinoma.

- *Other types of breast cancer.* Several other types of breast cancer may develop, but collectively they account for only 10% to 15% of all diagnoses. Inflammatory breast cancer is associated with edema, redness, and heat in the breast; this occurs because the tumors block lymphatic return. Inflammatory breast cancer usually has a poor prognosis. Paget's disease of the breast affects specifically the nipple and presents with specific eczema-like changes in the skin. Medullary breast cancer is a rare malignancy of the connective tissues in the breast.

Many types of breast cancer begin as in situ growths, which eventually develop malignant characteristics. It can take a long time for a tumor to become large enough to notice; it is estimated that it takes several years for a growth to reach a diameter of 1 cm.

As tumors grow, the risk of having some cells invade the circulatory or lymphatic system increases. The proximity of the axillary lymph nodes makes these a common site for the spread of malignant cells. Between 30% and 40% of all breast cancers have spread to the axillary nodes by the time the tumors are palpable.

Tumors are usually composed of several different types of cells. Some of them may be vulnerable to chemotherapeutic drugs; others are not. Unfortunately, when medications kill off the vulnerable tumor cells, they may then be replaced with drug-resistant cells.

Breast cancer usually metastasizes to nearby lymph nodes in the axilla and thoracic cavity first; invasion of chest muscles, bones, and skin then follows. Finally, distant metastatic sites include the liver, lung, and brain. If the cancer is not successfully treated, several complications may develop, including spinal cord pressure, bone fractures, pleural effusion, or bronchial obstruction.

Risk Factors

One of the most frustrating things about this disease is that no dependable profile of the women most likely to get it has ever been developed. Some cancers, such as lung, colon, and skin cancer, can be directly linked to diet or environmental factors; breast cancer cannot. Although some risk factors have been identified as increasing the chance that a woman may develop breast cancer, most women with these risk factors (outside of genetic predisposition) never develop the disease, and most breast cancer patients do not carry most of these risk factors.

Statistically, women who started having menstrual periods early in life, who had children after age 30 or not at all, who have late onset of menopause, and who are obese, especially after menopause, are at greater risk than the general population. Women who have more than two alcoholic drinks every day, or who have a history of proliferative breast disease (a type of nonmalignant breast change) are also at a slightly increased risk of developing breast cancer.

Women with a family or personal history of breast cancer have a significantly increased risk of developing the disease, but the reliable risk factor is the presence of two abnormal "breast cancer genes," BRCA 1 and BRCA 2. Approximately 80% of all women carrying these genes will develop breast cancer, but they account for only 5% to 10% of all diagnosed patients. For the other 90% the only dependable risk factor is age.

Signs and Symptoms

Early symptoms of breast cancer are subtle. Breast tissue is soft; tumors have ample room to grow without causing pain. Sometimes self-examination will find hard spots or lumps before a mammogram may show them, and sometimes a mammogram will reveal thickenings or minute calcifications that are too subtle to feel. Advanced cases of breast cancer show asymmetric breast growth, inverted nipples that may have discharge, and sometimes a characteristic "orange peel" texture of the skin on the breast. Advanced cases also may create symptoms in other parts of the body that are damaged by the growth of invasive tumors: bone pain, weight loss, spinal cord compression, and swelling in the arms may be the result of tumors far from the original site of the cancer. Specific protocols for breast cancer staging are discussed in sidebar, "Breast Cancer Staging."

Breast Cancer Staging

Although the progression of cancer from stage to stage has been categorized for the sake of convenience, it is impossible to predict accurately exactly how this disease will progress in each person. Every person who develops breast cancer will undergo a unique disease process, unlike anybody else's.

The most current staging protocol for breast cancer uses the TNM classification for tumor, node, and metastasis to quantify the progression of the disease into stages 0 to IV.

Tumor	Node	Metastasis
Tx: unassessable	Nx: unassessable	Mx: unassessable
T0: no tumors are present	N0: no nodes are involved	M0: no distant metastasis
T-IS: cancer in situ, with just the first layer of tissue involved	N1: 1–3 lymph nodes involved, with a sentinel node	M1: distant metastasis
T1: one or more tumors found, under 2 cm indiameter	N2: 4–9 nodes involved, all on the same side as the tumor(s)	
T2: one or more tumors found, between 2 and 5 cm in diameter	N3: 10 or more axillary nodes involved, *or* nodes are involved from other groups, i.e., the infra- or supra-clavicular, or internal mammary nodes	

Tumor	Node	Metastasis
T3: one or more tumors found, greater than 5 cm in diameter		
T4: tumors have invaded the chest wall or skin		

Stage	Tumor	Node	Metastasis	5-year survival rate
0	T-IS	N0	M0	100%
I	T1	N0	M0	98%
IIA	T0–T2	N0	M0	88%
IIB	T2–T3	N0–N1	M0	76%
IIIA	T0–T2	N2	M0	56%
IIIA	T2	N0–N2	M0	56%
IIIB	T4	N0–N2	M0	49%
IIIC	Any	N3	M0	
IV	Any	Any	M1	16%

Figure 10.5. Mammogram of breast cancer (note the irregular shape and borders of the growth).

Diagnosis

Breast cancer is usually detected first by a woman who notices a change in her breast, and then confirmed by mammogram (Figure 10.5), ultrasound, and tissue biopsy. These procedures may rule out nonmalignant breast changes. (See sidebar, "Fibrocystic Breast Changes.")

Biopsy procedures are becoming more sophisticated daily; several different techniques have been developed to offer the best chance of an accurate diagnosis, while doing the least amount of damage to the body.

If breast cancer is identified, it is then staged. If lymph node involvement is suspected, a search for the "sentinel node" may be conducted. This means that a *radioisotope* is

---

Fibrocystic Breast Changes

Nonmalignant Breast Growths

Not all breast growths are malignant. Most growths in breast tissue are cysts or benign tumors; many fall into the classification of what used to be called *fibrocystic breast disease*. It turns out these are so common (over 50% of all autopsied women show signs of fibrocystic breast growths) that this condition is no longer even called a disease; it is now referred to as *fibrocystic breast changes*. Some of these growths carry a risk of eventually becoming malignant, but they are, for the most part, not serious conditions that can easily be distinguished from malignancies with testing procedures that include mammograms, fine-needle aspiration (FNA), ultrasound, or biopsy.

- *Gross cysts*: In this situation "gross" means large, not ugly. Gross cysts are large enough to create a visible distortion of the breast. They grow most often in women in their 40s and can be reduced with fine-needle aspiration. They may recur, however, with the menstrual cycle.

- *Fibroadenomas*: These are smaller cysts, which may grow in clusters. They are most common in women in their 30s and 40s. *Fibroadenomas* are sensitive to estrogen; they tend to become enlarged and tender in the days that precede a menstrual period, and then they subside until the following month.

- *Atypical hyperplasia*: This is also called *proliferative breast disease*. It involves changes in the epithelial lining of both ducts and lobes. When it grows in the ducts, it can be difficult to differentiate from in situ ductal carcinoma. Of all the noncancerous breast changes, this one carries the highest risk for malignancy.

- *Fibrosis*: Sometimes the connective tissue framework for breast tissue, called the stroma, becomes thick and dense with excessive connective tissue. These areas of fibrosis have a characteristic hard, rubbery texture. They are firm and painless.

- *Phyllodes tumors*: These are relatively rare growths of both epithelium and connective tissue. Most are benign, but *Phyllodes tumors* carry a low risk of becoming cancerous.

- *Papillomas*: These are tiny warts, each less than a centimeter in diameter, which may grow inside the ductal tissue.

- *Other breast pathologic conditions*: Breasts can also be affected by infection (called *mastitis* if a woman is lactating, or *ductal ectasia* if she is not). Injury from trauma, surgery, or radiation may cause *fat necrosis*, a condition in which the fat cells, which make up the bulk of breast tissue, degenerate and die. Breast infections and fat necrosis can be serious situations that require medical intervention for the best outcomes.

injected near the breast, and clinicians examine where the substance is taken up; most usually flows into a single lymph node before moving on to other nodes. This first stop is the sentinel node. If this lymph node is clear of cancer cells, the likelihood is that all of the lymph nodes will be clear. Interestingly, various types of massage have been explored to aid in this process.

Prevention

Breast cancer is not a preventable disease. The two most dependable risk factors, age and genetics, are not controllable. Therefore, efforts toward prevention are targeted at early detection, which significantly increases the life expectancy of the breast cancer patient. The three main courses for early detection are self-examination, breast examination by a professional, and mammograms, which use radiation to look for unusually dense masses in the breast tissue.

Opinions vary over how frequently mammograms should be performed. This stems from the fact that the breast tissue of many women is too dense to yield dependable results before the age of 40 or even older. However, most health care agencies now recommend that women 40 and older should have yearly professional breast examinations and mammograms, and all women should learn to perform self-examinations. Breast self-examination seldom identifies new growths, but the self-awareness of what is "normal" for any individual woman gives her the tools to recognize when changes begin to occur. Women who have a personal or family history of breast cancer, who are positive for the breast cancer genes, or who are otherwise considered "high risk" for this disease may be counseled to test earlier and more often than the general public.

Understanding that a mammogram is not a definitive test for breast cancer is important. Mammogram interpretations can vary widely, and mammograms may miss the subtle changes in breast tissue that only women who perform monthly self-examinations may notice. Therefore, an "all clear" from a mammogram does not rule out the possibility of breast cancer.

Treatment

Treatment for breast cancer depends entirely on what stage the disease is in when it is found. Whatever treatment strategy is followed, every cancer patient should have access to support groups that will benefit her healing process.

Four main options for treatment are often used in combinations for best results.

- *Surgery:* Lumpectomies, partial mastectomies, total mastectomies, and modified mastectomies are surgical options for removing tumors and nearby lymph nodes. Lymph nodes are then examined for signs of further metastasis.
- *Radiation:* Radiation is aimed at tumors to slow or stop growth, or to shrink tumors to make them easier to remove surgically. Radiation may be applied externally or internally with radioactive pellets that are surgically placed around the tumors and then removed later.
- *Chemotherapy:* Chemotherapy is the treatment of cancer with highly toxic drugs that may slow or stop the growth of tumors.
- *Hormone therapy:* Some breast cancer tumors have been found to be sensitive to estrogen; they need access to this hormone to grow. A medication called *tamoxifen* binds up the estrogen receptors on tumors, which then prevents them from growing. Another drug, *letrozole*, has been found to significantly decrease the risk of breast cancer recurrence after tamoxifen has been used for 5 years.

Complications of Treatment

Cancer is a life-threatening disease that aggressively invades the body. Options to deal with cancer are similarly aggressive and often create serious side effects, which, though not as deadly as the disease itself, can be debilitating.

Surgery that removes part of the breast tissue and lymph nodes can also injure brachial plexus nerves, resulting in chronic pain in the shoulder and arm. If enough lymph nodes are removed, *lymphedema*, the accumulation of interstitial fluid in the arm, can be a serious problem. A variety of pumps and drainage devices have been developed, but all have limited success. Lymph drainage techniques can deal with this problem, but this is a very different approach from Swedish massage, and is not appropriate to practice without rigorous training. Fortunately, as diagnosticians are refining their skills, fewer lymph nodes are generally taken for analysis than in the past; this means that the incidence of lymphedema as a complication of breast cancer is on the decline.

Radiation therapy can cause skin problems, from drying and itchiness to burns and localized ulcerations.

Chemotherapy introduces highly toxic drugs into the body. These drugs can kill cancer cells, but they also cause hair loss, nausea, mouth sores, and immune suppression. Extremely high doses of chemotherapy can be successful at treating advanced cases of cancer but must be followed by bone marrow transplants to replace damaged tissue there as well.

Tamoxifen is effective at keeping hormone-sensitive tumors under control, but it is associated with several side effects, including menopause-like symptoms, an increased chance of uterine cancer, and, for some women, a tendency to form blood clots leading to *deep vein thrombosis*, *pulmonary embolism* (see Chapter 4), or *stroke* (see Chapter 3). Letrozole is associated with a low risk of *osteoporosis* (see Chapter 2).

Prognosis

If breast cancer is caught and removed before it spreads into the axillary lymph nodes, patients have a 97% chance of living 5 years or more. Overall, the 5-year survival rate is 83%, the 10-year survival rate is 65%, and the 15-year survival rate is 56%. Not surprisingly, women in whom cancer cells have been found in the lymph nodes have a much higher recurrence rate.

Breast cancer is not the kind of disease in which a person can ever say, "I'll never have to worry about that again." Because it can take many years for tumors to grow to palpable size, and because metastasis may occur before this point, even a radical mastectomy may miss far-flung cells that invade distant tissues. Breast cancer patients are obliged to be forever vigilant against the possibility of new growths.

Massage?

For many years, it was assumed that because Swedish massage increases circulation and lymph flow, it could contribute to cancer metastasis. Although conducting research to specifically explore this idea is ethically impractical, a closer look indicates some basic problems with this assumption. First, it takes years for tumors to reach palpable size; any tumor that is found after a massage has been in the making for a long time. Second, exactly how much massage increases blood and lymph movement, and for how long, are variables that have never been fully quantified. Does doing a 60-minute full-body Swedish massage move as much lymph or blood as taking a long, hot shower? How does it compare to a vigorous half-hour walk?

Obviously, a massage therapist needs to locally avoid tumor sites, especially if they are close to the surface of the skin, but most of the other cautions that surround massage and breast cancer have to do with respecting the challenges brought about by the treatment these clients must deal with, more than with the disease itself. Massage therapists can gauge their choices to provide the maximum benefit for cancer patients (anxiety and pain reduction, immune system strengthening, better appetite and sleep quality, along with general support and informed nurturing touch) while minimizing the risks of over-challenging a client who is already struggling to keep up with the demands of surgery, chemotherapy, radiation, or a combination of all three.

If a decision is made to include massage as part of a treatment program for a cancer patient, certain cautions must be observed: radiation and tumor sites are local contraindications; chemotherapy compromises immune system reactions, making the client vulnerable to a variety of infections that may contraindicate massage; changes in the health of the tissues may make clients susceptible to blood clots, bruising, or other damage that healthy people would not sustain. Because the severity of cancer treatment symptoms vary widely, it is impossible to predict what is appropriate for all clients. Rather, the therapist should work as part of a well-informed healthcare team to provide the best care and support possible.

Regardless of whether massage therapists choose to work with women who have breast cancer, one thing they *can* do is encourage their women clients to perform self-examinations. It is not within the scope of practice to do this for clients, or even to teach them how, but stressing the importance of self-examinations is a meaningful way that all massage therapists can support their clients.

Case History 10.1

Breast Cancer

Carol E., Age 60: "When You Have Had Breast Cancer, the Thought of Possible Recurrence Is Always With You. It Makes You Look at What Is Really Important in Life."

It was in July, right before my 57th birthday, when I found a lump in my left breast while doing a breast exam in the shower. We were just getting ready to leave on a vacation with friends, so I did not say anything. My annual mammogram was already scheduled in about 3 weeks.

When I went in for my mammogram, I told the doctor about the lump. He said he couldn't feel a lump. The mammogram was normal. A subsequent ultrasound did not reveal anything, and the technician also could not feel what I felt. So, even though I knew better, because of a medical background, this gave me a sense of security that all was well.

Until January. I could still feel the lump and by now my husband could also—so I was not imagining it. I talked with our daughter, an RN involved in risk management. She said, "You could have a normal mammogram and ultrasound and still have breast cancer. You have to go by what you know is normal for you." So I made an appointment with a surgeon for the week I returned from a previously planned trip to Florida.

I returned on Valentine's Day, and my appointment was on February 16th. The surgeon not only felt what I had felt (which was a thickening, more than a lump), but in checking my previous mammogram, he found pinpoints of calcium in the right breast, which are sometimes indicators of cancer. Three days later I had bilateral biopsies.

Breast Cancer, *continued*

During the biopsies, a frozen section was done on the thickening on the left side, which meant the pathologist could tell right away whether the tissue was malignant. (The tissue from the right breast biopsy went through routine pathology, and I had to wait for several days for those results). So there I was, in the recovery room, when the doctor came in and told me that the left breast biopsy was malignant. Then he left to talk to my husband and I was by myself. The greatest feeling I had was just incredible sadness. I don't know why I wasn't angry or anything else; I was just so sad. After a few minutes I was able to join my husband and we both cried.

When something like this happens to you, you begin by wondering, how bad is it? Are you going to die soon? Then you go home and do the waiting game again—for the results of the other biopsy—and this was absolutely, incredibly stressful. You are already facing surgery on one breast, and now you are wondering if you will lose both breasts. After 3 days, the call came saying the second biopsy was not malignant. By that time I was thankful that only one breast had a malignancy. Strange thing for which to be thankful.

My diagnosis was a stage 1 infiltrated ductal carcinoma, upper medial quadrant, left breast. After getting a second opinion, surgery was scheduled for the following Monday. Before that, I had to have chest x-rays, bone scan, and a radiation oncology consult as I had opted to have conservative surgery (a lumpectomy followed by 6 weeks of radiation).

The surgeon performed a lumpectomy and also did an axillary dissection—removal of some lymph nodes in the armpit. It is during this surgery that a nerve in my armpit was either severed or damaged. This produces numbness in the underarm and inner upper arm that can be permanent. The lymph nodes removed (16 in my case) were tested for malignancy, and later I learned that they showed no cancer. Chances were that the cancer had been confined to the breast tissue. Good news indeed!

However, the next Thursday, the surgeon called and said that the margins of the tissue removed were not clean—meaning that there were still some cancer cells in the breast. So, back to surgery the next Monday for a re-resection of the breast. My surgeon did not usually do this, but he felt that there was very little cancer left, and a mastectomy could still be avoided.

After a few days of recuperation, I returned home after being out to find my husband in bed with a bad headache. This was very rare, so I didn't bother him. The telephone rang and it was my surgeon again, saying (in a very upset and sad tone) that the margins on the last tissue sample still were not clean. He had spoken with the radiation oncologist and she felt she could kill the remaining cancer cells with radiation. However, the surgeon felt he could give me even better odds by performing a total mastectomy. Of course, I opted for the better odds against recurrence, and the following Monday again found me in surgery having a total mastectomy. Three major surgeries in 3 weeks with general anesthetic each time are a lot to cope with, but you do what you have to do.

Because I had a mastectomy, I did not have to have any radiation, and because my lymph nodes were negative for cancer cells, I also did not have to have chemotherapy. A big relief!

I do take tamoxifen, an anti-breast cancer drug used in certain circumstances to guard against recurrence. The standard commitment to this is 5 years. I also take amitriptyline, a mild anti-depressant, to help break the cycle of chronic nerve pain that I have had in my left arm—an unusual and difficult complication. About 8 months ago I also started on Neurontin, an anti-seizure drug that can also work on nerve pain, and in my case it has really helped. So, after almost 2 years, the pain in my arm is under control. I have no lymphedema (swelling of the arm due to a compromised lymph system). However, this could happen at any time.

I do not feel that the doctors emphasize enough how vulnerable the affected arm is. Infections can develop very easily and I have to be really careful, especially working in the garden. It seems that little burns and scratches take forever to heal. I should not lift more than 10 pounds with the affected arm and should not have any needle sticks or have blood pressure taken on that arm. Once I awoke after minor surgery to find a blood

Breast Cancer, *continued*

pressure cuff on my left arm, and was I upset! I thought that I had taken enough precautions that this should not have happened. The prescription for postsurgery medication had been clipped over the warning note! The next time I had an anesthetic, I wrote on my left arm with a surgical pen, and that did not come off!

When you have had breast cancer, the thought of possible recurrence is always with you. Breast cancer does not follow the 5-year rule; it can come back at any time. It is a lifelong commitment to always be on the watch and take really good care of yourself. This makes you look at what is really important in life. You try not to put off things that you want to say or do. Life is precious, and I am glad to still have it!

As a part of her recovery process, Carol became active in several breast cancer support groups. One of the groups of **Bosom Buddies** that she helped to co-facilitate still meets every month to have fun and draw support from each other. Through **Reach to Recovery**, Carol does hospital and home visits to new breast cancer patients, teaching them about their options, telling them what they might expect, and giving them guidance in getting more information. She would like to see women become their own advocates as they deal with the complexities of this disease.

Ovarian Cancer in Brief

What is it?
Ovarian cancer is the development of malignant tumors on the ovaries that may metastasize to other structures in the pelvic or abdominal cavity.

How is it recognized?
Symptoms of ovarian cancer are generally extremely subtle until the disease has progressed to life-threatening levels. Early symptoms include a feeling of heaviness in the pelvis, vague abdominal discomfort, occasional vaginal bleeding, and weight gain or loss.

Is massage indicated or contraindicated?
As with all cancers, the appropriateness of massage depends on what treatment measures the client chooses. Massage therapists working with clients who have ovarian cancer should be part of a fully informed health care team.

Ovarian Cancer

Definition: *What Is It?*

Ovarian cancer is the growth of malignant tumors on the ovaries. Several varieties of ovarian cancer have been identified, but most of them begin in the epithelial lining of these organs. The tumors may take a long time to become established, but once they do, some types may grow quickly and metastasize readily to the peritoneum and other organs in the abdomen.

Demographics: *Who Gets It?*

Ovarian cancer can affect any woman of any age, but it is most common in women who are 60 years of age or older. Ovarian cancer is diagnosed in approximately 25,000 women each year; that means about one out of every 60 to 70 women in the United States will have this disease. Although the incidence of this disease is low compared with other cancers, its mortality rate is high; ovarian cancer kills approximately 15,000 women every year.

Etiology: *What Happens?*

Three specific types of tumors have been found to grow on ovaries: tumors of germ cells, tumors of stromal cells, and tumors of epithelial cells. As with most types of cancers, epithelial tumors are the most common and often the most invasive. Epithelial tumors, or *adenocarcinomas*, constitute approximately 90% of all ovarian cancers.

Epithelial tumors of the ovaries fall into several different categories, each with different growth patterns and prognoses. Some of these tumors are slow-growing and may never become malignant. Early identification and removal of these growths may leave the reproductive system intact if the woman wishes to have more children. However, many types of epithelial ovarian tumors aggressively invade not only the ovaries, but other pelvic and abdominal organs as well. These tumors are life threatening, partly because they are so prone to metastasis, but also because they create few (if any) noticeable symptoms in their early stages. Usually by the time a woman is concerned enough to consult a doctor, ovarian cancer has progressed into advanced stages that are difficult or impossible to treat.

Ovarian cancer metastasizes through direct extension of tumors or through the lymph or circulatory systems. The most common route for the spread of ovarian cancer, however, is dissemination through peritoneal fluid: cancer cells from a malignant tumor may land on other areas in the pelvis, directly on the peritoneum, or up in the abdomen, to colonize and invade other tissues.

Risk Factors

Although the specific triggers for the formation of tumors on the ovaries are unknown, some of the most important risk factors for developing the disease have been identified.

- *Familial history:* A significant risk factor for ovarian cancer is having it in the family. Women who have a first-degree relative (mother, sister, daughter) with ovarian cancer could have up to a 50% chance of developing the cancer themselves. Having a second-degree relative (grandmother, aunt, half-sister) with ovarian cancer also increases the chance of developing the disease. Families with a history of *breast cancer* (this chapter) also have statistically higher rates of ovarian cancer than the general population.

- *Reproductive history:* Any woman who has never had a child or taken birth control pills, or who has experienced multiple miscarriages, is at increased risk for developing ovarian cancer. This association points to the theory that ovarian cancer may have something to do with poor healing after ovulation. Women who never have a break in their menstrual cycle are at significantly increased risk for this disease. In addition, women who have taken fertility drugs without conceiving and bearing a child also may be at increased risk, although the statistics for these women have been inconsistent.

- *Health history:* Women who have a history of breast or colon cancer themselves have approximately twice the chance of developing ovarian cancer as the rest of the population. Women who carry the breast cancer genes BRCA 1 and BRCA 2, or the genes for hereditary nonpolyposis colorectal cancer syndrome (see *colorectal cancer*, Chapter 7), are at especially high risk.

- *Estrogen replacement therapy:* Women who have employed ERT against *osteoporosis* (see Chapter 2) for more than 4 years have a higher chance of developing ovarian cancer than others.

- *Other:* Other risks involve exposure to radiation or asbestos, the use of talcum powder on the genitals, a high-fat diet, and age; the chance of developing ovarian cancer goes up considerably between ages 40 and 60.

Signs and Symptoms

The feature that makes ovarian cancer such a dangerous disease is that early symptoms are practically nonexistent, or so subtle that they are easily passed over. Then when the cancer is finally identified, it has often metastasized beyond the point of control.

Early symptoms of ovarian cancer include a feeling of heaviness in the pelvis, vague abdominal discomfort including bloating, nausea, diarrhea, and constipation, vaginal bleeding, a change in menstrual cycles, and weight gain or loss. Because the most common age for women to be affected by ovarian cancer is also the time when symptoms of menopause develop, these signals are easily ignored. Later symptoms can include a palpable abdominal mass, increased girth around the abdomen, and ascites: the accumulation of fluid in the peritoneum.

Diagnosis

Ovarian cancer is difficult to diagnose early. A pelvic examination may show unusual abdominal masses, but only a fourth of these turn out to be cancerous. Other tests that may be conducted include ultrasound tests conducted through the vagina, CT scans, and MRIs. Barium enemas and pyelograms (a process that stains urine in the kidneys to see how it moves down the ureters into the bladder) may be conducted to look for structures that may be pressing on other abdominal organs. A blood test called CA-125 looks for a particular tumor marker in the bloodstream. This has been useful in confirming a diagnosis, but it occasionally yields false-positive and false-negative results, so it is not a definitive test. Ultimately, a *laparotomy* must be conducted to take a tissue sample from the ovaries for analysis.

Ovarian cancer is found in stages I or II only 25% of the time. Most diagnoses come when the cancer has advanced to stage III or IV, when the chances for survival fall drastically. The overall 5-year survival rate for ovarian cancer is 50%, but those women who find their disease in stage I have close to a 100% chance of reaching that goal. For more information on ovarian cancer staging protocol, see sidebar, "Ovarian Cancer Staging."

Ovarian Cancer Staging

Different professionals use slightly different protocols to stage ovarian cancer. What follows is a simplified version of the TNM protocol that is predominantly used in the United States.

Tumor	Nodes	Metastasis
Tx: unassessable	Nx: unassessable	Mx: unassessable
T1: tumor(s) is confined to the ovaries; cells may be present in peritoneal fluid	N0: no nodes involved	M0: no distant metastasis
T2: tumors are found in pelvic tissues or in peritoneal fluid	N1: only regional lymph nodes are affected	M1: distant metastasis
T3: tumors have spread to abdominal peritoneum or organs		

These guidelines are used to quantify the progression of ovarian cancer into stages I through IV as follows:

Stage	Tumor	Node	Metastasis	5-year survival
I a, b, c	One or both ovaries are affected; the outside surface may be ruptured; cells may be present in the peritoneum	N0	M0	80%–90%
II a, b, c	Ovaries and pelvic organs are affected; cells may be found in peritoneal fluid	N0	M0	65%–70%
III	Ovaries, pelvic organs, or lymph nodes are affected	N0–N1	M0	30%–60%
IV	Ovaries, pelvic, and abdominal organs are affected; cells in pleural fluid may be found	N1	M1	20%

Treatment

Ovarian cancer is generally treated with surgery and chemotherapy. Surgery is done to remove the ovaries (*oophorectomy*), and sometimes the uterine tubes and uterus as well. Chemotherapy can be conducted orally at home or intravenously in a hospital. One method delivers the cytotoxic drugs directly into the peritoneum, where it can have immediate access to malignant tumors.

Radiation therapy is not usually used for ovarian cancer.

Massage?

As with any kind of cancer, the appropriateness of massage for ovarian cancer is a matter of personal choice. A client who is recovering from ovarian cancer may find that massage can ameliorate the challenges of surgery and chemotherapy. If a client wishes to include massage in her treatment program, she and her massage therapist should consult with her oncologist and other health care team members for the best and safest results.

Mittelschmerz:

This is a term derived from German for "middle pain." This refers to the sensation some women have when the leading follicle on an ovary ruptures, and the egg is released into the pelvic cavity. It is called "middle" because it occurs precisely in the middle (about day 14) of the menstrual cycle.

Ovarian Cysts

Definition: What Are They?

A variety of cysts may grow on the ovaries. They may be related to endometriosis (this chapter), or they may be varieties of precancerous growths that may develop into *ovarian cancer* (this chapter). The cysts under discussion in this article, however, are *functional cysts*, that is, they arise from normal ovaries, usually as a result of hormonal imbalance or dysfunction.

Demographics: Who Gets Them?

Ovarian cysts have been found in females of all ages, from prenatal babies to elderly women. Most of functional cysts are found in women between the onset of menstruation (*menarche*) and the onset of menopause. In other words, women who ovulate are at greatest risk for functional ovarian cysts.

Functional cysts are very common among fertile women. Up to 30% of all women with regular menstrual cycles develop an ovarian cyst at least once; up to 50% of women with irregular cycles develop at least one ovarian cyst.

When ovarian cysts are found in premenarchal girls or postmenopausal women, the chances of malignancy are much higher than among other patients. Abnormal growths among these populations are treated much more aggressively than those among women of childbearing age.

Etiology: What Happens?

A follicle is a small sac or cavity that produces a secretion. Every month a fertile woman develops several follicles on one of her ovaries. As her cycle progresses, a single follicle becomes dominant, and the others recede. At the appropriate hormonal signal, the follicle ruptures, releasing a mature egg, or *oocyte*, into the pelvic cavity, where it is drawn into the uterine tubes for the journey toward the uterus.

Each follicle that develops is a potential cyst. Sometimes the hormonal signal (a surge in leuteinizing hormone) does not occur, and the follicle does not rupture completely.

Ovarian Cysts in Brief

What are they?
Most ovarian cysts are fluid-filled growths on the ovaries. Some types of cysts are associated with ovarian cancer or other reproductive disorders, but the cysts under discussion in this article are benign.

How are they recognized?
The symptoms of ovarian cysts may be nonexistent, or they may cause a disruption in the menstrual cycle. Constant or intermittent pain in the pelvis, pain with intercourse, or symptoms similar to early pregnancy may arise from different types of ovarian cysts.

Is massage indicated or contraindicated?
Ovarian cysts that have been diagnosed locally contraindicate massage.

Consequently, a blister forms on the ovary. Sometimes the ruptured follicle (now called the *corpus luteum*) seals up behind the discharged ovum but traps the hormones that should flow freely from it. This kind of blister may eventually break and bleed into the pelvic cavity. Some other cysts arise in conjunction with abnormal pregnancies, or as a result of hormonal imbalances that may begin in the pituitary gland.

Most ovarian cysts are not dangerous, but they have the potential to become large and painful, and they may develop dangerous complications.

Types of Cysts

Several types of cysts can form on the ovaries. Three of the most common kinds are discussed here:

- *Follicular cysts*: When a follicle that holds a mature egg does not rupture completely, a blister forms at the site. Follicular cysts rarely get bigger than 2 to 3 inches across, and they usually spontaneously recede within two menstrual cycles (Figure 10.6). Follicular cysts are the most common of all ovarian cysts.

- *Corpus luteum cysts*: Blisters can form over the corpus luteum, which blocks the hormones that should be secreted from the ovaries. Corpus luteum cysts will delay subsequent ovulations and produce pregnancy-like symptoms (nausea, vomiting, breast tenderness) until they spontaneously resolve, usually within a month or two. Corpus luteum cysts are less common than follicular cysts, but they can be more serious, because they may create bleeding into the peritoneal space.

- *Polycystic ovaries*: Also called **Stein-Leventhal syndrome**, this condition involves enlarged ovaries with multiple small cysts (Figure 10.7). The interference in hormone secretion that this condition creates may lead to obesity, loss of menstrual cycle, *acne* (see Chapter 1), and **hirsutism** (increased body hair). Polycystic ovary disease (PCOD) is also closely linked with poor use of insulin, high triglycerides, and low high-density lipoproteins, and other signs associated with *metabolic syndrome* (Chapter 8).

Other cysts that may grow on the ovaries may be a part of endometriosis, **cystadenomas**, which are usually benign tumors but can occasionally become cancerous, and dermoid cysts or **teratomas**. In these cysts, some primitive cells have been isolated from

Figure 10.6. Ovarian cyst.

Figure 10.7. Polycystic ovary.

the rest of the body and have developed into different types of tissues. Dermoid cysts have been found that contain teeth, hairs, bone fragments, and other types of tissue. They are usually harmless in women. Men can develop them too, but for males teratomas are a much more serious condition that may involve *testicular cancer* (this chapter).

Signs and Symptoms

Most ovarian cysts have no symptoms until the cyst is injured in some way. Some women, however, will experience a constant dull ache in the lower abdomen on the affected side. A firm, painless swelling may develop in the pelvis, and occasionally an ovarian cyst will cause pain with intercourse. Large cysts may create low back pain, or, through pressure on the lumbar plexus, pain into the legs. Corpus luteum cysts and polycystic ovaries have special symptoms of their own, which are described above. In the absence of these signs, a person would never know a cyst was there unless it grew big enough to interfere with other functions, or if it ruptured.

Complications

Size is the major factor that determines whether ovarian cysts are going to cause any trouble. They can grow big enough to interfere with blood flow; they may also rest on the bladder. In rare cases, they can grow to incredible dimensions. An ovarian cyst that hangs from a stalk may sometimes get twisted. If that happens, acute abdominal pain, nausea, and fever will develop; medical intervention is necessary because the tissue may die and become necrotic. Similar symptoms will be present if the cyst ruptures. The risk of *peritonitis* (Chapter 7) is high in this situation.

Perhaps the most serious complicating factor of ovarian cysts is that their early symptoms, subtle as they may be, mimic an *advanced* case of *ovarian cancer* (this chapter). This is a highly dangerous cancer that has few early symptoms. By the time a person can feel a firm painless swelling in her pelvis, the disease is dangerously advanced. Therefore, if a client displays any of these symptoms but has not been examined, urge her to get checked out as soon as possible.

Diagnosis

Ovarian cysts are frequently found as a swelling or mass during a routine pelvic examination. Ultrasound pictures generally confirm the diagnosis. If the patient is at high risk for cancer, or if the cyst looks to have a solid rather than liquid core, a laparoscopy may be performed to take a tissue sample for analysis. Follow-up on cyst-like symptoms that last for more than 60 days is important because follicular and corpus luteum cysts, the two most common and benign varieties, will usually have been resolved within this period.

Treatment

Follicular and corpus luteum cysts are often treated with oral contraceptives. Birth control pills alter hormonal secretions and allow the cysts to recede completely, or to shrink to a size that is easily removed. Ovarian cysts that do not spontaneously resolve may be aspirated, but more often surgery is performed to remove them. The affected ovary is usually taken as well. In some cases, a complete removal of the ovaries and uterus will be recommended because some types of cysts tend to recur and can develop into cancer.

Massage?

Ovarian cysts locally contraindicate massage. Be aware that ovarian cysts also can displace the pelvic contents, so deep abdominal work done where it would be safe on a woman without cysts may lead to bruising of the ovaries or even rupture of the cyst on someone who has this condition. Massage elsewhere on the body is appropriate.

DISORDERS OF THE MALE REPRODUCTIVE SYSTEM

Benign Prostatic Hyperplasia

Benign Prostatic Hyperplasia in Brief

What is it?
Benign prostatic hyperplasia (BPH) is a condition in which the prostate gland of a mature man begins to grow for the first time since the end of puberty. It is not related to cancer, which is why this condition is called "benign."

How is it recognized?
The primary symptoms of BPH have to do with mechanical obstruction of the urethra. This leads to problems with urination, including a feeling of frequency, difficulties with initiating flow, leaking, and the sensation that the bladder is never emptied. Many men with BPH never develop these symptoms, however. For them, BPH is a silent condition.

Is massage indicated or contraindicated?
BPH is a common condition among mature men, and it does not usually involve cancer or infection. Massage is perfectly appropriate for these clients, as long as no signs of urinary tract infection or kidney disorders are present.

Definition: What Is It?

Benign prostatic hyperplasia (BPH) is a condition in which the prostate gland of mature men becomes enlarged. This growth late in life is not related to *prostate cancer* (this chapter), hence the name "benign."

Demographics: Who Gets It?

The single greatest risk factors for developing BPH are simply being a male and being mature. Although not all men with BPH experience symptoms, its incidence is remarkably high. Nearly 50% of all men over 60 years of age have some level of BPH; 70% of men over 70 have it; 80% of men over 80 have it, and so on.

Etiology: What Happens?

The prostate gland of a preadolescent male is very small. As a boy enters puberty, this pea-sized gland that wraps around the urethra just below the bladder grows approximately to the size of a walnut. It stays that size until a man is approximately 40 years old, and then some prostates begin to grow again.

Why some prostate glands grow and others do not is unclear. Theories about triggers for late prostate growth involve hormonal changes with maturity. One possible factor may be the formation of ***dihydrotestosterone***, or DHT. This hormone is a form of testosterone that has been seen to increase prostate size. Another theory is that as men age they produce less testosterone to balance out their normal levels of estrogen; this may lead to hyperplasia, because estrogen is also associated with prostate growth.

Regardless of the cause of prostate growth, BPH may lead to mechanical pressure on the urethra (Figure 10.8). This occurs for two reasons: the prostate is surrounded by a tough fascial capsule that does not allow it to expand outwardly, and the tissue usually affected by BPH is in the periurethral and transitional sections of the gland. (This helps to distinguish BPH from prostate cancer, which typically begins on the outer borders of the prostate.)

The extent of growth does not always correspond with the amount of pressure on the urethra; some men have advanced BPH with no urinary symptoms at all, and others have minimal amounts of prostate growth and severe urethral constriction.

Mechanical pressure on the urethra makes it difficult to expel urine from the body (see Figure 10.8). Long-term consequences can lead to pathologic changes in the bladder, which can become stiff, inelastic, and irritable. The risk of *urinary tract infections*, *pyelonephritis* (see Chapter 9) and bladder stones is much higher in men who cannot urinate easily; these are common complications of BPH.

Signs and Symptoms

Signs and symptoms of BPH, when any develop at all, involve difficulties with urination. Weak flow, interrupted flow, frequency, and a feeling that the bladder is never completely emptied are often reported. Leaking or dribbling urine between visits to the bathroom is common. Some men find it difficult to initiate urination, and they must strain or push to start their flow. Other men find that they need to urinate more frequently, especially at night. BPH does not typically cause pelvic pain, which distinguishes it from *prostatitis* (this chapter).

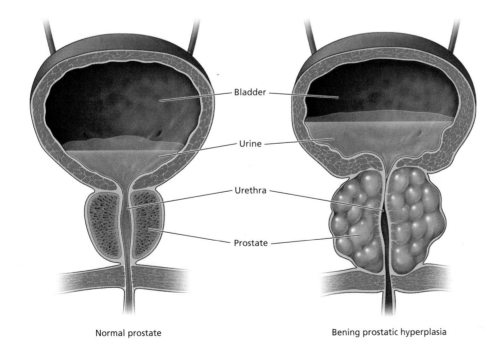

Normal prostate   Bening prostatic hyperplasia

Figure 10.8. Benign prostatic hyperplasia.

One rare but serious symptom of BPH is an abrupt obstruction of the urethra, called *acute urinary retention*. In this situation, the urethra is suddenly completely obstructed, and urine has no way to get out of the body. This is a medical emergency, and must be treated in a hospital.

Diagnosis

BPH is diagnosed in a number of ways, to identify exactly where and how seriously the urethra is obstructed. Palpation through the wall of the rectum yields information about the size and quality of the growths; BPH usually feels like overall enlargement or smooth, deep nodules, whereas prostate cancer involves harder, more superficial growths. Tests may measure the speed and completeness of urination, pressure in the bladder, or how much urine is left in the bladder after urination.

Because the symptoms of BPH are so similar to those of prostate cancer, part of any screening for BPH includes a PSA (prostate-specific antigen) blood test.

Treatment

BPH is treated according to severity. If it does not seriously impact a man's ability to urinate, it may be left untreated but closely monitored for signs of further growth. A number of options have been developed to limit prostate growth, including medications and a variety of surgeries.

Medications for BPH include drugs designed to lower levels of DHT, the testosterone derivative believed to stimulate prostate growth, and alpha-blockers, a group of medications that help the prostate and bladder to relax. The side effects of these medications can be severe, however, including the inability to achieve erection, lowered sex drive, lowered sperm counts, and others. Several herbal preparations may be recommended to prevent or limit prostate growth. Saw palmetto has been seen in clinical trials to be as effective as some medications, while creating fewer side effects. The challenge with this option is finding a source in which potency and dosage is consistent.

Surgical options for BPH include a variety of techniques that cut away, vaporize, burn, microwave, or otherwise remove small sections of the prostate gland to relieve pressure on the urethra. This field is rapidly expanding because the American population is aging, and it is estimated that 25% to 30% of all American men may need surgical intervention to help with BPH symptoms at some time. Tissue removed with prostate surgery is routinely examined for signs of cancer. Approximately 10% of all men who undergo surgery for BPH have developed early signs of prostate cancer.

Massage?

Massage can have little (if any) impact on prostate growth, and the prostate itself is located in an area that most bodyworkers do not access. Although massage will not improve this situation, it can certainly improve the quality of life of the patient; therefore, BPH indicates massage systemically, if not locally. If a client reports any symptoms of a urinary tract or kidney infection, however, it is important that he get appropriate care as soon as possible.

Prostate Cancer

Definition

Prostate cancer is the growth of malignant tumor cells in the prostate gland. This cancer often grows slowly, but some versions of it can be aggressive. Prostate cancer can metastasize to other parts of the body, most often the bladder, rectum, and bones of the pelvis.

Demographics: Who Gets It?

Each year, approximately 212,000 cases of prostate cancer are diagnosed in this country, and an estimated 29,000 men die of the disease. With the aging of the baby boomers, those numbers are expected to at least double in the next 20 years. Prostate cancer is rarely found in men younger than 40 years, but microscopic precancerous changes are found in approximately 25% of men over the age of 50, and approximately 50% of men over 80. The incidence of prostate cancer rises with increasing age; the average age at diagnosis is 70 to 72 years. The lifetime risk of developing prostate cancer for all males in this country is approximately 10%. Prostate cancer is the second most commonly diagnosed cancer in men (skin cancer is first), and the second leading cause of death by cancer in men (lung cancer is first).

African American men are approximately twice as likely to develop prostate cancer as whites; they are also about twice as likely to die of this disease. Asians and Pacific Islanders have the statistically lowest rates of this disease.

Prostate Cancer in Brief

What is it?
Prostate cancer is the growth of malignant cells in the prostate gland, which may then metastasize, usually to nearby bones or into inguinal lymph nodes.

How is it recognized?
The symptoms of prostate cancer include problems with urination: weak stream, frequency, urgency, nocturia, and other problems arising from constriction of the urethra.

Is massage indicated or contraindicated?
Prostate cancer patients may face any combination of surgery, radiation, chemotherapy, and hormonal therapy to deal with their disease. Bodywork that accommodates for these challenges while minimizing risks can be helpful and supportive, as long as the massage therapist is working as part of a fully informed health care team.

Etiology: What Happens?

The prostate is a donut-shaped gland that lies inferior to the bladder and encircles the male urethra. It produces the fluid that allows for the motility and viability of sperm. The prostate also controls release of the urine from the bladder. Some enlargement of the prostate in later years is almost a guarantee for men. Simple enlargement with no malignant cells is called BPH, or benign prostatic hyperplasia (this chapter). However, sometimes the growth and thickening of the prostate gland is not benign; it indicates prostate cancer.

When cancerous cells begin to form a tumor in the prostate, they can exert direct pressure on the urethra. This can lead to a number of different problems, from difficulty in urinating to urgency, frequency, *nocturia*, painful ejaculation, and bladder infections. Because the symptoms of prostate cancer are so similar to those of BPH, these signs may be ignored until the urethra is seriously restricted. Prostate cancer grows slowly, and it can stay silent long enough for cells to metastasize before it is detected.

The precise genetic mutations that lead to prostate cancer are under intense scrutiny. At this point, the disease seems to be related to several contributing factors: the activation of *oncogenes* that stimulate the growth of new cells; the inhibition of tumor-suppressor genes that limit new growth; and the absence of a key enzyme that works to bind up and neutralize free radicals that have been seen to damage prostate cells.

Causes

The precise causes of prostate cancer are unknown. It has been observed, however, that for tumors to grow they must have access to testosterone from fully functional testes. This disease is unknown in men who have been castrated, and removal of the testes has also been shown to shrink cancerous tumors.

Men with prostate cancer in their immediate family are more likely than others to develop this disease; heredity is estimated to account for approximately 10% of all prostate cancer cases. Men whose diets are high in animal fats have higher rates of prostate cancer than others. And, as discussed before, advanced age and being African American are two other risk factors for this disease. It is important to point out however, that risk factors are only general tendencies. As with many other types of cancers, many prostate cancer patients do *not* fit the profile, and being free from these identified risk factors does not mean a person can automatically avoid this problem.

Signs and Symptoms

Symptoms of prostate cancer are exactly the same as those for BPH: an enlarged, hard prostate, obstruction of the urethra with resulting difficulty in urination, and susceptibility to *urinary tract* and *kidney infections* (see Chapter 9). In addition, men with prostate cancer may also experience pain while urinating or ejaculating, blood in the urine, and the inability to maintain an erection. Low back pain and pain that refers into the upper thighs may follow as the growths become large enough to put mechanical pressure on pelvic nerves.

Diagnosis

Historically prostate cancer has been difficult to diagnose in the early stages, because its only signs and symptoms are so close to BPH, a disorder experienced by most elderly men. However, the advent of some early detection tests has made prostate cancer much easier to find before it has spread beyond the prostate.

A digital rectal exam (DRE) is the first step in prostate cancer detection. Prostate cancer tends to grow first on the periphery of the prostate gland, in hard, palpable nodules; this feature distinguishes it from BPH, which tends to involve deeper and smoother nodules.

A blood test to look for prostate-specific antigen (PSA) is another early detection device. Its usefulness is somewhat debatable because many variables may cause PSA levels to rise or fall, but when levels are higher than normal, this blood test can serve as a warning sign to consider the possibility of prostate cancer. PSA tests can be further clarified to examine whether the PSA is "free" or "attached." Some research now associates free PSA with BPH, whereas PSA that is attached to blood proteins may indicate more aggressive forms of prostate cancer.

The American Cancer Society recommends that most men have a yearly DRE and PSA test after age 50 and that black men and men with other family members who have prostate cancer should start by age 40 or 45.[4]

If the DRE or PSA turn up any specific concerns, further exploration is conducted through a transrectal ultrasound and the biopsy of suspicious tissue.

Prostate cancer is staged by advancement and by the aggressiveness of the growths. Early detection methods have made it possible to find close to 80% of all cases before the cancer has spread beyond the prostate; the 5-year survival rate for these patients approaches 100%. For more information on staging prostate cancer, see sidebar, "Prostate Cancer Staging."

Prostate Cancer Staging

Several different staging protocols for prostate cancer have been developed, but they all follow a similar, relatively simple pattern:

- Stage I (Stage A): The tumor is impalpable, completely confined to the prostate, and is probably found as a result of treatment for BPH or as part of an elevated PSA test.
- Stage II (Stage B): The tumor is palpable with a digital rectal examination; high PSA levels are noted; a tissue biopsy is positive. The growth is still confined to the prostate gland.
- Stage III (Stage C): Tumors have metastasized to nearby tissues, including the bladder, colon, rectum, or sacrum.
- Stage IV (Stage D): Nearby lymph nodes have been invaded; distant metastasis has developed.

[4] Can Prostate Cancer Be Found Early? Copyright © 2004 American Cancer Society, Inc. Available at: http://www.cancer.org/docroot/CRI/content/CRI_2_4_3X_Can_prostate_cancer_be_found_early_36.asp?rnav=cri.

Treatment

Treatment options for prostate cancer include radiation from internal or external sources, surgery to remove part or all of the prostate or the testes, and hormone therapy: estrogen counteracts elevated levels of testosterone. Chemotherapy is generally reserved for very advanced cases. Most treatment options for prostate cancer involve serious complications including incontinence, impotence, and the development of feminine characteristics. Elderly men or men with other health problem who have slow-growing tumors may simply opt not to treat their disease because their quality of life would be so seriously impacted.

New treatment options for treating prostate cancer are in continuing development. These include drugs that inhibit angiogenesis so that tumors cannot grow, and other substances that interrupt the replication of any cell that produces PSA.

Massage?

Most massage therapists who have elderly men as part of their clientele have some clients who live with the threat of prostate cancer. It is important to know how the client keeps his condition under observation, and what treatment options he chooses. Massage therapists working as part of a health care team can certainly improve the quality of these clients' lives by providing supportive, informed touch during a time of great stress and challenge.

Prostatitis

Definition: What Is It?

Prostatitis is a condition in which the prostate becomes enlarged and possibly inflamed. Unlike benign prostatic hyperplasia (BPH, this chapter), prostatitis usually involves significant pain throughout the pelvis and groin. Although occasionally connected to a specific infection, the causes of prostatitis are often difficult to clearly identify and treat.

Demographics: Who Gets It?

Prostatitis is a common disorder; it is responsible for 25% of all visits to urologists: approximately 2 million doctor visits per year. An estimated 10% to 50% of all men between 20 and 74 years of age will have symptoms at least once. It is the most common urologic problem in men younger than 50 years.

Certain types of prostatitis are linked to specific demographic groups. Acute bacterial prostatitis, for instance, is often associated with *sexually transmitted diseases* (this chapter) and is seen most often in younger men with multiple partners.

Etiology: What Happens?

The prostate gland is a walnut-sized gland that surrounds the urethra just distal to the urinary bladder. It is composed of ducts and channels into which epithelial cells secrete seminal fluid, a constituent of semen. The seminal fluid is expressed into the urethra during ejaculation.

Prostatitis in Brief

What is it?
Prostatitis is the inflammation of the prostate gland, from either bacterial or nonbacterial causes.

How is it recognized?
Symptoms of prostatitis vary according to their cause. Acute prostatitis involves fever, extremely painful urination, urinary frequency and urgency, and pain in the penis, testicles, perineum, and low back. Chronic prostatitis involves similar symptoms, but they tend to be less severe, and they do not include fever.

Is massage indicated or contraindicated?
Judgments about massage in the context of prostatitis need to be made according to the causative factors. An acute bacterial infection contraindicates circulatory bodywork, but a low-grade, noninfectious, chronic situation may not carry the same cautions. "Prostate massage" is a procedure performed by a doctor through the rectal wall and is not within the scope of practice of massage therapists.

The draining channels in the prostate are arranged in a basically horizontal plane around the periphery of the organ. This allows material to become stagnant within the gland if it is not frequently expelled. Furthermore, bladder reflux, in which urine collects in the prostate, can cause irritation or even direct bacterial exposure to these delicate epithelial tissues, leading to a risk of prostate stones, and acute or chronic infections that may be difficult to treat.

Prostatitis is an umbrella term that covers four basic types of problems. These classes of prostatitis were outlined by the National Institutes of Health in 1995 to create a framework for more efficient study of this often mysterious and difficult problem.[5]

- *Type 1: Acute bacterial prostatitis* is an acute infection of the prostate. This may be accompanied by an abscess, which requires surgery to remove.

- *Type 2: Chronic bacterial prostatitis* is a recurrent infection of the prostate.

- *Type 3: Chronic nonbacterial prostatitis/chronic pelvic pain syndrome* (CPPS) is prostate enlargement with no demonstrable infection. Subgroups of this class are:
   - 3.1. *Inflammatory chronic pelvic pain syndrome*, in which white blood cells are found in the semen, expressed prostatic secretions, or urine.
   - 3.2. *Noninflammatory chronic pelvic pain syndrome*, in which white cells are *not* found in semen, expressed prostatic secretions, and urine.

- *Type 4: Asymptomatic inflammatory prostatitis* (AIP) has no subjective symptoms; however, white blood cells are found in prostate secretions or in prostate tissue during an evaluation for other disorders.

When prostatitis is related to an acute or recurrent infection (types 1 or 2), the most common agent is *E. coli*, although *Klebsiella* or *Proteus mirabilis* may be involved. It is not always clear how bacteria get into the prostate; leading theories suggest that they could move up the urethra after unprotected sexual intercourse or the use of a contaminated catheter, or bacteria could migrate to the prostate through the circulatory or lymph systems.

Type 3 prostatitis (chronic pelvic pain syndrome, or CPPS) is by far the most commonly reported condition, accounting for up to 90% of all prostatitis diagnoses. This mysterious condition is not well understood because no specific causative factors have ever been identified. Some researchers suggest that CPPS is indeed a bacterial infection; however, the pathogens are of a type that do not culture on standard tests. Others have found that the pelvic pain that accompanies CPPS may be as much attributable to chronic hypertonicity of the perineal muscle as to any prostate dysfunction; this moves CPPS into a category of myofascial pain.

Signs and Symptoms

Acute bacterial prostatitis has all of the signs and symptoms of a *urinary tract infection* (Chapter 9): pain and burning with urination; urinary frequency and urgency; pain in the pelvis, perineum, testicles, and penis; penile discharge; painful ejaculation; low back pain; and fever. The prostate, felt through the wall of the rectum, is exquisitely painful and palpably hot. Chronic bacterial prostatitis, which indicates recurrent low-grade infection, shares the same symptoms, but with less severity. Chronic pelvic pain syndrome has the same profile, without the element of fever, and palpation of the prostate may show it to be enlarged and soft, but only mildly painful.

---

[5] Chronic Prostatitis Workshop. National Institute of Diabetes and Digestive and Kidney Diseases, National Institutes of Health. Available at: http://kidney.niddk.nih.gov/kudiseases/pubs/chronicprostatitis/index.htm. Accessed winter 2004.

Complications

The most common complication for any type of prostatitis is the risk of urethral obstruction. If enough pressure is exerted deeply on the urethra, acute urinary retention may develop. This is a medical emergency and requires immediate intervention.

Diagnosis

The first goal in diagnosis of prostate dysfunction is to rule out *BPH* and *prostate cancer* (this chapter). After that, bacterial infection is often assumed, although seldom actually cultured.

Urologists who specialize in these disorders frequently conduct a multi-step series of tests to try to confirm the presence or absence of bacteria. Urine is analyzed from three different stages: the initial stream (which may be contaminated with material from the urethra), midstream (when the urine should be sterile), and after prostate massage: a procedure in which the prostate is manipulated through the rectal wall by a doctor to express some fluid through the penis for examination. A semen sample also may be analyzed to look for the presence of bacteria or white blood cells that indicate inflammation in the urogenital tract.

Biopsies of prostate tissue are not recommended if infection is a possibility, to avoid the risk of inadvertently spreading any pathogens.

Treatment

Acute bacterial prostatitis (type 1) responds well to antibiotics. Unfortunately, type 2 (chronic bacterial prostatitis) does not. It may take 6 weeks or more of antibiotic therapy to address this issue, and it frequently recurs.

If prostate stones are identified during the diagnostic process, these are surgically removed, typically through laser surgery conducted through the urethra.

Type 3 prostatitis is often treated with a short or long course of antibiotics "just in case" some bacteria were missed but then dealt with symptomatically. Alpha-blockers relax the smooth muscle tissue in the bladder for easier urination; anti-inflammatories, frequent ejaculations, and sitz baths (a bath just for the pelvic area) to help relax the perineal muscle are also recommended. Biofeedback techniques to increase awareness of tightness in the perineal muscle have some success, as well as a dietary supplement called *quercetin* (a bioflavonoid found in red wine, onions, and green tea). For many men, however, chronic pelvic pain syndrome is a stubborn disorder with no simple answers; it can have a long-term negative impact on the quality of life.

Massage?

Massage is only peripherally influential on prostate problems, because the gland is located in an area to which massage therapists have no access. Nonetheless, when acute infection is present, with fever and inflammation, massage is obviously inappropriate. For men who struggle with chronic problems, however, massage may be part of a useful coping mechanism as long as the client is comfortable on the table.

Testicular Cancer

Definition: What Is It?

Testicular cancer is the growth of malignant cells in the testicles. These cells usually grow slowly, but they may metastasize through the lymph or blood systems.

Testicular Cancer in Brief

What is it?
Testicular cancer is the growth of malignant cells in the testicles, which may then metastasize all over the body.

How is it recognized?
Early signs of testicular cancer include a painless lump in the scrotum, a dull ache in the low abdomen or groin, a sense of heaviness in the scrotum, and enlarged or tender breasts.

Is massage indicated or contraindicated?
Guidelines about massage in the context of testicular cancer follow the same rules as for other types of cancer. This particular variety of cancer usually has an excellent prognosis and responds well to radiation or chemotherapy. Massage may be a useful adjunct to these therapies to improve tolerance and shorten recovery time, but it must be conducted within the client's tolerance, and as part of a fully integrated health care effort.

Demographics: Who Gets It?

Testicular cancer accounts for 1% of all male cancers. It is diagnosed approximately 7,500 times per year, and causes approximately 400 deaths per year in this country. It is eight times more common in whites than in other races. Testicular cancer is unusual in that it targets young men; it is the leading cause of cancer among males from 15 to 35 years of age. Although it is comparatively rare, some research indicates that rates of testicular cancer climbed 51% between 1973 and 1995.

Etiology: What Happens?

The causes or contributing factors for testicular cancer are not well understood. The only consistent risk factor is that males who were born with an undescended testicle (a condition called *cryptorchidism*) have a somewhat higher risk of developing this disease.

Testicular cancer is typically discussed as germ cell tumors or stromal cell tumors.

- *Stromal cell tumors:* These are growths within the supportive tissue for the testicle. They are quite rare and account for only 5% or less of all testicular cancers. They are called *Sertoli cell tumors* or *Leydig cell tumors*.

- *Germ cell tumors:* These are tumors that arise within the sperm and hormone-producing cells of the testicle. Germ cell tumors are further classified into seminomas and non-seminomas.

  - *Seminomas: Seminomas* are the most common single variety of testicular cancer, accounting for 40% to 45% of all diagnoses. They tend to grow slowly and are highly sensitive to radiation.

  - *Non-seminomas:* These are several different types of testicular tumors, some of which are more aggressive than others. Some types of non-seminomas are diagnosed among young boys and are not classified as malignant, but they can change if neglected. *Embryonic carcinomas*, *yolk sac tumors*, and *teratomas* are growths in which tissues resemble the growth pattern of embryos. In teratomas, the cells may even differentiate into different types of tissue cells, including glands, nerve tissue, and bones. One type of non-seminoma is called *choriocarcinoma*. Of all the types of testicular cancer, this one is the most aggressive and has the poorest prognosis.

Signs and Symptoms

Testicular cancer usually begins with a painless lump on the testicle. It may be accompanied by a feeling of fullness or heaviness or fluid in the scrotum. A dull ache in the low abdomen or groin may develop, along with enlargement and tenderness at the breasts. If any of these symptoms persist for more than 2 weeks, the person should consult his doctor as soon as possible.

Diagnosis

The first step in diagnosing any testicular dysfunction is to rule out the possibility of infection or injury. Ultrasound tests then may be recommended; these are highly sensitive to growths in the testicles. Blood tests may show specific markers of non-seminoma tumors. If a suspicious area is found, an *inguinal orchiectomy* (the removal of the testicle through the abdomen) is performed so the testicle can be examined for signs of cancer. This procedure is conducted through the abdomen rather than through the scrotum to avoid the possibility of inadvertently spreading any malignant cells.

If cancerous cells are found in the testicle, they are identified for type, and deep abdominal lymph nodes may be extracted to look for signs of metastasis. For more information on testicular cancer staging, see sidebar, "Testicular Cancer Staging."

Treatment

The treatment options for testicular cancer begin with surgery to remove the affected testicle and any secondary tumors that might be found. If the cancer is identified as a seminoma, radiation therapy follows surgery; these cancer cells are extremely sensitive to radiation, and this protocol is usually completely successful.

If the cancer was a mixed tumor or a non-seminoma, chemotherapy may be used after surgery. Recent developments of new chemotherapeutic agents have significantly improved the prognosis for non-seminoma cancer.

Follow-up care after testicular cancer treatment is critical, to make sure no metastases were missed. Furthermore, testicular cancer survivors have a small but significant risk of developing cancer in the other testicle.

Survival rates for most cases of testicular cancer are excellent. The 5-year survival rate for seminomas found in stages I or II is close to 95%. Most non-seminomas have a 5-year survival rate of 70% to 85%. The exception to this rule is choriocarcinoma, which has a near-zero 5-year survival rate.

The survival rate for testicular cancer is so high, and the treatments available are so effective, that no invasive early screening protocols for this disease have been developed or recommended. Nonetheless, many men are taught to conduct testicular self-examinations, just as women are taught to do breast self-examinations. In this way, any changes that occur in the tissue may be identified and investigated as quickly as possible.

Massage?

A person who is fighting testicular cancer is probably undergoing cycles of radiation or chemotherapy. Massage may improve the tolerance for these demanding treatments, as long as the client is resilient enough to keep up with the changes massage brings about. Many testicular cancer patients are encouraged to exercise; this is a good sign that massage is appropriate as well. Massage may improve appetite and quality of sleep: two features that are especially important for patients undergoing treatment for cancer.

Massage therapists working with clients who have testicular cancer (or any other kind of cancer) must be sure to keep the rest of the client's health care team informed so that everyone can work together for the best possible outcome.

Testicular Cancer Staging

Testicular cancer is staged differently from most other cancers; instead of progressing from stage 0 through stage IV, it is usually discussed as stages 0 through III. Specialists use highly defined and detailed staging protocols to make appropriate treatment plans and prognoses; these often include measurements of cancer markers in the blood along with tumor, node, and metastatic progress. The following is a simplified version of testicular cancer staging:

- *Stage 0:* This is cancer in situ: preinvasive germ cell cancer.
- *Stage I:* The testicle and spermatic cord are affected; no spread to lymph nodes; blood tests are normal.
- *Stage II:* The lymph nodes below the diaphragm are invaded.
  - *Stage IIA:* The nodes show signs of microscopic invasion. This is sometimes called "nonbulky stage II."
  - *Stage IIB:* The nodes are larger than 5 cm; this can be called "bulky stage II."
- *Stage III:* Lymph nodes and other tissues above the diaphragm are invaded.
  - *Stage IIIA:* Only lymph nodes are invaded, but growths are smaller than 2 cm ("nonbulky stage III").
  - *Stage IIIB:* Other tissues are invaded, usually the CNS or lungs. Lymph node metastases are larger than 2 cm ("bulky stage III").

OTHER REPRODUCTIVE SYSTEM CONDITIONS

Menopause

Definition: What Is It?

Menopause refers to a specific event: the moment the ovaries permanently stop secreting enough hormones to initiate a menstrual cycle. The time leading up to this event is called *perimenopause*, and many of the symptoms associated with declining hormone secretion occur during this period. Menopause itself is not conclusively identified until menstruation has completely stopped for a full year.

Demographics: Who Gets It?

All women who live long enough will experience a decline in ovarian function. In 1900, the average female life expectancy was 51 years, and menopause was not a significant health care issue. In 2000, the average female life expectancy was close to 80. Women today can expect to live one third to one half of their lives after menopause.

The average age for the onset of perimenopausal symptoms is 47.5 years; the average age at which the transition is final is 51.4 years. These average ages have not changed since records on menopause have been kept, but some factors such as cigarette smoking or genetic predisposition appear to be associated with an earlier onset of perimenopausal symptoms.

As the U.S. population ages, increasing numbers of women now live with the consequences of menopause. Today approximately 40 million women are postmenopausal. By 2020, an estimated 46 million living American women will have gone through menopause.

Etiology: What Happens?

In addition to ripening several eggs each month, and releasing at least one for the possibility of fertilization, the ovaries have the job of secreting a variety of chemicals into the bloodstream. Estrogen and its chemical predecessor progesterone are two of these. It is somewhat misleading to refer to estrogen and progesterone as only two hormones; both of these substances are produced in various chemical formats, each of which is metabolized and used in different ways.

Estrogens and progesterones work on sex organs to either support a pregnancy or shed the endometrial lining of the uterus. When the ovaries lose function, either as a normal part of aging or because their function has been interrupted by surgery, radiation, or drugs (this is called "induced menopause"), these processes come to a stop. A woman no longer ovulates, she no longer grows an endothelial lining in her uterus, and she no longer sheds that lining during menstruation: she is infertile. These ovarian hormones also work on many other tissues in the body, however, in ways that are only just beginning to be explored.

- *Bone density:* The role of estrogens and progesterones in maintaining bone density is complex. It seems clear that estrogen inhibits osteoclast activity; that is, it helps to prevent the thinning of bone tissue. Some forms of progesterone are involved in maintaining bone density as well: this class of chemicals appears to stimulate osteoblast activity. In other words, estrogen prevents bone from being dissolved, and progesterone helps it to build up. (See more in *osteoporosis*, Chapter 2.)

- *Cardiovascular health:* When women go through menopause, one of the many changes that occur is in the types of cholesterol that are present in the blood. It has been dependably observed that postmenopausal women have higher levels of low-density lipoproteins and triglycerides (the "bad" types of cholesterol) than premenopausal women. It has been assumed that because estrogens influence the metabolism of fats, lowering estrogen levels could be reflected in these pathologic changes, but the precise chain of events has not been thoroughly explored. Although it has traditionally been assumed that estrogen supplementation reduced the risk of cardiovascular disease in postmenopausal women, recent research indicates exactly the opposite (see sidebar, "Hormone Replacement Therapy"). The mechanisms for these changes are not yet understood.

- *Protection from some types of cancer:* This is an extremely complex issue that reflects just how little is understood about the effects of different types of estrogens and progesterones on different types of tissues. High levels of some types of estrogen have a statistical link with lower rates of colon cancer, but higher rates of some other types of cancer, including breast and ovarian cancers. Ultimately, it may be found that whether hormone levels are dangerous or protective depends on the chemical variation of the hormone, where it comes from, how it is metabolized, where it is used, and other variables that have not even been considered yet.

- *Central nervous system functions:* Estrogen seems linked in ways that are not clearly understood to mood, depression, and basic cognitive function. Supplementing low doses of estrogen has been seen to be effective for dealing with the mild depression, insomnia, and short-term memory loss that may accompany menopause, but it is not effective for more severe depressive disorders (see *depression*, Chapter 3).

Hormone Replacement Therapy

Recently, a major research project called the Women's Health Initiative set out to study several long-term health trends in 161,809 postmenopausal American women between 50 and 79 years of age.[6] The goal was to track these participants over 8 years to gather information about health trends for older women. One question they asked concerned the benefits and risks of the most common version of hormone replacement therapy (HRT): concentrated equine estrogens (Premarin) plus medroxyprogesterone acetate (progestin) on women who had not had a hysterectomy. This hormone supplement regimen has traditionally been prescribed for menopausal and postmenopausal women to reduce perimenopausal symptoms such as hot flashes and vaginal dryness, and to reduce the risk of heart disease and osteoporosis.

After 5 years of following the study participants, some surprising results were found. Although the relative risk of osteoporosis and colorectal cancer went down as expected, all other health issues being tracked actually increased, as follows:

Heart attack	Increased	29%
Breast cancer	Increased	26%
Stroke	Increased	41%
Blood clot in leg or lung	Increased	111%
Dementia	Increased	105%
Hip fractures (as a measure of osteoporosis)	Decreased	33%
Colorectal cancer	Decreased	37%

The cardiovascular risks occurred within 2 years of beginning HRT, whereas the breast cancer risk was found after 4 years. Protection against osteoporosis was lost when HRT stopped. These findings were so significant that it was considered unethical to keep women on HRT without informed consent, and this branch of the study was concluded in July 2002.

Other branches of the study are continuing, including the use of estrogen replacement therapy (ERT, without progestin) in women who have had hysterectomies. ERT is not appropriate for women who still have a uterus because estrogen uncontrolled by progesterone stimulates endometrial growth and increases the risk of uterine cancer.

The use of natural hormone supplementation, or supplementation by means other than pills, has not been studied.

[6] Menopause One Woman's Story, Every Woman's Story. National Institute on Aging, National Institutes of Health. Available at: http://www.niapublications.org/pubs/menopause/menopauseupdate2003.pdf. Accessed winter 2004

When the ovaries decrease hormonal production, a woman becomes dependent on other tissues to secrete enough estrogens and progesterones to provide for her daily function. Some fat cells and other tissues continue to produce these hormones after the ovaries atrophy, but at a fraction of previous levels. In addition, although a postmenopausal woman may have to get by on 30% to 40% of her previous estrogen levels, her progesterone may fall to as low as 1/20th of her premenopausal levels. This has implications for general health, because estrogens and progesterones are designed to balance each other in their effects on a variety of tissues. Add the fact that environmental estrogens can enter the body through hormone-supplemented meats and exposure to many common toxins (see sidebar, "What Is This Thing Called Estrogen?"), and it is easy to see how precarious is the balance of hormones in a postmenopausal woman.

Historically, much of the common wisdom about the effects of hormones on the body is based on conclusions drawn from observing what happens when those hormones are in short supply. This is a clumsy way to try to understand such a complex subject. As our ability to trace the subtle interplay of hormone subtypes, metabolic pathways, and target tissues improves, our general concepts about menopause as a potential threat to health also may change.

Signs and Symptoms

Menopause itself is simply the event in which ovaries permanently cease to secrete hormones or to produce eggs. Menopause is not identified until a full year after a woman has stopped having menstrual cycles. Ovaries can take several years to slow down, during which their function becomes irregular but does not entirely cease. This time leading up to menopause is referred to as perimenopause, and the symptoms women experience during this time have to do with sudden changes in hormone secretion. Symptoms generally subside when hormone levels stabilize.

The signs and symptoms of menopause vary with each individual, but some of the most common are hot flashes (some women call them "power surges"), night sweats, insomnia, mood swings, decreased sex drive, vaginal dryness or itchiness, confusion, short-term memory loss, and poor concentration. Some of these symptoms may be interrelated; for instance, insomnia may have to do with night sweats and hot flashes; depression and decreased sex drive may have to do with a change in self-perception as a woman enters a time in her life when she is no longer fertile. For some women, however, the symptoms of perimenopause are directly linked to hormonal disruption, and taking steps to smooth out the hormonal shifts can alleviate a lot of discomfort.

The long-term consequences of menopause include pathologic thinning of bones and decreased resistance to heart disease, although these phenomena are certainly controllable.

Treatment

Treatment options for the symptoms of perimenopause and the long-term consequences of reduced estrogen/progesterone secretion are many and varied. Estrogen replacement therapy (ERT) provides supplements of various types of estrogens. This seems to be adequate for some women, but it does not address the lost balance between estrogens and progesterones that are implicated in many health issues. Furthermore, it is only appropriate for women who have had a hysterectomy, because estrogen stimulates potentially dangerous endometrial growth.

Hormone replacement therapy (HRT) supplements both estrogen and progesterone, in varying levels and in varying forms, but traditional HRT is also associated with increased risk of heart disease, stroke, and some types of cancer, especially if it is used for more than 2 years. Many studies have been conducted and are ongoing to try to decipher how to get the best out of hormone supplementation, while reducing possible risks.

It is also possible to supplement hormones in the form of a topical cream, which allows access to the bloodstream without processing in the liver. Many women successfully treat their perimenopausal symptoms with these applications, although they must also be used with care, as the potency from one brand or even one batch to another may vary.

Massage?

Bodywork is a wonderful idea for a woman who is experiencing symptoms of perimenopause. This condition is not a disease; it is a natural process. Although many women feel that entering this phase of life is a liberating, exciting time, others may feel that their role in life must change so fundamentally that they lose touch with their own self-definition. Massage, because it involves supportive, nurturing, informed touch, can reinforce the positive aspects of a woman's physical experience and help her through what can be a difficult period.

Pelvic Inflammatory Disease

Definition: What Is It?

Pelvic inflammatory disease (PID) refers to infections anywhere in the upper reproductive tract of women. Infection of the uterus (*endometritis*), infection of the uterine tubes (*salpingitis*), or abscesses on the ovaries (*oophoritis*) can all fall under the umbrella term of PID.

Demographics: Who Gets It?

PID is usually a disorder of young women. It is most common among women between 15 and 25 years of age who have had multiple sexual partners; it is rare in women older than 35. Over 1 million cases of PID are reported in the United States every year; it accounts for 250,000 hospitalizations, and between $4 and $7 billion in medical costs in the United States every year. Outside of human immunodeficiency virus (HIV), PID is considered the most frequent and most serious sexually transmitted infection affecting women today.

Pelvic Inflammatory Disease in Brief

What is it?
Pelvic inflammatory disease, or PID, is an infection of female reproductive organs. It starts at the cervix and can move up to infect the uterus, fallopian (uterine) tubes, ovaries, and entire pelvic cavity.

How is it recognized?
The symptoms of acute PID include abdominal pain, fever, chills, headache, nausea, and vomiting. Chronic PID may produce no symptoms or may involve chronic pain, lassitude, and pain during urination and intercourse.

Is massage indicated or contraindicated?
Acute PID systemically contraindicates massage until all signs of infection have subsided. Chronic PID may be appropriate for massage if the woman is aware of her condition and is treating it appropriately. Deep work in the lower abdomen or pelvis is not appropriate for women with PID.

Etiology: What Happens?

Pelvic inflammatory disease is usually the result of a bacterial infection that begins in the vagina. The infectious agents are often a combination of chlamydia or gonorrhea (see *sexually transmitted diseases*, this chapter), but irritation from an intrauterine device (IUD) or incomplete elective or spontaneous *abortions* (this chapter) also can be precipitators for PID. Although it usually begins in the vagina, the infection may spread to the uterus, the fallopian tubes, the ovaries, and into the pelvic cavity.

Other agents that have been found in PID infections include mycoplasma, some anaerobic bacteria, and some forms of bacteria that occur naturally in the lower reproductive tract. It is not clear how or why these bacteria change their characteristics to cause these serious infections.

Signs and Symptoms

PID may be an acute or chronic infection. Acute PID is, as its name implies, a serious and severe condition. Its symptoms include abdominal pain, low back pain, fever, chills, nausea, vomiting, painful intercourse, heavy irregular periods, and heavy, pus-laden vaginal discharge. Chronic PID has low-grade, long-term symptoms that seldom flare up into an acute situation, but that can ultimately cause the same kind of internal damage and complications as acute PID. Its symptoms include mild abdominal pain, backache, heavy menstrual periods, painful intercourse, and general lethargy.

Complications

If an infection backs up from the vagina to the uterus and into the fallopian tubes, it can start growing in the open pelvic cavity. Occasionally PID causes the growth of tubo-ovarian abscesses. If an abscess ruptures, it releases infectious material into the pelvis. In either case, life-threatening *peritonitis* (Chapter 7) is the result.

More common complications of PID include infertility, ectopic pregnancy, and chronic pelvic pain. Infertility arises from the accumulation of scar tissue that may block fallopian tubes. Women with a history of three PID infections have a 40% to 60%

chance of becoming infertile; this disease is estimated to cause 75,000 to 225,000 cases of infertility each year. Women with a history of PID have ectopic pregnancies approximately 6 times more frequently than women who have not; these pregnancies can result in severe internal bleeding and always involve the loss of the fetus (see more in *pregnancy*, this chapter). Approximately 18% of all women diagnosed with PID experience chronic pelvic pain that may outlast their infection by many years.

Diagnosis

Diagnosis of this disorder is based on several different signs: abdominal tenderness, pain at the uterine cervix, ovaries, and fallopian tubes. These are palpated during a standard pelvic examination. In addition to these symptoms, a high white blood cell count is present, pelvic abscesses may develop, and an analysis of vaginal or cervical secretions shows signs of infection. A laparoscopy may be performed to look for abscesses and internal adhesions that may interfere with reproductive function.

Treatment

Most of the time, PID is a fairly simple bacterial infection. Caught early, it responds well to antibiotics and bed rest, although approximately 25% of women require hospitalization and IV antibiotics. Sexual activity needs to be curtailed for several weeks, and the woman's sexual partner(s) should also be treated for gonorrhea or chlamydia, if those are involved in the infection.

Massage?

PID is a potentially dangerous infection that can complicate into peritonitis. Acute cases systemically contraindicate massage until the client has completed a course of antibiotics and has been cleared by her doctor. Chronic PID patients also need to be under a doctor's care and treating their infection appropriately before receiving massage.

Pregnancy in Brief

What is it?
Pregnancy is the state of carrying a fetus.

How is it recognized?
The symptoms of advanced pregnancy are obvious, but symptoms that specifically pertain to massage include loose ligaments, muscle spasms, clumsiness, and fatigue.

Is massage indicated or contraindicated?
All stages of uncomplicated pregnancy indicate massage, with specific cautions relating to each trimester.

Pregnancy

Definition: What Is It?

Pregnancy, obviously, is the condition a woman is in when she is carrying a fetus. Most of the general information about pregnancy is skipped in this discussion, but it is worthwhile to look at some of the aspects of this condition in the context of massage.

Signs and Symptoms

Pregnancy creates a wide array of symptoms, and some of them have specific implications for massage. Here are some of the symptomatic complaints of pregnant women that bodyworkers can influence:

- *Loose ligaments*: One of the hormones secreted during pregnancy is relaxin. Its job is to loosen the ligaments so that the pelvis is elastic enough to allow the baby to emerge. Relaxin starts working very early in pregnancy, however, making all of the ligaments in the body looser and more mobile. This can cause numerous problems from unstable vertebrae to asymmetric sacroiliac joints. Muscles then tighten to stabilize the joints, causing *spasm* (see Chapter 2) and pain.

- *Fatigue*: Pregnant women carry a lot of extra weight. The baby itself is only a tiny part of the whole load, which includes the placenta, amniotic fluid, 40% more blood, and any extra body fat cells she may accumulate during her pregnancy. In addition to carrying extra weight, a pregnant woman secretes hormones that require her to get a lot of rest. This is a command that many pregnant women do not have the luxury of obeying, at least while they are trying to hold down a job and grow a baby at the same time.

- *Shifting proprioception*: Pregnant women change their size every day. This is especially true in the last trimester, when the baby grows at an astounding rate. The result is that a pregnant woman never knows exactly how much room she takes up. Her sense of where in space her body ends and the rest of the world begins is very shaky. This tends to make a pregnant woman clumsy and prone to injury. Massage provides an extraordinary sense of where bodies are in space. It can improve proprioceptive senses by giving continuous and positive feedback about boundaries.

Complications

In the vast range of things that could possibly go wrong in a pregnancy, three conditions are especially important for massage therapists to watch out for: *gestational diabetes*, *pregnancy-induced hypertension*, and *ectopic pregnancy*.

- *Gestational diabetes*: Pregnancy-related diabetes develops in about 4% of all pregnancies. It is diagnosed through a glucose tolerance test, in which the woman drinks a sweet beverage and then her urine is examined for elevated levels of glucose. Gestational diabetes is usually identified in the fifth or sixth month of pregnancy (between 24 and 26 weeks of gestation).

  If diabetes develops during pregnancy, risks to the baby and mother are serious. The incidence of birth defects (especially *spina bifida* [Chapter 3] and Down syndrome) and stillbirths with diabetic mothers is three times greater than with nondiabetic mothers. The rerouting of nutrients in the blood can cause babies to grow abnormally large, requiring a cesarean section. A woman who develops prenatal diabetes *must* be under a doctor's care and get clearance before receiving circulatory massage; her blood pressure may be higher than is otherwise healthy.

- *Pregnancy-induced hypertension (PIH)*: This is a condition that generally starts mildly but can quickly become life-threatening both for the baby and the mother. It occurs in three categories: hypertension alone; *preeclampsia*, which is hypertension along with elevated proteins in the urine and possible systemic edema; and *eclampsia*, which is the same situation along with convulsions.

  The exact causes of PIH are unknown. Some postulate that it may be an autoimmune problem, or even an allergic reaction to the baby; others suggest that in processing waste products for two people the mother's system is simply overloaded. In any case, increased blood pressure makes it harder for the placenta to deliver nutrients to the baby.

  Most cases of PIH occur during a first pregnancy. Other women at risk include those who are obese before pregnancy, those who have a personal or family history of chronic high blood pressure, women younger than 20 or over 40 years old, women carrying multiple babies, and women who have underlying diseases that can affect the circulatory system, including diabetes, *lupus* (Chapter 5), and *scleroderma* (Chapter 2). Treatment includes medication to bring down the blood pressure, strict bedrest, and where appropriate, cesarean section.

  A condition related to PIH but that may eventually be addressed by experts as a separate issue, is *HELLP*: **h**emolysis with **e**levated **l**iver enzymes and **l**ow **p**latelet count. Some women with PIH develop this version of the disorder, which, because it involves damaged blood cells and impaired liver function, can result in severe damage to the liver.

Complications of PIH for mothers include *renal failure* (Chapter 9), cerebral hemorrhage (see *stroke*, Chapter 3), liver damage, and retinal detachment leading to blindness. Risks to the baby include reduced growth from circulatory impairment, and *placenta abruptio*, a condition in which the placenta prematurely separates from the uterus.

- *Ectopic pregnancy*: An ectopic pregnancy is a fertilized egg that implants outside of the uterus. Most ectopic pregnancies develop in the fallopian tubes; others may implant in the peritoneum, on the ovaries, or on the cervix. Extrauterine implantation occurs in approximately 1% to 2% of all pregnancies.

  Risk factors for ectopic pregnancy include IUD use, a history of *pelvic inflammatory disease*, *endometriosis*, or *sexually transmitted diseases* (all in this chapter), and adhesions from previous abdominal surgeries. Ectopic pregnancies cannot come to term; the fallopian tube inevitably ruptures, killing the fetus and endangering the life of the mother. Ectopic pregnancies that are recognized early (usually by ultrasound and testing for hormone levels) may be terminated by laparoscopic surgery, preserving fertility for the chance of another successful pregnancy.

Massage?

For pregnancies that are *not* complicated by diabetes, hypertension, or other disorders, massage is a wonderful gift for someone whose body does not quite belong to herself for a while.

Special training is available to learn pregnancy and prenatal massage, but for more general purposes, here are some guidelines and cautions to preserve the pregnant client's comfort and safety:

- *1st trimester*: From the moment a woman knows she is pregnant to several days after she has delivered, deep abdominal work is contraindicated. The first and last trimesters are the times when the fetal attachment is most fragile, and massage therapists must respect that fragility. Practitioners of Eastern techniques would add that other cautions for massage in the first trimester include deep specific point work on the heels and Achilles tendons (reflexology abortion points), and on the *hoku* point in the web of the thumb.

- *2nd trimester*: This is the safest, easiest part of the pregnancy. Very often a woman's energy levels will be up while her nausea levels will be down. She probably has not yet gained enough weight to be very uncomfortable. However, connective tissue changes begin to show during this time: ligaments begin to loosen, and muscles may go into spasm in response. Massage at this stage centers on making sure the client is comfortable. Bolsters and other physical support tools will be useful. Somewhere in this trimester, often around week 22, she will no longer want to be face down; then the therapist is limited to doing work from the side or supine, unless extensive bolstering is employed.

- *3rd trimester*: A midwife once said, "God invented the third trimester of pregnancy to make labor look like a pretty good deal." Massage therapists are more limited in what they do in this trimester than any other, but their work is more important than ever. Prone work is out of the question at this point, and supine work probably needs to be limited or modified, according to the mother's comfort. Being fully reclined allows the fetus to rest directly on the big abdominal blood vessels, which may either limit blood flow to the legs, leading to cramping in the gastrocnemius, or limit blood flow up the vena cava, leading to dizziness and unconsciousness (Figure 10.9). It may be best to do a lot of side work unless the client can be in a semi-reclined position.

Figure 10.9. Pregnancy: a late-term fetus can obstruct blood flow through the iliac arteries or the vena cava.

Aorta   Vena cava

Another caution for this stage is limited blood return from the legs, leading to edema. Watch for varicose veins as well, which, combined with long-standing edema and the increased number of red blood cells that is a normal part of being pregnant, can be ideal environments for clot formation (see *deep vein thrombosis*, Chapter 4). Some people suggest that to be completely safe, the medial calf and thigh (in other words, the area around the great saphenous vein) should be a local contraindication for massage during the third trimester regardless of whether edema or varices are present.

If *pitting* edema, coupled with fever, dizziness, headache, and nausea are present, the client may be in preeclampsia and needs immediate medical referral. Massage is contraindicated until she has medical clearance.

Premenstrual Syndrome

Definition: What Is It?

Premenstrual syndrome (PMS) is a collection of signs and symptoms that combine to interfere with a woman's ability to function normally during the luteal phase of the menstrual cycle: the time between ovulation and menstruation.

Demographics: Who Gets It?

Up to 85% of all women between the onset of menarche and menopause report some symptoms of PMS. Approximately 20% to 40% of those women believe that their symptoms create a problem, but only 5% to 10% of them are significantly impacted by PMS.

Whereas symptoms of PMS have been seen to be more severe among women who have high-fat diets, no other particular risk factors or target populations have been identified.

Menarche, menstruation, menses, menopause:

What are all these *men* doing in women's health issues? The root word is *mēn*, which is Greek for "month."
Menarche is "*mēn*" plus "*arche*," or "beginning."
Menstruation is "*mēn*" plus "*atus*," meaning "to be menstruant."
Menses is the plural for "*mēn*", meaning many months.
Menopause is "*mēn*" plus "*pausis*," or "cessation."

Premenstrual Syndrome in Brief

What is it?
Premenstrual syndrome (PMS) is a collection of many signs and symptoms that occur in the time between ovulation and menstruation and then subside after menstruation begins. It may have several different causes and triggers.

How is it recognized?
Signs and symptoms of PMS are often divided into physical and emotional features. Physical symptoms include breast tenderness, bloating, digestive upset, fatigue, changes in appetite, backache, and many others. Emotional signs include irritability, anxiety, depression, mood swings, and other possible problems.

Is massage indicated or contraindicated?
Although the specific causes of PMS are not clearly understood, it is clear that this condition is not related to infection, structural problems, or neoplasm. Therefore, PMS indicates bodywork, which may help to reestablish balance in the endocrine and nervous systems.

Etiology: What Happens?

PMS is one of the most common and least well-understood conditions that women experience. It has been described since ancient times; it was recognized as a specific pattern in 1931, and finally named in 1953. Nonetheless, the cause of this condition remains mysterious. Several different factors seem to contribute to this problem, and each woman's experience is unique. This makes it difficult to predict or treat, because no single approach is universally successful.

Some of the theories for the causes or triggers of PMS include the following:

- *Hormonal imbalance*: During the luteal phase of the menstrual cycle, the body prepares to shed the endometrial lining that has accumulated for the implantation of a fertilized egg. Estrogen and progesterone levels rise as the lining thickens, and then just before menstruation begins, these hormones suddenly and rapidly drop in production. One theory behind PMS is that this precipitous drop in hormones is difficult to accommodate, and that exposure to environmental estrogens (in animal fats and toxic exposures) may cause the endometrial lining to become overactive, thus requiring an even more extreme fluctuation in hormonal levels. In addition to problems with estrogen and progesterone levels, some women with PMS report problems with adrenal function.

- *Nutritional deficiencies*: Some women with PMS are deficient in specific areas, notably calcium, vitamin B$_6$, and some essential fatty acids.

- *Neurotransmitter imbalance*: Plunging estrogen and progesterone has been seen to suppress the secretion of serotonin, a neurotransmitter that is strongly related to mood swings and depression. Opioid peptides are other brain chemicals that appear to be adversely affected by hormone disruption. These chemicals also help to determine mood.

- *Other factors*: Some factors that may contribute to PMS are more vague but are definitely a part of the picture for many women. Genetic predisposition may be a factor, but no genetic mutation has been isolated for PMS; whether the condition is passed on through heredity, or the likelihood to seek help for the condition is passed on through environmental influence, is unclear. Cultural expectations, general stress, and a number of unrelated disorders also may contribute to signs and symptoms of PMS.

Signs and Symptoms

More than 150 different signs and symptoms have been documented among PMS patients. These have been loosely categorized into physical and emotional indicators of this disorder.

- *Physical symptoms*: The most common physical symptoms associated with PMS include bloating, breast tenderness, acne, salt and sugar cravings (along with binge eating), headaches, backaches, insomnia, and digestive upset: diarrhea or constipation. Less common physical symptoms can include sinus problems, heart palpitations, dizziness, asthma, and seizures.

- *Emotional symptoms*: These include confusion, depression, anxiety, panic attacks, mood swings, and general irritability.

Another disorder, called ***premenstrual dysphoric disorder*** (PMDD) is essentially like PMS but with the added factor of extremely depressed mood or anxiety (see *depression, anxiety disorders*, Chapter 3). PMDD also occurs cyclically, just as PMS does, but it is typically treated with antidepressants and anti-anxiety medications rather than with birth control pills.

Diagnosis

It seems clear that PMS has several different causes and creates a different experience for every woman who has it. The one constant in this condition is that symptoms appear after ovulation and subside when menstruation begins. The most important diagnostic test for PMS is a diary in which a woman records her experiences and finds that this pattern is consistent with her menstrual cycle.

Several other conditions create overlapping symptoms with PMS, including *diabetes* or *hypothyroidism* (see Chapter 8), *eating disorders* or *depression* (see Chapter 3), *chronic fatigue syndrome* (see Chapter 5), *irritable bowel syndrome* (see Chapter 7), or any combination of these disorders. Only PMS will show a cessation of symptoms during and after menstruation, however.

Treatment

Because PMS is not understood as a distinct disease process, it is treated symptomatically. Women who consult allopathic physicians for this disorder may be prescribed low-dose birth control pills to control estrogen and progesterone levels, diuretics to control water retention, or antidepressants to address serotonin levels. Most women are also strongly recommended to make sure that they get best quality sleep they can muster during their difficult time and to exercise regularly.

Health professionals who focus on nutritional aspects of this disorder often recommend that patients follow a low-fat vegetarian diet to avoid excessive estrogen exposure, and that they avoid salt, sugar, caffeine (specifically in soda, coffee, tea, and chocolate), and alcohol. Many herbal remedies have been reputed to help PMS; few of them have been accepted by the medical mainstream. Some of the more common herbal recommendations include borage or evening primrose (for essential fatty acids), black cohosh, and dong quai.

Ultimately, PMS is a condition that can usually be successfully managed so that a woman does not have to lose function for 10 days every month, but it seldom spontaneously disappears until the onset of menopause.

Massage?

PMS is a condition in which symptoms are not related to circulatory dysfunction, neoplasm, structural problems, infection, or any other situation that might make bodywork impractical. PMS definitely indicates massage and other kinds of bodywork, which have been shown to reduce depression and anxiety and to help ameliorate some of the fluid retention that makes PMS so physically uncomfortable.[7]

Sexually Transmitted Diseases

Definition: What Are They?

Sexually transmitted diseases (STDs) are contagious conditions that are spread through intimate contact. The primary mode of transmission is through vaginal, oral, or anal sex, although an infected mother carries a risk of infecting her baby either through the blood or through direct contact in the birth process.

[7] Field T. Touch Therapy. Churchill, Livingstone, 2000, p. 78.

Sexually Transmitted Diseases in Brief

What are they?
Sexually transmitted diseases (STDs) are contagious conditions that are spread through intimate contact. The three major diseases discussed here are all bacterial infections: chlamydia, gonorrhea, and syphilis. Most other STDs are viral infections, including genital herpes, molluscum contagiosum, and genital warts.

How are they recognized?
The major bacterial STDs all share some common signs, when any signs are present at all. These include penile or vaginal discharge, painful urination, and painful intercourse. Other more specific symptoms vary by causative agent.

Is massage indicated or contraindicated?
Bacterial STDs are responsive to antibiotic therapy. Once an infection has been identified and controlled, massage is perfectly appropriate. Silent conditions that are untreated may lead to serious complications that contraindicate massage, depending on the severity of the infection.

Demographics: Who Gets Them?

The vast majority of STDs are diagnosed among adolescents and young adults. People ages 15 to 25 are most at risk for these conditions. Because people tend to become sexually active at an earlier age, and marry at a later age than in previous generations, the average number of sex partners a person has is increasing. This trend also increases the risk of exposure to many STDs, some of which frequently occur concurrently, and many of which have dangerous and even life-threatening complications.

Approximately 13 million people are diagnosed with some kind of STD each year, at a cost of roughly $10 billion health care dollars for treatment. More information about the infection rates of specific STDs is included in the discussions below.

Types of STDs

More than 20 different infectious diseases are spread through intimate contact. Several have been discussed elsewhere in this book; they include *herpes simplex* (Chapter 1), *HIV/AIDS* (Chapter 5), and *hepatitis B and C* (Chapter 7). This discussion has been reserved for the most common bacterial STDs: chlamydia, gonorrhea, and syphilis, followed by a brief look at some other conditions.

Chlamydia Definition   Chlamydia is a bacterial infection with the agent *Chlamydia trachomatis.*

Chlamydia Demographics   Statistics on the rate of new infection with this bacterium are hard to gather, because it is often completely asymptomatic in women, so it is difficult to project exactly how many people might be infected. The Centers for Disease Control and Prevention document that in 2002 new chlamydia infections were reported in over 800,000 people[8], but that it actually may cause over 3 million new infections each year.[9]

Chlamydia Etiology   The bacteria that cause chlamydia have an affinity for columnar mucus-producing cells. These infections can develop at any site of sexual contact: the reproductive tract, the mouth and throat, and the anus.

The real danger with chlamydia is that while it is silently attacking columnar mucus cells in the reproductive tract, it can progressively invade the uterus and uterine tubes, where a chronic low-grade infection and inflammatory response may lead to permanent scarring and infertility. This is one variety of *pelvic inflammatory disease* (this chapter). Furthermore, chlamydia bacteria also may infect the eye. Worldwide, chlamydia is the leading cause of new blindness.

Chlamydia Signs and Symptoms   Chlamydia is often a silent disorder; three quarters of all infected women and approximately half of all infected men report no symptoms. When symptoms are present, they include vaginal or penile discharge, pain and burning during urination, and painful intercourse. If the infection invades the upper female reproductive tract, signs of PID (fever, abdominal and low back pain, inflamed lymph nodes) may be present.

---

[8] Rates of STD's. Centers for Disease Control and Prevention. Available at: http://www.cdc.gov/std/stats/tables/table1.htm. Accessed winter 2004
[9] Chlamydia. Disease Information. Centers for Disease Control and Prevention, National Center for HIV, STD and TB Prevention. Available at: http://www.cdc.gov/nchstp/dstd/Fact_Sheets/FactsChlamydiaInfo.htm. Accessed winter 2004

Chlamydia Complications   The primary complication of a chlamydia infection for a woman is PID and the risk of lifelong infertility. An infection in a man may cause epididymitis, swelling of the testicles, and a risk of infertility. A baby born to a woman with undiagnosed chlamydia has a risk of exposure in the birth canal that may lead to conjunctivitis or pneumonia. A chlamydia infection also increases the rate of HIV transmission; the virus crosses from one partner to another more easily when a bacterial infection is present.

Chlamydia Diagnosis and Treatment   Chlamydia is typically diagnosed by taking a culture from the cervix or penis. (This is not the same as a Pap smear, which scrapes cells off the cervix to examine them for signs of dysplasia.) If tests come back positive for an active chlamydia infection, a course of antibiotics is usually successful, as long as the person and all of his or her sex partners are treated completely. Chlamydia often appears with gonorrhea, which requires a different antibiotic treatment, so it is important to get a thorough diagnosis. Exposure and treatment for chlamydia does *not* impart immunity, so any future exposure to this pathogen will lead to a new infection and requirement for treatment.

Gonorrhea Definition   Gonorrhea is infection with a bacterium called *Neisseria gonorrhoeae*. This is a diplococcal bacterium: a spherical cell that tends to clump together in characteristic pairs.

Gonorrhea Demographics   Gonorrhea is reported as a new infection approximately 400,000 times per year in this country. It is most prevalent among people who are 15 to 29 years old, especially those with multiple sex partners, a history of other STDs, and who live in a low socioeconomic status with limited access to health care.

Gonorrhea Etiology   Gonorrhea is spread through intimate contact; it can infect the throat, vagina, and rectum. It is rarely transmitted in any contact other than sex; it is rare for a pregnant mother with gonorrhea to pass it to her child. Once inside the body, gonorrhea may infect tissues other than mucous membranes; it often affects joints in a condition called gonococcal arthritis. This is a type of *septic arthritis* (Chapter 2).

Gonorrhea Signs and Symptoms   Like chlamydia, gonorrhea is often silent, especially in women. If symptoms do appear for a woman, they typically develop 2 to 5 days after exposure, when they might include vaginal discharge, urinary discomfort, and painful intercourse. An infection from oral sex may lead to sores in the mouth and a sore throat.

Male symptoms of gonorrhea include burning on urination, a yellow-white discharge from the penis, and *orchitis*.

Gonorrhea Complications   Like chlamydia, gonorrhea has a high risk of developing into PID; this happens with 10% to 15% of women who are untreated for this infection. As mentioned above, gonorrhea can infect joints, causing septic arthritis. And like chlamydia, the presence of gonorrhea increases the transmission rate of HIV.

Gonorrhea Diagnosis and Treatment   Gonorrhea is diagnosed through a culture of mucus from the rectum, cervix, throat, or penis. It is responsive to antibiotics, although it has developed resistance to penicillin. A number of powerful, single-dose antibiotic therapies have been developed that can successfully and quickly eradicate a gonorrhea infection. This condition frequently appears with chlamydia, which requires a different antibiotic.

A person with septic arthritis from gonorrhea also benefits from careful stretching and mobilization of the affected joints once the infection has been eradicated. Massage may be appropriate at this time as well.

Syphilis Definition   Syphilis is an infection with a spirochetal bacterium called *Treponema pallidum*.

Syphilis Demographics   Statistics on syphilis infection have changed significantly in recent years. They nearly doubled from 1980 to 1990, but aggressive public health efforts and campaigns to treat not only the diagnosed person but all of that person's partners led to an 89% drop in rates of syphilis infection from 1990 to 2000. The rates have begun to climb again, but not at the same speed as we saw in the 1980s. Approximately 32,000 new cases of syphilis are reported per year.

Syphilis Etiology   Syphilis spreads through sexual contact and from mother to unborn child. This bacterium is very fragile outside of a host and does not last when exposed to air or sunlight.

Syphilis moves through the system in specific stages. It is communicable only in the first two stages of infection. In the late stage, although it may cause very serious problems in the infected person, it is no longer contagious.

This bacterium is transmitted when an infected lesion comes in contact with microscopic openings in another person's skin. Syphilis travels through the blood and may affect joints, bones, blood vessels, and the central nervous system if it is untreated.

Syphilis Signs and Symptoms   Primary syphilis is detectable 10 days to 3 months after exposure, when a characteristic chancre, or open ulcer, appears. A chancre is usually not acutely painful, and if it appears inside the vaginal canal a woman may not be aware of its presence. The tissue in chancres is very contagious. A typical chancre heals in 3 to 6 weeks.

Secondary syphilis takes the form of a rash of open brownish sores that appear several weeks after the chancre heals. This rash is often on the soles of the feet or palms of the hands, but may be anywhere. These lesions are also highly infectious. The rash associated with secondary syphilis may come and go for 1 to 2 years before the infection becomes latent.

In some people, syphilis becomes a silent infection after the secondary stage, and may produce no further symptoms. No skin lesions appear, and the infection is no longer contagious. However, approximately one third of all people with secondary syphilis develop tertiary syphilis: a condition in which the bacteria invade other body systems. At this point, the infection may attack the bones and joints, causing rheumatic pain, or the blood vessels, causing a risk of *aneurysm* (Chapter 4). Most significantly, syphilis may attack the central nervous system leading to a range of problems, including blindness, loss of hearing, *stroke*, *meningitis* (Chapter 3), or psychosis.

Syphilis Complications   Like other bacterial STDs, syphilis significantly increases the transmission rate of HIV. A pregnant woman with syphilis, if she does not miscarry, has a nearly 100% chance of spreading the disease to her newborn through the bloodstream. Babies born with syphilis may not have symptoms immediately but may develop vision or central nervous system problems, along with syphilitic rhinitis; their mucus secretions are highly contagious.

Other complications of tertiary syphilis are listed above.

Syphilis Diagnosis and Treatment   The good news is that syphilis is simple to diagnose and to treat. It can be diagnosed by examining a scraping of a chancre or secondary rash, or through a blood test. Syphilis is sensitive to penicillin, and a single dose is typically adequate. Treatment must be administered before organ damage takes place, however.

Syphilitic damage to the central nervous system (CNS), blood vessels, and other structures is irreversible.

Other STDs

- *Nongonococcal urethritis (NGU):* This is a bacterial infection of the urinary tract from agents other than gonorrhea. It is often related to chlamydia, **Ureaplasma urealyticum**, or adenovirus. NGU is usually an STD, but it also can be related to *prostatitis* (this chapter), *urinary tract infection* (Chapter 9), or catheterization. If NGU is identified as a bacterial infection, it can be successfully treated with antibiotics.

- *Molluscum contagiosum virus (MCV):* This is a generally benign condition that is commonly seen among children, when it is not an STD. It has increasing incidence among adults, however, as a result of skin-to-skin contact. MCV also may be transmissible through other surfaces, however; it may spread through contact with towels or other cloth, or possibly even through water, as in a shared bath. When MCV appears as an STD, it appears on the thighs, buttocks, groin, external genitalia, and anus. It is treated by removing the growths with topical chemicals or cryotherapy.

- *Genital warts (human papilloma virus, or HPV):* Genital warts are also called **condylomata acuminata**. They affect more than 5 million people each year, and can grow on the vulva, the walls of the vagina, the perineum, or cervix of a woman, or on the penis, scrotum, or anus of a man. Oral infections may grow in the mouth or throat. They have a high transmission rate; exposure leads to infection approximately two thirds of the time.

  Genital warts are typically small but can grow in large clusters. They may grow large enough interfere with a pregnancy. Many types of HPV can cause genital warts, and some of them are associated with *cervical cancer* (this chapter) or penile or vulvar cancer.

  Genital warts can be removed, but over-the-counter medications that treat common *warts* (Chapter 1) are inappropriate for these lesions, which grow on more sensitive, delicate tissues.

Prevention

The transmission of STDs can be prevented, but the only completely consistent method is to practice abstinence. Having sex only with one partner who is known to be uninfected is of course highly recommended. Barrier methods of birth control (male or female condoms) provide protection from some but not all STDs: molluscum contagiosum, genital warts, and syphilis may be spread to areas not covered by condoms. And of course, other methods of birth control (spermicidal cream, birth control pills, or other hormonal applications) provide no protection from STDs.

Massage?

Most STDs are only spread through sexual contact, which makes communicability for massage therapists a non-issue. Exceptions to this rule include molluscum contagiosum, genital warts, and open syphilis lesions, which only require skin-to-skin contact, and the lesions may not be confined to the genitalia.

If a client knows that he or she is positive for any type of STD, the first priority is to treat the infection. Because most of these clear within days of the administration of antibiotics, it is not a great hardship to postpone a massage until after the infection has resolved.

CHAPTER REVIEW QUESTIONS

1. Why is the incidence of advanced cervical cancer a fraction of what it was in the first half of the 20th century?

2. Is the risk factor profile a very useful guideline for breast cancer? Why or why not?

3. What are prostaglandins, and how are they involved in dysmenorrhea?

4. Describe how stress can exacerbate menstrual pain.

5. Under what circumstances may fibroid tumors cause symptoms?

6. How can endometriosis or pelvic inflammatory disease lead to sterility?

7. An elderly client has been diagnosed with prostate cancer. He has opted not to treat it. Is he a good candidate for bodywork? What modalities, and why?

8. Discuss the relationship between certain hormonal changes that occur in pregnancy and muscle spasm.

9. Why may it be uncomfortable to work with a late-term pregnant woman in a fully supine position?

10. A client has been diagnosed with endometriosis but has no particular symptoms at the time of her appointment. To help with her low back pain, her massage therapist works deeply on the psoas. Within a few hours the client has sharp shooting pains low in her abdomen, and cannot stand up straight. What may have happened?

 Answers to these questions can be found on the Student Recource CD-ROM that accompanies this book.

Bibliography

General Resources, Reproductive System

1. de Dominico G, Wood E. Beard's Massage. Philadelphia: WB Saunders, 1997.
2. Damjanou I. Pathology for the Health-Related Professions. Philadelphia: WB Saunders, 1996.
3. Travell J, Simons DG. Myofascial Pain and Dysfunction: The Trigger Point Manual. Baltimore: Williams & Wilkins, 1983.
4. Clemente CD. Anatomy: A Regional Atlas of the Human Body. 3rd Ed. Baltimore: Urban & Schwarzenburg, 1987.
5. Tortora GJ, Anagnostakos NP. Principles of Anatomy and Physiology. 6th Ed. New York: Harper & Row, 1990.
6. Taber's Cyclopedic Dictionary. 14th Ed. Philadelphia: FA Davis, 1981.
7. Stedman's Medical Dictionary. 26th Ed. Baltimore: Williams & Wilkins, 1995.
8. Memmler RL, Wood DL. The Human Body in Health and Disease. 5th Ed. Philadelphia: JB Lippincott, 1983.
9. Juhan D. Job's Body: A Handbook for Bodywork. Barrytown, NY: Station Hill Press, 1987.
10. Kunz JRM, Finkel AJ, eds. The American Medical Association Family Medical Guide. New York, NY: Random House, 1987.
11. Marieb EM. Human Anatomy and Physiology. Redwood City, CA: Benjamin/Cummings, 1989.
12. Field T. Touch Therapy. London: Churchill Livingstone; 2000.

Abortion, Spontaneous and Elective

1. Gaufberg SV. Abortion, Complications. Copyright © 2004, eMedicine.com, Inc. Available at: http://www.emedicine.com/emerg/topic4.htm. Accessed winter 2004.
2. Fact Sheet Abortion Surveillance, 2000. Centers for Disease and Control and Prevention. Available at: http://www.cdc.gov/reproductivehealth/surv_abort00.htm. Accessed winter 2004.
3. Shermer CD, Valley VT. Miscarriage. Copyright © 2004, eMedicine.com, Inc. Available at: http://www.emedicine.com/aaem/topic307.htm. Accessed winter 2004.
4. Scientific Advances in Reproductive Health: Non-Surgical Abortion and Emergency Contraception. NARAL Pro-Choice America Foundation. Available at: http://www.naral.org/facts/loader.cfm?url=/commonspot/security/getfile.cfm&PageID=1973.

Cervical Cancer

1. Cervical Cancer. American Cancer Society. Available at: http://www.cancer.org/downloads/PRO/CervicalCancer.pdf. Accessed winter 2004.
2. Garcia AA, Bia J. Cervical Cancer. Copyright © 2004, eMedicine.com, Inc. Available at: http://www.emedicine.com/med/topic324.htm. Accessed winter 2004.
3. Human Papillomavirus and Genital Warts. National Institute of Allergy and Infectious Diseases, National Institutes of Health. Available at: http://www.niaid.nih.gov/factsheets/stdhpv.htm. Accessed winter 2004.
4. Cervical Cancer Overview. Copyright © 1998–2004 Mayo Foundation for Medical Education and Research (MFMER). Available at: http://www.mayoclinic.com/invoke.cfm?id=DS00167. Accessed winter 2004.
5. Ruffin MT. Family Physicians' Knowledge of Risk Factors for Cervical Cancer. Copyright © 2003 Mary Ann Liebert, Inc. Available at: http://www.medscape.com/viewarticle/461569_1. Accessed winter 2004.
6. Staging. Copyright © 2002 American Society of Clinical Oncology. Available at: http://www.peoplelivingwithcancer.org/plwc/MainConstructor/1,1744,_04-0026-00_12-001043-00_17-001029-00_18-0026061-00_19-000-00_20-001-00_21-008,00.asp. Accessed winter 2004.
7. Cervical Cancer Prevention. Copyright © 1992–2004 the Author(s) and The University of Iowa. Available at: http://www.vh.org/adult/patient/cancercenter/

cancertips/cervical.html. Accessed winter 2004.

8. What You Need To Know About™ Cancer of the Cervix. National Cancer Institute. Available at: http://www.cancer.gov/cancerinfo/wyntk/cervix. Accessed winter 2004.

Dysmenorrhea

1. Clark AD, Steele T.Ü Dysmenorrhea. Copyright © 2004, eMedicine.com, Inc. Available at: http://www.emedicine.com/emerg/topic156.htm. Accessed winter 2004.
2. Dysmenorrhea Overview. Copyright © 1998–2004 Mayo Foundation for Medical Education and Research (MFMER). Available at: http://www.mayoclinic.com/invoke.cfm?id=DS00506. Accessed winter 2004.
3. Barnard ND. Nutritional Factors in Menstrual Pain and Premenstrual Syndrome. Physicians Committee for Responsible Medicine. Available at: http://www.pcrm.org/health/clinres/menstrual.html. Accessed winter 2004.

Endometriosis

1. Causes of Endometriosis. Copyright © 2000 Inlet Medical Inc. Available at: http://www.dyspareunia.org/html/endometriosis_causes.htm. Accessed winter 2004.
2. Endometriosis. National Institute of Child Health and Human Development, National Institutes of Health. Available at: http://www.nichd.nih.gov/publications/pubs/endometriosis.pdf. Accessed winter 2004.
3. Endometriosis Overview. Copyright © 1998–2004 Mayo Foundation for Medical Education and Research (MFMER). Available at: http://www.mayoclinic.com/invoke.cfm?id=DS00289. Accessed winter 2004.
4. What is Endometriosis? Copyright © 2003 by IVF.com, Atlanta, GA, USA. Available at: http://www.ivf.com/endoassn.html. Accessed winter 2004.

Fibroid Tumors

1. Fast Facts about Uterine Fibroids. National Institute of Child Health and Human Development, National Institutes of Health. Available at: http://www.nichd.nih.gov/publications/pubs/fibroids/index.htm. Accessed winter 2004.
2. Uterine Fibroids. Copyright 2000–2002 National Uterine Fibroids Foundation. Available at: http://www.nuff.org/health_uterinefibroids.htm. Accessed winter 2004.
3. Thomason P. Leiomyoma, Uterus (Fibroid). Copyright © 2004, eMedicine.com, Inc. Available at: http://www.emedicine.com/radio/topic777.htm. Accessed winter 2004.
4. Miethke MC, Raugi GJ. Leiomyoma. Copyright © 2004, eMedicine.com, Inc. Available at: http://www.emedicine.com/derm/topic217.htm. Accessed winter 2004.

Breast Cancer

1. Breast Cancer. Copyright © 2003 American Cancer Society, Inc. Available at: http://documents.cancer.org/104.00/104.00.pdf. Accessed winter 2004.
2. Updated Breast Cancer Screening Guidelines Released. Copyright © 2003 American Cancer Society, Inc. Available at: http://www.cancer.org/docroot/NWS/content/NWS_1_1x_Updated_Breast_Cancer_Screening_Guidelines_Released.asp. Accessed winter 2004.
3. Benign Breast Conditions. Copyright © 2003 American Cancer Society, Inc. Available at: http://www.cancer.org/docroot/cri/content/cri_2_6x_benign_breast_conditions_59.asp?sitearea=CRI&viewmode=print&. Accessed winter 2004.
4. Breakthrough: Letrozole Cuts Breast Cancer Recurrences Almost in Half. Copyright © 2003 American Cancer Society, Inc. Available at: http://www.cancer.org/docroot/NWS/content/NWS_1_1x_Breakthrough_Letrozole_Cuts_Breast_Cancer_Recurrences_in_Half.asp. Accessed winter 2004.
5. Haynes G, Garske D, Case D, et al. Effect of massage technique on sentinel lymph node mapping for cancer of the breast. Copyright © 1995–2003 Doctor's Guide Publishing Limited. Am Surg. 2003 Jun;69(6):520–2. PMID: 12852511 [PubMed - indexed for MEDLINE]. Accessed winter 2004.
6. HRT Trial Stopped Early Due to Breast Cancer Risk. Copyright © 2003 Reuters. Available at: http://www.nlm.nih.gov/medlineplus/news/fullstory_15883.html. Accessed winter 2004.
7. Williams AF, Vadgama A, Franks PJ, ET AL. A randomized controlled crossover study of manual lymphatic drainage therapy in women with breast cancer-related lymphedema. Copyright © 1995–2003 Doctor's Guide Publishing Limited. Available at: http://www.blackwell-synergy.com/openurl?genre=article&sid=nlm:pubmed&issn=0961-5423&date=2003&volume=11&issue=4&spage=254. Accessed winter 2004.

Ovarian Cancer

1. Ovarian Cancer. Copyright © 2004 American Cancer Society, Inc. Available at: http://documents.cancer.org/114.00/114.00.pdf. Accessed winter 2004.
2. How Is Ovarian Cancer Staged? Copyright © 2004 American Cancer Society, Inc. Available at: http://www.cancer.org/docroot/CRI/content/CRI_2_4_3X_How_is_ovarian_cancer_staged_33.asp?sitearea=CRI. Accessed winter 2004.
3. Garcia AA. Ovarian Cancer. Copyright © 2004, eMedicine.com, Inc. Available at: http://www.emedicine.com/med/topic1698.htm. Accessed winter 2004.
4. What You Need To Know About™ Ovarian Cancer. National Cancer Institute

(NCI). Available at: http://www.cancer.gov/cancerinfo/wyntk/ovary. Accessed winter 2004.

Ovarian Cysts

1. Ovarian cysts Overview. Copyright © 1998–2004 Mayo Foundation for Medical Education and Research (MFMER). Available at: http://www.mayoclinic.com/invoke.cfm?id=DS00129. Accessed winter 2004.
2. Ovarian Cysts. Copyright © April 1999 The American College of Obstetricians and Gynecologists. Available at: http://www.medem.com/medlb/article_detailb.cfm?article_ID=ZZZEB8EN97C&sub_cat=9. Accessed winter 2004.
3. Ovarian Cysts. Available at: http://www.4woman.gov/faq/ovarian_cysts.htm. Accessed winter 2004.
4. Polycystic Ovary Syndrome. Copyright © 2000 The InterNational Council on Infertility Information Dissemination, Inc. Available at: http://www.inciid.org/faq/pcos2.html. Accessed winter 2004.
5. Polycystic Ovary Syndrome (PCOS). Available at: http://www.4woman.gov/faq/pcos.htm. Accessed winter 2004.

Benign Prostatic Hypertrophy

1. Rajavel S, Kao RY-K. Nephrology and Urology: Benign Prostatic Hypertrophy. Copyright © 1992–2004 the Author(s) and The University of Iowa. Available at: http://www.vh.org/adult/provider/familymedicine/FPHandbook/Chapter08/06-8.html. Accessed winter 2004.
2. Prostate Enlargement: Benign Prostatic Hyperplasia. National Institute of Diabetes and Digestive and Kidney Diseases, National Institutes of Health. Available at: http://kidney.niddk.nih.gov/kudiseases/pubs/prostateenlargement/index.htm. Accessed winter 2004.
3. Leveillee RJ, Patel V. Prostate Hyperplasia, Benign. Copyright © 2003, eMedicine.com, Inc. Available at: http://www.emedicine.com/med/topic1919.htm. Accessed winter 2004.
4. Smith IM. The Prostate Gets Bigger With Aging. Copyright © 1992–2004 the Author(s) and The University of Iowa. Available at: http://www.vh.org/adult/patient/internalmedicine/aba30/1995/prostate.html. Accessed winter 2004.
5. Rubenstein J, McVary KT. Transurethral Microwave Thermotherapy of the Prostate (TUMT). Copyright © 2003, eMedicine.com, Inc. Available at: http://www.emedicine.com/med/topic3070.htm. Accessed winter 2004.

Prostate Cancer

1. Can Prostate Cancer Be Found Early? Copyright © 2004 American Cancer Society, Inc. Available at: http://www.cancer.org/docroot/CRI/content/CRI_2_4_

3X_Can_prostate_cancer_be_found_early_36.asp?rnav=cri. Accessed winter 2004.
2. Prostate Cancer: The Public Health Perspective. Centers for Disease Control and Prevention. Available at: http://www.cdc.gov/cancer/prostate/prostate.htm. Accessed winter 2004.
3. Prostate cancer Overview. Copyright © 1998–2004 Mayo Foundation for Medical Education and Research (MFMER). Available at: http://www.mayoclinic.com/invoke.cfm?id=DS00043. Accessed winter 2004.
4. What You Need To Know About™ Prostate Cancer. National Cancer Institute (NCI). Available at: http://www.cancer.gov/cancerinfo/wyntk/prostate. Accessed winter 2004.
5. Questions and Answers about the Prostate-Specific Antigen (PSA) Test. National Cancer Institute (NCI). Available at: http://cis.nci.nih.gov/fact/5_29.htm. Accessed winter 2004.
6. Prostate Cancer. Copyright © 2003 Johns Hopkins Medicine. Available at: http://urology.jhu.edu/diseases/prostate/prostate.html. Accessed winter 2004.
7. Stages of Prostate Cancer. U.S. Food and Drug Administration. Available at: http://www.pueblo.gsa.gov/cic_text/health/prostate-no1answer/prosdiag.html. Accessed winter 2004.

Prostatitis

1. Piesman M, Costabile RA. Acute Bacterial Prostatitis and Prostatic Abscess. Copyright © 2003, eMedicine.com, Inc. Available at: http://www.emedicine.com/med/topic2845.htm. Accessed winter 2004.
2. Ahuja SK. Chronic Bacterial Prostatitis. Copyright © 2003, eMedicine.com, Inc. Available at: http://www.emedicine.com/med/topic3571.htm. Accessed winter 2004.
3. Zermann D-H, Ishigooka M, Doggweiler R, et al. Chronic Prostatitis: A Myofascial Pain Syndrome? Copyright © 1999 Cliggott Publishing, Division of SCP Communications. Available at: http://www.medscape.com/viewarticle/416999. Accessed winter 2004.
4. Prostatitis—chronic. Copyright © 2002 A.D.A.M., Inc. Available at: http://www.nlm.nih.gov/medlineplus/ency/article/000523.htm. Accessed winter 2004.
5. Nickel JC. Chronic Prostatitis: An Infectious Disease? Copyright © 2000 Cliggott Publishing, Division of SCP Communications. Available at: http://www.medscape.com/viewarticle/410204. Accessed winter 2004.
6. Prostatitis Overview. Copyright © 1998–2003 Mayo Foundation for Medical Education and Research (MFMER). Available at: http://www.mayoclinic.com/invoke.cfm?id=DS00341. Accessed winter 2004.
7. New Study Offers Hope for Chronic Prostatitis Treatment. Copyright © 2000 Medscape. Available at: http://www.

medscape.com/viewarticle/411511. Accessed winter 2004.
8. Chronic Prostatitis Workshop. National Institute of Diabetes and Digestive and Kidney Diseases, National Institutes of Health. Available at: http://kidney.niddk.nih.gov/kudiseases/pubs/chronicprostatitis/index.htm. Accessed winter 2004.
9. Ahuja SK. Nonbacterial Prostatitis. Copyright © 2003, eMedicine.com, Inc. Available at: http://www.emedicine.com/med/topic3405.htm. Accessed winter 2004.
10. Pais V Jr, Wagner A. Prostatitis, Tuberculous. Copyright © 2003, eMedicine.com, Inc. Available at: http://www.emedicine.com/med/topic1921.htm. Accessed winter 2004.
11. Prostatitis. Copyright © 1996–2003 MedicineNet, Inc. Available at: http://www.medicinenet.com/prostatitis/article.htm. Accessed winter 2004.
12. Prostatitis—nonbacterial. Copyright © 2002 A.D.A.M., Inc. Available at: http://www.nlm.nih.gov/medlineplus/ency/article/000524.htm. Accessed winter 2004.

Testicular Cancer

1. Testicular Cancer (Cancer of the Testicle). Copyright © 1996–2003 MedicineNet, Inc. Available at: http://www.medicinenet.com/testicular_cancer/article.htm. Accessed fall 03.
2. Pathology of the Testis, Male Genital Tract Pathology, IV. Neoplasms. Copyright © 1998–2001 by the Rector and Visitors of the University of Virginia. Available at: http://hsc.virginia.edu/med-ed/path/gu/testis4.html. Accessed fall 2003.
3. Light D. Testicle, Malignant Tumors. Copyright © 2003, eMedicine.com, Inc. Available at: http://www.emedicine.com/radio/topic680.htm. Accessed fall 2003.
4. Testicular Cancer. Harvard Medical School. Available at: http://www.intelihealth.com/IH/ihtPrint/WSIHW000/9339/10848.html?hide=t&k=basePrint. Accessed fall 2003.
5. Testicular cancer. Copyright © 1998–2003 Mayo Foundation for Medical Education and Research (MFMER). Available at: http://www.mayoclinic.com/invoke.cfm?id=DS00046. Accessed fall 03.

Menopause

1. About Estrogen and Estrogen Dominance. Copyright © 1999–2000 Progesterone Advocates Network. Available at: http://www.progestnet.com/documents/estrogen.html. Accessed winter 2004.
2. Shangold MM, Sherman C. Exercise and Menopause: A Time for Positive Changes. Copyright © 1998. The McGraw-Hill Companies. Available at: http://www.physsportsmed.com/issues/1998/12dec/shangold.htm. Accessed winter 2004.
3. Hormone replacement therapy (HRT). Copyright © 2002 A.D.A.M., Inc. Available at: http://www.nlm.nih.gov/medlineplus/ency/article/007111.htm. Accessed winter 2004.

4. Menopause Overview. Copyright © 1998–2004 Mayo Foundation for Medical Education and Research (MFMER). Available at: http://www.mayoclinic.com/invoke.cfm?id=DS00119. Accessed winter 2004.
5. Hormones and the Menstrual Cycle. Copyright © 2000–2002, ICBS, Inc. Available at: http://www.holistic-online.com/Remedies/hrt/hrt_menstr_hormone.htm. Accessed winter 2004.
6. Marcus EN. Menopause. Copyright © 2004, eMedicine.com, Inc. Available at: http://www.emedicine.com/aaem/topic305.htm. Accessed winter 2004.
7. Menopause One Woman's Story, Every Woman's Story. National Institute on Aging, National Institutes of Health. Available at: http://www.niapublications.org/pubs/menopause/menopauseup-date2003.pdf. Accessed winter 2004.
8. Questions and Answers about Black Cohosh and the Symptoms of Menopause. National Center for Complementary and Alternative Medicine, National Institutes of Health. Available at: http://ods.od.nih.gov/factsheets/blackcohosh.html. Accessed winter 2004.
9. Risks and Benefits of Estrogen Plus Progestin in Healthy Postmenopausal Women. Copyright © 2002 American Medical Association. Available at: http://jama.ama-assn.org/cgi/content/abstract/288/3/321. Accessed winter 2004.
10. Hormone Replacement Therapy (HRT). Copyright © 1997–2002 Imaginis Corporation. Available at: http://imaginis.com/breasthealth/hrt.asp?mode=1. Accessed winter 2004.

Pelvic Inflammatory Disease

1. Meiner EM, Shoff WH. Salpingitis. Copyright © 2003, eMedicine.com, Inc. Available at: http://www.emedicine.com/MED/topic2059.htm. Accessed winter 2004.
2. Pelvic Inflammatory Disease Overview. Copyright © 1998–2004 Mayo Foundation for Medical Education and Research (MFMER). Available at: http://www.mayoclinic.com/invoke.cfm?id=DS00402. Accessed winter 2004.
3. Abbuhl S, Reyes I. Pelvic Inflammatory Disease. Copyright © 2004, eMedicine.com, Inc. Available at: http://www.emedicine.com/EMERG/topic410.htm. Accessed winter 2004.
4. Pelvic Inflammatory Disease. National Institute of Allergy and Infectious Diseases, National Institutes of Health. Available at: http://www.niaid.nih.gov/factsheets/stdpid.htm. Accessed winter 2004.

Pregnancy

1. Ectopic Pregnancy. American Society for Reproductive Medicine. Available at: http://www.asrm.org/Patients/patientbooklets/ectopicpregnancy.pdf. Accessed winter 2004.

2. Gestational Diabetes: What It Means for Me and My Baby. Copyright © 2001–2003 American Academy of Family Physicians. Available at: http://familydoctor.org/075.xml. Accessed winter 2004.

3. Padden MO. HELLP Syndrome: Recognition and Perinatal Management. Copyright © 1999 by the American Academy of Family Physicians. Available at: http://www.aafp.org/afp/990901ap/829.html. Accessed winter 2004.

4. High Blood Pressure in Pregnancy. National Heart, Lung, and Blood Institute (NHLBI), National Institutes of Health (NIH). Available at: http://www.nhlbi.nih.gov/health/public/heart/hbp/hbp_preg.htm. Accessed winter 2004.

5. Mackenzie S. Obstetrics: Hypertension in Pregnancy, Preeclampsia, and Eclampsia. Copyright © 1992–2004 the Author(s) and The University of Iowa. Available at: http://www.vh.org/adult/provider/familymedicine/FPHandbook/Chapter14/12-14.html. Accessed winter 2004.

Premenstrual Syndrome

1. PMS: What You Can Do to Ease Your Symptoms. Copyright © 2003 American Academy of Family Physicians. Available at: http://familydoctor.org/x5126.xml?printxml. Accessed winter 2004.

2. Premenstrual syndrome Overview. Copyright © 1998–2004 Mayo Foundation for Medical Education and Research (MFMER). Available at: http://www.mayoclinic.com/invoke.cfm?id=DS00134. Accessed winter 2004.

3. Moline ML, Kahn DA, Ross RW, et al. Premenstrual Dysphoric Disorder: A Guide for Patients and Families. A postgraduate medicine special report. Available at: http://www.psychguides.com/DinW%20PMDD.pdf. Accessed winter 2004.

4. Premenstrual Syndrome (PMS). Copyright © 1996–2003 Aetna InteliHealth Inc. Available at: http://www.intelihealth.com/IH/ihtIH/WSIHW000/9339/23664.html. Accessed winter 2004.

5. Dickerson LM, Mazyck PJ, Hunter MH. Premenstrual Syndrome. Copyright © 2003 by the American Academy of Family Physicians. Available at: http://www.aafp.org/afp/20030415/1743.html. Accessed winter 2004.

6. Ransom S, Moldenhauer J. Premenstrual Syndrome: Systematic Diagnosis and Individualized Therapy. Copyright © 1998. The McGraw-Hill Companies. Available at: http://www.physsportsmed.com/issues/1998/04apr/ransom.htm. Accessed winter 2004.

Sexually Transmitted Diseases

1. Genital warts Overview. Copyright © 1998–2003 Mayo Foundation for Medical Education and Research (MFMER). Available at: http://www.mayoclinic.com/invoke.cfm?id=DS00087. Accessed winter 2004.

2. Molluscum Contagiosum. Copyright © 2001, American Social Health Association. Available at: http://www.ashastd.org/stdfaqs/molcon.html. Accessed winter 2004.

3. Nongonococcal Urethritis (NGU). Copyright © 2001, American Social Health Association. Available at: http://www.ashastd.org/stdfaqs/ngu.html. Accessed winter 2004.

4. An Introduction to Sexually Transmitted Infections. National Institute of Allergy and Infectious Diseases, National Institutes of Health. Available at: http://www.niaid.nih.gov/factsheets/stdinfo.htm. Accessed winter 2004.

5. Rates of STD's. Centers for Disease Control and Prevention. Available at: http://www.cdc.gov/std/stats/tables/table1.htm. Accessed winter 2004.

Chlamydia

1. Chlamydia. Disease Information. Centers for Disease Control and Prevention, National Center for HIV, STD and TB Prevention. Available at: http://www.cdc.gov/nchstp/dstd/Fact_Sheets/FactsChlamydiaInfo.htm. Accessed winter 2004.

2. Chlamydia infections in women. Copyright © 2002 A.D.A.M., Inc. Available at: http://www.nlm.nih.gov/medlineplus/ency/article/000660.htm. Accessed winter 2004.

3. Grella M. Chlamydial Infections. Copyright © 2003, eMedicine.com, Inc. Available at: http://www.emedicine.com/ped/topic378.htm. Accessed winter 2004.

4. Chlamydia Overview. Copyright © 1998–2003 Mayo Foundation for Medical Education and Research (MFMER). Available at: http://www.mayoclinic.com/invoke.cfm?id=DS00173. Accessed winter 2004.

5. Chlamydial Infection. National Institute of Allergy and Infectious Diseases, National Institutes of Health. Available at: http://www.niaid.nih.gov/factsheets/stdclam.htm. Accessed winter 2004.

Gonorrhea

1. Medical Encyclopedia: Gonorrhea—female. Copyright © 2002 A.D.A.M., Inc. Available at: http://www.nlm.nih.gov/medlineplus/ency/article/000656.htm. Accessed winter 2004.

2. Gonorrhea. Centers for Disease Control and Prevention, National Center for HIV, STD and TB Prevention. Available at: http://www.cdc.gov/nchstp/dstd/Fact_Sheets/FactsGonorrhea.htm. Accessed winter 2004.

3. Grella M. Gonorrhea. Copyright © 2003, eMedicine.com, Inc. Available at: http://www.emedicine.com/ped/topic886.htm. Accessed winter 2004.

4. Gonorrhea. Copyright © 1995–2003 Merck & Co., Inc. Available at: http://www.merck.com/mrkshared/mmanual/section13/chapter164/164b.jsp. Accessed winter 2004.

5. Gonorrhea Overview. Copyright © 1998–2003 Mayo Foundation for Medical Education and Research (MFMER). Available at: http://www.mayoclinic.com/invoke.cfm?id=DS00180. Accessed winter 2004.

6. Gonorrhea. National Institute of Allergy and Infectious Diseases, National Institutes of Health. Available at: http://www.niaid.nih.gov/factsheets/stdgon.htm. Accessed winter 2004.

Syphilis

1. Syphilis. National Institute of Allergy and Infectious Diseases, National Institutes of Health. Available at: http://www.niaid.nih.gov/factsheets/stdsyph.htm. Accessed winter 2004.

2. Syphilis Overview. Copyright © 1998–2003 Mayo Foundation for Medical Education and Research (MFMER). Available at: http://www.mayoclinic.com/invoke.cfm?id=DS00374. Accessed winter 2004.

3. Some facts about Syphilis. Centers for Disease Control and Prevention, National Center for HIV, STD and TB Prevention. Available at: http://www.cdc.gov/nchstp/dstd/Fact_Sheets/Syphilis_Facts.htm. Accessed winter 2004.

4. Waseem M. Syphilis. Copyright © 2003, eMedicine.com, Inc. Available at: http://www.emedicine.com/ped/topic2193.htm. Accessed winter 2004.

MISCELLANEOUS CONDITIONS

Chapter Objectives

After reading this chapter, you should be able to . . .

- Name the most common type of cancer reported.
- Identify the leading cause of death in patients with cancer.
- Name three carcinogenic chemicals.
- Describe five of the seven leading signs and symptoms of cancer.
- Identify the meaning of "T, N, and M" in cancer staging.
- Identify a caution for massage when a client is receiving radiation treatment.
- Identify a caution for massage when a client is receiving chemotherapy treatment.
- Identify a caution for massage when a client has had some lymph nodes removed for staging purposes.
- Describe three stimulants in a massage setting that might irritate a person with multiple chemical sensitivity syndrome.
- Identify two cautions for massage and recent open surgery.

MISCELLANEOUS CONDITIONS

Cancer, General
Cysts
Fatigue

Multiple Chemical Sensitivity
Syndrome

Postoperative Situations

Metastasis:

Meta means "beyond" (e.g., the metacarpals are beyond the carpals). *Stasis* means "staying the same." meta-stasis, then, means "beyond staying the same," or in other words, *changing what should not be changed.*

 # MISCELLANEOUS CONDITIONS

Cancer, General

Definition: What Is It?

Cancer is a variety of more than 100 different diseases that have one thing in common: normal body cells mutate slightly and begin to replicate uncontrollably. These new cells form masses called tumors, or if they are blood cells, they simply circulate but provide no useful function. At some point in the process, some cells may break off the initial growth and travel elsewhere in the body, where they colonize new tissue.

Demographics: Who Gets It?

One half of all men and one third of all women in the United States will develop some sort of cancer in their lifetime.[1] Cancer kills more than 550,000 people in the United States every year. Overall, both the incidence of new cases and the death rate of most cancers have begun to decline. This is probably due to a number of issues, including slowing tobacco use, better education about the risks of sunlight exposure, more sensitive screening procedures, and better chances of finding cancers in early stages. Nonetheless, the improvement in cancer statistics also reflects inequities in health care access. The incidence and death rates of cancer are better among white upper-income citizens than they are among non-white citizens who have lower incomes.

Skin cancer is the most common variety of cancer reported (and these statistics do not even reflect the countless moles that are removed as a safeguard against melanoma development), but lung cancer is the leading cause of death by cancer for both men and women. Other leading causes of death include breast and ovarian cancer for women, prostate cancer for men, and cancer of the pancreas, colon, and rectum for both genders.

Etiology: What Happens?

No one is positive about what causes a healthy cell to change into a malignant cell. One thing that all cancers have in common is that the DNA of a cell mutates in a way that the cell acquires certain growth properties. As researchers learn more about the process of metastasis, new ways to interrupt the process and limit the ability of cancer cells to invade and destroy healthy tissue are being discovered.

The following is a simplified version of the process of metastasis, as it is currently understood:

- *Oncogene activation.* An **oncogene** is a gene that initiates malignant characteristics within a cell. Oncogene activation is the beginning of the changes that cause certain

Cancer in Brief

What is it?
Cancer is the mutation of normal cells into cells with particular characteristics, including the tendency to proliferate into distinguishable growths and to spread through the body to other areas where they may colonize new tissues.

How is it recognized?
In early stages, many cancers are difficult to detect. Later signs depend on what part of the body is being affected but can include things such as unusual bleeding, susceptibility to infection, changes in skin lesions, a persistent cough or hoarseness, changes in bladder or bowel habits, painless lumps or swellings, or pain where tumors have grown to the point that they erode into or compress delicate tissue.

Is massage indicated or contraindicated?
The decision about whether to include massage as part of a treatment plan with cancer is complicated. Some types of bodywork are said to boost circulatory and lymph flow, which could be interpreted as increasing the risk of metastasis. Research shows, however, that it can take several years for many tumors to reach a palpable size. In light of this, it seems unlikely that a 60-minute session could have a serious impact on this disease process, as long as the therapist is not rubbing directly on the tumor.

Many cancer patients seek massage as a way to help them cope with the challenges of cancer treatments. Massage and other bodywork modalities offered in this context can be beneficial, as long as the risks of working with clients who are undergoing surgery, chemotherapy, radiation, or other procedures are respected, and the therapist works as part of a well-informed health care team.

[1] Who Gets Cancer? Copyright © 2004 American Cancer Society, Inc. Available at: http://www.cancer.org/docroot/CRI/content/CRI_2_4_1x_Who_gets_cancer.asp?sitearea=CRI. Accessed winter 2004.

cells to become malignant. The trigger for activation may be toxic environmental exposures, diet, a genetic predisposition, or some combination of the above, but it is often not clear.

- *Proliferation.* The mutated cells proliferate without control, often piling up into distinct masses. As they do this, they may secrete enzymes that allow them to survive a normal immune system attack against perceived invaders.

- *Angiogenesis. Angiogenesis* is the growth of blood vessels to supply the tumor. Any growth of more than 1 or 2 cm^3 requires a specific blood supply. Some cancer cells seem well supplied with the chemical messengers that command the body to build new capillaries. The more highly invested a tumor is with blood vessels, the more likely it is to have metastasized.

- *Invasion.* As a tumor grows, it must convince the local extracellular matrix to make room for it without stimulating an inflammatory response. Again, special enzymes secreted by cancer cells are at the center of this process. These enzymes help to dissolve the connective tissue that provides the support for epithelium, where most cancers grow.

- *Migration.* Some cancer cells break off the primary tumor and travel through the lymphatic or circulatory capillaries to new areas. This is a complicated process involving the penetration of capillary walls to enter them and a second penetration to exit them.

- *Colonization.* When cancer cells land in a new target tissue, they must begin the process over again, starting with proliferation. This requires that the cells be able to adhere to the new tissue and that they can secrete the correct enzymes to suppress an immune system attack, create new blood vessels, and erode the extracellular matrix. The first tumor that grows in the disease process is called the primary tumor; other tumors that grow from metastasis of the primary tumor are called secondary tumors. In other words, a tumor in the bladder that metastasized from the ovary is not bladder cancer—it is secondary ovarian cancer in the bladder.

How often cells become malignant in an average human life is unclear. It may be a fairly common occurrence, which simply is not successful as long as immune system mechanisms prevent the growth of abnormal new cells. This raises some interesting questions about the connections among cancer, stress, and immune system efficiency.

Causes

Triggers for oncogene activation vary by tissue type and individual. Causes of cancer are slowly being narrowed to some identifiable factors. These are generally discussed as internal or external factors.

Internal Factors   Every cell in the body has a built-in capacity for self-destruction. This is a natural and healthy process called *apoptosis*. A specific gene in some cancer cells has been found to inhibit apoptosis. Therefore, some cancers may be as much caused by cells that *refuse to die* as it is by new cells coming to life.

Some cancers are brought about by or connected to inherited characteristics. This means an inherited gene is likely to cause cellular mutations some time in the future (such genes have been identified for a small percentage of breast and colon cancers). It could also mean that a person may have a genetic susceptibility to environmental factors that would not be a threat to someone else. Some inborn hormonal problems or immune system dysfunctions also can increase the risk for developing cancer.

External Factors   Carcinogens are chemical or environmental agents that have been identified as cancer-causers. The hydrocarbons in cigarette smoke are carcinogens, as is ultraviolet radiation from the sun, especially for fair-skinned people. Radiation from excessive x-rays and exposure to certain substances such as asbestos, benzene, nickel, cadmium, uranium, and vinyl chloride have also been found to be carcinogenic.

Some viruses can cause certain types of cancer. Others simply have a strong statistical link with the development of various cancers, but the cause-and-effect relationship has not been defined. Some cancer-related viruses include:

- *Human immunodeficiency virus (HIV)*. This virus can cause Kaposi's sarcoma, a type of skin cancer (see *HIV/AIDS*, Chapter 5).

- *HTLV-1*. This is a virus in the same family as HIV; it has been linked to *leukemia* (Chapter 4) and *lymphoma* (Chapter 5).

- *Hepatitis B (HBV) and hepatitis C (HCV)*. These infections have been linked to *liver cancer* (see *hepatitis* and *liver cancer*, Chapter 7).

- *Epstein-Barr virus (EBV)*. This has been linked to Burkitt's *lymphoma* and Hodgkin's disease (Chapter 5).

- *Human papilloma virus (HPV)*. This is implicated in nearly all cases of *cervical cancer* (Chapter 10).

- *Herpes simplex type II (genital herpes)*. This has been linked to cervical and uterine cancer. (See *herpes*, Chapter 1.)

Often a combination of external and internal factors tip the scales in favor of developing cancer. Exposure to carcinogens in certain combinations also can be dangerous. For example, heavy smoking combined with excessive alcohol consumption is an especially potent combination for developing cancers of the mouth or upper gastrointestinal tract. Very often many years, even decades, may pass between the initial exposure to a carcinogen and the development of distinguishable tumors. This makes it difficult to pin down precise causes of cancer that will be consistent from person to person.

Signs and Symptoms

Symptoms of cancer vary widely, depending on the site. One of the most insidious features of this disease is that it is often painless until it is too late to do anything about it. Tumors begin to cause pain when they place pressure on nerve endings, or when they cause a blockage in a tube or duct that will in turn put pressure on nerve endings. The American Cancer Society has compiled a list of common signs that are red flags for the possibility of cancer.[2] They include:

- A change in bowel or bladder habits
- A sore that does not heal
- Unusual bleeding or drainage
- Thickening or lump in the breast or elsewhere
- Indigestion or swallowing difficulty
- A change in a wart or mole
- Persistent cough or hoarseness
- Unexplained weight loss
- Fatigue, anemia
- Fever
- Skin changes, including darkening, yellowing, reddening, or sudden hair growth

[2] Signs and Symptoms of Cancer. Copyright © 2004 American Cancer Society, Inc. Available at: http://www.cancer.org/docroot/CRI/content/CRI_2_4_3X_What_are_the_signs_and_symptoms_of_cancer.asp?rnav=cri. Accessed winter 2004.

Diagnosis

Cancers are found by a variety of methods, depending on the affected part of the body. Many cancers are found by either self or clinical examinations; this is true for breast, cervical, colorectal, and prostate cancers. Other tumors are found by imaging techniques such as radiographs, computed tomography (CT) scans, magnetic resonance imaging (MRI), endoscopies, and ultrasound. Barium swallows and enemas can reveal tumors in the gastrointestinal tract.

If suspicious changes are noted, tissue samples are taken and analyzed for the presence of malignant cells; this is called a biopsy. If these tests are positive, further examinations of the patient follow to determine how far the cancer has developed.

Staging

Most types of cancer develop in predictable enough patterns that they can be staged or given a label that indicates how far the cancer has advanced. Staging is often done with the TNM system, which is then used to rate the cancer numerically.

The TNM classification system rates tumors by:

- *(T)* Tumor size or area of involvement
- *(N)* Nodal involvement: how many nodes and where they are
- *(M)* Extent of metastasis: local or distant

Staging may be further qualified by the use of "A" and "B" delineations to allow for differences in patterns of progression.

Cancers of the lymph nodes and bone marrow have a different growth pattern than other cancers. Because they do not involve primary tumors, their staging systems refer to blood counts and symptoms.

Findings of the TNM status are then often translated into Stages 0 to IV, depending on the type of cancer. The purpose of staging is to evaluate the progression of the disease, with the intention of designing a treatment approach with the best chance of success.

Treatment

Decisions for how to treat cancer depend on the stage it is in, the age and general health of the patient, and what kind of cancer is present. Within each tumor, different kinds of cells may require different modes of attack. This makes the successful treatment of cancer a matter of finding the correct combination of surgery, chemotherapy, hypothermia, radiation, hormones, and biologic therapies.

- *Surgery.* Cancer surgeries are performed to remove malignant tumors and a margin of healthy tissue around them, when possible. A sample of nearby lymph nodes is often taken as well to examine them for signs of metastasis. If a "sentinel" node can be identified (this is a node through which most or all of the lymph entering an area passes before going on to other nodes), it can be taken alone for examination. This refinement has led to a reduction in some of the side effects of cancer surgery.

- *Radiofrequency thermal ablation.* This is a procedure in which instruments are inserted through the skin to the depth of a targeted tumor, and an electrical current essentially "microwaves" cancerous material. This method is being used for tumors that are not easily accessible for traditional surgery, especially in liver cancer.

- *Chemotherapy.* A variety of cytotoxic drugs have been developed for use in cancer treatment. These drugs specifically target any fast-growing cells in the body, so in addition to killing cancer cells they also may attack the skin (resulting in hair loss), the gastrointestinal tract (leading to chronic nausea and mouth sores), and the blood cells (causing easy bruising and bleeding disorders as well as white blood cell suppression).

- *Autologous bone marrow transplant.* **Autologous bone marrow transplant** is a procedure in which some healthy bone marrow is harvested from the patient and stored. Then a very extreme course of cytotoxic drugs is administered. This kills the cancer cells but kills most white blood cells too. After chemotherapy, the stored bone marrow is replanted in the patient, where it replaces the immune system cells killed by chemotherapy. This procedure is for use only in very extreme cases; it has a number of dangerous side affects and serious complications, but it can be a life-saver if nothing else works. **Allogenic bone marrow transplants** use the marrow of a closely matched donor.

- *Radiation.* With this type of therapy, high-energy rays are focused on tumors to kill them or at least slow their growth. The radiation may be applied from an external machine, which requires daily outpatient visits for several weeks, or it may come from small radioactive pellets that are temporarily implanted close to the tumor.

- *Hormones.* Breast and prostate cancer tumors both depend on the presence of certain hormones to grow. Therapies to limit the secretion of these hormones or to change the way they affect the body are used in the treatment of these cancers.

- *Hypothermia.* In some cases, specifically with cervical cancer and actinic keratosis (see *skin cancer,* Chapter 1), potentially malignant cells may be killed by freezing them off the affected structure.

- *Biologic therapy.* Recently found weaknesses in the process of metastasis have led to the development of more refined cancer treatments. Cancer cells are able to limit immune system responses because of their particular enzyme secretions, but that could be overcome with specialized treatments that enhance an immune system response to cancer cell antigens. Several cancer "vaccines" are currently being explored to sensitize immune system agents to these antigens. An exciting aspect of this research is that it targets *only* cancer cells, which could keep the side effects of treatment to a minimum. These highly specialized treatments may eventually reach the same prevalence as traditional cancer treatments.

- *Stem cell implantation.* The implantation of stem cells specifically for leukemia patients carries promise as an effective cancer treatment. These "cellular blanks" have the potential to grow into whatever kinds of cells the body needs to replace.

Prevention

Most resources that study cancer publish a list of simple lifestyle choices that can reduce the risk of developing this disease. Whereas different aspects are emphasized for different types of cancer, a basic approach would follow these guidelines:

- Eat more fruit, vegetables, and whole grains, while controlling dietary fat.

- Exercise regularly, and control weight

- Use sunscreen or clothing to protect the skin from UV radiation

- Stop smoking and other tobacco use

- Use alcohol moderately

- Practice safe sex (Note: this is as a precaution against contracting human papilloma virus, which is associated with cervical cancer. Research shows, however, that barrier methods such as condoms do *not* protect against the spread of this virus.[3] Therefore, "safe sex" in this context means to have relations with an uninfected partner.)

- Use early cancer screening methods (see sidebar, "Cancer Screening: Who, What, Where, When, Why?").

[3] Human Papilloma Virus (HPV). Copyright © 2004 American Cancer Society, Inc. Available at: http://www.cancer.org/docroot/cri/content/cri_2_6x_human_papilloma_virus_hpv.asp?sitearea=cri. Accessed spring 2004.

Cancer Screening—Who, What, Where, When, Why?

The science of early cancer detection is far from fully developed or universally accepted. A survey of several different medical agencies yields significantly different guidelines for individuals to follow in the attempt to be vigilant against early signs of cancer. One of the concerns with making screening recommendations is the high risk of many "false positives" leading to unnecessary interventions and even dangerous surgeries. Screening recommendations are further complicated by differences for low-risk and high-risk populations.

The following is a brief synopsis of the leading ideas about early cancer detection. Any of these is subject to change as research reveals whether specific testing procedures actually reduce the mortality rate from the types of cancer they target.

Type of Cancer	Recommendations for Low-Risk Populations	Recommendations for High-Risk Populations
Breast cancer	*Self-examination.* Monthly from age 20 onward. *Clinical examination.* Every 3 years from ages 20–39, and annually from 40 onward. *Mammogram.* Opinions vary, but most suggest examinations every 1–3 years from age 40 or 50 onward.	High-risk populations include women with the identified breast cancer genes, women who have first-degree relatives with breast cancer, or women who have had breast cancer or other types of cancer before. Screening schedules need to be matched to individual cases.
Cervical cancer	When a woman becomes sexually active, she should have a yearly pelvic examination and Pap test; when she has had three normal tests in a row, she can cut back on frequency to once every 3 years, or by her doctor's recommendation, for as long as she has a cervix. Some studies suggest that testing can be suspended after age 65.	High-risk populations for cervical cancer are women who have shown signs of cervical dysplasia in pelvic examinations or Pap tests. Screening should continue on a yearly basis until patients have three normal tests in a row. Screening can be discontinued if a patient has had a hysterectomy, *unless* the surgery was related to cervical cancer.
Skin cancer	Several agencies recommend a monthly self-examination for changes in skin, with a clinical visual examination every 3 years from age 20 to 40, and annually from age 40 onward; counseling for avoiding sun exposure and the use of sunblock is also a part of skin cancer prevention and early detection.	High-risk populations include persons previously diagnosed with any type of skin cancer or precancerous condition; clinical examinations should be scheduled on an as-needed basis.
Prostate cancer	A PSA test and annual digital rectal examination (DRE) are recommended yearly for men over 50 years old with no risk factors for prostate cancer.	African American men, and men with a first-degree relative (father, brother, son) who have prostate cancer should begin testing at age 40–45.
Colon cancer	Beginning at age 50, men and women should do the following: have a fecal occult blood test (FOBT) every year; a sigmoidoscopy or colonoscopy every 5 to 10 years.	Persons with a history of colon polyps, inflammatory bowel disease, or a family history of hereditary colorectal cancer should begin screening procedures before age 50.
Lung, ovarian, and endometrial cancer	No effective noninvasive screening measures have been developed to detect these cancers in early stages; therefore, it is not practical to make recommendations for low-risk populations.	Some screening techniques may find these cancers, but they tend to be invasive procedures that are reserved for patients with a high risk for developing them.

Massage?

For many years, it has been assumed that circulatory types of massage carry the risk of aiding the process of metastasis by boosting blood and lymph flow. Research shows, however, that cancerous growths can take years to become established before they are detectable by palpation. It seems farfetched to suppose that a 60-minute massage could contribute to that process any more significantly than a brisk walk around the block or a long hot shower. Nonetheless, it is obviously inappropriate to rub on a tumor or any undiagnosed swelling or thickening of tissue.

Massage for persons undergoing cancer treatment, however, has a vital and useful role. It can assist in pain control, decrease perceived stress levels, and create a general parasympathetic state through reduced blood pressure and decreased muscle tension. It can improve appetite and the quality of sleep. Perhaps most of all, it provides for a basic human need: nurturing, caring, informed touch at a time when many cancer patients feel isolated and dehumanized. The benefits massage has to offer are so well accepted that many hospitals are now including massage treatments for their cancer patients.[4]

It is important, however, to bear in mind the complications associated with various cancer treatments, because they can have serious implications for the choices of bodywork modalities, especially when multiple treatments are employed.

- *Surgery*. The most obvious caution for recent cancer surgery to remove tumors and lymph nodes is the open scar and risk of infection that goes along with it. Other complications of surgery can include nerve damage and lymphedema (see sidebar, "Lymphedema", Figure 11.1).

- *Chemotherapy*. Chemotherapy has many serious side effects, including a drastically impaired immune system, nausea, fatigue, and ulcers in the mouth and mucous membranes. Chemotherapy is usually administered in stages, so a patient may undergo a course of treatment, take some time to recover, and then have another course. Massage therapists working with clients undergoing chemotherapy must be especially conscious of their own health so as not to expose their clients to dangerous pathogens. Some experts recommend that patients receive massage during breaks between chemotherapy treatments; others suggest that therapists might want to use gloves if they are working with clients who are suffused with cytotoxic drugs. These decisions must be made on a case-by-case basis. It would be wise to share any such concerns with the client's health care team.

- *Radiation*. Externally applied radiation can result in burns on the skin as well as fatigue, impaired immunity, and lymphedema if lymph nodes are destroyed in the

Lymphedema

Part of cancer staging is the removal and examination of local lymph nodes for signs of metastasis. If cancer cells are found, the remaining nodes may be treated with radiation therapy. Both the surgery to remove sample nodes and the treatment to kill cancer that might be growing in remaining nodes can lead to a serious complication called lymphedema.

Lymphedema describes the accumulation of protein-rich fluid in the interstitial spaces as a result of lymph system dysfunction. (This distinguishes it from simple edema, which is typically related to venous insufficiency.) The chemistry of interstitial fluid is such that when it does not flow freely into nearby lymph vessels, it attracts water. That is, a small amount of fluid retention can become a significant problem in a short period.

Lymphedema can develop in the days or weeks after cancer surgery or radiation treatment, or it can suddenly appear decades later; all that is required is an insufficiency in lymph node function. Patients most at risk for this problem are those who have had nodes removed, had radiation after surgery, who are overweight, and who are sedentary. Once the shift in tissue proteins occurs, the symptoms may subside, but the risk of recurrence is always high.

Signs and symptoms of lymphedema can include redness, heat, and pain; these signs indicate infection along with fluid retention. Often, however, it is simply the deep ache and loss of function of a limb that grows to huge proportions (Figure 10.2). Pitting edema (Figure 5.2 a and b) is another indicator. Lymphedematous limbs

are particularly vulnerable to bacterial and fungal infections, and must be cared for very carefully.

Long-standing lymphedema can lead to fibrosclerotic changes in the interstitial spaces of the superficial fascia. In other words, the tissue and skin on the affected limb become indurated, or hardened. Once this stage is reached, it is very difficult to reverse.

Standard treatment options for lymphedema are limited. Compression machines, bandages, and supportive clothing are first options but are often unsatisfactory. Lymphedema is of particular relevance for massage therapists, because it would seem tempting to use Swedish massage, well known for its ability to move fluid, to help resolve this situation. However, because of the chemical imbalance in the interstitial spaces, any kind of work that compresses blood vessels only makes lymphedema worse. Various kinds of bodywork techniques have been developed to address lymphedema, but they are very light, and they employ extensive knowledge of the anatomy and physiology of the lymph system to maximize benefits while minimizing risks. In other words, they are advanced techniques that require extensive training to do responsibly. Practitioners who learn these techniques, however, are likely to find an eager group of clients hoping to benefit from their work, and various types of manual lymph drainage or lymph drainage technique find acceptance in the medical community.

Clients with a history of lymphedema live with a lifetime risk of repeated episodes. Although massage to the rest of the body may be fine, massage to the affected arm or leg must be conducted very conservatively.

[4] Massage Benefits Hospitalized Cancer Patients. Articles from Massage Magazine. Available at: http://www.amtafoundation.org/or_article_massagemag105B.html. Accessed winter 2004.

Figure 11.1. Lymphedema: this occurs most frequently in arms or legs where lymph nodes have been removed for staging purposes.

process. Massage therapists must avoid skin lesions and the possibility of sharing pathogens with clients who have very limited capacity to fight back. Radiation can cause significant burns on the skin, which of course must be avoided (Figure 11.2).

- *Other cautions.* The side effects of other cancer treatments are variable. Applications of liquid nitrogen to freeze off actinic keratosis lesions can injure the skin. Tamoxifen, a hormone-like drug for breast cancer, is associated with an increased risk of blood clotting. The potential side effects of biologic cancer treatments and stem cell implants have yet to be discovered.

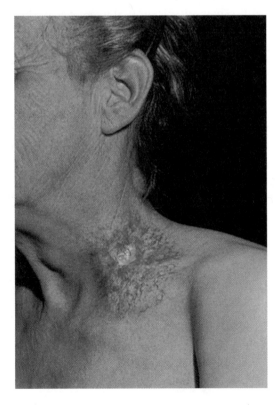

Figure 11.2. Radiation burn.

No matter what kind of cancer or cancer treatments a person is going through, it is vital for his or her massage therapist to keep in communication with the rest of the client's health care team to provide the best benefits that bodywork has to offer with minimum risks.

Cysts

Cysts in Brief

What are they?
Cysts are layers of connective tissue that surround and isolate something that should not be in the body (e.g., a piece of shrapnel or a localized infection).

How are they recognized?
Palpable cysts are generally small, painless, distinct masses that move slightly under the skin.

Is massage indicated or contraindicated?
Cysts locally contraindicate massage.

Definition: What Are They?

When something that does not really belong gets inside or grows inside the body, a remarkable reaction occurs. Like an oyster covering a grain of sand with layers of pearl, humans cover their "grains of sand" with layers of connective tissue, making an easily discernible and isolated cyst. The notable exception to this habit is *cancer* (this chapter).

Etiology: What Happens?

A wide variety of cysts may develop in the body. *Baker's cysts* (Chapter 3) are outpouchings of the synovial joint in the popliteal fossa. *Ganglion cysts* (Chapter 3) are pouches formed by tendinous sheaths. *Ovarian cysts* (Chapter 10) are usually harmless self-limiting growths on the ovaries at the site of egg release. Layers of connective tissue also form around any foreign material that gets into the body. Unremoved shrapnel is encysted, for example, as are localized infections of *tuberculosis* (Chapter 6).

The most common kinds of cysts that massage therapists encounter are sebaceous cysts and lipomas, which are the focus of the rest of this discussion. Sebaceous cysts are a bit like a pimple gone bad (see *acne*, Chapter 1). A sebaceous gland fills up with sebum and waste, but instead of draining or being consumed by macrophages, the debris from this localized infection is walled off and "removed" from the body by a tough layer of dense connective tissue. There it generally stays until it is surgically removed or the body eventually (and this can take months or years) gets around to reabsorbing it.

Lipomas are benign fatty tumors surrounded by a connective tissue capsule. They are common in the skin but may occur in virtually any tissue in the body, including the intestines, the liver, and the reproductive tract.

Signs and Symptoms

Sebaceous cysts are small, usually painless bumps under the skin that may move slightly, depending on the mobility of the fascia. They are most common on the scalp, neck, or shoulders (sites of acne infections).

Lipomas in the skin are similar in presentation, but they are not preceded by acne or any other infection. They may be present at birth, or develop during childhood or adulthood. Some lipomas are very small and easy to palpate through the skin; others may be quite large.

Complications

Staphylococcus bacteria can sometimes attack sebaceous cysts, resulting in an acute infection. Other cysts are generally not vulnerable to infection but may be situated in a place to become snagged or irritated by normal day-to-day activities.

The main complications associated with lipomas occur when they block important passageways in the gastrointestinal (GI) tract, respiratory tract, or reproductive tract.

Treatment

Most cysts require no treatment unless they are in a place that causes pain or they are removed for cosmetic reasons. If the connective tissue wrapping has isolated the cyst adequately, it can generally be removed with simple surgery. Infected sebaceous cysts are treated with systemic antibiotics.

Massage?

Cysts locally contraindicate massage. In the extremely unlikely event that a massage therapist could pop one, its contents could cause a dangerous immune reaction. It is more likely, however, that massage would simply irritate the surrounding tissues and cause soreness. If a client has a questionable or new cyst that has not been diagnosed, the therapist should recommend that the client have it diagnosed before the next appointment. Most painless bumps under the skin are not dangerous, but diagnosis is not within the scope of practice of massage therapy.

Fatigue

Definition: What Is It?

Here is a condition with which most people are familiar. Fatigue is a state in which the body does not function at its best levels because of lack of recovery time. For the purposes of simplicity, the world of fatigue will be divided here into two types: *mental/emotional* fatigue and *physical* fatigue brought about by overexertion.

Etiology: What Happens?

The two varieties of fatigue are usually inextricably blended with each other. For example, living in chronic stress (mental/emotional fatigue) can throw the neck and jaw muscles into chronic contraction, leading to physical fatigue. This person always feels more tired than if those muscles were able to release their unnecessary tension. The feeling of always being tired is a self-fulfilling prophecy; the perception that a person is tired causes him to move less efficiently, which exacerbates that loss of energy.

> ### Fatigue in Brief
>
> **What is it?**
> Fatigue is a state of having less than optimal energy as a result of inadequate rest and recovery time. Fatigue can be brought about by mental or physical exertion or by any combination of both.
>
> **How is it recognized?**
> A person living with mental or physical fatigue feels tired, moves inefficiently, and may be more prone to injury.
>
> **Is massage indicated or contraindicated?**
> In the absence of other conditions, fatigue indicates massage.

Complications

Fatigue is often related to *sleep disorders* (Chapter 3), which can create long-lasting problems in the body. Fatigue can cause a person to move inefficiently or clumsily, thus increasing the chance of accident or injury. Fatigue that is not relieved with a reasonable amount of rest and recovery time may be a warning sign of some other conditions. *Chronic fatigue syndrome* (Chapter 5) is a possibility, as are *anemia* (Chapter 4) and *hypothyroidism* (Chapter 8).

Massage?

As long as more serious pathologic conditions are ruled out, physical and emotional fatigue both indicate massage. After a good session, a client can get off the table and feel like he or she has just been infused with several hours' worth of sleep. That is the extra measure of energy available when it is not being wasted on counterproductive muscular contractions. Massage can also provide an hour-long vacation from the stress that was stimulating the hypertonicity and inefficient muscle use.

For fatigue brought on by mental or emotional stress, massage can reestablish the lost balance between sympathetic and parasympathetic reactions. Massage sessions provide a rare opportunity for a client to listen and pay attention to what is happening in his or her body, which provides tools for coping with similar problems in the future.

For physical fatigue from exhaustion or overexertion, massage works on a mechanical level by reducing hypertonicity, flushing out waste products, improving local circulation, and speeding recovery time.

Ultimately, ongoing fatigue is a reflection of the continuous circle between emotions that are expressed in bodies through muscular tension and muscular tension that interferes with rest and recovery and thus causes emotional upset. For massage therapists, it is a chicken-or-the-egg proposition, and frankly, it does not matter which came first. The bodyworker's job is to address whatever symptoms are present and to be sensitive to the more subtle signals about underlying tensions that may exacerbate those symptoms.

Multiple Chemical Sensitivity Syndrome

Multiple Chemical Sensitivity Syndrome in Brief

What is it?
Multiple chemical sensitivity syndrome (MCSS) is a situation in which a history of toxic exposure initiates a variety of different responses.

How is it recognized?
MCSS can involve headaches, disorientation, cognitive difficulties, joint pain, respiratory problems, and other symptoms.

Is massage indicated or contraindicated?
People with MCSS need to be careful about massage lubricants, essential oils, perfumes, candles, and other equipment that therapists often use that may trigger a reaction.

Definition: What Is It?

Multiple chemical sensitivity syndrome (MCSS) is also called "idiopathic environmental intolerance." It is a condition in which a history of exposure to a trigger (usually an environmental toxin) results in a variety of possible reactions that become progressively more severe with repeated exposures.

Demographics: Who Gets It?

Multiple chemical sensitivity syndrome develops most often in people who undergo prolonged exposure to toxic substances. The exposure may be sudden and extreme, as with a chemical spill, or ongoing in smaller amounts, as with a poorly ventilated building. Gulf War veterans are diagnosed with MCSS approximately 3 times more often than the general population.

Etiology: What Happens?

MCSS has been described since the 1940s, but its definition continues to evolve. The currently accepted description of MCS is a set of objectively observable signs and symptoms that are acquired after documentable exposure to a triggering substance; symptoms affect multiple body systems; the severity of symptoms occurs in relation to measurable (but not usually toxic) levels of chemical triggers; chemically unrelated substances can trigger symptoms; symptoms leave no objective evidence of permanent organ damage.

A few of the most common triggers for MCS include cigar and cigarette smoke; colognes, perfumes, and deodorants; diesel and gasoline exhaust; household and laundry detergents and cleaners; varnish, shellac, and lacquer; and tar fumes from roof or roadwork.

Researchers disagree as to whether MCSS is an allergic reaction, a neurobiologic problem, or a cumulative toxicity problem. Significant overlap of MCSS with *fibromyalgia* (Chapter 2) and *chronic fatigue syndrome* (Chapter 5) further clouds the issue.

Signs and Symptoms

Multiple chemical sensitivity symptoms vary widely but include chronic headaches, joint pain, cognitive difficulties, weakness, dizziness, and heat intolerance. Exposure to one trigger may permanently exacerbate symptoms for future exposures, even to different chemical triggers.

Diagnosis

Diagnosis of MCSS is controversial because not all specialists recognize the same criteria. Some consistent signs that are highly indicative of MCSS are an elevated number of mast cells, deficiencies in some blood enzymes, and markers of poisoning by pesticides or heavy metals as observed in tests of hair, stool, urine, blood, or fat. No single test is conclusive for MCSS, however, so diagnoses are often based on clinical observations in combination with ruling out other possible disorders such as fibromyalgia, chronic fatigue syndrome, *candidiasis* (Chapter 7), and others.

Treatment

MCSS is somewhat problematic to treat, because many patients are hypersensitive to drugs. Furthermore, because patients often cannot work, they may have limited access to health care. Mainstream and complementary practitioners may recommend gentle detoxification programs combined with avoidance of known triggers. This is a challenge for persons sensitive to plastics (including the plastic bottles that hold filtered water), pesticides, hormones, and fertilizers found in most foods, synthetic fabrics, the chemicals used to treat building materials, any kind of air pollution, and possibly the heavy metal amalgams that may be part of their own dental work.

Acupuncture, dietary adjustments, and careful exercise regimens may be recommended to help restore lost balance and resilience in overtaxed systems. Ultimately the most realistic goal of a person with MCSS may be to *manage* his or her disease, rather than to "get over it."

Massage?

A person with MCSS may receive massage if the facility in which it is performed is a safe and comfortable place to be. Detergents or bleach used to launder massage linens may be a trigger, as may be any candles, scents, incense, or the perfume worn by the client who just left. Any lubricant needs to be evaluated carefully not only for allergenic ingredients, but for the risk of contamination from pesticides or the plastic bottles in which it may be stored. If these hurdles can be overcome, or if the client with MCSS can tolerate whatever levels are present in a massage room, bodywork may be a supportive, strengthening, and preciously rare time for a person to feel that his or her body is a good place in which to live.

Postoperative Situations

Definition: What Are They?

Until recently, most surgeries involved systemic anesthesia, large incisions, and major trauma to the body. These were followed by prolonged hospital stays and a wide variety of possible complications ranging from infection, to blood clots, to the discovery that a sponge or clamp had been left inside the body.

<table>
</table>

Postoperative Situations in Brief

What are they?
Postoperative situations are conditions in which clients are recovering from any kind of surgery.

How are they recognized?
Surgeries may be major and invasive, or they may be conducted through tiny holes in the abdomen or through long tubes inserted into blood vessels to get to a destination far away.

Is massage indicated or contraindicated?
Massage can be appropriate for persons recovering from surgery, depending on the reason for the surgery and the danger of possible complications.

Today the world of surgery has changed with lasers, balloons, and procedures that are conducted with microscopic cameras and tools through tiny incisions in the skin. Many surgeries that used to involve general anesthesia and hospital stays are now being performed on an outpatient basis.

Massage?

The rapid development of new less invasive surgical techniques is good news for massage therapists, because the risks involved with major surgery are very serious and frequently make doing many kinds of bodywork impractical. Obviously, the appropriateness of massage for someone recovering from any kind of surgery depends on the scope and predisposing cause of the surgery and how much of the body has been affected.

Massage is finding increasing usage in hospital settings, because it is consistently found to compare favorably with other types of pain-relieving interventions.[5] When massage was compared with other modalities (vibrations from a special machine and usual hospital postsurgical care) after laparoscopic surgery, patients reported significantly favorable results from Swedish massage.[6]

The two major cautions for massage with clients recovering from open surgery are immunosuppressant drugs and blood clots (see *thrombophlebitis/deep vein thrombosis*, Chapter 4). Immunosuppressant drugs are usually used with a client recovering from an organ transplant or cancer surgery. A client taking these medications is at risk for infection from anyone else's pathogens.

Blood clots are a lurking threat for anyone who has just been through major surgery, especially surgery involving the leg, hip, or pelvis. A safe plan is to avoid circulatory types of bodywork until the threat of clotting has passed. The therapist should consult with the client's health care team to identify when that might be (6 weeks is a commonly suggested waiting period). Reflexive and energetic workup until then will not only be safe and appropriate, but very welcomed as well.

In the absence of contraindications, carefully applied frictions around the edges of a new scar can have positive influence on the localized healing process. It is important not to stretch the skin beyond tolerance or to work near an open wound. Therapists also can teach their clients how to mobilize their own scar tissue to minimize hypertrophy and adhesions.

CHAPTER REVIEW QUESTIONS

1. Briefly describe the staging process for cancer. What are the labels and what do they mean?
2. What are the possible risks of massaging a client who is living with cancer?

[5] Survey Shows Many Hospitals Using Massage Therapy: Used Mostly for Stress Relief and Pain Management. Copyright 2003 American Massage Therapy Association. Available at: http://www. amtamassage.org/news/AHA%20survey%20statement.pdf. Accessed winter 2004.
[6] Massage for Postoperative Pain and Distress. Copyright © American Massage Therapy Association Foundation. Available at: http://www.amtafoundation.org/or_article_massagemag105C.html. Accessed winter 2004.

3. What are the possible benefits of massaging a client who is living with cancer?

4. Name three external factors that may contribute to the risk of developing cancer.

5. Describe the circular relationship between mental/emotional fatigue and physical fatigue.

6. How have recent innovations in surgical techniques changed the way massage applies to postoperative patients?

7. Name two important risks to bear in mind for patients recovering from open surgery.

8. Your client has multiple chemical sensitivity syndrome. Name two accommodations that you may have to make for her.

9. A client has a small (5 cm) undiagnosed lump on her upper back. It is dense but not painful, and moves slightly on palpation. What is it most likely to be, and what should a responsible massage therapist do about it?

 Answers to these questions can be found on the Student Recource CD-ROM that accompanies this book.

Bibliography

General Resources

Cancer, General

1. Walton T. Clinical thinking and cancer. Massage Ther J 2000;39(3):66.
2. Curties D. Could massage therapy promote cancer metastasis? Massage Ther J 2000; 39(3):83.
3. Malloy J. Do the benefits of massage outweigh the risks? Massage Ther J 2001; 39(4):60.
4. MacDonald G. How cancer spreads. Massage Ther J 2001;39(4):74.
5. Curties D. Cancer therapies. Massage Ther J 2001;39(4):80.
6. Chapman C. Lymphedema 101: What every therapist should know. Massage Ther J 2001;39(4):86.
7. Comprehensive Cancer Control. Centers for Disease Control and Prevention. Available at: http://www.cdc.gov/cancer/ncccp/about.htm. Accessed winter 2004.
8. Massage Benefits Hospitalized Cancer Patients. Articles from Massage Magazine. Available at: http://www.amtafoundation.org/or_article_massagemag105B.html. Accessed winter 2004.
9. Can Cancer Be Prevented? Copyright © 2004 American Cancer Society, Inc. Available at: http://www.cancer.org/docroot/CRI/content/CRI_2_4_2x_Can_cancer_be_prevented.asp?sitearea=CRI. Accessed winter 2004.
10. What Is Cancer? Copyright © 2004 American Cancer Society, Inc. Available at: http://www.cancer.org/docroot/CRI/content/CRI_2_4_1x_What_Is_Cancer_72.asp?sitearea=CRI. Accessed winter 2004.
11. Zoorob R, Anderson R, Cefalu C, et al. Cancer Screening Guidelines. Copyright © 2001 by the American Academy of Family

Physicians. Available at: http://www.aafp.org/afp/20010315/1101.html. Accessed winter 2004.
12. Gates TJ. Screening for Cancer: Evaluating the Evidence. Copyright © 2001 by the American Academy of Family Physicians. Available at: http://www.aafp.org/afp/20010201/513.html. Accessed winter 2004.
13. Cancer Screening Guidelines. Copyright © 2003 The Siteman Cancer Center at Barnes-Jewish Hospital and Washington University School of Medicine. Available at: http://www.siteman.wustl.edu/patient/other_specialized/detect_guidelines.shtml. Accessed winter 2004.
14. Cancer Facts & Figures 2004. Copyright © 2004, American Cancer Society, Inc. Available at: http://www.cancer.org/downloads/STT/CAFF2004PWSecured.pdf. Accessed winter 2004.
15. Complementary and Alternative Therapy. Copyright © 2004 American Cancer Society, Inc. Available at: http://www.cancer.org/docroot/CRI/content/CRI_2_4_4X_Complementary_and_Alternative_Therapy.asp?rnav=cri. Accessed winter 2004.
16. Signs and Symptoms of Cancer. Copyright © 2004 American Cancer Society, Inc. Available at: http://www.cancer.org/docroot/CRI/content/CRI_2_4_3X_What_are_the_signs_and_symptoms_of_cancer.asp?rnav=cri. Accessed winter 2004.
17. Wood BJ, Winkler MT. The ABCs of Complementary and Alternative Therapies and Cancer Treatment. Copyright © 2001 Association of Community Cancer Centers. Available at: http://www.medscape.com/viewarticle/421548_print. Accessed winter 2004.
18. What Are the Risk Factors for Cancer? Copyright © 2004 American Cancer Society, Inc. Available at: http://www.

cancer.org/docroot/CRI/content/CRI_2_4_2x_What_are_the_risk_factors_for_cancer_72.asp?sitearea=CRI. Accessed winter 2004.
19. What Is Staging? Copyright © 2004 American Cancer Society, Inc. Available at: http://www.cancer.org/docroot/CRI/content/CRI_2_4_3X_What_is_staging.asp?rnav=cri. Accessed winter 2004.
20. Who Gets Cancer? Copyright © 2004 American Cancer Society, Inc. Available at: http://www.cancer.org/docroot/CRI/content/CRI_2_4_1x_Who_gets_cancer.asp?sitearea=CRI. Accessed winter 2004.
21. What Is Cancer? National Cancer Institute (NCI). Available at: http://www.cancer.gov/cancerinfo/wyntk/overview. Accessed winter 2004.
22. Human Papilloma Virus (HPV). Copyright © 2004 American Cancer Society, Inc. Available at: http://www.cancer.org/docroot/cri/content/cri_2_6x_human_papilloma_virus_hpv.asp?sitearea=cri. Accessed spring 2004.

Lymphedema

1. Breast Reconstruction. Copyright © 2000, American Massage Therapy Association. Available at: http://www.amtamassage.org/journal/fa_00_journal/mastectomy_3.html. Accessed winter 2004.
2. Massage Techniques for Mastectomy. Copyright © 2000, American Massage Therapy Association. Available at: http://www.amtamassage.org/journal/fa_00_journal/mastectomy_4.html. Accessed winter 2004.
3. Lymphedema. National Cancer Institute. Available at: http://www.cancer.gov/templates/page_print.aspx?viewid=41bbe94a-4a76-45ed-98c1-12c08b2fc906&version=patient. Accessed winter 2004.

4. Revis DR. Lymphedema. Copyright © 2003, eMedicine.com, Inc. Available at: http://www.emedicine.com/med/topic2722.htm. Accessed winter 2004.
5. Lymphedema. Harvard Medical School. Available at: http://www.intelihealth.com/IH/ihtPrint/WSIHW000/9339/23829.html?hide=t&k=basePrint. Accessed winter 2004.
6. Massage Away Lymphedema. Available at: http://abclocal.go.com/kfsn/health/healthwatch/print_health_080603_massage.html. Accessed winter 2004.
7. Lymphedema. Available at: http://www.merck.com/mrkshared/mmanual_home2/sec03/ch037/ch037b.jsp. Accessed winter 2004.

Cysts

1. Cysts. Copyright © 1997–2003 New Zealand Dermatological Society. Available at: http://www.dermnetnz.org/. Accessed winter 2004.
2. Radebold K. Lipomas. Copyright © 2003, eMedicine.com, Inc. Available at: http://www.emedicine.com/med/topic2720.htm. Accessed winter 2004.

3. Dermoid cysts. Copyright © 2003 New Zealand Dermatological Society. Available at: http://www.dermnetnz.org/. Accessed winter 2004.

Multiple Chemical Syndrome

1. Abnormal Medical Tests and Physical Signs Associated with Multiple Chemical Sensitivity. Copyright © 2000, MCS Referral & Resources. Available at: *http://www.mcsrr.org/resources/biomarkers.html*. Accessed winter 2004.
2. Multiple Chemical Sensitivities Syndrome (MCSS). National Institute of Environmental Health Sciences, National Institutes of Health. Available at: http://www.niehs.nih.gov/external/faq/mcss.htm. Accessed winter 2004.
3. Magill MK, Suruda A. Multiple Chemical Sensitivity Syndrome. Copyright © 1998 by the American Academy of Family Physicians. Available at: http://aafp.org/afp/980901ap/magill.html. Accessed winter 2004.
4. Multiple Chemical Sensitivity: A 1999 Consensus. Available at: http://heldref.org/html/Consensus.html. Accessed winter 2004.

5. Ross GH. Treatment Options in Multiple Chemical Sensitivity. Available at: http://www.aehf.com/articles/treatment_options_mcs.html. Accessed winter 2004.

Postoperative Situations

1. Survey Shows Many Hospitals Using Massage Therapy: Used Mostly for Stress Relief and Pain Management. Copyright © 2003 American Massage Therapy Association. Available at: http://www.amtamassage.org/news/AHA%20survey%20statement.pdf. Accessed winter 2004.
2. Massage for Postoperative Pain and Distress. Copyright © American Massage Therapy Association Foundation. Available at: http://www.amtafoundation.org/or_article_massagemag105C.html. Accessed winter 2004.
3. Canaday BR, Mays TA. Avoiding Misconceptions in Pain Management. Copyright © 1994–2003 by Medscape. Available at: http://www.medscape.com/viewprogram/560_pnt. Accessed winter 2004.

APPENDIX I

QUICK REFERENCE CHARTS

Read This First!

This appendix provides a reference for massage students and practitioners who need fast answers to simple questions. It is not intended as a substitute for reading the complete article for each condition and will not provide enough information to make a highly informed decision without that background.

Several things are important to remember while using these quick reference charts

- The label "indicated" does not mean that a condition will always be improved by massage. It means that massage will not make the situation worse, and the support comfort massage gives can certainly be beneficial to the client, if not to the particular condition.

- The term "massage" refers to circulatory-based massage that has a direct effect on blood and lymph flow. If a condition is labeled "contraindicated," it is usually because the influence of massage on circulation would have a negative impact on the client. This does not necessarily rule out touch altogether, however, and many conditions that contraindicate vigorous circulatory massage are perfectly appropriate for less mechanically based bodywork modalities.

- When massage is considered appropriate or indicated, it is a systemic recommendation. When massage is contraindicated, guidelines for whether those cautions are local or systemic have been provided.

- The specific kind of impact that massage may have on various conditions is discussed in the complete articles rather than here in the abbreviated version.

  The most important thing to remember is that it is impossible to make a foolproof judgment about whether massage is a good choice strictly from a book. Every client is different; every practitioner has a unique approach. These recommendations are just that: recommendations that may help to sort out the variables that contribute to the decision-making process.

Abortion, Spontaneous and Elective in Brief (p. 532)

What are they? Spontaneous and elective abortions are pregnancies that are ended, unintentionally or intentionally, before the fetus is born naturally.

How are they recognized? Generalized or pelvic pain may be present, along with vaginal bleeding. Often, however, no outward signs may show that a woman is recovering from a spontaneous or elective abortion.

Is massage indicated or contraindicated? Massage is locally contraindicated (no deep abdominal work) for women recovering from a recent spontaneous or elective abortion until her bleeding has stopped and she is free of any signs of infection. Bodywork elsewhere can be supportive and helpful.

Acne Rosacea in Brief (p. 24)

What is it? Acne rosacea is a chronic condition involving inflammation and damage to the skin of the face.

How is it recognized? Acne rosacea occurs in stages of severity, starting with occasional flushing and continuing through general inflammation of the face and eyes, the formation of papules and pustules, and finally to permanent thickening and distortion of facial skin, especially around the nose.

Is massage indicated or contraindicated? Acne rosacea has no contraindications for massage, although some clients may be sensitive to some lubricants.

Acne Vulgaris in Brief (p. 25)

What is it? Acne is a bacterial infection of sebaceous glands usually found on the face, neck, and upper back. It is closely associated with adolescence or liver dysfunction that results in excess testosterone in the system.

How is it recognized? It looks like raised, inflamed pustules on the skin, sometimes with white or black tips.

Is massage indicated or contraindicated? Acne locally contraindicates massage because of the risk of spreading infection, causing pain, and exacerbating the symptoms with the application of an oily lubricant.

Acromegaly in Brief (p. 490)

What is it? Acromegaly is a condition involving the excessive secretion of growth hormone, often related to a benign tumor on the pituitary gland.

How is it recognized? This disorder usually appears in the patient's 20s or 30s; patients find that their hands, feet, and face have gradually grown and become distorted. Joint pain with bony deformation is common. Debilitating headaches, visual problems, or cranial nerve damage may occur if the tumor presses on sensitive tissue in the central nervous system (CNS). Ultimately, cardiovascular weakness develops as the heart tries to pump blood to new tissues.

Is massage indicated or contraindicated? The primary risk for most acromegaly patients is that their cardiovascular system cannot keep up with the demands of their suddenly growing bodies. High blood pressure, enlargement of the heart, and heart failure are common complications of this disorder. As long as those concerns are respected and the therapist does not challenge the circulatory system of the client too vigorously, massage may be appropriate for acromegaly patients, who often also experience joint pain. Massage therapists should work with these clients as part of a well-informed health care team.

Acute Bronchitis in Brief (p. 383)

What is it? Acute bronchitis is an infection and inflammation of the bronchial tree anywhere between the trachea and the bronchioles. If inflammation extends into the bronchioles and alveoli, it is called bronchopneumonia.

How is it recognized? The hallmark of acute bronchitis is a persistent productive cough along with sore throat, nasal congestion, fatigue, and fever. Whereas other symptoms generally subside within 10 days, the cough may last for several weeks while the bronchi heal.

Is massage indicated or contraindicated? Acute bronchitis, like all acute infections, contraindicates circulatory massage. If the infection has passed and the cough is the only lingering symptom, massage may be appropriate as long as the client is comfortable on the table.

Allergic Reactions in Brief (p. 357)

What are they? Allergic reactions are immune system mistakes in which an inflammatory immune system response becomes potentially dangerous as it overreacts or reacts inappropriately to a variety of triggers.

How are they recognized? The most dangerous acute sign of an allergic reaction is swelling around the face and throat that may obstruct airflow. This may be accompanied by decreased blood pressure and bronchospasm. Other signs can include hives and other rashes, gastrointestinal discomfort with food allergies, and, in the case of multiple chemical sensitivity, headache, disorientation, cognitive difficulties, joint pain, and other symptoms.

Is massage indicated or contraindicated? Most hypersensitivity reactions contraindicate massage in the acute stage because blood flow to areas that are already congested is counterproductive. Between episodes, persons with allergies need to be careful about massage lubricants, essential oils, perfumes, candles, and other equipment that therapists often use, but that may trigger a reaction.

Alzheimer's Disease in Brief (p. 187)

What is it? Alzheimer's disease is a degenerative disorder of the brain involving shrinkage and death of neural tissue.

How is it recognized? Alzheimer's disease is difficult to definitively diagnose in a living person, but signs and symptoms include progressive memory loss, deterioration of language and cognitive skills, disorientation, and lack of ability to care for oneself.

Is massage indicated or contraindicated? If an Alzheimer's disease patient feels comfortable and nurtured while receiving touch, then massage is very much indicated. But if the patient feels disoriented and threatened, the therapist will have to change tactics. Alzheimer's patients may not be able to communicate verbally, so therapists must be sensitive to nonverbal cues.

Amyotrophic Lateral Sclerosis in Brief (p. 191)

What is it? Amyotrophic lateral sclerosis (ALS) is a progressive disease that begins in the central nervous system. It involves the degeneration of motor neurons and the subsequent atrophy of voluntary muscles.

How is it recognized? Symptoms of ALS include weakness, fatigue, and muscle spasms. It appears most frequently in patients between 40 and 70 years of age.

Is massage indicated or contraindicated? ALS indicates massage, with caution, when a massage therapist works as part of a health care team.

Anemia in Brief (p. 287)

What is it? Anemia is a symptom rather than a disease in itself. It indicates a shortage of red blood cells, or of hemoglobin, or of both.

How is it recognized? Symptoms of anemia include pallor, shortness of breath, fatigue, and poor resistance to cold. Other symptoms may accompany specific varieties of anemia.

Is massage indicated or contraindicated? Anemia that is idiopathic or attributable to nutritional deficiency may indicate massage, as long as no neurologic damage has occurred. Anemia related to bone marrow suppression (i.e., cancer), chronic disease or inflammation, or premature destruction of red blood cells may contraindicate rigorous bodywork, although some types of energy work may be appropriate.

Aneurysm in Brief (p. 308)

What is it? An aneurysm is a bulge or outpouching in a vein, artery, or the heart. They usually occur in the thoracic or abdominal aorta or in the arteries at the base of the brain.

How is it recognized? Symptoms of aneurysms are determined by their location. Thoracic aneurysms may cause chronic hoarseness; abdominal aneurysms may cause local discomfort, reduced urine output, or severe backache. Cerebral aneurysms may be silent, or they may cause extreme headache when they are at very high risk for rupture.

Is massage indicated or contraindicated? If a client has been diagnosed with an aneurysm, circulatory massage is contraindicated. Massage is also strongly cautioned for clients who fit the profile for aneurysms but who have not been diagnosed.

Ankylosing Spondylitis in Brief (p. 97)

What is it? Ankylosing spondylitis (AS) is a progressive inflammatory arthritis of the spine.

How is it recognized? It generally begins as stiffness and pain around the sacrum, with occasional referred pain down the back of the buttocks and into the legs. It has acute and subacute episodes. In advanced AS, the vertebrae fuse together in a flexed position.

Is massage indicated or contraindicated? Massage is indicated in the subacute stages of AS, where, along with exercise and physical therapy, it may be useful in maintaining flexibility.

Anxiety Disorders in Brief (p. 216)

What are they? Anxiety disorders are a group of mental disorders that have to do with exaggerated, irrational fears and the attempts to control those fears. Some anxiety disorders come and go, some are chronic progressive problems, and others reach a peak and then sometimes recede or remain stable. All anxiety disorders begin as emotional responses that create inappropriate sympathetic reactions.

How are they recognized? Although triggers for individual cases may vary, many anxiety disorders involve sympathetic reactions in the body, including fast heart rate, sweating, dizziness, faintness, nausea, and other symptoms. In addition, some disorders bring about feelings of impending death, a sense of physical detachment, unwelcome or frightening thoughts, and other reactions.

Is massage indicated or contraindicated? If the stimulus of bodywork is perceived as something safe and welcome, then massage can have a useful place in dealing with a variety of anxiety disorders.

Appendicitis in Brief (p. 444)

What is it? Appendicitis is inflammation of the vermiform appendix. It is usually a result of infection following a blockage at the opening of the appendix. The blockage may be caused by a hardened piece of fecal matter or by lymphatic inflammation.

How is it recognized? The symptoms of appendicitis are widely variable, but they include general abdominal pain that gradually settles in the lower right quadrant. Rebound pain is usually severe. Fever, nausea, vomiting, food aversion, constipation, and diarrhea may be present.

Is massage indicated or contraindicated? Acute appendicitis contraindicates massage. This condition may complicate into peritonitis if it is neglected.

Asthma in Brief (p. 400)

What is it? Asthma is the result of spasmodic constriction of bronchial smooth muscle tubes in combination with chronic local inflammation and excessive mucus production.

How is it recognized? Asthma attacks are sporadic episodes involving coughing, wheezing, and difficulty with breathing, especially exhaling.

Is massage indicated or contraindicated? Massage is indicated for anyone with asthma who is not in the throes of an attack. Between episodes, massage can be useful to reduce stress and to deal with some of the muscular problems that accompany difficulty with breathing.

Atherosclerosis in Brief (p. 311)

What is it? Atherosclerosis is a condition in which the arteries become inelastic and brittle because of atherosclerotic plaques.

How is it recognized? Atherosclerosis has no symptoms until it is very advanced. However, it is connected to several other types of circulatory problems, including hypertension, arrhythmia, coronary artery disease, cerebrovascular disease, and peripheral vascular disease.

Is massage indicated or contraindicated? Advanced atherosclerosis systemically contraindicates rigorous circulatory massage, but other modalities may offer many benefits with a minimum of risks.

Attention Deficit Hyperactivity Disorder in Brief (p. 214)

What is it? Attention deficit hyperactivity disorder (ADHD) is a neurobiochemical imbalance in the brain, resulting in problems with focus, impulse control, and motor activity. It occurs among children and adults.

How is it recognized? ADHD is recognized by the behavior changes it brings about: inattention, inappropriate impulsivity, and, when hyperactivity is present, difficulty with controlling movement. The diagnostic criteria for ADHD depend on the observations of people close to the patient, along with ruling out other possible sources for the problems.

Is massage indicated or contraindicated? ADHD indicates massage, although the preference for the type of bodywork and the length of time it can be administered may vary greatly from one client to another.

Avascular Osteonecrosis in Brief (p. 86)

What is it? Avascular osteonecrosis (AVN) is a situation in which blood supply to an area of bone is interrupted and the bone tissue consequently dies. It occurs most frequently at the head of the femur.

How is it recognized? AVN may be silent in early stages. Later stages show pain at the affected area, along with signs of arthritis and the risk of total joint collapse if the damage is near an articulation.

Is massage indicated or contraindicated? AVN can be brought about by several underlying disorders. Decisions about the appropriateness of massage must be made according to contributing factors. Generally speaking, massage may exacerbate pain and damage local to the affected area but may be appropriate elsewhere.

Baker Cysts in Brief (p. 130)

What are they? Baker cysts are fluid-filled extensions of the synovial membrane at the knee. They protrude into the popliteal fossa, usually on the medial side.

How are they recognized? Baker cysts are usually painless sacs that are palpable deep to the superficial fascia in the popliteal fossa. They may cause pain or a feeling of tightness in the knee in flexion.

Is massage indicated or contraindicated? Massage is locally contraindicated in the popliteal fossa, especially if a Baker cyst is present. In addition, if any signs of distal circulatory disruption (coldness, clamminess, edema) distal are visible distal to the cyst, that whole area is a contraindication, and the client needs to be cleared of the possibility of thrombosis.

Bell's Palsy in Brief (p. 236)

What is it? Bell's palsy is a flaccid paralysis of one side of the face caused by inflammation or damage to cranial nerve VII, the facial nerve.

How is it recognized? Symptoms of Bell's palsy include drooping of the muscles on the affected side, difficulty with drinking and eating, and difficulty in closing the eye on one side. Pain, headaches, hypersensitivity to sound, and drooling also may occur.

Is massage indicated or contraindicated? Bell's palsy indicates massage to maintain flexibility and good circulation in the affected muscles. It is important, however, to rule out causes for the nerve damage that may contraindicate massage.

Benign Prostatic Hyperplasia in Brief (p. 558)

What is it? Benign prostatic hyperplasia (BPH) is a condition in which the prostate gland of a mature man begins to grow for the first time since the end of puberty. It is not related to cancer, which is why this condition is called "benign."

How is it recognized? The primary symptoms of BPH have to do with mechanical obstruction of the urethra. This leads to problems with urination, including a feeling of frequency, difficulties with initiating flow, leaking, and the sensation that the bladder is never emptied. Many men with BPH never develop these symptoms, however. For them, BPH is a silent condition.

Is massage indicated or contraindicated? BPH is a common condition among mature men, and it does not usually involve cancer or infection. Massage is perfectly appropriate for these clients, as long as no signs of urinary tract infection or kidney disorders are present.

Bladder Cancer in Brief (p. 520)

What is it? Bladder cancer is the growth of malignant cells in the urinary bladder. Most bladder cancer starts in the superficial layer of transitional epithelium.

How is it recognized? The earliest sign of bladder cancer is the appearance of blood in the urine, which may be red or rust colored. Bladder cancer is painless at this point. In later stages, the bladder may become irritable. Painful urination, reduced urination, or increased urinary frequency all may occur.

Is massage indicated or contraindicated? As with most varieties of cancer, massage with its parasympathetic effects and immune system support has a place in the recovery process. Bladder cancer has a high recurrence rate, and most patients undergo surgery at some point. As long as these issues are respected and the massage therapist works as part of a well-informed health care team, bodywork may be appropriate for these patients.

Boils in Brief (p. 4)

What are they? Boils are localized bacterial infections of the skin. The causative agent is usually *Staphylococcus aureus.*

How are they recognized? Boils involve painful, red, hot pustules on the skin. They may occur singly or in interconnected clusters called carbuncles.

Is massage indicated or contraindicated? Boils contraindicate massage at least locally, and care should be taken to make sure the infection is not systemic (screen the client for other symptoms such as swelling, fever, or discomfort other than at the site of the lesion). The bacteria that cause boils are extremely virulent and communicable. The sheets of a client with boils should be isolated and treated with bleach.

Breast Cancer in Brief (p. 544)

What is it? Breast cancer is the growth of malignant tumor cells in breast tissue; these cells can invade skin and nearby muscles and bones. If they invade lymph nodes, they can metastasize to the rest of the body.

How is it recognized? The first sign of breast cancer is a small painless lump or thickening in the breast tissue or near the axilla. The lump may be too small to palpate, but it may show on a mammogram. Later the skin may change texture, the nipple may change shape, and discharge from the nipple may be present.

Is massage indicated or contraindicated? Breast cancer patients undergo treatment options that are extremely taxing on general health and physical and emotional well-being. As long as bodywork choices are made that respect these challenges, massage can be a wonderful, supportive, important coping mechanism for many breast cancer patients.

Bronchiectasis in Brief (p. 404)

What is it? Bronchiectasis is a condition in which the bronchial tubes become structurally damaged, leading to permanent dilation and excessive production of mucus.

How is it recognized? This condition usually follows congenital diseases or repeated severe lung infections. Its symptoms include chest pain, shortness of breath, productive coughing, and possible clubbing of the fingers.

Is massage indicated or contraindicated? Bronchiectasis contraindicates massage if acute infection is present, but otherwise massage (with percussion on the chest) may be appropriate if the client is comfortable and if the therapist works as part of a well-informed health care team.

Bunions in Brief (p. 132)

What are they? A bunion is a protrusion at the metatarsal–phalangeal joint of the great toe that occurs when the toe is laterally deviated.

How are they recognized? Bunions are recognizable by the large bump on the medial aspect of the foot. If they are inflamed, they will be red, hot, and possibly edematous.

Is massage indicated or contraindicated? Massage is locally contraindicated at the point of a bunion regardless, and especially when or if it is inflamed. Massage elsewhere on the foot or body is very much indicated within pain tolerance to help with compensation patterns that occur when it is difficult to walk.

Burns in Brief (p. 47)

What are they? Burns are caused by damage to the skin that causes the cells to die. They can be caused by fire, overexposure to the sun, dry heat, wet heat, electricity, radiation, extreme cold, and toxic chemicals.

How are they recognized? First-degree burns involve mild inflammation. Second-degree burns also involve blistering and damage at the deeper levels of the epidermis. Third-degree burns go down into the dermis itself and will often show white or black charred edges. In the post-acute stage, serious burns will often involve shrunken, contracted scar tissue over the area of skin that has been affected.

Is massage indicated or contraindicated? All burns (except, perhaps, mild sunburns) contraindicate massage in the acute stage. In the subacute and post-acute stages, massage may be performed around the damaged area within pain tolerance of the client.

Bursitis in Brief (p. 134)

What is it? A bursa is a fluid filled-sack that acts as a protective cushion at points of recurring pressure, eases the movement of tendons and ligaments moving over bones, and cushions points of contact between bones. Bursitis is the inflammation of a bursa.

How is it recognized? Acute bursitis is painful and will be aggravated by both passive and active motion. Muscles surrounding the affected joint will often severely limit range of motion. It may be hot or edematous if the bursa is superficial enough to be palpated.

Is massage indicated or contraindicated? Acute noninfectious bursitis locally contraindicates massage. Massage elsewhere on the body during an acute phase, and directly on the muscles of the affected joint (within pain limits) in a sub-acute phase, is perfectly appropriate.

Cancer in Brief (p. 588)

What is it? Cancer is the mutation of normal cells into cells with particular characteristics, including the tendency to proliferate into distinguishable growths and to spread through the body to other areas where they may colonize new tissues.

How is it recognized? In early stages, many cancers are difficult to detect. Later signs depend on what part of the body is being affected but can include things such as unusual bleeding, susceptibility to infection, changes in skin lesions, a persistent cough or hoarseness, changes in bladder or bowel habits, painless lumps or swellings, or pain where tumors have grown to the point that they erode into or compress delicate tissue.

Is massage indicated or contraindicated? The decision about whether to include massage as part of a treatment plan with cancer is complicated. Some types of bodywork are said to boost circulatory and lymph flow, which could be interpreted as increasing the risk of metastasis. Research shows, however, that it can take several years for many tumors to reach a palpable size. In light of this, a 60-minute session seems unlikely to have a serious impact on this disease process, as long as the therapist is not rubbing directly on the tumor. Many cancer patients seek massage as a way to help them cope with the challenges of cancer treatments. Massage and other bodywork modalities offered in this context can be beneficial, as long as the risks of working with clients who are undergoing surgery, chemotherapy, radiation, or other procedures are respected, and the therapist works as part of a well-informed health care team.

Candidiasis in Brief (p. 478)

What is it? Candidiasis is a condition in which the normally occurring *Candida albicans* fungi that colonize the gastrointestinal (GI) tract become invasive and disrupt normal function of the digestive system and other systems in the body.

How is it recognized? Signs and symptoms of candidiasis can be severe and acute, involving mouth and skin lesions as well as systemic blood infections, or subtle and chronic, involving fatigue, impaired mental ability, food and chemical sensitivities, and several other symptoms in varying degrees of severity.

Is massage indicated or contraindicated? Chronic candidiasis indicates massage, but therapists should understand that many acute candidiasis patients experience compromised immune system function and so should take care to protect clients from the threat of infection.

Carpal Tunnel Syndrome in Brief (p. 161)

What is it? Carpal tunnel syndrome (CTS) is irritation of the median nerve as it passes under the transverse carpal ligament into the wrist. It can have several different causes.

How is it recognized? CTS can cause pain, tingling, numbness, and weakness in the part of the hand supplied by the median nerve. Pain also may radiate proximally up the forearm.

Is massage indicated or contraindicated? Depending on the underlying factors, some CTS cases may respond well to massage. Work on or around the wrist must stop immediately if any symptoms are elicited. It is necessary to get a medical diagnosis to know which type of CTS is present.

Celiac Disease in Brief (p. 424)

What is it? Celiac disease is a condition in which a damaging inflammatory response follows the consumption of any food with gluten. This leads to the destruction of intestinal villi and poor access to ingested nutrients.

How is it recognized? Celiac disease can develop in childhood or adulthood, and its symptoms vary greatly from one person to another. Most symptoms are related to malabsorption (many nutrients are not absorbed and so pass through the stools) or malnutrition (complications related to vitamin and nutrient deficiencies).

Is massage indicated or contraindicated? Celiac disease is not directly affected by bodywork, although as with all situations involving intestinal discomfort, clients should be encouraged to seek a diagnosis if symptoms are persistent—even if massage provides temporary relief.

Cellulitis in Brief (p. 6)

What is it? Cellulitis is a Streptococcus infection that kills skin cells, leading to painful inflammation of the skin. It usually occurs on the face or lower leg.

How is it recognized? This condition is marked by redness and tenderness at the initial site of infection, along with fever, headache, malaise, and other signs of systemic infection.

Is massage indicated or contraindicated? This is a bacterial infection that can invade both the lymph and circulatory systems. Cellulitis systemically contraindicates massage until the infection has completely passed.

Cerebral Palsy in Brief (p. 239)

What is it? Cerebral palsy (CP) is an umbrella term used to refer to a variety of central nervous system injuries that may occur prenatally, at birth, or in early infancy. These injuries usually result in motor impairment, but they also may lead to sensory and cognitive problems.

How is it recognized? Cerebral palsy is usually diagnosed early in infancy, when voluntary motor skills are expected to begin to develop. CP patients may have hypertonic or hypotonic muscles, suppressed or extreme reflexes, poor coordination, and they may show random, involuntary movement.

Is massage indicated or contraindicated? As long as sensation is intact and the patient is able to communicate with the therapist in some way, massage is appropriate and potentially very useful for persons with CP, as they work to maintain muscular elasticity and improve motor skills.

Cervical Cancer in Brief (p. 534)

What is it? Cervical cancer is the development of cancerous cells in the lining of the cervix. These may spread to affect the whole cervix, the rest of the uterus, and other pelvic organs.

How is it recognized? Early stages of cervical cancer are virtually silent; this disease is detected by Pap tests before symptoms develop. Later signs and symptoms include bleeding or spotting outside a normal menstrual period, vaginal discharge, and pelvic pain.

Is massage indicated or contraindicated? Most cases of cervical cancer are caught and eradicated before the woman is in serious danger of metastasis. These patients are good candidates for any kind of bodywork. For a woman dealing with advanced stages of cervical cancer, the massage therapist must make adjustments for the radiation, chemotherapy, or surgical procedures that may be part of her experience.

Chemical Dependency in Brief (p. 220)

What is it? Chemical dependency is the use of material in methods or dosages that result in damage to the user and people whom the user contacts. The issue of chemical dependency covers the use of both legal and illegal substances.

How is it recognized? Specific symptoms of chemical dependency are determined by what substances are being consumed. Generally speaking, the symptoms of dependence include a craving for the substance in question, an inability to voluntarily limit use, unpleasant or dangerous withdrawal symptoms, and increasing tolerance of the substance's effects.

Is massage indicated or contraindicated? People who are recovering from chemical dependency can benefit from massage, as long as no contraindicating conditions have developed as part of the abuse. Massage is contraindicated for people who are intoxicated at the time of their appointment.

Chronic Bronchitis in Brief (p. 405)

What is it? Chronic bronchitis is one of the lung disorders classified as chronic obstructive pulmonary disease (COPD). It involves long-term inflammation of the bronchi with or without infection, leading to permanent changes in the bronchial lining. Chronic bronchitis frequently occurs as a prelude to or simultaneously with emphysema.

How is it recognized? Chronic bronchitis is diagnosed when a person experiences a productive cough that occurs most days for 3 months or more, for at least 2 consecutive years. Other common signs are a susceptibility to respiratory tract infections, cyanosis, and pulmonary edema.

Is massage indicated or contraindicated? Massage can be appropriate for chronic bronchitis patients, as long as they are not fighting acute respiratory infection at the time, and as long as heart function is not compromised.

Chronic Fatigue Syndrome in Brief (p. 360)

What is it? Chronic fatigue syndrome (CFS) is a collection of signs and symptoms that affect many systems in the body and result in debilitating fatigue.

How is it recognized? The central symptom to CFS is fatigue that is not restored by rest. It may be accompanied by swollen nodes, slight fever, muscular and joint aches, headaches, excessive pain after mild exercise, and non-restorative sleep.

Is massage indicated or contraindicated? Massage is indicated for CFS and can be a very helpful part of a treatment plan.

Cirrhosis in Brief (p. 458)

What is it? Cirrhosis is a condition in which normal liver cells become disorganized and dysfunctional; many of them are replaced or crowded out by scar tissue. Cirrhosis is often the final stage of chronic or acute liver diseases.

How is it recognized? Early symptoms of cirrhosis include loss of appetite, nausea, vomiting, and weight loss. Later complications may include muscle wasting, jaundice, ascites, vomiting blood, and mental and personality changes.

Is massage indicated or contraindicated? Advanced cirrhosis involves difficulties with fluid flow in the body. Bodywork that challenges this ability may not be appropriate. Some cirrhosis patients experience muscle wasting as their ability to metabolize proteins diminishes. Exercise and physical therapy are recommended for these patients for maintenance of strength and function, and massage as part of a health care team may have a role in this process as well.

Colorectal Cancer in Brief (p. 446)

What is it? Colorectal cancer is the development of malignant tumors in the colon or rectum. Growths can block the bowel or metastasize to other organs, particularly the liver.

How is it recognized? Colorectal cancer creates different symptoms depending on what part of the bowel is affected. The most dangerous symptoms are extreme changes in bowel habits, including diarrhea or constipation lasting more than 10 days. Other symptoms include blood in the stool, iron-deficiency anemia, and unintentional weight loss.

Is massage indicated or contraindicated? If a client is diagnosed with colon or rectal cancer in the early stages, some types of massage may be a useful supportive therapy to help deal with the side effects of cancer treatment. Colorectal cancer survivors are good candidates for massage, although the presence of a colostomy bag requires some adjustments.

Common Cold in Brief (p. 384)

What is it? The common cold (or upper respiratory tract infection: URTI) is a viral infection from any of about 200 different types of viruses.

How is it recognized? The symptoms of colds are nasal discharge, sore throat, mild fever, dry coughing, and headache. Symptoms last anywhere from 2 days to 2 weeks.

Is massage indicated or contraindicated? Colds indicate circulatory massage only when the acute stage has passed, and even then massage may exacerbate symptoms as the healing process may be accelerated. Energetic types of bodywork may be supportive and helpful if a person has a hard time getting past the peak of a cold.

Crohn Disease in Brief (p. 427)

What is it? Crohn disease is a progressive inflammatory condition that may affect any part of the GI tract. It involves the development of deep ulcers, blockages, and the formation of abnormal passageways (fistulas) in the small and large intestine.

How is it recognized? The primary symptom of Crohn disease is abdominal pain, especially in the lower right quadrant (the distal end of the ileum). Cramping, diarrhea, and pain at the anus may also accompany active flares of this disease.

Is massage indicated or contraindicated? Massage is appropriate for Crohn disease patients when their condition is in remission. During flares they also may benefit from noncirculatory work, but abdominal work will be uncomfortable.

Cystic Fibrosis in Brief (p. 412)

What is it? Cystic fibrosis is a congenital disease of exocrine glands that causes their secretions (mainly mucus, digestive enzymes, bile, and sweat) to become abnormally thick and viscous.

How is it recognized? Cystic fibrosis is a multisystem disease, but its effects on the respiratory system are typically the most common and most acute. Symptoms include chronic lung infections, shortness of breath, productive cough, along with digestive difficulties and failure to thrive in very young children.

Is massage indicated or contraindicated? Persons with cystic fibrosis receive intensive physiotherapy to dislodge mucus from the lungs, and they are recommended to exercise within tolerance to build lung capacity and immune system resilience. Massage certainly does not tax the body any more than these measures, but day-by-day judgments must be made based on the client's health and the presence of acute or chronic infection.

Cysts in Brief (p. 596)

What are they? Cysts are layers of connective tissue that surround and isolate something that should not be in the body (e.g., a piece of shrapnel or a localized infection).

How are they recognized? Palpable cysts are generally small, painless, distinct masses that move slightly under the skin.

Is massage indicated or contraindicated? Cysts locally contraindicate massage.

Decubitus Ulcers in Brief (p. 50)

What are they? Bedsores are ulcers caused by impaired circulation to the skin. Lack of blood supply leads to irreplaceable tissue death.

How are they recognized? Unlike other sores, ulcers do not crust over; they remain open wounds that are highly vulnerable to infection.

Are they indicated or contraindicated for massage? Bedsores are indicated for massage only before they happen. Once the tissue has been damaged, it is too late, and they locally contraindicate massage until they have completely healed over.

Depression in Brief (p. 224)

What is it? Depression is an umbrella term covering a number of mood disorders that can result in persistent feelings of sadness, guilt, or hopelessness.

How is it recognized? Symptoms vary according to the type of depression and the individual, but they usually include a loss of enjoyment derived from usual hobbies and activities, disappointment with oneself, hopelessness, irritability, and a change in sleeping habits.

Is massage indicated or contraindicated? Most types of depression indicate massage, which can work in several ways to alleviate symptoms both temporarily and in the long run.

Dermatitis/Eczema in Brief (p. 29)

What is it? Dermatitis is an umbrella term for inflammation of the skin. Eczema is a noncontagious skin rash usually brought about by an allergic reaction. Contact dermatitis is an inflammation brought about by irritation or allergic responses on the skin.

How is it recognized? Allergic or contact dermatitis presents in various ways, depending on what type of skin reactions are elicited. Exposure to poison oak or poison ivy results in large inflamed wheals; metal allergies tend to be less inflamed and more isolated in area. Eczema may appear as very dry and flaky skin, coin-shaped lesions, yellowish oily patches, or blistered, weepy skin.

Is massage indicated or contraindicated? The appropriateness of massage depends completely on the source of the problem and the condition of the skin. If the skin is very inflamed or has blisters or other lesions, massage is at least locally contraindicated until the acute stage has passed. If a rash could spread (e.g., poison oak), massage is systemically contraindicated while the irritation is present. If the skin is not itchy and the affected area is highly isolated, as with a metal allergy to a watchband or earrings, massage is only locally contraindicated.

Diabetes Mellitus in Brief (p. 491)

What is it? Diabetes is a group of metabolic disorders characterized by glucose intolerance and disturbances in carbohydrate, fat, and protein metabolism.

How is it recognized? Early symptoms of diabetes include frequent urination, thirstiness, and increased appetite, along with weight loss, nausea, and vomiting. These symptoms are often subtle enough that the first signs of disease are the complications it can cause: neuropathy, impaired vision, kidney dysfunction, or other problems.

Is massage indicated or contraindicated? Diabetes indicates massage as long as tissues are healthy and circulation is unimpaired. Many people with advanced or poorly treated diabetes experience numbness, cardiovascular problems, or kidney failure. Circulatory massage in these situations would not be appropriate.

Disc Disease in Brief (p. 165)

What is it? A herniated disc is a situation in which the nucleus pulposus or the surrounding annulus fibrosis of an intervertebral disc protrudes in such a way that it puts pressure on nerve roots, the cauda equina, or on the spinal cord itself.

How is it recognized? The symptoms of nerve pressure include radiculopathy (pain along the dermatome), specific muscle weakness, paresthesia, and numbness.

Is massage indicated or contraindicated? Herniated discs that are not acutely painful indicate massage.

Dislocations in Brief (p. 100)

What are they? Dislocations are traumatic injuries to joints in which the articulating bones are forcefully separated.

How are they recognized? Acute (new) dislocations are extremely painful. The bones may be visibly separated, and there will be total loss of function at the joint.

Is massage indicated or contraindicated? Dislocations indicate massage in the subacute stage, as long as work is conducted within pain tolerance. As the area heals, massage may be useful for managing scar tissue accumulation and muscle spasm around the affected joint.

Diverticular Disease in Brief (p. 450)

What is it? Diverticulosis is the development of small pouches that protrude from the colon or small intestine. Diverticulitis is the inflammation that happens when these pouches become infected. Collectively, these disorders are known as diverticular disease.

How is it recognized? Diverticulosis is generally silent, or symptomless. It occurs much more often in the colon than the small intestine. When inflammation (diverticulitis) is present, lower left side abdominal pain, cramping, bloating, constipation, or diarrhea may occur.

Is massage indicated or contraindicated? Deep abdominal massage is locally contraindicated if the client knows diverticula have developed. Acute infection of diverticula systemically contraindicates circulatory massage.

Dupuytren Contracture in Brief (p. 137)

What is it? Dupuytren contracture is an idiopathic shrinking and thickening of the fascia on the palm of the hand.

How is it recognized? This is a painless condition that usually affects the ring and little fingers, pulling them into permanent flexion.

Is massage indicated or contraindicated? Massage is indicated for Dupuytren contracture as long as sensation is present, although it may do little to reverse the process if it has gone too far.

Dysmenorrhea in Brief (p. 537)

What is it? Dysmenorrhea is the technical term for menstrual pain that is severe enough to interfere with and limit the activities of women of childbearing age. It may be a primary problem, or secondary to some other pelvic pathology.

How is it recognized? The symptoms of dysmenorrhea are dull aching or sharp severe lower abdominal pain preceding or during menstruation. Nausea and vomiting may accompany very severe symptoms. Secondary dysmenorrhea may create pelvic pain outside normal periods as well.

Is massage indicated or contraindicated? Massage is appropriate for primary dysmenorrhea, although the abdomen locally contraindicates deep work during days of heavy menstrual flow. The appropriateness of bodywork for secondary dysmenorrhea depends of the type of pathologic condition involved, along with stage, severity, treatment, and other variables.

Eating Disorders in Brief (p. 231)

What are they? Eating disorders are a group of psychological problems involving compulsions around food and weight gain or loss. Anorexia, bulimia, and compulsive overeating are each distinct problems, although overlap between them frequently occurs.

How are they recognized? Signs and symptoms of anorexia and bulimia may be hard to recognize in early stages, because these behaviors are usually done in private. Long-term consequences include esophageal and colon damage, tooth damage, arrhythmia and low cardiac stroke volume, electrolyte imbalance, hormonal disturbance, osteoporosis, and many other problems. Compulsive overeating is recognizable by eating habits, in combination with significant weight gain, often in a short period.

Is massage indicated or contraindicated? Massage may be very supportive and appropriate for all types of eating disorders, as long as the body's chemistry can keep up with the changes bodywork brings about. If a client is in an advanced stage of anorexia or bulimia, bodywork choices may need to change to respect the delicacy of her system.

Edema in Brief (p. 347)

What is it? Edema is the retention of interstitial fluid because of electrolyte or protein imbalances, or because of mechanical obstruction in the circulatory or lymphatic systems.

How is it recognized? Edematous tissue is puffy or boggy. It may be hot, if associated with local infection, or quite cool, if it is cut off from local circulation.

Is massage indicated or contraindicated? Most edemas contraindicate circulatory massage. This is especially true of pitting edema, where the tissue does not immediately spring back from a touch. Edemas that indicate massage include those caused by subacute soft tissue injury or temporary immobilization caused by some factor that does not contraindicate massage.

Embolism, Thrombus in Brief (p. 291)

What are they? Thrombi are stationary clots; emboli are clots that travel through the circulatory system. Emboli are usually composed of blood, but may also be fragments of plaque, fat globules, air bubbles, tumors, or bone chips.

How are they recognized? If venous thrombi break loose or embolize, they can only land in the lungs, causing pulmonary embolism (PE). Symptoms of PE include shortness of breath, chest pain, and coughing up sputum that is streaked with blood. Many venous thrombi and pulmonary emboli are silent; that is, they cause no symptoms until the damage has been done. Clots that form on the arterial side of the system can lodge anywhere their artery carries them. Some of the most common (and dangerous) locations for arterial clots to land are in the coronary arteries (heart attack), the brain (transient ischemic attack or stroke), and the kidneys (renal infarction).

Is massage indicated or contraindicated? Any disorder than involves the potential for lodged or traveling clots contraindicates circulatory massage.

Emphysema in Brief (p. 408)

What is it? Emphysema is a condition in which the alveoli of the lungs become stretched out and inelastic. They merge with each other, decreasing surface area, destroying surrounding capillaries, and limiting oxygen–carbon dioxide exchange.

How is it recognized? Symptoms of emphysema include shortness of breath with mild or no exertion, a chronic dry cough, rales, cyanosis, and susceptibility to secondary respiratory infection.

Is massage indicated or contraindicated? Emphysema indicates massage with caution for circulatory complications, secondary infection, and positioning the client for maximum comfort.

Encephalitis in Brief (p. 205)

What is it? Encephalitis is inflammation of the brain usually brought about by a viral infection.

How is it recognized? Signs and symptoms of encephalitis include fever, headache, confusion, and personality and memory changes. In rare cases, encephalitis may cause permanent neurologic damage or even death.

Is massage indicated or contraindicated? Acute encephalitis contraindicates massage, but if a client has had it in his history with no signs of present infection or neurologic damage, massage is perfectly acceptable.

Endometriosis in Brief (p. 539)

What is it? Endometriosis is the implantation and growth of endometrial cells in the peritoneal cavity (and possibly elsewhere) that grow and then decay with the menstrual cycle.

How is it recognized? Endometriosis may have no symptoms. When it does, they generally include heavy, painful menstruation, pelvic and abdominal pain, difficulties with urination or defecation, painful intercourse, and other problems, depending on which tissues have been affected. Symptoms are worst during menstruation. Infertility is a frequent complication of endometriosis.

Is massage indicated or contraindicated? If a client knows she has endometriosis, deep abdominal or pelvic work may be painful, especially when it is close to her menstrual cycle. The supportive effects of massage, however, can be an important part of the coping mechanisms that women with this disorder must develop.

Esophageal Cancer in Brief (p. 431)

What is it? Esophageal cancer is the growth of malignant cells in the esophagus. It is classified as squamous cell carcinoma, which usually occurs at the proximal end of the esophagus, and adenocarcinoma, which occurs at the distal end, near the lower esophageal valve.

How is it recognized? Esophageal cancer is rarely recognized in early stages. In later stages, a growth may obstruct the esophagus, leading to a feeling of food or liquid "getting stuck" on the way to the stomach. Pain and difficulty with swallowing along with unintended weight loss are the symptoms that usually prompt people to seek a diagnosis.

Is massage indicated or contraindicated? As with other cancers, the guidelines for massage and esophageal cancer are determined largely by what stresses or complications cancer treatments may cause. Surgery, radiation, chemotherapy, and other options all carry specific cautions and concerns for massage therapists.

Fatigue in Brief (p. 597)

What is it? Fatigue is a state of having less than optimal energy as a result of inadequate rest and recovery time. Fatigue can be brought about by mental or physical exertion or by any combination of both.

How is it recognized? A person living with mental or physical fatigue feels tired, moves inefficiently, and may be more prone to injury.

Is massage indicated or contraindicated? In the absence of other conditions, fatigue indicates massage.

Fever in Brief (p. 363)

What is it? Fever is a controlled increase in core temperature, usually brought about by immune system reactions, often in response to pathogenic invasion.

How is it recognized? Fever is identifiable by readings on a thermometer.

Is massage indicated or contraindicated? Most fever contraindicates massage, as it is an indication that the body is fighting an infection and should be allowed to do its work undisturbed.

Fibroid Tumors in Brief (p. 542)

What are they? Fibroid tumors are benign growths in the muscle or connective tissue of the uterus.

How are they recognized? Fibroid tumors are often asymptomatic. Some, however, cause heavy menstrual bleeding or may put mechanical pressure on other structures in the pelvis.

Is massage indicated or contraindicated? Large, diagnosed fibroid tumors contraindicate deep abdominal massage. However, most fibroids are quite small and virtually symptomless, and massage will not have any impact on them at all. In these cases, massage is indicated for the benefit of the client, if not for the possibility of changing the state of her fibroid tumors.

Fibromyalgia in Brief (p. 64)

What is it? Fibromyalgia syndrome (FMS) is a chronic pain syndrome involving sleep disorders and the development of a predictable pattern of tender points in muscles and other soft tissues.

How is it recognized? Fibromyalgia syndrome is diagnosed when other diseases have been ruled out, and when 11 active tender points are found distributed among all quadrants of the body.

Is massage indicated or contraindicated? Fibromyalgia syndrome indicates massage. Care must be taken not to over-treat, however, because clients are extremely sensitive to pain and may have accumulations of waste products in the tissues that are difficult to flush out adequately.

Fractures in Brief (p. 87)

What are they? A fracture is any kind of broken or cracked bone.

How are they recognized? Most fractures are painful and involve loss of function at the nearest joints, but some may be difficult to diagnose without an x-ray or other imaging techniques.

Is massage indicated or contraindicated? Acute fractures locally contraindicate massage, but work done on the rest of the body can yield reflexive benefits. Massage is indicated for people in later stages of recovery from fractures.

Fungal Infections in Brief (p. 7)

What are they? Fungal infections of human skin, also called mycoses, are caused by fungi called dermatophytes. The characteristic lesions caused by dermatophytes are called tinea. Several types of dermatophytes cause tinea in different areas; they are typically named by location.

How is it recognized? Most tinea lesions begin as one reddened circular itchy patch. Scratching the lesions spreads them to other parts of the body. As they get larger, they tend to clear in the middle and keep a red ring around the edges. Athlete's foot, another type of mycosis, involves moist blisters and cracking between the toes. Fungal infections of toenails or fingernails involve thickened, pitted, discolored nails that may detach.

Is massage indicated or contraindicated? Fungal infections locally contraindicate massage in all stages. If the affected areas are very limited, for instance, only the feet are involved, or only one or two small, covered lesions on the body are present, massage may be administered elsewhere. If a large area is involved, and especially if the infection is acute (i.e., not yet responding to treatment), then it systemically contraindicates massage.

Gallstones in Brief (p. 462)

What are they? Gallstones are crystallized formations of cholesterol or bile pigments in the gallbladder. They can be as small as grains of sand or as large as a golf ball.

How are they recognized? Most gallstones do not cause symptoms. When they do, pain that may last several hours develops in the upper right side of the abdomen. Pain may refer to the back between the scapula and the right shoulder. Gallstones stuck in the ducts of the biliary system may cause jaundice or pancreatitis.

Is massage indicated or contraindicated? Silent (symptomless) stones have little impact on overall health and function, so massage for these clients is certainly appropriate, although draining strokes over the liver are contraindicated. Clients recovering from gallbladder surgery may need some special considerations. A client with a history of gallstones but no current symptoms is fine for massage.

Ganglion Cysts in Brief (p. 138)

What are they? Ganglion cysts are small fluid-filled synovial sacks that are attached to tendinous sheaths, or joint capsules.

How are they recognized? Ganglion cysts form small bumps that usually appear on the hand, wrist, or ankle. They are not usually painful, unless they are in a place to be injured by normal wear and tear.

Is massage indicated or contraindicated? Ganglion cysts locally contraindicate massage. Friction or direct pressure will not make them go away and may irritate them by stimulating excessive fluid flow.

Gastroenteritis in Brief (p. 433)

What is it? Gastroenteritis is any form of gastrointestinal inflammation. This may be due to a viral or bacterial infection, a parasite, fungus, food intolerance, or other cause.

How is it recognized? The symptoms of gastroenteritis are nausea, vomiting, and diarrhea. Fever, blood in the stools, and other signs may be present, depending on the cause.

Is massage indicated or contraindicated? Acute gastroenteritis contraindicates massage, especially when it is caused by an infectious agent. Chronic situations may be appropriate for bodywork, as long as the cause of the problem is clearly understood.

Gastroesophageal Reflux Disease in Brief (p. 435)

What is it? Gastroesophageal reflux disease (GERD) is a condition involving a weak or impaired esophageal sphincter, and the chronic splashing of acidic stomach secretions into the unprotected esophagus.

How is it recognized? Most people experience occasional "heartburn": the sensation of having corrosive gastric juices enter the esophagus. GERD is diagnosed when heartburn symptoms have been present long enough to cause structural changes to the esophageal lining, which could lead to serious complications.

Is massage indicated or contraindicated? People with GERD often find that lying down exacerbates their symptoms, especially if it is within a couple of hours of eating. Clients may therefore wish to use bolsters that will allow them to be in a reclining position, or to have the head-end of the table elevated by several inches, or to work with a massage chair, rather than lying flat on a table.

Glomerulonephritis in Brief (p. 511)

What is it? Glomerulonephritis is a condition in which the glomeruli (small structures that are part of the nephron–capillary unit) become inflamed and cease to function efficiently.

How is it recognized? Early signs and symptoms of glomerulonephritis include high blood pressure, dark or rust-colored urine, or foamy urine. Later symptoms indicate chronic renal failure and include systemic edema, fatigue, headaches, decreased urine output, rashes and discoloration of the skin, and general malaise.

Is massage indicated or contraindicated? Symptomatic glomerulonephritis systemically contraindicates circulatory massage. This is an inflammatory condition that impairs the body's ability to manage fluid exchanges. Bodywork that does not significantly impact circulation may be appropriate.

Gout in Brief (p. 102)

What is it? Gout is an inflammatory arthritis caused by deposits of sodium urate (uric acid) in and around joints, especially in the feet.

How is it recognized? Acute gout causes joints to become red, hot, swollen, shiny, and extremely painful. It usually has a sudden onset.

Is massage indicated or contraindicated? Gout systemically contraindicates massage when it is acute. Gouty joints locally contraindicate massage at all times.

Guillain-Barré Syndrome in Brief (p. 261)

What is it? Guillain-Barré syndrome (GBS) is a demyelinating disorder of peripheral nerves. It usually begins in the feet, and moves proximally. It is probably autoimmune in nature, but the specific triggers have not been identified.

How is it recognized? Guillain-Barré syndrome is marked by its sudden onset (symptoms usually begin quickly and peak within 2 weeks) followed by its gradual remission (most patients have full or nearly full recovery within 18 months). Furthermore, Guillain-Barré syndrome affects limbs symmetrically, and moves proximally toward the trunk, which distinguishes it from other peripheral nerve problems.

Is massage indicated or contraindicated? When a person has reached the peak of his or her GBS attack, physical and occupational therapy are often employed to speed recovery and prevent muscle atrophy. Massage may be useful at this stage as well, to improve circulation and to reduce fatigue and anxiety.

Headaches in Brief (p. 263)

What are they? Headaches are pain caused by any number of sources. Muscular tension, vascular spasm and dilation, and chemical imbalances all can contribute to headache. Headaches only rarely indicate a serious underlying disorder.

How are they recognized? Tension-type headaches are usually bilateral and steadily painful. Vascular headaches are often unilateral and have a distinctive "throbbing" pain from blood flow into the head. Headaches brought about by central nervous system injury or disease are extreme, severe, and prolonged. They can have a sudden or gradual onset

Is massage indicated or contraindicated? Headaches caused by infection or CNS injury contraindicate massage. Persons experiencing vascular headaches generally avoid stimuli such as massage, but massage is definitely indicated for tension-type headaches.

Heart Attack in Brief (p. 327)

What is it? A heart attack, or myocardial infarction (MI), is damage to the myocardium caused by a sudden obstruction in blood flow through the coronary arteries, which results in permanent myocardial damage.

How is it recognized? Symptoms of most heart attacks include a sensation of great pressure on the chest, spreading pain, and lightheadedness, dizziness, and nausea. Sometimes symptoms vary, and occasionally a minor heart attack may occur with no symptoms at all.

Is massage indicated or contraindicated? Patients recovering from recent heart attacks are not candidates for circulatory massage. After they have completely recovered, they may be able to receive massage, depending on the rest of their cardiovascular health.

Heart Failure in Brief (p. 334)

What is it? Heart failure is a condition in which the heart no longer can function well enough to keep up with the needs of the body. It is usually slowly progressive, developing over a number of years before any changes in function may be noticeable.

How is it recognized? Different symptoms are present, depending on which side of the heart is working inefficiently. Left-sided heart failure results in fluid congestion in the lungs with general weakness and shortness of breath. Right-sided heart failure results in fluid back-ups throughout the system, which shows as edema, especially in the ankles and legs. Both varieties of heart failure will lead to chest pain; cold, sweaty skin; a fast, irregular pulse; coughing, especially when the person is lying down; and very low stamina.

Is massage indicated or contraindicated? Circulatory massage is inappropriate for clients with heart failure because it has the goal of pushing fluid through a system that is incapable of adjusting to those changes. Energetic work may be more appropriate to help clients lower stress and to cope with the challenges of severely restricted circulation.

Hematoma in Brief (p. 295)

What is it? A hematoma is a deep bruise (leakage of blood) between muscle sheaths.

How is it recognized? Superficial hematomas are simple bruises. Deep bleeds may not be visible, but they will be painful, and if extensive bleeding has occurred, a characteristic "gel-like" feel will develop in the affected tissue.

Is massage indicated or contraindicated? Massage is at least locally contraindicated for acute hematomas because of the possibility of blood clots and pain. In the subacute stage (at least 2 days later), when the surrounding blood vessels have been sealed shut and the body is in the process of breaking down and reabsorbing the debris, gentle massage around the perimeter of the area and hydrotherapy can be helpful.

Hemophilia in Brief (p. 296)

What is it? Hemophilia is a genetic disorder in which certain clotting factors in the blood are either insufficient or missing altogether.

How is it recognized? Hemophilia can cause superficial bleeding that persists for longer than normal, or internal bleeding into joint cavities or between muscle sheaths with little or no provocation.

Is massage indicated or contraindicated? Severe cases of hemophilia contraindicate bodywork that can mechanically stretch, manipulate, or accidentally injure delicate tissues. Milder cases of hemophilia may be safer for circulatory massage.

Hepatitis in Brief (p. 465)

What is it? Hepatitis is inflammation of the liver, usually due to viral infection.

How is it recognized? All types of hepatitis produce the same symptoms, with variable severity. Symptoms, when any occur at all, include fatigue, abdominal pain, nausea, diarrhea, and jaundice.

Is massage indicated or contraindicated? Acute hepatitis contraindicates circulatory massage. For clients with chronic hepatitis, the appropriateness of massage will depend on their general health.

Hernia in Brief (p. 139)

What is it? A hernia is a hole or rip in the abdominal wall or the inguinal ring through which the small intestines may protrude.

How is it recognized? Abdominal hernias usually show some bulging and mild to severe pain, depending on whether a portion of the small intestine is trapped.

Is massage indicated or contraindicated? Untreated hernias locally contraindicate massage. If the hernia is accompanied by fever or other signs of infection, it systemically contraindicates massage. Recent hernia surgeries fall under the category of postsurgical situations. Old hernia surgeries with no complications are fine for massage.

Herpes Simplex in Brief (p. 12)

What is it? Herpes simplex is a viral infection resulting in cold sores or fever blisters on the face or around the mouth, or blisters around the genitals, thighs, or buttocks.

How is it recognized? Herpes outbreaks are often preceded by 2 to 3 days of tingling, itching, or pain. Then blisters appear gathered around a red base. The blisters gradually crust and disappear, usually within 2 weeks.

Is massage indicated or contraindicated? Any kind of herpes in the acute stage locally contraindicates massage. Massage is systemically contraindicated if the client is showing any signs of systemic infection. The sheets of clients with herpes must be isolated and bleached. Massage for clients with a history of herpes but no active symptoms is indicated.

Herpes Zoster in Brief (p. 207)

What is it? Herpes zoster, or shingles, is a viral infection of sensory neurons from the same virus that causes chickenpox.

How is it recognized? Shingles creates rashes and extremely painful blisters unilaterally along the affected dermatomes. The trunk or buttocks are the most common areas, but it occasionally affects the trigeminal nerve.

Is massage indicated or contraindicated? This is an extraordinarily painful condition, and it contraindicates massage in the acute stage. After the blisters have healed and the pain has subsided, massage is appropriate.

HIV/AIDS in Brief (p. 365)

What is it? Acquired immune deficiency syndrome (AIDS) is a disease caused by the human immunodeficiency virus (HIV), which attacks and disables the immune system. This leaves a person vulnerable to a host of diseases that are usually not a threat to uninfected people.

How is it recognized? Most people with HIV experience a week or 2 of flu-like symptoms within several weeks of being infected, followed by an interval with no symptoms. When the virus has successfully inactivated the immune system, infection by opportunistic pathogens such as herpes simplex and zoster, cytomegalovirus, or *Pneumocystis carinii* occurs.

Is massage indicated or contraindicated? All stages of HIV infection indicate massage as long as the practitioner is healthy and does not pose any risk to the client, and the client is able to keep up with the changes that massage brings about in the body.

Hives in Brief (p. 33)

What are they? Hives are an inflammatory skin reaction to an allergen or emotional stressor.

How are they recognized? Hives range from small red spots to large wheals, which are pink to red, warm, and itchy. Individual lesions generally subside within a few hours, but successive hives may appear; the cycle can continue for several weeks at a time.

Is massage indicated or contraindicated for hives? Hives systemically contraindicate massage during the acute stage and locally contraindicate it in the subacute stage. Massage would bring even more circulation to the skin, making a bad situation worse.

Hypertension in Brief (p. 318)

What is it? Hypertension is the technical term for high blood pressure.

How is it recognized? High blood pressure has no dependable symptoms. The only way to identify it is by taking several blood pressure measurements over time.

Is massage indicated or contraindicated? For borderline or mild high blood pressure, massage may be useful as a tool to control stress and increase general health, but other pathologic conditions having to do with kidney or cardiovascular disease must be ruled out. High blood pressure that accompanies other cardiovascular disease may be inappropriate for circulatory massage, but it may respond well to other modalities.

Hyperthyroidism in Brief (p. 497)

What is it? Hyperthyroidism is a condition in which the thyroid gland produces too much of its hormones that stimulate metabolism of fuel into energy. It is usually related to an autoimmune attack against the whole thyroid gland, but it can be caused by small, localized hyperactive nodules or infection.

What does it look like? Signs and symptoms of hyperthyroidism involve too much production of energy from available fuel: restlessness, sleeplessness, irritability, dry skin and hair, rapid heartbeat, tremor, unintended weight loss, and for women, irregularity of menstrual periods. Some hyperthyroid patients experience complications involving eye problems or skin rashes. A severe and acute episode of hyperthyroidism is called a thyroid storm.

Is massage indicated or contraindicated? Most people with hyperactive thyroid glands respond well to massage, which may help, at least temporarily, to ameliorate some of the stress-related symptoms that they experience.

Hypoglycemia in Brief (p. 500)

What is it? Hypoglycemia is the condition of having abnormally low levels of blood glucose, so cells have no access to important fuel.

What does it look like? Signs and symptoms of a hypoglycemic episode include dizziness, confusion, chills and sweating, hunger, headache, and pallor. Symptoms pass when a person eats or drinks something with available glucose.

Is massage indicated or contraindicated? A person in a hypoglycemic episode needs to replace glucose first, get a massage second. Once the symptoms have passed, bodywork is a fine choice. If a person experiences ongoing hypoglycemic symptoms, or frequent acute episodes, he or she should find out why.

Hypothyroidism in Brief (p. 501)

What is it? Hypothyroidism is a condition in which the thyroid gland produces an inadequate supply of the hormones that regulate metabolism of fuel into energy. Some cases of hypothyroidism are the result of an autoimmune attack on the thyroid gland, but others are related to the long-term complications of treatment for hyperthyroidism or other factors.

What does it look like? Symptoms of hypothyroidism are subtle and often missed. They include fatigue, weight gain, depression, intolerance of cold, and for women, heavy menstrual periods.

Is massage indicated or contraindicated? One of the complications of hypothyroidism, especially in elderly patients, is the accelerated development of atherosclerosis. As long as this condition is recognized and respected, massage can be a supportive and positive experience for hypothyroidism patients.

Ichthyosis in Brief (p. 54)

What is it? Ichthyosis is pathologically dry skin: much more severe than average dry skin.

How is it recognized? Ichthyosis creates distinctive diamond-shaped "scales" on the skin, usually on the lower legs.

Is massage indicated or contraindicated? When ichthyosis appears independently of other conditions, it certainly indicates massage. It probably will not be a permanent solution to this problem, but massage can certainly make it better in the short run. Take care to avoid areas where deep cracking may expose blood supply.

Impetigo in Brief (p. 15)

What is it? Impetigo is a bacterial (Staphylococcus or Streptococcus) infection of the skin.

How is it recognized? Streptococcal impetigo is marked by a rash with fluid-filled blisters and honey-colored crusts. It usually begins somewhere on the face, but it can appear anywhere on the body. Staphylococcal impetigo involves large, delicate blisters that may appear anywhere on the body.

Is massage indicated or contraindicated? Until the lesions have completely healed, this highly contagious condition strictly contraindicates massage.

Inflammation in Brief (p. 370)

What is it? Inflammation is a protective device in response to injury or infection. It involves localized vascular, cellular, and chemical reactions to isolate the area and to resolve the damage through immune system response.

How is it recognized? The signs of inflammation are redness, pain, swelling, heat, and loss of function. These can be localized or systemic.

Is massage indicated or contraindicated? Acute inflammation contraindicates circulatory massage, but bodywork may be appropriate for subacute situations, depending on the causative factors. Inflammation due to infection obviously carries a higher risk to the client and the practitioner than inflammation in response to musculoskeletal injury.

Influenza in Brief (p. 386)

What is it? Influenza ("flu") is a viral infection of the respiratory tract.

How is it recognized? The symptoms of flu include high fever and muscle and joint achiness that may last for up to 3 days, followed by a runny nose, coughing, sneezing, and general malaise.

Is massage indicated or contraindicated? Massage is indicated for the flu in the subacute stage only.

Interstitial Cystitis in Brief (p. 523)

What is it? Interstitial cystitis (IC) is a chronic inflammation of the bladder involving scar tissue, stiffening, decreased capacity, pinpoint hemorrhages, and sometimes ulcers in the bladder walls.

How is it recognized? Symptoms of IC are very much like those of urinary tract infections: burning, increased frequency, and urgency of urination; decreased capacity of the bladder; and pain, pressure, and tenderness.

Is massage indicated or contraindicated? IC is a poorly understood condition that seems to be exacerbated by stress. Bodywork may be a helpful and supportive choice for IC patients, although it probably does not work to reverse the situation.

Irritable Bowel Syndrome in Brief (p. 453)

What is it? Irritable bowel syndrome (IBS) is a collection of signs and symptoms that indicate a functional problem with the digestive system, specifically with the colon. It is aggravated by stress and diet.

How is it recognized? The symptoms of IBS include alternating bouts of constipation and diarrhea, bloating or abdominal distension, and moderate to severe cramping abdominal pain that is relieved with defecation.

Is massage indicated or contraindicated? IBS indicates massage, as long as bodywork does not exacerbate symptoms.

Jaundice in Brief (p. 470)

What is it? Jaundice is a symptom of liver dysfunction, involving the presence of excess bilirubin in the blood. The bilirubin is then distributed and dissolved in subcutaneous fat, mucous membranes, and the sclera of the eyes.

How is it recognized? Jaundice gives the skin, eyes, and mucous membranes a yellowish cast.

Is massage indicated or contraindicated? The presence of jaundice is not enough information on which to base a decision about bodywork. The underlying cause for the jaundice must be understood before a decision can be made, based on the comparative risks and benefits of bodywork in the context of that condition.

Kidney Stones in Brief (p. 513)

What are they? A kidney stone is a solid deposit of crystalline substances inside the kidney.

How are they recognized? Small stones may create no symptoms at all, but when larger stones enter the ureters, they can cause blood in the urine and extreme pain called renal colic. Renal colic may be accompanied by nausea and vomiting. Fever and chills indicate that infection is part of the problem. Pain may refer from the back into the groin.

Is massage indicated or contraindicated? Acute renal colic contraindicates massage, although any kind of bodywork is appropriate for people with a history of stones but no current symptoms.

Leukemia in Brief (p. 298)

What is it? Leukemia is a collection of blood disorders involving the production of nonfunctioning white blood cells in bone marrow.

How is it recognized? Different types of leukemia have slightly different profiles, but all varieties include signs brought about by interference with the production of normal blood cells: anemia, easy bruising from lack of platelets, and low resistance to infection.

Is massage indicated or contraindicated? Leukemia is usually treated with chemotherapy. Both the disease and the treatment wreak havoc with the immune system. Although some types of bodywork may be supportive during this time, care must be taken to protect the client from any threat of infection.

Liver Cancer in Brief (p. 471)

What is it? Primary liver cancer is the growth of malignant cells within hepatocytes. Liver cancer is aggressive and usually silent in early stages, leading to late diagnoses and a generally poor prognosis.

How is it recognized? Liver cancer is silent in early stages, but as tumors grow and interfere with function symptoms may include vague to intense abdominal pain, ascites, muscle wasting, fever, unintended weight loss, and jaundice.

Is massage indicated or contraindicated? A person with liver cancer may undergo extensive and intrusive treatment options; any bodywork must be adjusted to respect the challenges of these treatments. Other liver cancer patients may be in the process of dying, and massage may be an important and welcome comfort measure in this situation.

Lung Cancer in Brief (p. 414)

What is it? Lung cancer is the development of malignant cells in the lungs. These cells have easy access to blood and lymph vessels, and they quickly spread to other organs in the body.

How is it recognized? The early symptoms of lung cancer are virtually indistinguishable from normal irritation from cigarette smoke: a chronic cough, blood-stained sputum, and recurrent bronchitis or pneumonia.

Is massage indicated or contraindicated? Sadly, most people diagnosed with lung cancer will not survive. Massage has a place in cancer recovery care, as well as in terminal care, but these situations call for specific precautions to achieve maximum benefit with minimal risk.

Lupus in Brief (p. 373)

What is it? Lupus is an autoimmune disease in which antibodies attack various types of tissue throughout the body. Three distinct types of lupus exist, but systemic lupus erythematosus (SLE) is both the most common and the most serious.

How is it recognized? Eleven specific criteria have been determined for a diagnosis of lupus. They include, among other things, arthritis in two or more joints, pleurisy, pericarditis, kidney, and nervous system dysfunction.

Is massage indicated or contraindicated? When lupus is in a state of acute flare, circulatory massage could exacerbate symptoms. When the condition is in remission, bodywork of any kind could be very helpful to reduce pain and anxiety and to help maintain flexibility.

Lyme Disease in Brief (p. 106)

What is it? Lyme disease is a bacterial infection spread by the bites of specific species of ticks. The immune response to the bacteria causes inflammation of large joints, along with neurologic and cardiovascular symptoms.

How is it recognized? The hallmark early symptom of Lyme disease is a circular "bull's eye" rash at the site of the tick bite. The skin will be red, itchy, and hot, but not usually raised. The rash may be accompanied by fever, fatigue, and joint pain. Later symptoms may include acute intermittent inflammation of one or more large joints, numbness, poor coordination, Bell's palsy, and irregular heartbeat.

Is massage indicated or contraindicated? The inflammation associated with Lyme disease runs in acute and subacute phases. During subacute phases, massage may be appropriate to maintain joint function and relieve pain. In this situation, it is important to be working as part of a health care team for the maximum benefit and minimum risk to the infected person.

Lymphangitis in Brief (p. 349)

What is it? Lymphangitis is an infection of lymph capillaries. If it gets into the nodes, it is called lymphadenitis. If it gets past the lymphatic system it is called blood poisoning (septicemia), and it can be life threatening.

How is it recognized? Lymphangitis has all the signs of local infection: pain, heat, redness, and swelling. It also may show red streaks from the site of infection running toward the nearest lymph nodes.

Is massage indicated or contraindicated? Lymphangitis contraindicates circulatory massage until the infection has been completely eradicated.

Lymphoma In Brief (p. 351)

What is it? Lymphoma is any variety of cancer that grows in lymph nodes. Several types have been identified, some of which are aggressive and very threatening, others of which may progress more slowly.

How is it recognized? Painless swelling of lymph nodes is the cardinal sign of lymphoma, along with the possibility of anemia, fatigue, low-grade fever, night sweats, itchiness, abdominal pain, and loss of appetite, all of which last for 2 weeks or more.

Is massage indicated or contraindicated? Rigorous circulatory massage is generally not recommended for a person who is fighting lymphoma, although this may be a case-by-case decision. Persons who have been free from lymphoma for 5 years or more are considered "cured." Noncirculatory types of massage may be appropriate for lymphoma patients, although it is recommended that the therapist participate as part of an integrated health care team.

Marfan Syndrome in Brief (p. 141)

What is it? Marfan syndrome is a genetic defect leading to problems in the construction of fibrillin, a connective tissue fiber. Consequently, connective tissues are systemically affected, with the most serious problems occurring in the skeleton, cardiovascular system, and the eyes.

How is it recognized? Marfan syndrome patients are often taller than average, with very long fingers. Joints tend to be hypermobile. Listening to the heart may show signs of valve problems. Many Marfan syndrome patients are myopic, and up to half experience a dislocated lens in the eye.

Is massage indicated or contraindicated? Marfan syndrome patients must adjust their daily activities to accommodate for fragility in their connective tissues. Massage likewise must be adjusted to meet the reduced capacity to adjust to changes in their environment.

Meningitis in Brief (p. 209)

What is it? Meningitis is an infection of the meninges, specifically the pia mater and the arachnoid layers.

How is it recognized? Symptoms of acute meningitis include very high fever, rash, photophobia, headache, and stiff neck. Symptoms are not always consistent, however; they may appear in different combinations for different people.

Is massage indicated or contraindicated? Meningitis, a contagious and inflammatory disease, strictly contraindicates massage in the acute phase. People who have recovered from meningitis with no lasting damage are perfectly fine to receive massage.

Menopause in Brief (p. 568)

What is it? Menopause refers to the moment when functioning ovaries become nonfunctioning ovaries. Although this usually happens as a normal part of aging, menopause can be induced through surgery, radiation, or medication.

How is it recognized? The symptoms associated with a decline in ovarian function ("perimenopause") include night sweats, hot flashes, insomnia, mood swings, decreased sex drive, vaginal itchiness or dryness, and poor concentration and memory. Longer-term symptoms include an increased risk for osteoporosis and cardiovascular disease.

Is massage indicated or contraindicated? Bodywork is highly indicated for a woman who is going through the transition of losing ovarian function. Although for some women this is a liberating, exciting time, for others it involves radical and not always welcome changes in self-definition and self-perception. Massage gives powerful positive feedback about physical experience, and can help to ameliorate some of the psychological and physical disruptions that menopause can bring about.

Metabolic Syndrome in Brief (p. 504)

What is it? Metabolic syndrome is a collection of problems that indicates a high risk of several serious diseases, including diabetes, heart attack, atherosclerosis, and stroke.

How is it recognized? Metabolic syndrome is recognized though its combined associated conditions, including disruptions in cholesterol, hypertension, central obesity, and others.

Is massage indicated or contraindicated? The appropriateness of massage for a person with metabolic syndrome depends on his or her cardiovascular health. If exercise is recommended for weight loss and improved insulin function, then massage is probably also safe. If, however, these conditions have led to severe cardiovascular problems, massage must be adjusted to accommodate circulatory weakness.

Mites and Lice in Brief (p. 35)

What are they? Lice and mites are tiny animals that drink blood. They are highly contagious and spread through close contact with skin or infested sheets or clothing.

How are they recognized?

- The mites that cause scabies are too small to see, but they leave itchy trails where they burrow under the skin. They prefer warm, moist places such as the axillae or between fingers.

- Head lice are easy to see, but they can hide. A more dependable sign is their eggs: nits are small white rice-shaped flecks that cling strongly to hair shafts.

- Body lice look very similar to head lice, but they live primarily in clothing and only visit the host for blood meals.

- Pubic lice look like tiny white crabs in pubic and coarse body hair. All of these parasites create a lot of itching through allergic reactions to the toxins they produce.

Is massage indicated or contraindicated? Massage is contraindicated for all three infestations, until the infestation has been completely eradicated. If a massage therapist is exposed to any of these parasites, every client he or she works on subsequently will also be exposed even before the therapist shows any symptoms.

Moles in Brief (p. 35)

What are they? Moles are isolated areas in which the pigment cells in the epidermis have produced excess melanin.

How are they recognized? Moles can range in color from light tan to blackish-blue. Their color is usually uniform throughout. Moles are usually circular or oval. Are they indicated or contraindicated for massage? Massage will not help or hurt moles, but massage therapists may be able to see changes in a mole of which their client may be unaware.

Is massage indicated or contraindicated? Massage will not help or hurt moles, but massage therapists may be able to see changes in a mole that their client may be unaware of.

Mononucleosis in Brief (p. 354)

What is it? Mononucleosis is an infection, usually with the Epstein Barr Virus (EBV) but occasionally with cytomegalovirus (CMV) or other agents. The virus attacks B-cells in the epithelial tissue in the salivary glands and throat first, and then invades the liver, spleen, and lymph nodes.

How is it recognized? The three leading symptoms for mononucleosis are fever, swollen lymph nodes, and sore throat. Other symptoms may include profound fatigue, low stamina, enlarged spleen, and enlarged liver.

Is massage indicated or contraindicated? Mononucleosis contraindicates circulatory massage in the acute stage when the body is fighting hard to beat back this viral attack. In later stages, as long as circulation is healthy and the spleen and liver are not congested, circulatory massage may improve recovery time. Noncirculatory types of bodywork may be appropriate, as long as the possibility of lymphatic congestion is considered.

Multiple Chemical Sensitivity Syndrome in Brief (p. 598)

What is it? Multiple chemical sensitivity syndrome (MCSS) is a situation in which a history of toxic exposure initiates a variety of different responses.

How is it recognized? MCSS can involve headaches, disorientation, cognitive difficulties, joint pain, respiratory problems, and other symptoms.

Is massage indicated or contraindicated? People with MCSS need to be careful about massage lubricants, essential oils, perfumes, candles, and other equipment that therapists often use that may trigger a reaction.

Multiple Sclerosis in Brief (p. 193)

What is it? Multiple Sclerosis (MS) is an idiopathic disease that involves the destruction of myelin sheaths around both motor and sensory neurons in the CNS.

How is it recognized? MS has many symptoms, depending on the nature of the damage. These can include fatigue, eye pain, spasticity, tremors, and a progressive loss of vision, sensation, and motor control.

Is massage indicated or contraindicated? Massage is indicated in subacute stages of MS, when the client is in remission, rather than during acute periods where function is diminishing.

Muscular Dystrophy in Brief (p. 74)

What is it? Muscular dystrophy is a group of related inherited disorders, all of which involve the degeneration and wasting of muscle tissue.

How is it recognized? Different varieties of muscular dystrophy destroy different areas of skeletal muscles. The age of onset, initial symptoms, and long-term prognosis depend on what kind of genetic problem is present.

Is massage indicated or contraindicated? The early signs of muscular dystrophy often involve muscles that become tight and constrictive. Physical therapy is often used to prevent or minimize contractures as long as possible; massage can fit in this context as well, as long as the massage therapist is working as part of a health care team.

Myasthenia Gravis in Brief (p. 170)

What is it? Myasthenia gravis (MG) is a neuromuscular disorder in which an autoimmune attack is launched against acetylcholine receptors at the neuromuscular junction. This makes it difficult to stimulate a muscle to contract, leading to fatigue and weakness.

What does it look like? Myasthenia gravis can develop at any age, but it is most common in women in their 20s, and in men in their 50s. It often begins with weakness in facial muscles and in the muscles used in speech, eating, and swallowing. MG is a progressive disease, but it is usually treatable with medical intervention.

Massage? Massage can be appropriate for persons with MG because this disease does not affect sensation. Massage may not impact acetylcholine uptake in any positive way, but it will not make it worse either. Care must be taken to respect the side effects that accompany medications used to treat MG.

Myofascial Pain Syndrome in Brief (p. 68)

What is it? Myofascial pain syndrome (MPS) is a collection of signs and symptoms that indicate trauma to muscles and leads to a cycle of chronic spasm, ischemia, and pain.

How is it recognized? MPS is recognized mainly through the development of trigger points in predictable locations in affected muscles. Trigger points are highly painful both locally and in specific patterns of referred pain.

Is massage indicated or contraindicated? MPS indicates massage, which can "break through" the pain–spasm cycle and help to eradicate the irritating metabolic wastes that accumulate around trigger points.

Myositis Ossificans in Brief (p. 76)

What is it? This is the growth of a bony deposit in soft tissues. It usually follows trauma that involves significant leakage of blood between fascial sheaths.

How is it recognized? An x-ray is the best way to see this problem, but it is palpable as a dense mass where, anatomically, no such thing should be.

Is massage indicated or contraindicated? Massage is always a local contraindication for myositis ossificans, but work around the edges of the area may stimulate the reabsorption of the bone tissue without doing further damage.

Open Wounds and Sores in Brief (p. 51)

What are they? Open wounds and sores are skin injuries that have not completely healed.

How are they recognized? Unhealed lesions may be marked by bleeding, crusts, exuding pus, or other signs of regenerative activity.

Is massage indicated or contraindicated? Any opening in the skin is an open invitation for infection. At the very least, open wounds and sores locally contraindicate massage. They may systemically contraindicate massage if they appear as a sign of serious systemic disease.

Osgood-Schlatter Disease in Brief (p. 143)

What is it? Osgood-Schlatter disease is the result of chronic or traumatic irritation at the insertion of the quadriceps tendon, in combination with adolescent growth spurts.

How is it recognized? When Osgood-Schlatter disease is acute, the tibial tuberosity will be hot, swollen, and painful. The bone may grow a large protuberance at the site of the tendinous insertion.

Is massage indicated or contraindicated? An acute flair of Osgood-Schlatter disease locally contraindicates circulatory massage, which could exacerbate inflammation. Techniques for reducing lymphatic retention, and work elsewhere on the body, are certainly appropriate. A client with a history of Osgood-Schlatter disease but no current inflammation at the knee may benefit from the pain relief and reduction in quadriceps muscle tone that massage can supply.

Osteoarthritis in Brief (p. 109)

What is it? This is joint inflammation brought about by wear-and-tear causing cumulative damage to articular cartilage.

How is it recognized? Affected joints are stiff, painful, and occasionally palpably inflamed. Osteoarthritis most often affects knees, hips, and distal joints of the fingers.

Is massage indicated or contraindicated? Arthritis contraindicates massage if it is acutely inflamed. It indicates massage in the subacute stage, when bodywork can contribute to muscular relaxation and mobility of the affected joint.

Osteoporosis in Brief (p. 89)

What is it? This is loss of bone mass and density brought about by endocrine imbalances and poor metabolism of calcium.

How is it recognized? Osteoporosis in the early stages is identifiable only by x-ray and bone-density tests. In later stages, compression or spontaneous fractures of the vertebrae, wrists, or hips may be present. Kyphosis brought about by compression fractures of the vertebrae is a frequent indicator of osteoporosis.

Is massage indicated or contraindicated? Gentle massage is indicated for persons with osteoporosis, with extra caution for the comfort and safety of the client. Massage will not affect the progression of the disease once it is present, but it may significantly reduce associated pain. Massage for acute fractures, however, is contraindicated.

Ovarian Cancer in Brief (p. 552)

What is it? Ovarian cancer is the development of malignant tumors on the ovaries that may metastasize to other structures in the pelvic or abdominal cavity.

How is it recognized? Symptoms of ovarian cancer are generally extremely subtle until the disease has progressed to life-threatening levels. Early symptoms include a feeling of heaviness in the pelvis, vague abdominal discomfort, occasional vaginal bleeding, and weight gain or loss.

Is massage indicated or contraindicated? As with all cancers, the appropriateness of massage depends on what treatment measures the client chooses. Massage therapists working with clients who have ovarian cancer should be part of a fully informed health care team.

Ovarian Cysts in Brief (p. 555)

What are they? Most ovarian cysts are fluid-filled growths on the ovaries. Some types of cysts are associated with ovarian cancer or other reproductive disorders, but the cysts under discussion in this article are benign.

How are they recognized? The symptoms of ovarian cysts may be nonexistent, or they may cause a disruption in the menstrual cycle. Constant or intermittent pain in the pelvis, pain with intercourse, or symptoms similar to early pregnancy may arise from different types of ovarian cysts.

Is massage indicated or contraindicated? Ovarian cysts that have been diagnosed locally contraindicate massage.

Paget's Disease in Brief (p. 93)

What is it? This is a chronic bone disorder in which healthy bone is rapidly reabsorbed and replaced with fibrous connective tissue that never fully calcifies.

How is it recognized? Paget's disease is often silent. When it does cause symptoms, they usually include deep bone pain, local heat, and sometimes visible deformation of the affected bones. The risk of fractures is also high.

Is massage indicated or contraindicated? Paget's disease is often treated with exercise and physical therapy to maintain flexibility. Massage may fit into this context as well, with caution for the extreme fragility of the affected bones.

Pancreatic Cancer in Brief (p. 474)

What is it? Pancreatic cancer is the growth of malignant cells in the pancreas. It is usually a cancer of the exocrine cells, which normally produce digestive enzymes, but it occasionally grows in the islets cells where hormones are produced.

How is it recognized? Early signs of pancreatic cancer are subtle and not usually alarming: abdominal discomfort, unintended weight loss, and loss of appetite are frequently reported. Later signs may include jaundice, hepatomegaly or splenomegaly, ascites, and signs of distant metastasis, which vary according to location.

Is massage indicated or contraindicated? Pancreatic cancer is almost always fatal within a few months of diagnosis. Massage is appropriate as a comfort measure, particularly as part of a health care team working for pain relief and palliative effects.

Pancreatitis in Brief (p. 476)

What is it? Pancreatitis is the inflammation of the pancreas. It has an acute and chronic form.

How is it recognized? Constant or episodic pain high in the abdomen is the leading sign of pancreatitis. This pain often refers into the back. Other signs have to do with pancreatic dysfunction: poor absorption of food leading to weight loss, secondary diabetes mellitus, and jaundice are all possible signs of pancreatitis.

Is massage indicated or contraindicated? Undiagnosed abdominal pain that persists for more than a few days requires medical attention. Massage is unlikely to make pancreatitis worse unless a therapist works deeply high in the abdomen, but this is a potentially dangerous disease, it is important that a temporary relief in symptoms that massage might bring about not delay a person's getting an accurate diagnosis. After an episode of pancreatitis has passed and the client, doctor, and therapist have a clearer idea of the cause of symptoms, massage may be more appropriate so long as it does not cause pain.

Parkinson's Disease in Brief (p. 199)

What is it? Parkinson's disease is a degenerative disease of the substantia nigra cells in the brain. These cells produce the neurotransmitter dopamine, which helps the basal ganglia to maintain balance, posture, and coordination.

How is it recognized? Early symptoms of Parkinson's include general stiffness and fatigue; resting tremor of the hand, foot, or head; stiffness; and poor balance. Later symptoms include a shuffling gait, a "mask-like" appearance to the face, and a monotone voice.

Is massage indicated or contraindicated? Parkinson's disease indicates massage, with caution. Care must be taken for the physical safety of these clients, who cannot move freely or smoothly.

Patellofemoral Syndrome in Brief (p. 113)

What is it? Patellofemoral syndrome (PFS) is an overuse disorder that can lead to damage of the patellar cartilage.

How is it recognized? PFS causes pain at the knee, stiffness after immobility, and discomfort in walking down stairs.

Is massage indicated or contraindicated? PFS indicates massage, as long as the knee is not acutely inflamed. Massage may or may not be useful to correct this problem, but it will certainly do no harm and can address issues of muscle tightness and imbalance.

Pelvic Inflammatory Disease in Brief (p. 571)

What is it? Pelvic inflammatory disease, or PID, is an infection of female reproductive organs. It starts at the cervix and can move up to infect the uterus, fallopian (uterine) tubes, ovaries, and entire pelvic cavity.

How is it recognized? The symptoms of acute PID include abdominal pain, fever, chills, headache, nausea, and vomiting. Chronic PID may produce no symptoms, or may involve chronic pain, lassitude, and pain during urination and intercourse.

Is massage indicated or contraindicated? Acute PID systemically contraindicates massage until all signs of infection have subsided. Chronic PID may be appropriate for massage if the woman is aware of her condition and is treating it appropriately. Deep work in the lower abdomen or pelvis is not appropriate for women with PID.

Peripheral Neuropathy in Brief (p. 202)

What is it? Peripheral neuropathy is damage to peripheral nerves, usually of the hands and feet, often as a result of some other underlying condition such as alcoholism, diabetes, or lupus.

How is it recognized? Sensory damage, motor damage, or both may be present. Symptoms include burning or tingling pain beginning distally and slowly moving proximally, loss of movement or control of movement, hyperesthesia, and eventual numbness.

Is massage indicated or contraindicated? Peripheral neuropathy contraindicates massage when numbness interferes with the client's ability to give accurate feedback. In other cases, therapists will need to make case-by-case judgments about whether massage fits in the context of the underlying factors.

Peritonitis in Brief (p. 480)

What is it? Peritonitis is inflammation, usually caused by bacterial infection, of the peritoneal lining of the abdomen.

How is it recognized? Acute peritonitis usually shows the signs of systemic infection: fever and chills, along with abdominal pain, rigidity of abdominal muscles, distension, nausea, and vomiting.

Is massage indicated or contraindicated? Acute peritonitis is a medical emergency and contraindicates massage.

Pes Planus in Brief (p. 145)

What is it? These are the medical terms for flat fleet or jammed arches.

How is it recognized? In pes planus, the feet lack any arches. Pronation of the ankle also may be present. Persons with pes cavus have extremely high arches with little or no mobility between the tarsal bones.

Is massage indicated or contraindicated? Pes planus and pes cavus indicate massage. In some cases, the health of intrinsic foot muscles and ligaments can be improved to the point where alignment in the foot is also improved. In cases in which the ligaments are lax through genetic or other problems, massage may not correct the situation, but neither will it make it worse.

Plantar Fasciitis in Brief (p. 147)

What is it? Plantar fasciitis is the pain and inflammation caused by injury to the plantar fascia of the foot.

How is it recognized? Plantar fasciitis is acutely painful after prolonged immobility. Then the pain recedes, but it comes back with extended use. It feels sharp and bruise-like, usually at the anterior calcaneus or deep in the arch, but the pain can appear almost anywhere the plantar fascia goes.

Is massage indicated or contraindicated? Massage is indicated for plantar fasciitis. It can help release tension in deep calf muscles that put strain on the plantar fascia; it also can help to affect the development of scar tissue at the site of the tear.

Pneumonia in Brief (p. 389)

What is it? Pneumonia is an infection in the lungs brought about by bacteria, viruses, or other pathogens.

How is it recognized? The symptoms of pneumonia include coughing that may be dry or productive, high fever, pain on breathing, and shortness of breath. Extreme cases may show cyanosis, or a bluish caste to the skin and nails.

Is massage indicated or contraindicated? Depending on the causative factor and the general resiliency of the person, massage may indicate massage in the subacute stage.

Polio, Postpolio Syndrome in Brief (p. 211)

What is it? Polio is a viral infection, first of the intestines, and then (for approximately 1% of exposed people) the anterior horn cells of the spinal cord. Postpolio syndrome (PPS) is a group of signs and symptoms common to polio survivors, particularly those who experienced significant loss of function in the acute stage of the disease.

How is it recognized? The destruction of motor neurons leads to degeneration, atrophy, and finally paralysis of skeletal muscles in polio patients. Later in life they may develop a sudden onset of fatigue, achiness, and weakness. Breathing and sleeping difficulties also may occur.

Is massage indicated or contraindicated? The polio virus does not affect sensation or cognition. Therefore, massage is appropriate for polio survivors, as long as acute phase of the infection has passed. PPS also indicates massage.

Postoperative Situations in Brief (p. 599)

What are they? Postoperative situations are conditions in which clients are recovering from any kind of surgery.

How is it recognized? Surgeries may be major and invasive, or they may be conducted through tiny holes in the abdomen or through long tubes inserted into blood vessels to get to a destination far away.

Is massage indicated or contraindicated? Massage can be appropriate for persons recovering from surgery, depending on the reason for the surgery and the danger of possible complications.

Postural Deviations in Brief (p. 95)

What are they? Postural deviations are overdeveloped thoracic or lumbar curves (kyphosis and lordosis) or an S-curve in the spine (scoliosis).

How are they recognized? Extreme curvatures are easily visible, although x-rays are used to pinpoint exactly where the problems begin and end.

Is massage indicated or contraindicated? All postural deviations indicate massage as long as other underlying pathologic conditions have been ruled out. Bodywork may or may not be able to reverse any damage, but it can certainly provide relief for the muscular stress that accompanies spinal changes.

Pregnancy in Brief (p. 572)

What is it? Pregnancy is the state of carrying a fetus.

How is it recognized? The symptoms of advanced pregnancy are obvious, but symptoms that specifically pertain to massage include loose ligaments, muscle spasms, clumsiness, and fatigue.

Is massage indicated or contraindicated? All stages of uncomplicated pregnancy indicate massage, with specific cautions relating to each trimester.

Premenstrual Syndrome in Brief (p. 575)

What is it? Premenstrual syndrome (PMS) is a collection of many signs and symptoms that occur in the time between ovulation and menstruation, and then subside after menstruation begins. It may have several different causes and triggers.

How is it recognized? Signs and symptoms of PMS are often divided into physical and emotional features. Physical symptoms include breast tenderness, bloating, digestive upset, fatigue, changes in appetite, backache, and many others. Emotional signs include irritability, anxiety, depression, mood swings, and other possible problems.

Is massage indicated or contraindicated? Although the specific causes of PMS are not clearly understood, it is clear that this condition is not related to infection, structural problems, or neoplasm. Therefore, PMS indicates bodywork, which may help to reestablish balance in the endocrine and nervous systems.

Prostate Cancer in Brief (p. 560)

What is it? Prostate cancer is the growth of malignant cells in the prostate gland, which may then metastasize, usually to nearby bones or into inguinal lymph nodes.

How is it recognized? The symptoms of prostate cancer include problems with urination: weak stream, frequency, urgency, nocturia, and other problems arising from constriction of the urethra.

Is massage indicated or contraindicated? Prostate cancer patients may face any combination of surgery, radiation, chemotherapy, and hormonal therapy to deal with their disease. Bodywork that accommodates for these challenges while minimizing risks can be helpful and supportive, as long as the massage therapist is working as part of a fully informed health care team.

Prostatitis in Brief (p. 563)

What is it? Prostatitis is the inflammation of the prostate gland, from either bacterial or nonbacterial causes.

How is it recognized? Symptoms of prostatitis vary according to their cause. Acute prostatitis involves fever, extremely painful urination, urinary frequency and urgency, and pain in the penis, testicles, perineum, and low back. Chronic prostatitis involves similar symptoms, but they tend to be less severe, and they do not include fever.

Is massage indicated or contraindicated? Judgments about massage in the context of prostatitis need to be made according to the causative factors. An acute bacterial infection contraindicates circulatory bodywork, but a low-grade, noninfectious, chronic situation may not carry the same cautions. "Prostate massage" is a procedure performed by a doctor through the rectal wall and is not within the scope of practice of massage therapists.

Psoriasis in Brief (p. 37)

What is it? Psoriasis is a noncontagious chronic skin disease involving the excessive production of new skin cells that pile up into isolated lesions.

How is it recognized? The most common variety of psoriasis looks like pink or reddish patches, sometimes with a silvery scale on top. It occurs most frequently on elbows and knees, but it can develop anywhere.

Is massage indicated or contraindicated? Psoriasis locally contraindicates massage during the acute stage, because the extra stimulation and circulation massage provides can make a bad situation worse. In subacute stages, however, as long as the skin is intact, massage is a good idea.

Pyelonephritis in Brief (p. 516)

What is it? Pyelonephritis is an infection of the kidney or renal pelvis.

How is it recognized? Symptoms of acute pyelonephritis include burning pain with urination, back pain, fever, chills, nausea, and vomiting. Chronic infections may show no symptoms.

Is massage indicated or contraindicated? Kidney infections systemically contraindicate circulatory massage until the infection has been completely eradicated.

Raynaud's Syndrome in Brief (p. 321)

What is it? Raynaud's syndrome is defined by episodes of vasospasm of the arterioles, usually in fingers and toes, and occasionally in the nose, ears, and lips.

How is it recognized? Affected areas will often go through marked color changes of white or ashy gray for dark-skinned people, to blue to red. Attacks can last for less than a minute or several hours. Numbness or tingling may follow during recovery.

Is massage indicated or contraindicated? Massage is indicated for Raynaud's syndrome that is not associated with underlying pathologic conditions. Otherwise, follow the guidelines for the precipitating condition.

Reflex Sympathetic Dystrophy Syndrome in Brief (p. 242)

What is it? Reflex sympathetic dystrophy syndrome (RSDS) is a chronic pain condition in which an initial trauma causes pain that is more severe and longer lasting than is reasonable to expect. The pain can become a self-sustaining phenomenon that becomes a lifelong affliction.

How is it recognized? RSDS moves in stages, although symptoms may overlap. In early stages, it involves redness, heat, sweating, and severe burning pain. In later stages, the skin may turn bluish, and the nearby joints and muscles may atrophy. Bones in the area thin and become vulnerable to breakage. Late-stage RSDS can involve irreversible changes to the affected area and symptoms that spread to other parts of the body.

Is massage indicated or contraindicated? Most RSDS patients have little or no tolerance for touch of any kind, at least in the area where the pain syndrome began. Physical therapy is often recommended to keep the affected joints moveable and functioning; massage may help to relieve some of the pain associated with this therapy. Massage within tolerance in other parts of the body may be welcome and supportive.

Renal Failure in Brief (p. 518)

What is it? Renal failure is a situation in which the kidneys are incapable of functioning at normal levels. It may be an acute or a chronic problem, and it is potentially life-threatening.

How is it recognized? Symptoms of acute and chronic renal failure differ in severity and type of onset, but some things they have in common are reduced urine output, systemic edema, and changes in mental state brought about by the accumulation of toxins in the blood.

Is massage indicated or contraindicated? Acute and chronic renal failure systemically contraindicate circulatory massage.

Rheumatoid Arthritis in Brief (p. 114)

What is it? Rheumatoid arthritis (RA) is an autoimmune disease in which immune system agents attack synovial membranes, particularly of the joints in the hands and feet. Other structures, such as muscles, tendons, and blood vessels, also may be affected.

How is it recognized? In the acute phase, affected joints are red, swollen, hot, and painful. They often become gnarled and distorted. It tends to affect the body symmetrically, and it is not determined by age.

Is massage indicated or contraindicated? Massage is indicated in the subacute stages of RA only. At that point, it may be used to reestablish mobility and to reduce the stresses that can trigger another flare.

Scar Tissue in Brief (p. 52)

What is it? Scar tissue is the growth of new tissue—skin or fascia—after injury.

How is it recognized? Scar tissue on the skin often lacks pigmentation and hair follicles.

Is massage indicated or contraindicated? Massage is contraindicated during the acute stage of any injury in which the skin has been damaged. In the sub-acute stage, massage may improve the quality of the healing process.

Scleroderma in Brief (p. 149)

What is it? Scleroderma is a chronic autoimmune disorder involving damage to small blood vessels that leads to abnormal accumulations of scar tissue in the skin. Internal organs also may be affected.

How is it recognized? Scleroderma can have many varied symptoms, depending on which tissues are involved. The most common outward signs are edema followed by hardening and thickening of the skin, usually of the hands and face.

Is massage indicated or contraindicated? Scleroderma may indicate massage if circulatory and kidney damage is not advanced. Clients whose systems are not capable of keeping up with the changes circulatory massage brings about may benefit from bodywork with less mechanical impact.

Seizure Disorders in Brief (p. 269)

What are they? Seizure disorders are any condition that causes seizures. They are often related to some kind of neurologic damage in the shape of tumors, head injuries, or infection, although it may be impossible to delineate exactly what that damage is. Epilepsy is a subtype of seizure disorder.

How are they recognized? Seizures may take very different forms for different people; they range from barely noticeable to life-threatening. Seizure disorders are diagnosed through physical examination, a description of symptoms, computed tomography (CT) scans, magnetic resonance imaging (MRI) scans, and electroencephalograms (EEGs).

Is massage indicated or contraindicated? Seizure activity itself contraindicates massage, but bodywork is certainly appropriate for patients with most kinds of seizure disorders at any other time.

Septic Arthritis in Brief (p. 118)

What is it? Septic arthritis is joint inflammation caused by infection inside the joint capsule.

How is it recognized? This conditions shows the cardinal signs of inflammation: pain, heat, redness, and swelling, although these symptoms may be mild. It is often accompanied by fever.

Is massage indicated or contraindicated? Massage is contraindicated for septic arthritis until the infection is completely gone from the joint. At that time, massage may be useful to help restore function.

Sexually Transmitted Diseases in Brief (p. 577)

What are they? Sexually transmitted diseases (STDs) are contagious conditions that are spread through intimate contact. The three major diseases discussed here are all bacterial infections: chlamydia, gonorrhea, and syphilis. Most other STDs are viral infections, including genital herpes, molluscum contagiosum, and genital warts.

How are they recognized? The major bacterial STDs all share some common signs, when any signs are present at all. These include penile or vaginal discharge, painful urination, and painful intercourse. Other more specific symptoms vary by causative agent.

Is massage indicated or contraindicated? Bacterial STDs are responsive to antibiotic therapy. Once an infection has been identified and controlled, massage is perfectly appropriate. Silent conditions that are untreated may lead to serious complications that contraindicate massage, depending on the severity of the infection.

Shin Splints in Brief (p. 77)

What are they? "Shin splints" refers to a collection of lower leg injuries including compartment syndromes, muscle tears, periostitis, hairline fractures, and other problems. They are usually brought about by overuse or misalignment in the ankle.

How are they recognized? Pain along the tibia may be superficial or deep, mild or severe. The pattern of pain differs with the specific structures that are injured.

Is massage indicated or contraindicated? Muscle injuries indicate massage, but it must be used with caution for periostitis or stress fractures. Acute exertional compartment syndrome contraindicates massage.

Sinusitis in Brief (p. 392)

What is it? Sinusitis is inflammation of the paranasal sinuses from allergies, infection, or physical obstruction.

How is it recognized? Symptoms include headaches, localized tenderness over the affected area, runny or congested nose, facial or tooth pain, headache, fatigue and, if it is related to an infection, thick opaque mucus, fever, and chills.

Is massage indicated or contraindicated? Acute infections contraindicate massage, but in chronic or noninfectious situations, it can be appropriate for bodywork as long as the client is comfortable on the table.

Skin Cancer in Brief (p. 39)

What is it? Skin cancer is cancer in the stratum basale of the epidermis (basal cell carcinoma or BCC); cancer of the keratinocytes in the epidermis (squamous cell carcinoma or SCC); or cancer of the melanocytes (pigment cells) of the epidermis (malignant melanoma).

How is it recognized? For BCC and SCC, look for the cardinal sign: sores that never heal. These sores can resemble blisters, warts, pimples, or simple unexplained bumps and abrasions. They are usually painless, but they may bleed or become slightly itchy as the cells become active. For malignant melanoma, look for a mole that exhibits the ABCDEs of melanoma.

Is massage indicated or contraindicated? For BCC, which does not metastasize, massage is a local contraindication, as long as a dermatologist has diagnosed the lesion. SCC and malignant melanoma carry the risk of metastasis. Therefore, any decisions about massage must be made according to the treatments the client is having, weighing possible benefits with possible risks.

Sleep Disorders in Brief (p. 271)

What are they? Sleep disorders are a collection of problems including insomnia, sleep apnea, restless leg syndrome, narcolepsy, and circadian rhythm disruption that make it difficult to get enough sleep or to wake up feeling rested and refreshed.

How are they recognized? The primary symptom of sleep disorders is excessive daytime sleepiness. If this continues for a prolonged period, a weakened immune system, memory and concentration loss, and an increased risk of automotive or on-the-job accidents may occur.

Is massage indicated or contraindicated? Sleep disorders indicate massage. Bodywork may not correct a mechanical or psychological dysfunction that leads to sleep deprivation, but it can improve the quality of sleep and can reduce the mental and physical stresses that may interfere with sleep.

Spasms, Cramps in Brief (p. 80)

What are they? Spasms and cramps are involuntary contractions of skeletal muscle. Spasms are considered to be low-grade long-lasting contractions, whereas cramps are short-lived, very acute contractions.

How are they recognized? Cramps are extremely painful, with visible shortening of muscle fibers. Long-term spasms are painful and may cause inefficient movement, but they may not have acute symptoms.

Is massage indicated or contraindicated? Acutely cramping muscle bellies do not invite massage, although stretching and origin/insertion work can trick the proprioceptors into letting go. Muscles that have been cramping respond well to massage, which can reduce residual pain and clean up chemical wastes. Underlying cramp-causing pathologic conditions must be ruled out before massage is applied. Massage is indicated for long-term spasm because it can break through the ischemia-spasm-pain cycle to reintroduce circulation to the area, as well as reduce muscle tone and flush out toxins.

Spina Bifida in Brief (p. 245)

What is it? Spina bifida is a neural tube defect resulting in an incompletely formed vertebral arch, damage to the meninges or spinal cord, and a high risk of distal paralysis and infection.

How is it recognized? Spina bifida can be detected through prenatal testing, but the most obvious sign is a protrusion, sometimes covered by skin, of a cyst containing the dural and arachnoid layers of the meninges, and, usually, the spinal cord as well.

Is massage indicated or contraindicated? Infants recovering from spina bifida surgery are given rigorous physical therapy to establish and maintain function, especially in the abdomen and legs. Massage is appropriate in this context as well. For adults with spina bifida, the judgment about massage depends on the extent of the damage, complicating factors, and the presence or absence of sensation.

Spinal Cord Injury in Brief (p. 248)

What is it? Spinal cord injury (SCI) is a situation in which some or all of the fibers in the spinal cord have been damaged, usually by trauma, but occasionally from other problems such as tumors or bony growths in the spinal canal.

How is it recognized? The signs and symptoms of spinal cord injury vary with the nature of the injury. Loss of motor function follows destruction of motor neurons, but that paralysis may be flaccid or spastic depending on the injured area. Loss of sensation follows the destruction of sensory pathways. If the injury is not complete, some motor or sensory function may remain in the affected tissues.

Is massage indicated or contraindicated? Mechanical types of massage are appropriate only where sensation is present and no underlying pathologic conditions may be exacerbated by the work. Areas without sensation contraindicate massage that intends to manipulate and influence the elasticity of tissue.

Spondylosis in Brief (p. 120)

What is it? Spondylosis is osteoarthritis of the spine.

How is it recognized? It is identifiable by x-ray, which shows a characteristic thickening of the affected vertebral bodies, facets, and ligamentum flava. Pain will be present only if pressure is exerted on nerve roots, causing pain, numbness, paresthesia, and specific muscle weakness. Otherwise, the only sign of spondylosis may be slow, progressive loss of range of motion in the spine.

Is massage indicated or contraindicated? Spondylosis indicates massage with caution. Muscle splinting to protect against movement that may be dangerous is often a feature of this condition; massage therapists should not interfere with this mechanism.

Sprains in Brief (p. 123)

What are they? Sprains are injured ligaments. Injuries can range from a few traumatized fibers to a complete rupture.

How are they recognized? In the acute stage pain, redness, heat, swelling, and loss of joint function will be evident. In the sub-acute stage, these symptoms will be abated, although perhaps not entirely absent. Passive stretching of the affected ligament will be painful until all inflammation has subsided.

Is massage indicated or contraindicated? Subacute sprains indicate massage. Bodywork can influence the healthy development of scar tissue and reduce swelling and damage due to edematous ischemia. Therapists must take care to rule out bone fractures or other injuries that sprains may temporarily mask.

Stomach Cancer in Brief (p. 438)

What is it? Stomach cancer is the development of malignant tumors in the stomach, which may then metastasize directly to other abdominal organs, or through blood and lymph flow to distant places in the body.

How is it recognized? Symptoms of stomach cancer include a feeling of fullness after only a little food, heartburn, unintentional weight loss, blood in the stools, vague abdominal pain above the navel, and occasionally vomiting, constipation, or diarrhea.

Is massage indicated or contraindicated? The prognosis for stomach cancer, which is rarely found before metastasis, is generally not promising. Most clients who know that they have stomach cancer will probably be undergoing a series of treatments including surgeries, chemotherapy, and radiation. Bodywork to alleviate the discomforts of cancer treatment may be appropriate, as long as the risks involved with each type of intervention are respected.

Strains in Brief (p. 82)

What are they? Strains are injuries to muscles.

How are they recognized? Pain, stiffness, and occasionally palpable heat and swelling are all signs of muscle strain. Pain may be exacerbated by passive stretching or resisted contraction of the affected muscle.

Is massage indicated or contraindicated? Muscle strains indicate massage, which can powerfully influence the production of useful scar tissue, reduce adhesions and edema, and reestablish range of motion.

Stroke in Brief (p. 252)

What is it? A stroke is damage to brain tissue caused either by a blockage in blood flow or by an internal hemorrhage.

How is it recognized? The symptoms of stroke include paralysis, weakness, or numbness on one side; blurry or diminished vision on one side with asymmetrically dilated pupils; dizziness and confusion; difficulty in speaking or understanding simple sentences; sudden extreme headache; and possibly loss of consciousness.

Is massage indicated or contraindicated? Most people who survive strokes are at high risk for other cardiovascular problems. Rigorous circulatory massage should probably be avoided with this group, although they may certainly benefit from other types of bodywork to augment their rehabilitative physical therapy.

Temporomandibular Joint Disorders in Brief (p. 126)

What are they? Temporomandibular joint disorders arise when constant strain, stress, and malocclusion of the jaw lead to pain and loss of function of the temporomandibular joint.

How is it recognized? Symptoms of TMJ disorder include head, neck, and shoulder pain, ear pain, mouth pain, clicking or locking in the jaw, and loss of range of motion in the jaw.

Is massage indicated or contraindicated? Massage can be useful for TMJ problems, if intervention is begun before bony deformation begins. However, this condition can be difficult to diagnose, so it is important to be working with other medical professionals in these situations.

Tendinitis in Brief (p. 152)

What is it? Tendinitis is inflammation of a tendon, usually caused by injury at the tenoperiosteal or musculotendinous junction.

How is it recognized? Pain and stiffness are usually present, and in acute stages palpable heat and swelling will occur. Pain is exacerbated by resisted exercise of the injured muscle–tendon unit.

Is massage indicated or contraindicated? Tendinitis indicates massage. In the acute stage, lymph drainage techniques may help to limit and resolve inflammation. In the subacute stage, massage may influence the production of useful scar tissue, reduce adhesions and edema, and reestablish range of motion.

Tenosynovitis in Brief (p. 153)

What is it? Tenosynovitis is the inflammation of a tendon or its surrounding tenosynovial sheath. It can happen wherever a tendon passes through a sheath, but it is especially common in the wrist and hand.

How is it recognized? Pain, heat, and stiffness mark the acute stage of tenosynovitis. In the sub-acute stage, only stiffness and pain may be present. The tendon may feel or sound gritty as it moves through the sheath. It is difficult to bend fingers with tenosynovitis, but even harder to straighten them.

Is massage indicated or contraindicated? Tenosynovitis contraindicates massage in the acute stage of inflammation and indicates massage when the swelling has subsided.

Testicular Cancer in Brief (p. 565)

What is it? Testicular cancer is the growth of malignant cells in the testicles, which may then metastasize all over the body.

How is it recognized? Early signs of testicular cancer include a painless lump in the scrotum, a dull ache in the low abdomen or groin, a sense of heaviness in the scrotum, and enlarged or tender breasts.

Is massage indicated or contraindicated? Guidelines about massage in the context of testicular cancer follow the same rules as for other types of cancer. This particular variety of cancer usually has an excellent prognosis and responds well to radiation or chemotherapy. Massage may be a useful adjunct to these therapies to improve tolerance and shorten recovery time, but it must be conducted within the client's tolerance, and as part of a fully integrated health care effort.

Thoracic Outlet Syndrome in Brief (p. 172)

What is it? Thoracic outlet syndrome (TOS) is a collection of signs and symptoms brought about by occlusion of nerve and blood supply to the arm.

How is it recognized? Depending on which structures are compressed, TOS will show shooting pains, weakness, numbness, and paresthesia ("pins and needles") along with a feeling of fullness and possible discoloration of the affected arm from impaired circulation.

Is massage indicated or contraindicated? This depends on the source of the problem. If it is related to muscle tightness, massage is indicated. TOS symptoms due to muscle degeneration or some other disorder such as spondylosis or herniated disc will not respond well to massage.

Thrombophlebitis, Deep Vein Thrombosis in Brief (p. 304)

What is it? Thrombophlebitis and deep vein thrombosis (DVT) are inflammations of veins due to blood clots.

How is it recognized? Symptoms for thrombophlebitis may or may not include pain, heat, redness, swelling and local itchiness, and a hard cord-like feeling at the affected vein. Symptoms for DVT may be nonexistent, or they can be more extreme: possibly pitting edema distal to the site, often with discoloration, and intermittent or continuous pain that is exacerbated by activity or standing still for a long period.

Is massage indicated or contraindicated? Thrombophlebitis and deep vein thrombosis contraindicate any kind of bodywork that may disrupt clots, which could lead to a pulmonary embolism.

Torticollis in Brief (p. 155)

What is it? Torticollis is a unilateral spasm of neck muscles. It can be caused by a variety of factors, including mild musculoskeletal injury, congenital abnormalities, or CNS problems.

How is it recognized? Flexion and rotation of the head are the main symptoms. The spasm may be constant or intermittent. Torticollis may also cause pain in the neck, shoulders, and back.

Is massage indicated or contraindicated? This depends on the cause of the problem. Simple wryneck from trigger points, cervical misalignment, ligament sprain, or trauma may be appropriate for massage if no acute inflammation is present. Spasmodic torticollis patients may benefit from pain relief offered by massage, but work should be done in cooperation with the patient's health care team. If symptoms do not improve, or if signs of systemic infection are present, a more thorough diagnosis should be sought.

Traumatic Brain Injury in Brief (p. 257)

What is it? Traumatic brain injury (TBI) is damage to the brain brought about by trauma rather than congenital or chronic degenerative disease.

How is it recognized? Symptoms of TBI vary according to the location and severity of the injury. Long-term effects range from mild cognitive impairment, learning problems, and motor control difficulties to varying types of coma or persistent vegetative state.

Is massage indicated or contraindicated? Many TBI patients undergo intensive physical, occupational, and speech therapy to preserve or recover motor function. Carefully administered massage is also appropriate, as long as it is incorporated within the patient's health care plan and does not pose any risk in the presence of spasticity, numbness, or psychiatric disturbance.

Tremor in Brief (p. 204)

What is it? Tremor is rhythmic, involuntary muscle movement. It can be a primary disorder (unrelated to other problems), or it can be a symptom of other neurologic diseases.

How is it recognized? Tremor is identified through uncontrolled fine or gross motor movements.

Is massage indicated or contraindicated? Tremor may indicate massage, as long as no contraindicating conditions are contributing factors.

Trigeminal Neuralgia in Brief (p. 259)

What is it? Trigeminal neuralgia (TN) is a condition involving sharp electrical or stabbing pain along one or more branches of the trigeminal nerve (cranial nerve V), usually in the lower face and jaw.

How is it recognized? The pain of TN is very sharp and severe. Patients report stabbing, electrical or burning sensations that occur in brief episodes, but that repeat with or without identifiable triggers. A muscular tic is often present as well.

Is massage indicated or contraindicated? TN is intensely painful, and even very light touch may trigger an attack. It therefore contraindicates massage on the face, unless the client specifically guides the therapist into what feels safe and comfortable. Massage elsewhere on the body is appropriate, although TN clients may prefer not to be face down.

Tuberculosis in Brief (p. 396)

What is it? Tuberculosis is a bacterial infection that usually begins in the lungs but may spread to bones, kidney, lymph nodes, or elsewhere in the body. It is a highly contagious airborne disease.

How is it recognized? Infection with the tuberculosis bacterium may produce no initial symptoms. If the infection turns into the active disease, symptoms may include coughing, bloody sputum, fatigue, weight loss, and night sweats.

Is massage indicated or contraindicated? Active tuberculosis disease contraindicates massage, unless the client has been on consistent medication for several weeks and has medical clearance. Massage for clients with tuberculosis infection but no disease is fine, but these people should be under medical supervision as well.

Ulcerative Colitis in Brief (p. 456)

What is it? Ulcerative colitis is a condition in which the mucosal layer of the colon becomes inflamed and develops shallow ulcers.

How is it recognized? Symptoms of acute ulcerative colitis include abdominal cramping pain, chronic diarrhea, blood and pus in stools, weight loss, and mild fever.

Is massage indicated or contraindicated? Acute ulcerative colitis contraindicates circulatory massage at least locally; massage is systemically contraindicated in the presence of fever. In subacute situations, gentle abdominal massage may be helpful, but only within the tolerance of the client.

Ulcers in Brief (p. 441)

What are they? Ulcers are sores that for various reasons do not go through a normal healing process; they remain open and vulnerable to infection. Peptic ulcers occur in the esophagus, stomach, or duodenum: the proximal portion of the small intestine.

How are they recognized? The symptoms of peptic ulcers include general burning or gnawing abdominal pain between meals that is relieved by taking antacids or eating. Other symptoms can include bloating, burping, gas, and consistent vomiting after meals.

Is massage indicated or contraindicated? Specific work on the abdomen may exacerbate symptoms of peptic ulcers, so they are at least a local contraindication for mechanical types of bodywork. Other modalities, and massage away from the upper abdomen are certainly indicated for ulcer patients.

Urinary Tract Infection in Brief (p. 524)

What is it? A urinary tract infection (UTI) is an infection of the urinary tract, usually from bacteria that live harmlessly in the digestive tract.

How is it recognized? Symptoms of UTI include pain and burning sensations during urination, increased urinary frequency, urgency, and cloudy or blood-tinged urine. Abdominal, pelvic, or low back pain may occur. In the acute stage, fever and general malaise may be present.

Is massage indicated or contraindicated? Acute UTIs contraindicate circulatory massage, as do all acute infections. Massage may be appropriate in the subacute stage, although deep work on the abdomen is still locally cautioned until all signs of infection are gone.

Varicose Veins in Brief (p. 324)

What are they? Varicose veins are distended veins, usually in the legs, caused by vascular incompetence and a reflux of blood returning to the heart.

How are they recognized? Varicose veins are ropey, slightly bluish, elevated veins that twist and turn out of their usual course. They happen most frequently in branches of the saphenous veins on the medial side of the calf, although they are also found on the posterior aspects of the calf and thigh.

Is massage indicated or contraindicated? Massage is locally contraindicated for extreme varicose veins, and anywhere distal to them. Mild varicose veins contraindicate deep, specific work, but they are otherwise safe for massage.

Warts in Brief (p. 21)

What are they? Warts are neoplasms that arise from the keratinocytes in the epidermis; they are caused by extremely slow-acting viruses.

How are they recognized? Typical warts (verruca vulgaris) look like hard, cauliflower-shaped growths. They usually occur on the hands. They can affect anyone, but teenagers are especially prone to them.

Is massage indicated or contraindicated? Massage is a local contraindication for warts. The virus is contained in the blood and shedding skin cells, and it is possible to get warts from another person.

Whiplash in Brief (p. 157)

What is it? Whiplash is an umbrella term referring to a collection of soft tissue injuries that may occur with cervical acceleration/deceleration. These injuries include sprained ligaments, strained muscles, damaged cartilage and joint capsules, and temporomandibular joint (TMJ) problems. Although whiplash technically refers to soft-tissue injury, damage to other structures, including vertebrae, discs, and the CNS, frequently occurs at the same time.

How is it recognized? Symptoms of whiplash vary according to the nature of the injuries. Pain at the neck and referring into the shoulders and arms along with chronic headaches are the primary indicators.

Is massage indicated or contraindicated? An acute whiplash injury contraindicates circulatory or mechanically based massage. In the subacute and mature phases of scar tissue formation, however, massage along with chiropractic or manipulation can contribute greatly to a positive resolution to the problem.

APPENDIX II

TAKING A CLIENT HISTORY

Taking a thorough client health history is a delicate art, especially if it is to be done in less than 1 hour. Many people have uncomplicated backgrounds and simple complaints and disorders, but as massage moves into the medical mainstream, therapists will need to be prepared to deal responsibly and professionally with clients whose lists of diseases, conditions, accidents, surgeries, and medications can make a person's head swim.

Massage therapists go to school to learn how to touch people in ways that are beneficial to their health. They also go to massage school to learn whom *not* to touch, or at least not to touch in certain ways. The health history is the first conversation a therapist has with a potential client about his or her body; this is the time to make that all-important judgment about the appropriateness of massage. The time will come for most therapists when they will have to turn someone away, at least temporarily. It is not easy to do, but knowing that it is, above all, for the client's safety and benefit, makes it an easier task.

A successful client–therapist relationship is a partnership in which both parties work together toward specific goals. The most important quality for massage therapists to cultivate as they learn how to establish this relationship is careful, patient listening. This skill is a rare one, but it is critical for a successful practice. Massage therapy clients put themselves in very vulnerable, intimate relationships with virtual strangers. If massage therapists are good listeners and show understanding about clients' experiences, the relationship can be one of warmth, safety, and productivity rather than disconnection or even anxiety.

What follows is a sample client history form that might be used in a massage clinic specializing in circulatory-based bodywork. Relevant questions are discussed to see how some answers might influence the decision-making process. Finally, some ideas for creating possible treatment plans are offered.

This is a longer, more detailed intake form than many therapists use. Nevertheless, it can provide a great deal of valuable information not only about a client's present status, but about his or her past experiences and current attitudes about health. It is often a good idea to schedule an extra-long appointment for a therapist and client to go through this form together.

It is utterly impossible to create a comprehensive guideline for taking client histories; there are simply too many variables. The way some conditions connect to or hint at others; whether a client is taking various kinds of medications; a client's occupation, working conditions, and living conditions; and the way sleep, diet, and exercise habits can influence overall health all influence the decision about whether certain types of massage may be appropriate, or whether, perhaps, the client should seek help elsewhere.

Sample Client History Form

Name

Address

Billing Information

General Information

Age

Occupation

Describe your exercise habits:

Describe your general diet:

Describe how well you sleep:

Describe your general health:

Health History

Have you ever had any surgery or hospitalization?
    More than 10 years ago:
    5 to 10 years ago:
    Less than 5 years ago:

Have you ever been involved in an injury or an accident?
    More than 10 years ago:
    5 to 10 years ago:
    Less than 5 years ago:

What kind of care did you receive?

Do you consider that you have recovered from these events?

Do you have any chronic, ongoing conditions that you deal with on a regular basis? Explain.

Are you taking any medication? Explain.

Are you currently seeing a doctor for any reason? Explain.

Do you have any skin rashes or other skin problems right now?

Check off any of the following conditions that you have experienced:

Skin
Boils
Fungal infections
Herpes simplex
Warts
Eczema
Psoriasis
Skin cancer

Musculoskeletal
Fibromyalgia
Rheumatoid arthritis
Osteoarthritis
TMJ dysfunction
Strains, sprains or tendinitis
Carpal tunnel syndrome
Thoracic outlet syndrome

Nervous
Depression
Multiple sclerosis
Postpolio syndrome
Headaches
Stroke
Seizure disorders
Reduced sensation
Sleep disorders
Chemical dependency

Circulatory
Anemia
Thrombophlebitis
Deep vein thrombosis
High blood pressure
Heart disease
Varicose veins
Clotting disorders

Lymph/Immune
Edema
Leukemia/lymphoma
HIV/AIDS
Chronic fatigue syndrome
Lupus
Other autoimmune disorders

Respiratory
Asthma
Emphysema
Sinusitis
Tuberculosis

Digestive
GERD (reflux)
Ulcers
Crohn disease
Ulcerative colitis
Irritable bowel syndrome
Gallstones
Cirrhosis
Hepatitis

Endocrine
Diabetes
Hypothyroidism
Hyperthyroidism

Urinary
Kidney stones
Renal failure

Reproductive
Breast cancer
Endometriosis
Ovarian cysts
Prostate cancer
Painful menstruation
Are you pregnant?

Other:
Explanation:

Treatment Goals:
Why are you here? What do you hope to accomplish?

Please indicate where you have pain:

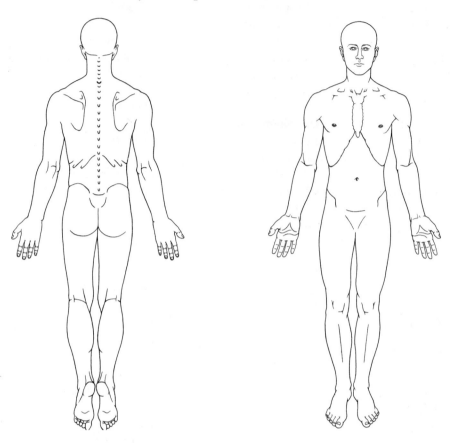

Describe what you do that causes pain and what activities tend to make it worse:

Do you have any questions about massage?

Disclaimer

General Questions

Age

Age is a pertinent question because some conditions are particularly prevalent in certain age groups. Of course, it is fairly easy to tell whether a client is within a reasonable age expectation for these conditions just by sight, but getting it in writing anyway is a good idea.

Occupation

This is a key piece of information, particularly for clients who come in with specific pain patterns or injuries that they want to address. This question can lead to a brief discussion of the physical demands that a job may place on a person. The massage therapist should not hesitate to try to "act out" any repetitive or stressful motions a client describes, in an attempt to understand how these activities might contribute to pain and dysfunction.

Exercise, Sleeping, Eating Habits

These descriptions can reveal how a client sees her health efforts. This is not the time to pass judgment or make recommendations; it is rather a chance to add information to the whole picture.

General Health Description

Many people will describe themselves as basically healthy, but some will come seeking massage to help them cope with ongoing difficult physical situations. How a client perceives her own health is a useful piece of information.

Health History

Surgeries and Hospitalizations

For convenience, these are broken into three time periods. Knowing about long-ago events is useful because they may influence what is currently happening. However, knowing what has been going on in more recent history is usually more crucial.

Injuries and Accidents

As with surgeries and hospitalizations, recent events are usually more pertinent than ancient history, but the complete picture can reveal important patterns. This question should elicit information about on-the-job injuries, sports injuries, car accidents, and any other kinds of trauma that caused significant pain or loss of function.

Care and Recovery

The follow-up questions about accidents and injuries give information about the client's perspective of her healing process.

Ongoing, Chronic Conditions

This question will be asked again in a different way with the check-off list of diseases, but it is always good to give clients an extra chance to reveal important information.

Seeing a Doctor

If a client is under a doctor's care, she probably has at least a moderately serious condition that massage may influence for better or worse. It is never a bad idea to inform a primary care physician that a particular patient wishes to include massage as part of her health care.

Taking Medication

If the answer to this question is yes, it is vitally important to know *why*. If a client is unsure why, then a consultation with the primary care physician is called for.

Medications for cardiovascular problems, high blood pressure, kidney dysfunction, antibiotics, pain killers, muscle relaxants, and antidepressants all have implications for massage. A discussion of why a client may need them and how to fit massage into the picture will keep both client and therapist on safe ground.

Skin Rashes

This is a self-defensive question for massage therapists, as well as an important part of the health picture. If the answer is yes, again it is important to know *why*. A skin rash may be just a local caution, or it may suggest that a client needs to reschedule.

Check-off List

If everything has gone well, nothing will appear on this list that has not already been discussed. This is by no means a complete list of every condition a person is likely to encounter, but the conditions included here are either chronic, ongoing, or repetitive situations, or they have special significance to massage therapists. This list is simply a suggestion. As therapists develop their own client history forms, they may have other conditions they wish to include, and some they prefer to leave out.

Disclaimer

Many people recommend including a disclaimer explaining that a massage therapist does not diagnose conditions or treat them medically and that it is the client's responsibility to seek medical care appropriately and to keep the therapist updated on her health status.

Treatment Plan

The difference between an outstanding massage therapist and a so-so one is intention. Good massage therapists always know why they are doing what they are doing, and though those goals and methods may change from moment to moment, the consciousness of working with purpose should always be present. Treatment plans are important tools for therapists and clients. They provide a basis for "before and after" comparisons and reminders of intentions for future work. Even clients who are just seeking massage as a once-in-a-while treat can benefit from the clarification of goals that a treatment plan can offer.

Having a human figure drawing that a client can mark with painful spots is a useful visual guide that will accompany a therapist's own sensitivities. Some people recommend that a client mark this figure with numbers from 1 to 10, indicating how painful certain areas might be.

Problems areas can change, move, and even disappear. Treatment goals also may change as a person's health status evolves. Having clients redo this portion of the history form every few appointments can provide useful progress reports for the client–therapist team.

Some massage therapists use a standard "SOAP" format to accompany the general health information with a client history. It can be used with each appointment, or updated as needed. This format is as follows:

Subjective Findings

That is, what does the client report—what hurts, where, when, and under what circumstances.

Objective Findings

That is, what does the therapist find—are there different areas from the client's description that are painful? Does the tissue have varying qualities of elasticity and resilience in different areas? Are there hot spots? Cold areas? Limited range of motion?

Assessment

This is the therapist's interpretation of findings. It is *not* a diagnosis, but rather a pulling together of information to create an understanding of why a client is experiencing her symptoms.

Plan

This is the strategy the client and therapist will use together to achieve their goals. It might be as simple as "Swedish massage for relaxation of muscles, improved circulation, and pain relief in upper back" or as complex as "Cross fiber friction to specific tendon insertions with range of motion gymnastics followed by ice and a referral to a physical therapist for strengthening exercises to overcome a chronic tendinitis."

An example of a client intake form is included here. This client is a real person, whose long-ago problems have recurring influence on her everyday living.

Sample Client History Form

Name *Janet M.*

General Information

Age *34*

Occupation: *Accounting. I sit at the computer and on the phone for 8 hours a day. I have a cordless headset.*

Describe your exercise habits: *I walk two times a day, for fifteen minutes. Some days are more vigorous than others. From July to October I coach cheer-leading, and I never ask the girls to do something I'm not willing to do.*

Describe your general diet: *I have a quick breakfast: a bagel or something like that. Lunch depends on how busy I am. It could be some yogurt, or a microwave meal. Sometimes I have* *leftovers from last night's supper. Dinner is always a sit-down meal. We eat lots of fruit and veggies.*

Describe how well you sleep: *I usually sleep for six hours, but I never feel rested. I can always remember my dreams. I never seem to get past the dream stage.*

Describe your general health: *It's pretty good. I seldom get sick, although it's happened more this year than ever before. I have to make myself do a lot of things—I have very low energy. And depression is a factor in all of this too.*

Health History

Describe any surgery or hospitalization:
    More than 10 years ago:
1988: childbirth, followed by cryosurgery for dysplasia.
    5 to 10 years ago:
1990: I had a kidney stone while I was pregnant. I finally passed it, soon before my daughter was born. If I hadn't, they would have taken it out right after labor.
    Less than 5 years ago:
Four years ago I had two surgeries for thoracic outlet syndrome. In the first one, they went in through the axilla on the left side. They took out the cervical rib and the first rib. A month later they did the same thing on the right side, but they only took the first rib. The cervical rib was too small to worry about.

Describe any injuries or accidents:
    More than 10 years ago:
I was in a VW in the middle of a 5-car pile up. My little car ended up looking like an accordion.
    5 to 10 years ago:
    Less than 5 years ago:

What kind of care did you receive?
No care for the whiplash following the car wreck. Lots of physical therapy following my surgeries.

Do you consider that you have recovered from these events? Please explain:
Oh, yes. Before I had surgery, I couldn't even hold my hands above my shoulders.

Do you have any chronic, ongoing conditions that you deal with on a regular basis? Explain.
Sure. I have pain, fatigue, stress, and depression. Several months ago I was diagnosed with fibromyalgia.

Are you taking any medication? Please explain:
I take Zoloft, an anti-depressant.

Are you currently seeing a doctor for any reason? Please explain:
Yes, I see an MD for fibromyalgia and a chiropractor as needed.

Do you have any skin rashes or other skin problems right now?
No.

Check off any of the following conditions that you have experienced:

Skin
Boils
Fungal infections
Herpes simplex
Warts
Eczema
Psoriasis
Skin cancer

Musculoskeletal
✓ Fibromyalgia
Rheumatoid arthritis
Osteoarthritis
TMJ dysfunction
Strains, sprains or tendinitis
Carpal tunnel syndrome
✓ Thoracic outlet syndrome

Nervous
Depression
Multiple sclerosis
Postpolio syndrome
✓ Headaches
Stroke
Seizure disorders
Reduced sensation
Sleep disorders
Chemical dependency

Circulatory
Anemia
Thrombophlebitis
Deep vein thrombosis
High blood pressure
Heart disease
Varicose veins
Clotting disorders

Lymph/Immune
Edema
Leukemia/lymphoma
HIV/ AIDS
✓ Chronic fatigue syndrome
Lupus
Other autoimmune disorders

Respiratory
Asthma
Emphysema
Sinusitis
Tuberculosis

Digestive
GERD (reflux)
Ulcers
Crohn disease
Ulcerative colitis
✓ Irritable bowel syndrome
Gallstones
Cirrhosis
Hepatitis

Endocrine
Diabetes
Hypothyroidism
Hyperthyroidism

Urinary
✓ Kidney stones
Renal failure

Reproductive
Breast cancer
Endometriosis
Ovarian cysts
Prostate cancer
Painful menstruation
Are you pregnant?

Other: *My hands swell up at night. I had severe dizziness and headaches for several months at the onset of the fibromyalgia.*

Explanation: *The chronic fatigue and irritable bowel syndrome are part of the fibromyalgia.*

Treatment Goals:
Why are you here? What do you hope to accomplish?
I was told this would help with stress and muscle pain.

Please indicate where you have pain:

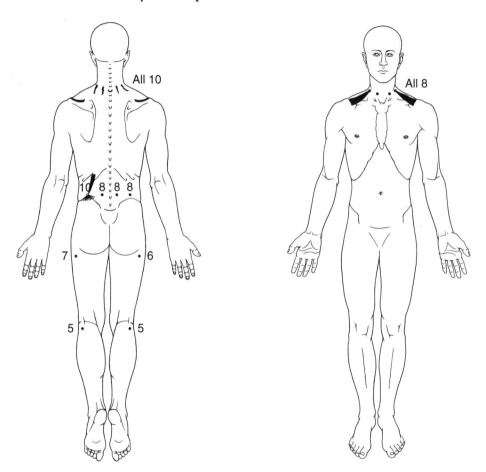

Describe what you do that causes pain, and what activities tend to make it worse:
At the onset of my fibromyalgia, I was working full time, I went to school two nights a week, I was on the PTA, and I helped to run Brownies. I've found that overdoing in general makes everything much worse, but so does doing nothing. I also have to be careful about overexercising.

What questions do you have about massage or this massage session?
How badly is it going to hurt and how often should I do it?

Subjective Findings

These are recorded on the image of the human body, above.

Objective Findings

Janet's tissues are generally mobile and elastic superficially, although there is a sense of brittleness or fragility when the deeper layers are palpated. Circulation is good. The area over and above the scapula on the right side is particularly unyielding; it feels like a piece of cardboard under skin. By the end of our time together, it had begun to give, but just a little.

When she lies supine, Janet's shoulders rise up off the table by several inches. The tissue on the anterior aspect of the shoulder girdle is tender and not clearly definable through touch.

Assessment

I suspect that as a result of Janet's thoracic outlet surgery, her pectoralis minor and major are bound up with significant scar tissue. This accounts for the rolling of the shoulders anteriorly, and the chronic pain she feels in her upper back—she marked these areas with "10"s on her chart. I would not be at all surprised if her diagnosis of fibromyalgia related to the muscular imbalances caused by her surgeries, although the headaches and dizziness she experienced may be connected to a different aspect of that disease.

Plan

I recommend regular sessions (every week or every other week, depending on time constraints) of gentle Swedish massage, focussing on the muscular relationships surrounding the shoulder girdle: pectoralis minor and major, the deltoid, trapezius, rhomboids, levator scapulae, etc.

I encourage Janet to do the exercises taught by her physical therapist to stretch the anterior shoulder girdle muscles.

I plan to focus on the paraspinals and quadratus lumborum, perhaps in relationship to the iliopsoas, in future appointments.

I plan to work slowly and conservatively and to encourage Janet to drink a lot of water after each appointment so that she can minimize any soreness that may follow.

APPENDIX III

HYGIENIC METHODS FOR MASSAGE THERAPISTS

Massage therapists work with a physical intimacy unmatched by practically any other health care profession. How many health professionals, outside of surgeons, spend an hour or more devoting the total of their concentration and focus, as well as their touch, to the well-being of their clients?

Working in physically intimate circumstances carries the risk of spreading infection. Infection can move from the therapist to the client, but also from the client to the therapist (who can transfer it to the next client, and so on). For this reason, massage therapists have to be very familiar with the most common types of infectious agents to recognize them when possible and to guard against them always.

The guidelines provided here are probably more conservative than most practicing therapists observe. Massage is a quickly growing profession, however, and massage therapists will be increasingly at risk for professional liability if stringent standards of cleanliness and professionalism are not followed.

This discussion focuses on three aspects of keeping therapists and clients healthy: the infectious agents to guard against, methods by which to keep free of infection, and practical implications for massage therapists.

Infectious Agents

Millions of pathogens can make people sick. The main groups discussed here are not a comprehensive list but cover the agents that are most common in industrialized countries. They include bacteria, viruses, fungi, and animal parasites.

Bacteria

These are divided into saprophytes (the "good guys" that live off dead material) and parasites (the "bad guys" that live off living material—such as human bodies).

Parasitic bacteria include the following groups:

- Cocci (round-shaped bacteria), which appear in these configurations:

  - *Staphylococcus* bacteria are shaped like bunches of grapes. They are responsible for most local skin infections and boils.

  - *Streptococcus* bacteria are in chains. They are involved in many systemic infections such as strep throat and blood poisoning.

  - *Gonococcus* bacteria cause gonorrhea.

  - *Diplococcus* bacteria cause bacterial pneumonia.

Everybody has colonies of bacteria growing on their skin. Hosts do not usually become sick because their immune system can develop resistance to resident pathogens. However, clients, especially clients who are in any way immune suppressed, will not be so resistant to a therapist's personal colonies of bacteria. This why it is so important to avoid touching areas where the skin is not intact: these lesions are an infection waiting to happen.

Staphylococcus and Streptococcus are the two most important bacteria to know about. These have mutated into thousands of tough varieties that can be difficult to treat.

Other types of bacteria are less common, but it is a good idea to be familiar with them. They include:

- *Bacilli.* These rod-shaped bacteria are the spore-makers. They have a tough outer shell that protects them from the environment and many chemicals that would kill other bacteria. Bacilli bacteria are responsible for anthrax, tuberculosis, typhoid, tetanus, and diphtheria.
- *Spirochetes.* These spiral-shaped bacteria cause syphilis and Lyme disease.

Viruses

Viruses are not, technically speaking, alive. They are tiny (much smaller than bacteria) collections of proteins with genetic coding. Once inside a host cell, the virus changes the function of that cell to be a virus factory. When that factory is full of inventory, it ruptures, releasing the new viruses to search for new host cells.

Viruses outside bodies usually disintegrate fairly quickly. Some of them, however, are tougher to get rid of than others. The two main adversaries of massage therapists are herpes simplex and hepatitis B.

- *Herpes simplex.* This is the virus that causes oral and genital herpes. It is a sturdy virus that can linger on tables, doorknobs, and other surfaces for several hours. It is highly contagious in the acute (blistering) stage. If a client has fever blisters or suspicious sores around their thighs and buttocks, consider them at least locally contraindicated and isolate sheets, face pads, or other equipment in a special laundry container for bleaching.
- *Hepatitis B.* This virus is not easy to catch (it requires some sort of intimate contact or fluid exchange), but it has a serious impact on the body and is strongly associated with liver cancer. Hepatitis B is transmissible through shared fluid, including saliva, lymph, and blood. The virus is extremely sturdy and very virulent. It is the leading killer of nurses in the United States. In some places, it is considered to be an epidemic.

A vaccine for hepatitis B has been developed. People who are in blood-exposure professions are required to get it, and massage therapists can, too.

Fungi

The chief enemies here are dermatophytes, specifically the fungi that cause tinea corporis (body ringworm), tinea capitis (head ringworm), tinea cruris (jock itch), or tinea pedis (athlete's foot). Tinea lesions look like red, slightly raised rings on the skin. They are very common and very contagious, especially for people with weak immune systems.

Fungal infections can have a gestation period of 2 to 3 weeks, during which time the infected person can transmit the fungus to others.

Animal Parasites

Three main species constitute the majority of animal parasites that can spread from one person to another.

- *Head lice.* These are arthropods that live on the scalp. They spread from one person to another very easily, either by moving from one head to the next or by lurking on coat hooks, chair backs, or in shared hats. Lice are often identified by the presence of nits—lice eggs—which are white and cling to hair shafts.

- *Crab lice.* These are relatives of head lice. They usually live in pubic hair but also can be found in body hair, eyebrows, and eyelashes. They drink blood and cause a great amount of itching. Crab lice usually spread through intimate contact, as in sharing a bed or massage sheets.

- *Scabies.* These are lesions caused by microscopic mites that burrow under the skin, drinking blood, laying eggs, and leaving irritating wastes. They can be hard to diagnose because actual bugs are not always picked up in skin samples. Scabies lesions are itchy, especially at night, and they often appear in warm, sweaty places such as the groin, armpits, crooks of elbows and knees, and between fingers and toes.

Consider the sheets and other linens of any client who shows signs of parasitical infestation as "hot." Separate them from other sheets and wash them in hot water with extra bleach.

Aseptic Methods: Keeping Free from Infection

Asepsis means absence of infection. Aseptic methods are techniques to keep massage therapists and their clients as free as possible from infectious agents.

Antiseptics

Antiseptic substances are the weakest of the aseptic methods. They create a hostile environment for many bacteria, although they may not actually kill them. Antiseptics are ineffective against bacteria that are encased in spores and many viruses. Antiseptics are safe to use on skin. Some antiseptics (rubbing alcohol, iodine, hydrogen peroxide) used to be considered disinfectants (a stronger class of germ-killer), but now, because germs have become so much tougher, they can no longer dependably kill what they used to.

Antiseptics include:

- *Hand soap.* Some hand soaps include special germ-killers in their formulae. These may increase the soap's effectiveness at killing easily accessible pathogens, but this does not mean that hands washed with special antiseptic soap are completely germ-free.

- *Rubbing alcohol.* Rubbing alcohol works best in a 70% solution (as it is packaged) because a 100% solution makes the germs' membranes thicker and less permeable. Rubbing alcohol is effective against bacteria but not viruses or spores.

- *Hydrogen peroxide.* This is a mild antiseptic that is used in 3% solution for skin and mucous membranes.

Disinfectants

These are agents that should be effective against all viruses and bacteria except those with spores. Many disinfectants are marketed with target pathogens. They can also be called *germicides* or *bactericides*.

Disinfectant techniques are too strong to be used on skin, but as a rule, they *do not* kill spores.

Examples include:

- *Bleach.* A 10% solution is used for surfaces, and 1 cup/wash is used for laundry. Bleach is effective against staphylococcus, streptococcus, fungus, hepatitis, HIV, and herpes. It is still the industry standard for disinfecting most surfaces.

- *Phenol.* A 10% solution of phenol can be used for surfaces. It is caustic to skin and lungs. Phenol is effective against bacteria, fungus, herpes, and flu virus.

- *Quaternary ammonium compounds (Quats)*. These substances are available through medical or janitorial supply outlets. Although they are useful for killing pathogens, they do not necessarily remove dirt or other debris. Quats are used for "cold sterilization" of items that cannot be subjected to an autoclave.

Sterilization

These methods kill every living thing within a field. Massage therapists cannot sterilize themselves or their clients, but they can sterilize some of their tools and work surfaces, if absolutely necessary.

Some sterilization methods include:

- *Baking*. At 350°F for 1 hour.
- *Boiling*. The item should be completely immersed in water at 212°F for 20 minutes.
- *Autoclave (steam cabinet)*. Items should be under 15 psi, at 250°F for 30 minutes.

Microwave ovens do not sterilize items because the heat is unevenly distributed.

Practical Applications for Massage Therapists

Massage therapists should be especially aware of the dangers of pathogens and parasites. They carry the risks of contracting disease themselves and of spreading disease from client to client. It is important for massage therapists to use aseptic methods wisely and regularly.

Personal Cleanliness

- *Washing hands*. It is impossible to say this too often. Hands should be washed between clients and after handling tissues or other bodily fluid–bearing items. Remember that cold and flu viruses are transmitted by hands far more efficiently than by floating randomly in the air. The friction of hands rubbing together is the most important part of handwashing.
- *Keep fingernails short and clean*. Imagine getting a massage from someone with longish or slightly dirty nails. How relaxed could a person be, imagining all those cooties crawling around on the skin?
- *Attend to clothing*. Uniforms, jackets, or aprons should be scrupulously clean. If a style of massage is practiced in which the client's skin comes in contact with the therapist's clothing (e.g., when arms are being treated), then that clothing should be treated in the same way as sheets. Care should be taken so that one client does not come in contact with cloth or materials that may have been contaminated by a previous client.
- *Broken skin*. Broken skin is an open invitation to infection. Massage therapists should avoid it on their clients and keep it covered on themselves. Rubber "finger cots" are extremely useful items when a therapist has a scraped knuckle or a hangnail.

Linen

Laws regarding linen storage for health care professionals vary from state to state. Some states require professionals to store their dirty linen in closed containers and clean linen in closed cabinets. It is a good idea to have a second container available for "hot" sheets that need to be treated with special care. In addition to sheets, a massage therapist's laundry may include uniforms or aprons, pillowcases, face hole covers, heating pad covers, towels, bolster covers, and anything else that contacts a client's skin.

Beware of stuffing oily sheets into baskets or boxes and letting them sit. Oil will go rancid and smell, or it has been known to spontaneously combust. The moral: wash sheets promptly!

Some massage therapists or clinics hire a laundry service to take care of their linens. In this case, sheets probably will be rented from the service. These sheets are typically washed and rinsed repeatedly at 180°F. They are bleached and then subjected to anti-bleachers to reduce the chemical aftermath. Even so, some people may have a reaction to the chemicals left in the fabric.

Extra blankets, mattress pads, sheepskins, etc., do not need to be washed unless they come in contact with clients. It is a good idea to wash them once a month or so anyway, just for freshness.

Storage and Dispensation of Oil, Lotion, and Creams

All lubricants need to be kept in clean containers and dispensed in a way that prevents contamination. For instance, if a therapist has a tub of coconut oil, he or she must dip out what is going to be used into a paper cup (using a spatula, not the fingers). Then the therapist must *not* put the leftovers back into the tub—it is contaminated and must be thrown away.

Remember that if a client has a contagious condition—herpes, for example—the therapist may transmit the virus to the outside of the oil bottle. That same oil bottle may be used for the next client, and the virus is lurking on the surface just waiting for a chance to get on another potential host's skin. In other words, it is a good idea to wash oil bottles at the same time as washing hands.

Care of Massage Tables and Other Equipment

If a client who shows signs of a communicable disease has been on a table, it is time to swab. A 70% concentration of rubbing alcohol is the standard, although it is drying to vinyl and of questionable impact against sturdy viruses such as herpes and hepatitis B. (It will remove those annoying oily hand prints, though.) Regardless, it is a good habit to swab the table once a week or so, especially the face cradle.

Any other surfaces that clients contact should be cleaned regularly. Most items such as heat or cold packs are probably covered by cloth that can be laundered, but therapists must be ever vigilant against possible contaminated surfaces.

APPENDIX IV

CLIENT ENDANGERMENTS

Endangerments are sites where massage therapists can cause damage to some of the body's most delicate tissues. Structures particularly at risk are nerves, blood vessels, organs, and lymph nodes. This list covers the most basic endangerments; although if a massage therapist tries hard enough, he or she could cause injury to almost any part of the body.

Nerves

Pinning or compressing nerves can bruise, irritate, or otherwise damage them. Clients can experience sharp shooting, tingling, electric, or hot sensations when this happens. It is important to know the pathways of the most vulnerable nerves because, unfortunately, massage therapists cannot always count on clients, some of whom expect massage to hurt, to give accurate feedback about whether the pain they are feeling is "good" pain or bad pain.

Blood Vessels

The general risk of arterial entrapment is the blocking of circulation, causing numbness, discomfort, and even blackouts. Entrapment of veins, since they are weaker, can injure them, creating varicosities, hemorrhages, or clots.

Organs

A few organs can be trapped and impaired by massage therapy. They are generally at risk because they are close to the surface, or they are anchored in a way that makes them vulnerable to being pinned or compressed.

Lymph Nodes

Lymph nodes are epithelial cells within a connective tissue framework. They are especially palpable when they are inflamed; being able to feel lymph nodes, especially around the neck or the back of the head, often indicates that they are working overtime, and the client may be fighting off an infection.

Head and Face Endangerments

- *Eyes.* Obviously, eyes are a local caution for massage. Special care must also be taken with clients who wear contact lenses. If a client wears hard contacts, the therapist should suggest that they be removed during a treatment (potential problems include drying out and lacerations to the sclera). If a client wears soft or extended wear contacts, removing them probably will not be an issue. Some therapists keep a bottle of distilled water and a lens case in their office, just in case a client decides to remove their contact lenses.

- *Nerve foramina.* Three pairs of foramina allow the mental, the infraorbital, and the supraorbital nerves to exit from the skull. These nerves supply the face with sensation and motor control. Heavy pressure on these spots can be extremely painful and may even damage the nerves as they emerge (Fig. 1).

- *Temporomandibular joint (TMJ).* Branches of both the trigeminal and the facial nerves are accessible near the TMJ. Whether massage therapy could actually cause an attack of Bell's palsy or trigeminal neuralgia is not clear, but it is the responsibility of every therapist to know how to avoid even the possibility of putting a client at risk for these problems.

This is not to say that the whole TMJ area and jaw muscles are off-limits to massage. On the contrary, massage can be an important part of reducing habitual muscle tone in persons prone to jaw-clenching. Nevertheless, massage practitioners who work in this area must know where the nerves are vulnerable and how to avoid putting them at risk.

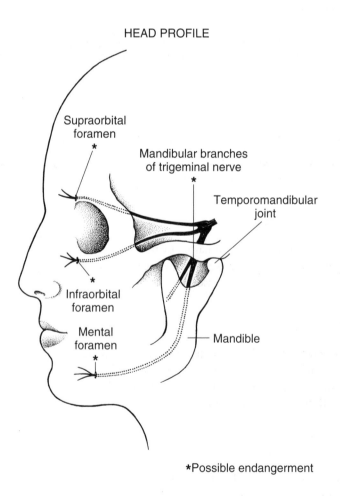

HEAD PROFILE

Supraorbital foramen

Mandibular branches of trigeminal nerve

Temporomandibular joint

Infraorbital foramen

Mental foramen

Mandible

*Possible endangerment

Figure 1. Head profile.

Anterior Trunk and Neck Endangerments

For all structures in the anterior triangle of the neck and the anterior trunk, see Figure 2.

- *Anterior triangle of the neck.* The anterior triangle of the neck is defined by the sternal fibers of the left and right sternocleidomastoid muscles and the mandible. Many structures contained in this area are vulnerable to damage, and not much musculature that is easily accessible for massage. Some therapists make a specialty of working

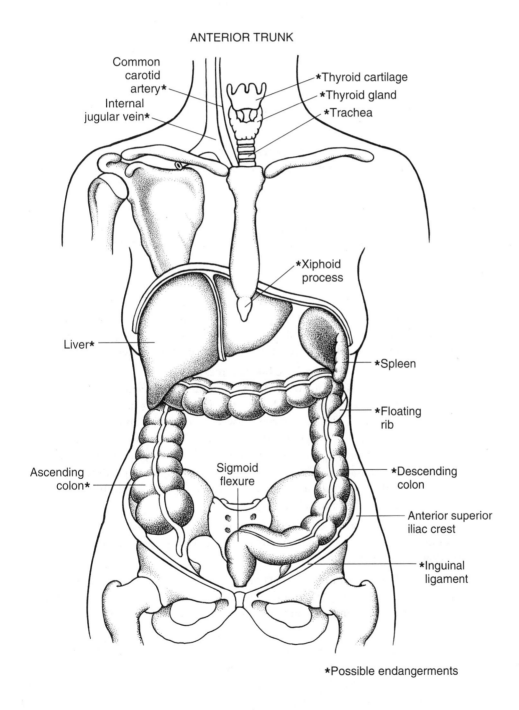

ANTERIOR TRUNK

Common carotid artery*
Internal jugular vein*
*Thyroid cartilage
*Thyroid gland
*Trachea
*Xiphoid process
Liver*
*Spleen
*Floating rib
Ascending colon*
Sigmoid flexure
*Descending colon
Anterior superior iliac crest
*Inguinal ligament

*Possible endangerments

Figure 2. Anterior trunk.

on the muscles of the anterior neck with good results, but they, along with all other massage practitioners, must be very familiar with the complicated anatomy of this area to stay out of harm's way. Structures in the anterior triangle of the neck that must be respected include:

- *Common carotid artery*

  This huge artery runs deep to the sternocleidomastoid muscles and carries most of the blood supply to the head. Approximately level with the thyroid cartilage, the common carotid artery splits into the internal and external carotid artery. The point of division, the carotid sinus, is equipped with special sensory nerves that measure blood pressure to maintain appropriate blood flow to the head. External pressure applied here can alter that blood flow, leading to dizziness and faintness. Atherosclerotic plaque also can accumulate in the carotid artery, making this area a local contraindication for clients with a high risk of cardiovascular disease.

- *Jugular vein*

  The jugular vein lies superficial to the common carotid. It is less vulnerable to damage but still does not need to be stretched or compressed in any way.

- *Trachea*

  This cartilaginous tube is part of the respiratory system and leads to the lungs. It is quite strong and resilient, but pressure directly on the tube will cause a choking feeling for the client.

- *Thyroid cartilage*

  The thyroid cartilage is a moveable piece of material that bobs up and down with the swallowing reflex. The most prominent part of the thyroid cartilage is the laryngeal prominence, or Adam's apple.

- *Thyroid gland*

  The thyroid gland is a butterfly-shaped piece of epithelium that wraps around the trachea. It is an endocrine gland, secreting hormones that control metabolism. Embedded within the thyroid gland are much smaller parathyroid glands. This whole structure is primarily epithelial, with little connective tissue protection.

- *Brachial plexus: neck and shoulder.* The brachial plexus is made up of spinal nerves C5 to T1. They criss-cross and interweave with each other before separating into the different nerves that supply the arm. Most of this interweaving happens between the neck and the shoulder. The nerves run between the medial and posterior scalene muscles, under the clavicle and coracoid process, and then wrap around the humerus. They are larger than they seem; coming out of the neck they are actually about the same thickness as shoelaces. They can be pinned against several different bones or other tissues on their way to the arm, so massage therapists should be very familiar with the pathways of the brachial plexus nerves.

- *Xiphoid process.* The inferior edge of the sternum has a small piece of bone that protrudes out over the liver. This prominence, the xiphoid process, can be broken off if sharp, downward pressure is exerted on it.

- *Floating ribs.* Massage is unlikely to actually damage floating ribs. Tracing or outlining the ribcage can cause ticklishness or even pain if a therapist does not know exactly where the floating ribs are and how to avoid pinning soft tissue against them.

- *Liver.* A massage therapist would have to be working much too deep and hard than is usually called for to bruise a healthy liver. However, it is good to know both where it is located and how big it is. Clients with enlarged livers due to hepatitis, jaundice, cirrhosis, or other problems may be particularly sensitive in this area.

- *Spleen.* The spleen is tucked up way under the left ribs. For most people, the spleen is not a significant endangerment, but if it is enlarged for any reason, the whole area can be uncomfortable.

- *Colon.* The colon is at special risk for entrapment and bruising because it is anchored at the flexures and cannot simply move out of the way like the small intestine can. Care must be taken when doing deep abdominal work to respect both that the colon can be pinned and that material should move through it in a clockwise direction. Pressure should not be exerted contrary to this direction of flow.

- *Ovaries.* The ovaries are normally located so low and central in the pelvis that they are inaccessible to massage therapists. Sometimes, though, endometriosis, an ovarian cyst, or other anomaly can cause the ovaries to move into areas where they may be pinned and bruised.

Posterior Trunk and Neck Endangerments

For all structures in the posterior trunk and neck, see Figure 3.

- *Kidneys.* The kidneys are vulnerable to damage because they are only partially protected by the rib cage. The right kidney sits a bit lower than the left. An easy way to remember this is that it looks like the right kidney is pushed downward by the liver. Both can be bruised if vigorous tapotement is performed over the mid-back area.

- *Spinous processes.* These are listed as endangerments because massage therapists can cause pain by pressing or frictioning paraspinal muscles in toward the spinous processes, rather than out and away from them. Pressure toward the spine can be appropriate, as long as soft tissues are not being impaled or ground into hard ones.

Arm Endangerments

For structures in the arms, see Figures 4 and 5.

- *Brachial plexus: arm.* By the time the brachial plexus has reached the arm, it has separated into its five different components: the axillary nerve, the musculocutaneous nerve, and the radial, median, and ulnar nerves. It is useful to know the basic pathways of all these structures, although they may vary slightly from one person to another. Specific endangerment spots include the axilla, the medial aspect of the upper arm, and the cubital fossa. The ulnar nerve is vulnerable medial to the olecranon: it causes the "funny bone" sensation when it is knocked or irritated.

- *Axillary lymph nodes.* Lymph nodes should not be specifically isolated or massaged. They have the important job of filtering pathogens from the blood and should be left alone.

- *Cephalic and basilic veins.* Veins, perhaps more than any other structure discussed here, run in pathways that are unique from one person to the next, so it is impossible to state categorically where they might be vulnerable. One thing that is consistent, however, is that they run at least part of the way up the medial side of the upper arm. Conveniently, this is already an area to avoid because some of the brachial plexus nerves are also vulnerable here. The cephalic vein also can be trapped where it runs along the edges of the anterior deltoid and pectoralis major.

POSTERIOR TRUNK

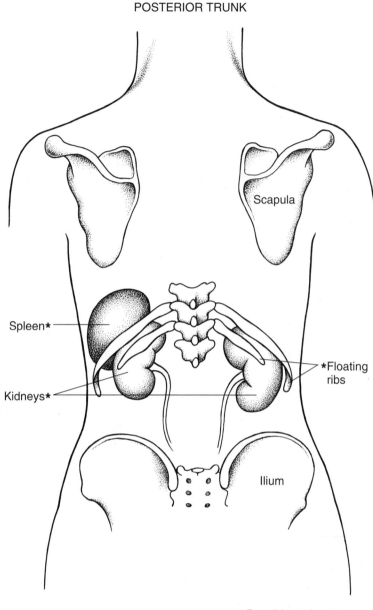

Figure 3. Posterior trunk.

Leg Endangerments

For structures of the legs, see Figures 6, 7, 8, and 9.

- *Femoral triangle.* The femoral triangle, defined by the inguinal ligament and the sartorius muscle, is a particularly rich area for vulnerable structures. The femoral artery and vein are both accessible here, as are the inguinal lymph nodes and the femoral nerve. Deep, specific work on the adductors must be conducted with special care to avoid damaging these structures (see Figure 6).

- *Sciatic nerve.* The sciatic nerve, the thickest nerve in the body, runs through the deep lateral rotators and down the back of the leg, where it splits into the common per-

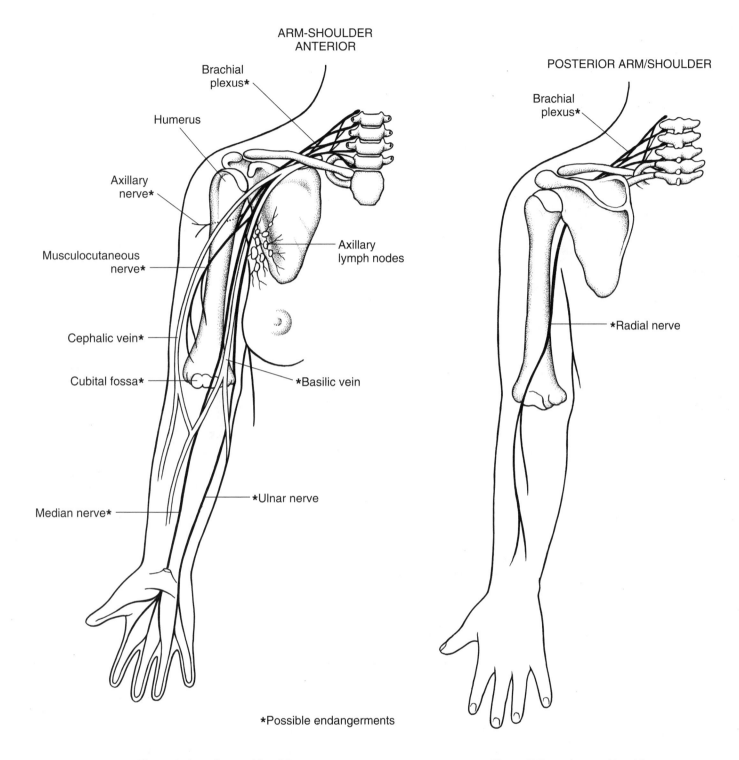

ARM-SHOULDER
ANTERIOR

Brachial
plexus*

Humerus

Axillary
nerve*

Musculocutaneous
nerve*

Cephalic vein*

Cubital fossa*

Median nerve*

Axillary
lymph nodes

*Basilic vein

*Ulnar nerve

*Possible endangerments

POSTERIOR ARM/SHOULDER

Brachial
plexus*

*Radial nerve

Figure 4. Anterior arm/shoulder.

Figure 5. Posterior arm/shoulder.

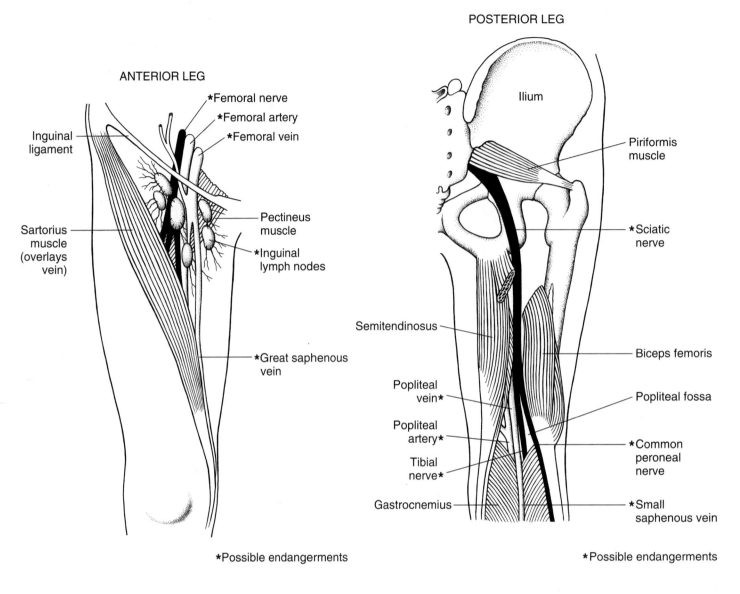

ANTERIOR LEG

Inguinal ligament

Sartorius muscle (overlays vein)

*Femoral nerve
*Femoral artery
*Femoral vein

Pectineus muscle

*Inguinal lymph nodes

*Great saphenous vein

*Possible endangerments

Figure 6. Anterior leg.

POSTERIOR LEG

Ilium

Piriformis muscle

*Sciatic nerve

Semitendinosus

Biceps femoris

Popliteal vein*

Popliteal fossa

Popliteal artery*

*Common peroneal nerve

Tibial nerve*

Gastrocnemius

*Small saphenous vein

*Possible endangerments

Figure 7. Posterior leg.

oneal nerve and the tibial nerve. The sciatic nerve is difficult to pin or damage because the musculature surrounding it is so thick, but if the nerve is irritated for any reason, massage may exacerbate the situation (see Figure 7).

- *Popliteal fossa.* The popliteal fossa is the area on the posterior aspect of the knee that is defined by the heads of the gastrocnemius below, and the edges of the biceps femoris and the semitendinosus above. In this hollow area, there are several structures to know about, including the small saphenous vein, the popliteal vein, the popliteal artery, and the lower branches of the sciatic nerve: the tibial and common peroneal nerves (see Figure 7).

- *Great saphenous vein.* The great saphenous vein runs up the medial side of the calf, where there is little to protect it from being pinned to the tibia (see Figure 8). On the upper leg, the vein runs along the edge of the sartorius, but the quadriceps are bulky enough that pinning the great saphenous to the femur is not generally possible.

LATERAL LEG

MEDIAL LEG

Saphenous nerve

*Great saphenous vein

Biceps femoris

Common peroneal nerve*

*Possible endangerments

*Possible endangerments

Figure 8. Medial leg.

Figure 9. Lateral leg.

- *Common peroneal nerve.* The common peroneal nerve is vulnerable for a short distance just inferior to the head of the fibula. Specific pressure or friction on the peroneus longus can sometimes irritate this nerve, which will send shocky, electrical sensations down into the foot (see Figure 9).

APPENDIX V

MEDICATIONS

Massage therapists are always encouraged to ask about what medications, prescription or otherwise, their clients might be taking. Traditionally this has been to help discover what conditions a client might have that could influence the way massage needs to be conducted. However, the possible interactions between bodywork and medications themselves are a related but separate topic.

The following is a *very* short collection of classes of medications that are commonly prescribed for chronic conditions. Massage therapists must balance the effects of medications, medical interactions, all possible side effects, and the potential for bodywork to tip the scales in one direction or another. In many cases, a conversation with the primary care provider is in order—not so much to ask permission to do massage as to investigate whether the generally parasympathetic changes massage brings about carry any concern or risk in the presence of prescription drugs.

Recently some excellent resources about bodywork in the context of pharmaceuticals have been developed. I recommend these resources:

Wible J. *Pharmacology for Massage Therapy*, Lippincott Williams & Wilkins, 2004.
Persad R. *Massage Therapy and Medications*. Curties-Overzet Publications, 2001.

In addition, massage offices would do well to have a general reference about medications on hand. In this way, when a client enters "doxercalciferol" on her intake form and neither one of you are sure what it is for, you will have a way to find out. A good option is:

Springhouse Nurse's Drug Guide 2005, 6th Ed. Lippincott Williams & Wilkins.

The short list of medication classes under discussion here includes the following:

Anti-inflammatories/analgesics   Anti-depressants
Muscle relaxants   Anti-anxiety medications
Cardiovascular disease management   Diabetes management
Clot management   Thyroid supplements

Within each description, the following information is provided:

- Basic mechanism of the drug

- Bodywork cautions associated with the medication or the condition it treats

- Common name brands: please be aware that this information is perhaps the most changeable of all and requires that every therapist get accurate and current information from every client.

Anti-Inflammatories and Analgesics

Inflammation is frequently a source of nerve irritation at acute or chronic sites of tissue damage. Consequently, many analgesics work to reduce pain sensation by reducing or inhibiting the inflammatory process. Other analgesics alter pain perception in the central nervous system and do not affect inflammation.

Regardless of the site of drug activity, analgesics and anti-inflammatories change tissue response. It is important to work extremely conservatively with clients who take these medications, because information therapists gather about temperature, muscle guarding, local blood flow, and other signs will be altered, and over-treatment is a significant risk. Although it is inappropriate to suggest that clients skip or change their medication for massage, it is preferable to work with clients when these drugs are at their lowest level of activity so that therapists may collect the most accurate information about tissue response.

Classes of Drugs

Salicylates
Acetaminophen
NSAIDs
Steroidal anti-inflammatories
Narcotics and mixed narcotics

Salicylates	Aspirin, Bayer, Empirin, Doan's pills
Basic mechanism	Salicylates inhibit prostaglandin synthesis, which then reduces pain sensitivity and inflammatory response. They also reduce fever by acting on the hypothalamus and promoting peripheral vasodilation. (They will not reduce a normal temperature.) In addition, aspirin works to inhibit platelet aggregation (see *anticoagulants*).
Implications for massage	Reduced pain perception and inhibited inflammation means that compromised tissue may not send a strong signal about pain; bodywork needs to be conducted conservatively to avoid over-treatment. Also, the tendency for peripheral vasodilation raises the risk for hypotension (dizziness and lethargy) and chilling during and after a massage.
Acetaminophen	Tylenol, Anacin
Basic mechanism	The mechanism for acetaminophen is not thoroughly understood. It is clear that these medications act on the heat-regulating center of the hypothalamus to reduce fever. These drugs reduce pain sensation but do *not* influence inflammation.
Implications for massage	As with other pain medications, caution must be used to avoid over-treatment.
NSAIDs	Celebrex, Lodine, Advil, Excedrin, Nuprin, Relafen, Indomethacin, Aleve, Vioxx
Basic mechanism	All of these medications work to inhibit prostaglandin synthesis at sites of tissue damage to reduce inflammation and the pain associated with it.
Implications for massage	NSAIDs are effective for pain and inflammation, but they are also associated with stomach and kidney damage; clients need to consult their doctor if they have any discomfort (bear in mind that kidney pain may present as low back pain). Massage therapists carry the responsibility to avoid over-treatment, even if the client does not report feeling pain.

Steroidal anti-inflammatories	Cortisone, Compound E, Beconase, Propaderm, H-Hydrocort, Hydrocortone, Depo-Medrol, Prednisol, Prednisone, Decadron, and Methotrexate
Basic mechanism	These synthetic analogs to glucocorticoids produced in the adrenal cortex all work to undo the main symptoms of inflammation: they reduce pain, heat, redness, and edema in the short run. The mechanism by which they do this is not well understood, although some researchers suggest that they change local cellular activity leading to suppressed production of prostaglandins, histamine, and other inflammatory substances.
Implications for massage	Steroidal anti-inflammatories are powerful but have several serious side effects. In addition to altering tissue response (which requires extra caution with massage), they suppress immune system activity. Long-term use is associated with weakened connective tissues, fat deposition, muscle wasting, reduced bone density, fluid retention, hypertension, and easy bruising. Topical applications of steroid creams can lead to thinning skin. All of these features influence bodywork choices. Steroidal anti-inflammatories also may be prescribed in inhalant form for the treatment of asthma. Although these medications specifically target the lung, long-term use may have negative impact on other tissues.
Narcotics and mixed narcotics	Codeine, Demerol, Oxycontin, Darvon, Percocet, Lortab, Vicodin
Basic mechanism	Narcotics bind to opiate receptors in the brain to mimic the action of pain-killing endorphins. This leads to a reduced sensation of pain without loss of consciousness, along with suppression of the cough reflex, and GI tract sluggishness. Narcotics are potentially addictive; mixed narcotics were developed to minimize the risk of dependence, but have proved to be addictive also.
Implications for massage	A client taking these medications has a problem that is too extreme to be managed with less intrusive analgesics. Interference with pain perception is more complete, and appropriate caution is called for. Furthermore, clients taking narcotic analgesics may be prone to mood swings and difficulties with accurate communication.

Muscle Relaxants

Muscle relaxants are prescribed to deal with acute spasms related to trauma or anxiety, or to help with chronic spasticity from central nervous system damage as seen with multiple sclerosis, stroke, spinal cord injury, or cerebral palsy. They can act on the brain, the spinal cord, or in the muscle tissue itself.

A client who takes muscle relaxants is *not* inherently relaxed, although his or her tissues may seem that way. These drugs interfere with muscle protection reflexes, and so the risk of over-treatment with deep tissue work, range of motion exercises, or stretching is significant.

Classes of Drugs

Centrally acting skeletal muscle relaxants
Peripherally acting skeletal muscle relaxants

Centrally acting skeletal muscle relaxants	Soma, Paraflex, Flexeril, Skelaxin, Norflex, Baclofen, Valium, Robaxin, Zanaflex
Basic mechanism	These medications are central nervous system depressants. They suppress reflexes that would tighten muscles in response to stretching or damage. They are used to control painful acute spasms related to trauma or anxiety.
Implications for massage	These drugs enforce a parasympathetic state, which may then be intensified by massage. Therapists should take care that clients are not overly exhausted at the end of a session. In addition, the protective stretch reflex is inhibited under these medications; therapists should not try to create an increased range of motion while the client is in this altered state.
Peripherally acting skeletal muscle relaxants	Dantrium
Basic mechanism	This drug interferes with calcium release at the sarcoplasmic reticulum of muscle cells, leading to weaker contractions. It is used to treat chronic spasticity associated with central nervous system damage, but the overall weakness that ensues makes it a questionable choice for patients whose strength is borderline.
Implications for massage	A client taking Dantrium will have a compromised stretch reflex and falsely hypotonic muscles; massage must be conducted conservatively.

Cardiovascular Disease Management

Most of the drugs used to treat cardiovascular disease work in some way to minimize a sympathetic response or to dilate peripheral blood vessels. The overriding rule when a client uses these substances is that their slide into a parasympathetic state may be intensified by massage, leaving the client dizzy, fatigued, and lethargic. Ending a session with strokes that are more stimulating may help to ameliorate these effects, as long as they fit into a protocol that is suitable for a person with compromised cardiovascular health. Clients should be instructed to sit up and move slowly after their massage, to minimize dizziness or discomfort.

Hydrotherapeutic techniques can present a greater challenge to maintain homeostasis than many other modalities. Many clients with cardiovascular diseases should avoid total immersions in favor of smaller, localized hydrotherapy applications.

Classes of Drugs

Beta-blockers
Calcium channel blockers
ACE inhibitors
Digitalis

Anti-angina drugs
Antilipemic drugs
Diuretics

Beta-blockers	Inderal, Normodyne, Levatol, Corgard, Tenormin, Metoprolol, Toprol, Sotalol
Basic mechanism	These affect beta receptors at the heart, bronchi, blood vessels, and the uterus. They lower blood pressure and cardiac output. They are used to treat angina, hypertension, anxiety, and some other disorders. Beta-blockers may be selective for action on the heart only, or nonselective for a more general effect.
Implications for massage	Beta-blockers can lead to excessively low blood pressure, especially when the client is in a relaxed state. Hydrotherapy is generally safer with local applications than systemic immersions in hot tubs, saunas, or other facilities.

Calcium channel blockers	Norvasc, Cardizem, Cardene, Isoptin, Adalat, Plendil, Verapamil
Basic mechanism	These drugs block the movement of calcium ions in smooth and cardiac muscle tissue. The result is vasodilation and more efficient myocardial function. They are used for hypertension and long-term (not acute) angina.
Implications for massage	Side effects of these drugs include flushing, dizziness, and hypotension. Massage should be conducted to minimize the risk of exacerbating these: less emphasis on big, draining strokes and more emphasis on smaller, less circulatory strokes is appropriate.

ACE Inhibitors	Lotensin, Captopril, Vasotec, Monopril, Accupril
Basic mechanism	Angiotensin-converting enzyme (ACE) inhibitors work by limiting the action of an enzyme that is employed in the renin–angiotensin system: the loop between blood pressure and kidney function. They promote the excretion of sodium and water, reducing load on the heart. They are used to control hypertension and heart failure.
Implications for massage	As with other drugs for cardiovascular disease, excessive hypotension is a possible side effect. Clients may experience fatigue, dizziness, and lethargy if gently invigorating strokes are not administered toward the end of the session.

Digitalis	Digitek, digoxin, Lanoxicaps, Lanoxin
Basic mechanism	Digitalis increases the force of the heartbeat by boosting calcium in cardiac muscle cells; it also slows the heartbeat through action in the CNS. It is used to treat arrhythmia and heart failure.
Implications for massage	Clients who take any form of digitalis to control heart failure are not good candidates for rigorous circulatory massage. Invigorating strokes to conclude a session must be chosen to support alertness rather than circulatory flow.

Antilipemic drugs	LoCholest, Lopid, Prevalite, Questran, Lipitor, Lescol, Zocor, Crestor, Mevacor, Pravachol, Zetia, Lopid, Tricor, Niaspan.
Basic mechanism	Cholesterol-lowering drugs work by sequestering bile or by inhibiting cholesterol synthesis. Bile-sequestering drugs promote the excretion of bile in stool, requiring the liver to use more cholesterol in bile manufacturing; this lowers blood cholesterol. Cholesterol synthesis inhibitors interfere with enzyme activity in the liver that leads to cholesterol synthesis. Both approaches lead to lower LDL levels.
Implications for massage	A common side effect for all these drugs is constipation, as they influence the GI tract. Massage may help to relieve this symptom, but if a client has abdominal pain and has had no bowel movement for several days, an acute bowel impaction is possible; this is a medical emergency.
	Other side effects (which are not always listed) may include muscle soreness, cramping, and weakness. If a client taking an antilipemic drug has these problems, the prescribing doctor should be consulted before the massage therapist works to resolve them.
Diuretics	Thalidone, Kaluril, Lasix, Bumex, Lozide, Lozol, Spirono-lactone, Chlorthalidone, Demadex, Zaroxolyn, Dyazide, Maxzide, HCTZ (hydrochlorothiazide)
Basic mechanism	Some diuretics prevent sodium from being reabsorbed in the kidney. As it is processed into urine, it pulls water along with it. Other medications target specific parts of the nephron to prevent water and salt reabsorption, but can control the loss of other electrolytes more carefully
Implications for massage	Rigorously applied massage may put an extra load on the kidneys. Resting hypotension may also be a problem for people taking these medications. General diuretics may cause a loss of potassium that can contribute to muscle cramps. This needs to be addressed by a doctor rather than by a massage therapist.
Anti-angina medication	Apo-ISDN, Cedocard, IMDUR, Monoket, Nitrodisc, Nitrostat, Transderm-Nitro
Basic mechanism	Anti-angina drugs reduce myocardial oxygen demand, or they increase the supply of oxygen to the heart, or both. Chronic angina is treated with beta-blockers or calcium channel blockers, discussed elsewhere. Acute angina is typically treated with various nitrates. These cause vasodilation, especially of veins, leading to decreased load on the heart. They are typically dissolved under the tongue for fast action, or applied with a skin patch or ointment for longer-lasting effect.
Implications for massage	If a client has a transdermal patch for anti-anginal medication, that area and the adjacent tissue must be avoided so that dosage is not influenced. Clients taking these medications have the same risk of hypotension, flushing, and dizziness seen with other cardiovascular drugs.

Clot Management

Medications to manage blood clots come in three basic forms: anticoagulants to prevent the formation of new clots by acting on clotting factors; antiplatelet medications prevent the clumping of platelets to form new clots; and thrombolytics, which are used to dissolve preexisting clots. Thrombolytics are used only in emergency situations (i.e., in early treatment for heart attack or ischemic stroke), and so are not discussed here. Other clot management drugs are used for chronic problems or to lower the risk of future clots.

Classes of Drugs

Anticoagulants
Antiplatelet drugs

Anticoagulants	Heparin, Lovenox, Coumadin
Basic mechanism	Heparin and Lovenox are injected anticoagulants; Coumadin is an oral medication. All of them alter the formation of clotting factors in the liver to prevent the formation of new clots, although they do not help to dissolve pre-existing clots. These medications are used for people with atrial fibrillation, a high risk of deep vein thrombosis (DVT), or for people using hemodialysis. Heparin also may be used in orthopedic surgery to reduce the risk of postsurgical DVT.
Implications for massage	All blood-clotting medications carry a risk for bruising, even with relatively light massage. Furthermore, the need for these medications indicates a tendency to form blood clots that may contraindicate all but the lightest forms of bodywork.
Antiplatelet drugs	Aspirin, Empirin, Pletal, Plavix
Basic mechanism	These drugs prevent platelets from clumping at the site where a clot might otherwise form.
Implications for massage	Although these are typically less powerful than anticoagulants, the risk of bruising must still be respected for clients who take antiplatelet drugs.

Antidepressants

The exact causes of depression remain under dispute, and so do the exact working mechanisms of antidepressant medications. Three main classes have been developed: tricyclics, MAOIs, and SSRIs, although some newer drugs have recently been added to the market. As a whole, these drugs prolong the availability of various types of neurotransmitters in synapses in the brain, although why exactly this makes a difference is still an issue of some contention. It takes time for the body to adapt to these changes; however, 2 weeks or more are often needed for the drugs to take effect.

Antidepressants all have some side effects, although these are usually temporary and mild. Agitation at the beginning of treatment is common, along with increased anxiety, headaches, and insomnia; these often fade quickly. Other side effects include dry mouth, constipation, reduced sexual function, bladder problems, increased heart rate, and dizziness. If these symptoms do not subside, or if they become a significant issue, patients should consult with their prescribing doctors as soon as possible.

Two types of antidepressants are associated with significant health risks: MAOIs have dangerous interactions with decongestants and some food groups that lead to dangerously high blood pressure and a risk of stroke; and Serzone has been associated with liver toxicity.

Dizziness, drowsiness, and lightheadedness are common side effects to many antidepressants. Massage may exacerbate these symptoms, so the therapist should take care not to over-treat, especially when a client is just starting new course of drugs.

Classes of Medications

Tricyclics
Monamine oxidase inhibitors
Selective serotonin reuptake inhibitors
Other antidepressants

Tricyclics **Basic mechanism**	Imipramine, Amitriptyline, Nortriptyline, Desipramine, Elavil Tricyclics block the reuptake of norepinephrine and serotonin at synapses; this leads to "down-regulation" and more normal function of the postsynaptic receptors, but it may take 2 weeks or more before improvement is noticed.
Implications for massage	Like other antidepressants, tricyclics may have dizziness as a side effect. Clients may need some gently stimulating strokes at the end of the session to come back to full alertness. Of all the antidepressants, tricyclics tend to have the most extreme side effects.
Monamine Oxidase Inhibitors (MAOIs)	Nardil, Parnate, Marplan
Basic mechanism	MAOIs work like tricyclics but are used less often than other antidepressants because of the risk of dangerous interactions with some substances, notably decongestants, and aged cheeses, red wine, pickles, and other foods with tyramine.
Implications for massage	MAOIs and other antidepressants have the tendency to cause excessive drowsiness and dizziness; massage must be performed and concluded appropriately.
Selective Serotonin Reuptake Inhibitors (SSRIs)	Prozac, Zoloft, Luvox, Paxil, Celexa, Lexapro
Basic mechanism	These drugs all work to keep serotonin present in CNS synapses for a longer period. The theory is that this will lead to a more normalized uptake of serotonin from presynaptic neurons and a decrease in symptoms. SSRIs are used to treat various types of anxiety disorders and eating disorders as well as depression.

Implications for massage	SSRIs often have fewer side effects than other antidepressants, but therapists should be alert for signs of excessive dizziness or drowsiness and compensate appropriately.
Others	Effexor, Serzone, Wellbutrin
Basic mechanism	These drugs are similar to other antidepressants, although they focus on serotonin and norepinephrine uptake.
Implications for massage	In addition to the general guidelines about massage and antidepressants, Serzone, in particular, is associated with a risk of liver toxicity. Clients with signs of jaundice, chronic nausea, or other abdominal discomfort should immediately consult their primary caregiver.

Anti-Anxiety Medications

These medications are used to alter the sympathetic "flight or fight" response that is so prevalent for many people with anxiety disorders. They act on the central nervous system, but their effects may be far-reaching. Common side effects of anti-anxiety medications include bleeding, CNS depression, poor reflexes, and feeling unusually exhausted. All of these side effects impact decisions about bodywork. Although most of the time side effects are mild and easily tolerated, they can become a medical emergency. Clients should be encouraged to report any troubling symptoms to their primary physician.

Classes of Drugs

Benzodiazepines
Buspirone HCl

Benzodiazepines	Valium, Ativan, Xanax, Loftran, Halcion
Basic mechanism	It is believed that these medications mimic the inhibitory action of the neurotransmitter GABA, making neurons harder to activate. Benzodiazepines are used for short-term anxiety, seizures, and convulsions. They are potentially addictive.
Implications for massage	When a person's sympathetic response is suppressed, she is more prone to slide into a deep parasympathetic state. This is fine, until she tries to sit up, and falls off the table because of orthostatic hypotension. Massage in the presence of these drugs must be conducted conservatively to respect the client's reduced ability to adapt to external changes.
Buspirone HCl	BuSpar
Basic mechanism	The mechanism of this medication is not well understood. It appears to bind up serotonin and dopamine receptors in the brain, leading to calmer affect without the CNS side effects seen with benzodiazepines. It is less addictive as well. BuSpar is used for short-term anxiety, and for chronic problems such as general anxiety disorder.
Implications for massage	The systemic side effects with BuSpar are less than those with other anti-anxiety medications, but the rules are the same: clients need to move carefully after a session because of sympathetic suppression.

Diabetes Management

Because type 2 diabetes is so prevalent in the United States, the chances that a massage therapist might have diabetic clients are excellent. When type 2 diabetes cannot be managed by diet and exercise alone, other interventions are used. They often start with diabetes management drugs and may eventually culminate with the supplementation of insulin in various forms.

The implications for diabetes and massage therapists are many and complicated. Although many diabetics manage their disease well and minimize their risk for secondary complications, others are prone to several problems that pose serious cautions for massage: systemic atherosclerosis, an increased risk of stroke, diabetic ulcers, and peripheral neuritis to name a few.

Furthermore, massage lowers blood glucose. Although this is an advantage to diabetic clients, this challenge to homeostasis may sometimes be overwhelming enough to trigger a hypoglycemic episode. Massage therapists with diabetic clients should be aware of signs of hypoglycemia and hyperglycemia and should consult with those clients about how best to address their needs in an emergency.

Classes of Drugs

Insulin
Oral glucose management drugs

Insulin	Humulin, Humalog, Lantus, NovoLog
Basic mechanism	Insulin is a protein-based hormone that would be destroyed by digestive juices if taken orally. Consequently, it is administered by injection, either through multiple daily injections or through an insulin pump. It decreases blood glucose by helping to deliver glucose to cells that need this clean-burning fuel to do their jobs.
Implications for massage	Clients who supplement insulin vary their injection sites; these areas need to be locally avoided so as not to interfere with normal uptake of the drug. Because blood glucose stability is an issue for diabetic clients, it is best for them to receive massage in the middle of their insulin cycle, rather than at the end or at the beginning. It might also be useful for a new client to check blood glucose before and after the session, so that if he or she needs to take in sugar in an easily accessible form, the therapist can plan ahead and have some juice, milk, or candy available.
Oral glucose management drugs	Diabinase, Glucotrol, Glucophage, Precose
Basic mechanism	These drugs work in a variety of ways to inhibit the production of sugar in the liver, to improve the output of insulin in the pancreas, and to increase the sensitivity of insulin receptors on target cells.
Implications for massage	Of these drugs, Glucophage may have the least risk for setting up a hypoglycemic episode. Nonetheless, any clients who manage their diabetes with any combination of drugs and insulin must be monitored carefully for blood glucose stability. As with insulin, it is safest to work with these clients *after* the peak of drug activity.

Thyroid Supplements

Hypothyroidism is typically treated with supplements to replace thyroid secretions T3 and T4. Levothyroxine sodium is chemically identical to the thyroid secretion T4 and is meant to be converted to bioactive T3. Although many hypothyroidism patients successfully treat their disease with levothyroxine sodium, some supplement T3 instead of or in addition to T4. This substance is only available in the form of desiccated animal glands.

Classes of Drugs:

Levothyroxine sodium
Desiccated extract

Levothyroxine sodium	Synthroid, Eltroxin, Levo-T, Levothroid, Levoxyl
Basic mechanism	Synthetic thyroid hormones mimic the action of naturally occurring thyroid hormones to boost protein synthesis in cells, promote the use of glycogen stores, increase heart rate and cardiac output, and increase urine output.
Implications for massage	New users of synthetic thyroid supplements may go through a period of nervousness, agitation, and insomnia, which massage may help to improve. If these symptoms persist, the dosage may not be correct, and the person should consult with the prescribing physician.
	Someone who has been taking synthetic thyroid supplements for a long time probably has no significant side effects and no implications for massage therapy.
Desiccated extract	Armour Thyroid, Nature-Throid, Thyroid USP, Westhroid
Basic mechanism	These forms of thyroid hormone have the same action as synthetic supplements: they mimic the action of naturally occurring thyroid hormones to boost protein synthesis in cells, promote the use of glycogen stores, increase heart rate and cardiac output, and increase urine output. The difference is that the potency of these dosages is more difficult to predict, so users may experience significant fluctuation of symptoms.
Implications for massage	As with synthetic hormones, a new user may experience increased anxiety, insomnia, or agitation, all of which indicate massage. If symptoms persist, the person needs to consult with the physician. Otherwise, massage is perfectly appropriate for clients who supplement thyroid hormones.

GLOSSARY

Pronunciation Key

You can use this glossary to learn how to pronounce medical terms. The pronunciation appears in parentheses between the term and the beginning of its definition. The pronunciation of terms defined in this glossary is indicated with letters of the English alphabet rather than with phonetic symbols. The following key shows the sounds represented by these letters.

Vowels

ă	day, care, trait, gauge	ë	erythrocyte, genesis, system, lower	ū	prune, fruit, genu, food
a	mat, damage, far			yū	cube, urine, beauty, value
ă	about, hepatitis, data, tartar	ī	isle, lie, pyre, bacilli		
		i	igloo, hip, irritate	u	put, wool
ah	father, what	ĭ	pencil, circus	ŭ	upset, putt, murmur, tough
aw	raw, fall, cause	ō	oval, form, go		
ē	ego, here, bead, beet, artery	o	got, bought		
		ö	oven, bottom, motor		
e	bed, head, therapy, teratoma	ow	cow, hour		
		oy	boy, oil		

Consonants

b	bad, tab		English is found in the word 'zone' wherein the ending of that word is pronounced as if swallowed.	n	no, tender, run
ch	child, itch			ng	ring
d	dog, bad			p	pan, upset, top
dh	this, smooth (cf, th)			r	rot, atropy, tar
f	fit, defect; phase, hyphen; tough			s	so, distill, mess (cf z); center, council (cf k)
		j	jade; gender, rigid, edge (cf. g)		
g	got, bag			sh	show, wish; social
h	hit, behold	k	cut, tlc; tachycardia (cf, ch)	t	ten, batter, put
[h]	Denotes an approximation of a tone used in French words whereby the sound is pulled to the back of the tongue. The closest equivalent in			th	thin, with (cf dh)
		ks	extra, tax	v	vote, oven, nerve
		kw	quick, aqua	w	we, awake, tow
		l	law, kill	y	yes, payload
		m	me, timid, bum	z	zero; disease, faces (cf s); xiphoid (cf ks)
				zh	azure, vision, measure

GLOSSARY

Ablate (ab-lāt′): To remove or destroy function.

Abrasion: A scrape involving injury to the epithelial layer of the skin or mucous membranes.

Absence seizure (ab′sen sē′zhŭr): A type of seizure characterized by lack of activity with occasional clonic movements.

Acanthosis nigricans (ak-an-thö′sis nīgri-kanz): An eruption of velvet warty benign growths and hyperpigmentation occurring in the skin of the axillae, neck, anogenital area, and groins; may be associated with endocrine disorders. (See *metabolic syndrome*)

Acetaminophen (as-et-ă-mē′nö-fen): A drug with anti-fever and analgesic effects similar to aspirin, but with limited anti-inflammatory action.

Acetylcholine (as-e-til-kö′lēn): The neurotransmitter at cholinergic synapses, which causes cardiac inhibition, vasodilation, gastrointestinal peristalsis, and other parasympathetic effects.

Acral lentiginous melanoma (ak′răl len-tij′i-nēz mel′ă-nö′mă): Pigmented lesions usually on the nail-bed, fingers, palms, soles, or between toes. (See *skin cancer*)

Acromegaly (ak-rö-meg′ă-lē): A disorder marked by progressive enlargement of peripheral parts of the body, linked to excessive secretion of growth hormone.

Acromioclavicular joint sprain (ă-krö′mē-ö-kla-vik′ū-lăr joynt): An injury to the ligaments that support the acromioclavicular joint.

Actinic cheilitis (ak-tin′ik kī-lī′tĭs): Actinic keratosis lesions that appear on the lip. (See *skin cancer*)

Actinic keratosis (ak-tin′ik ker-ă-tö′sis): A premalignant warty lesion occurring on the sun-exposed skin of the face or hands in aged light-skinned persons. (See *skin cancer*)

Acute (ă-kūt): A stage of injury or infection: short-term, severe.

Acute exertional compartment syndrome: A serious injury involving excessive swelling of leg muscles that may dangerously compress blood vessels and peripheral nerves. (See *shin splints*)

Acute granulocytic leukemia (ă-kyŭt′ gran′yū-lö-sit′ik lū-kē′mē-ă): Synonym for acute myelogenous leukemia. (See *leukemia*)

Acute idiopathic polyneuritis (ă-kyūt′ id′ē-ö-path′ikpol′ē-nū-rī′tis): Synonym for Guillain-Barré syndrome.

Acute lymphoblastic leukemia: Synonym for acute lymphocytic leukemia. (See *leukemia*)

Acute lymphoid leukemia: Synonym for acute lymphocytic leukemia. (See *leukemia*)

Acute myelocytic leukemia: Synonym for acute myelogenous leukemia. (See *leukemia*)

Acute myelogenous leukemia: Aggressive cancer of the myeloid class of blood cells. (See *leukemia*)

Acyclovir (ā-sī′klö-vir): An antiviral agent often used in the treatment of herpes simplex.

Adenocarcinoma (ad′ĕ-nö-kar-si-nö′mă): A malignant neoplasm of epithelial cells in glandular or gland-like pattern.

Adenoma (ad-ĕ-nö′mă): A benign neoplasm, usually occurring in epithelial tissue. (See *colon cancer*)

Adhesion (ad-hē′zhūn): The adhering or uniting of two surfaces. Layers of connective tissue may adhere, which limits its movement and increases the risk of injury.

Adhesive capsulitis (ad-hē′siv kap′soo-lī′tis): A condition involving inflammatory thickening of a joint capsule, usually at the shoulder, leading to loss of range of motion. Also known as "frozen shoulder."

Adson's test (ad′son): A test for thoracic outlet syndrome. The patient is seated with his or her head extended and rotated toward the affected side. With deep inspiration there is a diminution or total loss of radial pulse on that side.

Adventitia (ad-ven-tish′ă): The outermost connective tissue layer that covers organs and vessels.

Aerobic metabolism (ār-ö′bik mĕ-tab′ö-lizm): Metabolism that occurs in the presence of adequate oxygen, which reduces the overall production of toxic waste products.

Aflatoxin B1: A toxin produced by some strains of *Aspergillus flavus* that causes cancer in some animals. (See *liver cancer*)

Agglutination (ă-gloo-ti-nā′shŭn): The process by which suspended red blood cells or other particles are caused to adhere and form clumps. (See *chemical dependency*)

Agoraphobia (ag′ör-ă-fö′bē-ă): A mental disorder characterized by an irrational fear of leaving the familiar setting of home, or venturing into the open; often associated with panic attacks. (See *anxiety disorders*)

Albumin (al-bū′min): Any of several naturally occurring blood proteins, some of which contribute to blood clotting capacity.

Alcoholism (al′kö-hol-izm): Chronic alcohol abuse, dependence, or addiction; chronic excessive drinking of alcoholic beverages resulting in impairment of health and/or social or occupational functioning, and increasing adaptation to the effects of alcohol, requiring increasing doses to achieve and sustain a desired effect. (See *chemical dependency*)

Aldosterone (al-dos′ter-ön): A hormone manufactured in the adrenal cortex. It helps to maintain appropriate fluid balance by influencing sodium reabsorption in the kidneys. The principal mineralocorticoid.

Alkaline phosphatase (al′kă-lĭn fos′fă-tās): A phosphatase with an optimum pH of above 7.0 present in many tissues; low levels of this enzyme are seen in cases of hypophosphatasia. (See *Paget's disease, osteoporosis*)

Allergen (al′er-jen): A substance that elicits an allergic reaction.

Allergic rhinitis (ă-lĕr′jik rī-nī′tis): Synonym for hay fever. (See *sinusitis*)

Allogenic transplant: A graft transplanted between genetically nonidentical individuals of the same species.

Alpha-1 antitrypsin: A protein that protects the inner lining of alveoli. (See *emphysema, bronchiectasis*)

Alpha-blockers: A class of medications employed to help control hypertension.

Alpha-fetoprotein: An antigen present in the fetus, associated with neural tube defects. (See *spina bifida*)

Alveolus (al-vē′ö-lŭs), alveoli: A small cavity or socket. Specifically, the terminal epithelial structures in the lungs where gaseous exchange takes place.

Alzheimer's disease (awlz′hī-mĕrz): Progressive mental deterioration manifested by loss of memory, ability to calculate, and visual–spatial orientation; confusion; disorientation.

Amantadine (ă-man′tā-dēn): An antiviral agent sometimes used to treat influenza.

Ambulatory (am′bū-lă-tör-ē): Able to walk about; not confined to bed or a wheelchair.

Amenorrhea (ă-men-ö-rē′ă): Absence or abnormal cessation of menses.

Amine (ă-mēn′): A positively charged ion found only in association with negatively charged ions; amines combine with acids to form salts.

Amino acid (ă-mē′nö): An organic acid in which one of the hydrogen atoms on a carbon atom has been replaced by NH$_2$. A building block of proteins.

Amniocentesis (am′nē-ö-sen-tē′sis): Transabdominal aspiration of fluid from the amniotic sac for diagnostic purposes.

Amphiarthrosis (am′fi-ar-thrö′sis), amphiarthroses: A form of joint in which the two bones are joined by fibrocartilage.

Amyotrophic lateral sclerosis (ă-mī-ö-trö′fik lat′ĕr-ăl sklĕrö′sis): A disease of the motor tracts of the lateral columns and anterior horns of the spinal cord, causing progressive muscular atrophy, increased reflexes, fibrillary twitching, and spastic irritability of muscles. Also called Lou Gehrig's disease.

Anaerobic metabolism (an-ār-ö′bik mĕ-tab′ö-lizm): Metabolism that takes place without adequate supplies of oxygen, which may result in the excessive buildup of toxic waste products.

Anaphylaxis (an′ă-fī-lak′sis): An immediate, transient allergic reaction characterized by contraction of smooth muscle and dilation of capillaries.

Androgen (an′drö-jen): A hormone that stimulates activity of sex organs.

Aneurysm (an′ū-rizm): Circumscribed dilation of an artery or a cardiac chamber, a direct communication with the lumen, usually caused by an acquired or congenital weakness of the wall of the artery or chamber.

Angina (an′ji-nă): A severe, often constricting pain. Usually refers to angina pectoris.

Angioedema (an′jē-ö-ĕ-dē′mă): Recurrent large circumscribed areas of subcutaneous edema of sudden onset, usually disappearing within 24 hours, frequently seen as an allergic reaction to foods or drugs. (See *allergic reactions*)

Angiogenesis (an′jē-ö-jen′ĕ-sis): Development of new blood vessels.

Angiogram (an′jē-ö-gram): Radiograph of blood vessels after the injection of contrast material.

Angioneurotic edema (an-jē-ö-nū-rot′ik e-dē′mă): A situation in which hives appear on the face and neck and swelling occurs to the point that breathing becomes difficult.

Angioplasty (an′jē-ö-plas-tē): Recanalization of a blood vessel, usually by means of balloon dilation or the placement of a stent.

Ankylosing spondylitis (ang-ki-lö′sing spon-di-lī′tis): Arthritis of the spine; the disease is more common in the male, often with the rheumatoid factor absent and the HLA antigen present. The strong familial aggregation suggests an important genetic factor.

Annulus fibrosis: Fibrous ring of tissue in an intervertebral disc.

Anoxia (an-ok′sē-ă): Absence of oxygen.

Anterior knee pain syndrome: Synonym for patellofemoral syndrome.

Antibody (an′tē-bod-ē): An immunoglobulin molecule produced by B-cells and designed to react with specific antigens.

Anticholinergic (an′tē-kol-i-ner′jik): Antagonistic to the action of parasympathetic or other cholinergic nerve fibers (e.g., atropine).

Anticoagulant (an′tē-kö-ag′ū-lant): An agent that prevents or inhibits coagulation of the blood.

Antidiuretic hormone (an′tē-dī-yū-ret′ik hör′mön): Also called vasopressin, a hormone that suppresses the output of urine.

Antigen (an′ti-jen): Any substance that, as a result of coming into contact with appropriate cells, elicits a state of immune response.

Antinuclear antibody (an-tē-nū′klē-ăr an′tē-bod-ē): An antibody showing an affinity for cell nuclei, demonstrated by exposing a cell substrate to the serum to be tested, followed by exposure to an antihuman-globulin serum; found in the serum of a high proportion of patients with systemic lupus erythematosus, rheumatoid arthritis, and certain collagen diseases, in some of their healthy relatives, and in approximately 1% of normal individuals.

Antrectomy (an-trek′tö′mē): Removal of the antrum (distal half) of the stomach in treatment of peptic ulcer.

Aphasia (ă-fā′zē-ă): Impaired or absent comprehension or production of, or communication by, speech, writing, or signs; due to an acquired lesion of the dominant cerebral hemisphere. (See *stroke*)

Aphtha (af′thă), aphthae: Small ulcer on a mucous membrane, usually in the mouth.

Aplastic (ā-plas′tik): Referring to conditions characterized by defective regeneration (i.e., varieties of cancer).

Apnea (ap′nē-ă): Absence of breathing.

Aponeurosis ap′ö-noo-rö′sis): A fibrous sheet or flat, expanded tendon, giving attachment to muscular fibers and serving as the means of origin or insertion of a flat muscle; it sometimes serves as a fascia for other muscles.

Apoptosis (ap′op-tö′sis): Programmed cell death.

Arachidonic acid: An essential fatty acid associated with hypersensitivity reactions on the skin.

Arachnoid (ă-rak′noyd): A delicate membrane of spider-web–like filaments that lies between the dura mater and the pia mater.

Arrhythmia (ă-rith′mē-ă): Irregularity of the heartbeat.

Arteriogram (ar-tēr′ē-ö-gram): Radiographic demonstration of an artery after the injection of a contrast medium.

Arteriole (ar-tēr′ē-öl): A minute artery continuous with a capillary network.

Arteriosclerosis (ar-tēr′ē-ö-skler-ö′sis): Hardening of the arteries; types generally recognized are: atherosclerosis, Mönckeberg arteriosclerosis, and arteriolosclerosis.

Ascites (ă-sī′tēz): The accumulation of serous fluid in the peritoneal cavity. (See *cirrhosis*, *liver cancer*)

Aspergillosis (as′per-ji-lö′sis): The presence of *Aspergillus* (a genus of fungi) in the tissues or on a mucous surface of humans and animals, and the symptoms produced thereby. (See *bronchiectasis*)

Asphyxia (as-fik′sē-ă): Impaired or absent exchange of carbon dioxide and oxygen in the respiratory system.

Ataxic (ă-tak′sik): Unable to coordinate muscle activity for smooth movement.

Atelectasis (at-ĕ-lek′tă-sis): Absence of gas from a part or whole of the lung; pulmonary collapse.

Atherosclerosis (ath′er-ö-skler-ö′sis): Hardening of the arteries characterized by the formation of lipid deposits in the intima of large arteries. Deposits lead to fibrosis and calcification, and a narrowing of the lumen.

Athetoid (ath′ĕ-toyd): Referring to slow, writhing, involuntary movement of fingers and hands, sometimes of toes and feet. (See cerebral palsy)

Atopic (ă-top′ik): Relating to an allergic reaction.

Atrial fibrillation (a′trē-ăl fi-bri-lā′shŭn): Fibrillation in which the normal rhythmical contractions of the cardiac atria are replaced by rapid irregular twitchings of the muscular wall. (See *embolism*)

Atrium (ā′trē-ŭm), atria: A chamber or cavity connected to other cavities. Specifically, the superior chambers of the heart.

Atrophic (ă-trof′ik): Denoting atrophy.

Atrophy (at′rö-fē): A wasting of tissues from a number of causes, including diminished cellular proliferation, ischemia, malnutrition, and death.

Auscultation (aws-kŭl-tā′shŭn): Listening to sounds made by various body parts as a diagnostic tool.

Autoantibody (aw-tö-an′ti-bod-ē): Antibody occurring in response to antigenic constituents of the host's tissue, and which reacts with the inciting tissue component.

Autodigestion (aw′tö-dī-jes′chŭn): Enzymatic digestion of cells (especially dead or degenerate) by enzymes present within them. (See *pancreatitis*)

Autogenic transplant: The transplantation of a substance that originated within the patient's body, as in bone marrow cells. Also called autologous transplant.

Autoimmune (aw-tö-i-mūn′): Arising from and directed against the individual's tissues.

Autologous transplant: Synonym for autogenic transplant.

Autonomic hyperreflexia (aw-tö-nom′ik hī pĕr-rē-flek′sē-ă): A syndrome occurring in some persons with spinal cord lesions and resulting from functional impairment of the autonomic nervous system. Symptoms include hypertension, bradycardia, severe headaches, pallor below and flushing above the cord lesion, and convulsions.

Avascular (ă-vas′kū-ler): Without blood or lymphatic vessels.

Avulsion (ă-vŭl′shŭn): A tearing away or forcible separation.

Axon (ak′son): The process of a nerve cell that conducts impulses away from the cell body.

Babesiosis (bă-bē′zē-ö′sis): An infection with a species of protozoan parasites, transferred to humans by tick bites.

Barrel chest (ba′rĕl chest): An occasional symptom of emphysema, in which the intercostal muscles hold the rib cage out as widely as possible.

Barrett's esophagus (bar′et ē-sof′ă-gŭs): Chronic ulceration of the lower esophagus, often associated with gastroesophageal reflux disorder (GERD); sometimes a precursor to adenocarcinoma of the esophagus.

Basal ganglia (bā′săl gang′lē-a): Large masses of gray matter at the base of the cerebral hemispheres.

Basal layer (bā′săl lā′ĕr): Also called the stratum basale: the deepest layer of the epidermis.

Basophil (bā'sö-fil): A phagocytic leukocyte.

Bell's law (bel): The ventral spinal roots are motor, whereas the dorsal spinal roots are sensory.

Benign (bē-nīn'): Denoting the mild character of an illness or nonmalignant character of a neoplasm.

Benign prostate hypertrophy (BPH) (bē-nīn' pros-tat'ik hī-per'trö-fē): A nodular hyperplasia of the prostate; the gland thickens in a way that may obstruct the urethra.

Benzene (ben'zēn): A highly toxic hydrocarbon from light coal tar oil, used as a solvent.

Benzodiazepine: Any of a group of psychotropic drugs with sedative action; used as anti-anxieties or sleeping aids. (See *anxiety disorders*)

Beta amyloid (bā'tă am'i-loyd): A type of protein associated with the formation of plaque in the brain. (See *Alzheimer's disease*)

Beta blocker: A type of drug that limits sympathetic reactions, specifically as they relate to the cardiovascular system.

Beta cell: Cell in the pancreas that secretes insulin.

Bile (bīl): Yellowish-brown or green fluid produced in the liver, stored in the gallbladder, and released into the duodenum to aid in the digestion of fats.

Biliary colic (bil'ē-ăr-ē kol'ik): Intense spasmodic pain felt in the right upper quadrant of the abdomen from impaction of a gallstone in the cystic duct.

Bilirubin (bil-i-roo'bin): A dark bile pigment formed from the hemoglobin of dead erythrocytes.

Biphosphate: A group of medications that inhibit reabsorption of bone; often recommended in the treatment of osteoporosis.

Bipolar disease (bī-pö'ler di-zēz'): Synonym for manic depression.

Bismuth (biz'mŭth): A metallic element used in several medicines, specifically in those designed to affect stomach acidity.

Blood-brain barrier (bŭd-brān bar'ē-er): A selective filter that prevents or inhibits the passage of ions or large compounds from the blood to the brain tissue; located in a continuous layer of endothelial cells connected by tight junctions.

Bolus (bö'lŭs): A masticated morsel of food or other substance ready to be swallowed.

Bone scan (bön skan): A diagnostic test to look for bone cancer or infections, to evaluate unexplained pain, or to diagnose fractures.

Borrelia burgdorferi (bö-rē'lē-ă bŭrg-dör'fĕr-ī): A species of bacteria that causes Lyme disease; transferred to humans through tick bites.

Botulinum (bot-yū-lī'nŭm): A potent neurotoxin from *Clostridium botulinum.*

Bovine spongiform encephalitis (bö'vīn spön'ji-förm en-sef-ă-lop'ă-thē): A disease of cattle first reported in 1986 in Great Britain; characterized clinically by apprehensive behavior, hyperesthesia, and ataxia, and histologically by spongiform changes in the gray matter of the brainstem; caused by a prion, like spongiform encephalopathies of other animals (e.g., scrapie) and human beings (Creutzfeldt-Jakob disease). (See *Alzheimer's disease*)

Bowen's disease (bö'wen di-zēz): A form of intraepidermal carcinoma characterized by the development of slowly enlarging pinkish or brownish papules or eroded plaques covered with a thickened horny layer. (See *skin cancer*)

Bowman's capsule (bö'măn): The beginning of a nephron that surrounds the glomerulus.

Bradykinesia (brad-ē-kin-ē'zē-ă): A decrease in the spontaneity of movement.

Bronchiectasis (brong-kē-ek'tă-sis): Chronic dilation of the bronchi or bronchioles, often as a consequence of inflammatory disease or obstruction.

Bruxism (brŭk'sizm): Jaw clenching that results in rubbing and grinding of teeth, especially during sleep.

Buerger's disease (bĕr'gĕr di-zēz): Inflammation of the intima of a blood vessel, with thrombosis. (See *Raynaud syndrome*)

Bulla (bul'ă), bullae: A bubble-like structure, specifically the air-filled blisters on the lung formed by fused alveoli in emphysema.

Burkitt's lymphoma (bĕr'kit): A form of malignant lymphoma frequently involving the jaw and abdominal lymph nodes. Geographic distribution of Burkitt's lymphoma suggests that it is found in areas with endemic malaria. It is primarily a B-cell neoplasm and is believed to be caused by Epstein-Barr virus, a member of the family *Herpesviridae*.

Bursectomy (ber-sek'tö-mē): Surgical removal of a bursa.

Calcitonin (kal-si-tö'nin): A hormone that increases the deposition of calcium and phosphate in bone.

Calcium channel blockers: A class of medications that prevents the passage of calcium through membranes; used to treat hypertension, angina pectoris, and arrhythmia.

Calcium oxalate (kal'sē-ŭm ok'să-lāt): A sediment in urine and renal calculi. (See *kidney stones*)

Calcium phosphate: Calcium salts of phosphoric acid.

Calcium pyrophosphate dehydrate (kal'sē-ŭm pī-rö-fos'făt dī-hī'drāt): Substance deposited in pseudogout, leading to acute attacks of joint inflammation. (See *gout*)

Callus (kal'ŭs): A thickening of the keratin layer of the epidermis as a result of repeated friction or intermittent pressure.

Campylobacter jejuni (kam'pi-lö-bak'tĕr je-jū'nī): A species that causes an acute gastroenteritis of sudden onset with constitutional symptoms (malaise, myalgia, arthralgia, and headache) and cramping abdominal pain.

Campylobacter pylori (kam'pi-lö-bak'tĕr pī-lör'ī): Synonym for *Helicobacter pylori*. (See *ulcers*)

Candida albicans (kan'dĭ-ă al-bi'kanz): A genus of yeast-like fungi.

Carbuncle (kar'bŭng-kl): A group of localized infections of hair follicles, with the formation of connecting sinuses. A group of boils.

Cardiomyopathy (kar'dē-ō-mī-op'ă-thē): Disease of the myocardium; a primary disease of heart muscle in the absence of a known underlying cause.

Cataplexy (kat'ă-plek-sē): A transient attack of extreme generalized muscular weakness, often precipitated by an emotional state such as laughing, surprise, fear, or anger. (See *sleep disorders*)

Catheter atherectomy (kath'ĕ-ter ath-e-rek'tō-mē): Removal of atherosclerotic plaque through a catheter; usually applied to carotid arteries.

Cauda equina (kaw'dă ē-kwī'nă): Bundle of spinal nerve roots that runs through the lumbar cistern; it comprises the roots of all the spinal nerves below L₁. From Latin, "horse tail." (See *ankylosing spondylitis, disc disease*)

Causalgia (kaw-zal'jē-ă): Persistent severe burning sensation, usually after partial injury of a peripheral nerve, accompanied by trophic changes (thinning of skin, loss of sweat glands and hair follicles). (See *reflex sympathetic dystrophy syndrome*)

Celiac sprue (sē'lē-ak sproo): Chronic inflammation and atrophy of the mucosa of the small intestine, related to an allergy to gluten. (See *celiac disease*)

Cellular immunity (sel'yū-lăr i-myū'ni-tē): Also called cell-mediated immunity. Immune responses that are initiated by T-cells and mediated by T-cells, macrophages, or both.

Cervical rib (ser'vi-kăl rib): An abnormally wide transverse process of a cervical vertebra, or a supernumerary rib that articulates with a cervical vertebra but does not articulate with the sternum. C₇ is the vertebra most often affected.

Cervical spondylitic myelopathy (ser'vĭ-kal spon-di-lit'ik mī-ĕ-lop'ă-thē): Damage to the spinal cord due to osteophytic pressure. (See *spondylosis*)

Chancre (shan'ker): The primary lesion of syphilis, which begins at the site of infection after an interval of 10 to 30 days as a papule or area of infiltration, of dull red color, hard, and insensitive; the center usually becomes eroded or breaks down into an ulcer that heals slowly after 4 to 6 weeks. (See *sexually transmitted diseases*)

Chemonucleolysis (kem'ö-noo-klē-ol'i-sis): Injection of chymopapain into the nucleus pulposus of a herniated disc.

Chemotherapy (kem'ö-thăr-ă-pē): The treatment of disease by chemical means (i.e., drugs).

Chimeric (kī-mēr'ik): Any macromolecule fusion formed by two or more macromolecules from different species or from different genes. (See *scleroderma*)

Chlamydia (kla-mid'ē-ă): A genus of bacteria that is a causative factor for pelvic inflammatory disease and other infections; the chief agent of bacterial sexually transmitted diseases in the United States.

Chlamydia trachomatis (kla-mik'ē-yă trak-ö'măt-ĭs): Spherical organisms that cause a variety of infections, including conjunctivitis, pelvic inflammatory disease, and others.

Cholangitis (kö-lan-jī'tis): Inflammation of the bile duct or biliary tree.

Cholecyst (kö'le-sist): Synonym for gallbladder.

Choledocholithiasis (kö-led'ö-kö-lith-ī'ă-sis): Presence of a gallstone in the common bile duct.

Cholelithiasis: Presence of stones in the gallbladder or bile ducts.

Cholinesterase inhibitors: Class of drugs that improves myoneural function; used for myasthenia gravis, Alzheimer's disease.

Chondroitin sulfate: One of the substances present in the extracellular matrix of connective tissue.

Chondromalacia patellae (kon'drö-mă-lā'shē-ă pa-tel'ē): Degenerative condition in the articular cartilage of the patella caused by abnormal compression or shearing forces at the knee joint; may cause patellalgia (knee pain).

Choriocarcinoma (kö'rē-ö-kar-si-nö'mă): A highly malignant neoplasm. Hemorrhagic metastases are found in the lungs, liver, and brain, and vagina; choriocarcinoma may follow any type of pregnancy, especially hydatidiform mole, and occasionally originates in teratoid neoplasms of the ovaries or testes. (See *testicular cancer*)

Christmas disease (krist'mas diz'ēz): Synonym for hemophilia B, involving a deficiency in clotting factor IX.

Chronic (krŏn'ik): Referring to a health-related state: low intensity, lasting a long time.

Chronic exertional compartment syndrome: The accumulation of fluid pressure in one or more of the tough fascial compartments of the lower leg. (See *shin splints*)

Chronic granulocytic leukemia (kron'ik gran'yū-lö-sit'ik lū-kē'mē-ă): Synonym for chronic myelogenous leukemia. (See *leukemia*)

Chronic myeloid leukemia (kron'ik mī'ĕ-loyd lū-kē'mē-ă): Synonym for chronic myelogenous leukemia. (See *leukemia*)

Chyme (kīm): Semifluid mass of partly digested food in the stomach or small intestine.

Cilium (sil'ē-ŭm), cilia: Hair-like extension of the surface of certain epithelial cells.

Circadian rhythm (ser-kā'dē-ăn): Relating to biologic variations or rhythms that last approximately 24 hours. From Latin *circa* (about) and *dies* (day).

Cirrhosis (sir-rö'sis): Progressive disease of the liver characterized by damage to hepatocytes and the accumulation of scar tissue.

Clonic spasm (klon′ik spa′zm): Alternating involuntary contraction and relaxation of a muscle.

Coagulability: Capable of being coagulated or clotted.

Cobalamine (kō-bal′ă-min): General term for compounds containing the nucleus of vitamin B₁₂.

Cognitive–behavioral therapy: A technique in psychotherapy that uses guided self-discovery, imaging, self-instruction, and other elicited cognitions as the principal mode of treatment.

Colchicine (kol′chi-sin): An alkaloid obtained from autumn crocus used for the treatment of gout.

Colic (kol′ik): An abnormal contraction of smooth muscle, particularly in the digestive tract.

Collagen (kol′lă-jen): A major protein forming the white fibers of connective tissue.

Collagenase (kol-ă′jēn-năs): A proteolytic (dissolving) enzyme that acts on one or more of the collagens.

Colonoscopy (kō-lon-os′kŏ-pē): A visual examination of the internal surface of the colon by means of a colonoscope.

Colostomy (kō-los′tō-mē): The establishment of an artificial opening from the skin to the colon.

Colposcopy (kol-pos′kŏ-pē): Examination of the vagina and cervix by means of an endoscope.

Comedo (kom′ē-dö): A dilated hair follicle filled with bacteria; the principal lesion of acne vulgaris. (plural: comedos, comedones)

Comminuted (kom′i-noo-ted): Broken into several pieces; denoting especially a fractured bone.

Complement (kom′plĕ-ment): A combination of many serum proteins that react with each other in various ways to disable antigens and assist immune system response.

Complex regional pain syndrome: A term used to describe a chronic pain syndrome; sometimes called reflex sympathetic dystrophy syndrome.

Condyle (kon′dīl): A rounded articular surface at the extremity of a bone.

Condylomata acuminatum: A warty growth on the external genitals or at the anus, consisting of fibrous overgrowths covered by thickened epithelium showing koilocytosis, due to sexually transmitted infection with human papilloma virus; malignant change is associated with particular types of the virus. (See *sexually transmitted diseases*)

Congenital (kon-jen′i-tăl): Referring to mental or physical traits that exist at birth.

Congenital nevus (kon-jen′i-tăl nē′vŭs): A benign localized overgrowth of melanin-forming cells of the skin present at birth or appearing early in life. (See *moles*)

Consolidation (kon-sol-i-dā′shŭn): Solidification into a firm, dense mass, specifically with cellular exudate in the lungs during pneumonia.

Constriction (kon-strik′shŭn): A narrowed portion of a luminal structure.

Contact inhibition (kon′takt in-hi-bish′yŭn): The tendency of basal cells involved in healing to stop reproducing when they encounter cells from the other side of the wound.

Contralateral (kon-tră-lat′er-ăl): Relating to the opposite side, as when pain is felt or paralysis occurs on the side opposite to that of the lesion.

Cor pulmonale (kör pul-mö-nā′lā): Right-sided ventricular hypertrophy, often arising from diseases of the lungs.

Corpus callosum (kör′pŭs ka-lö′sŭm): The plate of nerve fibers interconnecting the cortical hemispheres.

Corpus luteum (kör′pŭs lū′tē-ŭm): The site of egg release on follicles of the ovaries immediately after ovulation.

Corticosteroid injection: An injection of a specific steroid into an injured area for its anti-inflammatory or connective tissue–dissolving properties.

Cortisol (kör′ti-sol): A glucocorticoid secreted by the adrenal cortex. It acts on carbohydrate metabolism and influences the growth and nutrition of connective tissue.

Cortisone (kör′ti-sön): A form of cortisol that may be injected into specific areas to act as an anti-inflammatory or to help dissolve connective tissue.

Coup-contrecoup: Pattern of brain injury involving a primary impact on one side of the skull, and a secondary impact as the brain bounces to the opposite side of the cranium. (See *traumatic brain injury*)

Cox 2 inhibitors: A class of NSAIDS that work by blocking COX-2 enzyme, which is involved in the inflammation pathway.

Coxsackie virus (kok-sak′ē vī′rŭs): A group of viruses first isolated in Coxsackie, New York. They may be responsible for several human diseases, including meningitis and juvenile diabetes.

C-reactive protein (rē-ak′tiv prö′tēn): A β-globulin found in the serum of various persons with certain inflammatory, degenerative, and neoplastic diseases. (See *heart attack, atherosclerosis*)

Creatine kinase (krē′ă-tēn kī′nās): An enzyme used in muscle contraction that allows the transformation of adenosine diphosphate (ADP) into adenosine triphosphate (ATP) and creatine; levels of creatine kinase are sometimes elevated after a heart attack. (See *muscular dystrophy*)

Crepitus (krep′i-tŭs): A crackling sound resembling the noise heard on rubbing hair between the fingers.

CREST syndrome (krest sin′dröm): *C*alcinosis, *R*aynaud phenomenon, *e*sophageal motility disorders, *s*clerodactyly, and *t*elangiectasia. (See *scleroderma*)

Crisis (krī′sis): A sudden change, usually for the better, in the course of an acute disease.

Cruciate ligament sprains: Major ligaments that crisscross the knee in the anteroposterior direction, providing stability in that plane.

Crust (krŭst): A hard outer covering; a scab.

Cryomyolysis: A procedure using liquid nitrogen to freeze uterine fibroid tumors.

Cryptococcus neoformans: A genus of yeastlike fungi that reproduce by budding. (See *HIV/AIDS*)

Cryptorchism (krip-tör'kizm): Failure of one or both of the testes to descend. (See *testicular cancer*)

Cryptosporidium (krip'tö'spö-rid'ē-ŭm): A genus of sporozoans that are common parasites of humans with impaired immunity. (See *gastroenteritis*)

Cyanosis (sī-ă-nö'sis): A bluish or purplish coloration of the skin and mucous membranes due to deficient oxygenation of the blood. (See *Raynaud syndrome*; *anemia*)

Cyclooxygenase-2: see Cox-2 inhibitors.

Cystadenoma (sist'ad-ĕ-nö'mă): A benign neoplasm derived from glandular epithelium. (See *ovarian cysts*)

Cystine (sis'tīn): A type of acid that can create deposits of crystals in the urine or in the kidneys.

Cystoscope (sis'tö-sköp): A lighted tubular endoscope for examining the interior of the bladder.

Cytokine (sī'tö-kin): Hormone-like proteins secreted by many different cells, involved in cell-to-cell communication.

Cytomegalovirus (sī-tö-meg'ă-lö-vī'rŭs): A group of viruses in the Herpesviridae family infecting humans and animals. (See *mononucleosis*)

Cytotoxic drug (sī-tö-tok'sik): A drug that is detrimental or destructive to certain cells.

De Quervain tenosynovitis (dĕ kār-vā'): Inflammation of the tendons of the first dorsal compartment of the wrist, which includes the extensor pollicis brevis and the abductor pollicis longus.

Debridement (dā-brēd-mawn'): Excision of dead tissue and foreign matter from a wound.

Decubitus ulcer (dē-kyū'bi-tŭs ŭl'sĕr): Focal ischemic necrosis of skin and underlying tissues at sites of constant pressure or recurring friction in persons confined to bed or immobilized by illness.

Degeneration (dē-jen-er-ā'shŭn): A retrogressive pathologic change in tissues, in consequence of which their functions may be impaired or destroyed.

Degenerative joint disease (dē-jen'ĕr-ă-tiv joint di-zēz): Synonym for osteoarthritis.

Dementia (dē-men'shē-ă): The loss, usually progressive, of cognitive and intellectual functions, without impairment of perception or consciousness.

Dendrite (den'drīt): The process of a nerve cell that carries impulses toward the cell body.

Dermabrasion (der-mă-brā'zhŭn): Procedure to remove acne scars or pits from the skin using sandpaper, rotating wire brushes, or other abrasive materials.

Dermatitis herpetiformis (dĕr'mă-tī'tis hĕr-pe-ti-fŏr'mis): A chronic disease of the skin marked by a symmetric itching eruption of vesicles and papules that occur in groups; relapses are common; associated with gluten-sensitive enteropathy. (See *celiac disease*)

Dermatome (der'mă-töm): The area of skin supplied by cutaneous branches from a single spinal nerve.

Dermatophyte (der'mă-tö-fīt): A fungus that causes superficial infections of the skin, hair, and nails.

Dermatophytosis (der'mă-tö-fī-tö'sis): An infection of the hair, skin, or nails caused by any one of the dermatophytes. The lesions are characterized by erythema, small papular vesicles, fissures, and scaling. (See *fungal infections*)

Dermoid cyst (dĕr'moys sist): A tumor consisting of displaced ectodermal structures along lines of embryonic fusion, the wall being formed of epithelium-lined connective tissue, including skin appendages and containing keratin, sebum, and hair. (See *testicular cancer*, *ovarian cysts*)

Dextroamphetamine: A medication for central nervous system stimulation.

Diabetes insipidus (dī-ă-bē'tēz in-sip'i-dŭs): Chronic excretion of very large amounts of pale urine of low specific gravity, causing dehydration and extreme thirst; ordinarily results from inadequate output of pituitary antidiuretic hormone.

Diaphoresis (dī-ă-fö-rē'sis): Perspiration.

Diaphysis (dī-af'i-sis): The shaft of a long bone.

Diarthrosis (dī-ar-thrö'sis), diarthroses: Also called synovial joint. A joint in which articulating surfaces are covered by articular cartilage and held together by a capsular ligament, which is lined with a synovial membrane. Some degree of freedom of movement is possible with diarthrotic joints.

Diastole (dī-as'tö-lē): Normal post-systolic dilation of the heart cavities, during which they fill with blood.

Diethylstilbestrol: An estrogenic compound sometimes used in birth control pills.

Diffuse axonal injury (di-fyūs' ax-on'ăl in-jū-rē): Injury to white matter in the central nervous system that is frequently associated with a persistent vegetative state. (See *traumatic brain injury*)

Diffuse large cell lymphoma: A type of intermediate-grade lymphoma.

Diffuse mixed cell lymphoma: A type of intermediate-grade lymphoma.

Diffuse scleroderma (di-fūs sklēr-ö-der'mă): A form of systemic scleroderma involving sudden onset and early involvement of internal organs.

Diffusion (di-fū'zhŭn): Random movement of small particles in solution to a uniform distribution within a closed space.

Dihydrotestosterone (DHT) (dī-hī'drö-tes-tos'ter-ön): An androgenic hormone with the same uses and actions as testosterone. Elevated levels are associated with an increased risk of benign prostatic hyperplasia.

Dilation (dī-lā′shŭn): The enlargement of a hollow structure or opening.

Dilation and curettage (dī-lā′shŭn kū-rĕ-tahzh′): Dilation of the cervix and curettement of the endometrium.

Dimethyl sulfoxide (DMSO) (dī-meth′il): A penetrating solvent enhancing absorption of therapeutic agents through the skin.

Dioxin (dī-oks′in): A contaminate in some herbicides, associated with toxicity, some forms of cancer, and birth defects.

Diphtheria (dif-thē-r′ĕă): A highly infectious bacterial disease that begins in the nose and throat; can resemble symptoms of mononucleosis.

Diplegia (dī-plē′jē-ă): Paralysis of corresponding parts on both sides of the body.

Discoid lupus erythematosus (dis′koyd lū′pŭs er′ă-thē-mă-tō′sŭs): Autoimmune disease involving lesions on the skin. (See *lupus*)

Discectomy (dis-kek′tö-mē): Excision, in part or whole, of an intervertebral disc. (See *disc disease*)

Diuretic (dī-ū-ret′ik): A chemical agent that increases urine output.

Diverticulum (dī-ver-tik′ū-lŭm)/diverticula: A pouch or sac opening from a tubular or saccular organ (e.g., the colon or urinary bladder).

Dopamine (dö′-pă-mēn): A neurotransmitter present in the basal ganglia.

Double crush syndrome (dŭb′ĕl krŭs sin′dröm): A situation in which peripheral nerves may be irritated at multiple sites, leading to confusing signs and symptoms. (See *carpal tunnel syndrome*)

Ductal ectasia (dŭk′tăl ek-tā′zē-ă): Inflammation of the ducts of the breast. (See *breast cancer*)

Dupuytren contracture (doo-pwē-trah′): A disease of the palmar fascia resulting in thickening and shortening of fibrous bands on the palmar surface of the hand and fingers resulting in a characteristic flexion deformity of the fourth and fifth digits.

Dura mater (doo′ră mā′ter): A tough, fibrous membrane forming the outer covering of the central nervous system.

Dyshidrosis (dis-i-drö′sis): A skin eruption involving blisters and itching that usually appears on the volar surface of the hands or feet.

Dysmotility: Inefficient or uncoordinated peristalsis in the gastrointestinal tract. (See *scleroderma*)

Dyspepsia (dis-pep′sē-ă): "Upset stomach," resulting in pain, burning, nausea, and gas.

Dysphagia (dis-fā′jē-ă): Difficulty in swallowing.

Dysplasia (dis-plā′zē-ă), dysplastic: Abnormal tissue development.

Dysplastic nevus (dis-plas′tik nē′vŭs): Atypical moles with an increased risk for developing into malignant melanoma. (See *moles*)

Dyspnea (disp-nē′ă): Shortness of breath.

Dysthymia (dis-thī′mē-ă): Chronic mood disorder involving long-term, low-grade depression.

Dystonia (dis-tö′nē-ă): A state of abnormal (too much or too little) muscle tone.

Dystrophic (dis-trof′ik): Relating to progressive changes that may result from defective nutrition of a tissue or organ.

Dystrophin (dis-trö′fin): A protein found in the sarcolemma of normal muscle tissue; it is missing in individuals with some forms of muscular dystrophy.

E. coli: *Escherichia coli*, a genus of bacteria linked with infections of the gastrointestinal or urinary tracts.

Ecchymosis (ek-i-mö′sis): A purplish patch caused by blood leaking into the skin; a bruise.

Echocardiogram (ek-ö-kar′dē-ö-gram): The record obtained by the use of ultrasound in the investigation of the heart and great vessels and diagnosis of cardiovascular lesions.

Eclampsia (ek-lamp′sē-ă): The occurrence of one or more convulsions not attributable to other cerebral conditions. In this case, related to pregnancy-induced hypertension.

Eczema (ek′zĕ-mă): Generic term for inflammatory conditions of the skin, particularly with blistering in the acute stage, often accompanied by sensations of itching and burning.

Edema (e-dē′mă): An accumulation of an excessive amount of watery fluid in cells, tissues, or serous membranes.

Ehrlichiosis (er-lik-ē-ö′sis): A tick-borne bacterial infection of humans and dogs. (See *Lyme disease*)

Elastin (ĕ-las′tin): A yellow, elastic fibrous protein that contributes to the connective tissue of elastic structures.

Electrocauterization (ē-lek′trö-caw′ter-i-zā′shŭn): Cauterization by passage of high-frequency current through tissue, or by metal that has been electrically heated.

Electroencephalogram (EEG) (ē-lek′trö-en-sef′ă-lö-gram): A recording of electrical potentials of the brain, derived from electrodes attached to the scalp.

Electrolyte (ē-lek′trö-līt): Any compound that, in solution, conducts electricity and is decomposed by it.

Electromyography (EMG) (ē-lek′trö-mī-og′ră-fē): A recording of electrical activity in muscle tissue.

ELISA test: Enzyme-linked immunosorbent assay. (See *HIV/AIDS*)

Embolization (em′bol-i-zā′shun): Therapeutic introduction of various substances into the circulation to occlude vessels, either to arrest or prevent hemorrhaging or to devitalize a structure or organ by occluding its blood supply.

Embryonic carcinoma (em-brē-on′ik kar-si-nö′mă): A type of testicular cancer.

Emery-Dreifuss muscular dystrophy: A generally benign

type of muscular dystrophy that typically begins in the shoulder girdle and then spreads distally; an X-linked inherited disorder.

Emollient (ē-mol′ē-ent): An agent that softens the skin or soothes irritation of the skin.

Encephalitis (en-sef-ă-lī′tis): Inflammation of the brain.

Endarterectomy (end-ar-ter-ek′tö-mē): Excision of the diseased layers of an artery along with atherosclerotic plaques.

Endemic (en-dem′ik): Present in a community or among a group of people; said of a disease prevailing continually in a region.

Endo-: A prefix indicating within, inner, absorbing, or containing.

Endocarditis (en′dö-kar-kī′tis): Inflammation of the innermost tunic of the heart.

Endogenous (en-doj′ĕ-nŭs): Originating or produced within the organism or one of its parts.

Endometritis (en′dö-mē-trī′tis): Inflammation of the endometrium.

Endometrium (en′dö-mē′trē-ŭm): The inner layers of the uterine wall.

Endomysium (en′dö-miz′ē-ŭm): The connective tissue sheath surrounding muscle fibers.

Endoscopic retrograde cholangiopancreatography (ERCP) (en-dö-skop′ik ret′rö-grādkö-lan′jē-ö-pan-krē-ă-tog′ră-fē): A diagnostic procedure to detect problems in the liver, gallbladder, bile ducts, or pancreas. (See *gallstones*)

Endosteum (en-dos′tē-ŭm): A layer of cells lining the inner surface of bone in the central medullary cavity of long bones.

Endovascular: Referring to procedures conducted within blood vessels.

Enterovirus (en′ter-ö-vī′rŭs): Any of a diverse group of viruses that attack the intestines.

Enzyme (en′zīm): A protein that acts as a catalyst to induce chemical changes in other substances while remaining unchanged itself.

Eosinophil (ē-ö-sin′ö-fil): A class of phagocytic white blood cells with anti-parasitic functions.

Ephelis (ef-ē′lis), ephelides: Freckles.

Epi-: Prefix indicating upon, following, or subsequent to.

Epicondylitis (ep′i-kon-di-lī′tis): Infection or inflammation of an epicondyle.

Epidermis (ep-i-derm′is): The superficial epithelial portion of the skin.

Epidermophyton (ep′i-der-mof′i-ton): A genus of fungi whose macroconidia are clavate and smooth-walled. The only species, *Epidermophyton floccosum*, is a common cause of tinea pedis and tinea cruris. (See *fungal infections*)

Epididymis (ep-i-did′i-mis): A tube on the posterior aspect of the testes in which sperm mature.

Epimysium (ep-i-mis′ē-ŭm): The connective tissue membrane surrounding a skeletal muscle.

Epinephrine (ep′i-nef′rin): The chief hormone of the adrenal medulla; a potent stimulant of the sympathetic response.

Epistaxis (ep′i-stak′sis): Profuse bleeding from the nose.

Epithelium (ep-i-thē′lē-ŭm): A purely cellular avascular layer covering all free surfaces, including skin, mucous, and serous glands.

Epstein–Barr virus (ep′stīn băr): A herpesvirus that causes infectious mononucleosis and is implicated in Burkitt's lymphoma.

Ergot (er′got): The resistant, overwintering stage of the parasitic ascomycetous fungus *Claviceps purpurea*. Ergot induces uterine contractions, controls bleeding, and alleviates certain localized vascular disorders (migraine headaches).

Ernest syndrome: A condition involving a weakened and irritated stylomandibular ligament; frequently mistaken for temporomandibular joint disorder. (See *temporomandibular joint disorder*)

Erysipelas (er-i-sip′ĕ-las): A specific, acute, cutaneous inflammatory disease caused by β-hemolytic streptococci and characterized by hot, red, edematous, brawny, and sharply defined eruptions; usually accompanied by severe constitutional symptoms. (See *cellulitis*)

Erythema migrans: A type of rash, usually seen as an early symptom of Lyme disease.

Erythema (er-ĭ-thē′mă): Redness of the skin due to capillary dilation.

Erythrocyte (ĕ-rith′rö-sīt): A mature red blood cell.

Erythrodermic psoriasis (ĕ-rith-rö-der′mik sö-rī′ă-sis): A generalized form of psoriasis that can cover 85% or more of the body.

Erythropoietin (EPO) (ĕ-rith-rö-poy′ĕ-tin): A hormone secreted by the kidneys and possibly other tissues that stimulates the formation of red blood cells.

Essential (ĕ-sen′shăl): Of unknown cause, specifically in reference to hypertension.

Estradiol (es-tră-dī′ol): The most potent naturally occurring estrogen in mammals.

Estriol (es′trē-ol): Estrogenic metabolite of estradiol; usually the predominant estrogenic metabolite found in urine, especially during pregnancy.

Estrogen replacement therapy (ERT) (es′trö-jen rē-plās′ment ther′ă-pē): A treatment for the prevention or slowing of osteoporosis by replacing some of the hormones that are lost or diminished with the onset of menopause.

Estrogen (es′trö-jen): A group of hormones secreted by the ovaries, placenta, testes, and possibly other tissues. Estrogens influence secondary sexual characteristics and the menstrual cycle.

Estrone (es′trön): A metabolite of estradiol.

Exenteration (eks-en-ter-ā′shŭn): Removal of internal organs and tissues, usually performed to ablate cancer.

Exogenous (eks-oj′ĕ-nŭs): Originating or produced outside the organism.

Exophthalmus: Protrusion of one or both eyeballs.

External scar tissue: Scar tissue that develops outside of the injured structure, often binding that structure to other nearby structures in adhesions.

Extracorporeal shockwave lithotripsy (eks′tră-kör′pö′rē0ăl shŏk wāv lith′ö-trip′sē): Breaking up of renal or ureteral calculi by focused ultrasound energy.

Exudate (eks′oo-dāt): Any fluid that has seeped out of a tissue or its capillaries because of inflammation or injury.

Facioscapulohumeral dystrophy: A relatively benign, slowly progressive type of muscular dystrophy involving the muscles of the face, shoulders, and arms.

Familial adenomatous polyposis (fa-mil′ē-ăl ad-ĕ-nö′mă-tŭs pol-i-pö′sis): An inherited trait involving the formation of epithelial polyps in the colon; may be associated with an increased risk of colon cancer.

Fascicle (fas′i-kl), fasciculi: A band or bundle of fibers, specifically muscle fibers.

Fasciculation (fa-sik-ū-lā′shŭn): Involuntary contractions or twitchings of fasciculi.

Fat necrosis (fat nĕ-krö′sis): The death of fat cells, often in the breast.

Fecalith (fē′kă-lith): A hard mass composed of solidified or petrified feces. (See *appendicitis, diverticular disease*)

Festinating gait (fes-tĭ-nā′ting gāt): Gait in which the trunk is flexed, legs are stiff but flexed at the knees and hips, and the steps are short and progressively more rapid.

Fetal alcohol syndrome (fē′tăl al′kö-hol sin′dröm): A specific pattern of fetal malformation and health problems among offspring of mothers who are chronic alcoholics.

Fibrillation (fī-bri-lā′shŭn): Exceedingly rapid contractions or twitching of muscular fibrils.

Fibrillin (fī′bril′in): A protein of connective tissue. (See *Marfan syndrome*)

Fibrin (fi′brin): An elastic filamentous protein that aids in coagulation of the blood.

Fibrinogen (fibrin′ö-jen): A globulin of the blood plasma that is converted into fibrin by the action of thrombin in the presence of ionized calcium to produce coagulation of the blood.

Fibroadenoma (fī′brö-ad-ĕ-nö′mă): A benign neoplasm of glandular epithelium, in which fibroblasts and other connective tissue proliferate. (See *breast cancer*)

Fibroblast (fī′brö-blast): A cell capable of forming collagen fibers.

Filtration (fil-trā′shŭn): The process of passing a liquid or gas through a filter.

Fimbria (fim′brē-ă), fimbriae: Any fringe-like structure. Ovarian fimbriae extend over the ovaries.

Fistula (fis′tū′lă), fistulae: An abnormal passage from one epithelial surface to another.

Fixation (fik-sā′shŭn): The condition of being firmly attached or set. In regard to the spine, being excessively limited in movement between individual vertebrae.

Flaccid paralysis (flak′sid pă-ral′i-sis): Paralysis with a loss of muscle tone, although sensation is present.

Focal dystonia (fö′kăl dis-tö′nē-ă): A movement disorder that affects only one region of the body. (See *torticollis*)

Folate (fö′lāt): A form of folic acid.

Folic acid (fö′lik): Member of the vitamin B complex necessary for the normal formation of red blood cells.

Follicular cleaved-cell lymphoma: A type of low-grade lymphoma.

Follicular large-cell lymphoma: A type of intermediate-grade lymphoma.

Follicular mixed-cell lymphoma: A type of low-grade lymphoma.

Frozen shoulder: See *adhesive capsulitis*.

Fundoplication (fŭn′dö-pli-kā′shŭn): Suture of the fundus of the stomach around the esophagus to prevent reflux with hiatal hernia.

Furuncle (fū′rŭng-kl): A localized bacterial infection in a hair shaft. A boil.

Gamma-aminobutyric acid (GABA) : A principal inhibitory neurotransmitter.

Gamma globulin: A preparation of proteins of human plasma, containing the antibodies of normal adults.

Gastritis (gas-trī′tis): Inflammation, especially mucosal, of the stomach.

Gastrostomy (gas-tros′tö-mē): Establishment of a new opening into the stomach.

Geniculate ganglion (je-nik′yū-lāt gang′glē-on): A ganglion of the fibers conveyed by the facial nerve, located within the facial canal, containing the sensory neurons innervating the taste buds on the anterior two thirds of the tongue and a small area on the external ear. (See *Bell's palsy*)

Giardia (jē-ar′dē-ă): A genus of parasitic flagellates that parasitize the gastrointestinal tract of many mammals.

Gigantism (jī′gan-tizm): A condition of abnormal size or overgrowth of the entire body or of any of its parts. (See *acromegaly*)

Gliadin (glī′ă-din): A class of protein, separable from wheat and rye glutens. (See *celiac disease*)

Globus pallidus (glö′bŭs pal′i-dŭs): The inner and lighter gray portion of the lentiform nucleus. (See *Parkinson's disease*)

Glomerular filtration rate (glö-mer′yūlăr fil-trā′shun rāt): The amount of fluid that passes from the glomeruli to the nephron within a given amount of time.

Glomerulonephritis (glö-măr′ū-lö-nef-rī′tis): Inflammation of the glomerulus and Bowman's capsule.

Glomerulus (glö-măr′ū-lŭs): A tuft of capillary loops surrounded by the Bowman's capsule at the beginning of each nephric tubule in the kidney.

Glucagon (gloo′kă-gon): A hormone secreted by the pancreas, which elevates blood sugar concentration.

Glucocorticoid (gloo-kö-kör′ti-koyd): Any steroid-like compound capable of influencing metabolism; also exerts an anti-inflammatory effect. Cortisol is the most potent of the naturally occurring glucocorticoids.

Glucosamine sulfate (gloo′kö-să-mēn sŭl′fāt): An amino sugar used to support cartilaginous repair in osteoarthritis.

Glutamate (gloo′tă-māt): A salt or ester of glutamic acid, an amino acid that occurs in proteins; the sodium salt is monosodium glutamate. (See *amyotrophic lateral sclerosis*)

Gluten (gloo′těn): The insoluble protein constituent of wheat and other grains.

Gluten-sensitive enteropathy: Synonym for celiac disease.

Glycogen (glī′kö-jen): A substance found primarily in the liver and muscles that is easily converted into glucose.

Goiter (goy′ter): Chronic enlargement of the thyroid gland not due to a neoplasm. May be related to both hyperthyroidism and hypothyroidism.

Golfer's elbow: Synonym for medial epicondylitis.

Golgi tendon organ (gōl′jē): A proprioceptive sensory nerve ending embedded in tendon fibers. It is activated by changes in tendon tension.

Grand mal (grahn mahl): Also called generalized tonic–clonic seizure. Characterized by a sudden onset of tonic contraction of the muscles, giving way to clonic convulsive movements.

Granulocyte (gran′ū-lö-sīt): A mature granular leukocyte.

Granulomatosis enteritis (gran′ū-lö-mă-tö′sis en-ter-ī′tis): A term that was once used to refer to Crohn disease.

Grave disease (grāvz di-zēz′): An organ-specific autoimmune disease of the thyroid gland. (See *hyperthyroidism*)

Grave ophthalmopathy: Exophthalmos caused by increased water content of retroocular orbital tissues; associated with thyroid disease, usually hyperthyroidism.

Greater omentum (grā′těr ö-men′tŭm): A fold of peritoneum holding fat cells that hangs like an apron in front of the intestines.

Growth hormone (GH) (grōth hör′mön): See *somatotrophin*.

Guaifenesin (gwī-fen-′ě-sin): An expectorant that reduces the viscosity of sputum; sometimes recommended in the treatment of fibromyalgia syndrome.

Guillain-Barré syndrome: A self-limiting demyelinating syndrome related to autoimmune dysfunction, surgical complication, some vaccines, Hodgkin's disease, and some types of drug reactions. Motor or sensory dysfunction begins in the extremities and moves proximally, sometimes leading to respiratory failure, before function is restored within weeks or months.

Guttate psoriasis (gŭt′tāt sö-rī′ă-sis): A type of psoriasis that appears in round small patches, often following streptococcal infections.

HAART: Highly active antiretroviral therapy. (See *HIV/AIDS*)

Haemophilus influenzae (hē-mof′i-lŭs in-flū-en′zē): A species found in the respiratory tract that causes acute respiratory infections, including pneumonia, acute conjunctivitis, bacterial meningitis, and purulent meningitis in children, rarely in adults.

Hallux valgus (hal′ŭks val′gŭs): A deviation of the great toe toward the lateral side of the foot. (See *bunion*)

Hansen's disease: Synonym for leprosy. (See *ichthyosis*)

Hashimoto's thyroiditis (hah-shē-mö′tö): Diffuse infiltration of the thyroid gland with lymphocytes, resulting in diffuse goiter, progressive destruction of the parenchyma, and hypothyroidism. (See *hypothyroidism*)

Haustrum (hos′trŭm), haustra: One of a series of sacs or pouches, as seen in the colon.

Helicobacter pylori (hel′i-kö-bak′ter pī-lör′ī): Species of bacteria associated with peptic ulcers.

HELLP: A mnemonic for *h*emolysis, *e*levated *l*iver enzymes, *l*ow *p*latelet count; associated with pregnancy-induced hypertension.

Hematoma (hē-mă-tö′mă): A localized mass of extravasated blood that is relatively or completely confined within an organ or tissue, a space, or a potential space; the blood is usually clotted, and, depending on how long it has been there, may manifest various degrees of organization and decolorization.

Hematuria (hē-mă-too′-rē-ă): Any condition in which the urine contains blood or red blood cells.

Heme (hēm): The oxygen-carrying, color-bearing group of hemoglobin.

Hemiplegia (hem-ē-plē′jē-ă): Paralysis of one side of the body.

Hemo-: A prefix denoting anything to do with blood.

Hemochromatosis (hē′mö-krö-mă-tö′sis): A genetic disorder involving the absorption of too much iron in the blood. Sometimes associated with liver cancer.

Hemodialysis (hē′mö-dī-al′i-sis): Dialysis of soluble substances and water from the blood by diffusion through a semipermeable membrane.

Hemoglobin (hē-mö-glö′bin): Red protein of erythrocytes that binds to oxygen.

Hemoglobin A1c test: A test of blood glucose that reflects trends over a 3-month period. (See *diabetes*)

Hemolysis (hē-mol′i-sis): Destruction of blood cells.

Hemolytic uremic syndrome (yū-rē′mikk sin′dröm): Hemolytic anemia and thrombocytopenia occurring with acute renal failure.

Hemolytic (hē-mö-lit′ik): Destructive to blood cells.

Hemophilia (hē-mö-fil′ē-ă): An inherited disorder of blood

coagulation characterized by a permanent tendency to hemorrhages, spontaneous or traumatic, caused by a defect in the blood coagulating mechanism.

Hemoptysis (hē-mop′ti-sis): Expectoration of blood derived from the lungs or bronchi as a result of pulmonary or bronchial hemorrhage.

Hemorrhage (hem′ŏ-rij): An escape of blood through ruptured vessels.

Hemorrhoid (hem′ŏ-royd): A varicose condition of the external or internal rectal veins causing painful swellings at the anus.

Hepatocellular carcinoma (hep′ă′tö-sel′yū-lăr kar-si-nö′mă): A carcinoma derived from parenchymal cells of the liver. (See *liver cancer*)

Hepatorenal syndrome (hep′ă-tö-rē′năl sin′dröm): Occurrence of acute renal failure in patients with disease of the liver or biliary tract, apparently due to decreased renal blood flow.

Hereditary nonpolyposis colorectal cancer syndrome: A genetic condition that predisposes some people toward the development of colorectal and other cancers.

Herniated disc (hĕr′nē-ā-tĕd disk): Protrusion of a degenerated or fragmented intervertebral disk into the intervertebral foramen with potential compression of a nerve root or into the spinal canal with potential compression of the cauda equina in the lumbar region or the spinal cord at higher levels. (See *disc disease*)

Heterophile (het′er-ö-fīl): A neutrophilic leukocyte. (See *mononucleosis*)

Heterotopic ossification (het′ĕr-ö-top′ik os′i-fi-kā′shŭn): The formation of calcium deposits in soft tissues, particularly seen with spinal cord injury patients. (See *myositis ossificans*, *spinal cord injury*)

Hidradenitis suppurativa (hī-drad-ĕ ni′tis sŭp-yŭr-ă-tī′vă): Chronic suppurative folliculitis of apocrine sweat-gland–bearing skin, producing abscesses with scarring. (See *boils*)

High-density lipoprotein (HDL): A compound in plasma containing both lipids and proteins; HDLs are associated with a reduced risk of cardiovascular disease.

Hirsutism (her′soo-tizm): Presence of excessive bodily and facial terminal hair, in a male pattern, especially in women; may develop in children or adults as the result of androgen (male hormone) excess caused by tumors, drugs, or medications. (See *ovarian cysts*)

Histamine (his′tă-mēn): A secretion of some cells that is a powerful stimulant of gastric secretion, a constrictor of bronchial smooth muscle, and a vasodilator.

Hobnailed liver (hob′nāl liv′ĕr): Characteristically knobby, bumpy appearance of a liver with advanced cirrhosis.

Homans' sign (hö′mĕnz): A pain at the back of the knee or calf when the ankle is slowly dorsiflexed with the knee bent. This test indicates incipient or established thrombosis in the veins of the leg.

Homeostasis (hö′mē-ö-stā′sis): A state of equilibrium in the body with respect to various functions and the chemical compositions of fluids and tissues.

Human herpesvirus 6 (hyū′măn hĕr′pēz-vī-rŭs): A herpesvirus found in certain lymphoproliferative disorders. (See *mononucleosis*)

Human papilloma virus (HPV) (hyū′măn pap-i-lö′mă vī-rŭs): Class of DNA viruses that cause genital and cutaneous warts.

Human T-cell lymphotropic virus: A group of viruses (subfamily Oncovirinae, family Retroviridae) that are lymphotropic with a selective affinity for the helper/inducer cell subset of T lymphocytes and that are associated with adult T-cell leukemia and lymphoma.

Humoral immunity (hyū′mör-ăl i-myū′ni-tē): Immunity associated with circulating antibodies, as opposed to cellular immunity.

Hunner ulcer (hun′ĕr): A focal and often multiple star-shaped lesion involving all layers of the bladder wall; a sign of interstitial cystitis.

Hyaluronic acid (hī′ă-loo-ron′ik): A gelatinous material in tissue spaces that acts as a lubricant and shock absorber.

Hydrocephalus (hī-drö-sef′ă-lŭs): A condition marked by an excessive accumulation of cerebrospinal fluid resulting in dilation of the cerebral ventricles and raised intracranial pressure; also may result in enlargement of the cranium and atrophy of the brain. (See *cerebral palsy*)

Hyper-: A prefix denoting excessive, above normal.

Hyperacusis (hī′per-ă-koo′sis): Abnormal acuteness of hearing caused by irritability of sensory nerves. (See *Bell's palsy*)

Hyperglycemia (hī′per-glī-sē′mē-ă): An abnormally high concentration of glucose in the circulating blood.

Hyperkinesia (hī′pĕr-ki-nī′zē-ă): Excessive muscular activity.

Hyperosmolality (hī′per-oz′mö′lal′i-tē): Increased concentration of a solution expressed as osmoles of solute per kilogram of serum water. (See *diabetes*)

Hyperplasia (hī-per-plā′zhī-ă): An increase in the number of cells in a tissue or organ, outside of tumor formation.

Hyperreflexia (hī′per-rē-flek′sē-ă): A condition in which the deep tendon reflexes are exaggerated.

Hypersensitivity (hī′per-sen-si-tiv′i-tē): An exaggerated response to the stimulus of a foreign agent.

Hyperthermia (hī-per-ther′mē-ă): High body temperature; fever.

Hypertonic (hī-per-ton′ik): Having a greater degree of tension.

Hypertrophic scar: An elevated scar resembling a keloid but that does not spread into surrounding tissues.

Hypertrophy (hī-per′trö-fē): General increase in bulk of a part or organ, due to increase in size, but not in number, of the individual tissue elements.

Hyperuricemia (hī-per-ū-rē-sē′mē-ă): Enhanced blood concentrations of uric acid.

Hypnagogic hallucinations (hip-nă-goj′ik ha-lū-si-nā′shŭn): Vivid hallucinations that occur when wakening from sleep; occurs with narcolepsy. (See *sleep disorders*)

Hypnic myoclonia: The startling sensation that a person is about to fall; it often occurs while nearly asleep.

Hypo-: A prefix denoting deficient, below normal.

Hypoglycemia (hī′pö-glī-sē′mē-ă): An abnormally low concentration of glucose in circulating blood.

Hypokinesia (hī′pö-ki′nē′zē-ă): Diminished or slowed movement.

Hypothermia (hī′pö-ther′mē-ă): A body temperature significantly below 98.6°F (37°C).

Hypotonic (hī-pö-ton′ik): Having a lesser degree of tension.

Hypoxia (hī-pok′sē-ă): Below normal levels of oxygen.

Ichthyosis (ik-thē-ö′sis): Congenital disorders of keratinization characterized by noninflammatory dryness and scaling of the skin, often associated with other defects and with abnormalities of lipid metabolism.

IDDM: Insulin-dependent diabetes mellitus.

Idiopathic (id′ē-ö-path′ik): Denoting a disease of unknown cause.

Immunoblastic lymphoma: A type of high-grade lymphoma.

Impetigo (im-pe-tī′gö): A contagious superficial pyoderma, caused by *Staphylococcus aureus* or group A streptococci, that begins with a superficial flaccid vesicle that ruptures and forms a thick yellowish crust, most commonly occurring on the faces of children.

In situ (in sī′too): At the site only; refers to early stages of cancer development.

Incision (in-sizh′ŭn): A cut or surgical wound.

Indomethacin (in-dö-meth′ă-sin): A nonsteroidal analgesic agent used in the treatment of various types of arthritis.

Induction (in-dŭk′shŭn): The introduction of chemotherapeutic drugs into the central nervous system.

Infantile paralysis (in′făn-tīl pă-ral′i-sis): Synonym for polio.

Infarction (in-fark′shŭn): Sudden insufficiency of arterial or venous blood supply caused by emboli, thrombi, vascular torsion, or necrosis.

Inflammatory bowel disease: Umbrella term for Crohn disease and ulcerative colitis.

Infundibulum (in-fŭn-dib′ū-lŭm): Funnel-shaped structure or passage; the link between the pituitary gland and the hypothalamus.

Inguinal orchiectomy (ing′gwi-năl ör-kē-ek′tö-mē): Removal of one or both testes through the abdominal cavity. (See *testicular cancer*)

Insulin (in′sŭ-lin): A hormone secreted by beta cells in the pancreas that promotes the utilization of glucose in tissue cells.

Integumentary (in-teg-ū-men′tă-rē): Relating to the skin.

Interferon (in-ter-fēr′on): A class of proteins with anti-viral properties.

Interleukin-1 (in-ter-loo′kin): A cytokine that enhances the proliferation of T-helper cells and the growth and differentiation of B-cells.

Internal scar tissue: Scar tissue that accumulates within the injured structure (e.g., tendon, muscle, or ligament).

Interstitial (in-ter-stish′ăl): Relating to spaces within a tissue or organ but excluding such spaces as body cavities or potential space.

Intrathecal pump (in′tră-thē′kăl pŭmp): Device for introducing drugs directly into the central nervous system. (See *reflex sympathetic dystrophy syndrome*)

Intravenous pyelography: Radiologic study of the kidney, ureters, and usually the bladder, performed with the aid of a contrast agent injected intravenously.

Intrinsic factor (in-trin′sik fak′tŏr): A mucoprotein in the stomach necessary for the absorption of vitamin B_{12}.

Inverse psoriasis: Psoriasis in which lesions are red and thickened and focused around skin folds.

Iritis (ī-rī′tis): Inflammation of the iris of the eye.

Ischemia (is-kē′mē-ă): Local anemia due to a mechanical obstruction of the blood supply.

IUD: Intrauterine device.

Ixodes (ik-sö′dēz): A genus of hard ticks, many of which are parasitic to humans and which may be the vector for the spread of some diseases. (See *Lyme disease*)

Jumper's knee: Synonym for patellofemoral syndrome.

Kaposi's sarcoma (kah-pö′sē): A malignant neoplasm occurring in the skin and sometimes in lymph nodes or viscera; clinically manifested by cutaneous lesions consisting of reddish-purple to dark-blue macules, plaques, or nodules; seen most commonly in men over 60 years of age and, in AIDS patients.

Keloid scar: A nodular mass of scar tissue that may occur after surgery, a burn, or cutaneous diseases.

Keratin (ker′ă-tin): A substance present in cuticular structures (e.g., hair, nails, and horns).

Keratinocyte (ke-rat′i-nö-sīt): A cell of the epidermis that produces keratin.

Ketoacidosis (kē′tö-as-i-dö′sis): Acidosis caused by the enhanced production of ketonic acids.

Ketogenic (kē-tö-jen′ik): Giving rise to ketones in metabolism.

Ketone (kē′tön): A potentially toxic product of metabolism; the most recognized ketone is acetone.

Klebsiella (kleb-sē-el′ă): A genus of bacteria that may or may not be pathogenic, depending on the individual type.

Kupffer cells: Phagocytic cells found in the liver.

Kyphosis (kī-fö′sis): A deformity of the spine, characterized by extensive flexion. (See *postural deviations*)

Laceration (las-er-ā′shŭn): A torn or jagged wound.

Lactobacilli (lak-tö-bă-sil′ī): A genus of bacteria that are part of the normal flora of the mouth, intestinal tract, and vagina.

Lamivudine: A reverse transcriptase inhibitor used to treat HIV and hepatitis B.

Lanugo (lă-noo′gö): Fine, soft, lightly pigmented hair, associated with fetal development and advanced anorexia nervosa.

Laparoscopy (lap-ă-ros′kŏ-pē): Examination of the abdominal contents with a scope passed through the abdominal wall.

Laparotomy (lap′ă-rot′ö-mē): Incision into the abdominal wall.

Legg-Calve-Perthes disease (leg′kal-vă′per′tĕz diz′ēz): Epiphysial necrosis of the upper end of the femur. (See *avascular necrosis*)

Leiomyoma (lī′ö-mī-ö′mă): A benign neoplasm derived from smooth muscle tissue. (See *fibroid tumors*)

Lentigo (len-tī′gö): A brown macule or spot, resembling a freckle.

Leprosy (lep′rö-sē): A chronic bacterial infection caused by *Mycobacterium leprae* affecting the cooler body parts, especially the skin, peripheral nerves, and testes. Leprosy is classified into two main types, lepromatous and tuberculoid, representing extremes of immunologic response. Also called Hansen's disease.

Lesion (lē′zhŭn): A wound or injury; a pathogenic change in tissues.

Letrozole: A medication used to reduce the risk of recurrent breast cancer.

Leukocyte (loo′kö-sīt): A type of blood cell formed in several different types of tissues, involved in immune reactions. A white blood cell.

Leukoplakia (loo-kö-plā′kē-ă): A white patch of oral mucous membrane that cannot be wiped off and cannot be diagnosed clinically; biopsy may show malignant or premalignant changes. (See *skin cancer*)

Levodopa (lē-vö-dö′pă): The biologically active form of dopa; a precursor of dopamine.

Levulose (lev′ū-lös): Fructose: fruit sugar.

Leydig cell tumors (lī-dig): A type of testicular cancer.

Lhermitte's sign (lăr-mēt′): Sudden electric-like shocks extending down the spine on flexion of the head. (See *muscular dystrophy*, *multiple sclerosis*)

Ligamentum flava: A pair of yellow elastic fibrous structures that bind the laminae of adjoining vertebrae.

Limb-girdle dystrophy (lim-gĭr′dĕl dis′trö-fē): One of the less well-defined types of muscular dystrophy. Characterized by weakness and wasting, usually symmetrical, of the pelvic girdle muscles, the shoulder girdle muscles, or both, but not the facial muscles.

Limbic system (lim′bik sis′tĕm): A group of brain structures and their connections that exert important influence on the endocrine and autonomic nervous systems. The limbic system is associated with motivational and mood states.

Limited systemic scleroderma (sis-tem′ik sklĕr-ö-der′mă): A form of scleroderma that carries a lower risk of internal organ involvement.

Linea alba (lin′ē-ă al′bă): Fibrous band that runs vertically from the xiphoid process to the pubis; site of attachment for abdominal muscles.

Lipoprotein (lip-ö-prö′tēn): Complexes or compounds containing lipid and protein. Plasma lipoproteins are characterized as very-low-density (VLDL), intermediate-density (IDL), low-density (LD), high-density (HDL), or very-high-density (VHDL). Levels of lipoproteins are important in assessing the risk of cardiovascular disease.

Lithium (lith′ē-ŭm): An element of the alkali metal group, used to treat depression and other mood disorders.

Lithotripsy (lith′ö-trip-sē): The crushing of a stone in the renal pelvis, ureter, or bladder, by mechanical force or sound waves.

Lordosis (lör-dö′sis): A deformity of the spine, characterized by excessive extension. (See *postural deviations*)

Low-density lipoprotein (LDL): A compound in plasma containing both lipids and proteins; LDLs are associated with an increased risk of cardiovascular disease.

Lumen (loo′men): The space in the interior of a tubular structure.

Lymphadenitis (lim′-fad′ĕ-nī′tis): Inflammation of a lymph node or nodes.

Lymphadenoma (lim-fad′ĕ-nö′mă): Enlarged lymph node; may be associated with cancer.

Lymphangion (lim-fan′jē-on): A lymphatic vessel.

Lymphedema (limf′e-dē′mă): Swelling as a result of obstruction or damage to lymph nodes.

Lymphoblastic lymphoma (lim-fö-blas′tik lim-fö′mă): A type of high-grade lymphoma.

Lymphocyte (lim′fö-sīt): A white blood cell formed in lymphatic tissues.

Lymphocytic lymphoma (lim-fö-sit′ik lim-fö′mă): A type of low-grade lymphoma.

Lymphokines (lim′fö-kīnz): A group of hormone-like substances, released by lymphocytes, that mediate immune responses.

Macrophage (mak′rö-fāj): A type of phagocytic white blood cell.

Magnetic resonance imaging (MRI) (rez′ö-năns im′ă-jing): A diagnostic modality in which the magnetic nuclei of a patient are aligned in a strong, uniform magnetic field. The signals they emit are converted into images that permit three-dimensional reference to soft tissues.

Malaise (mă-lāz′): A feeling of general discomfort or uneasiness.

Malar rash (mā′lăr): A rash of the cheeks or cheekbones, often associated with lupus or erysipelas.

Malignant (mă-lig′nănt): Having the property of locally invasive and destructive growth and metastasis.

Malignant hypertension (mă-lig′nănt hī′per-ten′shŭn): Severe hypertension that runs a rapid course, causing necrosis of arteriolar walls in kidney and retina, hemorrhages, and death most frequently caused by uremia or rupture of a cerebral vessel.

Malocclusion (mal-ö-kloo′zhŭn): Any deviation from a physiologically acceptable contact of opposing dentitions.

Mast cell (mast sel): A white blood cell found in connective tissue that contains heparin and histamine.

Mastitis (mas-tī′tis): Infection of the breast.

Matrix (mā′triks): The intercellular substance of a tissue.

Medial tibial stress syndrome: Pain at the posteromedial border of the tibia that occurs in conjunction with exercise. (See *shin splints*)

Melanin (mel′ă-nin): Dark brown to black pigment formed in the skin and some other tissues.

Melanocyte (mel′ă-nö-sīt): A pigment-producing cell located in the basal layer of the epidermis.

Melatonin (mel-ă-tön′in): A substance secreted by the pineal gland that suppresses some glandular function; associated with circadian rhythm.

Menarche (me-nar′kē): A woman's first menstrual period.

Meningitis (men-in-jī′tis): Inflammation of the membranes of the brain or spinal cord.

Meniscus (mĕ-nis′kŭs): A crescent-shaped fibrocartilaginous structure of the knee, the acromioclavicular and sternoclavicular and the temporomandibular joints.

Menses (men′sēz): Periodic hemorrhage from the uterine mucosa; usually preceded by ovulation but not by fertilization.

Mesangial glomerulonephritis (mes-an′jē-ăl glö-măr′ū-lö-nef-rī′tis): A type of glomerulonephritis associated with immune system abnormalities and the loss of erythrocytes into the urine.

Mesentery (mes′en-ter-ē): A double layer of peritoneum attached to the abdominal wall and enclosing a portion of the abdominal viscera.

Metabolite (mĕ-tab′ö-līt): Any product of metabolism, especially catabolism.

Metastasis (mĕ-tas′tă-sis): The spread of a disease process from one part of the body to another, as with the spread of cancer.

Methylphenidate (meth-il-fen′i-dāt): A central nervous system stimulant often used to treat attention deficit hyperactivity disorder.

Microaerophilic (mī-′krö-ār-ö-fil′ik): Referring to a type of bacteria that requires oxygen, although less than is available in the air.

Microbe (mī′kröb): Any very minute organism.

Micrographia: Handwriting that grows progressively smaller and more cramped. (See *Parkinson's disease*)

Microsporum (mI-kros″pŏ-rŭm): A genus of pathogenic fungi causing dermatophytosis. (See *fungal infections*)

Mineralocorticoid (min′er-al-ö-kör′ti-koyd): One of the steroids from the adrenal cortex that influence salt metabolism.

Mitochondria: An organelle of the cell cytoplasm; mitochondria are the principal energy source of the cell.

Mittelschmerz (mit′el-schmärts): Abdominal pain occurring at the time of ovulation.

Molluscum contagiosum (mo-lŭs′kŭm kon-tā′jĕ ŏ′sŭm): A contagious disease of the skin caused by proliferation of a virus of the family Poxviridae and characterized by the appearance of small, pearly, epidermal growths. In adults it typically occurs on or near the genitals and is sexually transmitted. (See *sexually transmitted diseases*, *warts*)

Monoamine oxidase inhibitor (MAOI) (ok′si-dās in-hib′i-tŏr): A class of antidepressants that inhibit the breakdown of certain neurotransmitters.

Monocyte (mon′ö-sīt): A relatively large leukocyte; normally comprises 3% to 7% of the leukocytes in circulating blood.

Mononeuropathy (mon′ö-noo-rop′ă-thē): Disorder involving a single nerve.

Mononucleosis (mon′ö-noo-klē-ö′sis): Presence of abnormally large numbers of mononuclear leukocytes in the circulating blood, especially with reference to forms that are not normal.

Movie-goer's knee: Synonym for patellofemoral syndrome.

Mucolytic (mū-kö-lit′ik): Capable of dissolving, digesting, or liquefying mucus.

Mucopolysaccharide (mūkö-pol-ē-sak′ă-rīd): Protein–polysaccharide complex, obtained from proteoglycans. (See *hyperthyroidism*)

Mucosal-associated lymphoid type lymphoma: A type of cancer associated with *H. pylori*. (See *ulcers*)

Muscle spindle: Proprioceptor that wraps around specialized muscle fibers to relay information about the relative length of the muscle fibers.

Myalgic encephalomyelitis (mī-al′jik en-sef′ă-lö-mī-ĕ-lī′tis): Inflammation of the brain and spinal cord characterized by muscle pain. (See *chronic fatigue syndrome*)

Myasthenia gravis (mī-as-thē′nē-ă gra′vis): Immunologic disorder of neuromuscular transmission, marked by fluctuating weakness, especially of the oculofacial muscles and the proximal limb muscles.

Mycobacterium tuberculosis (mī′kö-bak-tēr′ē-ŭm tū-bĕr-kyū-lö′sis): Species of bacteria that causes tuberculosis in humans.

Mycoplasma (mī′kö-plaz-mă): A specialized type of bacteria that do not possess a true cell wall but are bound by a three-layered membrane.

Mycosis (mī-kö′sis): Any disease caused by a fungus.

Myelin (mī′ĕ-lin): A membrane composed of fat and protein molecules that surrounds nerve fibers.

Myelodysplastic anemia: A primary, neoplastic, stem-cell disorder characterized by peripheral blood cytopenias and prominent maturation abnormalities in the bone marrow. The disease evolves progressively and may transform into leukemia.

Myeloid cell: Any cell that develops into a granulocyte of blood; also refers to any bone marrow cell.

Myocardial infarction (mī-ö-kar′dē-ăl in-fark′shŭn): Synonym for heart attack.

Myoclonic (mī-ö-klon′ik): Related to one or a series of shocklike contractions of a group of muscles, of variable regularity, synchrony, and symmetry, generally caused by a central nervous system lesion.

Myofibril (mī-ö-fī′bril): One of the fine longitudinal fibers occurring in skeletal or cardiac muscle fiber.

Myopia (mī-ö′pē-ă): Optical condition in which only rays from a finite distance from the eye focus on the retina; nearsightedness. (See *Marfan syndrome*)

Myositis ossificans (mī-ö-sī′tis os′sif′ĭ-kanz): Ossification of inflammatory tissue within a muscle, usually at the site of a hematoma caused by blunt trauma.

Myotonia (mī-ö-tö′nē-ă): Delayed relaxation of a muscle after a strong contraction.

Myxedema coma (mik-se-dē′mă): A state of profound unconsciousness related to extreme hypothyroidism.

Narcolepsy (nar′kö-lep-sē): A sleep disorder involving recurring episodes of sleep during the day and interrupted sleep at night.

Necrosis (nĕ-krö′sis): Pathologic death of one or more cells or of a portion of tissue or organ.

Neisseria gonorrhoeae: A species that causes gonorrhea and other infections in humans; the type species of the genus *Neisseria*.

Neisseria meningitides: A bacterial species found in the nasopharynx; the causative agent of meningococcal meningitis.

Neoplasm (nē′ö-plazm): An abnormal tissue that grows by cellular proliferation, more rapidly than normal, and continues to grow after the stimuli that initiated the new growth cease.

Nephrolithiasis (nef′rö-li-thī′ă-sis): Presence of renal calculi.

Nephron (nef′ron): A long convoluted tubular structure; the functional unit of the kidney.

Nerve growth factor: A protein that helps to control the development of sympathetic neurons and other nerve tissue; associated with heightened pain sensitivity.

Neuralgia-inducing cavitational osteonecrosis (NICO): A situation in which there is tissue death at the site of extracted teeth, which causes pain in the face. Also called osteomyelitis.

Neurilemma (noor-i-lem′ă): A cell that enfolds one or more axons of the peripheral nervous system.

Neuroendocrine (noor-ö-en′dö-krin): Descriptive of cells that release hormones in response to a neural stimulus. (See *pancreatic cancer*)

Neurofibrillary tangle: Intraneural accumulations of filaments with twisted, contorted patterns; associated with Alzheimer's disease.

Neurogenic bladder (nūr-ö-jen′ik blad′er): Bladder dysfunction that originates with nervous system damage.

Neuroma (noo-rö′mă): General term for any neoplasm derived from cells of the nervous system, especially Morton's neuroma. (See *pes planus, pes cavus*)

Neuron (noor′on): The functional unit of the nervous system consisting of the nerve cell body, the dendrites, and the axon.

Neuropeptide (noor-ö-pep′tīd): Any of a variety of peptides found in neural tissue; e.g., endorphins, enkephalins.

Neutrophil (noo′trö-fil): A type of mature white blood cell formed in the bone marrow.

Neutrophilic (noo-trö-fil′ik): Characterized by the presence of neutrophils.

Nevus (nē′vŭs), nevi: A malformation of the skin, colored by hyperpigmentation or increased vascularity.

NIDDM: Non–insulin-dependent diabetes mellitus.

Nit (nĭt): The ovum of a head or body louse.

Nociceptor (nö-si-sep′ter): A peripheral nerve organ or mechanism for the reception and transmission of painful or injurious stimuli.

Nocturia (nok-too′rē-ă): Urinating at night.

Nodular (nod′yu-lăr): Having nodes or knot-like swellings.

Non-Burkitt's lymphoma: A type of high-grade lymphoma.

Non-gonococcal urethritis: Urethritis not from gonococcal infection; chlamydia trachomatis is the most common agent. (See *sexually transmitted diseases*)

Non-seminoma: A type of testicular cancer.

Nonsteroidal anti-inflammatory drug (NSAID): Aspirin, ibuprofen. Any collection of anti-inflammatory drugs that do not include steroidal compounds. Examples include aspirin, acetaminophen, ibuprofen, and naproxen.

Nontropical sprue non-trop′ĭk-ăl sprū): Synonym for celiac disease.

Noradrenaline (nor-ă-dren′ă-lin): See norepinephrine

Norepinephrine (nör′ep-i-nef′rin): A hormone produced in the adrenal medulla, secreted in response to hypotension and physical stress.

Norovirus: Genus name for the group of viruses provisionally described as "Norwalk-like viruses" (NLV).

Nosocomial (nos-ö-kö′mē-ăl): Denoting a new disorder that develops while being treated in a hospital; specifically applied to some varieties of pneumonia.

Noxious (nok′shŭs): Injurious, harmful.

Nucleus pulposus: The soft fibrocartilage central portion of an intervertebral disk.

Numb-likeness: A condition characterized by reduced sensation but not total numbness.

Nummular eczema (nŭm'yū'lăr ek'zĕ-mă): Discrete, coin-shaped patches of eczema.

Occult (ŏ-kŭlt'): Hidden; concealed; not manifest.

Oculopharyngeal muscular dystrophy (ok-ū'lö-fă-rin-jē-ăl dis'trö'fē): An inherited progressive form of muscular dystrophy that often involves ptosis and problems with swallowing.

Oligodendrocyte (ol'i-gö'den'drö-sīt): One of the three types of glia cells (the other two being astrocytes and microglia) that, together with nerve cells, compose the tissue of the central nervous system.

Oncogene (ong'kö-jēn): Any of a family of genes that may foster malignant processes if mutated or activated by certain viruses.

Onycholysis (on-i-kol'i-sis): Loosening of the nails, beginning at the free border, and usually incomplete. (See *psoriasis*)

Onychomycosis (on'i-kö-mī-kö'sis): Fungal infection of the nails.

Oocyte (ö'ö-sīt): The female sex cell.

Oophorectomy (ö-of-ör-ek'tö-mē): Surgical removal of the ovaries.

Oophoritis (ö-of-ör-ī'tis): Inflammation of an ovary. (See *pelvic inflammatory disease*)

Orchiectomy (ör-kē-ek'tö-mē): Removal of one or both testes.

Orchitis (ör-kī'tis): Inflammation of the testes.

Organic brain syndrome (brān sin'dröm): A group of behavioral or psychological signs and symptoms caused by transient or permanent dysfunction of the brain; associated with chronic alcoholism.

Orthotics (ör-thot'iks): The science concerned with the making and fitting of orthopedic appliances. Also used to refer to orthopedic appliances that are made to adjust the alignment and weight-bearing stress in the feet.

Os coxae: The fused unit containing the ilium, ischium, and pubis.

Oscillation (os-i-lā'shŭn): A to-and-fro movement. (See *tremor*)

Osgood-Schlatter disease (oz'good shlaht'ere dī-zēz'): Inflammation or partial avulsion of the tibial tuberosity due to traction forces.

Osteoblast (os'tē-ö-blast): A bone-forming cell.

Osteoclast (os'tē-ö-klast): A cell functioning in the absorption and removal of osseus tissue.

Osteomalacia (os'tē-ö-mă-lā'shē-ă): A disease characterized by progressive softening and bending of the bones.

Osteomyelitis (os'tē-ö-mī-ĕ-lī'tis): Inflammation of the bone marrow and adjacent bone tissue.

Osteonecrosis (os'tē-ö-ne-krö'sis): The death of bone en masse, as distinguished from caries ("molecular death") or relatively small foci of necrosis in bone.

Osteophyte (os'tē-ö-fīt): A bony outgrowth or protuberance.

Osteotomy (os-tē-ot'ö-mē): Cutting bone, usually using a saw or chisel.

Over-utilization syndrome: Synonym for patellofemoral syndrome.

Oxygen free radical: An atom or atom group carrying an unpaired electron and no charge. They may promote heart disease, cancer, Alzheimer's disease, and other progressive disorders.

Pain–spasm cycle: Self-perpetuating cycle of pain, which causes spasm, which increases pain, ad infinitum.

Palliative (pal'ē-ă-tiv): Denoting the alleviation of symptoms without curing the underlying disease.

Palmar fasciitis (pawl'măr fas-ē-ī'tis): Synonym for Dupuytren contracture.

Palpable (pal'pă-bl): Perceptible to touch.

Palpitation (pal-pi-tā'shŭn): Forcible or irregular pulsation of the heart perceptible to the patient, usually with an increase in frequency or force, with or without an irregularity in rhythm.

Pap test (pap): Microscopic examination of cells scraped (usually from the uterine cervix) and stained with Papanicolaou stain to look for signs of cancer.

Paraplegia (par-ă-plē'jē-ă): Paralysis of both lower extremities and generally the lower trunk.

Parathyroid hormone (PTH) (par-ă-thī'royd hör'mön): A hormone secreted by the parathyroid glands that raises serum calcium levels by causing bone resorption.

Paresis (pă-rē'sis): Partial or incomplete paralysis.

Paresthesia (par-es-thē'zē-ă): An abnormal sensation, such as burning, prickling, tickling, or tingling.

Patellar tendonitis (pa'tel'ăr ten-dö-nī'tis): Injury to the insertion of the quadriceps group.

Pathogen (path'ö-jen): Any virus, microorganism, or substance causing disease.

Pediculosis (pĕ-dik'ū-lö'sis): The state of being infested with lice.

Pediculus (pĕ-dik'ū-lŭs): A genus of parasitic lice that live in the hair and feed periodically on blood. Important species include *Pediculus humanus* var. *capitis*, the head louse of man; *Pediculus humanus* var. *corporis* (also called *Pediculus corporis*), the body louse or clothes louse, which lives and lays eggs (nits) in clothing and feeds on the human body.

Pedunculate (pĕ-dŭng'kū-lāt): Having a pedicle; suspended by a stalk.

Peptide (pep'tīd): A compound of two or more amino acids.

Percutaneous nephrolithotomy (per-kū-tā'nē-ū-tā'nē-ŭs

nef′rö-li-thot′ö-mē): Incision through the skin directly to the kidney for the removal of a renal calculus.

Percutaneous transluminal coronary angioplasty (PCTA) (pĕr-kyū-tā-nā-yŭs tranz′lū-men′ăl an′jē-ö-plas-tē): A surgical procedure for enlarging a narrowed coronary vessel by inflating and withdrawing through the narrowed region a balloon on the tip of a catheter.

Perforation (per-fö-rā′shŭn): Abnormal opening in a hollow organ.

Perfusion (per-fū′shŭn): The forcing of fluid to flow through the vascular bed of a tissue or through the lumen of a hollow structure.

Peri-: Prefix denoting around, about, or near.

Pericarditis (per′i-kar′dī′tis): Inflammation of the pericardium.

Perimenopause (per′i-men′ö-paws): The 3- to 5-year period before the final cessation of the menstrual cycle, during which estrogen levels begin to drop.

Perimysium (per-i-mis′ē′ŭm): The fibrous sheath enveloping each of the primary bundles of skeletal muscle fibers.

Periodic limb movement disorder (PLMD): A disorder characterized by periodic episodes of repetitive and highly stereotyped limb movements that occur during sleep. (See *sleep disorders*)

Periosteum (per-ē-os′tē-ŭm): The thick fibrous membrane covering every surface of a bone except the articular cartilage.

Periostitis (per′ē-os-tī′tis): Inflammation of the periosteum. (See *shin splints*)

Pes cavus (pes kă′vŭs): Condition characterized by increased height of the foot's medial longitudinal arch.

Pes planus (pes plā′nŭs): A condition in which the longitudinal arch is broken down, the entire sole touching the ground.

PET scan: Positron emission tomography scan, a device using nuclear medicine and digital imaging to observe chemical and electrical activity in living tissue.

Petit mal (pĕ-tē′): A brief seizure characterized by arrest of activity and occasional clonic movements.

Phalen maneuver (fā′lĕn): Maneuver in which the wrist is maintained in flexion for 60 seconds or more; the sensation of paresthesia or other symptoms may indicate carpal tunnel syndrome.

Phlebectomy (fle-bek′tö-mē): Excision of a segment of a vein, especially to treat varicose veins.

Phlegm (flem): Abnormal amounts of mucus, especially as expectorated from the mouth.

Photodynamic therapy (fö-tö-dī-nam-ik′thăr-ah-pē′): A treatment option that destroys some types of cancer cells through the use of a fixed-frequency laser light in combination with a photosensitizing agent.

Photosensitivity (fö′tö′-sen′si-tiv′i-tē): Abnormal sensitivity to light, especially of the eyes.

Phyllodes tumors: A low-grade, rarely metastasizing form of breast neoplasm. (See *breast cancer*)

Phyto-: Having to do with plants.

Phytoestrogen: Plant-based chemical that has estrogenic effect on the body.

Pia mater (pī′ă mā′ter): A delicate fibrous membrane firmly adherent to the brain and spinal cord.

Pilonidal cysts: An abscess in the sacral region containing hair, which may act as a foreign body leading to chronic inflammation. (See *boils*)

Pinna (pin′ă): A feather, wing, or fin—used to describe the ear.

Pitting edema (pit′ing e-dē′mă): Edema that retains for a time the indentation produced by pressure.

Placenta abruptio: Premature separation of the placenta.

Plaque (plak): A small differentiated area on a surface; atheromatous plaques form well-defined yellow areas or swellings on the intimal surface of an artery.

Plasmapheresis (plaz′mă-fĕ-rē′sis): Removal of whole blood from the body, separation of its cellular elements, and reinfusion of them suspended in saline or another plasma substitute.

Platelet (plāt′let): An irregularly shaped fragment of a megakaryocyte that aids in blood clotting.

Pleurisy (ploor′i-sē): Inflammation of the pleurae.

Plexus (plek′sŭs): A network or interjoining of nerves, blood vessels, or lymphatic vessels.

Pneumococcus (noo-mö-kok′ŭs): Synonym for *Streptococcus pneumoniae.*

Pneumocystis carinii pneumonia: Pneumonia resulting from infection with *Pneumocystis carinii*, frequently seen in the immunologically compromised, such as persons with AIDS, or steroid-treated individuals, the elderly, or premature or debilitated babies.

Pneumothorax (noo-mö-thör′aks): The presence of air or gas in the pleural cavity.

Poliomyelitis (pö′lē-ö-mī′ē-lī′tis): An inflammatory process involving the gray matter of the spinal cord.

Poly-: Many; multiplicity.

Polyarteritis nodosa (pol′ē-ar-tĕr-ī′tis nö-dö′să): A disease involving segmental inflammation and necrosis of medium- and small-sized arteries.

Polycythemia (pol′ē-sī-thē′mē-ă): An increase above normal in the number of red cells in the blood.

Polydipsia (pol-ē-dip′sē-ă): Excessive thirst that is relatively prolonged. (See *diabetes*)

Polyneuropathy (pol′ē-noo-rop′ă-thē): A disease process involving a number of peripheral nerves.

Polyphagia (pol-ē-fā′jē-ă): Excessive eating. (See *diabetes*)

Polysomnography (pol′ē-som-nog′ră-fē): Continuous monitoring of normal and abnormal physiologic functioning during sleep.

Polyuria (pol-ē-ū′rē-ă): Excessive excretion of urine. (See *diabetes*)

Popliteal fossa (pop-lit′ē-ăl fos′ă): The diamond-shaped space posterior to the knee joint bounded superficially by the diverging biceps femoris and semimembranosus muscles above and inferiorly by the two heads of the gastrocnemius muscle.

Portal hypertension (pör'tăl hī'per-ten'shŭn): Elevation of pressure in the hepatic portal circulation due to cirrhosis or other fibrotic change in liver tissue.

Postherpetic neuralgia: A pain that lasts after the lesions related to herpes zoster have healed.

Prednisone (pred'ni-sōn): An analog of cortisol; used as a steroidal anti-inflammatory.

Preeclampsia (prē-ē-klamp'sē-ă): Development of hypertension with proteinuria or edema, or both, due to pregnancy.

Premenstrual dysphoric disorder (PMDD) (prē-men-strū'ăl dis-ör'dĕr): A pervasive pattern occurring during the last week of the luteal phase in most menstrual cycles for at least a year and remitting within a few days of the onset of the follicular phase; the symptoms are comparable in severity to those seen in a major depressive episode, distinguishing this disorder from the far more common premenstrual syndrome.

Pretibial myxedema (prē-tĭb'ē-ăl mik-se-dē'mă): A rash that occurs in the tibial region, specifically associated with hyperthyroidism.

Prodromic (prö-drö'mik): Relating to the early or premonitory symptom of a disease, especially herpes simplex.

Progestin (prö-jes'tin): A hormone of the corpus luteum.

Proliferants: Injected substances that are designed to stimulate the growth of new collagen fibers, which, with appropriate stretching and exercise, then lay down in alignment with the original fibers.

Prophylaxis (prö-fi-lak'sis): Prevention of a disease or of a process that can lead to a disease.

Proprioceptor (prö-prē-ö-sep'ter): Sensory end organs that relay information about position and muscle tension.

Proptosis (prop-tö'sis): Protruding eyes, exophthalmos. (See *hyperthyroidism*)

Prostaglandin (pros-tă-glan'din): Several substances present in many tissues with effects such as vasodilation, vasoconstriction, and stimulation of smooth muscle tissue.

Prostate-specific antigen (PSA) (pros'tāt'spe-sif'ik an'tijen): A glycoprotein found in normal seminal fluid and produced in prostate epithelial cells. Elevated levels of PSA are associated with prostatic enlargement and an increased risk of prostate cancer.

Protease inhibitor (prö'tē-ās in-hib'i-tör): A group of acquired immune deficiency syndrome (AIDS) drugs that work to interrupt the maturing phase of the virus.

Pruritus: Itchiness.

Pseudogout (soo'dö-gowt): Acute episodes of synovitis caused by calcium pyrophosphate crystals as opposed to urate crystals, as in true gout.

Pseudohypertrophy (soo'dö'hī-per'trö-fē): Increase in size

of an organ or a part, due not to increase in size or number of the specific functional elements but to that of some other tissue, fatty or fibrous. (See *muscular dystrophy*)

Pseudomonas aeruginosa: Species of aerobic bacteria that sometimes infect humans, especially when the host is otherwise compromised. (See *cystic fibrosis*)

Psoralen (sör'ă-len): A phototoxic drug used in the treatment of psoriasis.

Psoriasis (sö-rī'ă-sis): A common inherited condition characterized by the eruption of reddish, silvery-scaled maculopapules, predominantly on the elbows, knees, scalp, and trunk.

Psychodynamic therapy: Therapy based on the psychological forces that underlie human behavior.

Psychoneuroimmunology (sī'kö-noo-rö-im'ū-nol'ö-jē): An area of study that focuses on emotional or other psychological states that affect the immune system, rendering an individual more susceptible to a disease or the course of a disease.

Pthirus pubis (thī'rŭs pyu'bis): Pubic or crab lice.

Ptosis (tö'sis): A sinking down or prolapse of an organ, specifically the eyelid. (See *myasthenia gravis*)

Pugilistic parkinsonism: A disorder of professional boxers who receive multiple blows to the head and in whom symptoms progress even after they stop fighting. (See *Parkinson's disease*)

Pustular psoriasis: Psoriasis with pustule formation in the normal and psoriatic skin.

Pustule (pŭs'chool): A small, circumscribed elevation of the skin containing purulent material.

PUVA: Oral administration of *p*soralen and subsequent exposure to long wavelength ultraviolet light (UVA); used to treat psoriasis.

Pyelogram (pī'el-ö-gram): A radiograph of the kidneys and ureters after the injection of a contrast medium.

Pyelography (pī'ĕ-log'ră-fē): Radiologic study of the kidneys, ureters, and bladder.

Pyrogen (pī'rö-jen): A fever-inducing agent that causes a rise in temperature.

Q-angle: The angle formed by the line of traction of the quadriceps tendon on the patella and the line of traction of the patellar tendon on the tibial tubercle. (See *patellofemoral syndrome*)

Quadriplegia (kwah'dri-plē'jē-ă): Paralysis of all four limbs.

Quercetin (kwer'sē-tin): A bioflavonoid with antihistamine and anti-inflammatory properties. (See *prostatitis*)

Radiation (rā'dē-ā'shŭn): The sending forth of light, short radio waves, ultraviolet or x-rays, or any other waves for treatment, diagnosis, or other purpose.

Radicular pain (ra-dik'yū-lăr pān): Pain felt along the pathway of a spinal nerve.

Radiculopathy (ra-dik'ū-lop'ă-thē): Any disorder of the spinal nerve roots.

Radioimmunotherapy: The use of radiation with medication to target specific tumor cells.

Radioisotope (rā′dē-ö-ī′sö-töp): An isotope that changes to a more stable state by emitting radiation.

Rales (rahls): Term for an extra sound heard on auscultation of breath sounds.

Ramsay-Hunt syndrome type 1 (ram′sē-hunt): Facial paralysis, ear pain, and herpes zoster resulting from viral infection of the seventh cranial nerve and geniculate ganglion.

Raynaud's syndrome (rā-nö′): Idiopathic bilateral cyanosis of the digits due to arterial and arteriolar contraction.

Reduction (fē-dŭk′shŭn): The restoration, by surgical or manipulative procedures, of a part to its normal anatomic relation.

Reed–Sternberg cells (rēd-stern′berg sel): Large transformed lymphocytes, indicative of Hodgkin's disease.

Regional enteritis (rē′jŭn-ăl en-tĕr-ī′tis): Synonym for Crohn disease.

Reiter's syndrome (rī-tĕr): A combination of symptoms, including urethritis, cutaneous lesions, arthritis, and diarrhea. One or more of these symptoms may recur at intervals, but the arthritis may be persistent.

Relaxin (rē-lak′sin): A hormone secreted during pregnancy that allows the softening and lengthening of the pubis symphysis, along with other connective tissues.

Renal calculus (rē′năl kal′kyū-lŭs): A stone or pebble formed in the kidney collection system. (See *kidney stones*)

Renal colic: Severe pain caused by the impaction or passage of a calculus in the ureter or renal pelvis.

Renin (rē′nin): An enzyme produced by the kidneys that is involved in vasoconstriction and hypertension.

Repetitive stress injury: Any injury related to wear-and-tear brought about by repeated, especially percussive, movements. (See *carpal tunnel syndrome*)

Restenosis (rē′sten-ö-sis): Recurrence of stenosis after corrective surgery on the heart valve; narrowing of a structure (usually a coronary artery) after the removal or reduction of a previous narrowing.

Restless leg syndrome: A sense of uneasiness, twitching, or restlessness that occurs in the legs after going to bed. (See *sleep disorders*)

Reticulocyte (re-tik′ū-lö-sīt): An immature red blood cell.

Retinoin: A class of keratolytic drugs derived from retinoic acid and used for treatment of severe acne and psoriasis.

Retinopathy (ret-i-nop′ă-thē): Noninflammatory degenerative disease of the retina.

Retrovirus (re′trö-vī′rŭs): A virus in the family of Retroviridae. They possess RNA, which serves as a template for the synthesis of DNA in the host cell.

Rheumatoid spondylitis (rū′mă-toyd spon-di-lī′tis): (See *ankylosing spondylitis*)

Rhinitis (rī-nī′tis): Inflammation of the nasal mucous membrane.

Rhinophyma (rī′nö-fī′mă): Hypertrophy of the nose with follicular dilation, resulting from hyperplasia of sebaceous glands with fibrosis and increased vascularity. (See *acne rosacea*)

Rickettsia rickettsii (ri-ket′sē-ă- ri-ket′sē-ī): The agent of Rocky Mountain spotted fever and its geographic variants; transmitted by infected ixodid ticks, especially *Dermacentor andersoni* and *D. variabilis*. (See *Lyme disease*)

Rimantadine (rĭ-man′tă-dēn): An antiviral agent that closely resembles amantadine but is often better tolerated.

Ringworm (ring′werm): A fungal infection of the keratin component of hair, skin, or nails. Tinea.

Rodent ulcer (rö′dent ŭl′sĕr): A slowly enlarging ulcerated basal cell carcinoma, usually on the face. (See *skin cancer*)

Rosacea (rö-zā′shē-ă): Chronic vascular and follicular dilation involving the nose and contiguous portions of the cheeks with erythema, hyperplasia of sebaceous glands, deep-seated papules and pustules, and telangiectasia.

Rotator cuff tears: See *tendinitis/injury sidebar*

Rotavirus: A group of RNA viruses that infect the human gastrointestinal tract.

Rubella (roo-bel′ă): An acute exanthematous disease caused by rubella virus (*Rubivirus*), with enlargement of lymph nodes, but usually with little fever or constitutional reaction; a high incidence of birth defects in children results from maternal infection during the first several months of fetal life (congenital rubella syndrome). (See *mononucleosis*)

S-adenosyl-methionine (SAM-e) (a-den′ö-sil-me-thī′ö-nēn): An amino acid associated with mood improvement. (See *depression*)

Salmonella (sal′mö-nel′ă): A group of bacteria associated with gastrointestinal tract infections and food poisoning.

Salpingitis (sal-pin-jī′tis): Inflammation of the fallopian (uterine) tube.

Sarcolemma (sar′kö-lem′ă): The plasma membrane of a muscle fiber.

Sarcomere (sar′kö-mēr): The segment of a myofibril between Z lines; the functioning contractile unit of striated muscle.

Sarcoptes scabiei (sar-kop′tēz skā′bē-ī): The itch mite, varieties of which are distributed worldwide and affect humans and many animals. The mite burrows into the skin and lays eggs within the burrow; intense itching and rash develop near the burrow in about a month.

Sauriasis (saw-rī′ă-sis): Synonym for ichthyosis.

Sauriosis (saw-ri-ö′sis): Synonym for ichthyosis.

Sauroderma (saw′rö-der′mă): Synonym for ichthyosis.

Scheuermann's disease (shoi′ĕr-mahn di-zēz′): Epiphysial osteonecrosis of adjacent vertebral bodies in the thoracic spine. (See *postural deviations*)

Schistosoma haematobium (skis-tö-sö′mă hē-mă′tă′tö′bē-yŭm): The vesical blood fluke, a species that occurs as a parasite in the portal system and mesenteric veins of the bladder (causing human schistosomiasis haematobium) and rectum; found throughout Africa and the Middle East. (See *bladder cancer*)

Schwann cells (shvahn): Cells forming a continuous envelope around each fiber of peripheral nerves.

Sclerodactyly (sklēr-ö-dak′ti-lē): Stiffness and tightness of the skin of the fingers, with atrophy of the soft tissue and osteoporosis of the distal phalanges of the hands and feet; a limited form of progressive systemic sclerosis. (See *scleroderma*)

Scleroderma (sklēr-ö-der′mă): Thickening and induration of the skin caused by new collagen formation; either a manifestation of progressive systemic sclerosis or localized (morphea).

Scoliosis (skö-lē-ö′sis): Abnormal lateral curve of the vertebral column.

Seasonal affective disorder (SAD) (af-fek′tiv dis-ör′dĕr): A depressive disorder that is exacerbated by reduced daylight hours and subsides in spring and summer.

Sebaceous gland (sē-bā′shŭs): Gland in the dermis that usually opens into hair follicles and secretes an oily semifluid: sebum.

Seborrheic keratosis (seb-ö-rē′ik ker-ă-tö′sis): Superficial benign skin lesions of proliferating epithelial cells.

Seborrheic (seb-ö-rē′ik): Relating to overactivity of the sebaceous glands resulting in an excessive amount of sebum. (See *eczema*)

Sebum (sē′bŭm): The secretion produced by sebaceous glands.

Selective serotonin reuptake inhibitor (SSRI) (sě-lek′tiv sĕr-ö-tön′in rē-up′tăk in-hib′i-tör): A class of drugs used in the treatment of depression that selectively prevent the reuptake of serotonin in the brain.

Self-limiting: Denoting a disease that tends to cease after time.

Seminiferous tubules: The glandular part of testicles that contain the sperm-producing cells.

Seminoma (sem-i-nö′mă): A type of germ cell tumor. (See *testicular cancer*)

Sentinel lymph node (limf nöd): The first lymph node to receive lymph drainage from a malignant tumor; if it is found clear of metastasis, all the other nearby nodes are clear as well.

Septicemia (sep-ti-sē′mē-ă): Systemic disease caused by the spread of microorganisms and their toxins in the circulating blood. (See *cellulitis, lymphangitis*)

Serotonin (sēr-ö-tö′nin): A chemical found in many different tissues. In the brain it is a neurotransmitter associated with mood disorders; in the body it can be a vasoconstrictor, it can stimulate smooth muscle contraction, and it can inhibit gastric secretion.

Sertoli cell tumors (sir-tö′lē): A testicular tumor containing Sertoli cells, which may cause feminization. (See *testicular cancer*)

Shigella (shē-gel′lă): A genus of bacteria associated with gastrointestinal infection.

Shoulder–hand syndrome: Synonym for reflex sympathetic dystrophy syndrome

Sigmoidoscopy (sig′moy-dos′kŏ-pē): An inspection, through an endoscope, of the sigmoid flexure of the colon.

Sine scleroderm: An unusual form of systemic scleroderma with significant organ involvement and minimal effect on the skin.

Sinoatrial node (sī-nö-ā′trē-ăl nöd): The mass of specialized cardiac fibers that act as the "pacemaker" for the heart.

Sitz bath (sitz bath): Immersion of only the perineum and buttocks, with the legs being outside the tub.

Sjögren's syndrome: An autoimmune disorder with a collection of signs and symptoms, including conjunctivitis, dryness of mucous membranes, and bilateral enlargement of the parotid glands. (See *rheumatoid arthritis, lupus, scleroderma*)

Sleep paralysis (slēp pă-ral′i-sis): Brief episodic loss of voluntary movement that occurs when falling asleep (hypnagogic sleep paralysis) or when awakening (hypnopompic sleep paralysis). (See *sleep disorders*)

Sodium urate (sö′dē-ŭm ūr′āt): Uric acid.

Somatomedin C (sö′mă-tömē′din): A peptide that stimulates growth in bone and cartilage. (See *acromegaly*)

Somatotrophin: A hormone produced in the anterior pituitary that promotes body growth, fat mobilization, and the inhibition of glucose utilization.

Sonogram (son′ö-gram): A diagnostic technique that uses ultrasound waves to create a computerized image.

Spastic paralysis: Central nervous system damage resulting in permanent muscle contraction; combines aspects of hypertonia, hypokinesia, and hyperreflexia.

Spasticity (spas-tis′i-tē): A state of increased muscle tone with exaggerated muscle tendon reflexes. (See *cerebral palsy, spinal cord injuries*)

Specific immunity (spě-sif′ik i-myū′ni-tē): The immune state in which there is an altered reactivity directed solely against the antigens that stimulated it.

Specific muscle weakness: Degeneration and weakening of muscles supplied by specifically damaged motor neurons; as opposed to general muscle weakness, which may not be related to nerve damage.

Sphincter (sfingk′ter): A muscle that encircles a duct, tube, or orifice.

Sphygmomanometer (sfig′mö-mă-nom′ě-ter): Blood pressure cuff.

Spina bifida meningocele (spī′nă bĭ′fi-dă mě-ning′gö-sēl): Protrusion of the membranes of the brain or spinal cord through a defect in the skull or vertebral column.

Spina bifida myelomeningocele (spī′nă bĭ′fi-dă mī′ě-lö-mě-ning′gö-sēl): Protrusion of the spinal cord and its membranes through a defect in the vertebral column.

Spina bifida occulta (spī'nă bĭ'fi-dă ö'kult-a): Spina bifida in which there is a spinal defect, but no protrusion of the cord or its membrane, although there is often some abnormality in their development.

Spirochete (spī'rö-kēt): A type of bacteria shaped like undulating spiral-shaped rods. (See *ulcers, Lyme disease, syphilis*)

Spirometry (spī-rom'ĕ-trē): A test to measure respiratory gases using a spirometer.

Splenomegaly (splē-nö-meg'ă-lē): Enlargement of the spleen. (See *mononucleosis, anemia*)

Spondylolisthesis (spon'di-lö-lis-thē'sis): Forward movement of the body of one of the lumbar vertebrae on the vertebra below it, or on the sacrum.

Spondylolysis (spon-di-lol'i-sis): Degeneration of the articulating part of the vertebra.

Spondylosis (spon-di-lö'sis): Stiffening of the vertebrae; often applied nonspecifically to any lesion of the spine of a degenerative nature.

Sporadic (spö-rad'ik): Occurring irregularly, haphazardly.

Sputum (spū'tŭm): Expectorated matter, especially mucus or mucopurulent matter expectorated in diseases of the air passages.

Squamous: Relating to or covered with scales.

Staghorn calculus: A calculus occurring in the renal pelvis, with branches extending into the calices. (See *kidney stones*)

Staging: The classification of distinct phases or periods in the course of a disease.

Staphylococcus: A type of bacteria formed of spherical cells that divide to make irregular clusters.

Starling's equilibrium (stahr'ling ē-kwi-lib'rē-ŭm): Also called Starling's hypothesis: the principle that the amount of fluid squeezed out of circulatory capillaries should be almost equal to the amount being drawn into lymphatic capillaries.

Status epilepticus: Repeated seizure or a seizure prolonged for at least 30 minutes; may be convulsive (tonic–clonic), nonconvulsive (absence or complex partial) or partial (epilepsia partialis continuous), or subclinical (electrographic status epilepticus). (See *seizure disorders*)

Stein-Leventhal syndrome: Synonym for polycystic ovary disease. (See *ovarian cysts*)

Stenosis: A stricture or narrowing of any canal.

Stent: A device to hold tissue in place or provide support.

Steroids: A large group of chemical compounds including some hormones and drugs of a particular molecular composition. Some steroids include gonadal and adrenal hormones.

Stomatitis: Inflammation of the mucous membrane of the mouth.

Strabismus: A lack of parallelism in the visual axes of the eyes. (See *cerebral palsy*)

Stratum basale: The deepest layer of the epidermis, composed of dividing stem cells and anchoring cells.

Streptococcus pneumonia (strep-tö-kok'ŭs nū-mö'nē-ā): A species of diplococci frequently occurring in pairs or chains. Normal inhabitants of the respiratory tract, and the cause of lobar pneumonia, otitis media, meningitis, sinusitis, and other infections.

Streptococcus: A type of bacteria formed of spherical cells that occur in pairs or in long or short chains.

Stroma (strö'mă): The framework, usually made of connective tissue, of an organ, gland, or other tissue.

Stromal cell tumor (strö'măl sel too'mŏr): A tumor that arises of connective tissue stroma rather than epithelium. (See *breast cancer*)

Struvite (stroo'vīt): A compound of magnesium ammonium phosphate, found in some renal calculi. (See *kidney stones*)

Subacute (sŭb-ă-kūt'): Between acute and chronic, denoting a mild duration or severity.

Subcutaneous (sŭb-koo-tā'nē-ŭs): Beneath the skin.

Subluxation (sŭb-lŭk-sā'shŭn): An incomplete dislocation; although a relationship is altered, contact between joint surfaces remains.

Substance P (sŭb'stăns): A neurotransmitter that is primarily involved in pain transmission and is one of the most potent compounds affecting smooth muscle tissue. (See *fibromyalgia*)

Substantia nigra (sŭb-stan'shē-ă nī'gră): A large mass composed of pigmented cells located in the brainstem. The site of dopamine synthesis.

Sudeck's atrophy: Synonym for reflex sympathetic dystrophy syndrome.

Superficial fascia (sū-pĕr-fish'ăl fash'ē-ă): A loose fibrous envelope of connective tissue under the skin containing fat, blood vessels, and nerves.

Superior vena cava syndrome (sū-pĕr'ē-ör vē'nă cā'vā sin'dröm): Obstruction of the superior vena cava by benign or malignant lesions that cause the engorgement of the blood vessels of the face, neck, and arms. (See *lung cancer*)

Sympathectomy (sim-pă-thek'tö-mē): Excision of a section of a sympathetic nerve or one or more of the sympathetic ganglia. See reflex sympathetic syndrome.

Synarthrosis (sin'ar-thrö'sis), synarthroses: A fibrous joint, sometimes said to be immovable.

Syncytial (sin-sish'ăl): Relating to a mass formed by the secondary union of originally separated cells.

Syndrome X: A synonym for metabolic syndrome.

Synovectomy (sin-ö-vek'tö-mē): The excision of part or all of the synovial membrane of a joint.

Synovial joint (si-nö'vē-ăl joynt): A diarthrosis or freely moveable joint.

Systemic lupus erythematosus (sis-tem'ĭk lū'pŭs ĕr-thē'mă-tö'sŭs): An inflammatory connective tissue disease with variable features including fever, weakness and fatigability, joint pains or arthritis resembling rheumatoid arthritis, and diffuse erythematous skin lesions on the face, neck, or upper extremities.

Systole (sis′tö-lē): The contraction of the heart, specifically of the ventricles.

Tachycardia (tak′i-kar′dē-ă): Rapid heartbeat, usually applied to rates greater than 100 beats per minute.

Tamoxifen: An anti-estrogen agent used in the treatment of breast cancer.

Tau (tau): A protein that helps to maintain the structure of the cytoskeleton; found in the plaques of persons with Alzheimer's disease.

Telangiectasia (tel-an′jē-ek-tā′zē-ă): Dilation of previously existing small vessels, most commonly in the skin. Also called "spider veins." (See *scleroderma, varicose veins, acne rosacea*)

Tender point (ten′dĕr poynt): One of many predictable bilateral pairs of points that produce a painful response with a minimum of pressure (4 kg); used to help diagnose fibromyalgia.

Tendinosis (ten-di-nö′sis): The condition of chronic tendon injury without inflammation. (See *tendinitis*)

Tennis elbow (tĕn′is el′bö): A synonym for lateral epicondylitis.

Tenosynovitis (ten′ö-sin-ö-vī′tis): Inflammation of a tendon and its enveloping sheath.

TENS (Transcutaneous electrical nerve stimulation) (tranz-kyū′tā-nē-us ē-lek′trik-al nĕrv stim-yū-la′shŭn): A device to control pain with electrical stimulation applied through the skin to the nerves.

Teratoma (ter-ă-tö′-mă): A neoplasm that contains tissues not normally found in the tissue in which it arises; usually found as benign ovarian cysts in women and malignant testicular growths in men. (See *testicular cancer, ovarian cysts*)

Terminal ileitis (tĕr′mi-năl il-ē′tis): Synonym for Crohn disease.

Testosterone (tes-tos′tĕ-rön): A naturally occurring androgen found in testes and other tissues.

Tetraplegia (tet′ră-plē′jē-ă): Quadriplegia.

Thenar (thē′nar): Referring to the fleshy mass on the lateral side of the palm; the ball of the thumb.

Thermal capsulorraphy (ther′măl kap-soo-lör′ă-fē): The use of heat to shrink and repair a joint capsule, specifically at the shoulder, to prevent future dislocations.

Thermography (ther-mog′ră-fē): The making of a regional temperature map of the body, obtained by using an infrared sensing device.

Thrombocyte (throm′bö-sīt): Platelet.

Thrombosis (throm-bö′sis): Formation or presence of a clot.

Thrush (thrŭsh): Infection of the oral tissues with *Candida albicans;* often an opportunistic infection in persons with AIDS or other conditions that depress the immune system. (See *HIV/AIDS, Candida*)

Thymoma (thī-mö′mă): A neoplasm originating in the thymus; usually benign. (See *myasthenia gravis*)

Thymosin (thī′mö-sin): A hormone that restores thymus function.

Thyroxin (thī-rok′sin): Tetraiodothyronine (T4); a secretion of the thyroid gland.

Tic douloureux (tik doo-loo-rĕ): A synonym for trigeminal neuralgia.

Tinea barbae (tin′ē-ă bar′bē): Tinea of the beard, occurring as a follicular infection or as a granulomatous lesion; the primary lesions are papules and pustules. (See *fungal infections*)

Tinea capitis (tin′ē-ă kap′i-tis): A common form of fungus infection of the scalp caused by various species of *Microsporum* and *Trichophyton* on or within hair shafts. (See *fungal infections*)

Tinea corporis (tin′ē-ă pör-is): A well-defined, scaling, macular eruption of dermatophytosis that frequently forms annular lesions and may appear on any part of the body. (See *fungal infections*)

Tinea cruris (tin′ē-ă kroo′ris): A form of tinea imbricata occurring in the genitocrural region, including the inner side of the thighs, the perineal region, and the groin. (See *fungal infections*)

Tinea manus: Ringworm of the hand, usually referring to infections of the palmar surface. (See *fungal infections*)

Tinea pedis (tin′ē-ă pē′dis): Dermatophytosis of the feet, especially of the skin between the toes, caused by one of the dermatophytes, usually a species of *Trichophyton* or *Epidermophyton;* the disease consists of small vesicles, fissures, scaling, maceration, and eroded areas between the toes and on the plantar surface of the foot. (See *fungal infections*)

Tinea unguium (tin′ē-ă un-gwī′yūm): Ringworm of the nails due to a dermatophyte. (See *fungal infections*)

Tinea versicolor (tin′ē-ă vĕr′si-kö′lor): an eruption of tan or brown branny patches on the skin of the trunk, often appearing white, in contrast with hyperpigmented skin after exposure to the summer sun; caused by growth of *Malassezia furfur* in the stratum corneum with minimal inflammatory reaction. (See *fungal infections*)

Tinea (tin′ē-ă): A fungal infection of the keratin component of hairs, skin, or nails.

Tinel's sign (tē-nel′): Distally radiating pain or tingling caused by tapping over the site of a superficial nerve, indicating inflammation or entrapment of that nerve; a test used to help identify carpal tunnel syndrome.

Tinnitus (ti-nī′tŭs): A sensation of noises (ringing, whistling, booming) in the ears.

TINS (Topical immunomodulators): A class of anti-inflammatory ointments used as an alternative to steroidal applications in the treatment of atopic dermatitis. (See *eczema*)

Tissue plasminogen activator (tPA) plaz-min′ö-jen ak′ti-vā-tŏr): A genetically engineered protein that acts as a powerful thrombolytic ("clot-busting") agent.

Titer: The standard of strength of a volumetric test solution; the assay value of an unknown measure by volumetric means.

Tonic spasm (ton′ik spazm): Continuous involuntary spasm of skeletal muscle.

Tonic–clonic seizure: The sudden onset of tonic contraction of muscles, giving way to clonic convulsive movements. Grand mal seizure.

Tophus (tö′fŭs), tophi: Deposits of uric acid and urates in tissue around joints and other areas, Seen with gout.

Torticollis (tör-ti-kol′is): A contraction, often spasmodic, of the muscles of the neck, chiefly those supplied by the spinal accessory nerve; the head is drawn to one side and usually rotated so that the chin points to the other side.

Toxic megacolon (tok′sik meg′ă-kö-lon): Acute nonobstructive dilation of the colon.

Transcriptase (tran-skrip′tās): An enzyme that converts RNA to DNA in the acquired immune deficiency syndrome (AIDS) virus.

Transcutaneous (trans-kū-tā′nē-ŭs): Denoting the passage of substances through unbroken skin.

Treponema pallidum (trep-ö-nē′mă pal′i-dŭm): A species of spirochetal bacteria that causes syphilis in humans.

Trichophyton (tri-kof′i-tŏn): A genus of pathogenic fungi that cause dermatophytosis in humans and animals. (See *fungal infections*)

Tricyclic antidepressants: A chemical group of drugs that share a three-ringed nucleus (e.g., amitriptyline, imipramine).

Trigger point (trĭg′ĕr poynt): A small area in which muscle fibers have suffered injury and not gone through a normal healing process. Pressure on a trigger point elicits moderate to severe pain in specific referring patterns.

Triiodothyronine: T3, a secretion of the thyroid gland. (See *hypothyroidism*)

Trophic ulcer (trof′ik ŭl′sĕr): Ulcer resulting from cutaneous sensory denervation.

Trophic (trof′ik): Relating to or dependent on nutrition.

Tubercle (too′ber-kl): A nodule or bump; may refer to bony prominences, elevations on the skin or other tissues, or to the lesions caused by infection with *Mycobacterium tuberculosis*.

Tumor necrosis factor (too′mŏr nĕ-krö′sis fak′tŏr): A polypeptide hormone, produced by activated macrophages, that has the ability to initiate fever.

Tumor (too′mŏr): Any swelling, usually denoting a neoplasm.

Tunica intima (too′ni-kă in′ti-mă): The innermost coat of a blood or lymphatic vessel.

Tunica media (tū′ni-kă mē′dē-ă): The middle, usually muscular coat of a blood vessel or lymphatic vessel.

Tyrosine (tī′rö-sēn): An amino acid present in most proteins.

Unilateral (oo-ni-lat′ĕ-răl): Confined to one side only.

Ureaplasma urealyticum: A species of bacteria that cause infections in the genitourinary tract. (See *sexually transmitted diseases*)

Uremia (ū-rē′mē-ă): An excess of urea and other nitrogenous waste in the blood.

Ureterolithiasis (ū-rē′ter-ö-li-thī′ă-sis): A kidney stone lodged in the ureter.

Ureteroscopic stone removal: Removal of a calculus in the mid-to-lower ureters with a ureteroscope.

Urogram (ūr′ö-gram): Radiographic record of any part of the urinary tract.

Urticaria (er′ti-kar′i-ă): An eruption of itching wheals; synonym for hives.

Uveitis (ū-vē-ī′tis): Inflammation of the uveal tract: iris, ciliary body, and choroid of the eye. (See *ulcerative colitis*)

Vagotomy (vā-got′ö-mē): Division of the vagus nerve.

Vapocoolant: A topical anesthetic aerosol spray used for pain relief and stretching of muscles affected by trigger points. (See *myofascial pain syndrome*)

Varicocele (var′i-kö-sēl): A condition manifested by abnormal dilation of the veins of the spermatic cord, caused by incompetent valves in the internal spermatic vein and resulting in impaired drainage of blood into the spermatic cord veins when the patient assumes the upright position.

Varix (var′iks), varices: A dilated vein.

Vas deferens (vas dif′ĕr-enz): The secretory duct of the testicle, running from the epididymis to the prostatic urethra, where it terminates as the ejaculatory duct.

Vasculitis (vas-kū-lī′tis): Inflammation of a blood or lymphatic vessel.

Venography (vē-nog′ră-fē): A radiographic demonstration of a vein after the injection of a contrast medium.

Ventricle (ven′tri′kl): A normal cavity, specifically in the brain or heart.

Venule (ven′ool): A venous branch continuous with a capillary.

Verruca (vĕ-roo′kă): A wart composed of a thickened keratitic layer of the epidermis.

Vesicle (ves′i-kl): A small, circumscribed fluid-filled elevation of the skin, a blister.

Vesicoureteral reflux: Backward flow of urine from bladder into ureter.

Villus (vilŭs), villi: A projection from the surface, especially of a mucous membrane.

Virulent (vir′oo-lent): Extremely toxic, denoting a markedly pathogenic microorganism.

Von Willebrand disease (vahn vil′ē-brahnt): A disease characterized by the tendency to bleed primarily from the mucous membranes and prolonged bleeding time.

Wheal (hwēl): A reddened, itchy, changeable edematous area of the skin that is caused by exposure to an allergenic substance in a susceptible individual.

Wolff's law (vŭlf): A law stating that every change in the form or function of a bone is followed by changes in internal and external architecture of the bone.

Wright's test: A thoracic outlet syndrome test in which the hand is placed over the head, and the head is turned toward the affected side. If this exacerbates symptoms or reduces the strength of the pulse of the affected side, impingement to the axillary artery and lower brachial plexus nerves is suspected.

Xeroderma (zēr′ö-der′mă): Excessively dry skin; a mild form of ichthyosis.

Yolk sac tumor: Malignant neoplasm occurring in the gonads. (See *testicular cancer*)

Yuppie flu: Vernacular for a set of signs and symptoms that may be diagnosed as chronic fatigue syndrome.

Zygapophyseal joint: Relating to a zygapophysis or articular process of a vertebra.

These glossary terms can also be found in the Audio Glossary on the Student Resource CD. Most terms are accompanied by sound files of the correct pronunciation.

ILLUSTRATION CREDITS

CHAPTER 1

1-2 Reprinted with permission from Rassner G. Atlas of Dermatology, 3rd ed. Philadelphia: Lea & Febiger; 1994:228.

1-3 Reprinted with permission from Rassner G. Atlas of Dermatology, 3rd ed. Philadelphia: Lea & Febiger; 1994:228.

1-4 Reprinted with permission from Rubin E, Gorstein F, Schwarting R, Strayer DS. Rubin's Pathology: Clinicopathologic Foundations of Medicine, 4th ed. Philadelphia: Lippincott Williams & Wilkins; 2005: 380.

1-5 Reprinted with permission from Rassner G. Atlas of Dermatology, 3rd ed. Philadelphia: Lea & Febiger; 1994:51.

1-6 Reprinted with permission from Willis MC. Medical Terminology: The Language of Health Care. 1st ed. Baltimore: Williams & Wilkins; 1996:100. Courtesy of Laurence J, and Richard D. Underwood, Mission Viejo, CA.

1-7 Reprinted with permission from Goodheart HP. A Photoguide of Common Skin Disorders: Diagnosis and Management. Baltimore: Lippincott Williams & Wilkins; 1999:160.

1-8 Reprinted with permission from Goodheart HP. A Photoguide of Common Skin Disorders: Diagnosis and Management. Baltimore: Lippincott Williams & Wilkins; 1999:132.

1-9 Reprinted with permission from Rassner G. Atlas of Dermatology, 3rd ed. Philadelphia: Lea & Febiger; 1994:65.

1-10 Reprinted with permission from Rassner G. Atlas of Dermatology, 3rd ed. Philadelphia: Lea & Febiger; 1994:42.

1-11 Reprinted with permission from Goodheart HP. A Photoguide of Common Skin Disorders: Diagnosis and Management. Baltimore: Lippincott Williams & Wilkins; 1999:90.

1-12 Reprinted with permission from Rassner G. Atlas of Dermatology, 3rd ed. Philadelphia: Lea & Febiger; 1994:49.

1-13 Reprinted with permission from Willis MC. Medical Terminology: The Language of Health Care. 1st ed. Baltimore: Williams & Wilkins; 1996:90.

1-14 Reprinted with permission from Goodheart HP. A Photoguide of Common Skin Disorders: Diagnosis and Management. Baltimore: Lippincott Williams & Wilkins; 1999:246.

1-16 From Goodheart HP. Goodheart's Photoguide of Common Skin Disorders, 2nd ed. Philadelphia: Lippincott Williams & Wilkins; 2003.

1-17 From Fleisher GR, Ludwig S, Baskin MN. Atlas of Pediatric Emergency Medicine. Philadelphia: Lippincott Williams & Wilkins; 2004.

1-18 Reprinted with permission from Goodheart HP. A Photoguide of Common Skin Disorders: Diagnosis and Management. Baltimore: Lippincott Williams & Wilkins; 1999:310.

1-19 Reprinted with permission from Rassner G. Atlas of Dermatology, 3rd ed. Philadelphia: Lea & Febiger; 1994:46.

1-20 Reprinted with permission from Rassner G. Atlas of Dermatology, 3rd ed. Philadelphia: Lea & Febiger; 1994:47.

1-21 Reprinted with permission from Rassner G. Atlas of Dermatology, 3rd ed. Philadelphia: Lea & Febiger; 1994:241.

1-22 From Goodheart HP. Goodheart's Photoguide of Common Skin Disorders, 2nd ed. Philadelphia: Lippincott Williams & Wilkins; 2003.

1-23 Reprinted with permission from Goodheart HP. A Photoguide of Common Skin Disorders: Diagnosis and Management. Baltimore: Lippincott Williams & Wilkins; 1999:60.

1-23 Reprinted with permission from Goodheart HP. A Photoguide of Common Skin Disorders: Diagnosis and Management. Baltimore: Lippincott Williams & Wilkins; 1999:53.

1-25 Reprinted with permission from Goodheart HP. A Photoguide of Common Skin Disorders: Diagnosis and Management. Baltimore: Lippincott Williams & Wilkins; 1999:44.

1-26 Reprinted with permission from Willis MC. Medical Terminology: The Language of Health Care.

Baltimore: Williams & Wilkins; 1996:1A5. Courtesy of American Academy of Dermatology, Schamburg, IL.

1-27 Reprinted with permission from Rassner G. Atlas of Dermatology, 3rd ed. Philadelphia: Lea & Febiger; 1994:196.

1-28 Reprinted with permission from Goodheart HP. A Photoguide of Common Skin Disorders: Diagnosis and Management. Baltimore: Lippincott Williams & Wilkins; 1999:49.

1-29 Reprinted with permission from Rubin E, Gorstein F, Schwarting R, Strayer DS. Rubin's Pathology: Clinicopathologic Foundations of Medicine, 4th ed. Baltimore: Lippincott Williams & Wilkins; 2005: 1217.

1-30 Reprinted with permission from Goodheart HP. A Photoguide of Common Skin Disorders: Diagnosis and Management. Baltimore: Lippincott Williams & Wilkins; 1999:49.

1-31 From Goodheart HP. Goodheart's Photoguide of Common Skin Disorders: Diagnosis and Management, 2nd ed. Philadelphia: Lippincott Williams & Wilkins; 2003.

1-32 Reprinted with permission from Rassner G. Atlas of Dermatology, 3rd ed. Philadelphia: Lea & Febiger; 1994:47.

1-33 Reprinted with permission from Rassner G. Atlas of Dermatology, 3rd ed. Philadelphia: Lea & Febiger; 1994:170.

1-34 Reprinted with permission from Rassner G. Atlas of Dermatology, 3rd ed. Philadelphia: Lea & Febiger; 1994:171.

1-35 Reprinted with permission from Rassner G. Atlas of Dermatology, 3rd ed. Philadelphia: Lea & Febiger; 1994:176.

1-36 Reprinted with permission from Rassner G. Atlas of Dermatology, 3rd ed. Philadelphia: Lea & Febiger; 1994:319.

1-37 Reprinted with permission from Rassner G. Atlas of Dermatology, 3rd ed. Philadelphia: Lea & Febiger; 1994:207.

1-39 Reprinted with permission from Rubin E, Gorstein F, Schwarting R, Strayer DS. Rubin's Pathology: Clinicopathologic Foundations of Medicine, 4th ed. Baltimore: Lippincott Williams & Wilkins; 2005: 1253.

1-40 From Goodheart HP. Goodheart's Photoguide of Common Skin Disorders, 2nd ed. Philadelphia: Lippincott Williams & Wilkins; 2003.

1-41 Reprinted with permission from Judd RI, Ponsell PP. Mosby's First Responder, 2nd ed. St. Louis, MO: Mosby-Year Book; 1988.

1-42 Reprinted with permission from Rassner G. Atlas of Dermatology, 3rd ed. Philadelphia: Lea & Febiger; 1994:82.

1-43 Reprinted with permission from Judd RI, Ponsell PP. Mosby's First Responder, 2nd ed. St. Louis, MO: Mosby-Year Book; 1988.

1-44 Reprinted with permission from Willis MC. Medical Terminology: The Language of Health Care. Baltimore: Williams & Wilkins; 1996:A5.

1-45 Reprinted with permission from Rubin E, Gorstein F, Schwarting R, Strayer DS. Rubin's Pathology: Clinicopathologic Foundations of Medicine, 4th ed. Baltimore: Lippincott Williams & Wilkins; 2005: 115.

1-46 Reprinted with permission from Rassner G. Atlas of Dermatology, 3rd ed. Philadelphia: Lea & Febiger; 1994:25.

CHAPTER 2

2-6   Reprinted with permission from Stedman's Concise Medical Dictionary for the Health Professions Illustrated, 4th ed. Baltimore: Lippincott Williams & Wilkins; 2001:653.

2-11 Reprinted with permission from Rubin E, Farber J. Pathology, 3rd ed. Philadelphia: Lippincott Williams & Wilkins; 1999:1357.

2-13 Reprinted with permission from Roentgen EJ. Diagnosis of Diseases of Bone, 3rd ed. Baltimore: Williams & Wilkins; 1981;2:841. Courtesy of Herbert M. Stauffer, Temple University Hospital, Philadelphia, PA.

2-14 Reprinted with permission from Rubin E, Gorstein F, Schwarting R, Strayer DS. Rubin's Pathology: Clinicopathologic Foundations of Medicine, 4th ed. Philadelphia: Lippincott Williams & Wilkins; 2005:1336.

2-15 Reprinted with permission from Agur AMR, Lee MJ. Grant's Atlas of Anatomy, 10th ed. Baltimore: Lippincott Williams & Wilkins; 1999:251.

2-16 Reprinted with permission from Brant WE, Helms CA. Fundamentals of Diagnostic Radiology, 2nd ed. Baltimore: Lippincott Williams & Wilkins; 1999: 1058.

2-18 Reprinted with permission from Rubin E, Farber J. Pathology, 3rd ed. Philadelphia: Lippincott Williams & Wilkins; 1999:1370.

2-21 Reprinted with permission from Baker CL. The Hughston Clinic Sports Medicine Book. Baltimore: Williams & Wilkins; 1995:365.

2-22 Reprinted with permission from Rubin E, Gorstein F, Schwarting R, Strayer DS. Rubin's Pathology: Clinicopathologic Foundations of Medicine, 4th ed. Philadelphia: Lippincott Williams & Wilkins; 2005: 1374.

2-23 Reprinted with permission from Rubin E, Gorstein F, Schwarting R, Strayer DS. Rubin's Pathology: Clinicopathologic Foundations of Medicine, 4th ed. Philadelphia: Lippincott Williams & Wilkins; 2005: 1375.

2-24 Reprinted with permission from Koneman EW, Allen SD, Janda WM, Schreckenberger PC, Winn WC Jr. Color Atlas and Textbook of Diagnostic Microbiology, 5th ed. Philadelphia: Lippincott Williams & Wilkins; 1997:Figure E.

2-25 Reprinted with permission from Goodheart HP. A Photoguide of Common Skin Disorders: Diagnosis and Management. Baltimore: Lippincott Williams & Wilkins; 1999:145.

2-27 Reprinted with permission from Harris JH Jr, Harris WH, Novelline RA. The Radiology of Emergency Medicine, 3rd ed. Baltimore: Williams & Wilkins; 1993:440.

2-28 Reprinted with permission from MacNab I, McCulloch J. Neck Ache and Shoulder Pain. Baltimore: Williams & Wilkins; 1994:45.

2-29 Reprinted with permission from MacNab I, McCulloch J. Neck Ache and Shoulder Pain. Baltimore: Williams & Wilkins; 1994:45.

2-31 Reprinted with permission from Barker LR, Burton JR, Zieve PD. Principles of Ambulatory Medicine, 4th ed. Baltimore: Williams & Wilkins; 1995:946.

2-32 Reprinted with permission from Barker LR, Burton JR, Zieve PD. Principles of Ambulatory Medicine, 4th ed. Baltimore: Williams & Wilkins; 1995:946.

2-36 From Moore KL, Dalley AF II. Clinically Oriented Anatomy, 4th ed. Baltimore, Lippincott Williams & Wilkins; 1999.

2-39 Reprinted with permission from Rubin E, Farber J. Pathology, 3rd ed. Philadelphia: Lippincott Williams & Wilkins; 1999:242.

2-40 Reprinted with permission from Yochum TR, Rowe LJ. Essentials of Skeletal Radiology, 2nd ed. Baltimore: Williams & Wilkins; 1996;2:1291, Figure 13-59B.

2-43 Reprinted with permission from Goodheart HP. A Photoguide of Common Skin Disorders: Diagnosis and Management. Baltimore: Lippincott Williams & Wilkins; 1999:366.

CHAPTER 3

3-3 A, B Reprinted with permission from Rubin E, Farber J. Pathology, 3rd ed. Philadelphia: Lippincott Williams & Wilkins; 1999:1511.

3-5 From Fleisher GR, Ludwig W, Baskin MN. Atlas of Pediatric Emergency Medicine. Philadelphia: Lippincott Williams & Wilkins; 2004.

3-9 Photo courtesy of Rober Schwarzmann, MD, Philadelphia, PA.

3-13 Reprinted with permission from Yochum TR, Rowe LJ. Essentials of Skeletal Radiology, 2nd ed. Baltimore: Williams & Wilkins; 1996;1:398, Figure 6-38.

CHAPTER 4

4-1 From Cohen BJ, Wood DL. Memmler's The Human Body in Health and Disease, 9th ed. Philadelphia: Lippincott Williams & Wilkins; 2000.

4-3 Reprinted with permission from Rubin E, Farber J. Pathology, 3rd ed. Philadelphia: Lippincott Williams & Wilkins; 1999:1081.

4-8 Reprinted with permission from Rubin E, Farber J. Pathology, 3rd ed. Philadelphia: Lippincott Williams & Wilkins; 1999:1466.

4-12 Reprinted with permission from Rassner G. Atlas of Dermatology, 3rd ed. Philadelphia: Lea & Febiger; 1994:271.

4-14 From Moore KL, Dalley AF II. Clinically Oriented Anatomy, 4th ed. Baltimore: Lippincott Williams & Wilkins; 1999.

CHAPTER 5

5-2 A, B Reprinted with permission from Rubin E, Gorstein F, Schwarting R, Strayer DS. Rubin's Pathology: Clinicopathologic Foundations of Medicine, 4th ed. Baltimore: Lippincott Williams & Wilkins; 2005:298.

5-3 Reprinted with permission from Fitzpatrick J, Aeling J. Dermatology Secrets in Color, 2nd ed. Philadelphia: Hanley & Belfus; 2000;191, Figure 8.

5-4 Reprinted with permission from Bickley LS. Bates' Guide to Physical Examination and History Taking, 7th ed. Baltimore: Lippincott Williams & Wilkins; 1999:660.

5-5 Reprinted with permission from Stedman's Medical Dictionary, 27th ed. Baltimore: Lippincott Williams & Wilkins; 2000.

5-6 From DeVita VT Jr, Hellaman S, Rosenberg S, Durran J, Essex M, Fauci AS. AIDS: Etiology, Diagnosis, Treatment, and Prevention, 4th ed. Philadelphia: Lippincott-Raven; 1997.

5-8 Reprinted with permission from Stedman's Medical Dictionary, 27th ed. Baltimore: Lippincott Williams & Wilkins; 2000:1036.

5-9 Reprinted with permission from Goodheart HP. A Photoguide of Common Skin Disorders: Diagnosis and Management. Baltimore: Lippincott Williams & Wilkins; 1999:356, Figure 25-20.

CHAPTER 6

6-3 Reprinted with permission from Rubin E, Farber J. Pathology, 3rd ed. Philadelphia: Lippincott Williams & Wilkins; 1999:607.

6-7 From Moore KL, Dalley AF II. Clinically Oriented Anatomy, 4th ed. Baltimore: Lippincott Williams & Wilkins; 1999.

CHAPTER 7

7-6 Reprinted with permission from Rubin E, Farber J. Pathology, 3rd ed. Philadelphia: Lippincott Williams & Wilkins; 1999:165.

7-9 From Sun T. Parasitic Disorders: Pathology, Diagnosis, and Management, 2nd ed. Baltimore: Lippincott Williams & Wilkins; 1999.

7-11 Reprinted with permission from Rubin E, Farber J. Pathology, 3rd ed. Philadelphia: Lippincott Williams & Wilkins; 1999:832.

7-12 Reprinted with permission from Rubin E, Farber J. Pathology, 3rd ed. Philadelphia: Lippincott Williams & Wilkins; 1999:762.

CHAPTER 8

8-1 Reprinted with permission from Rassner G. Atlas of Dermatology, 3rd ed. Philadelphia: Lea & Febiger; 1994:302.

8-2 Reprinted with permission from Rubin E, Farber J. Pathology, 3rd ed. Philadelphia: Lippincott Williams & Wilkins; 1999:1167.

CHAPTER 9

9-2 Reprinted with permission from Rubin E, Gorstein F, Schwarting R, Strayer DS. Rubin's Pathology: Clinicopathologic Foundations of Medicine, 4th ed. Philadelphia: Lippincott Williams & Wilkins; 2005:877.

CHAPTER 10

10-5 Reprinted with permission from Mitchell GW. The Female Breast and Its Disorders. Baltimore: Williams & Wilkins; 1990:140.

10-7 Reprinted with permission from Rubin E, Gorstein F, Schwarting R, Strayer DS. Rubin's Pathology: Clinicopathologic Foundations of Medicine, 4th ed. Philadelphia: Lippincott Williams & Wilkins; 2005:968.

CHAPTER 11

11-1 Reprinted with permission from Rubin E, Gorstein F, Schwarting R, Strayer DS. Rubin's Pathology: Clinicopathologic Foundations of Medicine, 4th ed. Philadelphia: Lippincott Williams & Wilkins; 2005:299.

11-2 Reprinted with permission from Rassner G. Atlas of Dermatology, 3rd ed. Philadelphia: Lippincott Williams & Wilkins; 1994:84.

INDEX

In this index, page numbers in *italic* designate figures; page numbers followed by "t" designate tables; entries preceded by "vs." designate Compare/Contrast boxes; *(see also)* designates related topics or more detailed subentries.